Second Edition

NEUROLOGICAL SURGERY
Volume 5

A Comprehensive Reference Guide to the Diagnosis and Management of Neurosurgical Problems

Edited by

JULIAN R. YOUMANS, M.D., Ph.D.

Professor, Department of Neurological Surgery,
School of Medicine, University of California
Davis, California

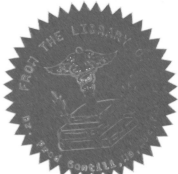

W. B. SAUNDERS COMPANY
Philadelphia • London • Toronto • Mexico City • Rio de Janeiro • Sydney • Tokyo

W. B. Saunders Company: West Washington Square
Philadelphia, PA 19105

1 St. Anne's Road
Eastbourne, East Sussex BN21 3UN, England

1 Goldthorne Avenue
Toronto, Ontario M8Z 5T9, Canada

Apartado 26370—Cedro 512
Mexico 4, D.F., Mexico

Rua Coronel Cabrita, 8
Sao Cristovao Caixa Postal 21176
Rio de Janeiro, Brazil

9 Waltham Street
Artarmon, N.S.W. 2064, Australia

Ichibancho, Central Bldg., 22-1 Ichibancho
Chiyoda-Ku, Tokyo 102, Japan

Library of Congress Cataloging in Publication Data

Youmans, Julian Ray, 1928–
  Neurological surgery.

  1. Nervous system—Surgery. I. Title.
[DNLM: 1. Neurosurgery. WL368 N4945]
RD593.Y68   1980   617'.48
ISBN 0-7216-9662-7 (v. 1)   80-21368

Volume 1	ISBN	0-7216-9662-7
Volume 2	ISBN	0-7216-9663-5
Volume 3	ISBN	0-7216-9664-3
Volume 4	ISBN	0-7216-9665-1
Volume 5	ISBN	0-7216-9666-X
Volume 6	ISBN	0-7216-9667-8
Six Volume Set	ISBN	0-7216-9658-9

Neurological Surgery—Volume Five

Last digit is the print number: 9   8   7   6   5   4   3   2

Contributors

JOHN R. BENTSON, M.D.

Acoustic Neuromas

Associate Professor of Radiology, University of California at Los Angeles. Chief of Section of Neuroradiology, University of California Los Angeles Medical Center, Los Angeles, California.

WILLIAM H. BROOKS, M.D.

Classification and Biology of Brain Tumors

Assistant Professor of Neurological Surgery, University of Kentucky College of Medicine. Chief of Neurological Surgery, Veterans Administration Hospital, Lexington, Kentucky.

ALBERT B. BUTLER, M.D.

Classification and Biology of Brain Tumors

Professor of Neurological Surgery, School of Medicine, University of Virginia. Attending Surgeon, University of Virginia Hospital, Charlottesville, Virginia.

SHELLEY N. CHOU, M.D., Ph.D., F.A.C.S.

Urological Problems; Scoliosis, Kyphosis, and Lordosis; Tumors of Skull

Professor of Neurological Surgery, Head of Department of Neurological Surgery, University of Minnesota Medical School. Chief of Neurological Surgery Service, University of Minnesota Hospitals; Consultant, Minneapolis Veterans Administration Hospital, Minneapolis, Minnesota.

CULLY A. COBB, III, M.D., F.A.C.S.

Glial and Neuronal Tumors, Lymphomas, Sarcomas and Vascular Tumors, Tumors of Disordered Embryogenesis

Assistant Clinical Professor of Neurological Surgery, University of California, School of Medicine at Davis, Davis, California. Attending Neurological Surgeon, Sutter Community Hospitals and University of California Davis Medical Center at Sacramento, Sacramento, California.

iii

WILLIAM M. COCKE, JR., M.D., F.A.C.S.

Scalp Injuries, Tumors of Scalp

Professor of Surgery, Chief of Plastic and Reconstructive Surgery, School of Medicine, Texas Technical University. Chief of Plastic Surgery, Health Sciences Center; Attending Staff, St. Mary's of the Plains, Lubbock, Texas; Consultant, Veterans Administration Hospital, Big Springs, Texas.

EDWARD S. CONNOLLY, M.D., F.A.C.S.

Spinal Cord Tumors in Adults

Clinical Professor of Neurological Surgery, Tulane University School of Medicine; Associate Professor of Neurological Surgery, Louisiana State University School of Medicine. Chairman of Department of Neurological Surgery, Ochsner Clinic, New Orleans, Louisiana.

GUY CORKILL, M.B., B.Ch., F.R.C.S., F.R.C.S.(E.), F.R.A.C.S.

Craniofacial Neoplasia

Professor of Neurological Surgery, University of California, School of Medicine at Davis, Davis, California. Attending Neurological Surgeon, University of California Davis Medical Center at Sacramento, Sacramento, California; Consultant in Neurological Surgery, Martinez Veterans Administration Hospital, Martinez, California; David Grant Medical Center, Travis Air Force Base, Travis, California.

DONALD D. DIRKS, Ph.D.

Acoustic Neuromas

Professor of Head and Neck Surgery, University of California at Los Angeles, School of Medicine. Staff, Head and Neck Surgery, University of California at Los Angeles Hospital, Los Angeles, California.

PAUL J. DONALD, M.D., F.R.C.S.(C.), F.A.C.S.

Craniofacial Neoplasia

Associate Professor of Otorhinolaryngology, Vice Chairman of Department of Otorhinolaryngology, University of California, School of Medicine at Davis, Davis, California. Attending Staff, Department of Otorhinolaryngology, University of California Davis Medical Center at Sacramento, Sacramento, California.

MICHAEL J. EBERSOLD, M.D.

Meningeal Tumors of Brain

Instructor in Neurological Surgery, Mayo Medical School. Consultant, Department of Neurological Surgery, Mayo Clinic; Attending Neurological Surgeon, St. Marys Hospital and Rochester Methodist Hospital, Rochester, Minnesota.

FRANCIS W. GAMACHE, JR., M.D.

Metastatic Brain Tumors

Assistant Professor of Neurological Surgery, Cornell University Medical College. Attending Neurological Surgeon, New York Hospital–Cornell Medical Center, New York, New York.

MELVIN GREER, M.D.

Pseudotumor Cerebri

Professor of Neurology, Chairman of Department of Neurology, University of Florida College of Medicine. Chief of Neurology, University of Florida Teaching Hospitals and Clinics, Gainesville, Florida.

E. B. HENDRICK, M.D., F.R.C.S.(C.)

Spinal Cord Tumors in Children

Professor of Surgery, University of Toronto. Neurosurgeon in Chief, The Hospital for Sick Children; Consultant in Neurological Surgery, Queensway General Hospital and Ontario Society for Crippled Children; Active Staff in Neurological Surgery, Toronto Western Hospital; Consultant Neurosurgeon, North York General Hospital, Toronto, Ontario.

SADEK K. HILAL, M.D., Ph.D

Interventional Neuroradiology, Tumors of Orbit

Professor of Radiology, Columbia University College of Physicians and Surgeons. Attending Radiologist, Presbyterian Hospital; Director of Neuroradiology, Neuroradiological Institute of New York, New York, New York.

STEPHEN F. HODGSON, M.D.

Empty Sella Syndrome

Assistant Professor of Medicine, Mayo Medical School. Consultant in Internal Medicine and Endocrinology, Mayo Clinic; Attending Physician, St. Marys Hospital and Rochester Methodist Hospital, Rochester, Minnesota.

HAROLD J. HOFFMAN, M.D., F.R.C.S.(C.), F.A.C.S.

Supratentorial Tumors in Children

Associate Professor of Surgery, University of Toronto Faculty of Medicine. Neurological Surgeon, The Hospital for Sick Children, Toronto, Ontario.

TAKAO HOSHINO, M.D., D.M.Sc.

Chemotherapy of Brain Tumors

Associate Professor of Neurological Surgery, School of Medicine, University of California at San Francisco. Research Associate, Laboratory of Radiobiology, School of Medicine, University of California at San Francisco, San Francisco, California.

EDGAR M. HOUSEPIAN, M.D., F.A.C.S

Tumors of Orbit

Professor of Clinical Neurological Surgery, Columbia University College of Physicians and Surgeons. Attending Neurological Surgeon, Columbia–Presbyterian Medical Center, New York, New York.

ROBIN P. HUMPHREYS, M.D., F.R.C.S.(C.)

Posterior Fossa Tumors in Children

Assistant Professor of Neurological Surgery, University of Toronto Faculty of Medicine. Neurological Surgeon, The Hospital for Sick Children; Consultant, North York General Hospital and Ontario Crippled Children's Center, Toronto, Ontario.

WARREN Y. ISHIDA, M.D.

Peripheral and Sympathetic Nerve Tumors

Attending Neurological Surgeon, Kapiolani Children's Hospital, Queen's Medical Center, St. Francis Hospital, and Kuakini Medical Center, Honolulu, Hawaii.

FREDERICK A. JAKOBIEC, M.D., D.Sc.

Tumors of Orbit

Professor of Ophthalmology and Pathology, Cornell University Medical College. Director of Laboratories, Manhattan Eye, Ear and Throat Hospital, New York, New York.

LUDWIG G. KEMPE, M.D., F.A.C.S.

Glomus Jugulare Tumors

Professor of Neurological Surgery and Anatomy, Medical University of South Carolina. Staff, Veterans Administration Medical Center, Charleston, South Carolina.

STEPHEN A. KIEFFER, M.D.

Tumors of Skull

Professor of Radiology, Chairman of Department of Radiology, State University of New York at Syracuse. Chief of Radiology, University Hospital, Syracuse, New York.

ALEX M. LANDOLT, M.D.

Sellar and Parasellar Tumors

Privatdozent, Neurosurgical Clinic, Kantonsspital, University of Zurich, Zurich, Switzerland.

EDWARD R. LAWS, M.D., F.A.C.S.

Empty Sella Syndrome

Professor of Neurological Surgery, Mayo Medical School. Neurological Surgeon, Mayo Clinic; Attending Neurological Surgeon, St. Marys Hospital and Rochester Methodist Hospital, Rochester, Minnesota.

VICTOR A. LEVIN, M.D.

Chemotherapy of Brain Tumors

Associate Professor of Neurological Surgery, Pharmacology and Pharmaceutical Chemistry, Schools of Medicine and Pharmacy, University of California at San Francisco. Associate Director, Brain Tumor Research Center; Chief, Neuro-Oncology Service, Department of Neurological Surgery, San Francisco, California.

CONTRIBUTORS

DONLIN M. LONG, M.D., Ph.D., F.A.C.S.

Tumors of Skull, Chronic Pain, Pain of Spinal Origin, Pain of Visceral Origin, Peripheral Nerve Pain

Professor of Neurological Surgery, Chairman of Department of Neurological Surgery, The Johns Hopkins School of Medicine. Neurological Surgeon-in-Chief, Johns Hopkins Hospital, Baltimore, Maryland.

COLLIN S. MacCARTY, M.D., F.A.C.S.

Meningeal Tumors of Brain

Emeritus Professor of Neurological Surgery, Mayo Medical School. Consultant, Department of Neurological Surgery, Mayo Clinic, Rochester, Minnesota.

DONALD E. MORGAN, Ph.D.

Acoustic Neuromas

Associate Professor of Head and Neck Surgery, University of California at Los Angeles, School of Medicine. Director of Audiology Clinic, University of California at Los Angeles Hospital, Los Angeles, California.

MARTIN G. NETSKY, M.D.

Classification and Biology of Brain Tumors

Professor of Pathology, Vanderbilt University School of Medicine. Attending Pathologist, Vanderbilt University Hospital, Nashville, Tennessee.

DWIGHT PARKINSON, M.D., F.R.C.S.(C.), F.A.C.S.

Cavernous Plexus Lesions

Professor of Neurological Surgery, University of Manitoba. Chief of Section of Neurological Surgery, Health Sciences Centre, Winnipeg, Manitoba.

RUSSELL H. PATTERSON, JR., M.D., F.A.C.S.

Extradural Dorsal Spinal Lesions, Metastatic Brain Tumors, Hypophysectomy by Craniotomy

Professor of Neurological Surgery, Cornell University Medical College. Attending Surgeon-in-Charge, Department of Neurological Surgery, The New York Hospital, New York, New York.

DAVID GEORGE PIEPGRAS, M.D.

Operative Management of Intracranial Occlusive Disease, Meningeal Tumors of Brain

Assistant Professor of Neurological Surgery, Mayo Medical School. Consultant, Department of Neurological Surgery, Mayo Clinic; Attending Neurological Surgeon, St. Marys Hospital and Rochester Methodist Hospital, Rochester, Minnesota.

JEROME B. POSNER, M.D.

Metastatic Brain Tumors

Professor of Neurology, Cornell University Medical College. Chairman of Department of Neurology, Memorial Sloan–Kettering Cancer Center, New York, New York.

ROBERT W. RAND, M.D., Ph.D., J.D., F.A.C.S.

Acoustic Neuromas

Professor of Neurological Surgery, University of California, Los Angeles, School of Medicine; Attending Neurological Surgeon, University of California Hospital, Los Angeles, California.

RAYMOND V. RANDALL, M.D., F.A.C.P.

Neuroendocrinology, Empty Sella Syndrome

Professor of Medicine, Mayo Medical School. Senior Consultant, Mayo Clinic; Consultant Physician, St. Marys Hospital and Rochester Methodist Hospital, Rochester, Minnesota.

GLENN E. SHELINE, Ph.D., M.D., F.A.C.R.

Radiation Therapy of Brain, Pituitary, and Spinal Cord Tumors

Professor of Radiation Oncology, Vice-Chairman of Radiation Oncology, University of California, School of Medicine at San Francisco. Attending Radiologist, Mount Zion Hospital, Franklin Hospital, and Ft. Miley Veterans Administration Hospital, San Francisco, California.

JOHN S. SILVERTON, M.D., F.R.C.S., F.R.C.S.(Ed.)

Tumors of Scalp

Assistant Clinical Professor of Plastic Surgery, University of California, School of Medicine at Davis, Davis, California. Consultant, Department of Plastic Surgery, University of California Davis Medical Center at Sacramento, Sacramento, California; Plastic Surgery Consultant, Veterans Administration Hospital, Martinez, California; Attending Staff, St. Joseph's Hospital and Dameron Hospital, Stockton, California; Lodi Memorial Hospital and Lodi Community Hospital, Lodi, California.

BENNETT M. STEIN, M.D., F.A.C.S.

Pineal Tumors

Byron Stookey Professor of Neurological Surgery, Chairman of Department of Neurological Surgery, Columbia University College of Physicians and Surgeons. Director of Neurological Surgery, The Neurological Institute, New York, New York.

STEPHEN L. TROKEL, M.D.

Tumors of Orbit

Associate Professor of Clinical Ophthalmology, Columbia University College of Physicians and Surgeons. Attending Ophthalmologist, Edward S. Harkness Eye Institute, Columbia–Presbyterian Medical Center, New York, New York.

WILLIAM M. WARA, M.D.

Radiation Therapy of Brain, Pituitary, and Spinal Cord Tumors

Associate Professor of Radiation Oncology, University of San Francisco, School of Medicine at San Francisco; Attending Radiologist, University of California Hospital, San Francisco, California.

MICHAEL WEST, M.D., Ph.D., F.R.C.S.(C.)

Cavernous Plexus Lesions

Lecturer in Physiology, Department of Physiology, University of Manitoba. Staff Neurosurgeon, St. Boniface General Hospital, Winnipeg, Manitoba.

CHARLES B. WILSON, M.D., F.A.C.S.

Dural Fistulae, Chemotherapy, Sellar and Parasellar Tumors, Indications for and Results of Hypophysectomy, Stereotaxic Hypophysectomy

Professor of Neurological Surgery, Chairman of Department of Neurological Surgery, University of California. School of Medicine at San Francisco. Chief of Neurological Surgery, University Hospital, San Francisco, California.

JULIAN R. YOUMANS, M.D., Ph.D., F.A.C.S.

Diagnostic Biopsy, Cerebral Death, Cerebral Blood Flow, Trauma to Carotid Arteries, Glial and Neuronal Tumors, Lymphomas, Sarcomas and Vascular Tumors, Tumors of Disordered Embryogenesis, Peripheral and Sympathetic Nerve Tumors, Parasitic and Fungal Infections.

Professor of Neurological Surgery, University of California, School of Medicine at Davis, Davis, California. Attending Neurological Surgeon, University of California Davis Medical Center at Sacramento, Sacramento, California; Consultant in Neurological Surgery, United States Air Force Medical Center, Travis Air Force Base, California; Veterans Administration Hospital, Martinez, California.

Contents

X
TUMORS

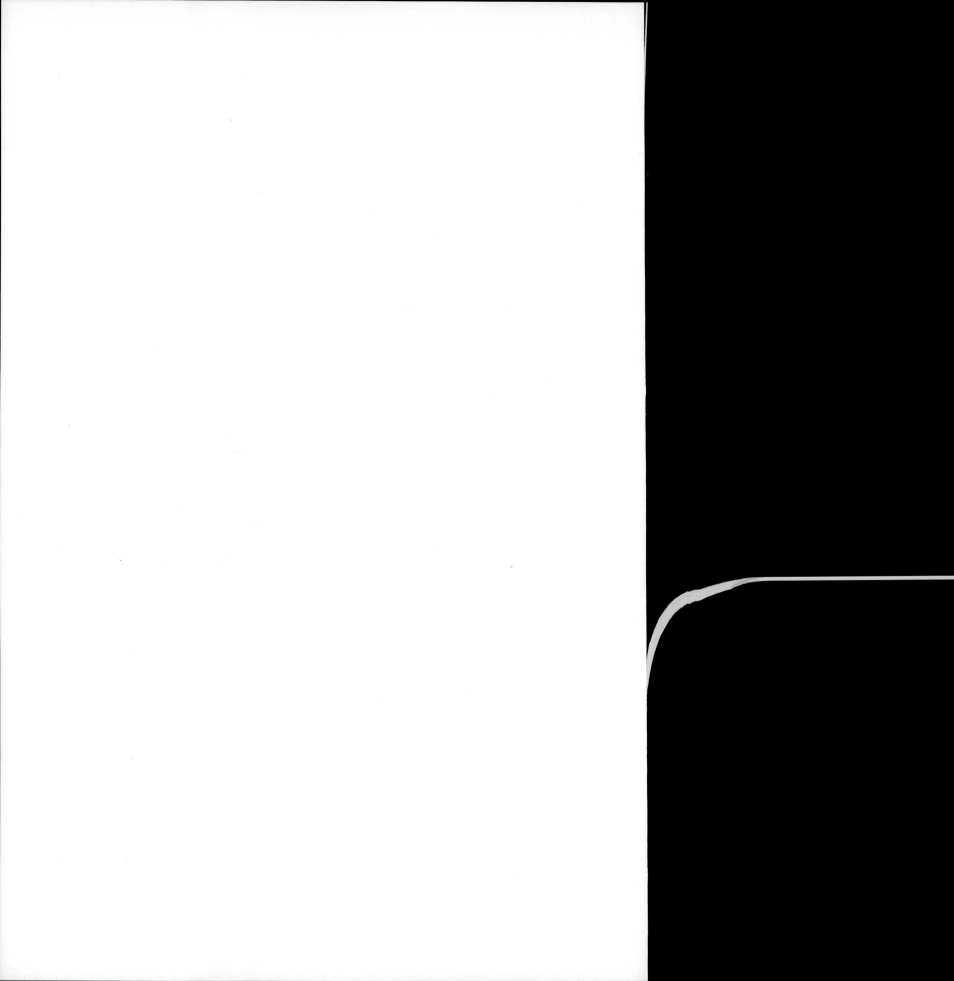

CLASSIFICATION AND BIOLOGY OF BRAIN TUMORS

CLASSIFICATION

Classification in its broadest sense is the division of individual things into groups or classes. Scientific classification additionally demands that the arrangement be systematic, that it be based on an important principle, that the classification be exhaustive, and that the categories be mutually exclusive. The most important feature of classification, however, is its clinical or theoretic usefulness.

Taxonomists may be classified as "lumpers" or "splitters." The "lumper" divides things into relatively large groups and accepts the fact that much variability will be encountered within these limits. The "splitter," at the extreme, regards every identifiable variant of living matter as a significant nameable natural unit.[248]

Early Schemes

Before the time of Virchow, pathologists and surgeons described brain tumors in great detail, according to external characteristics. Writing in 1839, Bressler was one of many authors who tried to create order with categories such as "induration of the brain," "blood tumors," and "bone tumors." He also recognized "brain cancers," of which he collected 45 cases, including three hypophyseal tumors.[26] In this same period, the epidermoid or "pearly" tumors were described, and gliomas were known as "medullary sarcoma" or "fungus medullare."

The present-day concept of classification of tumors was initiated by Virchow.[248] He recognized the supporting elements of the nervous system, labeled them neuroglia, and thus initiated the cytological approach to classification. Virchow created the term "glioma," and classified these tumors for the first time by the type of cell. Some descriptive terms from the older classifications were retained, such as soft, hard, telangiectatic, or hemorrhagic. He described ependymal tumors and eighth nerve neuromas, and offered an interpretation of dural neoplasms. He characterized gliomas as enormous tumors of firm, brain-like appearance, not clearly demarcated from the cerebrum, and resembling a hypertrophy of normal parts. Microscopically, the tumors were formed by glial cells, and on occasion contained fibers, clearly an account of astrocytic tumors.

He also described a hemorrhagic telangiectatic tumor that in places appeared well circumscribed and in others merged into surrounding tissues. Microscopically, it was hypercellular and contained some large cells. Fatty degeneration was prominent in the well-vascularized tumor. He thus gave one of the earliest descriptions of glioblastoma multiforme. Virchow distinguished between gliomas and sarcomas, although the latter group was established by predominantly gross criteria with little histological verification. His work was so well accepted that, for a time, only scattered attempts were made at further classification. More workers became interested in brain tumors and made rapid progress in histological techniques in the last half of the nineteenth century. Simon described the "spider-cell glioma," and Stroebe further contributed to the differentiation between sarcomas and gliomas begun by Virchow.[221,231]

New histological methods were devel-

A. B. BUTLER, W. H. BROOKS, AND M. G. NETSKY

oped in Spain by Ramon y Cajal and del Rio Hortega during the first quarter of the twentieth century. They used metallic impregnations on the cells of the brain, a work that had a strong influence on many surgeons and pathologists. Among these workers were Bailey and Cushing, who later concentrated on comparing types of tumor cells with cells in normal stages of development and extensively used these impregnation techniques.[13]

Tooth published a descriptive study of brain tumors collected at the National Hospital in London from 1902 to 1911.[241] This study comprised 500 cases, of which 258 were gliomas; for the first time, extensive neurosurgical material was studied histologically. In addition, he was one of the first to emphasize the correlation of morphological structure and clinical course. He discussed benign and malignant gliomas, and the presence of histologically different areas in the same glioma. He concluded that complete recovery from the diffuse form was "practically impossible."

In the meantime, Pick and Bielschowsky were classifying neuronal tumors according to the degree of maturation and resemblance to normal ganglion cells.[185] Ribbert studied gliomas and used the theory of Cohnheim pertaining to the development of tumors from embryonic rests.[191] Ribbert thought that morphological differences could be best explained by comparing the tumor cells with developmental stages of the glia. This concept was the foundation for many classifications used to the present time. It was influential in the systems proposed by Bailey and Cushing and by others who followed them. Ribbert contended that gliomas arose from cells *arrested* at different stages in their development. Although he did not use the newer metallic techniques, his work initiated a new phase of research on gliomas, placing emphasis on cytological studies.

Bailey and Cushing

The approach of Harvey Cushing to the study of tumors established a pattern of excellence. In his description of medulloblastoma, for example, Cushing thoroughly considered macroscopic appearance, point of origin, method of growth and spread, and life history, correlating these findings with the cellular architecture of the tumor.[12,48] In 1926 Bailey and Cushing proposed "A classification of the tumors of the glioma groups on a histogenetic basis with a correlated study of prognosis," from a study of more than 400 verified gliomas, including 167 necropsy specimens.[13] They used the metallic impregnation techniques of Cajal and Hortega as well as other staining methods. The histogenetic or cytogenetic concept of the types of glioma was based on the resemblance of tumor cells to embryonic cells in various stages of differentiation. In this regard, they differed from Cohnheim and Ribbert, who theorized that gliomas arose from "arrested" cells. Bailey and Cushing undoubtedly were influenced by this theory, but their writing makes it clear they were dealing with the resemblance of cells rather than with a theory of origin. They classified the tumors in terms of the morphological stages through which each cell was conceived to pass in embryogenesis. Twenty cell types were considered to arise from the medullary plate, from which they derived 14 tumors (Fig. 83–1). Bailey and Cushing were concerned about the awkward and probably unwarranted term neuroepithelioma, which might better have been called primitive spongioblastoma. They noted, perhaps as an afterthought, that the term "glioblast" could be used for bipolar and unipolar spongioblasts considered to be unipotential, that is, already determined as glial cells.

In making clinical correlations, Bailey and Cushing first considered modifying factors, such as position of the tumor, effect of radiation, age of the patient, and results of the surgical procedure itself. They found that tumors with less differentiated cells, resembling those of earlier embryonic stages, grew more rapidly than tumors composed of more differentiated cells. The groups of tumors were arranged in series according to the average survival period; longevity was significantly related to greater degree of differentiation of the neoplastic cells. The authors found later that certain groups, such as the cerebellar astrocytomas, did not fit into this scheme, and more was to be written on this at a later time. They concluded that the diagnosis, localization, and surgical treatment of a brain tumor was important, but also essential "is a clear understanding of the life history of the lesion treated, for on this depends more

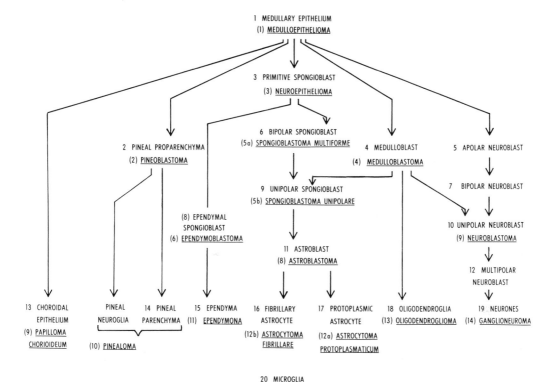

Figure 83–1 Diagram modified from Cushing and Bailey. Twenty types of cells identified in the development of the nervous system are numbered. The 14 types of glial tumors presumably derived from these cells are numbered in parentheses.

than anything else the nature of the procedure appropriate to the particular kind of tumor which happens to be disclosed.[13]

Although this classification was not universally accepted and lacked confirmation, particularly in the embryological scheme and the comparison with stages of histogenesis, it was a practical system bringing order to the existing confusion. Bailey and Cushing moreover created a classification of clinical value by correlating the types of tumor with survival times.

With increased use, Bailey decided to change the term "spongioblastoma multiforme" to "glioblastoma multiforme," reserving the term "spongioblastoma" for tumors related to the primitive spongioblast.[11] The term "glioblast" was used for the unipolar and bipolar spongioblast, and "glioblastoma" for the tumors in which they were found. He also proposed that the categories of medulloepithelioma, pineoblastoma, ependymoblastoma, and neuroblastoma be eliminated. Although originally Bailey and Cushing placed papillomas of the choroid plexus among the gliomas, Bailey did not include them because they "are

not usually considered as gliomas.[11,13] Little doubt exists as to the origin of the epithelial cells of the choroid plexus from the same ependymal cells as the remainder of the glia, hence these papillomas are properly viewed as gliomas.

The revised system was presented by Bailey and Cushing in 1920.[14] The 10 categories (plus papilloma of the choroid plexus) then were as follows: (1) medulloblastoma, (2) glioblastoma multiforme, (3) spongioblastoma, (4) astroblastoma, (5) astrocytoma, (6) neuroepithelioma, (7) ependymoma, (8) pinealoma, (9) ganglioneuroma, (10) oligodendroglioma, and (11) papilloma choroideum.

Other Classifications and Grading

Hortega published a classification similar to that of Bailey and Cushing, but it lacked correlation with patient survival.[90] Hortega was far removed from his material, being in Spain while the surgeon from whom he received the specimens was in Paris. Hortega excelled in cytological observation of brain tumors. He also used the histogenetic principle, but did not deal with the biological aspects of these tumors, such as location, age of the patient, and correlation of survival with tumor type, nor did he consider the architectural pattern of the tumors.

Roussy and Oberling modified the scheme originally proposed by Roussy, Lhermitte, and Cornil.[195,196] They attempted to consider clinical and anatomical factors as much as possible. They distinguished three main groups of tumors derived from supporting neural tissue: (1) glial, (2) ependymal and choroidal, and (3) those arising from neuronal elements. They proposed two additional groups, the neurospongiomas (medulloblastomas), and the neuroepitheliomas, which represented tumors similar to tissue at the earliest stages of development. They based their classification on similarity of the tumor to embryonic cells in stages of development and assumed that dedifferentiation of mature cells led to the production of neoplasms.

In the field of general pathology, the theory of embryonic cell rests has met with little enthusiasm in interpreting the pathogenesis of tumors, except for teratomas and congenital tumors. The idea that tumors develop from dedifferentiation of adult cells is more often accepted. Support for this theory was gained from the experimental induction of tumors in mature animals with carcinogens and radiation. That these adult cells stimulated by known or unknown agents to become neoplastic actually follow an embryological path is unproved, although it is often tacitly assumed.

Anaplasia (dedifferentiation) may be defined as "reversion of form of a cell or cells toward the embryonal."[22] This definition rests on the assumption of similarity between embryogenesis and carcinogenesis, and that the latter reverses the path of the former. Ewing thought that carcinogenesis is not a type of embryogenesis.[62] More recent evidence indicates that some tumors of the digestive tract have antigens in common with the fetal organ in which the tumor arises (carcinoembryonic antigens, or CEA).[72] These fetal antigens are not present in the adult organ unless the neoplasm occurs. Carcinoembryonic antigens were described in gliomas, but confirmation has been lacking.[242] Mahaley was unable to detect specific glioma antigens or specific antiglioma antibodies.[139] Common antigens

are not necessarily evidence of a common mechanism, hence the definition of anaplasia given by Dorland is currently preferable. Anaplasia is "a loss of differentiation of cells (dedifferentiation) and of their orientation to one another and to their axial framework and blood vessels, a characteristic of tumor tissue."[54] Anaplasia, then, is a measure of the loss of resemblance of tumor cells or tissue to the cells or tissue of origin; this definition has the advantage of being descriptive rather than related to an unproved theory.

General pathologists customarily divide tumors into two grades—benign or malignant. The division has its counterpart in the nomenclature of epithelial and mesodermal tumors—for example, adenoma and carcinoma, fibroma and fibrosarcoma, for benign and malignant versions respectively. It may be noted that a similar change of name is not available to categorize benign and malignant gliomas. Dividing tumors of the same cellular type into four grades of malignancy was suggested by Broders, a surgical pathologist, who in 1915 proposed the concept and then published a report in 1920.[28] The classification arose from histological examination of many epitheliomas in which he found similarities. The tumors were divided into four groups of different degrees of cellular anaplasia, on the theory that tumors were derived by dedifferentiation of mature cells. Broders stated that if about three fourths of the tumor were differentiated and one fourth dedifferentiated, it was graded I, and so on. Later, he changed this system by placing emphasis on the percentage rather than the proportion of anaplastic cells.[29] Grade I tumors thus contained cells in which differentiation ranged from almost 100 per cent to 75 per cent, but in grade IV tumors, differentiated cells constituted from 0 to 25 per cent of the total.

Kernohan and associates introduced a system of grading gliomas based on Broders' ideas, and correlated the findings with prognosis.[104,105] These authors proposed a scheme with four grades of malignancy, and applied these grades to astrocytomas, ependymomas, oligodendrogliomas, and "neuroastrocytomas." Medulloblastoma was considered a type in itself and was not graded. The most exact description was given for the four grades of astrocytoma. The authors proposed eliminating the terms "glioblastoma multiforme," "astroblastoma," and "polar spongioblastoma" because they were variants of astrocytoma. Their classification was based on the idea that "gliomas arise from pre-existing adult cells still capable of proliferation by a process of dedifferentiation or anaplasia." They found a direct relation between the degree of anaplasia and the postoperative survival period. Supporting their theory, they noted the occasional change in histological appearance from that of well-differentiated astrocytoma to glioblastoma, as shown by specimens obtained at succeeding operations on the same patient. Shein has shown experimentally that a single cell of astrocytoma can become a glioblastoma multiforme.[215] Kernohan and co-workers failed to note that oligodendrogliomas and ependymomas, when recurrent, may also finally appear as glioblastomas.[105]

Ringertz developed a similar system at the same time, but used three grades.[193] In 1950, he applied this classification to astrocytomas, ependymomas, and oligodendrogliomas. Ringertz compared the histopathological appearance and postoperative prognosis of the different types of gliomas. He stated that these gliomas could dedifferentiate into a common type of anaplastic glioma, and preferred the term "glioblastoma" for these anaplastic tumors without "recognizable special character." Ringertz probably is correct in his belief that, in adults, gliomas of many initial cell types may ultimately become glioblastomas. Medulloblastoma, as in Kernohan's classification, was not graded. Ringertz also showed that some astrocytomas of the cerebral hemispheres had the same histological appearance and prognosis as the cerebellar astrocytomas of childhood and adolescence.

Many objections have been raised to grading, none of them overwhelming in nature. The use of four grades is arbitrary: it cannot be applied to medulloblastoma; oligodendrogliomas do not differ so greatly as to require four grades; the varieties of astrocytoma could readily be divided into 10 or more grades by an enthusiastic "splitter." Nevertheless, any other subdivision may be equally arbitrary. A more important objection to grading is raised when, as in cerebral ependymoma, the histological findings are not correlated with prognosis.[118] The invasiveness of the tumor, a biological rather than a histological characteristic, is more important in determining the outcome. Furthermore, grade IV ependymomas are seldom encountered, and probably would be called glioblastomas by most nongrading neuropathologists.

The importance of considering factors other than histological has been re-emphasized by Zuelch.[283] He proposed five grades of malignancy based not only on the histological type but on overall behavior. Grade 0 thus would consist of completely resectable tumors, and grade IV of tumors associated with survival of a year or less.

The original system of two grades, benign or malignant, thus can be expanded into three (Ringertz), four (Kernohan et al.), or five (Zuelch). Each further split of the unknown adds additional complexity and calls for prophetic qualities of successively greater nature. Simplicity suggests that "benign versus malignant" is the easiest distinction to make, and that further subdivision could be made most usefully by dichotomy (more benign, less benign, and the like) if the pathologist thinks it necessary to satisfy his psychological needs or those of the surgeon.

Any ordering of tumors by degree of differentiation usually will have some statistical justification; usually, a patient with a better differentiated tumor will live longer than a patient with a poorly differentiated neoplasm. The individual patient, however, has the capability of transgressing the statistical conclusion; the wise clinician keeps in mind both the individual and the statistics.

If these classifications are considered apart from their theoretic base, we find that similar tumors may be given dissimilar names. If the various names indeed describe the same entity, it matters little whether a tumor is called glioblastoma multiforme or astrocytoma grade III or IV. When a spongioblastoma of the cerebellum, is called astrocytoma of the cerebellum, only the name has been changed. From the point of view of the patient or the practical neurosurgeon, the outcome is the same.

Present Views of Classification

A compromise has been offered by the Unio Internationalis Contra Cancrum.[84] Multiple names for a particular tumor are given in this system, and most of the common brain tumors are included. The classification has imperfections, such as the mixing of categories of cells (e.g., nerve cells, glia) with organs (e.g., nose, eye), but it is an attempt to obtain agreement on names used throughout the world, a desirable but difficult goal.

The presentation given in this text is a synthesis of various views, and is an attempt to simplify ("lump") a subject often made complex by "splitters." Astroblastoma is classified as either an ependymoma or a form of astrocytoma; careful examination will almost always disclose multiple processes on cells arranged in cartwheel fashion, and the need to imagine a relation to an embryonic cell is eliminated. Spongioblastoma polare is an astrocytoma in which the multiple processes are compressed as the cells grow in the tight spaces of the optic nerve or brain stem. This newer concept is in accord with the clinical fact that the duration of illness usually is long; a poorly differentiated cell, the "spongioblast," should not be associated with prolonged survival. Pinealoma is considered as a teratoma in accord with the findings of Russell; a teratoma is composed of two or more types of tissue foreign to the part in which they arise.[199] This view explains the instances in which "pinealoma" occurs although tumor is not seen in the presumed tissue of origin. The need to invoke aberrant pineal tissue is also obviated. Neoplasms arising from the stroma of the pineal body are tumors of glial cells, and are properly called astrocytoma, ependymoma, and so on. The possibility of a tumor of pineal tissue as such is not eliminated, but it is extremely small.

The modification of the original Bailey-Cushing scheme as shown in Table 83–1 is a reasonable one. The first three diagnoses may also contain the phrase "well differentiated" or "poorly differentiated" to serve as an additional guide to prognosis. The suffix "-blast" is generally avoided to prevent confusion with embryological forms. The degree of differentiation can be seen microscopically, but the analogy with embryological forms is a supposition.

Readers desiring an even simpler approach may be attracted to the suggestion that the first three diagnoses may be lumped into a single group. This concept does not violate clinical or anatomical facts. The life span of patients with these gliomas is generally measured in years, rather than months as with medulloblastoma or glioblastoma. Oligodendroglial cells are often present in ependymoma;[103] astrocytes are almost always found in oligodendrogliomas;[194] and ependymal cells in some places may not be distinguished from astrocytes except by processes radiating around blood vessels. Transitional cells abound in normal tissue;[189] it is often difficult to distinguish an astrocyte from an oligodendrocyte in either normal or neoplastic tissue. Radioautographic data and other findings indicate these cells may be interchangeable, and that different appearances are dependent on altered functional states.[114]

Any attempt to simplify complex matters must be counterbalanced by awareness of the complications. Therefore, "mixed" and "unclassified" have deliberately been added to Table 83–1. Mixed gliomas in the brain are of four varieties: mixtures of well-differentiated glial cells, of well- and poorly differentiated glial cells, of glial cells and neurons, and of glial and mesenchymal

TABLE 83–1 COMPARISON OF MODIFIED CUSHING-BAILEY CLASSIFICATION AND GRADING OF KERNOHAN ET AL.

MODIFIED BAILEY-CUSHING	KERNOHAN ET AL.
Astrocytoma	Astrocytoma, grades I and II
Oligodendroglioma	Oligodendroglioma, grades I to IV
Ependymoma	Ependymoma
Medulloblastoma	Medulloblastoma
Glioblastoma multiforme	Astrocytoma, grades III and IV
Pinealoma (teratoma)	Pinealoma
Ganglioneuroma (ganglioglioma)	Neuroastrocytoma, grade I
Neuroblastoma (sympathicoblastoma)	Neuroastrocytoma, grades II to IV
Papilloma of choroid plexus	
Mixed	
Unclassified	

cells. Further, mature oligodendrocytes, astrocytes, and ependymal cells mingle in many gliomas, a finding not related to anaplasia of the cells. In these cases, pathologists usually name the tumor for the predominant type of cell; hence clinicians are often unaware of the mixture. In a tumor containing both differentiated and anaplastic cells, neuropathologists conventionally name the tumor for the most histologically malignant feature, not by the largest number of cells identified. This usage gives the neurosurgeon the best approximation of the prognosis. If 98 per cent of a tumor is composed of mature astrocytes, but anaplastic cells and foci of necrosis are present, the appropriate diagnosis is glioblastoma multiforme. Glial cells and neurons may be mixed in a tumor in combinations ranging from a predominance of neurons (''ganglioneuroma''), an approximately equal mixture (''ganglioglioma''), to largely glial, so that the diagnosis of astrocytoma alone might be offered.

Combined gliomas and sarcomas have been reported increasingly in recent years. Rubinstein offered two possibilities to explain this mixture: either the invasive sarcoma produced a malignant change in the adjacent neuroglia or a sarcomatous change arose in the vascular proliferation of the glioblastoma.[198] More explicitly, experimental evidence from use of chemical carcinogens and viruses suggests that a single agent is capable of transforming cells of both glial and mesenchymal origin into neoplasms. The need to invoke the concept of *one* cell reacting to the presence of another stems largely from the commonly accepted but unproved assumption that all tumors arise from the neoplastic transformation of a single cell.

Table 83–1 also indicates that some brain tumors should be labeled ''unclassified.'' Each specific diagnosis is based on certain rules set by the pathologist, but criteria as well as interpretations differ. One problem is that few authors state specific criteria in writing, and diagnosis too often is an arbitrary process. For example, should the diagnosis of glioblastoma multiforme be made on cellular characteristics alone? Is the presence of necrosis necessary for this diagnosis? Should ependymoma be diagnosed when a few perivascular radiations of glial processes are seen, and if not, how many are needed? Another problem is that

criteria may need changing with new experience or added information, but old concepts tend to linger. The finding of blepharoplasts as a confirmation of the diagnosis of ependymoma, still cited in recent textbooks, offers an example. A small dark body near the surface often is found in tumor cells and may be a clump of chromatin or a precipitate of other protein as well as the blepharoplast (basal body) of a cilium. Electron microscopy has revealed that all cells in the nervous system are ciliated in embryonic life and that even adult neurons and glia may contain cilia.[53] Centrioles and cilia occur in meningiomas.[36] Indeed, rudimentary cilia have been found in smooth muscle cells and fibroblasts.[227]

Unclassified tumors occur more frequently if the cells are poorly differentiated. The diagnosis of tumors composed of small, round, and dark cells is influenced by the clinical data as well as by the microscopic appearance. Highly anaplastic tumors at times cannot be distinguished as to origin in glial, epithelial, or connective tissue.

Finally, the problem of classification should be approached clinically as well as by histological means. Pathologists classify tumors by a judgment as to the cells and tissues from which the neoplasm originated. Malignancy in the cranium, however, is not solely a function of cells of origin. For this reason, caution should be used in applying the terms ''benign'' and ''malignant'' to a histological classification of gliomas. The terms ''well-differentiated'' and ''poorly differentiated'' are preferable to ''benign'' and ''malignant.'' Decisions about prognosis, repeated surgical procedures, radiotherapy, and the like must take into account factors other than the histological diagnosis: the state of intracranial pressure, position and size of the tumor, age and general condition of the patient. The concept of ''total malignancy'' suggested by Zuelch, including not only the histological dedifferentiation but also the effect of location as in the case of a well-differentiated tumor in a critical position, is of importance in the clinical use of any classification.[284]

Ability to predict the biological activity of a tumor is limited at the present time. Tumors of the same cellular type and even in the same position may behave differently in different patients.[164] For example, one medulloblastoma responds promptly to ra diation, but another in the same location does not. The fate of a patient with a cerebral ependymoma is more dependent on its invasiveness than on its histological appearance. A histologically indistinguishable astrocytoma may be harbored for 20 years in one case, but in another, dedifferentiates to glioblastoma and the patient rapidly dies. The variable behavior of gliomas is not unique, however, and similar examples can be cited for systemic neoplasms.

BIOLOGY

Etiological Agents

Genetic Factors

Genetic predisposition is infrequent in tumors of the central nervous system, but unfortunately this information often is not obtained in sufficient detail. Some tumors have a hereditary component, exemplified by three developmental disorders of the group called phakomatoses: von Recklinghausen's neurofibromatosis, tuberous sclerosis, and von Hippel-Lindau disease. The evidence of hereditary influence is less striking in Sturge-Weber disease.

Multiple neurofibromatosis of von Recklinghausen is the major example of a tumor of the central nervous system with genetic influence. The frequency ranges from 1:2000 to 1:3000 in the general population. Inheritance is through an autosomal dominant or irregularly dominant gene. Sexual incidence is about equal, although Zuelch speaks of a female preponderance.[283] Neurofibromas of the spinal nerve roots and peripheral nerves are frequent, and the incidence of spinal ependymomas is increased. The most common associated intracranial tumors in this disease are schwannomas, gliomas, and meningiomas. The cutaneous and neural changes often occur in adolescence and adulthood, and a multiplicity of lesions is the common finding.

Tuberous sclerosis is less common than neurofibromatosis. The frequency is estimated between 1:30,000 to 1:150,000 in the general population. The sexual incidence is about equal. Transmission is as an autosomal dominant or irregularly dominant trait. The patients are usually children or adolescents. The cerebral lesions are firm hyper-

plastic nodules consisting of malformed and often extremely large glial cells. Most of the neoplasms are giant-cell astrocytomas of a benign nature. The estimated incidence of malignant changes is 1 to 3 per cent.

Von Hippel-Lindau disease has a dominant or irregularly dominant mode of inheritance. The disease most commonly includes hemangioblastoma of the cerebellum, and less frequently, of the brain stem and spinal cord. Another feature is angioma of the retina. The disorder usually becomes evident in adults.

Sturge-Weber disease is a combination of angioma of the brain and meninges, associated with an angioma on the same side of the face. Hereditary influence is less than in the other phakomatoses. Most instances are sporadic. The mode of transmission in the hereditary cases is occasionally dominant or irregularly dominant, and recessive inheritance has been reported. Chromosomal abnormalities have been found in some studies, a 22-trisomy in one case and a chromosomal translocation to a group D chromosome in another.[85,180] The fact that most patients have normal chromosomes suggests that these findings may be chance associations.

The phakomatoses thus are developmental defects in the mesoectoderm, and heredity often is important. The end-result is a group of disorders with considerable variation in penetrance of genetic factors and also in the clinical expression. Cases have been reported in which more than one of these diseases have occurred in the same individual or family.

The retina is embryologically related to the primary neural vesicle. Retinoblastoma, although not a primary intracranial tumor, may invade the cranial cavity. These tumors are of interest genetically. The incidence is estimated at from 1:20,000 to 1:34,000 live births. Most cases are detected before the age of 3 years. Sexual incidence is equal. Sporadic cases constitute about three quarters of the total. When the tumors are bilateral, other members of the family are likely to be affected. The hereditary cases have autosomal dominant transmission. Some authors have described an abnormal chromosome in group D.

These central nervous system tumors with a reasonably well-defined hereditary background are rare. Genetic relations in the remaining large group are still in question. Hague and Harvald selected 535 probands with glioblastoma, astrocytoma, medulloblastoma, and meningioma.[83] The study included the relatives of probands and a small number of controls and their relatives. The authors found that the number of deaths from intracranial tumor among the relatives of the probands did not significantly exceed those found in the controls.

Van der Wiel studied brain tumors occurring in the relatives of 100 probands from the Utrecht Neurological Clinic in whom the diagnosis of glioma had been established by biopsy or necropsy.[246] One hundred controls were randomly selected. In the relatives of the proband group, 14 cases of cerebral tumor were found in 12 families. The diagnosis was confirmed by histological examination in eight cases: six gliomas, one medulloblastoma, and one meningioma. None of the relatives of the control group died with intracranial tumors. The death rate from gliomas in the relatives of the proband group was four times as great as expected in the population of the Netherlands. Additionally, the control group had a 7.8 per cent incidence of dysrhaphic phenomena, but the incidence in the close relatives of the glioma probands was 20.8 per cent. Van der Wiel, therefore, suggested a hereditary factor in the genesis of gliomas.[246]

The contradictory results in these two studies may be related to the hospitals from which probands were collected. Koch contended that glioblastomas were encountered less frequently in neurosurgical clinics than in institutes of pathology and in neurological clinics.[113] He thought that gliomas, particularly, occur in families, and that the predilection depended on a factor associated with defective embryological development rather than specific inheritance. The familial incidence of gliomas was noted by van der Wiel in 31 cases from the medical literature. In this group, 23 cases involved parent-child or sibling relationships, and the other 8 were in more distant relatives. From 1950 to 1965, 41 families were reported in which isolated brain tumors were found in two or more members.[2]

Of interest also are reports of brain tumors in twins. The best known case was one reported by Leavitt in which identical twins developed medulloblastomas.[127] Three more cases of this tumor in twins were added later by others. Koch found reports of 12 pairs of twins affected with brain tumors.[112] Five were concordant for brain tumor, but were not identical. He added 20 pairs of twins discordant for brain tumor, including 3 identical, 7 fraternal, and 10 of uncertain nature. Hague and Harvald noted that eight probands were twins, all, discordant for intracranial tumor. Only two of the eight pairs were monozygotic. Twin studies have not been informative with respect to zygosity, and descriptions of family history are sparse. It seems likely that further studies of twins and the careful analysis of families with multiple intracranial tumors will contribute additional information on genetic mechanisms. At present, the genetic factor revealed by studies of families is weak but cannot be entirely ignored.

Cytogenetic Studies

Study of chromosomes in intracranial tumors is another method of investigating genetic mechanisms. Solid tumors and the leukemias have been analyzed extensively in the past, but recently attention has been directed to the central nervous system. These data have not been reviewed before, and hence are presented in detail.

Chromosomes may be studied only during cell division. A low mitotic index, that is, few cells in mitosis, is common in benign and even many malignant tumors of the central nervous system, decreasing the number of cells available for study. Culture methods therefore were developed largely to furnish more cells in mitosis. These methods of study have certain limitations. Analysis of chromosomes has improved since it was first introduced, but many artifacts still occur. Handling, diagnostic or therapeutic radiation, and cytotoxic drugs may alter cells, and spontaneous fragmentation also has been reported. In tumors of the central nervous system, as in other areas of the body, chromosomal analysis is performed either directly on tumor cells or after short- or long-term culture. Some described changes are related to these differences in preparation. When cells in culture are examined, the question arises whether in vitro findings can be translated to in vivo processes. The dividing cell cannot always be identified in cultured material, so that a diploid mode might represent an analysis of cells of nonneoplastic stroma, or blood vessels or leptomeninges in the case of a tumor of the central nervous system. In some cultures, especially long-term ones, stromal cells overgrow the tumor. The environment in tissue culture may in some way alter the tumor cell.

Some methods of culture selectively favor the growth of diploid cells. Although the presence of diploid karyotypes in cultured cells might then be normal, studies of other tumors in which most chromosome numbers were not diploid are against this idea.

In considering the differences between culture and direct examination of tumor cells, Conen and colleagues found predominance of aneuploidy on direct examination of chromosomes, but few aneuploid cells in cultures from the same malignant effusions of pleura and peritoneum.[42] Their comparison of cultured and noncultured central nervous system tumors, although not from the same patients, indicated that the methods of study affected the results. It was suggested that short-term cultures are more valid than long-term cultures with regard to consistency of chromosomal number in comparison with fresh material.

Sampling error, as in other statistical evaluations of biological data, is of importance. A small number of tumors may be insufficient to draw significant conclusions from, even though a large number of cells is examined. Sampling of a few cells within a tumor also may not allow adequate evaluation, as for example, when a bimodal population of cells is encountered but only one of the cellular components is represented.

The chromosomal pattern of three intracranial gliomas was directly analyzed by Lubs and Salmon.[132] A glioblastoma contained chromosomes with a bimodal (diploid and tetraploid) distribution. Acrocentric marker chromosomes were identical in both cell lines. Chromosome fragments were also observed, as well as variations in the number of chromosomes in cells of both lines. A 4500 R dose of radiation given before removal of the glioblastoma may have created the described alteration of chromosomal pattern. An oligodendroglioma contained several cells in which the chromosomes were tetraploid and of normal shape. The authors suggested that the findings indicated a tumor with a simple tetraploid mode. A medulloblastoma, reported in greater detail at a later date, was obtained

at craniotomy from an 8-year-old girl, and chromosomal analysis was done on the biopsy specimen.[133] Double minute chromosomes, probably chromosome fragments, were found in all mitoses, as were also an abnormal metacentric form and extra chromosomes in groups D and E. Cells in the bone marrow also contained the double minute fragments, abnormal metacentric forms, and extra chromosomes in groups D and E.

Cox and co-workers examined the chromosomes prepared directly from six neoplasms, five in children (medulloblastoma, rhabdomyosarcoma, and three neuroblastomas) and one carcinoma of the lung in an adult.[46] All cases had a similar feature: multiple small fragments in a structurally intact set of chromosomes. Each tumor had a different abnormal karyotype, but cells in the same tumor also varied. Nevertheless, these patients had not been previously treated, and the findings are similar to the case of medulloblastoma described by Lubs and Salmon.

Thirty-one fresh brain tumors were examined by Bicknell.[18] Cells satisfactory for analysis were obtained in only three: recurrent ependymoma, glioblastoma multiforme, and astrocytoma grade III (nomenclature of the author). The patient with ependymoma had been irradiated before chromosome study and had aneuploidy with extra chromosomes in group C and less frequently in groups D to G. Occasionally the chromosomes were abnormal and fragmented. Most chromosomal numbers were in the tetraploid range, but those in the glioblastoma were in the diploid range. Eleven of the cells in the grade III astrocytoma were tetraploid, six were hypertetraploid, and three were triploid. The greatest number of extra chromosomes was in group C, as in the recurrent ependymoma. It should be noted that group C of the karyotype has the largest number of chromosomal pairs, and the frequency of extra chromosomes in this group may be explained in this manner.

The chromosomal pattern was analyzed in 12 intracranial tumors in the fresh state, 8 of which had aneuploid or pseudodiploid patterns.[61] The chromosomes in five cases ranged closely around the diploid number (meningeal sarcoma with a pseudodiploid number, ependymoma, two grade IV astrocytomas, and a cerebellar sarcoma). Combined normal and abnormal cell lines were found in a grade III and a grade IV astrocytoma. Completely abnormal patterns were found in a grade IV astrocytoma (hypertetraploid) and a grade IV astrocytoma (triploid). A medulloblastoma had a normal pattern.

Conen and Falk later studied chromosomes after tissue culture on 12 tumors of the central nervous system from children aged one week to 13 years.[41] The patients had not received radiotherapy or chemotherapy before chromosomal studies. Tissue culture was used to provide an increased number of dividing cells because mitoses were infrequent in many of the tumors. The chromosomal analyses were normal in most cases, in contrast to those made in their earlier work in which abnormalities predominated, suggesting to these authors that stromal cells outgrew cultured tumor.

A study of 11 glioblastomas was made by Wilson and co-workers.[270] Cells satisfactory for direct study were obtained from three tumors, and the others were studied in cultures ranging from 5 to 236 days. Chromosome preparations were obtained at five different ages in one glioblastoma in an established cell line, the oldest more than five years. The most frequent karyotype was near-diploid; deviations occurred most often in group C. Two of the original tumors contained tetraploid cells (92 chromosomes), but the chromosomal number of the cultured cells was always 52 or less. The karyotype was hypotriploid in the established cell line of glioblastoma.

In general, benign tumors are difficult to study because the number of mitoses may be insufficient for analysis. Meningiomas are among the few benign tumors in the body to show aneuploidy. Porter and associates, for example, found a group G chromosome missing in each of three cases.[186]

The variation in chromosomal number in group C may represent a common denominator. It was found by Lubs and Salmon in a medulloblastoma and glioblastoma, and in an irradiated recurrent ependymoma and a grade III astrocytoma.[132] Wilson also identified variations in group C in glioblastomas.[270] The liability of group C to changes, however, may be only a reflection of a greater number of chromosomes. The work cited has, in addition, confirmed the finding of aneuploidy and polyploidy in many tumors

of the central nervous system, as found in systemic neoplasms.

Firm conclusions cannot be drawn from our present knowledge of the cytogenics of central nervous system tumors. Specific numbers or patterns of chromosomes are inconstant, as are excesses or deficiencies. Some similarities in number and karyotype exist, but consistent correlation cannot yet be made with the various types of intracranial tumors. Although these data relate to the extremely important process of formation of DNA and genetically coded information, they are largely descriptive. At this time, they offer little of clinical significance; they may become more valuable in the future.

Blood Groups

The ABO blood groups are genetically controlled and readily studied. The demonstration of associations between a blood group and a disease is a means of investigating genetic factors. Since about 1955, the relation between the blood groups and an increasing number of diseases has been reported. A study of 637 brain tumors revealed that the distribution of the ABO blood groups in the sample did not deviate significantly from that found in controls of a hospitalized population in Boston.[151] An excess of type O then was found in association with chromophobe adenomas in the Boston hospitals as well as in two hospitals in New York. This statistically significant finding was considered tentative because of the small size of the tumor group. Buckwalter and associates collected 565 brain tumors in patients of known blood type.[33] Voluntary donors were used as controls; the question may be raised whether these persons are a truly random population. Men with type A blood had an increased number of brain tumors, but not in any single diagnostic category.

A greater number of cases with type A also were found in a small series of 72 gliomas in children.[230] Considering that some of the previous reports might not have included a sufficient number of young persons, Yates and Pearce investigated 473 astrocytomas.[275] This tumor was used because it occurred in statistically useful numbers at all ages studied. The blood groups in patients less than 20 years of age were grossly disproportionate in cases diagnosed after 1945. This pattern was different from that noted in cases occurring before 1945. One possible explanation for this phenomenon is that patients with juvenile astrocytoma may have a weak A antigen not adequately detected by the grouping techniques used before 1945.

Selverstone and Cooper studied 139 consecutive patients with verified astrocytomas in which they found a significantly decreased prevalence of blood groups O and B in patients with this tumor.[213] A series of 630 consecutive patients undergoing craniotomy, including 132 cases of astrocytoma, was described by Garcia and coworkers.[69] They noted no statistical abnormality of blood group distribution in these cases of astrocytoma, compared with the distribution of blood types in patients with other cerebral tumors (279 cases), in patients undergoing operations for cranial trauma (124 cases), and in patients with nonneoplastic neurosurgical lesions (95 cases).

A still larger group of 3115 primary central nervous system tumors was analyzed by Pearce and Yates.[181] The only abnormal pattern was with astrocytoma, the proportion of type O cases being reduced. This finding, as reported by Yates and Pearce in 1960, was again particularly true in astrocytomas occurring in young people since 1945.

Many questions arise from these studies. The known rarity of type B in the populations of Europe and North America may complicate interpretation, as may the difference in frequency of blood groups in various races. Garcia's group found type B more common and type A less common in the American Negro than in the American Caucasian.[69] The frequency of type B in the region of Kings County Hospital Center in New York, where Negroes constitute 50 per cent of the inpatient population, was about twice as great as in the control group used by Yates and Pearce in England. Manuila noted that ABO frequencies differed greatly among the cities of Great Britain and often between districts of the same city.[143] This finding was confirmed by Wiener, who demonstrated considerable variation in the percentages of primary blood groups in geographic areas or ethnic groups.[264,265] These findings are of importance in evaluating the usual control groups. Technical errors are also a prob-

lem. Manuila stated that errors in grouping could be as high as 8.8 per cent. The histopathological criteria also must be considered in interpreting studies of tumors in relation to blood groups. Review of these data suggests that little has been accomplished with regard to establishing consistent statistical relation between the ABO blood groups and cerebral tumors.

Glossary of Terms in Genetics

Acrocentric—a chromosome with one long arm, the other small or imperceptible

Aneuploid—the condition when the number of chromosomes is not an exact multiple of the haploid number; if n designates the haploid number, the chromosomes may be represented by $2n + 1$, or $2n - 2$, or other combinations

Autosome—the somatic cell, not a germ cell; when referring to chromosomes, means all except the sex chromosomes, x and y

Centromere—the primary constriction of a chromosome and the point where the spindle fiber attaches; the position of the centromere determines whether a chromosome is acrocentric, metacentric, or submetacentric

Chromosome—a dark-staining body appearing in the nucleus at the time of cellular division; contains the genes and is composed of DNA

Chromosomal number—the total number of chromosomes in a cell, or, the arbitrary number assigned to identify each pair of chromosomes (see karyotype)

Concordant—twins sharing the same attribute

Deletion—the process whereby a fragment of a chromosome breaks off and is lost

Diploid—the full number of chromosomes in a somatic cell; the number in man is 46, also designated as $2n$, because it is twice the haploid number

Discordant—twins not sharing the same attribute, as when one twin has a brain tumor and the other does not

Euploid—a set of chromosomes in any balanced number, that is, an exact multiple of the haploid number; euploidy may thus be designated by n (haploid or monoploid, 23 chromosomes, the normal number in a human germ cell), $2n$ (diploid, 46 chromosomes, the normal number in a human somatic cell), $3n$ (triploid, 69 chromosomes) or $4n$ (tetraploid, 92 chromosomes)

Fragment—a small portion of a chromosome; often two homologous parts break off, as in double minute bodies described in the text

Haploid—only one set of chromosomes is present, as in germ cells; the number in normal human germ cells is 23, comprising 22 autosomal and 1 sex chromosome

Hypotetraploid—the number of chromosomes is less than $4n$

Hypertetraploid—the number of chromosomes is more than $4n$

Karyotype—the chromosomes arranged by size and shape. Seven groups are labeled A to G, according to a convention agreed upon by geneticists. Each group contains two to seven homologous chromosomal pairs, one paternal and one maternal in origin:

Group	Chromosomes
A	1, 2, 3 (metacentric)
B	4, 5 (submetacentric)
C	6, 7, 8, 9, 10, 11, 12, and X (submetacentric)
D	13, 14, 15 (acrocentric)
E	16, 17, 18 (submetacentric)
F	19, 20 (metacentric)
G	21, 22, and Y (acrocentric)

Marker chromosome—a chromosome of distinctive configuration allowing it to be identified by inspection; it is unpaired and can be transmitted from one cell generation to another

Metaphase—a stage in the mitotic process of cell division when the chromosomes are concentrated in a mid-position and are splitting into two chromatids

Monozygotic—developed from a single fertilized egg, or zygote, as in identical twins

Metacentric—the two arms of the chromosome are almost equal; hence the chromosome is X-shaped at metaphase

Proband—the starting point of a family pedigree

Pseudodiploid—having the full number of chromosomes ($2n$ or 46), but the grouping is abnormal; for example, group A contains two instead of three chromosomal pairs, but group B has three instead of two

Sex chromosomes—the X and Y chromosomes; the X chromosome is large and metacentric; the Y chromosome is small and acrocentric; two X chromosomes are present in women, one X and one Y in men

Submetacentric—a chromosome with unequal arms, one long and the other short

Tetraploid—having four haploid or two diploid sets of chromosomes; four times the normal number

Translocation—a segment of a chromosome changes position, either to a different chromosome, or another part of the same chromosome

Triploid—three times the normal haploid number

Trisomy—an abnormality in which three chromosomes of a given kind are present rather than two. The total number may then be 47, or, another chromosome may be lost and the total remains at 46 (pseudodiploid)

Zygote—the result of the union of two germ cells, the ovum and sperm; nonidentical twins develop from two zygotes

Physical Factors

Trauma

Trauma has long been considered a possible cause of meningeal or glial tumors. Two world wars and an increase in the destructive capability of the automobile have created a massive number of cerebral injuries, but an excess incidence of brain tumors has not been noted in this group. Head injuries were considered by Cushing and Eisenhardt to be of importance in the origin of some meningiomas; a history of head injury was obtained in 33 per cent of 313' cases.[49] They also noted depressed fracture in 24 instances of scar at the site of the tumor. Zuelch extensively reviewed cases causing physicians to consider trauma as an initiating factor.[283] He noted the work of Marburg and Helfand, who thought that trauma was significant in the genesis of intracranial tumors.[144] Zuelch suggested the following criteria for consideration of trauma as a causative factor:

1. The patient should have been healthy before the accident.
2. The trauma must have been adequate, that is, sufficient to injure a part of the brain or the meninges.
3. The site of tumor should correspond to that receiving the trauma.
4. The time between trauma and development of the tumor should be adequate.
5. The tumor should be proved histologically by biopsy or necropsy.

Little is known of the time necessary for development of intracranial neoplasms in man. Zuelch states that a tumor occurring a "few weeks" after an accident is unlikely to have been caused by the trauma. The statement seems reasonable, but data are unfortunately lacking on the time required for a cerebral neoplasm to appear after trauma.

Parker and Kernohan critically evaluated a series of brain tumors and found 4.8 per cent in which a connection between neoplasm and trauma to the head could be proposed.[179] They compared this group with two others. The first was a group of 431 patients with other diseases and of equivalent age, of whom 10.4 per cent had a history of head injury. The second was a series of healthy individuals of the same age, of whom 35.5 per cent had a history of trauma to the head. It was suggested that these data were against trauma as a cause of intracranial tumor.

A traumatic cause probably can be accepted for a small number of meningiomas, such as that in General Wood, reported by Cushing and Eisenhardt, and a few instances described by Zuelch.[49,283] In most cases, however, trauma probably initiates or aggravates clinical symptoms of a tumor already within the cranial cavity.

Radiation

Radiation-induced carcinoma of the skin is a well-known complication of the cumulative effect of radiation suffered by pioneer radiologists. Reports have also been made of fibrosarcomas of the lip, tongue, and esophagus, and of sarcomas of bone after various doses and types of radiation. Of interest is the finding on microscopic examination of bizarre stromal and parenchymal changes after therapeutic radiation of the nervous system. Russell and associates suggested that these alterations spread beyond the confines of the radiated area and that the changes were those of neoplasia.[202]

A single report is available of a meningioma induced by the presence of thorium dioxide.[124] Administration of x-rays to animals often causes sarcomas, but seldom results in gliogenous tumors of the central nervous system. An acceptable case of a glioma produced in a monkey after a heavy dose of x-rays to the head has been reported.[102] The symptoms began one year after radiation.

Glial tumors associated with radiation of human beings have not been described. Several authors have reported malignant mesodermal tumors in which radiation may have been causative. Zuelch reported a 15-year-old girl in whom complete removal of a hemispheric ependymoma was followed by radiation to the operative site for one year.[283] Necropsy six years later revealed a nodular fibrosarcoma in continuity with the dura in the region of the bone flap, but residual ependymoma was lacking. Russell and Rubinstein described an 18-year-old man who underwent removal of a circumscribed giant-cell glioblastoma of the frontal lobe.[201] A course of deep x-ray therapy was administered after the operation. Six years later, necropsy revealed a massive fibrosarcoma arising from the dura at the site

of operation. In another case, an astrocytoma of the optic nerve was removed from a 5-year-old girl, who then received radiotherapy postoperatively.[141] Five years later, a fatal malignant meningeal tumor appeared at the operative site. Noetzli and Malamud reported the case of a 10-year-old girl who received radiation after subtotal removal of a cerebellar medulloblastoma.[170] Eight years later, a large fibrosarcoma was found in the posterior part of the left cerebral hemisphere, unrelated to the operative site and not attached to dura. The medulloblastoma was not found at necropsy. The authors suggested that radiation had stimulated the cerebral blood vessels, and that the tumor arose from the adventitia. The lack of relation to the primary site, however, makes the case less acceptable than the others.

Malignant intracranial neoplasms arising within or adjacent to tissues exposed to radiation during treatment for acromegaly were reported by Goldberg and associates.[73] These cases included an anaplastic epidermoid carcinoma occurring 20 years after radiation, a hemangioendothelioma after 19 years, a fibrosarcoma after 10 years, and a malignant undifferentiated tumor resembling sarcoma 20 years after four months of radiation. The authors did not eliminate the possibility that acromegaly had a role in the genesis of these tumors. Intracranial meningioma occurred in five cases many years after radiation therapy of the scalp for tinea capitis.[160] Four of the tumors were histologically verified, and the fifth was considered most probably a meningioma on the basis of pneumoencephalography and angiography.

An important and well-controlled study of the ability of radiation to induce neoplasia was reported by Modan and co-workers.[156] About 11,000 children in Israel were irradiated for ringworm of the scalp. These children were retrospectively studied for periods from 12 to 23 years. The controls were two matched groups, one from the general population, and one of siblings. Neoplasms of the head and neck were increased in the radiated children, most strikingly in brain, parotid, and thyroid. Among brain tumors, meningioma was four times as frequent as "other" tumors of brain, which were also increased but unfortunately were not further described. The latent period for intracranial tumors ranged from 7 to 21 years. The mechanism of radiation-induced neoplasia is uncertain. Localized damage to tissues may provide a medium in which the direct action of a viral or chemical agent is more effective. Less is known as to why sarcomas are so frequent after radiation, carcinomas are rare, and gliomas are as yet unreported in man. The difference is not related only to the direct effect of radiation on blood vessels, glands, or glial tissue, because all are known to undergo cytological changes after radiation. Glial cells, however, are slower in reacting to some neoplastic stimuli, such as the insertion of a pellet of methylcholanthrene into the brain of a mouse (see next section); sarcomas may appear in a few weeks or months, but gliomas are not encountered until after a year. Viruses may induce both kinds of tumor in a month, and chemicals such as the nitroso compounds may produce gliomas in a few months. A patient surviving for 20 years or longer after radiation to the brain may ultimately develop a glioma, but this has not yet been described.

Chemical Factors

Anthracene Compounds

At present, neither genetic nor physical factors may be used to induce brain tumors regularly in animals. Chemical methods were introduced in an attempt to develop reproducible models. Tumors produced experimentally have been used to determine pathogenesis and growth rates, and as models for testing therapeutic agents.

Experimental brain tumors induced by chemical carcinogens were first reported in the late 1930's. Roussy and co-workers applied tar-impregnated gauze to the cortical surface of rats, causing only necrosis.[197] Oberling and co-workers applied crystals of benzpyrene to the cortex of rats, and found hypophyseal adenomas in three animals that survived 10 months or more.[171] They also injected benzpyrene-in-oil into the brain of one rat and found an epitheliomatous hypophyseal adenoma. Weil obtained epidermoid carcinomas in one of six rats after the intracerebral injection of methycholanthrene-in-lard.[256] Four of five rats developed sarcomas after injection of the same substance. He also reported the oc-

currence of tumors, resembling meningioma, glioma, and ependymoma in three of five rats after the injection of a quinoline derivative, styryl 430. Other investigators used widely different substances in several species without producing intracranial tumors.

Seligman and Shear placed pellets of methycholanthrene intracerebrally in 20 mice of the C3H strain.[212] Gliomas developed in 11 and meningeal fibrosarcomas in 2; no tumors were found in 7. The glial tumors resembled glioblastoma, spongioblastoma polare, fibrillary astrocytoma, medulloblastoma, ependymoma, oligodendroglioma, and pinealoma. One glioma and one fibrosarcoma grew when transplanted subcutaneously in other C3H mice.

Zimmerman and Arnold confirmed this work with intracerebral implants of methylcholanthrene, dibenzanthracene, and benzpyrene in C3H mice, and produced many glial tumors.[280-282] They found that the site of implantation was a partial determinant of the type of tumor produced. Tumors were also transplanted subcutaneously by Zimmerman and Arnold. Perese and Moore induced pinealoma and chromophobe adenoma of the pituitary with implantation of three different carcinogens.[182] These authors stated that glioblastomas transplanted subcutaneously in mice of the same strain were converted into sarcomas. The possibility that the "conversion" was the result of stromal overgrowth was not eliminated.

Factors related to the induction of tumor include species, strain, and individual variations. Dogs and monkeys are almost completely resistant to implantation of anthracene compounds. Chemical induction of gliomas is more difficult in the C57 black mouse than in the C3H strain. Few workers report a prevalence of brain tumors higher than 50 per cent, and rates are almost always lower when chemical carcinogens are implanted in the cerebrum in a large series of animals. Most animals of a susceptible strain of great genetic purity, then, are resistant to induction of brain tumors, even though the carcinogen lies in prolonged contact with glial cells.

Extracerebral tissue does not resist growth of gliomas in man or in animals. Cerebral gliomas in man on occasion may metastasize outside the central nervous system and have grown in the lung, lymph node, kidney, and elsewhere. Grace and associates transplanted gliogenous tumors from the brain to the subcutaneous tissue of the same patient and found growth in some cases.[77] Intravenous injection of gliomas in mice results in growth of tumor in many organs of the body.[164] The rate of growth of experimental gliomas under controlled conditions and with delivery of equal numbers of cells is extremely variable, representing undetermined growth factors. The histological appearance at times is poorly correlated with the rate of growth, as may be true of some human tumors.[164]

Zimmerman noted that because of the short life span of the mouse and the relatively long time required for development of glial tumors induced by chemical carcinogens, most gliomas occurred in mature animals.[278] Tumors have not been produced by this method in relatively young animals. It is therefore not possible to correlate these data with the higher frequency of astrocytomas of the benign type in young human beings. Glial cells chemically stimulated to proliferate to a tumor were adult cells, and Zimmerman therefore suggested that embryonic cell rests were not important factors in the genesis of gliomas. He saw no need for the concept of bipotential or multipotential cells in the nervous system producing a heterogeneous cell population after stimulation by carcinogens. Many adult cells were exposed to the chemical carcinogen, and the cells stimulated might be all of one type, or of several different varieties. His opinion was that mixed cell populations were the result of simultaneous stimulation and proliferation of more than one type of glial cell rather than dedifferentiation of a single glial cell. The possibility was not eliminated that daughter cells of similar parentage may appear in different form, depending on the environment. An epithelial cell growing in a compressed tissue space, for example, may lengthen and resemble a fibroblast or spongioblast. He did not encounter malignant proliferation of microglial or ganglion cells.

Zimmerman explained the occurrence of "pure" tumors in two ways. First, the carcinogen initiated proliferation of one cell, or of several cells of the same type. Second, what was at first a mixed glioma became in time a "pure" glioma because rapidly proliferating cells of one type predominated. Experience indicates that neither human nor animal tumors are often "pure."

Other Chemical Carcinogens

N-nitroso compounds have been used in the induction of neoplasms since 1956, when Magee and Barnes created systemic tumors with dimethylnitrosomine in rats.[136] Methylnitrosourea (MNU) was first of the nitroso compounds to be used for induction of a large number of nervous system tumors after systemic administration. This and other nitroso compounds have subsequently been shown to induce tumors of the central and peripheral nervous systems. Druckery and co-workers and Kleihues and co-workers have published comprehensive reviews of this work.[58,110] Important factors in the use of these neuro-oncogenic agents in tumor induction are the chemical structure and dosage, age and species of the animal, and mode of application.

Wechsler and co-workers have described the techniques, and noted a high incidence of central nervous system tumors when various nitroso compounds were administered by different routes.[255] The two nitroso compounds most frequently used for induction of neural tumors are methylnitrosourea (MNU) and ethylnitrosourea (ENU). These compounds yield many tumors of the brain, spinal cord, and cranial and peripheral nerves in adult rats. With methylnitrosourea the number of induced tumors is a function of the mode of application. Experimental data show that the incidence of nervous system tumors is greatest after intravenous injection and decreases with oral, intraperitoneal, and subcutaneous administration (see Table 1 in the review by Kleihues and associates).[110] In addition, tumors are found more frequently in the central than in the peripheral nervous system. Single doses given to adult rats yield few neural tumors; nonneurogenic tumors were more frequent. By contrast, repeated small doses caused a great prevalence of neural tumors, compared to tumors in other organs, in both young and adult animals.

There is evidence to suggest that the application of methylnitrosourea in perinatal rats enhances the oncogenic effect of this compound. The perinatal induction of tumors of the nervous system by ethylnitrosourea, first demonstrated in the rat by Druckery and Ivankovic and their co-workers, has proved to be the method most frequently used for inducing tumors of the nervous system at the present time.[55,93] The use of this method has demonstrated that, in the rat, the injection of ethylnitrosourea into pregnant animals does not yield tumors unless given after day 12 of gestation, suggesting that the fetal system must develop to a certain stage of maturity before it is capable of producing neoplasms. The yield of tumors is also high in the offspring when a single injection of ethylnitrosourea is given in the last week of gestation; thereafter, in the postnatal stage of development, the carcinogenic effect declines.[56,94] The route by which the carcinogen is applied seems to make little difference in the production of a high yield of tumors during the perinatal period.[111]

Different carcinogens administered systematically to different animals have predilection for certain sites within the nervous system. The induced tumors in the cerebral hemispheres develop most frequently within the subcortical white matter, in the hippocampus, and around the lateral ventricles. Tumors infrequently occur in cerebral structures contained within the posterior fossa. Neoplasms induced in the peripheral nervous system occur most frequently in the trigeminal nerve and brachial and lumbar plexuses.

Central and peripheral nervous system tumors induced chemically are primarily gliomas and schwannomas. Histological examination and classification of nitroso-induced central nervous system tumors has shown that these compounds produce a wide range of glial tumors including benign and anaplastic astrocytomas, oligodendrogliomas, ependymomas, and mixed glial tumors as well as glial-mesenchymal tumors.* Neoplasms of neuronal elements are uncommon. Carcinogen-induced tumors of the nervous system are most often typical schwannomas, ranging in degree of differentiation. Ultrastructural studies of these tumors have indicated, however, that the Schwann cells are neoplastic; the degree of differentiation depends on the carcinogenic agent used.[233]

These chemicals then can convert normal glial and Schwann cells into neoplasms. Particularly important is the fact that the induction is not by topical application, as

*See references 58, 98, 115, 233, 255.

with anthracene compounds. These drugs are administered at sites distant from the central nervous system, but many tumors are produced and may be specific for the nervous system. Furthermore, the induction period is months rather than a year or more, as when cholanthrenes are topically applied. The nitroso compounds also affect a wider range of species than the cholanthrenes; for example, rats are resistant to the cerebral implantation of methylcholanthrene, but are susceptible to production of brain tumors by nitroso compounds. The resistance of cells of the adult central nervous system to carcinogens is then relative, being high in the case of radiation or topical cholanthrenes, and lower for nitroso compounds and for some viruses.

Biological Factors

It is now well established that viruses, including many obtained from human tissues, are capable of inducing brain tumors when inoculated intracerebrally in a variety of animals. The susceptible species range from chickens to primates.

Experimentally, three groups of viruses have been used to create brain tumors: adeno-, papova-, and oncornaviruses.[19] The number and type of brain tumors produced depends on factors such as age of the animal and site of injection. Younger animals are more susceptible than older ones. Intracerebral injection is more effective than extrathecal. Different results are obtained from intracerebral inocula placed near the ependyma or in the meninges.

The three groups of viruses all can produce sarcomas, but oncornaviruses more often cause differentiated astrocytomas and glioblastomas; adenoviruses result in neurogenic tumors—neuroblastomas and retinoblastomas; and papovaviruses produce ependymomas, choroid plexus papillomas, and medulloblastomas. Results differ also depending on the subtype of virus: for example, the JC papovavirus is more likely to produce neural tumors than is the BK papovavirus.

The mechanism of production of tumor by a virus is by entrance of the microorganism into susceptible cells during the S phase of DNA synthesis (Fig. 83–2). Only the time for one cell cycle is necessary for the virus to be fixed. The need for a dividing cell may explain the greater susceptibil-

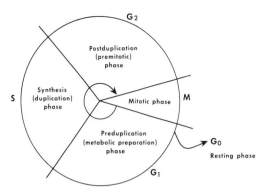

Figure 83-2 Diagram of cycle of cell division. The sectors are not necessarily accurate representations of the actual time of the phases.

ity of young animals to this method of tumor induction as well as the susceptibility of cells of the choroid plexus. The viral origin of tumors induced by direct application of chemical carcinogens was suggested by the observations of Ikuta and Zimmerman.[91] They found particles resembling viruses in electron micrographs of precancerous lesions in cells adjacent to the carcinogen, but not in cells of the growing tumor.

More importantly for those concerned with the care of human beings, information is accumulating to implicate viruses in the production of human neoplasms. The case for viruses as a cause of tumors in man, however, is not yet proved. A naturally occurring human tumor caused by a virus is not known, but the possibility cannot be dismissed.[276] Glial cells obtained from man and grown in culture may be made neoplastic by both DNA and RNA tumor viruses. The probability therefore exists that the human brain can undergo neoplasia as a result of viral stimulation. The demonstration in human brain tumors of particles resembling viruses, however, has not been convincing.[19] Viruses are rarely recovered from human tumors, and it is not certain that they are causative agents, even when found.[43] Viruses are, however, not retrievable from the experimental tumors they have induced. They may be "masked" by being incorporated into the genetic material of the host, or bound to antibody, or be in concentrations too low to be detected. "Molecular probes" may be used to detect the nucleic acid of viruses, as may various "unmasking" techniques.[225]

Another approach not yet used will be to determine the association of the histocompatibility antigen system (HL-A) with brain tumors. The HL-A antigens are specific proteins on the cell surface. They are controlled by the genetic composition of the individual. Susceptibility to various diseases has been shown to be related to these antigens.[52] Oncogenic viruses and the equivalent system of antigens are related in animals. Much more study is needed to determine the role of viruses in the production of brain and, indeed, other tumors in man.

Growth of Brain Tumors

Mechanisms of Growth: Expansion, Invasion, Cellular Proliferation

The growth of tumors is by expansion, infiltration, or both. Expansion is defined as enlargement around a central core. The adjacent tissue may be compressed or destroyed. Expanding growths therefore tend to have capsules of brain or connective tissue. Such growths are usually spherical unless the tumor is altered by external pressures, as when an angle tumor grows in the porus acusticus. Growth by expansion is dependent on proliferation rather than on enlargement of cells. In addition, fluid accumulation related to hemorrhage, increased permeability of blood vessels, or swelling and edema, may enlarge the mass. Benign tumors such as meningiomas seldom infiltrate, but grow by expansion, and are surrounded by capsules of connective tissue. Metastatic tumors also usually grow by expansion, but may be infiltrative, especially around blood vessels in the brain. The term "space-occupying lesion" is not strictly correct, because all lesions occupy space.

Infiltration or invasion is the spread of tumor into the interstices of surrounding tissue. Infiltrative growths may extend for long distances from the primary site. The characteristic mechanism of growth of gliomas in the central nervous system is by infiltration, but they also may expand to displace and replace normal tissue.

Infiltration is related to at least five properties of tumor cells: (1) progressive multiplication (proliferation), (2) mobility, (3) phagocytic powers, (4) elaboration of toxic or lytic substances, and (5) loss of growth restraints normally exercised by neighboring tissues.[267]

Progressive multiplication of cells does not fully explain invasion; rapidly growing tumors may simply expand, and some slowly growing tumors, such as diffuse astrocytoma, are highly infiltrative. Many types of glial tumor cells in tissue culture have ameboid movement.[200] Little is known, however, of the phenomenon in situ. The phagocytic power of gliogenous cells is poor, and this mechanism probably is not significant. The last two mechanisms are of potential interest, but unfortunately, little evidence is available. Scherer described aggregates of tumor cells at a distance from the advancing front of the main tumor.[209]

The process of division of tumor cells in the past was analyzed by observing mitotic figures and studying cells in tissue culture. Radioautography was developed as a research tool to augment these older methods. Thymidine, a specific precursor of deoxyribonucleic acid (DNA), is incorporated into the nucleus of the cell during the stage of DNA duplication (synthesis or S phase) in preparation for cellular division (see Fig. 83–2). The radioactivity of tritium incorporated in the thymidine then can be detected in photographic emulsions placed on a slide. After this stage, the cell enters the postduplication or "G_2" phase and further prepares for mitosis. The mitotic or "M" phase, when the appropriate chromosome complement is given to each daughter cell, is followed by the postduplication or "G_1" phase of the cell cycle. After mitosis, the cell may also enter a resting phase, G_0.

Cell populations of normal or neoplastic tissues in various organs may differ considerably with respect to type and number of cells proliferating at a given time. In a static group of cells, as in the neurons of the central nervous system, mitoses are not found. The epidermis, red blood cells, and digestive tract are examples of renewing cell populations in which mitoses are abundant, but cellular proliferation is balanced by an equivalent cell loss. Neoplastic cells, on the other hand, increase in number variably in different areas of the same tumor, but eventually produce an increased number of cells in some areas. Within the cranial cavity, these cells soon constitute a

neoplasm, the development of which also varies.

Several terms have been used in describing the proliferative potential of neoplastic cells. The "cell generation time" is that period between two successive cell divisions, and is known to vary in neoplastic tissues. The "tumor doubling time" is that period in which a tumor doubles in size or in number of cells. These times are the same only when all cells in a given population are proliferating uniformly without cell loss and are evenly distributed in the tumor. These conditions may not be fulfilled for several reasons: most cells in a tumor do not divide at an equal rate, some cells may be in a nonproliferative stage, portions of the tumor may be necrotic or filled with fluid, and the size of the tumor may influence the growth rate on the basis of circulatory deficit or lack of space in which to grow. These factors contribute to "biological variability."

Johnson and co-workers performed a radioautographic study of human glioblastoma after in vivo labeling with eight doses of tritiated thymidine.[97] Using the percentage labeling and an arbitrary DNA synthesis time, and applying these figures to cells growing exponentially, the authors determined the mean generation time of the tumor. They proposed this time to be equal to the doubling time of about one month. This value did not account for nonproliferating cells in the same area of tumor, and is excessively long. As mentioned before, in a neoplastic cell population, mean generation time is equal to tumor doubling time only when the cell population is homogenous and all cells are dividing. These conditions probably are not fulfilled in any tumor.

Another radioautographic study was made on specimens obtained at craniotomy, including four meningiomas, six astrocytic and two ependymal tumors, one chordoma, and one acoustic neuroma.[123] The authors used tritiated thymidine and measured uptake in vitro. In the astrocytic group, four of the six tumors were grade III or IV, and by our criteria would be considered glioblastomas. The labeling percentage in this group ranged between 3.6 and 7.4 per cent of cells counted, as compared with the 0.6 per cent found by Johnson's group.[97] The mean generation times ranged from 2 to 8 hours, based on DNA synthesis times of from 5 to 9 hours. Wilson and Hoshino reported cell generation times in the range of 24 hours, using tritiated thymidine and cinephotomicrography of glioblastoma in tissue culture.[269] Therefore, considering the cell generation time of one type of tumor, a range of 24 hours to one month is encountered in these studies. A period of some hours has been established as the generation time of almost all dividing cells in the human body; hence the estimate of a month is highly improbable. The discrepancy may be related to biological variability of the tumors studied, differences in technique involving in vitro and in vivo uptake of thymidine, differences in rate of proliferation in various areas of the same tumor, differences in tumor size and position, and technical factors such as the total time of exposure to thymidine, and inappropriate application of mathematical formulae for exponential growth to a system not truly exponential. Therefore, this method of study has serious limitations at the present time.

"Amitotic division" of tumor cells has been described as occurring in glial tumors, especially glioblastoma. Strictly, the term is incorrect because cellular division does not occur; biologists prefer the term "nuclear fragmentation," but the former term is widely used. Lapham found cells in glioblastoma with DNA content greater than the diploid number, indicating that the chromosomes may separate within a single cell.[126] These giant polyploid cells rarely take up tritiated thymidine.

Forms of Growth

Metastasis Within the Central Nervous System

A metastasis is a tumor growing separately from the primary focus as a result of transfer of detached tumor cells. Some authors customarily use "metastasis" to mean transfer of neoplastic cells by way of blood or lymphatic channels; "seeding" is applied to spread of cells in the cerebrospinal fluid. The distinction is arbitrary. Dissemination in a fluid medium, including the cerebrospinal fluid, is appropriately called metastasis, particularly when new growths occur at distant sites.

Cells of gliomas have the ability to separate from the original tumor and disseminate in the cerebrospinal fluid. These tumors then may spread throughout the subarachnoid space, and reinvade neural tissue elsewhere, further growth occurring at the new site. Metastasis by this route is most common with medulloblastoma, second with ependymoma, and less frequent with other gliomas. Zuelch suggested that a higher frequency of metastasis would be found if the spinal cord were examined routinely at necropsy.[283]

At least three inherent factors are important: proximity of tumor cells to the cerebrospinal fluid, paucity of stroma, and decreased cohesiveness of tumor cells. The lack of processes in medulloblastoma predisposes to decreased cohesiveness; hence, cells are more readily discharged into the cerebrospinal fluid. Cells of ependymoma, however, have numerous processes attached to each other and to blood vessels, thereby reducing the liability of cells to be free, although the tumor often is close to the ventricle. Little is known about other possible factors, such as the electrical charge on the surface of the cell. Metastases from intracranial tumors are being recognized increasingly, both within the central nervous system and elsewhere. This increase may be related to the greater number and longevity of patients undergoing operative procedures as well as other forms of therapy.

Metastasis Outside the Central Nervous System

Tumors of the central nervous system may reach distant parts of the body by several mechanisms. Surgical induction is the most common means of introducing tumor cells into cerebral blood vessels or dural sinuses, but entrance may be spontaneous. Other pathways include blood vessels or lymphatics in the scalp reached by tumor eroding through the bone or disseminated at craniotomy. Still other lymphatic channels may be in the perineurium and possibly in the dura.

If tumor is present both systemically and in the brain, the question arises as to the primary site. Weiss outlined the following criteria for a metastasizing tumor of the central nervous system: (1) a single histologically characteristic tumor of the central nervous system is present, (2) the appearances of the tumor of the central nervous system and the distant metastases are reasonably similar, (3) the history shows that the initial neurological symptoms were caused by the tumor, and (4) complete necropsy is reported in sufficient detail to rule out other primary sites.[262]

Several reviews of extracranial metastases have been published.[1,71] Glasauer and Yuan collected 89 cases, consisting of 35 meningeal tumors and 54 primary intracranial neoplasms, including 11 medulloblastomas and 27 other gliomas.[71] The lungs were most often affected. Metastatic lesions to the liver, lymph nodes, bones, pleura, and kidneys followed in descending order of frequency. Meningeal tumors metastasized primarily to the lungs and pleura, and less often to liver and lymph nodes. In the glioma group, the lungs, pleura, and lymph nodes were most frequently involved. The sites most favorable for metastasis of medulloblastoma were the vertebrae and other bones, and less frequently the lymph nodes. The authors found no difference in the favorite location of extracranial metastases as a result of craniotomy. Children constituted 26 per cent of the cases, but had 35 per cent of the cerebral tumors, and 11 per cent of the meningeal tumors. It is now clear that, under appropriate conditions, all types of intracranial neoplasms can spread out of the central nervous system. Gliomas, however, almost never metastasize except after craniotomy.

Metastasis of an intracranial tumor is favored by operative intervention, especially by multiple operations, and possibly by radiation. Abbott and Love proposed that operative intervention predisposed to metastasis by aspiration of tumor cells into opened veins.[1] A negative intraluminal pressure when a patient is in the sitting position may favor aspiration. It is also possible that the tumor, if not disseminated at the time of operation, may later spread by infiltrating the adjacent soft tissues. The predilection for meningiomas to metastasize may be related to the presence of these tumor cells in the dural sinuses.

At least two mechanisms may be invoked to explain the usual failure of intracranial gliomas to metastasize elsewhere in the body. The more generally accepted idea is that glial cells do not penetrate blood vessels in the brain, but some recent evidence is available that penetration may occur.[120,125] Those authors accepting the concept of inability of glial cells to enter vessels contend that larger vascular structures are enclosed in dense connective tissue, preventing easy penetration by neoplastic cells; that the thinner-walled veins often collapse because of increased pressure around the tumor; and finally that cerebral capillaries normally lack fenestrae and are enveloped by astroglial foot-plates.

Courville found tumor cells within the lumen of blood vessels in glioblastoma, the cells having penetrated a "weakened" vessel wall; they were usually confined to that position by an enveloping thrombus.[44] Kung and associates presented electron microscopic evidence of direct penetration of blood vessels by glioma cells.[120] Neoplastic cells were in the basal lamina of the vessel or between the endothelial cells or in the lumen. These findings were most common in glioblastoma and less frequent in astrocytoma.

The conditions necessary for a tumor cell to gain access to the vascular system were proposed by Potter and co-workers: decreased cohesiveness between adjacent tumor cells to facilitate detachment, increase in cell motility thought to be proportional to metastatic potential, and capability of transendothelial migration.[187,188] Kung's group showed these criteria were met, especially in the case of glioblastoma.[120] If it is assumed then that tumor cells gain access to the vascular system, realizing that glioblastoma rarely metastasizes spontaneously, one could propose that the life span of a patient with this tumor is not long enough to allow distal tumors to grow or that tumor cells are resisted in the bloodstream or end-organs, possibly on an autoimmune basis.

Shuangshoti and co-workers reviewed the literature on metastasizing meningioma.[218] They found 40 acceptable cases, of which 25 per cent had metastasized spontaneously. The higher frequency of spontaneous metastasis of meningioma as compared with glioma may be related to the greater potentiality of meningocytes to enter the dural sinuses and then be dislodged or to their more direct access to extracranial lymphatics.

The lymphatics have been proposed as a route by which cells may pass from the intracranial space, specifically through the perineural lymphatics and thus to the cervical lymphatic plexus directly, or through the thoracic duct to the mediastinal nodes. Some authors have contended that lymphatics drain the cerebrospinal fluid spaces in both normal and pathological conditions.[70,271] Tumor cells, however, have not been demonstrated in these pathways.

According to Millen and Woollam, the work of Rouviere suggested that the dura mater is traversed by a system of lymphatic spaces in communication with subarachnoid and subdural spaces. They concluded that "the cranial and the spinal dura mater . . . are undoubtedly drained by an important system of lymphatics."[155] Gyepes and D'Angio thought that "once the covering membranes are attained by the cells, lymphatic permeation becomes possible. These channels are also available to those tumors arising within the meninges themselves." They further proposed that dural tumors grow in a vascularized zone, "well equipped with lymphatics."[82]

The paucity of extraneural glial metastases has been explained by many workers as related to the "soil theory" that non-neural tissues are unable to support the growth of glial cells. Zimmerman and others have shown that carcinogen-induced glial tumors when transplanted to subcutaneous tissue, as well as to other extracranial locations, grow without difficulty.[283] They may enlarge enormously in these secondary sites, but still do not metastasize. Netsky demonstrated that homogenates of experimental gliomas, when injected into the tail veins of mice, disseminated widely in some animals, and widespread visceral deposits were found at necropsy.[164] Nevertheless, other animals similarly injected did not demonstrate lesions. Millions of circulating tumor cells thus were destroyed in some animals, but the mechanism of resistance is not known.

Spread of glial tumor through ventriculopleural shunts and subsequent widespread pleural growth has been reported.[273] Grace and co-workers described six patients with glioblastoma multiforme given subcutaneous grafts of their own tumors; two of the six had neoplastic proliferation.[77] The authors postulated that delayed hypersensitivity to antigens of the central nervous system might play a role in determining whether the autografts grew.

Diffuse Growth

The original concept of "tumor" was of a mass, which might be a neoplasm or a swelling of any other kind, visible grossly or microscopically. Current use restricts the word to mean a neoplasm. It is now recognized that neoplasms may infiltrate tissue spaces as multiple cells without forming a definite mass. Diffuse growths then are infiltrative or invasive. The term "diffuse" is sometimes used for multiple discrete masses, but it is best considered as applying to a tumor widely infiltrating the brain or subarachnoid space, without necessarily forming a definite swelling or multiple foci. If the cell type is known, diffuse tumors are identified by adding the suffix "-osis" to the cell type. The term thus includes gliomatosis, sarcomatosis, carcinomatosis, and central diffuse schwannosis.

Gliomas are the most common type of diffuse tumor. They include infiltrating tumors such as gliomas of the optic nerve and brain stem, considered as spongioblastoma polare by some authors and as piloid astrocytoma by others, and other widely infiltrating glial tumors in the cerebral hemispheres. Some of the latter cases have been designated as gliomatosis cerebri.[169] They are often associated with von Recklinghausen's disease. Scherer, in a systematic study of the growth of intracranial gliomas, estimated that "primary diffuse glioma without formation of a definite 'tumor' and without pronounced destruction of the preexisting tissue is encountered in about 25 per cent of gliomas in general."[209] This figure is higher than usually reported, but undoubtedly is related to his technique of examining many large sections. Scherer included the hemispheral infiltrating glial tumors, brain stem gliomas, certain rare glioblastomas, and a few unclassified tumors.[210]

Of interest also is Scherer's description of "secondary structures" associated with diffuse tumors. As the tumors infiltrated gray matter, the first manifestation was a "collection of glioma cells around all or a great number of nerve cells." He also described cellular aggregates in the subpial layer of the cortex, as well as extensive growths in the perivascular spaces. Tumor cells in the corona radiata and internal capsule were aligned in the direction of the tracts. Scherer considered the cellular aggregates in these areas to be indicative of early anaplasia. Whether the cellular collections represented dedifferentiation of cells already present (multicentricity) or migration of abnormal cells from another site (metastasis) was not determined.

Glioblastosis cerebri, also designated as diffuse spongioblastosis or glioblastosis, resembles grossly the diffuse cerebral astrocytomas. The term glioblast implies a poorly differentiated cell, but it is often difficult to exclude the possibility of a mature astrocyte growing in a small space and compressed to resemble a less well-differentiated cell. Some of these diffuse tumors may be anaplastic, but it seems probable that compression of astrocytes occurs more often.

Multiple and Multicentric Growth

The distinction is not always precise between multiple and multicentric tumors. Zuelch noted that "usually one speaks of 'multicentric' gliomas even if there is no cellular interconnection, but calls several meningiomas in one case multiple."[283] This usage may not be accurate, but is conventional. "Multiple" is a general term meaning more than one tumor: the implication of "multicentric" is that the masses arose in separate sites of origin rather than by extension of one tumor to another location. The question is: did the tumors arise independently or as a result of metastasis? Unfortunately, the answer often is not certain, and the decision may be arbitrary.

Courville found the frequency of multiple gliomas (he made no distinction between multiple and multicentric) was about 1.5 per 1000 autopsies or 0.15 per cent; they constituted 4.3 per cent of intracranial neoplasms in general, and 8 per cent of the glial tumors.[45] He also reported that about 10 per cent of glioblastomas and 6 per cent of astrocytomas were multiple. The cerebral hemispheres were most often involved when multiple tumors were present. Multiple astrocytomas usually occurred in cerebellum and thalamus. Multiple glioblastomas of the cerebellum were exceedingly rare.

Batzdorf and Malamud considered these routes of spread of tumor cells in the brain:

corpus callosum, fornix, or internal capsule; cerebrospinal fluid; and local extension with satellite formation in the immediate vicinity of the main tumor.[16] They defined multicentric gliomas as those widely separated lesions in different parts of one hemisphere or in different hemispheres, arising independently. The only evidence for independent growth, however, was the distance between tumors.

Scherer stated that about 10 per cent of all gliomas had multiple centers of growth, but only in half the cases were these areas found on gross examination.[209] Multiple growths were noted in about 20 per cent of glioblastomas. Moertel and associates, on the other hand, noted a 4.9 per cent prevalence of multiplicity in necropsies of gliomas at the Mayo Clinic.[157] Russell and Rubinstein reported a prevalence of 4.5 per cent multiplicity in glioblastoma on macroscopic examination, and 6 per cent on microscopic examination.[201] Scherer's extensive examinations, in which he thinly sliced the entire brain and studied large histological sections, were more likely to yield a higher percentage of multiple foci. His multiple aggregates of cells at a distance from the primary source, if considered as another focus of tumor, would also increase the percentage.

Stroebe first suggested that multiple foci of tumor are metastases from a single growth.[231] Courville theorized that glial tumors could spread by arterial embolization through the subarachnoid pathways, but judged from his experience that neither of these mechanisms explained multiplicity.[44] He concluded that in most cases multiple gliomas are "explained on the basis of the development of multiple primary foci," noting that many of the tumors were of about equal size and often were at opposite ends of the hemisphere. Willis proposed that multicentric lesions could develop by neoplastic transformation of a "field," some areas being more susceptible to tumor growth.[266] These foci would then continue to grow, yielding one or several tumors in different parts of the brain.

Multiple brain tumors of different histological types are common in von Recklinghausen's disease; multiple schwannomas and meningiomas often occur, as do glial tumors. Multiple hemangioblastomas are encountered in von Hippel-Lindau disease. Combinations of diverse primary brain tumors were reviewed by Madonick and co-workers.[135] Glioblastoma with meningioma was most frequent, a finding to be expected because the first is the most common malignant tumor in the cranium and the other is the most frequent benign neoplasm.

Incidence of Brain Tumors

The biological variability of tumors of the central nervous system is illustrated by the difference in characteristic location and incidence of tumors in different age groups. In children younger than 15 years of age, tumors of the central nervous system are the second most frequent type of cancer, exceeded only by leukemia. Fifteen to twenty per cent of all intracranial tumors occur during childhood. Odom and his colleagues reported that hospitalized children have an 0.42 per cent prevalence of brain tumors.[173] The prevalence in a hospitalized population of all ages ranges from 0.2 to 2.6 per cent.[283]

Many factors affect the validity of statistical data on intracranial tumors. The figures may be compiled from operative or necropsy series, or from death certificates. Operative series favor operable cases, and tend, for example, to reduce the number of metastatic lesions. The reputation of the surgeon or the hospital with regard to a particular operation can also weight the figures; the number of pituitary adenomas in Cushing's series is an example of this type of bias. Necropsy series favor diagnostic problems in a referral hospital and may include fewer resectable lesions. The number of metastatic tumors may be unduly high in a hospital for chronic diseases, as reported by Lesse and Netsky, who found that one third of metastases were clinically unsuspected.[130] Studies of hospitalized patients may be influenced by factors such as the racial or ethnic distribution of those admitted and the availability of special services. Death certificates contain many clinical diagnoses without pathological verification.

An inherent difficulty of reporting and interpreting statistical studies of central nervous system tumors is that of classification. The problems are noticeable when one hospital is compared with another in the United States, but they are magnified when the frequency of tumor groups in different countries is analyzed.

The incidence of brain tumor for all ages is estimated to be between 4.2 to 5.4 per 100,000 population.[122,283] Based on death certificates in the United States, the mortality rate from tumors of the central nervous system, both benign and malignant, was 0.45 per cent of all deaths in 1966. These tumors accounted for 2.7 per cent of the deaths from all cancers.[244]

Kurland and associates found that of the 2100 deaths among residents of Rochester, Minnesota, during a 10-year period, primary intracranial neoplasms were present in 1 per cent, but the percentage increased to 1.7 if metastatic brain tumors were included.[122] Kurland also noted an increase in age-specific incidence of neoplasms of the central nervous system in the older age group, in contrast to statistics compiled from death certificates throughout the United States, showing a gradual decline in incidence after the eighth decade (Fig. 83–3). He attributed the difference to a high necropsy rate in Rochester and the consequently higher percentage of the population in whom the cause of death was verified.

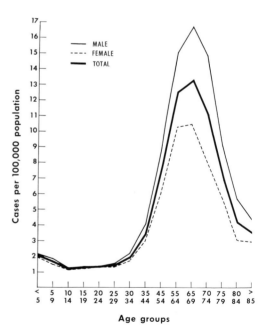

Figure 83–3 The incidence of all types of brain tumors in the United States in 1966 is shown by five-year age groups. Note the male predominance in adults. (Data from U.S. Department of Health, Education, and Welfare—Public Health Service: Vital Statistics Rates in the United States 1940–1960. Washington, D.C., 1968.)

The curve downward after 60 years of age was viewed with skepticism by the authors in the first edition of this book. It was based on data from death certificates in the United States and was therefore liable to error. Especially in the oldest age groups, death certificates may be unreliable.[166] Confirmation of the validity of the decreased incidence with age after the menopause came from an entirely different source, the Birmingham Regional Cancer Registry.[253] In another country (Great Britain), using an entirely different technique of gathering data (a registry of proved cases rather than death certificates), the data from the United States were confirmed. The peak incidence in British women was at 55 to 59 years, in men at 60 to 64.

The data therefore are evidence of an important biological difference between tumors of the brain and most other neoplasms in the body. The incidence of most neoplasms increases with age, with the exception of those clearly dependent on production of hormones (e.g., ovary and testis). Indeed, the incidence of "other endocrine tumors" (meaning largely pituitary tumors, but excluding cancer of the thyroid) also declines after the menopause.

Four possible explanations may account for the decreased incidence of brain tumors in old age. The possibility of an artifact is almost eliminated by the similar results derived from study of death certificates in the United States as shown in Figure 83–3 and data from the cancer registry in Great Britain.[147,244,253] Diminished exposure to exogenous stimuli is a second consideration, as when older people have smoked less, hence have had lesser rates of carcinoma of the lung. This explanation, applied to intracranial neoplasms, is unlikely in view of the minimal evidence of an exogenous cause of these tumors. Thirdly, the decline could be related to elimination of the susceptible population. Unfortunately, the factors determining susceptibility to cerebral neoplasia are not known. With our present knowledge, it is difficult to explain why some persons might be resistant to cerebral and other endocrine neoplasms, but not to most other tumors. This explanation has little support unless nongenetic factors of resistance are determined.

The most likely explanation for the decline in brain tumors with greater age is related to altered and decreased endocrine productivity. The brain is now well established as an endocrine organ. The entire curve of age incidence of brain tumors may be explained by endocrine mechanisms. Brain tumors most frequent in childhood decline in frequency during adolescence (Figure 83–4). A new group of tumors rise rapidly with onset of reproductive capacity. To these well-known data, the finding that brain and other endocrine tumors decline after reproductive ability diminishes is now added.[165] These observations have potential importance both diagnostically and

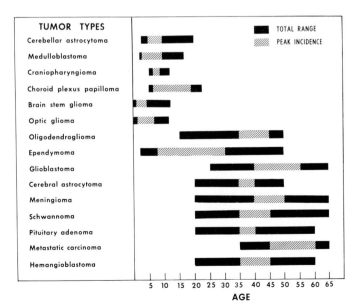

Figure 83–4 Chart showing approximate age distribution and peak incidence of major types of brain tumors, compiled from the literature. The clinical names are used in accord with cited reports. Most of these tumors occur predominantly either in children or in adults.

therapeutically, as well as in a new concept of pathogenesis.

Age

The age incidence of some principal brain tumors is shown in Figure 83–4. About two thirds of tumors occurring in childhood and adolescence (before the age of 16) are in the posterior fossa. Of all the masses in the cranium in this age group, approximately three quarters are gliomas. Ependymoma is most common above the tentorium, and cerebellar astrocytoma below the tentorium. The frequency of intracranial tumors decreases in adolescence, then gradually increases again in adult life. As previously stated, the frequency decreases in the oldest age groups (see Fig. 83–3).

In the middle decades, the prevalence of gliomas of the cerebral hemispheres rises. Glioblastoma is most frequent, but other gliomas except medulloblastoma often occur. Metastatic tumors are the most common infratentorial tumors in middle-aged persons. Pituitary adenomas, acoustic schwannomas, and meningiomas also increase during this period.

In old age, glioblastomas, meningiomas, acoustic schwannomas, and metastatic lesions constitute 80 to 90 per cent of all intracranial masses.[163] The benign gliomas—astrocytoma, ependymoma, and oligodendroglioma—decline in frequency in old age, but meningiomas and schwannomas increase proportionately. The malignancy of systemic tumors generally increases with age, but an old person harboring an intracranial mass has almost a 50 per cent chance of having a benign tumor, and a middle-aged person has only about a 25 per cent chance.

Sex

The sexual distribution of intracranial tumors has remained constant for many years. In 1889, Starr noted a male to female ratio of 55 to 45 in patients with all types of brain tumor.[228] This finding was confirmed by Zuelch in 1965 when he noted the same preponderance in men.[283] Death certificates in the United States for the year 1966 reveal a similar finding of 56 per cent in men, although the difference is most striking in adults rather than in children (see Fig. 83–3). Greater sexual predilection, moreover,

occurs with some tumors. Pinealomas are three times as common in men. Zuelch reports that the following tumors occur about twice as often in men: glioblastoma, angioblastoma, craniopharyngioma, epidermoid tumors, and medulloblastoma.[283] Those tumors with a slight male preponderance are astrocytoma, ependymoma, and metastases. The tumors occurring more frequently in women are schwannoma (twice the male incidence) and meningioma.

Localization

It has long been noted that infratentorial tumors in childhood significantly outnumber those above the tentorium. Fessard noted, however, in his study of intracranial tumors in infancy that 75 per cent occur above the tentorium in the first six months of life; tumors above and below the tentorium were equal in the next six months; and only after the first year were infratentorial tumors more common.[64] The number of cases was small, however; larger series are required for further study of these interesting findings.

The authors encountered 2700 brain tumors in children in the medical literature from 1942 to 1969, and found that 56 per cent were below the tentorium, and 44 per cent were above. This prevalence of infratentorial tumors is less than that encountered earlier by Cushing and others. Ingraham and Matson noted a 60 per cent prevalence of subtentorial tumors in 313 cases of brain tumors in children, but in 1969, Matson found 55 per cent in 750 patients.[92,150] The possibility that the intracranial location of childhood tumors is shifting with time is interesting but not yet certain.

The range of age of occurrence and the peak incidence of 15 common intracranial neoplasms are shown in Figure 83–4. Most tumors preferentially occur either in childhood or in adult life, but astrocytoma and ependymoma are unusual in having a high frequency in both age groups. Astrocytoma is more common below the tentorium in children, and in the cerebrum in adults. These regional predilections are further specified in Table 83–2 for three divisions of age. Additional details of localization of individual tumors may be found in the monograph by Zuelch.[283]

TABLE 83-2 SUBDIVISIONS OF MAJOR CEREBRAL TUMORS BY AGE OF OCCURRENCE AND LOCATION IN BRAIN*

Location	INFANCY AND ADOLESCENCE (0–20 YR.) Tumor Type	Per Cent of All Tumors	MIDDLE AGE (20–60 Yr.) Tumor Type	Per Cent of All Tumors	OLD AGE (>60 yr.) Tumor Type	Per cent of All Tumors
Supratentorial	Cerebral hemispheral glioma	10–14	Glioblastoma m.	25	Glioblastoma m.	35
	Craniopharyngioma	5–13	Meningioma	14	Meningioma	20
	Ependymoma	3–5	Astrocytoma	13	Metastases	10
	Choroid plexus papilloma	2–3	Metastases	10		
	Pinealoma	1.5–3	Pituitary tumors	5		
	Optic glioma	1–3.5				
	Total	16–25				
Infratentorial	Cerebellar		Metastases	5	Acoustic neuroma	20
	Astrocytoma	15–20	Acoustic neuroma	3	Metastases	5
	Medulloblastoma	14–18	Meningioma	1	Meningioma	5
	Brain stem glioma	9–12	Sarcoma	?		
	Ependymoma	4–8				
	Total	41–58				

* The percentages are estimates compiled from various sources. See text for further comments.

Geographic and Racial Factors

The population studied and the standards of reporting differ considerably around the world: adequacy of hospitals and staff, diagnostic criteria, and different methods of reporting contribute to the problems of comparative statistics. Some populations in rural communities and in parts of the Orient enter hospitals late in the clinical course, but many urban and Western patients tend to enter with minimal complaints; hence different aspects of the neoplastic process may be encountered. Indeed, hospitals in the same city may deal with different populations, as when a large city hospital and a more expensive private institution are available. In some countries, a clinical diagnosis of "cerebral tumor" may be reported on the basis of a bedside impression, without biopsy or necropsy. The diagnosis of brain tumor made in death certificates in a certain proportion of cases in all countries is without anatomical verification. A better indication of the incidence of central nervous system tumors is found in those series in which a large proportion of cases is verified histologically. Kurland and co-workers, in their study of intracranial tumors in Rochester, Minnesota, found twice as many cerebral neoplasms as were recorded in official mortality statistics.[122] They attributed the difference to the excellent diagnostic facilities available in the area and a high rate of necropsy.

Age-adjusted rates are also of importance, especially in analyses of deaths related to brain tumor among populations with different spans of life. Differences in the proportion of people at various ages can significantly change the incidence. In studying the biology of these tumors, therefore, comparisons of total incidence uncorrected for age are of less value. The most valid comparisons are those made of age-specific rates, that is, the number of cases occurring in one year in a given age group, divided by the entire population of that age group in that year and multiplied by 100,000.

Kurland's group analyzed the incidence of brain tumors in 27 countries for "several recent years."[122] The annual age-adjusted rate ranged from 4 to 5 per 100,000 population for the majority of countries reported. The figures were converted for a standard base population. Israel had the highest rate, but the authors suggested that the central bureau of statistics in that country changed the contributory cause of death to the underlying cause if they thought the referring physician had done it improperly. Other countries do not make such changes. Israel also has one of the highest ratios of physicians to patients, and the rate of detection may be higher.

Three countries had unusually low rates: Chile, Japan, and Mexico. Japan, for example had a rate of slightly more than 2 per 100,000. Kurland and associates state that

TABLE 83–3   NUMBER AND PERCENTAGE OF INTRACRANIAL TUMORS

	COUNTRY USA YEAR 1932 AUTHOR CUSHING		USA 1956 GRANT		GERMANY 1957 ZUELCH		SWEDEN 1958 OLIVECRONA		JAPAN 1959 KATSURA		INDIA 1966 RAMAMURTHRI With Granuloma	
TUMOR TYPE	No.	Per Cent	No.	Per Cent	No.	Per Cent	No.	Per Cent	No.	Per Cent	No.	Per Cent
Glioma	874	43.2	1169	50.3	2599	43.3	2816	50.1	1082	32.7	277	34.4
Meningioma	271	13.4	407	17.4	1079	18.0	1125	20.0	529	15.9	79	9.8
Metastatic	85	4.2	196	8.4	242	4.0	232	4.1	144	4.3	52	6.5
Pituitary adenoma	360	17.8	206	8.8	478	7.9	528	9.4	365	11.0	52	6.5
Schwannoma	176	8.7	110	4.7	451	7.5	469	8.3	399	12.1	84	10.4
Congenital	113	5.6	108	4.6	433	7.2	180	3.2	318	9.6	45	5.6
Vascular	41	2.0	64	2.7	78	1.3	140	2.5	132	4.0	16	1.9
Sarcoma	14	0.7	—	—	162	2.7	—	—	22	0.7	—	—
Calvarial	—	—	28	1.2	49	0.82	—	—	—	—	—	—
Tuberculoma	33	1.6	18	0.7	31	0.51			90	2.7	199	24.6
							54	0.96				
Other granuloma	12	0.6	5	0.2	14	0.23	2	0.03	13	0.4	2	0.24
Unclassified	44	2.2	15	0.6	375	6.2	74	1.3	218	6.6	—	—
Total	2023	100	2326	99.7	5991	99.7	5620	99.89	3312	100	806	99.9

neurology as a specialty is just beginning to come into its own in Japan, and that general surgeons perform much of the neurosurgery.[122] In addition, Netsky found that histological examination is often done by general pathologists without training in neuropathology, which perhaps explains the unusually high incidence of unspecified neoplasms as compared with benign or malignant neoplasms. The ratio was 6 to 1, higher for unspecified neoplasms than in any other country. Aside from Japan, reports of low rates of occurrence of brain tumors tend to come from the countries that are underdeveloped medically and economically.

The problems of standards of reporting are illustrated by these extreme cases, but it is remarkable that the overall rates are so similar in most of the rapidly developing countries. Striking differences in the incidence of particular tumors in any one country must be viewed with suspicion, unless full data and knowledge of the situation are available. For example, on the basis of the data of Katsura and associates, in Japan pinealoma constitutes 9 per cent of gliomas, as contrasted with 2 per cent in the United States and in most other countries (Table 83–3).[100] During an experience of four months of study in Japan during 1969, Netsky found reasons to doubt these figures. Some Japanese neurosurgeons stated that pinealoma in their experience occurred at the same rate as in the United States.

Suggested reasons for the discrepancy are:

1. Referral of patients to neurosurgical clinics in earlier times was largely based on hydrocephalus and the finding of relatively specific signs such as failure of upward gaze. Other patients did not enter the specialized hospitals.

2. Operative treatment is preferred by many Japanese surgeons. Radiation and shunting might be used in other countries.

3. Some Japanese pathologists diagnose any tumor in the pineal gland as pinealoma. For example, what would elsewhere be called an astrocytoma of this structure might be designated "pinealoma" in Japan.

One difference between east and west possibly is of more significance. Katsura and his colleagues found more infratentorial gliomas in Japan than in Western countries.[100] This finding has thus far been confirmed for glioblastoma and astrocytoma by Shuangshoti and co-workers in Thailand.[217,219] These reports also describe a higher percentage of brain tumors in children; glioblastoma in the brain stem, for example, is relatively common in Thai children. The number of cases, however, is still small; larger series are needed before these differences can be considered significant. The importance of such differences, if validated, is that they suggest racial or, more likely, environmental factors, and that these may become susceptible to study.

Whether yellow, black, or white races are indeed differentially susceptible to

REPORTED BY VARIOUS AUTHORS IN DIFFERENT COUNTRIES*

USA 1967 COURVILLE		INDIA 1968 DASTUR						USA 1968 ZIMMERMAN		ALL SERIES			
Without Granuloma				With Granuloma		Without Granuloma				All Series Including Granuloma		Excluding Granuloma	
No.	Per Cent	No.	Per Cent	No.	Per Cent	No.	Per Cent	No.	Per Cent	No.	Per Cent	No.	Per Cent
277	45.8	1259	42.1	370	37.4	370	48.1	1633	36.0	12,079	42.3	12,079	43.9
79	13.0	349	11.6	101	10.2	101	13.1	802	17.7	4,742	16.5	4,742	17.2
52	8.6	714	23.8	52	5.2	52	6.7	1056	23.3	2,773	9.6	2,773	10.1
52	8.6	103	3.4	67	6.7	67	8.7	229	5.0	2,388	8.4	2,388	8.6
84	13.9	78	2.6	76	7.7	76	9.9	79	1.7	1,922	6.7	1,922	7.0
45	7.4	104	3.4	58	5.8	58	7.5	84	1.8	1,443	5.0	1,443	5.2
16	2.6	235	7.8	38	3.8	38	4.9	99	2.2	843	2.9	843	3.0
—	—	8	0.26	1	0.10	1	0.13	216	4.7	423	1.4	423	1.5
—	—	—	—	5	0.50	5	0.65	—	—	82	0.28	82	0.29
—	—	—	—	215	21.7	—	—	—	—	1,023	3.5	—	—
—	—	49	1.63	—	—	—	—	334	7.4 *(See Tuberculoma and footnote)*		—	—	—	—
—	—	25	0.77	5	0.50	—	—	—	—	78	0.27	—	—
—	—	66	2.2	—	—	—	—	—	—	792	2.7	792	2.8
605	99.9	2990	99.6	988	99.6	768	99.6	4532	99.8	28,588	99.4	27,487	99.5

*Nonneoplastic cysts are not included. Papillomas of the choroid plexus are placed with gliomas. "Vascular tumor" does not include vascular malformations and aneurysms if information supplied by the author allowed this separation. Zimmerman placed only hemangioblastomas in this category and only craniopharyngiomas in the congenital group. Granulomas were not subdivided by him; hence all are listed as tuberculomas.

brain tumors cannot be stated with certainty. The contrast between rates for white and non-white in the United States illustrates the difficulty (Fig. 83–5). The white population has an excess at almost all ages, but the absolute difference is least from infancy through young adult life. Although the differences between the two curves are striking, the rates may actually be similar. The non-white population is generally undercounted, especially in the big cities where they have recently increased in number, but the magnitude of undercounting is not known. Second, the higher mortality rate of the non-white, especially in the perinatal period, removes some of the population from consideration. Third, the non-white person often receives a lower quality of medical care, is less prone to enter hospitals, undergoes necropsy less often; hence brain tumors may be missed more often.

A group of 16,311 cases of primary central nervous system tumors seen at the Armed Forces Institute of Pathology was studied with regard to ethnic distribution.[62a] The case ratio of Caucasian to Negro was 13.7 to 1, compared to a population ratio of 8.4 to 1. Gliomas were significantly more frequent in Caucasians than in Negroes, but Negroes had a proportionate excess of pituitary adenomas, meningiomas, and nerve sheath tumors. Similar findings were encountered in a group of 810 African Negroes. The similarity between American and African Negroes suggested the presence of genetic factors. These data lend support to the concept that brain tumors as a whole are less frequent in black people.

Examination of the records of death cer-

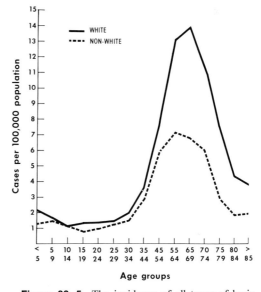

Figure 83–5 The incidence of all types of brain tumors in the United States is shown by age groups for white and non-white persons. The difference may be an artifact (see text). (Data from U.S. Department of Health, Education and Welfare—Public Health Service: Vital Statistics Rates in the United States 1940–1960. Washington, D.C., 1968.)

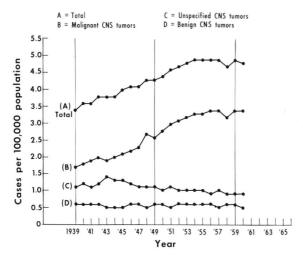

A = Total   C = Unspecified CNS tumors
B = Malignant CNS tumors   D = Benign CNS tumors

Figure 83–6 Incidence of tumors of the central nervous system in the United States from 1939 to 1960. The rise in incidence of the total is related to an increase in malignant tumors. (Data from U.S. Department of Health, Education and Welfare—Public Health Service: Vital Statistics Rates in the United States 1940–1960. Washington, D.C., 1968.)

tificates in the United States since 1939 reveals changes in the incidence of central nervous system tumors (Fig. 83–6). The categories examined are limited by the rubrics of the International Classification of Disease to benign, malignant, and unspecified tumors of the central nervous system. The rate for all neoplasms gradually rose between 1939 and 1960, because of an increased number of malignant neoplasms. Benign tumors remained almost unchanged, and unspecified types declined slightly. It is difficult to be certain of the interpretation of these data. They may be explained by an increased rate of detection of malignant tumors rather than a genuine increase. Improved neuropathological control is a factor in reducing the number of unspecified tumors. The possibility that an absolute increase has occurred, however, cannot be fully eliminated.

If "tumor" is used to include granulomas, the slowly developing countries with many infectious and parasitic diseases present a different statistical picture, resembling the United States at the turn of the century (see Table 83–3). At that time, Starr reported that 51 per cent of 300 brain tumors in children were tuberculomas, as were 14 per cent of 300 tumors of adults.[229] Dastur and co-workers in India found that 46.4 per cent of intracranial tumors in childhood were tuberculomas.[50,51] Parasitic disorders such as those of cerebral cysticercosis or schistosomiasis may be problems of significance in some countries.

Immunobiology of Brain Tumors

The treatment of patients with infiltrating malignant gliomas presents a difficult problem to the neurosurgeon. Although the average survival time can be increased with radiation and chemotherapy, these patients usually succumb rapidly to the disease. Nevertheless, patients may live for many years while harboring a malignant brain tumor.[168]

Specific immunity is a factor contributing to resistance to tumors. This concept implies that during neoplastic transformation (oncogenesis) specific alterations of the cell membrane and cytoplasm permit the normal, intact reticuloendothelial system to recognize and destroy cancerous cells. Qualitatively, the immunological response to tumor antigens resembles that involved in the rejection of homografts of normal tissue.

Early investigations of host immunity to intracranial tumors were impeded by the concept of the brain as an "immunologically privileged site."[81,153] Antigens originating within the brain were thought incapable of evoking an immune response. In addition, clear immunological differences between extracts of cells from glioblastoma and from normal adult brain were not detected.[222] The observations of Scheinberg and co-workers that tumors within the central nervous system *can* evoke an immune response indicate the privilege of the brain is partial rather than complete.[205–207] Furthermore, the finding that antibodies against malignant brain tumors of man are localized mainly within the tumor cells and blood vessels suggests differences in the antigenic composition of glioblastoma and of normal adult brain.[138] Neoplasms originating within the central nervous system are now known to be capable of inducing an immune response with some specificity.

The immunobiological response to human brain tumors, nevertheless, is not clear. Lymphocytic infiltration can be found in approximately a third of malignant gliomas.[192] The significance of this observation, however, is not known. These lymphocytes may be "killer cells," but confirmation is lacking. Circulating lymphocytes of patients with intracranial tumors are sensitized to tumor cells and, in the test tube, can be cytotoxic, that is, can destroy glioma cells.* Unfortunately, less than half these patients have a significant number of cytotoxic lymphocytes.

Wahlstrom and co-workers have shown that circulating lymphocytes react equally well to cells from normal brain of adults and fetuses.[249-252] The observed lymphocytic reactivity therefore may be directed toward the normal antigens of brain, and not only to tumor-specific or associated antigens. The mechanism of inducing sensitization to normal antigens of the central nervous system in patients with gliomas is uncertain. Circulating tumor cells have been found in the blood of these patients, but extracranial metastases are unusual.[159] It has been suggested that the rarity of these metastases can be explained by a strong immune response resulting from sensitization to both normal glia-specific antigens and tumor-specific antigens.[251]

In spite of the evidence that lymphocytes of patients with brain tumor are sensitized to normal brain, these individuals generally do not have signs of allergic encephalitis.[7] This failure to react may be related in part to the presence of protective factors in the serum. Kumar and others have demonstrated that the sera of patients with glioma are capable of blocking the lymphocytic cytotoxic response to the tumor.[30,31,119] The presence of these serum "blocking" factors may account for the lack of clinical evi-

dence supporting the laboratory observations of significant cytotoxicity by lymphocytes.

Kornblith and associates report that the sera of more than half the patients they studied were capable of killing glioma cells maintained in tissue culture.[116] The role of these cytotoxic factors in the serum of patients, however, remains to be elucidated.

Although not yet confirmed clinically, there is evidence that brain tumors influence immune responsiveness of the host.[30-32,237,277] Mahaley and co-workers found continued depression of lymphocyte counts throughout the course of the disease.[140] Furthermore, when compared to controls, these patients have significantly impaired ability to respond to various skin-test antigens. Although persistent elevations of the serum IgM content in patients with brain tumors have been reported, more exhaustive studies indicate that the IgM content actually falls during clinical deterioration of patients with glioblastoma.[140,239] Those patients with a stable clinical course or with benign intracranial tumors have normal IgM levels.

The report of Schneck and Penn that patients with renal transplants have a significant increase in intracranial tumors suggests that chronic immunosuppression under these conditions allows the occurrence of cancers that would normally be rejected.[211] The tumors most often are lymphomas, although these cerebral neoplasms are rare in the general population. Furthermore, lung and breast cancer are not increased in the immunodeficient patients, although these are the most common tumors in men and women, respectively. The temporal sequence of immunological deficiency in patients with glioma remains speculative. It is possible that suppression of host immunity follows rather than precedes the beginning of the neoplastic process.

Scheinberg and co-workers demonstrated that brain tumors could be prevented by prior immunization with glioma and adjuvant.[204,208] These investigators found that inbred mice receiving immunizations before cerebral implantation of tumor cells had significant inhibition and rejection of tumor growth. Immunizations after implantation were not beneficial. Application of these principles to human neoplasia de-

---

*See references 31, 37, 60, 63, 77, 119, 131, 225.

pends upon the demonstration of antigenicity specific to a single tumor, independent of other phenotypic or organ-specific variations.

Current techniques to identify and isolate these tumor-associated antigens generally employ antisera made by immunizing animals with extracts or whole cells of glial tumors. This "anti-glioma antibody" is purified, and its ability to react with individual tumor cells is measured. Malignant astrocytomas, meningiomas, and primitive neuroectodermal tumors have been reported to possess tumor-associated antigens.* Mahaley, however, demonstrated that labeled anti-glioblastoma antisera cross-reacted with normal blood vessels and neurons. Wahlstrom and co-workers and others found in vitro reactivity of glioma antibody with normal adult and fetal brain.[222,238,249] These observations indicate the lack of precise antigenicity of brain neoplasms, but further work is needed to settle this problem. An immunotherapeutic approach to gliomas is highly speculative. Considering the evidence of shared antigens between tumor cells, normal brain, and lymphoid tissue, immunotherapy may be detrimental to the patient.[74] Nevertheless, this treatment has been used with different results.

Takakura and co-workers transfused normal adult bone marrow into children who had various malignant intracranial tumors.[235] Approximately 50 ml of bone marrow aspirate was transfused into ABO- and Rh-compatible patients after operation, radiation, and chemotherapy. The average survival of these patients was 32 months. A control group was not reported. These investigators also reported the infusion of purified white blood cells into the tumor space created by operative removal.[236] The intratumoral instillation of 10^{10} cells was associated with an average survival of 25.7 months. These reports are difficult to interpret because immunotherapy was used with more conventional modes of therapy. In addition, the studies were neither well controlled nor randomized, and the investigation included more than one specific type of tumor. Nevertheless, the reports of Takakura stating that the addition of immunotherapy to operation, radiation, and chemotherapy increased the survival of patients

*See references 39, 40, 172, 203, 252, 272.

with "malignant brain tumors" from 49 days to one year should not be ignored.

Trouillas studied the efficacy of therapy supplemental to operation in a randomized study comparing immunotherapy, cobalt therapy, and combination therapy.[243] Postoperatively, patients receiving immunotherapy were given injections of a mixture of Freund's adjuvant and a saline extract of their own tumor. Four to ten injections were made, depending upon the amount of tumor tissue available. Supplemental immunotherapy increased survival from 3.4 months with operation alone to 7.4 months. There was no significant difference in length of survival between patients receiving radiation (7.1 months) or immunotherapy (7.4 months). The combination of operation, radiation, and immunotherapy increased the survival time of the group to 10.1 months. Although promising, this form of immunotherapy carries the inherent danger illustrated by the occurrence of one case of allergic encephalitis in the group. This complication is probably caused by antibodies cross-reacting between glioma and normal brain tissue.

Bloom and co-workers reported the results of a trial to assess the value of immunotherapy in patients receiving irradiation and chemotherapy.[24] One milliliter of irradiated tumor cells from the patient was injected into the thigh as soon as possible after craniotomy. During the course of radiation therapy, additional injections were made. Unlike the results obtained by Trouillas, this form of active specific immunotherapy did not improve the survival of patients treated by operation and radiotherapy.[243] Fourteen per cent of the patients receiving only operation and irradiation survived 36 months, but patients receiving immunotherapy were all dead by 30 months. Furthermore, one patient may have developed allergic encephalitis.

Nonspecific immunotherapy with BCG vaccine has been used to treat many solid tumors, but little has been done in patients with brain tumors. Ommaya and Albright are at present involved in a trial of combined chemotherapy and immunotherapy for malignant gliomas.[176]

Another facet of the study of the immunobiology of malignant gliomas is the need for an assay method comparable to the carcinoembryonic antigen (CEA) assay in patients with colonic and rectal carcinomas to detect the presence or recurrence of tumor.[72] Although fetal brain antigens have been studied and compared with gliomas, clinical application is not yet available.[268]

Biochemistry of Brain Tumors

The biochemical composition and reactivity of intracranial neoplasms has been investigated in the hope that detection of differences from normal brain might be diagnostic.[108, 148, 184] These studies also are of potential importance in the development of antitumor chemotherapy. Unfortunately, the analyses have provided little diagnostic aid to the clinician, and the therapeutic value has been small.

Investigations of the biochemical nature of gliomas pose many problems. Histological control of the material analyzed is important. A specimen of tumor may be contaminated by necrosis, hemorrhage, interstitial fluid, or normal brain. Nonneural elements such as macrophages, leukocytes, and blood vessels may be present. The histological and biochemical samples must be from the same area; otherwise, the magnitude of these contaminating factors is uncertain. Unfortunately, most studies lack direct histological control. Aside from contamination, biochemical variation may occur not only among different tumors of the same type but also in different parts of the same tumor.

These problems have resulted in many contradictory reports, and are discouraging in the quest for specific biochemical patterns. Nevertheless, recent advances in ultramicrochemical techniques provide some insight into the biology of intracranial tumors.[3-6,99,174,232]

During oncogenesis, biochemical alterations can be detected in all neoplastic cells. An early, essential feature is a defect in DNA and associated proteins. The replication and concentration of DNA per cell increases in preparation for accelerated cell division. As the neoplastic process continues, the rate of turnover of RNA is also quickened. Increased protein synthesis and degradation accompany tumor growth. Enzymes, particularly those required for specialized normal function, eventually become depleted, causing altered energy metabolism and increased glycolysis. Lysosomal enzymes, however, usually increase in activity.

In general, intracranial neoplasms behave biochemically as do cancers of other organs. These characteristics have been used to differentiate neoplasms from normal brain. For example, the concentration of DNA in brain tumors increases to two to eight times as much as found in normal brain.[86,162] The increased DNA content results from a block in the mitotic process with accumulation of replicating DNA.[126] The nature of this block, however, is not known.

The oxidative metabolism of most gliomas generally is less than that of gray matter by a factor of one tenth to one half.[108,129,247] The normal cortex has high levels of cytochrome oxidase; gliomas contain much less; white matter is intermediate.[3] The concentrations of other energy-related compounds such as phosphocreatine, adenosine triphosphate, adenosine monophosphate, and other substances are lower in brain tumors than in normal brain.[*] It has been suggested that loss of ability of tumor cells to accumulate these energy-rich compounds results from a diminished capacity for synthesis.

In regard to oxidative metabolism, oligodendroglioma is the only exception. These tumors have the highest oxygen consumption and glycolytic rate of the gliogenous neoplasms.[247] This observation, however, has not always been confirmed.[27,137] Cytochrome oxidase levels are approximately seven times as great as those in astrocytomas.[107] The higher oxidative rate of normal oligodendrocytes is related to the activity of maintaining large amounts of myelin in the normal central nervous system. The oxidative metabolism of neoplastic oligodendrocytes therefore may be similar to that of normal cells. The possibility of "contamination" with normal brain components, however, should be considered.

Proliferation of glial cells is also accompanied by increased lysosomal enzymes.[4,6,129] These enzymatic increases are nonspecific, occurring in both reactive and neoplastic glia.[146] Beta-glucuronidase has been more thoroughly studied than other lysosomal enzymes. Activity of this substance is generally greater in malignant tumors than in benign tumors or in normal tissue,

---

*See references 107, 109, 121, 129, 183, 245.

although exceptions have been reported.[6] In normal brain, β-glucuronidase is predominantly bound, but in gliomas it is significantly increased in the free form. Nevertheless, the intensified activity of this enzyme may be related to those processes that promote the release of lysosomal enzymes, such as division and death of cells, pinocytosis, and tissue necrosis.

Similar differences between tumor tissue and normal brain have been reported with respect to concentrations of other enzymes.[35,89,223,240] Those enzymes involved in metabolic processes are generally reduced in quantity and activity in gliomas, but oligodendroglioma, as noted, is an exception. Phosphodiesterase activity correlates better with the cell of origin than with the degree of malignancy. Greatest activity was noted in tumors of mesodermal origin, lowest values were in ectodermal tumors.[35,142] The value of this enzyme in distinguishing those tumors that are histologically mixed has not been determined.

Lipids are in higher concentration in brain than in other organs of the body.[25] The total content of lipids in gliomas, however, is lower than that of normal brain, but higher than in most normal nonneural organs. In gliomas, the concentration of the major classes of lipid (glycolipids, phospholipids, cholesterol) is decreased.[177,224,232] Cerebrosides and sulfatides, forms of glycolipids, however, have been detected in different amounts in brain tumors.[8,47,75,224] The discrepancies among these reports preclude satisfactory clinical correlation.[89]

Only desmosterol, the immediate precursor in the biosynthesis of cholesterol, has proved to be of value in detecting the presence of brain tumors. The concentration of desmosterol is elevated, as much as 5 per cent of the total sterols, in glioblastoma and oligodendroglioma, but not in nonglial tumors or astrocytoma.[68,108,258] The detection of this compound in the cerebrospinal fluid of patients with glial tumors has been used for diagnosis and follow-up, as is discussed later. Therapeutically, the synthesis of cholesterol in brain tumors has been altered in an attempt to interfere with neoplastic growth. Compounds blocking cholesterol synthesis were administered preoperatively to patients with gliomas. Although these tumors were then incapable of synthesis of cholesterol, the clinical course was not altered.[9]

Studies of amino acids and simpler chem-

ical substances including trace elements have produced conflicting results and are of little diagnostic value.[149,226,261]

In spite of the usual lack of clinical correlation, biochemical assays are valuable in the detection of neuroblastoma and ganglioneuroma. These tumors synthesize various intermediate compounds in the conversion of dihydroxyphenylalanine (DOPA) to norepinephrine and epinephrine. Other compounds of this metabolic chain include vanillylmandelic acid (VMA) and homovanillic acid (HVA). Although any of these compounds may appear in the urine of patients with neuroblastoma, high levels of vanillylmandelic and homovanillic acids are generally considered diagnostic.[21] Primary intracranial tumors, including medulloblastoma, do not use dopa metabolic pathways. The only other neural tumor associated with increased excretion of catecholamines is pheochromocytoma. The specificity of the biochemical diagnosis of neuroblastoma has led to the hope that other tumors may be similarly diagnosed.

Because the cerebrospinal fluid reflects the status of the central nervous system in many pathological conditions, the fluid obtained from patients with intracranial neoplasms has been extensively studied to detect specific abnormalities characteristic of brain tumors. Most reports deal with abnormally elevated concentrations of enzymes and sterols, but neither is clearly diagnostic.

Enzymes in the cerebrospinal fluid of patients with brain tumors may originate from the tumor, surrounding altered brain, blood, choroid plexus, or leukocytes in the fluid. The multiplicity of sources makes specific changes less likely, and interpretation of the findings is difficult. Glutamic oxaloacetic transaminase (GOT), lactate dehydrogenase (LDH), and other enzymes are increased in concentration in the cerebrospinal fluid of patients with intracranial neoplasms.* This elevation is most striking in cases of malignant tumors, but it is more consistent with metastases than with primary neoplasms, and additionally, similar elevated concentrations of enzymes are caused by nonneoplastic secondary alterations of the brain such as malacia and hemorrhage. The concentrations of various enzymes are elevated in the cerebrospinal fluid of patients with brain tumors, as well

---

*See references 79, 80, 88, 101, 106, 146, 154, 216.

as with cerebral destructive processes. These assays therefore are not useful in the diagnosis of intracranial tumors.

More recently, cerebrospinal fluid lipids have been used for diagnosis of brain tumors and in the study of patients undergoing treatment of tumors.[190,257] The most common test is for desmosterol, the precursor of cholesterol. This substance is found in developing brain and in malignant brain tumors, but not in normal adult brain. The test is based on the augmentation of cerebrospinal fluid desmosterol after five days of oral administration of triparanol to inhibit the conversion of desmosterol to cholesterol. Cerebrospinal fluid concentrations greater than 0.1 μg per milliliter are considered indicative of the presence of a brain tumor. Diagnostic accuracy greater than 75 per cent has been reported.[67,178] A false-positive test was uncommon. Concentrations of desmosterol have also been determined serially to evaluate patients after treatment. Presumably, these values can be used as a biochemical indicator of tumor activity.[259,260] Unfortunately, the results are inconsistent, leading some workers to declare this test a poor indicator of central nervous system neoplasia.[145]

Many other compounds are said to be increased in the cerebrospinal fluid of patients with intracranial tumors, but inconsistencies render the assays clinically useless.[79,142,146]

Although several clinical studies suggest the value of biochemical determinations in the diagnosis of intracranial neoplasms, the variability of other studies indicates that these assays are not useful at present. Neuroblastoma and related tumors are the only neoplasms consistently diagnosed biochemically. In spite of failure to fulfill the promise of diagnostic chemical determinations for primary intracranial tumors, elucidation of the biochemical properties may direct future chemotherapeutic trials and result in increased efficacy of these agents.

Acknowledgment. Dr. Brooks's work was supported in part by grant CA 18234 from the National Cancer Institute.

REFERENCES

1. Abbott, K. H., and Love, J. G.: Metastasizing intracranial tumors. Ann. Surg., *118*:343–352, 1943.

2. Aita, J. A.: Genetic aspects of tumors of the nervous system. Part I. Nebraska Med. J.,*53*:121–124, 1968.

3. Allen, N.: Cytochrome oxidase in human brain tumors. J. Neurochem., *2*:37–44, 1957.

4. Allen, N.: Dehydropeptidase I activities in human intracranial neoplasms. Exp. Neurol., *1*:155–165, 1959.

5. Allen, N.: Beta-glucuronidase activities in tumors of the nervous system. Neurology, *11*:578–596, 1961.

6. Allen, N., and Reagan, E.: Beta-glucuronidase activities in cerebrospinal fluid. Arch. Neurol., *11*:144–154, 1964.

7. Alvord, E. C.: The etiology and pathogenesis of experimental allergic encephalitis. *In* Bailey, O. T. ed.: The Central Nervous System, Williams & Wilkins, Baltimore, 1968, pp. 52–70.

8. Aruna, R. M., Balasubramanian, K. A., Mathai, K. V., and Vasu, D.: Isolation and characterisation of glycolipids and glycosaminoglycans from meningiomas. Indian J. Med. Res., *61*:1688–1693, 1973.

9. Azarnoff, D. L., Curran, G. L., and Williamson, W. P.: Incorporation of acetate-1-C[14] into cholesterol by human intracranial tumors in vitro. J. Nat. Cancer Inst., *21*:1109–1115, 1958.

10. Bader, J. P.: Metabolic requirements for infection by Rous sarcoma virus. I. The transient requirement for DNA synthesis. Virology, *29*:444–451, 1966.

11. Bailey, P.: Further remarks concerning tumors of the glioma group. Bull. Johns Hopk. Hosp., *40*:354–389, 1927.

12. Bailey, P., and Cushing, H.: Medulloblastoma cerebelli: a common type of midcerebellar glioma of childhood. Arch. Neurol. Psychiat., *14*:192–224, 1925.

13. Bailey, P., and Cushing, H.: A Classification of the Tumors of the Glioma Group on a Histogenetic Basis with a Correlated Study of Prognosis. Philadelphia, J. B. Lippincott Co., 1926.

14. Bailey, P., and Cushing, H.: Gwebsverschiedenheit der die Gliome und ihre Bedeutung fuer die Prognose. Jena, Fischer, 1930.

15. Battista, A. F., Bloom, W., Loffman, M., and Feigin, I.: Autotransplantation of anaplastic astrocytoma into the subcutaneous tissue of man. Neurology, *11*:977–981, 1961.

16. Batzdorf, U., and Malamud, N.: The problems of multicentric gliomas. J. Neurosurg., *20*:122–136, 1963.

17. Bell, R. L.: Concentration of labeled tri-iodothyronine and radioactive albumin in human cerebral neoplasms. J. Nucl. Med., *1*:180–185, 1960.

18. Bicknell, J. M.: Chromosome studies of human brain tumors. Neurology, *17*:485–490, 1967.

19. Bigner, D. D., and Pegram, C. N.: Virus-induced experimental brain tumors and putative associations of viruses with human brain tumors: A review. Adv. Neurol., *15*:57–83, 1976.

20. Bigner, D. D., Odom, G. L., Mahaley, M. S., Jr., and Day, E. D.: Brain tumors induced in dogs by the Schmidt-Ruppin strain of Rous sarcoma virus. J. Neuropath. Exp. Neurol., *28*:648–680, 1969.

21. Bill, A. H., Jr., and Koop, C. E.: Conference on the biology of neuroblastoma. J. Ped. Surg., *3*:103–194, 1968.

22. Blakiston's New Gould Medical Dictionary: Hoerr, N. L., and Osal, A., eds. 2nd Ed. New York, McGraw-Hill Book Co., 1956.

23. Bloom, W. H., Carstairs, K. C., Crompton, M. R., and McKissock, W.: Autologous glioma transplantation. Lancet, 2:77–78, 1960.

24. Bloom, H. J. G., Peckham, M. J., Richardson, A. E., Alexander, P. A., and Payne, P. M.: Glioblastoma multiforme: A controlled trial to assess the value of specific active immunotherapy in patients treated by radical surgery and radiotherapy. Brit. J. Cancer, 27:253–267, 1973.

25. Brante, G.: Studies on lipids in the nervous system with special reference to quantitative chemical determination and topical distribution. Acta Physiol. Scand., 18:suppl. 63, 1–189, 1949.

26. Bressler, H.: Die Krankheiten des Gehirns und der aeusseren Kopfbedeckungen. Berlin, Voss, 1839.

27. Brierley, J. B., and McIlwain, H.: Metabolic properties of cerebral tissues modified by neoplasia and by freezing. J. Neurochem., 1:109–118, 1956.

28. Broders, A. C.: Squamous cell epithelioma of the lip: a study of five hundred and thirty-seven cases. J.A.M.A., 74:656–664, 1920.

29. Broders, A. C.: The grading of carcinoma. Minn. Med., 8:76–730, 1925.

30. Brooks, W. H., Caldwell, H. D., and Mortara, R. H.: Immune responses in patients with gliomas. Surg. Neurol., 2:419–423, 1974.

31. Brooks, W. H., Netsky, M. G., Normansell, D. E., and Horwitz, D. A.: Depressed cell-mediated immunity in patients with primary intracranial tumors. J. Exp. Med., 136:1631–1647, 1972.

32. Brooks, W. H., Roszman, T. L., Mahaley, M. S., Woosley, R., and Bigner, D. D.: Immunobiology of primary intracranial tumors. II. Analysis of lymphocyte populations in patients with primary brain tumors. Immun., 29:61–66, 1977.

33. Buckwalter, J. A., Turner, J. H., Gambler, H. H., Raterman, L., Soper, R. T., and Knowler, L. A.: Psychoses, intracranial neoplasms and genetics. Arch. Neurol. Psychiat., 81:480–485, 1959.

34. Burnet, M. F.: Somatic mutation and chronic disease. Brit. Med. J., 1:338–342, 1965.

35. Canal, N., Frattola, L., Villani, R., and Bassi, S.: Adenyl cyclase and phosphodiesterase in human cerebral tumors. J. Neurol. Sci., 18:164–168, 1974.

36. Cervos-Navarro, J., and Vazquez, J.: Electronenmikroskopische Untersuchungen ueber das Vorkommen von Cilien in Meningiomen. Virchow Arch. Path. Anat., 341:280–290, 1966.

37. Ciembroniewicz, J., and Kolar, O.: Tissue culture study of glioblastoma cells with addition of autologous lymphocytes. Acta Cytol. (Balt.), 13:42–47, 1969.

38. Clarenburg, R., Chaikoff, I. L., and Morris, M. D.: Incorporation of injected cholesterol into the myelinating brain of the 17-day-old rabbit. J. Neurochem., 10:135–143, 1963.

39. Coakham, H. B.: Surface antigens common to human astrocytoma cells. Nature, 250:328–330, 1974.

40. Coakham, H. B., and Lakshmi, M. S.: Tumour-associated surface antigen(s) in human astrocytoma. Oncology, 31:233–243, 1975.

41. Conen, P. E., and Falk, R. E.: Chromosome studies on cultured tumors of nervous tissue origin. Acta Cytologica, 11:86–91, 1967.

42. Conen, P. E., Donahue, W. L., Falk, R. E., and Delarve, N. C.: Chromosome patterns of human malignant tumors and effusions. A comparison of results by direct examination and after tissue culture. Proc. Amer. Ass. Cancer Res., 4:12, 1963.

43. Cooper, J. R.: Tumor tissue growth. The growth of tumor tissue of the central nervous system in tissue culture. J. Kansas Med. Soc., 68:340–343, 1967.

44. Courville, C. B.: Multiple primary tumors of the brain: Review of the literature and report of twenty-one cases. Amer. J. Cancer, 26:703–731, 1936.

45. Courville, C. B.: Intracranial tumors. Notes upon a series of three thousand verified cases with some current observations pertaining to their mortality. Bull. Los Angeles Neurol. Soc., 32:1–80, 1967.

46. Cox, D., Yuncken, C., and Spriggs, A. I.: Minute chromatin bodies in malignant tumors of childhood. Lancet, 2:55–58, 1965.

47. Cristensen Lou, H. O., Clausen, J., and Bierring, F.: Phospholipids and glycolipids in tumours of the central nervous system. J. Neurochem., 12:619–627, 1965.

48. Cushing, H.: Experiences with the cerebellar medulloblastomas. Acta Path. Microbiol. Scand., 7:1–86, 1930.

49. Cushing, H., and Eisenhardt, L.: Meningiomas: Their Classification, Regional Behavior, Life, History, and Surgical End-Results, Springfield, Ill., Charles C Thomas, 1938.

50. Dastur, D. K., and Lalitha, V. S.: Pathological analysis of intracranial space-occupying lesions in 1000 cases including children. Part 2. Incidence, types and unusual cases of glioma. J. Neurol. Sci. 8:143–170, 1969.

51. Dastur, D. K., Lalitha, V. S., and Prabhakar, V.: Pathological analysis of intracranial space-occupying lesions in 1000 cases including children. Part I. Age, sex and pattern; and the tuberculomas J. Neurol. Sci., 6:575–592, 1968.

52. Dausset, J., Degos, L., and Hors, J.: The association of the HL-A antigens with diseases. Clin. Immun. Immunopath., 3:127–149, 1974.

53. del Cerro, M. P., and Snider, R. S.: The Purkinje cell cilium. Anat. Rec., 165:127–140, 1969.

54. Dorland's Illustrated Medical Dictionary. 25th Ed. Philadelphia, W. B. Saunders Co., 1974.

55. Druckery, H., Ivankovic, S., and Preussman, R.: Selektive Erzeugung maligner tumoren in Gehirn and Rückenmark von Ratten durch N-methyl-N-nitrosoharnstoff. Z. Krebsforsch., 66:389–408; 1965.

56. Druckery, H., Preussman, R., and Ivankovic, S.: N-nitroso compounds in organotypic and transplacental carcinogenesis. Ann. N.Y. Acad. Sci., 163:676–696; 1969.

57. Druckery, H., Ivankovic, S., and Preussman, R.: Teratogenic and carcinogenic effects in the offspring after single injection of ethylnitrosourea to pregnant rats. Nature, 210:1378–1379; 1966.

58. Druckery, H., Ivankovic, S., Preussmann, R.,

Zuelch, K. J., and Mennel, H. D.: Selective induction of malignant tumors of the nervous system by resorptive carcinogens. *In* Kirsch, W., Grossi-Paoletti, E., and Paoletti, P., eds.: The Experimental Biology of Brain Tumors. Springfield, Ill., Charles C Thomas, 1972, pp. 85–147.

59. Duffell, D., Hinz, R., and Nelson, E.: Neoplasms in hamsters induced by simian virus 40: light and microscopic observations. Amer. J. Path., 45:59–73, 1964.

60. Eggers, A. E.: Autoradiographic and fluorescence antibody studies of the human host immune response to gliomas. Neurology (Minneap.), 22:246–250, 1972.

61. Erkman, B., and Conen, P. E.: Chromosome constitution of 14 human malignant tumors. Proc. Amer. Ass. Cancer Res., 5:17, 1964.

62. Ewing, J.: Neoplastic Diseases. 4th Ed. Philadelphia, W. B. Saunders Co., 1940.

62a. Fan, K., Kovi, J., and Earle, K. M.: The ethnic distribution of primary central nervous system tumors. AFIP 1958 to 1970. J. Neuropath. Exp. Neurol., 36:41–49, 1977.

63. Febvre, H., Maunoury, R., Constans, J. P., and Trouillas, P.: Réactions d'hypersensibilité retardée avec des lignées de cellules tumorales humaines cultivées *in vitro* chez des malades porteurs de tumeurs cérebrales malignes. Int. J. Cancer, 10:221–232, 1972.

64. Fessard, C.: Cerebral tumors in infancy: 66 clinicoanatomical case studies. Amer. J. Dis. Child., 115:302–308, 1968.

65. Frattola, L., and Canal, N.: Research on aldolases in cerebrospinal fluid. Riv. Pat. Nerv. Ment., 81:133–140, 1960.

66. Fumagalli, R., Grossi, E., Paoletti, P., and Paoletti, R.: Studies on lipids in brain tumors. I. Occurrence and significance of sterol precursors of cholesterol in human brain tumors. J. Neurochem., 11:561–565, 1964.

67. Fumagalli, R., and Paoletti, P.: Sterol test for human brain tumors. Relationship with different oncotypes. Neurology (Minneap.), 21:1149–1156, 1971.

68. Galli, G., Galli-Kienle, M., Cattabeni, F., Fiecchi, A., Grossi-Paoletti, E., and Paoletti, R.: The sterol precursors of cholesterol in normal and tumor tissues. Advances Enzym. Regulat., 8:311–321, 1970.

69. Garcia, J. H., Okazaki, H., and Aronson, S. M.: Blood-group frequencies and astrocytomata. J. Neurosurg., 20:397–399, 1963.

70. Gatai, G., and Földi, M.: Lymphatic absorption of the CSF and its therapeutic use by hydrocephalus: the lymphatic shunt. 2nd Int. Congr. Neurol. Surg., Washington, D.C., 1961. Excerpta Med. No. 36:E77–E78, 1961.

71. Glasauer, F. E., and Yuan, R. H. P.: Intracranial tumors with extracranial metastases: case report and review of the literature. J. Neurosurg., 20:474–493, 1963.

72. Gold, P., and Freedman, S. O.: Specific carcinoembryonic antigens of the human digestive system. J. Exp. Med., 122:467–481, 1965.

73. Goldberg, M. B., Scheline, G. E., and Malamud, N.: Malignant intracranial neoplasms following radiation therapy for acromegaly. Radiology, 80:465–470, 1963.

74. Golub, E. S.: Brain-associated theta antigen. Reactivity of rabbit anti-mouse brain with mouse lymphoid cells. Cell. Immun., 2:353–361, 1971.

75. Gopal, L., Grossi, E., Paoletti, P., and Usardi, M.: Lipid composition of human intracranial tumors: A biochemical study. Acta Neurochir., 11:333–347, 1963.

76. Gowers, W. R.: A Manual of Diseases of the Nervous System. 3rd Ed. Philadelphia, Blakiston, 1903.

77. Grace, J. T., Perese, D. M., Metzgar, R. S., Sasabe, T., and Holdridge, B.: Tumor autograft responses in patients with glioblastoma multiforme. J. Neurosurg., 18:159–167, 1961.

78. Grant, F. C.: A study of the results of surgical treatment in 2,326 consecutive patients with brain tumor. J. Neurosurg., 13:479–488, 1956.

79. Green, J. B., and Perry, M.: Leucine aminopeptidase activity in cerebrospinal fluid. Neurology, 13:924–926, 1963.

80. Green, J. B., Oldewurtel, H. A., O'Doherty, D. S., Forster, F. M., and Sanchez-Longo, L. P.: Cerebrospinal fluid glutamic oxalacetic transaminase activity in neurologic disease. Neurology, 7:313–333, 1957.

81. Greene, H. S. N.: The transplantation of human brain tumors to the brains of laboratory animals. Cancer Res., 13:422–426, 1953.

82. Gyepes, M. T., and D'Angio, G. J.: Extracranial metastases from central nervous system tumors in children and adolescents. Radiology, 87:55–63, 1967.

83. Hague, M., and Harvald, B.: Genetics in intracranial tumors. Acta Genet., 7:573–591, 1957.

84. Hamperl, H., and Ackerman, L. V.: Illustrated Tumor Nomenclature. 2nd Ed. New York, Springer, 1969.

85. Hayward, M. D., and Bower, B. D.: Chromosomal trisomy associated with the Sturge-Weber syndrome. Lancet, 2:844–846, 1960.

86. Heller, I. H., and Elliott, K. A. C.: The metabolism of normal brain and human gliomas in relation to cell type and density. Canad. J. Biochem., 33:395–493, 1955.

87. Hess, H. H., Schneider, G., Warnock, M., and Pope, A.: Lack of effect of Na^+ plus K^{++} on Mg^{++} stimulated ATP phosphohydrolase activity of human astrocytomas. Fed. Proc., 22:333, 1963. (Abstract.)

88. Hildebrand, J., and Levin, S.: Enzymatic activities in cerebrospinal fluid in patients with neurological diseases. Acta Neurol. Belg., 73:229–240, 1973.

89. Hildebrand, J., and Van Houche, J.: Lipids of cerebrospinal fluid in patients with brain metastases. Acta Neurol. Belg., 73:25–30, 1973.

90. Hortega, del Rio P.: Estructura y sistematisación de los gliomas y paragliomas. Arch. Espan. Oncol., 2:411–677, 1932.

91. Ikuta, F., and Zimmerman, H. M.: Virus particles in reactive cells induced by intracerebral implantation of dibenzanthracene. J. Neuropath. Exp. Neurol., 24:225–243, 1965.

92. Ingraham, F. D., and Matson, D. D.: Neurosurgery of Infancy and Childhood. Springfield, Ill., Charles C Thomas, 1954.

93. Ivankovic, S., Druckery, H., and Preussman, R.: Erzeugung neurogener Tumoren bei den nachkommen nach einmaliger Injektion von Äthyl-

nitrosoharnstoff an schwangeren Ratten. Naturwissenschaften, 53:410, 1966.

94. Ivankovic, S., and Druckery, H.: Transplacentare erzeugung maligner Tumoren des Nervensystems. I. Acthyl-nitroso-harnstoff an BD IX-ratten. Z. Krebsforsch., 71:320–360, 1968.

95. Jelsma, R., and Bucy, P. C.: The treatment of glioblastoma multiforme of the brain. J. Neurosurg., 27:388–400, 1967.

96. Jelsma, R., and Bucy, P. C.: Glioblastoma multiforme: Its treatment and some factors affecting survival. Arch. Neurol., 20:161–171, 1969.

97. Johnson, H. A., Haymaker, W. E., Rubini, J. R., Fliedner, T. M., Bond, V. P., Cronkite, E. P., and Hughes, W. L.: A radioautographic study of a human brain and glioblastoma multiforme after the in vivo uptake of tritiated thymidine. Cancer, 13:636–642, 1960.

98. Jones, E. L., Searle, C. E., and Smith, W. T.: Tumors of the nervous system induced in rats by the neonatal administration of N-ethyl-N-nitrosourea. J. Path., 109:123–139, 1973.

99. Karlsson, K. A., Pascher, I., and Samuelsson, B. E.: Analysis of intact gangliosides by mass spectrometry. Comparison of different derivatives of a hematoside of a tumor and the major monosialoganglioside of brain. Chem. Phys. Lipids, 12:271–286, 1974.

100. Katsura, S., Suzuki, J., and Wada, T.: A statistical study of brain tumors in the neurosurgical clinics of Japan. J. Neurosurg., 16:570–580, 1959.

101. Katzman, R., Fishman, R. A., and Goldensohn, E. S.: Glutamic-oxalacetic transaminase activity in spinal fluid. Neurology (Minneap.), 7:853–855, 1957.

102. Kent, S. P., and Pickering, J. E.: Neoplasms in monkeys (Macaca mulatta): Spontaneous and irradiation induced. Cancer, 11:138–147, 1958.

103. Kernohan, J. W., and Fletcher-Kernohan, E. M.: Ependymomas. A study of 109 cases. In: Tumors of the Nervous System. Ass. Res. Nerv. Ment. Dis. Proc., 16:181–209, 1937.

104. Kernohan, J. W., and Sayre, G. P.: Tumors of The Central Nervous System. Atlas of Tumor Pathology, Section X, Fascicles 35 and 37. Washington, Armed Forces Institute of Pathology, 1952.

105. Kernohan, J. W., Mabon, R. F., Svien, H. J., and Adson, A. W.: A simplified classification of gliomas. Proc. Staff Meet. Mayo Clin., 24:71–75, 1949.

106. Kerr-Jakoby, R., and Jakoby, W. B.: Lactic dehydrogenase of cerebrospinal fluid in the differential diagnosis of cerebrovascular and brain tumor. J. Neurosurg., 15:45–51, 1968.

107. Kirsch, W. M.: Substrates of glycolysis in intracranial tumors during complete ischemia. Cancer Res., 25:432–439, 1965.

108. Kirsch, W. M., Grossi-Paoletti, E., and Paoletti, P.: Experimental Biology of Brain Tumors. Springfield, Ill., Charles C Thomas, 1971.

109. Kirsh, W. M., Schulz, D., and Leitner, J. W.: The quantitative histochemistry of the experimental glioblastoma: Glycolysis and growth. Acta Histochem., 28:51–85, 1967.

110. Kleihues, P., Lantos, P. L., and Magee, P. N.: Chemical carcinogenesis in the nervous system. In Richter, G. W., and Epstein, M. A., eds.: International Review of Experimental Pathology. New York, Academic Press, 1976, pp. 153–232.

111. Kleihues, P., Matsumoto, S., Wechsler, W., and Zuelch, K. J.: Morphologie und Wachstum der mit Äthylnitrosoharnstoff transplazentar erzeugten Tumoren des Nervensystems. Verh. (H) Deutsch. Ges. Path., 52:372–379; 1968.

112. Koch, G.: Beitrag zur Erblichkeit der Hirngeschwülste. Acta Genet. Med. Gemellol., 3:170–190, 1954.

113. Koch, G.: The genetics of cerebral tumors. In Classification of Brain Tumors. Acta Neurochir. Suppl. 10, 1965.

114. Koenig, H., Bunge, M. B., and Bunge, R. P.: Nucleic acid and protein metabolism in white matter: Observations during experimental demyelination and remyelination; a histochemical and autoradiographic study of spinal cord of the adult cat. Arch. Neurol., 6:177–193, 1962.

115. Koestner, A., Swenberg, J. A., and Wechsler, W.: Transplacental production with ethylnitrosourea of neoplasms of the nervous system in Sprague-Dawley rats. Amer. J. Path., 63:37–56, 1971.

116. Kornblith, P. L., Dohan, F. C., Wood, W. C., and Whitman, B. D.: Human astrocytoma: serum-mediated immunologic response. Cancer, 33:1512–1519, 1974.

117. Kotsilimbas, D. G., Levy, W. A., and Scheinberg, L. C.: Chloromerodrin Hg 203 and electrolyte distribution in murine brain tumors. Arch. Neurol., 13:525–532, 1965.

118. Kricheff, I. I., Becker, M., Schneck, S. A., and Taveras, J. M.: Intracranial ependymomas; factors influencing prognosis. J. Neurosurg., 21:7–14, 1964.

119. Kumar, S., Taylor, G., Steward, J. K., Waghe, M. A., and Morris-Jones, P.: Cell-mediated immunity and blocking factors in patients with tumors of the central nervous system. Int. J. Cancer, 12:194–205, 1973.

120. Kung, P. C., Lee, J. C., and Bakay, L.: Vascular invasion by glioma cells in man: An electron microscopic study. J. Neurosurg., 31:339–345, 1969.

121. Kurihara, T., Kawakami, S., Veki, K., and Takahashi, Y.: 2',3'-Cyclic nucleotide 3'-phosphohydrolase activity in human brain tumors. J. Neurochem., 22:1143–1144, 1974.

122. Kurland, L. T., Myrianthopoulos, N. C., and Leksell, S.: Epidemiologic and genetic considerations of intracranial neoplasms. In The Biology and Treatment of Intracranial Tumors. Springfield, Ill., Charles C Thomas, 1962.

123. Kury, G., and Carter, H. W.: Autoradiographic study of human nervous system tumors. Arch. Path., 80:38–42, 1965.

124. Kyle, R. H., Oler, A., Lasser, E. C., and Rosomoff, H. L.: Meningioma induced by thorium dioxide. New Eng. J. Med., 268:80–82, 1963.

125. Labitzke, H. G.: Glioblastoma multiforme with remote extracranial metastases. Arch. Path., 73:223–229, 1962.

126. Lapham, L. W.: Subdivision of glioblastoma multiforme on a cytologic and cytochemical

basis. J. Neuropath. Exp. Neurol., *18*:244–262, 1959.

127. Leavitt, F. H.: Cerebellar tumors occurring in identical twins. Arch. Neurol. Psychiat., *19*:617–623, 1928.

128. Lechner, H., Musil, A., Leb, D., Wawschinek, O., Beyer, W., Tagger, H. H., and Wielinger, H.: Untersuchungen über des Mengenund Spurenelementgehalt von Hirntumoren. Wien. Klin. Wschr., *76*:974–976, 1964.

129. Lehrer, G. M.: The quantitative histochemistry of human glial tumors. *In* Fields, W. S., and Sharkey, P. O., eds.: The Biology and Treatment of Intracranial Tumors. Springfield, Ill., Charles C Thomas, 1962.

130. Lesse, S., and Netsky, M. G.: Metastases of neoplasms to the central nervous system and meninges. A.M.A. Arch. Neurol. Psychiat., *72*:133–153, 1954.

131. Levy, N. L., Mahaley, M. S., and Day, E. D.: *In vitro* demonstration of cell-mediated immunity to human brain tumors. Cancer Res., *32*:477–482, 1972.

132. Lubs, H. A., and Salmon, J. H.: The chromosomal complement of human solid tumors: II. Karyotypes of glial tumors. J. Neurosurg., *23*:160–168, 1965.

133. Lubs, H. A., Salmon, J. H., and Flanigan, S.: Studies of a glial tumor with multiple minute chromosomes. Cancer, *19*:591–599, 1966.

134. Lumsden, C. E., and Pomerat, C. M.: Normal oligodendrocytes in tissue culture: A preliminary report on the pulsatile glial cells in tissue culture from the corpus callosum of the normal adult rat brain. Exp. Cell Res., *2*:103–114, 1951.

135. Madonick, M. J., Shapiro, J. H., and Torack, R. M.: Multiple diverse primary brain tumors: report of a case and review of literature. Neurology, *11*:430–436, 1961.

136. Magee, P. N., and Barnes, J. M.: The production of malignant primary hepatic tumors in the rat by feeding dimethylnitrosamine. Brit. J. Cancer, *10*:114–122, 1956.

137. Mahaley, M. S., Jr.: The *in vitro* respiration of normal brain and brain tumors. Cancer Res., *26*:195–197, 1966.

138. Mahaley, M. S.: Immunologic considerations and the malignant glioma problem. Clin. Neurosurg., *15*:175–189, 1968.

139. Mahaley, M. S.: Experiences with antibody production from human glioma tissue. Prog. Exp. Tumor Res., *17*:31–39, 1972.

140. Mahaley, M. S., Brooks, W. H., Woosley, R., Roszman, T. L., and Dudka, L.: Immunobiology of primary intracranial tumors. I. Studies of the cellular and humoral general immune competence of brain tumor patients. J. Neurosurg., *46*:467–476, 1977.

141. Mann, I., Yates, P. O., and Ainslie, J. P.: Unusual case of double primary orbital tumour. Brit. J. Ophthal., *37*:758–762, 1953.

142. Manno, N. J., McGuckin, W. F., and Goldstein, N. P.: Cerebrospinal fluid total polysaccharide in diseases of the nervous system. Neurology, *15*:49–55, 1965.

143. Manuila, A.: Blood groups and diseases—hard facts and delusions. J.A.M.A., *167*:2047–2053, 1958.

144. Marburg, O., and Helfand, M.: Injuries of the Nervous System Including Poisonings. New York, Veritas, 1939.

145. Marton, L. J., Gordan, G. S., Barker, M., Wilson, C. B., and Lubich, W.: Failure to demonstrate desmosterol in spinal fluid of brain tumor patients. Arch. Neurol., *28*:137–138, 1973.

146. Mason, D. Y., and Roberts-Thomson, P.: Spinal-fluid lysozyme in diagnosis of central nervous system tumors. Lancet, *2*:952–953, 1974.

147. Mason, T. J., McKay, F. W., Hoover, R., Blot, W. J., and Fraumeni, J. F., Jr.: Atlas of Cancer Mortality for U.S. Counties: 1950–1969. Washington, U.S. Department of Health, Education, and Welfare, 1975.

148. Maspes, P. E., and Paoletti, P.: Recent advances in chemical composition and metabolism of brain tumors. Prog. Neurol. Surg., *2*:203–366, 1968.

149. Massarelli, R., Ciesielski-Treska, J., Ebel, A., and Mandel, P.: Choline uptake in glial cell cultures. Brain Res., *81*:361–363, 1974.

150. Matson, D. D.: Neurosurgery of Infancy and Childhood. 2nd Ed. Springfield, Ill., Charles C Thomas, 1969.

151. Mayr, E., Diamond, L. K., Levine, P. R., and Mayr, M.: Suspected correlation between blood-group frequency and pituitary adenomas. Science, *124*:932–934, 1956.

152. McIlwain, H.: Biochemistry and the Central Nervous System. 3rd Ed. Boston, Little, Brown, and Co., 1966.

153. Medawar, P. B.: Immunity to homologous grafted skin. III. Fate of skin homografts transplanted to brain, to subcutaneous tissue, and to anterior chamber of the eye. Brit. J. Exp. Path., *29*:58–69, 1948.

154. Mellick, R. S., and Bassett, R. L.: The cerebrospinal fluid glutamic oxalacetic transaminase activity in neurological diseases. Lancet, *1*:904–906, 1964.

155. Millen, J. W., and Woollam, D. H. M.: The Anatomy of the Cerebrospinal Fluid. London, Oxford University Press, 1962.

156. Modan, B., Baidatz, D., Mart, H., Steinitz, R., and Levin, S. G.: Radiation-induced head and neck tumors. Lancet, *1*:277–279, 1974.

157. Moertel, C. G., Dockerty, M. B., and Baggenstoss, A. H.: Multiple primary malignant neoplasms. III. Tumors of multicentric origin. Cancer, *14*:238–248, 1961.

158. Morley, T. P.: The recovery of tumor cells from venous blood draining cerebral gliomas: A preliminary report. Canad. J. Surg., *2*:363–365, 1959.

159. Morley, T. P.: Discussion: Tumor autograft responses in patients with glioblastoma multiforme by Grace, J. T., Perese, D. M., Metzgar, R. S., Sasabe, T., and Holdridge, B.: J. Neurosurg., *18*:159–167, 1961.

160. Munk, J., Peyser, E., and Gruszkiewicz, J.: Radiation induced intracranial meningiomas. Clin. Radiol., *20*:90–94, 1969.

161. Napalkov, N. P.: Some general considerations on the problem of transplacental carcinogenesis. *In* Tomatis, L., and Mohr, U., eds.: Transplacental Carcinogenesis. Lyon, ARC Sci. Publ. No. 4, 1973, pp. 1–13.

162. Nayyar, S. N.: A study of phosphate, desoxyri-

bonucleic acid, and phospholipid fractions in neural tumors. Neurology, 13:287–291, 1963.

163. Netsky, M. G.: Diseases of the nervous system in the aged patient, arranged by common presenting symptoms. *In* Johnson, W., ed.: The Older Patient, New York, Hoeber, 1960, pp. 467–512.

164. Netsky, M. G.: Experimental induction and transplantation of brain tumors in animals. Acta Neurochir., suppl. 10:45–56, 1964.

165. Netsky, M. G., and Federspiel, C. F.: Aging, endocrines, and brain tumors. To be published.

166. Netsky, M. G., and Miyaji, T.: Prevalence of cerebral hemorrhage and thrombosis in Japan: Study of the major causes of death. J. Chronic Dis. 29:711–721, 1976.

167. Netsky, M. G., and Shuangshoti, S.: The Choroid Plexus in Health and Disease. Charlottesville, University Press of Virginia, 1974, pp. 250–254.

168. Netsky, M. G., August, B., and Fowler, W.: The longevity of patients with glioblastoma multiforme. J. Neurosurg., 7:261–269, 1950.

169. Nevin, S.: Gliomatosis cerebri. Brain, 61:170–191, 1938.

170. Noetzli, M., and Malamud, N.: Postirradiation fibrosarcoma of the brain. Cancer, 15:617–622, 1962.

171. Oberling, C., Guérin, M., and Guérin, P.: La production expérimentale de tumeurs hypophysaires chez le rat. C. R. Soc. Biol., 123:1152–1154, 1936.

172. Oda, Y., Takeuchi, J., and Handa, H.: Tumor specific antigens of brain tumors. Neurol. Surg., 1:27–35, 1973.

173. Odom, G. L., Davis, C. H., and Woodhall, B.: Brain tumors in children. Clinical analysis of 164 cases. Pediatrics, 18:856–870, 1956.

174. Olsson, J. E., Blomstrand, C., and Haglid, K. G.: Cellular distribution of beta-trace protein in the central nervous system and brain tumours. J. Neurol. Neurosurg. Psychiat., 37:302–311, 1974.

175. Deleted in proof.

176. Ommaya, A. K., and Albright, L. A.: Combined chemotherapy and immunotherapy for malignant gliomas. Presented to American Academy of Neurological Surgeons, 1975.

177. Onodera, Y., Masamichi, H., Yukio, Y., and Tetsuro, M.: Lipid and fatty acid composition of brain tumor. Biol. Abstr., 53:2083, 1972.

178. Paoletti, P., Vandenheuval, F. A., Fumagalli, R., and Paoletti, R.: The sterol test for the diagnosis of human brain tumors. Neurology, 19:190–197, 1969.

179. Parker, E. F., and Kernohan, J. W.: The relation of injury and glioma of the brain. J.A.M.A., 97:535–539, 1931.

180. Patau, K., Therman, E., Smith, D. W., Inhorn, S. L., and Picken, B. F.: Partial trisomy syndromes. I. Sturge-Weber's disease. Amer. J. Hum. Genet., 13:287–298, 1961.

181. Pearce, K. M., and Yates, P. O.: Blood groups and brain tumours. H. Neurol. Sci., 2:434–441, 1965.

182. Perese, D. M., and Moore, G. E.: Methods of induction and histogenesis of experimental brain tumors. J. Neurosurg., 17:677–699, 1960.

183. Perkins, J. P., Moore, M. M., Kalisker, A., and

184. Su, Y. F.: Regulation of cyclic AMP content in normal and malignant brain cells. Adv. Cyclic Nucleotide Res., 5:641–660, 1975.

184. Perria, L., and Viale, G. L.: A chemical approach to the problem of cellular malignancy in tumors of the nervous system. Acta Neurochir., 15:33–39, 1966.

185. Pick, L., and Bielschowsky, M.: Über das system der Neurone und Beobachtung an einem Ganglioneurom des Gehirns nebst Untersuchung über die Genese der Nervenfasern in "Neuromen." 2 schr. Neurol., 6:391–437, 1911.

186. Porter, I. H., Benedict, W. F., Brown, C. D., and Paul, B.: Recent advances in molecular pathology: A review: Some aspects of chromosome changes in cancer. Exp. Molec. Path., 3:340–367, 1969.

187. Potter, J. F., Franco, P. E., and Smith, J.: Motility characteristics of malignant cells. Surg. Forum, 16:104–106, 1965.

188. Potter, J. F., Wieneke, K., and Grisez, J.: Role of neoplastic intravasation in the development of hematogenous metastases in amelanotic melanoma tumors I and III. Ann. Surg., 161:400–405, 1965.

189. Ramon-Moliner, E.: A study on neuroglia: The problem of transitional forms. J. Comp. Neurol., 110:157–171, 1958.

190. Ramsey, R. B., and Davison, A. N.: Steryl esters and their relationship to normal and diseased human central nervous system. J. Lipid Res., 15:249–255, 1974.

191. Ribbert, H.: Ueber das spongioblastom und das Gliom. Virchow. Arch. Path. Anat., 225:195, 1918.

192. Ridley, A., and Cavanagh, J. B.: Lymphocytic infiltration in gliomas: evidence of possible host resistance. Brain, 94:117–124, 1971.

193. Ringertz, N.: "Grading" of gliomas. Acta Path. Microbiol. Scand., 27:51–64, 1950.

194. Roberts, M., and German, W. J.: A long term study of patients with oligodendrogliomas. Follow-up of 50 cases, including Dr. Harvey Cushing's series. J. Neurosurg., 24:697–700, 1966.

195. Roussy, G., and Oberling, C.: Histologic classification of tumors of the central nervous system. Arch. Neurol. Psychiat., 27:1281–1289, 1932.

196. Roussy, G., Lhermitte, J., and Cornil, L.: Essai de classification des tumeurs cérébrales. Ann. Anat. Path., 1:333–378, 1924.

197. Roussy, G., Oberling, C., and Raileanu, C.: Lésions expérimentales des centres nerveux provoquées par application locale de goudron. C. R. Soc. Biol., 104:762–764, 1930.

198. Rubinstein, L. J.: Morphological problems of brain tumors with mixed cell population. *In* Classification of brain tumors. Acta Neurochir. suppl., 10:141–165, 1964.

199. Russell, D. S.: The pinealoma: Its relation to teratoma. J. Path. Bact., 56:145, 1944.

200. Russell, D. S., and Bland, J. O. W.: A study of gliomas by the method of tissue culture. J. Path. Bact., 36:273–283, 1933.

201. Russell, D. S., and Rubinstein, L. J.: Pathology of Tumours of the Nervous System. 2nd Ed. London, Arnold, 1963.

202. Russell, D. D., Wilson, C. W., and Tansley, K.:

Experimental radio-necrosis of the brain in rabbits. J. Neurol. Neurosurg. Psychiat., *12*:187–195, 1949.

203. Sato, K., Raimondi, A. J., and Molinard, G. A.: Comparison of tumor-associated antigens on brain tumor-cells of children by a new immunocytoadhesion method. Presented to American Academy of Neurological Surgeons, 1976.

204. Scheinberg, L. C., Levine, M. C., Suzuki, K., and Terry, R. D.: Induced host resistance to a transplantable mouse glioma. Cancer Res., *22*:67–71, 1962.

205. Scheinberg, L. C., Edelman, F., Levy, W. A., and Kotsilimbas, D. G.: Is the brain "An immunologically privileged site"? 1. Studies on intracerebral tumor homotransplantation and isotransplantation to sensitized hosts. Arch. Neurol., *11*:248–264, 1964.

206. Scheinberg, L. C., Edelman, F., Levy, W. A., and Kotsilimbas, D. G.: Is the brain "An immunologically privileged site"? 2. Studies in induced host resistance to transplantable mouse glioma following irradiation of prior implants. Arch. Neurol., *13*:283–286, 1965.

207. Scheinberg, L. C., Kotsilimbas, D. G., Karpf, R., and Mayer, N.: Is the brain "An immunologically privileged site"? 3. Studies based on homologous skin grafts to the brain and subcutaneous tissue. Arch. Neurol., *15*:62–67, 1966.

208. Scheinberg, L. E., Levine, M. C., and Suzuki, K.: Studies in immunization against a transplantable cerebral mouse glioma. J. Neurosurg., *20*:312–317, 1963.

209. Scherer, H. J.: The forms of growth in gliomas and their practical significance. Brain, *63*:1–112, 1940.

210. Scherer, H. J.: A critical review: The pathology of cerebral gliomas. J. Belge Neurol. Psychiat., *3*:147–177, 1940.

211. Schneck, S. A., and Penn, I.: De-novo brain tumor in renal-transplant recipients. Lancet, *1*:983–986, 1971.

212. Seligman, A. M., and Shear, M. J.: Studies in carcinogenesis, VIII. Experimental production of brain tumors in mice with methyl cholanthrene. Amer. J. Cancer, *37*:364–373, 1939.

213. Selverstone, B., and Cooper, D. R.: Astrocytoma and ABO blood groups. J. Neurosurg., *18*:602–604, 1961.

214. Selverstone, B., and Moulton, M. J.: The phosphorus metabolism of gliomas: A study with radioactive isotopes. Brain, *80*:362–375, 1957.

215. Shein, H. M.: Neoplastic transformation of hamster astrocytes and choroid plexus cells in culture by polyoma virus. J. Neuropath. Exp. Neurol., *29*:70–88, 1970.

216. Sherwin, A. L., Norris, J. W., and Bulcke, J. A.: Spinal fluid creatine kinase in neurologic disease. Neurology (Minneap.), *19*:933–999, 1969.

217. Shuangshoti, S., and Tangchai, P.: Special features of intracranial glioblastoma multiforme in Thailand. Far East Med. J., *5*:19–31, 1969.

218. Shuangshoti, S., Hongsaprabhas, C., and Netsky, M. G.: Metastasizing meningioma. Cancer, *26*:832–841, 1970.

219. Shuangshoti, S., Tangchai, P., and Netsky, M. G.: Intracranial astrocytoma in Thailand. Far East Med. J., *5*:114–116, 1969.

220. Shuangshoti, S., Tangchai, P., and Netsky, M. G.: Primary adenocarcinoma of choroid plexus. Arch. Path., *91*:101–106, 1971.

221. Simon, T.: Das Spinnenzell-und Pinsel-zellen Gliom. Virchow Arch. Path. Anat., *61*:90–100, 1874.

222. Siris, J. H.: Concerning the immunological specificity of glioblastoma multiforme. Bull. Neurol. Inst. N.Y., *4*:597–601, 1936.

223. Slagel, D. E.: RNA polymerase activity in human brain tumors. Acta Neuropath. (Berl.), *30*:355–359, 1974.

224. Slagel, D. E., Dittmer, J. C., and Wilson, C. B.: Lipid composition of human glial tumor and adjacent brain. J. Neurochem., *14*:789–798, 1967.

225. Smith, K. O., Newman, J. T., Story, J. L., and Wissinger, J. P.: Viruses and brain tumors. Clin. Neurosurg., *21*:362–382, 1974.

226. Snodgrass, S. R., and Iversen, L. L.: Amino acid uptake into human brain tumors. Brain Res., *76*:95–107, 1974.

227. Sorokin, S.: Centrioles and the formation of rudimentary cilia by fibroblasts and smooth muscle cells. J. Cell Biol., *15*:363–377, 1962.

228. Starr, M. A.: Tumors of the brain in childhood; their variety and situation, with special reference to their treatment by surgical interference. Med. News, *54*:29–37, 1889.

229. Starr, M. A.: Brain Surgery. New York, Wood, 1903.

230. Steward, J. K.: 36th Annual Report of British Empire Cancer Campaign, 1959.

231. Stroebe, H.: Ueber Entstehung und Bau der Hirngliome. Beitr. Path. Anat., *18*:405–485, 1895.

232. Sun, G. Y., and Leung, B. S.: Phospholipids and acyl groups of subcellular membrane fractions from human intracranial tumors. J. Lipid Res., *15*:423–431, 1974.

233. Swenberg, J. A.: Chemical induction of brain tumors. Advances Neurol., *15*:85–99, 1976.

234. Deleted in proof.

235. Takakura, K.: Immunotherapy can aid in brain tumor treatment. Med. World News, *16*:39, 1975.

236. Takakura, K., Miki, Y., and Kubo, O.: Adjuvant immunotherapy for malignant brain tumors in infants and children. Child's Brain, *1*:141–147, 1975.

237. Thomas, D. G. T., Lannigan, C. B., and Behan, P. D.: Impaired cell-mediated immunity in human brain tumors. Lancet, *2*:1389, 1975.

238. Toh, B. H., and Cauchi, M. N.: Brain-associated tumour antigens demonstrated by immunofluorescence. Nature, *250*:597–598, 1974.

239. Tokumaru, T., and Catalano, L. W.: Elevation of serum immunoglobulin M(lgM) level in patients with brain tumors. Surg. Neurol., *4*:17–25, 1975.

240. Tomina, E. D., and Pevzner, L. F.: Protein content in nuclei of human tumor. Bull. Exp. Biol. Med., *60*:83–84, 1965.

241. Tooth, H. H.: Some observations on the growth and survival period of intracranial tumors. Brain, *35*:61–108, 1912.

242. Trouillas, P.: Immunologie des tumeurs cere-

brals: l'antigene carcinofetal-glial. Ann. Inst. Pasteur Lille, *122*:819–828, 1972.

243. Trouillas, P.: Immunology and immunotherapy of cerebral tumors. Current status. Rev. Neurol., *128*:23–38, 1973.

244. U. S. Department of Health, Education, and Welfare—Public Health Service: Vital Statistics of the United States 1966, Vol II; Vital Statistics Rates in the United States 1940–1960. Washington, D.C., 1968.

245. Uzunov, P., Shein, H. M., and Weiss, B.: Multiple forms of cyclic 3'-5'-AMP phosphodiesterase of rat cerebrum and cloned astrocytoma and neuroblastoma cells. Neuropharmacology, *13*:377–391, 1974.

246. Van der Wiel, H. J.: Inheritance of Glioma: The Genetic Aspects of Cerebral Glioma and Its Relation to Status Dysraphicus. Amsterdam, Elsevier, 1960.

247. Victor, J., and Wolf, A.: Metabolism of brain tumors. *In* Tumors of the Nervous System. Proc. Assoc. Res. Nerv. Ment. Dis., *16*:44–58, 1937.

248. Virchow, R.: Die Krankhaften Geschwuelste. Berlin, Hirschwald, 1863–1865.

249. Wahlstrom, T.: Sensitivity to normal brain antigens of blood lymphocytes from patients with gliomas. Acta Path. Microbiol. Scand., *81*:763–767, 1973.

250. Wahlstrom, T., Linder, E., and Saksela, E.: Glia-specific antigens in cell cultures from rabbit brain, human foetal, and adult brain, and gliomas. Acta Path. Microbiol. Scand., *81*:768–774, 1973.

251. Wahlstrom, T., Saksela, E., and Troupp, H.: Cell-bound anti-glial immunity in patients with malignant tumors of the brain. Cell. Immun., *6*:161–170, 1973.

252. Wahlstrom, T., Linder, E., Saksela, E., and Westermark, B.: Tumor-specific membrane antigens in established cell lines from gliomas. Cancer, *34*:274–279, 1974.

253. Waterhouse, J. A. H.: Cancer Handbook of Epidemiology and Prognosis. Edinburgh, Churchill Livingstone, 1974.

254. Webster's 3rd International Dictionary: Gove, P. B., ed. Springfield, Mass., Merriam, 1967.

255. Wechsler, W., Kleihues, P., Matsumoto, S., Zuelch, K. J., Ivankovic, S., Preussmann, R., and Druckrey, H.: Pathology of experimental neurogenic tumors chemically induced during prenatal and postnatal life. Ann. N.Y. Acad. Sci., *159*:360–408, 1969.

256. Weil, A.: Experimental production of tumors in the brain of white rats. Arch. Path., *26*:777–790, 1938.

257. Weiss, J. F.: Sterols and other lipids of the nervous system. Prog. Biochem. Pharmacol., *10*:227–268, 1975.

258. Weiss, J. F., Cravioto, H., and Ransohoff, J.: Desmosterol in rat central and peripheral nervous systems during normal and neoplastic growth. J. Nat. Cancer Inst., *54*:781–783, 1975.

259. Weiss, J. F., Kayden, H. J., and Ransohoff, J.: Evaluation of patients undergoing therapy for gliomas by examination of CSF sterols after triparanol treatment. Trans. Amer. Neurol. Ass. *96*:59–61, 1971.

260. Weiss, J. F., Ransohoff, J. R., and Kayden, H. J.: Cerebrospinal fluid sterols in patients undergoing treatment for gliomas. Neurology (Minneap.), *22*:187–193, 1972.

261. Wender, M., and Waligora, F.: Der Gehalt an Aminosaeuren der Eiweisskoerper in Hirngeschwuelsten. *In* Jacob, H., ed.: Proc. IV Inter. Congress Neuropath., Vol. 1, Stuttgart, Thieme, 1962.

262. Weiss, L.: A metastasizing ependymoma of the cauda equina. Cancer, *8*:161–171, 1955.

263. Wender, M., and Waligora, F.: Der Gehalt an Aminosaeuren der Eiweisskoerper in Hirngeschwuelsten. *In* Jacob, H., ed.: Proc. IV Intern. Congress Neuropath., vol. 1. Stuttgart, Thieme, 1962.

264. Wiener, A. S.: Modern blood group mythology. J. Forensic Med., *7*:166–176, 1960.

265. Wiener, A. S., and Wexler, I. B.: Blood group paradoxes. J.A.M.A., *162*:1474–1475, 1956.

266. Willis, R. A.: The Spread of Tumors in the Human Body. 2nd Ed. London, Butterworth, 1952.

267. Willis, R. A.: Pathology of Tumours. 3rd Ed. London, Butterworth, 1960.

268. Willson, C., Normansell, D. E., and Netsky, M. G.: Antigenicity of fetal and adult cerebral tissue of man. Neurology *24*:761–766, 1974.

269. Wilson, C. B., and Hoshino, T.: Current trends in the chemotherapy of brain tumors with special reference to glioblastomas. J. Neurosurg., *31*:589–603, 1969.

270. Wilson, C. B., Kaufmann, C., and Barker, M.: Chromosome analysis of glioblastoma multiforme. Neurology, *20*:821–838, 1970.

271. Winkelman, N. W., Cassel, C., and Schlesinger, B.: Intracranial tumors with extracranial metastases. J. Neuropath. Exp. Neurol., *7*:149–168, 1952.

272. Winters, W. P., and Rich, J. R.: Human meningioma antigens. Int. J. Cancer, *15*:815–822, 1975.

273. Wolf, A., Cowen, D., and Stewart, W. B.: Glioblastoma with extraneural metastases by way of a ventriculopleural anastomosis. Trans. Amer. Neurol. Ass., *79*:140–142, 1954.

274. Woosley, R., Mahaley, M. S., and Mahaley, J.: Immunobiology of primary intracranial tumors. III. Microcytotoxicity assays of specific immune responses of brain tumor patients. J. Neurosurg., *47*:871–885, 1977.

275. Yates, P. O., and Pearce, K. M.: Recent change in blood-group distribution of astrocytomas. Lancet, *1*:194–195, 1960.

276. Yohn, D. S.: Oncogenic viruses: Expectations and applications in neuropathology. Prog. Exp. Tumor Res., *17*:74–92, 1972.

277. Young, H. F., Sakalas, R., and Kaplan, A. M.: Inhibition of cell-mediated immunity in patients with brain tumors. Surg. Neurol., *5*:19–23, 1976.

278. Zimmerman, H. M.: Experimental brain tumors: The status of gliomas in man. *In* The Biology and Treatment of Intracranial Tumors. Springfield, Ill., Charles C Thomas, 1962.

279. Zimmerman, H. M.: Brain tumors: their incidence and classification in man and their experimental production. Ann. N.Y. Acad. Sci., *159*:337–359, 1969.

280. Zimmerman, H. M., and Arnold, H.: Experimental brain tumors: I. Tumors produced with methylocholanthrene. Cancer Res., *1*:919–938, 1941.

281. Zimmerman, H. M., and Arnold, H.: Experimental brain tumors: II. Tumors produced with benzypyrene. Amer. J. Path., *19*:939–955, 1943.

282. Zimmerman, H. M., and Arnold, H.: Chemical carcinogens and animal species as factors—experimental brain tumors. J. Neuropath. Exp. Neurol., *2*:416–417, 1943.

283. Zuelch, K. H.: Brain Tumors, Their Biology and Pathology. 2nd Ed. New York, Springer, 1965.

284. Zuelch, K. J., and Woolf, A. L., eds.: Classification of brain tumors. Acta Neurochir., *10*:suppl., 1965.

84

SUPRATENTORIAL BRAIN TUMORS IN CHILDREN

Prior to the documentation provided by Ingraham and Matson in 1954, statistics on brain tumors in childhood were buried in reports on brain tumors in populations consisting of adults and children.[26] Now, with increasing specialization in pediatric neurosurgery, it has become evident that brain tumors in childhood form a very significant proportion of all brain tumors seen. Brain tumors are among the most common causes of malignant disease in children. In the author's institution, they account for 25 per cent of the neoplasms seen in childhood, while in the general population, they account for only 1 to 2 per cent of all neoplasms.

Conventionally, one looks upon the posterior fossa as the usual site for a brain tumor in a child. This view seems to be substantiated by statistics provided by oncologists and radiotherapists, since so many of the posterior fossa tumors are malignant and are treated by radiotherapy and chemotherapy, whereas a very significant portion of the supratentorial tumors are benign and consequently are treated entirely by operation. In a review of brain tumors seen at the Hospital for Sick Children in Toronto between 1950 and 1975, it was found that 344 out of a total of 795 brain tumors (43.27 per cent) were situated entirely above the tentorium (Tables 84–1 and 84–2).[73] In this particular series, there was no sex predominance and the age group most frequently affected was between 1 and 6 years (Table 84–3).

Patients under 1 year of age numbered 21 and accounted for 6.0 per cent of the supratentorial tumors. Sato and co-workers found that 9 of the 10 neonatal tumors they treated were supratentorial in location.[60] In infancy, supratentorial tumors, although rare, seem to outnumber tumors located in the infratentorial compartment.

Many supratentorial tumors in childhood carry a good prognosis. Some, such as craniopharyngioma, arise from embryonic rests of cells, are extrinsic to the brain, and thus can frequently be totally removed, with resulting cure of the patient. Furthermore, because carcinoma elsewhere in the body is relatively rare in childhood, metastatic tumors, which form a very significant portion of the supratentorial tumors in the adult, are rarely seen in the child. In the Hospital for Sick Children series, they constituted only 0.6 per cent of supratentorial tumors (see Table 84–2).[73]

Because the infratentorial space is small and cramped, neoplasms growing there can quickly become symptomatic, while tumors in the supratentorial compartment are notorious for their gradual presentation. This is particularly true in the younger child, in whom open sutures allow for expansion of the head and thus for late presentation of signs of raised intracranial pressure. One important feature to bear in mind regarding brain tumors, and particularly children's supratentorial brain tumors, is that the length of history has no bearing on the rate of growth of the tumor. Small benign tumors may suddenly give rise to a seizure or hemorrhage, while large, slowly growing benign tumors can remain silent for years before eventually presenting in an acute fashion, either by obstructing cerebrospinal pathways and producing hydrocephalus or

H. J. HOFFMAN

Table 84–1 ANATOMICAL LOCATION OF SUPRATENTORIAL TUMORS*

LOCATION	NUMBER
Cerebral hemisphere	119
Pineal region	39
Suprasellar area	58
Third ventricle	3
Lateral ventricle	10
Hypothalamus	20
Thalamus and basal ganglia	30
Optic pathway	51
Pituitary	4
Dura	10
Total	344

* Data from study of 344 patients with supratentorial tumors treated at the Hospital for Sick Children, Toronto, 1950 through 1975.

Table 84–2 HISTOLOGICAL TYPES OF SUPRATENTORIAL TUMOR AND RESULTS OF TREATMENT*

TYPE OF TUMOR	NO. OF PATIENTS	Alive	Dead	Lost to Follow-Up
No histological verification	46	31	14	1
Astrocytoma				
Giant cell	4	2	2	0
Grades 1 and 2	83	52	27	4
Grade 3	34	10	24	0
Grade 4	31	6	25	0
Oligodendroglioma	2	0	2	0
Ependymoma	11	3	8	0
Ependymoblastoma	5	1	4	0
Mixed glioma	4	2	2	0
Ganglioglioma	6	6	0	0
Primitive neuroectodermal tumor	10	3	6	1
Schwannoma	2	2	0	0
Choroid plexus papilloma	8	4	4	0
Choroid plexus carcinoma	3	0	3	0
Craniopharyngioma	48	34	14	0
Dermoid	1	1	0	0
Teratoma				
Benign	2	1	1	0
Malignant	4	1	3	0
Germinoma	14	4	10	0
Pineoblastoma	7	1	6	0
Hemangioblastoma	1	1	0	0
Cavernous hemangioma	1	1	0	0
Lipoma	1	1	0	0
Pituitary adenoma	4	3	1	0
Hamartoma	2	1	1	0
Sarcoma	4	1	3	0
Meningioma	4	2	1	1
Metastatic	2	0	2	0
Totals	344	174	163	7

* Data from study of 344 patients with supratentorial tumors treated at the Hospital for Sick Children, Toronto, 1950 through 1975.

Table 84–3   AGE OF PRESENTATION OF SUPRATENTORIAL TUMORS*

| | AGE (YEARS) | | | | |
	< 1	1 to 6	7 to 12	> 13	TOTAL
Males	12	75	70	30	187
Females	9	81	49	18	157
Totals	21	156	119	48	344

* Data from study of 344 patients with supratentorial tumors treated at the Hospital for Sick Children, Toronto, 1950 through 1975.

by causing edema in the adjacent compressed brain.

CLINICAL MANIFESTATIONS

Increased Intracranial Pressure

In the young child, a rapidly growing supratentorial mass or a midline mass obstructing cerebrospinal fluid circulation will produce enlargement of the head and, in the infant, a bulging fontanelle. In the older child with relatively closed sutures, papilledema develops much earlier. In the series of 344 patients with supratentorial tumors, 142 (41 per cent) had papilledema.[73]

Because of its long intracranial course, the sixth cranial nerve is particularly vulnerable to stretching when intracranial pressure is raised, and accordingly, 66 patients (19 per cent) of the 344 patients presented with strabismus and diplopia due to sixth nerve palsy.[73]

Headaches are commonly associated with increased intracranial pressure. They tend to be intermittent and are particularly severe first thing in the morning when the child has been recumbent and intracranial pressure is high. The headache tends to remit and intensify, and is associated with irritability. Because the headache is made worse by straining at stool, constipation is common. The headaches tend to occur frontally or occipitally and are commonly accompanied by vomiting. Of the 344 patients with supratentorial tumors, 152 (44 per cent) presented with headaches.[73]

Seizures

Many physicians assume that seizures in children are the result of static lesions or metabolic factors. Tumors usually are not considered to be the cause. For this reason, an active investigation of seizures usually is not undertaken. The child is treated with anticonvulsant medication, and only if this treatment fails to deal with the seizure problem is further study done. The seizure due to a supratentorial brain tumor can be generalized, psychomotor, or focal motor or sensory or both in type. Seizures may be the initial symptom of a cerebral hemisphere neoplasm and in some instances they can persist for years before the development of other signs that make the diagnosis obvious. Now that computed tomography provides a benign method of investigation, an increased number of these "seizure" patients are found to be harboring intracranial tumors. In the Hospital for Sick Children series, 63 patients (18 per cent) presented with seizures as one of the early signs of their supratentorial tumors.[73]

Intracranial Hemorrhage

Intracranial hemorrhage—subarachnoid, intraventricular, or intracerebral—has been well described and documented as an initial presenting sign of a supratentorial tumor.[13,48,56,62,72] Although this is an uncommon presentation, one must be alert to the phenomenon. One patient with choroid plexus papilloma was initially treated, in another institution, for a traumatic subarachnoid hemorrhage (Fig. 84–1). Two patients with intracerebral tumor were initially believed to have massive intracerebral hematomas and presented without any preceding history suggestive of a cerebral hemisphere tumor.[73]

Phakomatoses

In a child presenting with signs that indicate an intracranial space-occupying lesion, a careful search must be made for cutaneous evidence of one of the phakomatoses. Of the 344 patients with supratentorial tumors, 20 had cutaneous evidence of von Recklinghausen's disease; 2 patients had adenomata sebaceum of tuberous sclerosis and presented with subependymal astrocytomas in the cerebral hemispheres, as shown in Figure 84–2; and 2 patients with

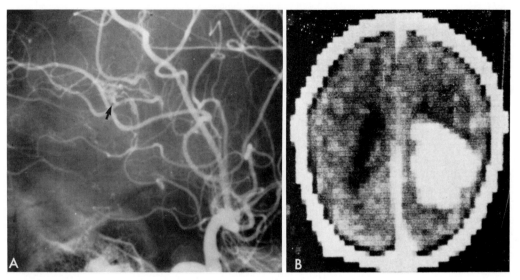

Figure 84–1 *A*. Lateral carotid angiogram showing tumor vessels (*arrow*) arising from anterior choroidal artery and feeding trigonal choroid plexus papilloma in a patient who presented with subarachnoid hemorrhage. *B*. Contrast enhanced CT scan of same patient showing large choroid plexus papilloma filling right lateral ventricle.

giant hairy nevi over their torsos presented with primary leptomeningeal melanomas extending both above and below the tentorium.[22,73]

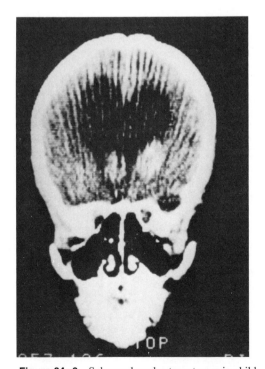

Figure 84–2 Subependymal astrocytomas in child with tuberous sclerosis as seen on CT scan.

Focal Neurological Signs

Personality changes often accompany tumors involving the frontal lobe, temporal lobe, and hypothalamus. Because of the personality changes associated with these tumors, the physical concomitants of the tumor have on occasion been regarded as functional.[71] One patient in the Hospital for Sick Children series was treated for hysterical blindness for several months by a psychiatrist, when in fact the blindness was due to infiltration of the chiasm and both optic nerves by a suprasellar germinoma (see Fig. 84–14).

The child's brain is remarkably plastic in regard to speech, and dominance can shift significantly up to the age of 10. The result is that aphasia is an infrequent sign of a cerebral hemisphere tumor. Of 119 patients with cerebral hemisphere tumors, only 5 presented with dysphasia, despite the fact that 64 of these patients had lesions in the left hemisphere.[73]

Impaired visual acuity, as well as visual field defects, is common in patients with suprasellar tumors. More than half the patients with craniopharyngiomas in the Hospital for Sick Children series presented with a visual field defect.[23] Visual acuity is significantly reduced in many patients with craniopharyngiomas as well as in patients with tumors of optic nerve and hypothalamus.

Oculomotor palsy can be seen with parasellar tumors, and typically the third cranial nerve is affected. With raised intracranial pressure, a sixth nerve palsy can be a false localizing sign.

Nystagmus is usually seen with posterior fossa lesions. A very unusual and clinically dramatic form of nystagmus, called seesaw nystagmus, is pathognomic of a suprasellar or parasellar lesion.[10] It may occur with tumors such as craniopharyngioma or optic nerve glioma. This type of nystagmus can be defined as disconjugate, vertical, and rotational eye movement in which one eye moves downward and the other eye upward —and vice versa—in continuous repetitive fashion. The eye that moves downward tends to rotate externally, while the eye that moves upward rotates internally. The seesaw nystagmus may be a prominent early sign of a craniopharyngioma; it can disappear once the tumor is totally removed.

Facial weakness and hemiparesis frequently associated with sensory loss and occasionally with a visual field defect reflect impingement on internal capsule or relevant cortex. In the series of 344 patients, 174 (51 per cent) presented with hemiparesis.[73]

Truncal ataxia is the hallmark of a midline posterior fossa tumor. When one sees truncal ataxia without nystagmus, however, the tumor is usually in the midline, impinging on the third ventricle. Patients with laterally placed massive tumors involving the parietal lobe may present with ataxia but frequently without focal disturbance. Twenty-one of the three hundred and forty-four patients with supratentorial tumors (6.1 per cent) presented with truncal ataxia.[73]

Endocrine dysfunction points to a hypothalamic-pituitary disturbance. Any neoplasm that impinges on the hypothalamic region can either depress or activate hypothalamic control centers and produce increased or diminished pituitary activity. More than 50 per cent of the craniopharyngioma patients in the Hospital for Sick Children series had symptoms of endocrine disturbance on presentation. Infants with hypothalamic neoplasms frequently present with the characteristic emaciation and euphoria of the diencephalic syndrome.[3,58]

Anterior pituitary tumors can suppress primary pituitary function, but if they are secreting tumors they can produce the clinical pictures of Cushing's syndrome, gigantism, or galactorrhea.

DIAGNOSTIC STUDIES

Plain Skull Radiography

Plain skull x-rays will show signs of raised intracranial pressure in the form of sutural splitting and increased digital markings. Tumors around the hypothalamus and chiasm will excavate the sella and produce in it a J shape. Calcification can be visible on plain skull films, particularly in tumors such as craniopharyngioma and oligodendroglioma. Localized calvarial enlargement, particularly of the middle fossa or the parietal region, can be seen with slowly growing hemispheric tumors.

Angiography

Carotid angiography has been one of the commonly used investigative tools for supratentorial tumors. Not only does it show the vascularity and vascular architecture of the tumor, but it locates the tumor within the supratentorial compartment (Fig. 84–3A). At the present time, we rely on cerebral angiography to define the position of major vessels in relation to a tumor as well as to demonstrate vascularity in potentially vascular tumors. More specifically, angiography is useful in tumors around the sella, such as craniopharyngioma, where the tumor must be carefully separated from the internal carotid artery. With vascular tumors such as choroid plexus papilloma, it is of great value to know the vascular supply of the tumor prior to operation and thus be prepared to deal with it (see Fig. 84–1A).

Air Encephalography and Ventriculography

Air encephalography is useful to define the basal cisterns in the case of a chiasmatic or optic nerve tumor, and ventriculography is of value with tumors in and about the third ventricle. But with these exceptions, air encephalography and ventriculography are now rarely part of the diagnostic investigation of supratentorial tumors.

Radioisotope Studies

Because they are benign these tests provided an extremely valuable service prior to the days of computed tomography (Fig. 84–3B). They are now used more as a means of confirmation rather than as a primary diagnostic study.

Echoencephalography

Echoencephalography was another benign, noninvasive test that was of value in showing the position of midline structures as well as ventricular size. Since the advent of computed tomography, this test is rarely

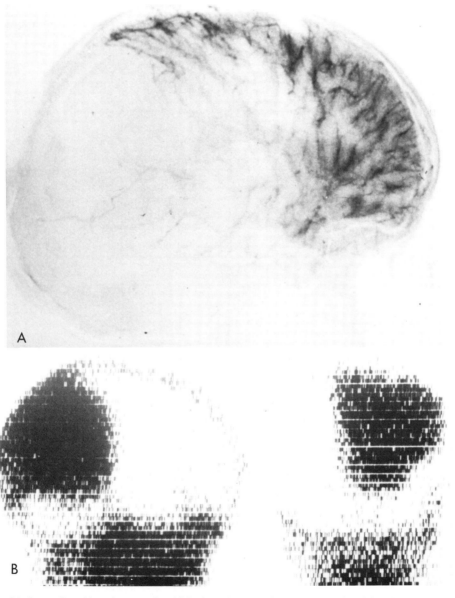

Figure 84–3 *A.* Carotid angiogram of a child with a large cystic astrocytoma involving the parieto-occipital region. *B.* Brain scan of same patient showing uptake of isotope by tumor.

used in the evaluation of supratentorial tumors.

Electroencephalography

The electroencephalogram is useful when seizures are a problem, particularly when a tumor has given rise to a seizure focus adjacent to it and treatment is aimed at removal of the seizure focus as well as of the tumor. In such cases, electrocorticography is utilized in the operating room to insure removal of the seizure focus.

Computed Tomography

Computed tomography has revolutionized the diagnosis of brain tumors in children. The test is noninvasive and painless, and can be performed on an outpatient basis. It shows not only the tumor location but also the form and size of the tumor. It is the supreme test for following the results of therapy in brain tumors, whether the treatment is operation, radiation, or chemotherapy.

TREATMENT

In 1958, Matson pointed out that there was a widespread impression among pediatric and general physicians as well as the lay public that with intracranial tumors in childhood the outlook for long-term survival as well as for normal growth and development was hopeless.[44] Because tumors such as medulloblastoma and brain stem glioma are common and continue to carry a relatively poor prognosis, this impression persists. Matson found, however, that in 46 per cent of his patients the brain tumors were benign; documentation of these tumors revealed that his operative mortality rate was 5.5 per cent and that the cure rate ranged between 80 and 87 per cent. Of his surviving patients, 92 per cent were normal neurologically or had only a mild neurological deficit. More than 20 years ago Matson suggested that the use of more precise diagnostic facilities together with improved methods of anesthesia, fluid and electrolyte and hormonal management, and the experience gained from a growing body of surgical knowledge accounted for his excellent results. Today, with the advances in diagnostic and operative techniques brought about by development of such facilities as the CT scanner, the operating room microscope, bipolar cautery, image intensification, and precise micro-operative tools, one can surely match if not surpass Matson's optimism about the efficacy of treatment of brain tumors in children.

Nonoperative Therapy

Radiotherapy has been used extensively for brain tumors, particularly for malignant gliomas and unverified deeply placed tumors. Recent emphasis on the consequences of radiotherapy, particularly in the child, has discouraged its indiscriminate use for brain tumors. Not only can radiation induce tumors but it can produce necrosis of the brain with consequent dementia and neurological deficits.[1,16,36,43,69] Irradiation that involves the hypothalamus and pituitary gland invariably impairs growth hormone production and may even have a more deleterious effect on the endocrine system of the developing child.

Consequently radiotherapy is restricted to treatment of gliomas that are malignant in nature and cannot be removed, or of those more benign gliomas that cannot be totally excised and that show evidence of growth, clinically and on CT scan.

Chemotherapeutic agents appear to be of limited use in treating patients with supratentorial tumors. There is no doubt that agents such as vincristine and CCNU will have some palliative effect in children with recurrent malignant gliomas. There is no evidence at present, however, that such agents, when given prophylactically, provide any significant benefit.

For many years neurosurgeons have noted that some patients harboring malignant gliomas can survive for years. This has been substantiated further in the Hospital for Sick Children series in which 16 of 125 patients (13 per cent) with verified malignant supratentorial tumors survived more than four years.[73] Immune mechanisms are now being credited with some of these long-term survivals, and this has given rise to immunotherapeutic techniques for treating intracranial tumors.[65]

Operative Therapy

The primary treatment of children's brain tumors is operative excision if that is at all possible. If only a partial excision is possible and the risk of early recurrence is small, careful monitoring with computed tomography is used before proceeding with more involved therapeutic procedures (radiotherapy or chemotherapy), which are reserved for the more malignant and aggressive tumors.

Anesthetic Management

Of paramount importance in reducing operative morbidity and mortality rates is proper neuroanesthesia. The anesthetists must be skilled not only in neurosurgical anesthesia but also in pediatric anesthesia, a very necessary combination in dealing with children's brain tumors.

Neuroleptanalgesia consists of a potent tranquilizer (droperidol) in combination with a potent analgesic (Fentanyl citrate), which together produce a state of indifference and analgesia.[53] These agents are used as the sole anesthetic when the patient must be conscious for stimulation and electroencephalographic recording during operative exploration adjacent to speech and motor centers.

Controlled ventilation is routinely employed during operations for supratentorial tumors. This technique has many advantages. Adequate oxygenation and elimination of carbon dioxide is assured, a light level of anesthesia is allowed, and adverse effects of posture are minimized.

Drug Management

Dexamethasone is routinely employed for all supratentorial tumor operations whenever cerebral edema occurs or is expected in the postoperative period. Corticosteroids tend to protect the brain from cerebral edema by reconstituting the blood-brain barrier as well as preventing its breakdown. Dexamethasone is given in a loading dose of 0.2 mg per kilogram (maximum 10 mg) and maintained with a dose of 0.1 mg per kilogram (maximum 4 mg).

Twenty per cent mannitol is given in a dose of 1.5 to 2.5 gm per kilogram to reduce brain bulk. Since this constitutes a considerable fluid load in a young child, half the total dose is given in the first 20 minutes and the remainder in the following 40 minutes. Urine is collected with an indwelling catheter. Although the urine produced by mannitol diuresis is low in electrolyte, it may be large in volume, and some electrolyte replacement is necessary.

Whenever the hemisphere is retracted for exposure or tumor excision, the possibility of inducing a seizure in the postoperative period exists. For this reason, all such patients are given prophylactic anticonvulsant medication, usually diphenylhydantoin (Dilantin) in a dose of 5 to 7 mg per kilogram every 24 hours. If there has been no incision into the hemisphere and the tumor is entirely extrinsic, anticonvulsants are discontinued after the first week or two. If the cerebral cortex has been incised, however, anticonvulsant medication is continued for at least six months.

CEREBRAL HEMISPHERE TUMORS

In the Hospital for Sick Children series, 119 (36 per cent) of the 344 supratentorial tumors were lodged in the cerebral hemispheres (Tables 84–4 and 84–5).[73] Fifty-four of these were in the right cerebral hemisphere, sixty-four in the left, and one was in the corpus callosum. Except for the oc-

Table 84–4 SITE OF CEREBRAL HEMISPHERE TUMORS*

	RIGHT	LEFT	MIDLINE	TOTAL
Frontal lobe	17	16		33
Temporal lobe	17	17		34
Parietal lobe	17	22		39
Occipital lobe	3	9		12
Corpus callosum	0	0	1	1
Totals	54	64	1	119

* Data from study of 344 patients with supratentorial tumors treated at the Hospital for Sick Children, Toronto, 1950 through 1975.

Table 84–5   HISTOLOGICAL TYPES OF CEREBRAL HEMISPHERE TUMORS
AND RESULTS OF TREATMENT*

TYPE OF TUMOR	NO. OF PATIENTS	RESULTS		
		Alive	Dead	No Follow-Up
No histological verification	2	1	1	0
Astrocytoma				
Giant cell	1	0	0	1
Grades I and II	28	18	9	1
Grade III	22	8	14	0
Grade IV	25	6	19	0
Oligodendroglioma	1	0	1	0
Ependymoma	8	3	5	0
Ependymoblastoma	5	1	4	0
Mixed Glioma	4	2	2	0
Ganglioglioma	6	6	0	0
Primitive neuroectodermal	10	3	6	1
Schwannoma	1	1	0	0
Hemangioblastoma	1	1	0	0
Cavernous hemangioma	1	1	0	0
Lipoma	1	1	0	0
Dermoid	1	1	0	0
Hamartoma	1	1	0	0
Metastatic	1	0	1	0
Totals	119	54	62	3

* Data from study of 344 patients with supratentorial tumors treated at the Hospital for Sick Children, Toronto, 1950 through 1975.

cipital lobe, where very few occurred, the distribution between the various lobes was relatively equal: 33 in the frontal lobe, 34 in the temporal lobe, 39 in the parietal lobe, 12 in the occipital lobe, and 1 in the corpus callosum (Fig. 84–4). In the age group most frequently affected, between 7 and 12 years, 51 of the 119 tumors presented. Another 48 presented between ages 1 and 6; 19 patients were older than 13 years of age and only 1 was an infant (Table 84–6).

Matson reported an almost 2:1 ratio of boys to girls in his series of cerebral hemisphere tumors.[45] In the Hospital for Sick Children series there were 75 boys and 44 girls, a distribution that closely approximates Matson's figures.

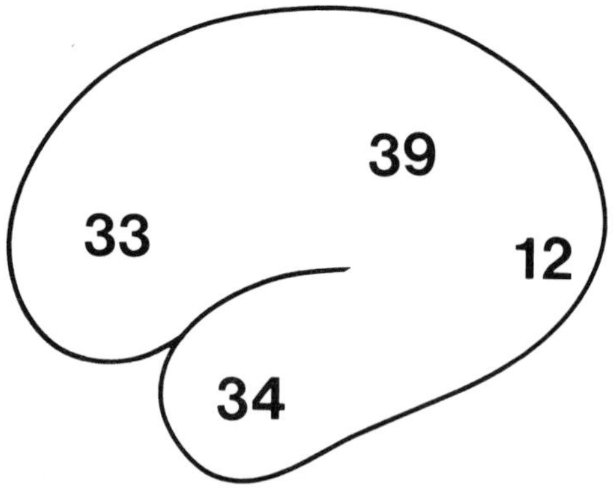

Epilepsy is one of the common presenting signs of these tumors. Low and coworkers reported that 40 percent of their children with cerebral hemisphere tumors presented with seizures.[39] In the Hospital for Sick Children series, 46 patients (39 per cent) had seizures at the time of initial presentation.[73]

Page and associates pointed out that a significant percentage of children with seizures unaccompanied by neurological deficits or signs of increased intracranial pressure may be harboring a cerebral glioma.[55] Furthermore, if the tumor is discovered early, operative excision is facilitated and control of the seizure disorder is rendered easy. One child in the Hospital for Sick Children series with an oligodendroglioma in the temporal lobe was treated for poorly controlled temporal lobe seizures for 10 years before an astute clinician obtained a plain skull x-ray that showed calcium in the tumor. With removal of her tumor, her epilepsy was cured. Now, with the facility of computed tomography, it is unnecessary to wait for calcification in a tumor to detect it by benign means. A child who develops seizures, particularly if they are focal, and especially if the electroencephalogram does not show a spike and

Figure 84–4   Diagrammatic sketch of location of hemispheral tumors in the author's series.

Table 84–6   AGE OF PRESENTATION OF CEREBRAL HEMISPHERE TUMORS*

SEX	< 1 YEAR	1 TO 6 YEARS	7 TO 12 YEARS	> 13 YEARS	TOTAL
Male	1	29	29	16	75
Female	0	19	22	3	44
Totals	1	48	51	19	119

* Data from study of 344 patients with supratentorial tumors treated at the Hospital for Sick Children, Toronto, 1950 through 1975.

wave pattern, deserves further investigation to rule out a remediable cause of the epilepsy, especially if that remediable cause is a tumor that can grow and do irreversible harm with the passage of time.

Because of open sutures, intrinsic tumors of the cerebral hemisphere can grow to enormous size before the child experiences difficulties, particularly if the tumor occurs in a silent area such as the frontal or occipital lobe. Even large parietal tumors can present without focal deficit, aside from the false localizing sign of ataxia, which was present in three patients in the series.[73] Furthermore, because of slow growth over a long period, these tumors can, in a young child, produce local deformity of the skull with a distinct bulge at the site of the tumor.

Despite the open sutures, however, raised intracranial pressure commonly accompanies this group of tumors. Sixty-one patients (51.3 per cent) with cerebral hemisphere tumors had headaches at the time of presentation, sixty-six (55.5 per cent) had papilledema, nine were drowsy, four were stuporous, and four were in coma.[73]

Most of the hemispheral tumors in this series impinged on motor strip or internal capsule, producing hemiparesis, as was evident in 98 (82.4 per cent) of 119 patients.[73]

Astrocytomas

Astrocytomas, by far the most common tumor of the cerebral hemispheres in childhood, accounted for 76 (64 per cent) of 119 hemispheral tumors.[73] These tumors typically grow to a very large size in the younger child with open sutures, and many of them contain large cysts, a fact pointed out by Gol in 1962.[18] Fifty-three (70 per cent) of the hemispheral astrocytomas in the Hospital for Sick Children series were cystic (Fig. 84–5).[73] Unlike the cystic astrocytomas of the cerebellum, however, the supratentorial cysts are usually lined entirely by tumor, and the entire cyst rather than a

mural nodule must be excised in an effort to prevent recurrence.

Despite their propensity for impinging on motor strip or internal capsule, astrocytomas can involve any portion of the cerebral hemisphere and, via the corpus callosum, may spread to the contralateral hemisphere in a butterfly fashion.

With astrocytomas of the cerebral hemisphere, as much tumor as possible should be removed without damaging the child. Whenever possible in frontal, temporal, or occipital lobe tumors, a lobectomy should be performed so that an en bloc removal of the tumor with the involved lobe can be accomplished. If epilepsy is a significant symptom, electrocorticography can be used and the epileptic focus excised with the tumor.[19] In the past, there was a tendency to irradiate all grades of gliomas. The practice in the author's institution now is to irradiate the more malignant varieties and follow more benign types of gliomas clinically and by CT scan. Those benign gliomas

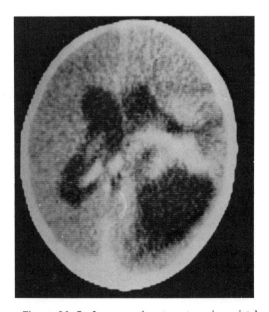

Figure 84–5   Large cystic astrocytoma in parietal and occipital lobes of 1-year-old child was seen on CT scan.

Table 84-7   RESULTS OF RADIOTHERAPY IN CEREBRAL
HEMISPHERE ASTROCYTOMAS*

ASTROCYTOMA	OPERATIVE TREATMENT	WITH RADIOTHERAPY		WITHOUT RADIOTHERAPY	
		Alive	*Dead*	*Alive*	*Dead*
Grades I and II	None	0	0	0	1
	Biopsy	6	4	5	4
	Gross tumor removal	3	0	5	0
	Total	9	4	10	5
Grades III and IV	None	0	0	0	1
	Biopsy	7	17	1	8
	Gross tumor removal	1	4	4	4
	Total	8	21	5	13
	Grand Total	17	25	15	18

* Data from study of 344 patients with supratentorial tumors treated at the Hospital for Sick Children, Toronto, 1950 through 1975.

that behave aggressively should, however, be treated with radiotherapy.

Review of the 28 patients with grade I and grade II astrocytomas in the cerebral hemisphere revealed that of the 13 treated by operation and radiotherapy, 9 were alive and 4 were dead.[73] Of the 13, however, 3 were treated by gross tumor removal and none of these succumbed to their disease. Furthermore, follow-up of the 15 patients treated without radiation showed that 10 were alive, of whom 5 had had a gross tumor removal. Thus, radiotherapy did not seem to make much difference to grade I and grade II astrocytomas (Table 84-7).[73]

Review of 47 patients with grade III and grade IV astrocytomas showed that of 29 treated with operation and radiation, 8 were alive, whereas of 18 treated without radiotherapy, 5 were alive. These figures do not

seem to favor radiotherapy; the series is too small, however, to produce statistically conclusive results (see Table 84-7).[73]

Study of the relation of tumor location to treatment results showed only that benign astrocytomas located in the frontal lobe had a very favorable prognosis, presumably because of the possibility of total excision (Table 84-8).

Ependymomas and Ependymoblastomas

There were 13 ependymomas and ependymoblastomas among the cerebral hemisphere tumors in the Hospital for Sick Children series.[73] These tumors arise from the ependymal surface of the ventricle and either fill the ventricle or spread intrinsically

Table 84-8   CORRELATION OF TREATMENT RESULTS AND LOCATION OF
CEREBRAL HEMISPHERE ASTROCYTOMAS*

ASTROCYTOMA	LOBE	NO. OF PATIENTS	
		Surviving > 4 years	*Dead*
Grades I and II	Frontal	5	1
	Temporal	6	5
	Parietal	3	7
	Occipital	1	1
	Total	15	14
Grades III and IV	Frontal	1	5
	Temporal	1	9
	Parietal	5	17
	Occipital	2	4
	Total	9	35

* Data from study of 344 patients with supratentorial tumors treated at the Hospital for Sick Children, Toronto, 1950 through 1975.

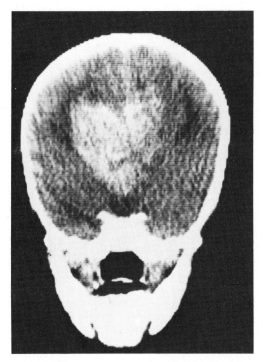

Figure 84–6   Large ependymoblastoma filling lateral ventricles and third ventricle, seen on contrast-enhanced CT scan of 3-month-old infant.

through the hemisphere. Both types of tumor can present with spontaneous hemorrhage. Ependymoblastomas tend to occur in the younger age group and can fill the ventricular system and extend into adjacent brain without causing major symptoms (Fig. 84–6). These tumors are treated by subtotal excision followed by radiotherapy.

Oligodendrogliomas

Oligodendrogliomas typically occur in adult life. The Hospital for Sick Children series includes only one cerebral hemisphere oligodendroglioma, which was situated in the temporal lobe. The tumor was calcified and had given rise to a long history of temporal lobe seizures before the child's problem was investigated and the tumor totally removed.[73]

Gangliogliomas

These tumors, although rare, occur most frequently in childhood and adolescence. The six gangliogliomas in the cerebral hem-

isphere in the Hospital for Sick Children series occurred in children ranging in age from 6 to 15. They have all followed a benign course. Three of the tumors were frontal in location, two temporal, and one parieto-occipital. Five were cystic. Subtotal excision was carried out in all, but only two have received postoperative radiotherapy. All the patients are alive and well, including the four who did not receive irradiation. These tumors do not appear to require irradiation. They should be followed with computed tomography postoperatively to determine whether the residual tumor is increasing in size.[73]

Primitive Neuroectodermal Tumors

Primitive neuroectodermal tumors histologically resemble medulloblastomas in the posterior fossa and behave in a very malignant fashion.[20] Of 10 patients with such tumors in the cerebral hemispheres in the Hospital for Sick Children series, 3 are still alive, the longest survival time being four years.[73] The survivors have all had radiotherapy.

Cavernous Hemangioma

The cavernous hemangioma is a rare and interesting tumor.[61] Despite its vascular appearance, it appears avascular on the arteriogram because of the extremely slow flow through it. It can, however, be seen on CT scan. The one patient in the series presented with a poorly controlled seizure disorder (Fig. 84–7). His tumor was totally extirpated, with consequent cure of his epilepsy.[73]

Corpus Callosum Lipoma

Lipomas of the corpus callosum are rare.[41] The child whose scan is shown in Figure 84–8 presented with a seizure disorder, and computed tomography made the diagnosis. He was neurologically intact. Electroencephalographically and clinically, his seizures were arising from the temporal lobe. It was elected to withold operative treatment and to manage him with anticonvulsant medication. He remains neurologi-

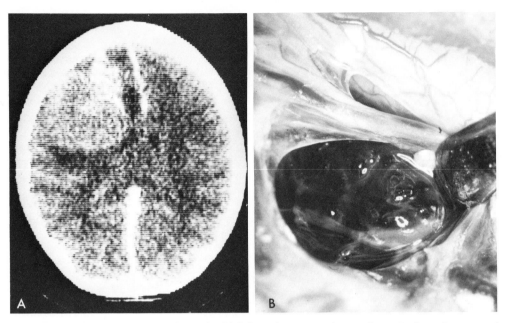

Figure 84–7*A*. CT scan (contrast-enhanced) of left frontal cavernous hemangioma. *B*. Operative removal of cavernous hemangioma.

cally intact, and his seizures are well controlled following two years of observation. These lipomas are not space-occupying lesions but may cause symptoms by irritating surrounding brain.

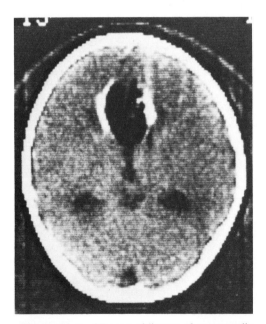

Figure 84–8   CT scan of lipoma of corpus callosum.

PINEAL REGION TUMORS

Expanding lesions at the back end of the third ventricle invariably lead to obstruction of the aqueduct of Sylvius and to development of hydrocephalus, with consequent signs of raised intracranial pressure. In addition, mass lesions in this area produce specific pressure on important adjacent structures and resultant clinical signs. Pressure on the superior colliculus, which lies just below the pineal gland, leads to loss of upward gaze (Parinaud's syndrome). Pressure on the third nerve nuclei leads to abnormalities of the papillary reflexes, pressure on the superior cerebellar vermis leads to ataxia, and pressure on the hypothalamus can produce hypersomnia and diabetes insipidus. In addition, about one third of the tumors of this region are germinomas of the pineal; these virtually always occur in males and frequently are associated with precocious puberty.

Dandy described his direct transcallosal approach to the pineal in 1921, and by 1943 Russell and Sachs documented 32 patients with tumors of the pineal who had been treated by direct attack upon the tumor.[9,59] Only three of these patients had survived the immediate postoperative period, an operative mortality rate of 90 per cent. Concerned by this dismal prognosis, in a 1948 paper titled "Should Extirpation Be Attempted in Cases of Neoplasm in or Near the Third Ventricle of the Brain?" Torkildsen answered "no."[66] He advocated inserting a shunt from the lateral ventricle to the cisterna magna and then applying postoperative radiotherapy to the lesion.

"Primum non nocere," or "first of all do no harm," was the plea made by Davidoff in 1967 in his masterful thesis on the treatment of pineal tumors when he said: "the direct surgical attack upon these tumors was, in the past, and still is, by and large—a harmful procedure."[11]

In 1965, Suzuki and Iwabuchi described their remarkable results with pineal region germinomas, achieved by following Dandy's original approach of direct operative attack.[64] Inspired by their report, the author's group approached their first pineal germinoma by a transcallosal route in 1967. Since then, they have routinely operated with little morbidity and no operative deaths. The advantages of magnification and illumination provided by the microscope, combined with preoperative shunting in those patients with hydrocephalus, has no doubt accounted for their results. They have continued to use Dandy's transcallosal approach (Figs. 84–9 and 84–10).

More recently, Stein has re-emphasized Krause's description of the infratentorial-

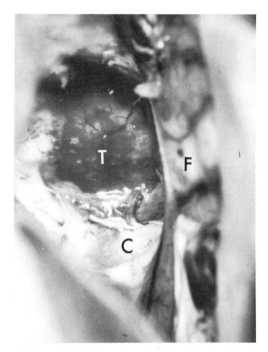

Figure 84–9 Operative view showing incision in corpus callosum for exposure of pineal germinoma. F, falx; C, corpus callosum; T, tumor.

supracerebellar exposure, and Jamieson has modified Poppen's approach by dividing the tentorium and allowing both a supracerebellar and a suboccipital approach simultaneously.[31,34,57,63] Because of the excellent success with the transcallosal ap-

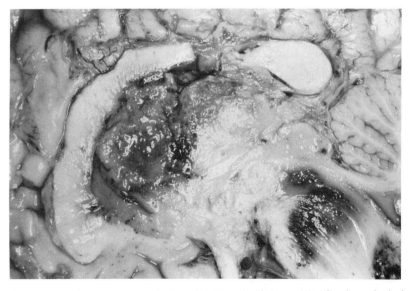

Figure 84–10 Postmortem specimen, sagittal section through third ventricle of patient who had transcallosal approach to malignant astrocytoma filling third ventricle. Note incision in corpus callosum.

proach, however, the author continues to favor it for pineal region tumors.

In the past, these tumors were investigated by ventriculography and angiography. Now the CT scan has replaced ventriculography (Fig. 84–11). Angiograms are still needed, however, for two reasons. A right-sided internal carotid anteriogram shows the parasagittal draining veins and therefore helps to plan the operative flap to avoid compromise of these veins. If the tumor is a germinoma or teratoma in the pineal region, the internal cerebral veins are humped over the dome of the tumor, whereas with an infiltrating astrocytoma, the internal cerebral veins frequently are not elevated and can even be depressed because the tumor infiltrates and surrounds them.

Between 1950 and 1975, 39 patients with posterior third ventricular or pineal region tumors were treated at the Hospital for Sick Children. These patients typically presented with signs of raised intracranial pressure due to obstruction of the third ventricle that had produced hydrocephalus. This was true in all except the first patient treated by Dandy's transcallosal approach 10 years ago. This particular patient pre-

Table 84–9   HISTOLOGICAL TYPES OF TUMORS OF PINEAL REAGION*

No histological verification	11
Astrocytoma	
Grades I and II	2
Grade III	3
Grade IV	1
Oligodendroglioma	1
Ependymoma	1
Teratoma	
Benign	1
Malignant	2
Germinoma	10
Pineoblastoma	7
Total	39

* Data from study of 344 patients with supratentorial tumors treated at the Hospital for Sick Children, Toronto, 1950 through 1975.

sented with only diabetes insipidus and had a small germinoma.

Of the 39 patients, 24 have been operated on through a transcallosal exposure. These procedures have all been done since 1967. Of the 15 patients whose tumors were not approached operatively, 6 are alive and 9 have died.

Histological confirmation was obtained in 28 patients: 24 at the time of operation and 4 at postmortem. Ten tumors were germinomas, seven were pineoblastomas, one was a benign teratoma, two were malignant teratomas, one was an ependymoma, one an oligodendroglioma, four were grade III or grade IV astrocytomas, and two were grade I or grade II astrocytomas (Table 84–9).[73]

Germinomas and Teratomas

All 10 germinomas occurred in males, eight of whom were between 7 and 12 years of age and two of whom were 13 or older. Six of these patients, of whom two were never treated, have died. Four are alive and well, and two of these have survived for more than four years. Both those with malignant teratomas have died; one was untreated and the other had biopsy and radiotherapy. The benign teratoma was totally removed, and the patient remains well.

Pineoblastomas

Pineoblastomas typically occur in infants. These tumors resemble the medulloblastoma of the cerebellar vermis and the primitive neuroectodermal tumor of the

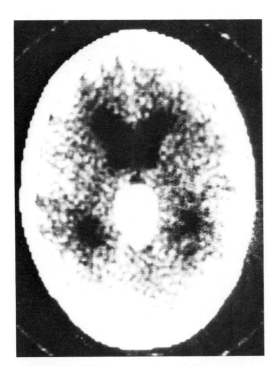

Figure 84–11 Contrast-enhanced CT scan showing pineal germinoma and attendant hydrocephalus.

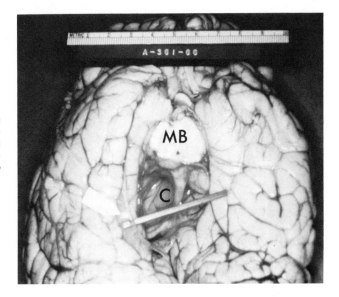

Figure 84–12 Huge collicular plate arachnoid cyst, C, producing marked midbrain, MB, compression and causing the patient's death. This infant was never investigated or treated and died a ''crib death.''

cerebral hemisphere, and can grow to enormous size. Three of the pineoblastomas in the series occurred in infants under 1 year and three in very young children, between 1 and 2 years, and only one in a 6-year-old. The only survivor with a pineoblastoma was a 6-year-old who had marked leptomeningeal spread and received total neural axis radiotherapy; he remains alive eight years following initial treatment.[73]

Discussion

In addition to the tumors already described, the pineal region also is subject to a host of benign lesions including arachnoid cysts, which can be treated easily by either a transcallosal approach or a Jamieson approach (Fig. 84–12).[31]

Most patients with pineal region tumors have hydrocephalus at the time of presentation. A ventriculoperitoneal shunt with a Millipore filter (to prevent shunting tumor cells into the peritoneal cavity—a definite risk with germinomas) should be inserted.* Seven to ten days after the shunt has been inserted, when the hydrocephalus is under control and the patient's clinical state has improved, craniotomy and tumor excision can be attempted.

Given modern methods of dealing with cerebral edema and hydrocephalus, and the

availability of the operating room microscope, the operative approach to the pineal region carries little risk. Benign tumors, cysts, thrombosed aneurysms of the vein of Galen, epidermoid tumors, and cavernous hemangiomas are all curable lesions that are amenable to the operative approach but do not respond to radiotherapy. It is important to establish a histological diagnosis. With the germinoma, there is the hazard of neural axis metastases. In 3 of the author's 10 cases of germinoma, spinal cord metastases did indeed develop. The incidence reported in the literature is somewhat less; Ishii and co-workers had only two cases of spinal cord metastases among 67 patients.[28] Jenkins and associates, however, believe that the risk of meningeal seeding is in the neighborhood of 10 to 15 per cent.[32] Since histological confirmation of pineal region tumors still remains a matter of controversy, the true incidence of leptomeningeal spread remains unknown, and until more data pertaining to the risk of spinal cord metastases are available, it is unwise to draw any firm conclusions about the benefit or hazard of total neural axis radiotherapy. On the basis of limited experience, however, it appears that radiotherapy of the neural axis should be done.

SUPRASELLAR TUMORS

Of the Hospital for Sick Children series of 344 patients, 58 (17 per cent) had supra-

* Manufactured by The Holter Company, Division of Extracorporal Medical Specialties, Inc., King of Prussia, Pennsylvania.

Table 84–10   SUPRASELLAR TUMORS*

Craniopharyngiomas	48
Germinoma	4
Teratoma	
Benign	1
Malignant	2
Astrocytoma grade I or II	1
No histological confirmation	2
Total	58

* Data from study of 344 patients with supratentorial tumors treated at the Hospital for Sick Children, Toronto, 1950 through 1975.

sellar tumors. Forty-eight were craniopharyngiomas, by far the most common tumor in the suprasellar area. In addition, there were four suprasellar germinomas and three teratomas. Two of these teratomas were malignant and one was benign. There was also one astrocytoma entirely confined to the suprasellar area and fungating out of the midbrain. The histological structure of two of the suprasellar tumors was never confirmed (Table 84–10).[73]

Craniopharyngiomas

Forty-eight of the suprasellar tumors were craniopharyngiomas. There was no sex predominance in this group of patients. Seventeen were aged 2 to 6, and thirty-one were 7 to 16. All but one had visual defects: papilledema was present in 13, bitemporal hemianopia in 25, homonymous hemianopia in 4, and unilateral temporal hemianopia in 4. Visual acuity was significantly reduced unilaterally in 17 cases and bilaterally in 11. Seesaw nystagmus was present in three cases.[10] More than 50 per cent of the patients had symptoms of endocrine disorder: six had diabetes insipidus, nine were excessively short, seven were excessively obese, two were hypothyroid, and four showed evidence of sex hormone deficiency. Plain skull radiographs revealed calcification in the tumor in 29 patients. In seven cases, severe hydrocephalus produced by the tumor necessitated shunting before the craniopharyngioma could be dealt with operatively. During the period 1950 to 1975, a variety of approaches was used to deal with craniopharyngioma. Patients whose tumors were treated by simple aspiration or partial excision did poorly, with 100 per cent of the tumors recurring and 63 per cent of the patients dying. When the tumor was subtotally resected, 40 per cent of the patients required no further therapy. When the tumors were totally excised, however, none recurred, and both the patients' vision and general neurological state were significantly better than the results achieved when the other two modes of operative therapy were used. Furthermore, the patients whose tumors were totally excised never required radiotherapy, thus avoiding the hazards concomitant with radiation.[69] It is clear that these tumors *can* and *should* be totally excised. Total excision of at least 80 per cent of craniopharyngiomas is possible, provided the attempt is made at the initial operative approach and microneuro-operative techniques are employed (Fig. 84–13). If the entire tumor cannot be removed, a subtotal excision should be performed and no further therapy done unless the tumor shows evidence of recurrence, either clinically or by CT scan,

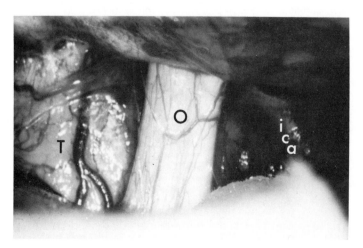

Figure 84–13 Operative view of craniopharyngioma, T, showing tumor elevating optic nerve, O, and pushing internal carotid artery, ica, out laterally.

at which time radiotherapy should be used.[23,73]

The remaining suprasellar tumors, which included four germinomas, three teratomas, and one astrocytoma, presented in a fashion indistinguishable from that of the craniopharyngiomas.

Germinomas

All four of the suprasellar germinomas in the series occurred in girls. Two of these were approached through a subfrontal route and, on operative examination, appeared to be intrinsic to the optic pathways (Fig. 84–14).[73] Cohen and associates pointed out this very deceptive appearance of suprasellar germinomas in 1974.[6] All the suprasellar germinoma patients in the series had some degree of visual impairment: two had visual field defects, and two had papilledema. In one of these, associated hydrocephalus necessitated a shunt. Three of the four presented with diabetes insipidus. Despite radiotherapy, all four died.[73]

Teratoma

Both patients with malignant suprasellar teratomas in the series received postoperative radiotherapy. One of these children has responded superbly, remains well four years after treatment, and has a normal CT scan. The child with the benign teratoma died without treatment.[73]

Astrocytoma

The single suprasellar astrocytoma in the series was first diagnosed as a solid cranio-pharyngioma at the time of operation, and therefore an attempt at total excision was made. It was only on discovery that the tumor appeared to blend with the midbrain that a halt was called to the operation. The tumor was a grade II astrocytoma. The child received a course of radiotherapy postoperatively, and except for a visual field defect he is well 10 years following treatment.

THIRD VENTRICLE TUMORS

Only three tumors in the Hospital for Sick Children series were entirely within the third ventricle. All three patients had hydrocephalus and raised intracranial pressure. Two of these patients had truncal ataxia. One patient, who had an ependymoma, was treated only with a bypass shunt and died within one year of diagnosis. One choroid plexus papilloma of the third ventricle was totally removed, and this patient has remained cured seven years after tumor excision. The third patient had a choroid plexus carcinoma, was treated with radiotherapy and a shunt, and subsequently died.[73]

LATERAL VENTRICLE TUMORS

In the Hospital for Sick Children series, these tumors consisted of one ependymoma, seven choroid plexus papillomas, and two choroid plexus carcinomas. All these patients presented under the age of 6 years, and five of the nine choroid plexus tumors were in patients younger than 1 year. All 10 patients had hydrocephalus,

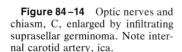

Figure 84–14 Optic nerves and chiasm, C, enlarged by infiltrating suprasellar germinoma. Note internal carotid artery, ica.

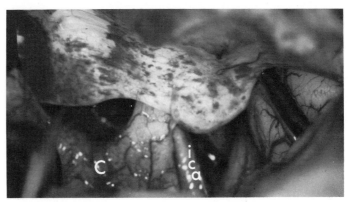

and 6 presented with increasing head size. All had hemiparesis.[73]

Choroid Plexus Papilloma and Carcinoma

Two choroid plexus papillomas were never diagnosed in life, and the patients died without treatment. Another patient had biopsy only and died. Four patients had the tumor totally removed; of these, only one has died. There were two patients with choroid plexus carcinoma, one of whom died without any form of treatment. The other underwent biopsy and radiation therapy; he also died.[73]

One of these choroid plexus papillomas in the lateral ventricle presented as a primary subarachnoid hemorrhage, and a subsequent CT scan made the diagnosis (see Fig. 84–1B). In 1973, Matsushima and co-workers reviewed this phenomenon of spontaneous hemorrhage from a choroid plexus papilloma.[48]

Removal of choroid plexus papillomas in the lateral ventricle has carried a high operative mortality rate because of uncontrolled blood loss due to the extreme vascularity of these tumors. De la Torre and associates pointed out in 1963 that the usual but incorrect approach to a lateral ventricle choroid plexus tumor is a vertical incision in the posterior parietal cortex.[67] This approach places the surgeon lateral, posterior, and superior to the tumor, making exposure of the main vascular pedicle difficult as an initial step. Because these tumors are closely applied to the glomus of the choroid plexus and are fed by either large anterior or large posterior choroidal arteries, the pedicle of the tumor lies inferior to the tumor. Thus, a horizontal transcortical incision along the posterior portion of the middle temporal gyrus permits the surgeon to elevate the tumor and clip the feeding vessels before removal (Fig. 84–15). Since 1963, the author has been using this approach, making the incision in the middle temporal gyrus, and has had no problems with uncontrolled hemorrhage.*

The association of choroid plexus papillomas and communicating hydrocephalus has long been recognized and is frequently ascribed to overproduction of cerebrospinal fluid. Even after removal of the papilloma, however, hydrocephalus frequently persists in these patients, presumably because adhesions cause obstruction of cerebrospinal fluid pathways. Furthermore, not all patients with choroid plexus papillomas develop hydrocephalus, and one of the author's patients had normal size ventricles (see Fig. 84–1B).[73]

---

* Fortunately the third ventricular choroid plexus papillomas are far less vascular and can be removed piecemeal through the foramina of Monro without undue hemorrhage.

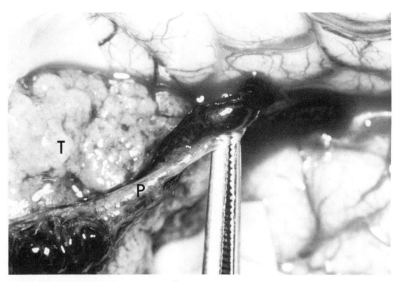

Figure 84–15 Trigonal choroid plexus papilloma, T, in process of excision through a middle temporal gyrus incision and showing tumor pedicle, P, consisting of choroidal artery and vein.

HYPOTHALAMIC TUMORS

The hypothalamus is a rather rare site for a supratentorial tumor in a child. In the Hospital for Sick Children series, there were 20 tumors whose primary location was in the hypothalamus, representing 6 per cent of the supratentorial tumors.[73] The diencephalic syndrome produced by tumors in the hypothalamus in infants has been a well-recognized entity since Russell's description in 1951.[58] In a review of the diencephalic syndrome by Burr and co-workers in 1976, the mean age for onset of symptoms in the syndrome was documented as 6.2 months, and the most common site of the tumor was in the floor of the third ventricle.[3] All the patients were emaciated despite an alert appearance and hyperkinesis. One third of them had hydrocephalus. The pathological nature of the tumors was varied, but the vast majority were astrocytomas. Five of the patients in the Hospital for Sick Children series presented with a diencephalic syndrome. Two of them were less than a year old and three were between 1 and 2 years.

Hydrocephalus produced by occlusion of the foramina of Monro is a common presenting problem in patients with hypothalamic tumors. In the series, seven had papilledema, two were drowsy, and one was in coma. The midline position of these tumors, together with the associated hydrocephalus, produced truncal ataxia in 4 of the 20 patients. Nine of the hydrocephalic patients had shunts inserted as the initial form of treatment; five of these had no further treatment. Four patients had operative excision of the tumor after insertion of the shunt, and three required a shunt after craniotomy had been performed for the tumor.[73]

Histological verification was obtained in 12 of the 20 cases. Eleven patients had a grade I or grade II astrocytoma and one had a hamartoma. Biopsy of nine of the astrocytomas was performed; seven of these patients went on to radiotherapy, and five of them are still alive. Two of the astrocytomas identified by biopsy were not irradiated, and one of these patients remains alive and shunt-reliant four years after treatment.[73]

Ten patients did not undergo exploration but received radiotherapy; six of these remain alive.[73]

The only hypothalamic hamartoma in the series was totally removed, but the patient died in the postoperative period. This particular child had a classic diencephalic syndrome and was slightly over 1 year of age at the time of presentation.

Tumors of the hypothalamus should be treated operatively, and tumor location and histological type should be verified. If the tumor proves to be a benign astrocytoma, as seems to be the case in the majority of instances, radiotherapy should be used only if the tumor shows evidence of further growth.

TUMORS OF THALAMUS AND BASAL GANGLIA

These deeply placed tumors are fortunately uncommon, but they occur more frequently in childhood than in adult life. In the Hospital for Sick Children series of tumors, the thalamic and basal ganglia tumors constituted a total of 30, representing 9 per cent of the supratentorial tumors (Table 84–11).[73] Patients with tumors within the thalamus and basal ganglia typically present with signs of raised intracranial pressure and associated hemiparesis. Both signs were common in the series: 15 of the patients had papilledema, 2 were drowsy, and 1 was stuporous; all 30 patients had some degree of hemiparesis. In addition, two of these patients had tuberous sclerosis, and two had von Recklinghausen's disease.

Associated hydrocephalus was common. In two patients, a shunt was inserted prior to craniotomy. Eight were treated with a shunt only and no further operation, and two others received a shunt following the craniotomy.

Table 84–11 TUMORS OF THALAMUS AND BASAL GANGLIA*

No histological verification	13
Astrocytoma	
Giant cell	3
Grades I and II	6
Grade III	3
Grade IV	5
Total	30

* Data from study of 344 patients with supratentorial tumors treated at the Hospital for Sick Children, Toronto, 1950 through 1975.

In the past, the thalamic and basal gangliar region was an almost forbidden area for the neurosurgeon, and consequently fewer than half of the tumors in this series received operative treatment. In recent years the policy has generally been to perform biopsy or to attempt removal of all these deeply placed tumors. Because one can approach this region transventricularly in a relatively benign fashion, biopsy of these tumors should be performed, particularly in view of the recent report by Chandler and co-workers of an intrathalamic epidermoid tumor and the report by Jain of a cavernous hemangioma appearing deep within the hemisphere, both being benign lesions that would not respond to radiotherapy and yet would be amenable to operative excision.[4,30]

In the series of 30 deeply placed tumors, 13 were never histologically verified, 3 were giant cell astrocytomas, 6 were grade I and II astrocytomas, and 8 were grade III and IV astrocytomas. Two of the astrocytomas were cystic.[73]

Because of the nature of the tumors that were encountered at operation, only biopsies were performed. There have been no operative deaths from the procedure. Following operation, most of the patients have been referred for radiotherapy. Two exceptions include one with a giant cell astrocytoma and one with a grade I astrocytoma. Biopsy was performed in both cases, and the tumors were not irradiated; both patients are alive and well. In addition, one patient whose grade I astrocytoma was irradiated remains alive. All eight patients with grade III and grade IV astrocytomas have died despite radiotherapy.[73]

In summary, 10 patients with tumors of the thalamus and basal ganglia remain alive and 20 are dead. Six of these ten were treated with radiotherapy and have now survived for more than four years.[73]

OPTIC PATHWAY GLIOMAS

In Matson's series, these tumors accounted for 3.6 per cent of all brain tumors.[46] In the Hospital for Sick Children series they number 51, which represents 15 per cent of the supratentorial tumors and 6 per cent of the total series of brain tumors.[73]

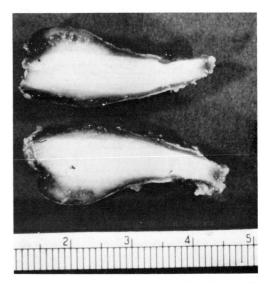

Figure 84–16 Sagittal section of excised optic nerve glioma in continuity with optic nerve, which has been transected just behind the tumor posteriorly and behind the globe anteriorly.

The most likely point of origin of these optic nerve astrocytomas is the optic canal. From the canal, the tumor tends to extend forward into the orbit as well as backward toward the chiasm (Fig. 84–16). Of 51 optic nerve astrocytomas, 16 lay in front of the optic chiasm, and all but one of these were unilateral. Thirty-five involved the chiasm and the optic tracts. Histological confirmation was obtained in 41 of these tumors: 35 were benign grade I and II astrocytomas, and six were grade III astrocytomas.[73]

The vast majority of these tumors presented between ages 1 and 6 and none presented beyond the age of 12. Boys outnumbered girls by two to one (Table 84–12).[73]

The presenting symptom of optic nerve tumors is usually visual loss.[5] This was found in all the patients and was of severe degree at the time of presentation in 39 of the 51. If the tumor extends forward into the orbit, proptosis is present in addition to visual loss. Nine of the fifteen patients with anteriorly placed optic nerve tumors had proptosis at the time of initial presentation.[73]

The close and frequent association of optic nerve tumors with von Recklinghausen's disease has been known since 1940, when it was described by Davies.[12] Of the 51 patients who had optic nerve tumors, 15 (29.4 per cent) also had von Recklinghausen's disease.[73]

**Table 84–12 OPTIC NERVE GLIOMAS: CORRELATION OF AGE OF
PRESENTATION AND SEX OF PATIENTS***

SEX	< 1 YEAR	1 TO 6 YEARS	6 TO 12 YEARS	> 13 YEARS	TOTAL
Male	2	11	4	0	17
Female	0	26	8	0	34
Total	2	37	12	0	51

* Data from study of 344 patients with supratentorial tumors treated at the Hospital for Sick Children, Toronto, 1950 through 1975.

Papilledema was present in 10 of the 51 patients, produced by compression of the drainage veins from the retina or due to increased intracranial pressure resulting from the tumor's obstructing cerebrospinal fluid pathways. Involvement of the optic tract was present in five patients who presented with either homonymous hemianopia or bitemporal hemianopia. Optic atrophy was obvious in 40 patients. Hydrocephalus, sufficiently severe to require shunting, was present in 14 patients, all of whom had posteriorly placed optic nerve tumors. Hypothalamic dysfunction, evidenced by obesity and lethargy, was present in six patients. Hemiparesis due to compression of the internal capsule was found in five patients: two presented with seizures, and four had increasing head size produced by the hydrocephalus.[73] In seven patients, nystagmus was present, and in one of these it was of the seesaw variety.[10]

One infant with an optic nerve glioma presented with a massive subdural effusion sufficiently large to be apparent on transillumination of the head. The diagnosis of optic nerve glioma was not established until the child's death some five years later (Fig. 84–17). A similar case was reported by Mori and co-workers in 1975.[51] Another patient in the series presented with unilateral nystagmus and hydrocephalus, and developed marked ascites following peritoneal shunting, although the tumor itself did not become evident until three years later.[73]

In 1925, Van der Hoeve introduced the radiological technique for demonstrating the optic foramen by which intracranial extension of an intraorbital mass can be determined.[68] The most common finding is a widened optic foramen without decalcification of its walls. An optic foramen 1 mm. larger than the contralateral foramen is abnormal, the width of a normal optic foramen varying between 4.1 and 4.65 mm (Fig. 84–18). In addition, the anterior wall of the sella and the ventral surfaces of the anterior clinoid processes may be eroded, and the sella may be J-shaped.

Tomographic cuts through the optic canals along the longitudinal axis, as described by Harwood-Nash, provide simultaneous visualization of both optic canals and can show signs of intracranial involve-

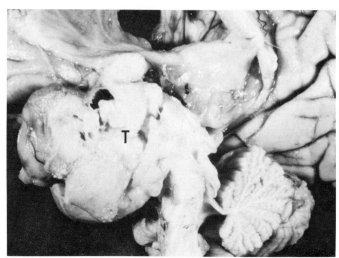

Figure 84–17 Huge optic nerve glioma, T, which led to child's death at age 5 years.

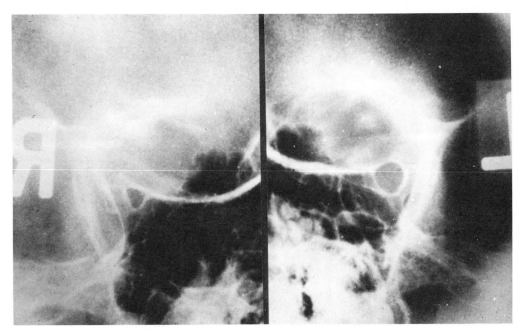

Figure 84–18 Optic foramen views demonstrating a pathologically enlarged optic foramen on the left in a patient with optic nerve glioma.

ment (Fig. 84–19).[21] With the advent of computer tomographic scanning, a simple noninvasive method of visualizing the orbital portion of the optic nerve has become available (Fig. 84–20). Not only is the intraorbital extent of the optic nerve demonstrated by computed tomography but any possible intracranial component is also detected (Fig. 84–21).

An operative technique introduced in 1888 by Krönlein allowed for resection of the intraorbital portion of an optic nerve glioma.[35] These tumors almost always involve the intracranial portion of the optic nerve, and as neurosurgery developed, a two-stage procedure emerged: The neurosurgeon resects the intracranial portion of the optic nerve tumor via a craniotomy and disengages the tumor from the optic canal; the ophthalmologist then approaches the

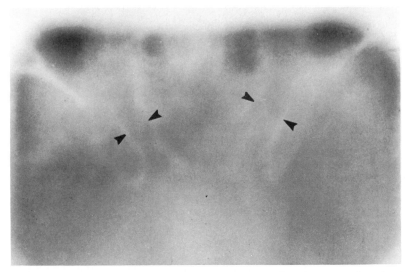

Figure 84–19 Optic canal tomograms showing a pathologically enlarged canal on the right.

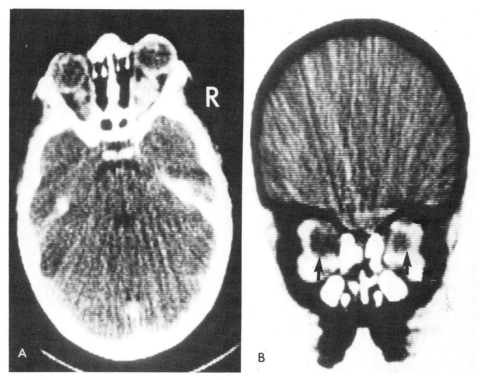

Figure 84-20 *A.* CT scan showing bilateral optic nerve gliomas in orbits. The larger one on the right is producing proptosis. *B.* Coronal CT scan of the same patient showing bilateral optic nerve gliomas (*arrows*).

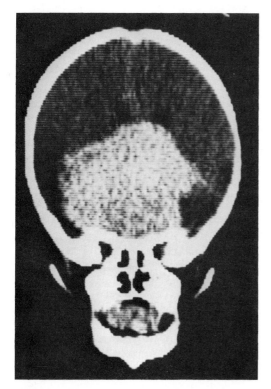

Figure 84-21 Huge contrast-enhanced optic nerve glioma on CT scan of a 6-week-old infant.

tumor through a Krönlein procedure and resects the intraorbital and canalicular tumor.

An entirely transcranial route, as advocated by Jackson and Housepian, allows access to the intracranial contents as well as to the orbital structures. The course of the fourth cranial nerve, however, is such that it may be damaged by the approach through the roof of the orbit, and the result may be an unsightly globe.[24,29]

The use of radiotherapy for these tumors remains controversial. Many neurosurgeons, including Matson, have not advocated radiotherapy in optic nerve tumors.[46]

Optic gliomas have an unpredictable course. The tumor will spread in one patient and lead to death (see Fig. 84-17), but will remain quiescent for many years in another patient. As a result, some clinicians advocate operative intervention; others advocate radiotherapeutic treatment; while yet others feel that no treatment is necessary, believing that the tumors are basically simple hamartomas that will not grow. Among the latter are Hoyt and Baghdassarian, who stated in 1969 that operative removal of optic nerve tumors did not affect

Table 84–13　RESULTS OF THERAPY OF OPTIC NERVE GLIOMAS*

OPERATIVE TREATMENT	NO RADIOTHERAPY		RADIOTHERAPY	
	Alive	*Dead*	*Alive*	*Dead*
Anterior tumors				
Total tumor removal	10	0	0	0
Partial removal or exploration	2	0	3	1
	12	0	3	1
Posterior tumors				
None	0	2	4	5
Biopsy or partial excision	3	2	16	3
	3	4	20	8

* Data from study of 344 patients with supratentorial tumors treated at the Hospital for Sick Children, Toronto, 1950 through 1975.

the prognosis for vision or survival.[25] They therefore advocated no treatment except measures to relieve unsightly proptosis or obstructive hydrocephalus.

Treatment of unilateral optic nerve tumors is perfectly straightforward: operative resection of the involved optic nerve (Table 84–13). In the one case of bilateral optic nerve tumor in the Hospital for Sick Children series the tumor producing the proptosis was resected and the other nerve left untouched (see Fig. 84–20). After three years, that child continues to show no change in visual acuity and no evidence of posterior involvement. Of the 16 anteriorly placed optic nerve tumors, 10 were treated by a two-stage resection. Approached transfrontally, the tumor was resected from behind, through the normal optic nerve and in front of the optic chiasm; a Krönlein procedure was then employed to remove the intraorbital tumor. In six patients, the entire tumor was removed through a transcranial approach in which the optic canal and orbit were unroofed. The fact that the tumor extended posteriorly was sometimes not ascertained until the time of operation or sometimes not until several years had passed and clinical progression or death made the diagnosis. One of these patients, originally reported in Lloyd's series as cured of a unilateral optic nerve tumor, presented 10 years later with evidence of tumor in the chiasm, optic tract, thalamus, and brain stem, and subsequently died.[38] All the other patients with anterior tumors are alive. Three of them received local irradiation because the tumor extended beyond the line of resection. Twelve patients were treated only by resection without radiotherapy and all of these are alive and well.[73]

Thirty-five of the fifty-one patients had posterior extension of their optic nerve gliomas.[73] Seven of these posteriorly placed tumors were never irradiated. Three of the patients are alive and four are dead. Of the 28 who did receive local radiotherapy, 20 are alive and 8 have died. Five of these surviving patients have severe neurological involvement: hemiplegia, dementia, and in one case clear evidence of radiation necrosis of the brain (Fig. 84–22).[73]

Radiotherapy has a role to play in the treatment of optic nerve gliomas. One must, however, consider that these tumors typically occur in young children, and that radiation of the brain in a young child carries some risk. Accordingly, radiotherapy is reserved for clinically progressive optic

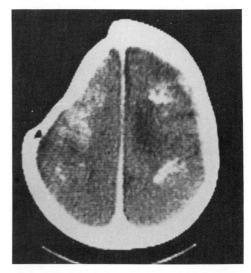

Figure 84–22 Nonenhanced CT scan of 8-year-old child who received radiotherapy for optic nerve glioma following craniotomy at age 3. Note bilateral cerebral calcification and sunken-in bone flap. The child is demented and hemiplegic but has no evidence of viable tumor.

nerve gliomas. This course of action is based on the assumption that exploration and biopsy have ruled out the occasional chiasmatic mass that turns out to be a radiosensitive germinoma or a benign craniopharyngioma. If the tumor is in one optic nerve, a transcranial approach, with resection behind the tumor posteriorly and in front of the tumor in the orbit appears to offer an excellent prognosis.

PITUITARY ADENOMAS

Pituitary adenomas are an extremely rare tumor in childhood. Ingraham and Matson reported only two pituitary adenomas out of a total of 313 intracranial tumors in children.[27] Koos and Miller had 10 pituitary adenomas in their series of 700 tumors in childhood.[33]

Physically these tumors enlarge the sella turcica and, as they emerge out of the sella, compress the optic chiasm and optic nerves, producing visual impairment and typically a bitemporal hemianopia. Headaches and endocrine dysfunction usually accompany these findings. In the Hospital for Sick Children series during the period of 1950 to 1975, four pituitary adenomas were encountered.[73] Three of these patients had chromophobe adenomas and presented with hypopituitarism in addition to their headaches and visual impairment, while one patient had a basophilic adenoma and presented with increased blood levels of cortisone and clinically was mildly obese and cushingoid.

Ortiz-Suarez and Erickson demonstrated that pituitary adenomas in children behaved in an aggressive fashion and that the incidence of extrasellar extension was high.[54] This was certainly true of two of the four adenomas in the Hospital for Sick Children series. One patient had rapid recurrence of her tumor and died. In the second patient, the recurrent tumor was irradiated and the patient has remained well for 10 years following therapy. The author feels that these tumors should be approached transsphenoidally in the child (Fig. 84-23).

The sphenoid sinus is well developed by adolescence, and all the pituitary adenomas seen at the Hospital for Sick Children occurred in children older than 10 years.

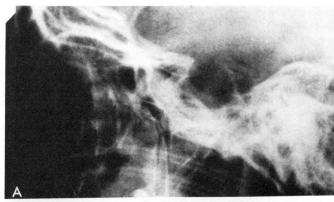
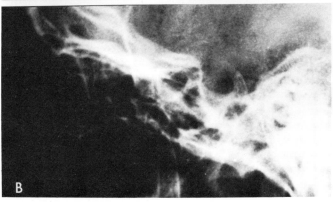

Figure 84-23 Views of the sella in a child with basophilic adenoma of the pituitary. *A.* Before transsphenoidal removal of the tumor. *B.* One year after removal of the tumor, showing reduction of sellar size.

Although Cushing attributed the syndrome to basophil tumors of the pituitary gland in 1932, the common form of treatment for Cushing's disease remained adrenalectomy or pituitary irradiation until very recently.[7,14,17,42]

Nelson and co-workers, in 1958, described the development of a pituitary gland tumor in a patient who had undergone previous bilateral adrenalectomy for Cushing's syndrome.[52] Since then, many patients have been reported to have "Nelson's syndrome" who presumably have had a small basophil pituitary tumor and have presented with hyperpigmentation, headaches, visual impairment, and an enlarging sella.[49,50] Recently, the first case of Nelson's syndrome in a child was described.[15]

The present operative treatment of Cushing's syndrome of primary pituitary origin is transsphenoidal removal of a microadenoma of the pituitary gland. Laws and Kern report cure of Cushing's syndrome in 10 of 11 patients so treated.[37] Wilson has found that even though the sella is perfectly normal, and particularly in a child, with Cushing's syndrome the pituitary gland will harbor a basophilic microadenoma.[70]

DURAL AND EXTRADURAL TUMORS

Meningiomas

Although these are relatively common tumors in adult life, they are extremely rare in childhood. Matson reported only three meningiomas among 750 tumors.[47] Koos and Miller had 19 meningiomas in their series of 700 tumors, making up 2.8 per cent of their brain tumors.[33] Cushing and Eisenhardt had only five patients in the preadolescent age group in their series of 295 patients with meningiomas.[8] In the Hospital for Sick Children series, they constitute 1 per cent of supratentorial tumors and 0.5 per cent of all brain tumors.[73]

Meningiomas are typically slow-growing tumors that tend to produce increased vascularization of the adjacent bone with hyperostosis of the skull and compression of the underlying brain. Total resection of the tumor, which always has a well-demarcated margin, is the treatment of choice and offers an excellent prognosis. Three of the meningiomas in the series were situated over the convexity of the cerebral hemisphere, and these could be radically removed, curing the patient. Meningiomas in children, however, although benign, tend to grow more quickly than do the adult meningiomas and they can infiltrate widely if they occur along the base of the skull. One patient had a massive sphenoidal wing meningioma that wrapped itself around the internal carotid arteries and infiltrated the cavernous sinus as well as spreading through the superior orbital fissure into the orbit so that only a subtotal removal was possible. This tumor rapidly recurred.[73]

Dural Sarcoma

Like meningiomas, dural sarcomas can occur in the supratentorial compartment. These tumors typically do not invade the underlying leptomeninges of brain.[2] Dural sarcomas should be radically excised, but frequently metastatic spread of the tumor precludes cure. Radiotherapy is always used following operative excision. In the Hospital for Sick Children series there were four dural sarcomas; of the four patients, three have died.[73]

Schwannomas

Schwannomas are tumors arising from the sheaths of Schwann cells of spinal and cranial nerves. In childhood, they are frequently associated with von Recklinghausen's disease. Although the common site for these tumors is on the eighth cranial nerve, on occasion they can arise from the Schwann cells of nerves within the orbit and present as an orbital mass, producing proptosis, and may spread back through the superior orbital fissure into the middle fossa. These tumors are well demarcated from their surroundings and enclosed by a capsule that may have numerous vessels. They are typically smooth or finely nodular in appearance and are benign and slowly growing. With total excision, a cure is achieved. In the Hospital for Sick Children series, one of the extradural tumors was indeed of this type, with a mass in middle fossa extending through the superior orbital

Table 84-14   SITE OF UNCONFIRMED SUPRATENTORIAL TUMORS*

LOCATION	NUMBER UNCONFIRMED	TOTAL NUMBER IN SITE
Cerebral hemisphere	2	119
Pineal	11	39
Suprasellar area	2	58
Hypothalamus	8	20
Thalamus and basal ganglia	13	30
Optic pathway	10	51
Totals	46	317

* Data from study of 344 patients with supratentorial tumors treated at the Hospital for Sick Children, Toronto, 1950 through 1975.

fissure into the orbit. The orbital and middle fossa schwannoma was subtotally removed, and the patient presented with a recurrence 10 years later.[73]

Metastatic Extradural Tumor

Since primary malignant tumors are relatively rare in children as compared with adults, metastatic extradural tumors are relatively rare in childhood. Although asymptomatic leukemic infiltration of the dura must be present in many children with leukemia, the neurosurgical service at the Hospital for Sick Children has encountered only one metastatic deposit of an osteogenic sarcoma in the extradural space in a child. The prognosis of these tumors is obviously bad, and only palliative therapy is recommended.

UNCONFIRMED TUMORS

Forty-six of the tumors in the author's series remain unconfirmed. The common sites in which operative confirmation was not obtained were the optic nerve, the thalamus and basal ganglia, the pineal region, and the hypothalamus (Table 84-14). Modern operative technique has brought all

these sites to within reasonable reach of the surgeon.

SUPRATENTORIAL ASTROCYTOMAS

Astrocytomas were the most common supratentorial tumor in the series, accounting for 152 of the 317 histologically confirmed tumors.[73]

The most common site for these supratentorial astrocytomas was the cerebral hemisphere, where 76 were found. There were 41 in the optic pathways, 17 in the thalamus and basal ganglia, 11 in the hypothalamus, 1 in the suprasellar area, and 6 in the pineal region (Table 84-15).

The prognosis for astrocytomas in nonvital and excisable areas, e.g., the frontal pole, is quite different from the prognosis for those situated in areas from which they cannot be totally extirpated, such as the posterior optic pathways, hypothalamus, thalamus and basal ganglia, and pineal region. Whenever possible, an attempt at total excision is recommended. If this is not feasible and if the tumor is of low grade, radiation is not used, but the patient is followed with repeated CT scans, and only if the tumor shows evidence of further growth

Table 84-15   SITE OF CONFIRMED SUPRATENTORIAL ASTROCYTOMAS*

ASTROCYTOMA	CEREBRAL HEMISPHERE	PINEAL	SUPRASELLAR AREA	HYPOTHALAMUS	THALAMUS AND BASAL GANGLIA	OPTIC PATHWAY	TOTAL
Giant cell	1				3		4
Grades I and II	28	2	1	11	6	35	83
Grade III	22	3			3	6	34
Grade IV	25	1			5		31
Totals	76	6	1	11	17	41	152

* Data from study of 344 patients with supratentorial tumors treated at the Hospital for Sick Children, Toronto, 1950 through 1975.

is radiotherapy used. With more malignant tumors (grades III and IV), radiotherapy is started after operative attack on the tumor.

CONCLUSIONS

The supratentorial region is frequently the site of children's brain tumors and in the Hospital for Sick Children series accounted for 43.27 per cent of all brain tumors.[73] Furthermore, a significant proportion of these tumors (18.3 per cent in the series) are benign and extrinsic, virtually assuring their successful total excision.

The development of a simple diagnostic study—the computed tomographic scan—should prevent seizures or disordered neurological function from being termed "epilepsy" or "encephalitis." Occasional children in the series whose disorders were so characterized were, on postmortem study, found to have an undiagnosed brain tumor.

Improvements in pediatric neuroanesthesia and neurosurgical instruments have made such previously forbidden areas as the pineal region and the hypothalamus safely accessible, and have enabled the neurosurgeon to remove completely tumors that, in the past, could only be subjected to biopsy or blindly irradiated in ignorance of their pathological nature. With histological verification of the tumor now a matter of course, a more rational and responsible approach to radiotherapy is also possible; accurate studies of the effects of radiotherapy on various tumor types, together with serial CT scans, will facilitate future treatment still further.

Modern methods of treating hydrocephalus with bypass shunts have removed much of the danger associated with tumors obstructing cerebrospinal fluid pathways and have no doubt contributed to the present aggressive approach to midline tumors: excisable tumors are removed, while benign tumors that cannot be excised are simply followed by serial CT scans and are not necessarily irradiated unless they show evidence of progressive growth.

In all areas of diagnosis and treatment, the approach to supratentorial tumors in children has become increasingly aggressive and positive. No longer are these patients regarded with despair but rather with confidence and optimism.

Acknowledgments: The author would like to express his thanks to Dr. Michael Feeley, Dr. Marilyn Craven, and Miss Stephanie Hill for their help in amassing and preparing the data presented in this chapter.

REFERENCES

1. Amine, A. R. C., and Sugar, O.: Suprasellar osteogenic sarcoma following radiation for pituitary adenoma. J. Neurosurg., *44*:88–91, 1976.
2. Bailey, O. T., and Ingraham, F. D.: Intracranial fibrosarcoma of the dura mater in childhood. Pathological characteristics and surgical management. J. Neurosurg., *2*:1–15, 1945.
3. Burr, I. M., Slonim, A. E., Danish, R. K., Gadoth, N., and Butler, I. J.: Diencephalic syndrome revisited. J. Pediat., *88*:439–444, 1976.
4. Chandler, W. F., Farhat, S. M., and Pauli, F. J.: Intrathalamic epidermoid tumor. J. Neurosurg., *43*:614–617, 1975.
5. Chutorian, A. M., Schwartz, J. F., Evans, R. A., and Carter, S.: Optic gliomas in children. Neurology (Minneap.), *14*:83–95, 1964.
6. Cohen, D. N., Steinberg, M., and Buchwald, R.: Suprasellar germinomas: Diagnostic confusion with optic gliomas. Case report. J. Neurosurg., *41*:490–493, 1974.
7. Cushing, H.: The basophil adenomas of the pituitary body and their clinical manifestations (pituitary basophilism). Bull. Johns Hopk. Hosp., *50*:137–195, 1932.
8. Cushing, H., and Eisenhardt, L.: Meningiomas, Their Classification, Regional Behaviour, Life History and Surgical End Results. Springfield, Ill., Charles C Thomas. 1938, p. 69.
9. Dandy, W. E.: An operation for the removal of pineal tumors. Surg. Gynecol. Obstet., *33*:113–119. 1921.
10. Daroff, B.: See-saw nystagmus. Neurology (Minneap.), *15*:874–877, 1965.
11. Davidoff, L. M.: Some considerations in the therapy of pineal tumors. Bull. N.Y. Acad. Med., *43*:537–561, 1967.
12. Davies, F. A.: Primary tumors of the optic nerve (a phenomenon of von Recklinghausen's disease); a clinical and pathological study with a report of five cases and a review of the literature. Arch. Ophthal., *23*:735–821, 957–1022, 1940.
13. Drake, C. G., and McGee, D.: Apoplexy associated with brain tumours. Canad. Med. Ass. J., *84*:303–305, 1961.
14. Edmonds, M. W., Simpson, W. J. K., and Meakin, J. W.: External irradiation of the hypophysis for Cushing's disease. Canad. Med. Ass. J., *107*:860–861, 1972.
15. Forni, C., and Giovanelli, M. A.: Nelson's syndrome in the paediatric age. Child's Brain, *3*:309–314, 1977.
16. Ghatak, N. R., and White, B. E.: Delayed radiation necrosis of the hypothalamus. Arch. Neurol., *21*:425–430, 1969.
17. Glenn, F., Karl, R. C., and Horwith, M.: The surgical treatment of Cushing's syndrome, Ann. Surg., *148*:365, 1958.
18. Gol, A.: Cerebral astrocytomas in childhood. A clinical study. J. Neurosurg., *19*:577–582. 1962.

19. Gonzalez, D., and Elvidge, A. R.: On the occurrence of epilepsy caused by astrocytoma of the cerebral hemispheres. J. Neurosurg., 19:470–482, 1962.
20. Hart, M. N., and Earle, K. M.: Primitive neuroectodermal tumors of the brain in children. Cancer, 32:890–897, 1973.
21. Harwood-Nash, D. C.: Axial tomography of the optic canals in children. Radiology, 96:367–374, 1970.
22. Hoffman, H. J., and Freeman, A.: Primary malignant leptomeningeal melanoma in association with giant hairy nevi. Report of two cases. J. Neurosurg. 26:62–71, 1967.
23. Hoffman, H. J., Hendrick, E. B., Humphreys, R. P., Buncic, J. R., Armstrong, D. L., and Jenkins, R. D. T.: Management of craniopharyngioma in children. J. Neurosurg., 47:218–277, 1977.
24. Housepian, E. M.: Surgical treatment of unilateral optic nerve gliomas. J. Neurosurg., 31:604–607, 1969.
25. Hoyt, W. F., and Baghdassarian, S. A.: Optic glioma of childhood. Natural History and rationale for conservative management. Brit. J. Ophthal., 53:793–798, 1969.
26. Ingraham, F. D., and Matson, D. D.: Neurosurgery of Infancy and Childhood. Springfield, Ill., Charles C Thomas, 1954.
27. Ibid: p. 223.
28. Ishii, R., Tsuchida, T., Honda, H., Ueki K., and Oyake, Y.: Radiation therapy and surgical management of pineal tumors—follow-up study of 96 patients. Neurol. Surg. (Tokyo), 4:263–270, 1976.
29. Jackson, H.: Orbital tumors. J. Neurosurg., 19:551–567, 1962.
30. Jain, K. K.: Intraventricular cavernous hemangioma of the lateral ventricle. Case report. J. Neurosurg., 24:762–764, 1966.
31. Jamieson, K. G.: Excision of pineal tumors. J. Neurosurg., 35:550–553, 1971.
32. Jenkins, R. D. T., Simpson, W. J. K., and Keen, C. W.: Pineal and suprasellar germinomas. Results of radiation treatment. J. Neurosurg., 48:99–107, 1978.
33. Koos, W. T., and Miller, M. H.: Intracranial tumors of infants and children. Stuttgart, Georg Thieme Verlag, 1971, p. 11.
34. Krause, F.: Operative Freilegung der Vierhügel, nebst Beobachtungen über hinndrude und Dekompression (mit Lichtbildern) Zbl. Chir., 53:2812–2819, 1926.
35. Krönlein, R. V.: Zur Pathologie und operativen Behandlung der dermoid Cysten der Orbita. Beitr. Z. Klin. Chir., 4:149–163, 1888.
36. Lampert, R., Tom, M. I., and Rider, W. D.: Disseminated demyelination of the brain following Co$_{60}$ (gamma) radiation. Arch. Path. (Chicago), 68:322–330, 1959.
37. Laws, E. R., and Kern, E. B.: Complications of trans-sphenoidal surgery. Clin. Neurosurg., 23:401–416, 1976.
38. Lloyd, L.: Gliomas of optic nerve and chiasm. Trans. Amer. Ophthal. Soc., 71:488–535, 1973.
39. Low, N. L., Correll, J. W., and Hammill, J. F.: Tumors of the cerebral hemispheres in children. Arch. Neurol. (Chicago), 13:547–554, 1965.
40. Mahaley, M. S., Gentry, R. E., and Bigner, D. D.: Immunobiology of primary intracranial tumors. The evaluation of chemotherapy and immunotherapy protocols using the avian sarcoma virus glioma model. J. Neurosurg., 47:35–43, 1977.
41. Manganiello, L. O. J., Daniel, E. F., and Hair, L. Q.: Lipoma of the corpus callosum. Case report. J. Neurosurg., 24:892–894, 1966.
42. Mannix, H., Jr., Karl, R., and Glenn, F.: Adrenalectomy for Cushing's syndrome. Amer. J. Surg., 99:449–457, 1960.
43. Martins, A. N., Johnston, J. S., Henry, J. M., Stoffel, T. J., and DiChiro, G.: Delayed radiation necrosis of the brain. J. Neurosurg., 47:336–345, 1977.
44. Matson, D. D.: Benign intracranial tumors of childhood. New Eng. J. Med., 259:330–337, 1958.
45. Matson, D. D.: Neurosurgery of Infancy and Childhood. 2nd Edition. Springfield, Ill., Charles C Thomas, 1969, p. 480.
46. Ibid: p. 523–536.
47. Ibid: p. 624.
48. Matsushima, M., Yamamoto, T., Motomochi, M., and Ando, K.: Papilloma and venous angioma of the choroid plexus causing primary intraventricular hemorrhage. J. Neurosurg., 39:666–670, 1973.
49. McKenzie, A. D., and McIntosh, H. W.: Hyperpigmentation and pituitary tumor as sequelae of the surgical treatment of Cushing's syndrome. Amer. J. Surg., 110:135–141, 1965.
50. Minagi, H., and Steinbach, H. L.: Roentgen aspects of pituitary tumors manifested after bilateral adrenalectomy for Cushing's syndrome. Radiology, 90:276–280, 1968.
51. Mori, K., Takeuchi, J., and Handa, H.: Subdural effusion and brain tumor. Surg. Neurol., 3:257–260, 1975.
52. Nelson, D. H., Meakin, J. W., Dealy, J. B., Matson, D. D., Emerson, K., and Thorn, G. W.: ACTH-producing tumor of the pituitary gland. New Eng. J. Med., 259:161–164, 1968.
53. Nilsson, E.: Origin and rationale of neuroleptanalgesia. Editorial views. Anesthesiology, 24:267–268, 1963.
54. Ortiz-Suarez, H., and Erickson, D. L.: Pituitary adenomas of adolescents. J. Neurosurg., 43:437–439, 1975.
55. Page, L. K., Lambroso, C. T., and Matson, D. D.: Childhood epilepsy with late detection of cerebral glioma. J. Neurosurg., 31:253–261, 1969.
56. Podt, J. P., DeRouck, J., and van der Eecken, H.: Intracerebral hemorrhage as initial symptom of a brain tumor. Acta Neurol. Belg., 73:241–251, 1973.
57. Poppen, J. L.: The right occipital approach to a pinealoma. J. Neurosurg., 25:706–710, 1966.
58. Russell, A.: A diencephalic syndrome of emaciation in infancy and childhood. Arch. Dis. Child., 26:274, 1951.
59. Russell, W. O., and Sachs, E.: Pinealoma: Clinicopathologic study of seven cases with a review of the literature. Arch. Path. (Chicago), 35:869–888, 1943.
60. Sato, O., Tamura, A., and Sano, K.: Brain tumors of early infants. Child's Brain, 1:121–125, 1975.
61. Schneider, R. C., and Liss, L.: Cavernous hemangiomas of the cerebral hemispheres. J. Neurosurg., 15:392–399, 1958.

62. Scott, M.: Spontaneous intracerebral hematoma caused by cerebral neoplasms. J. Neurosurg., *42*:338–342, 1975.

63. Stein, B. M.: The infratentorial supracerebellar approach to pineal lesions. J. Neurosurg., *35*:197–202, 1971.

64. Suzuki, J., and Iwabuchi, T.: Surgical removal of pineal tumors (pinealomas and teratomas). J. Neurosurg., *23*:565–571, 1965.

65. Takakura, K., Miki, Y., and Kubo, O.: Adjuvant immunotherapy for malignant brain tumors in infants and children. Child's Brain, *1*:141–147, 1975.

66. Torkildsen, A.: Should extirpation be attempted in cases of neoplasm in or near the third ventricle of the brain? J. Neurosurg., *5*:249–275, 1948.

67. de la Torre, E., Alexander, E., Jr., Davis, C. H., and Crandell, D. L.: Tumors of the lateral ventricles of the brain. Report of eight cases with suggestions for clinical management. J. Neurosurg., *20*:461–470, 1963.

68. Van der Hoeve, J.: Roentgenography of the optic foramen in tumors and diseases of the optic nerve. Amer. J. Ophthal., *8*:101–112, 1925.

69. Waga, S., and Handa, H.: Radiation-induced meningioma: With review of literature. Surg. Neurol., *5*:215–219, 1976.

70. Wilson, C.: Personal communication, 1977.

71. Withersty, D. J.: Brain tumors presenting with psychiatric symptomatology. W. Virginia Med. J., *70*:51–53, 1974.

72. Wyler, A. R., Hered, J., Smith, J. R., and Loeser, J. D.: Subarachnoid hemorrhage in infancy due to brain tumor. Arch. Neurol. (Chicago), *29*:447–448, 1973.

73. Series of brain tumors treated at The Hospital for Sick Children, Toronto, during the years 1950 to 1975.

POSTERIOR CRANIAL FOSSA BRAIN TUMORS IN CHILDREN

The management of posterior fossa tumors in children illustrates clearly the neurosurgeon's creed: "Always to comfort, often to alleviate, sometimes to cure."[56]

Intracranial neoplasms are the most common form of solid tumor that occurs in childhood. In one large children's hospital, brain tumors accounted for 25 per cent of all admissions for neoplastic diseases.[23] Among such diseases, cerebral tumors are exceeded in number only by those arising from the hematopoietic tissues.[24,31,55,61] The posterior cranial fossa contains approximately one quarter of the intracranial contents, yet in children it is the site of origin of 50 to 60 per cent of brain tumors.* The numbers cited in this chapter are derived from a study of 451 children with posterior fossa tumors, who constitute 56.7 per cent of all children with intracranial neoplasms in the group.

The posterior cranial fossa contents are cradled on all sides by bone—petrous temporals and occipital—and limited above by the tentorium. The tentorial incisura and foramen magnum are the sizable apertures at the rostral and caudal extremes of the posterior fossa through which major pathways pass and, on occasion, cerebellar tissue herniates. The congested brain stem traffic is vital and ultimately serves all other regions of the central nervous system. Despite the waterbag appearance of the cisterna magna, space in the posterior fossa is

* See references 24, 26, 31, 36, 51.

at a premium. Consequently, expansion of a subtentorial tumor is at the expense of the resident structures, and nowhere else in the nervous system can one better appreciate the aphorism "benign by histology, malignant by location."

This lack of space in which a neoplasm could expand is distressing to the children suffering from infratentorial tumors as well as to their families and the professionals caring for them. Yet the spectrum of tumors in this location encompasses both the laterally positioned benign cerebellar cystic tumor whose total removal can effect a lifetime cure and, at the other extreme, the highly malignant midline tumor that is sufficiently radiosensitive to permit a quiescent, symptom-free interval. Moreover, children, who tend to become ill quite quickly, also may improve with equal rapidity. Their marvelous but ill-defined "biological plasticity" usually permits a recovery that is better than originally anticipated.

CLINICAL PRESENTATION

The diagnosis of a posterior fossa neoplasm in a child can be accomplished at the bedside. The symptom complex is simple, almost classic, and apart from the inevitable past head injury, unburdened by other system complaints related to advancing years. Some children may keep the headache and failing vision from their parents for a considerable time until the illness becomes obvious to all.

R. P. HUMPHREYS

If the biological tempo of the symptoms is as expected, the briefer the history and the younger the child, the more rapidly growing the tumor will be. Similarly, the shorter the history, the more likely the tumor is to lie on or adjacent to the axial midline of the posterior fossa. The grouping of the appropriate symptoms and signs, like those of most other neurological disorders, is into one or more of four major categories —increased intracranial pressure, focal neurological signs, epilepsy, and meningismus.

Increased Intracranial Pressure

The symptoms of raised intracranial pressure—headache, vomiting, and double vision—are so exceedingly common in children with infratentorial tumors that they may be regarded as the hallmark for this disease. They represent the *indirect* consequences of such a tumor.

The cerebrospinal fluid channels lie in the mid-axis of the brain. Any process that obstructs circulation of the fluid not only alters this component of the intracranial contents, as implied in the Monro-Kellie doctrine, producing increased intracranial pressure, but also may do so without producing lateralizing findings. By virtue of the synergistic effects of tumor bulk and obstructed cerebrospinal fluid flow, posterior fossa or fourth ventricular tumors produce the classic features of raised intracranial pressure, also referred to as the "axial syndrome" or "midline syndrome" (Figs. 85–1 and 85–2).[48]

Headache

The *headache* pattern usually is characteristic. Beginning insidiously at first, the headache becomes more frequent and intense though not necessarily of longer duration. It is often present upon arising and may itself be the reason for early morning arousal. The antigravity effects of recumbency during sleep allegedly influence cardiac venous return and cerebrospinal fluid drainage, thereby increasing intracranial pressure and worsening its symptoms in the early morning hours. Upon arising, the child experiences relief from headache, which may dramatically abate after vomiting. There is no headache location specific

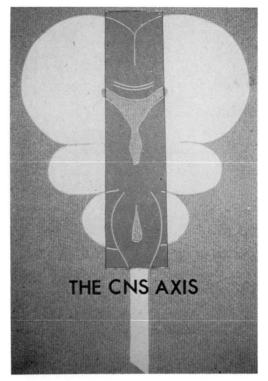

Figure 85–1　Lesions along the central nervous system axis produce the "axial syndrome" by their mass effect and obstruction of cerebrospinal fluid pathways.

for infratentorial tumor. Most children have bifrontal and bitemporal distress and many complain of occipital pain as well. The latter may blend in with neck pain and stiffness related to local meningismus.

Usually the headache is dull and throbbing, but with the passage of time it becomes sharp and intense. Regrettably, it has often been present continuously for weeks or months prior to diagnosis. One must resist the notion that children's headaches are emotional in origin or, like those in adults, of the "extracranial vascular" type; the child's complaint must be presumed to be due to an intracranial organic process until proved otherwise.

Vomiting

Vomiting frequently complements headache and may be the mechanism by which it is relieved. Presumably because of raised intracranial pressure generally, vomiting may be an intractable and relentless symptom, particularly in patients whose tumor (usually fourth ventricular ependymoma)

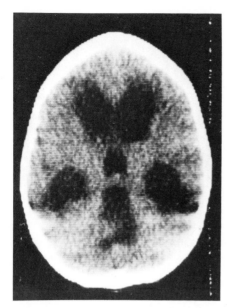

Figure 85-2 Computed tomogram. Marked hydrocephalus with dilatation of all cerebral ventricles from a fourth ventricular ependymoma. (See also Fig. 85-7.)

directly invades the floor of the fourth ventricle, compromising vagal nuclei. Eventually, the complaint claims its nutritional toll and results in weight loss, inanition, and dehydration.

Certain features distinguish this "central" form of vomiting from that related to intestinal disorders. Central vomiting usually occurs in the morning prior to or during breakfast, is not necessarily associated with warning nausea or anorexia, is forceful in nature, and frequently is associated with headache. Furthermore, upon completion of vomiting, the child often desires to finish eating.

Ocular Signs

The preceding symptoms may have been present for considerable time before the first objective evidence of increased intracranial pressure becomes apparent. When diplopia is complained of, the child's eyes are observed and show the characteristic strabismus. At last, the troubled parents can recognize an abnormality that they can demonstrate to medical personnel.

The commonest form of strabismus is related to nonlocalizing involvement of one or both abducens nerves. The result is paresis of the corresponding external rectus muscle. The child may describe the diplopia as doubled images in the horizontal plane and will show failure of lateral gaze to the affected side and perhaps a compensatory head rotation toward the involved eye.

The symptoms of the axial syndrome are common in children with posterior fossa tumors, and papilledema usually is present at the time of diagnosis. The funduscopic evaluation reveals retinal changes varying from congested, pulseless veins and pink, faintly blurred disc margins to florid disc swelling and obliteration with peripapillary hemorrhages. Unfortunately this examination often is unnecessarily delayed. Acute visual loss occasionally compounds the tragic symptom complex. When finally recognized, the papilledema galvanizes detailed neurological evaluation and investigation. As expected, the symptoms of the axial syndrome and attendant papilledema are more exaggerated with midline than with laterally positioned subtentorial tumors.[2]

Head Size

Expanding head size is an additional sign of intracranial hypertension in infants. There is nothing specific in the individual head circumference measurement, skull shape and symmetry, assessment of skull sutures, or scalp appearance to distinguish tumor-caused hydrocephalus from that due to other processes. But an infant suffering a subtentorial tumor with hydrocephalus has, historically, a skull of normal size and shape after birth. As time passes, the plotted head measurements cross growth percentiles to lie above the ninety-eighth. Infants with intracranial tumor have a disproportionate degree of anterior fontanelle enlargement and tension as contrasted with the relatively mild degree of clinical skull suture splitting.

Altered Neurological Function

The *direct* consequences of an infratentorial tumor are its effects on cerebellar nuclei and tracts and brain stem fiber bundles, cell stations, and issuing cranial nerves. For example, the clinical phenomena due to an intrinsic brain stem glioma are almost unique for this lesion and are therefore described separately.

Ataxia

The remaining mass lesions have at least a modicum of cerebellar involvement. Midline cerebellar compromise (a combination of anterior and posterior lobe involvement) accounts for truncal and gait ataxia, particularly noted in patients with medulloblastoma. The gait is broad-based and staggering or "drunken," and tandem walking is imperfectly performed. When erect, the child sways in all directions. When either standing or sitting, he may fall to the side with the lesion.[2] Yet when the child is tested in the supine position there is no abnormality of movement of the extremities.

Limb ataxia due to a defect of the timing of movement is manifested as dysmetria and dysdiadochokinesis, and usually it represents an abnormality of the cerebellar hemisphere. Often, the associated muscular hypotonia and hyporeflexia are less pronounced in children than in adults. Traditionally, ataxia of the extremities is detected in children with hemispheral cystic gliomas.

Nystagmus and Vertigo

By the time of diagnosis, tumor size, associated hydrocephalus, and connecting cerebellar tract involvement are such that nystagmus is usually present. This is to be expected, as there is little evidence for the phenomenon of isolated cerebellar nystagmus and most patients with cerebellar neoplasms who show nystagmus also have signs of brain stem involvement.[11,19] Horizontal gaze paretic nystagmus frequently is seen with lesions about the fourth ventricle. There is no unanimity of opinion regarding the lateralizing value of the fast and slow components as to tumor side.[2,11,31] On occasion, upbeat vertical nystagmus with the fast phase up and worsened by upward gaze is present in children with posterior fossa tumor.

Disabling vertigo may be associated with the nystagmus and appears to be more frequent with laterally positioned tumors.[2] The child finds all movement disturbing and prefers to lie on one side or the other, curled in the fetal position, and experiences less vertigo with the eyes closed.

Bulbar and Lower Cranial Nerve Function

Various disturbances of bulbar function may be present but apparent only when specifically searched for. The child may have difficulty swallowing, with nasal regurgitation of fluid, and impaired palatal and pharyngeal reflexes. Dysarthria characterized by speech that is slow, thick, and slurred is an inconstant feature in children with subtentorial tumors.

When the tumor breaks free of the brain stem, fourth ventricle, or cerebellum, the extra-axial portion of certain lower cranial nerves—facial, glossopharyngeal, vagal, and spinal accessory—may be enveloped by tumor and produce appropriate clinical signs.

In addition to these traditional signs of infratentorial tumor in children, characteristic disturbances of pyramidal and ascending sensory systems may result from secondary involvement of the brain stem.

Epilepsy

Epileptiform events of the classic variety seldom occur in children with posterior fossa tumors. If they do occur, then one should presume there is subarachnoid seeding of tumor (usually medulloblastoma) over the cerebral hemispheres and search for it.

"Cerebellar fits," perhaps not representative of true epilepsy, are a startling occurrence of grave prognostic significance. During such episodes, the child adopts sudden decerebrate posturing of all extremities. Opisthotonus is pronounced, consciousness is lost, respirations are slowed, and the Cushing reflex is invoked. The clinical implication usually is that acute and severe hydrocephalus has been produced by the obstructing effect of tumor bulk. Brain stem ischemia results, and the neuronal discharge likely originates in its reticular substance.[2]

Meningismus

This term usually connotes meningeal irritation due to subarachnoid blood or purulent debris. Neck stiffness, however, may also be detected in children harboring posterior fossa neoplasms. This is manifested in such children as a "fixed" neck posture when walking, a head tilt to one side, or resistance to passive neck flexion.

The posterior cranial fossa dura is innervated by ascending meningeal branches from the upper three cervical nerves, which enter the skull through the foramen magnum, jugular foramen, and hypoglossal canal.[59] The neck pain and rigidity in some children with subtentorial tumors represent dural irritation and stretch, especially at the cervicomedullary junction, by herniating cerebellar tonsils or tumor tissue.

Occasionally meningismus may manifest itself as a painful scoliosis or sciatic radiculopathy. These symptoms indicate that tumor (usually medulloblastoma or ependymoma) is spreading downward within the spinal canal.

In summary, the symptom complex of morning headache, vomiting, and diplopia is so very common in children with infratentorial tumors that almost nothing else need be considered. The presence of papilledema confirms the diagnosis. Altered cerebellar function, ocular movements, or focal cranial nerve signs are helpful in the search for tumor location. The diagnosis of subtentorial tumor whose symptoms have been present for weeks or months can be ratified with funduscopic assessment, clinical review, and computed tomography in a matter of minutes.

CONFIRMATORY STUDIES

Until recently, a surgeon could not rely upon diagnostic studies to inform him fully about the mass lesion that lurked in the posterior fossa. Consequently, the operation might be "exploratory," and accordingly the surgeon was advised to follow an orderly schema to identify and remove the neoplasm.[29] But tomographic air ventriculography and more particularly computed tomography are so astonishingly informative that the diagnosis of a posterior fossa tumor, its presence, location, and attendant phenomena, can be confirmed, though not, of course, its tissue type. A comment on orthodox radiographic studies still is justified, however.

Skull Radiography

On plain skull radiography the changes due to a subtentorial tumor usually are inferential, but this procedure should not be omitted in the preoperative evaluation of the patient. Evidence of raised intracranial pressure (most often seen as suture splitting or thinning of the occiput) may be all that is visualized on these films. But the surgeon also acquires from them a knowledge of the normal skull anatomy to assist in planning his operative approach and bony removal.

Radiopharmaceutical Brain Scanning

A persistent criticism of nuclear brain scanning is its failure to delineate posterior fossa neoplasms. In children, at least, this need not be so. The radiopharmaceutical [99m]technetium pertechnetate is administered to children in the dose of 210 μc per kilogram, and the radionuclide angiogram and blood pool images are obtained immediately and the delayed static scan two to four hours later.[21]

For suspected posterior fossa lesions, it is critical that neck flexion be sufficient to visualize the posterior fossa. Accumulations of abnormal radioactivity in this site must be confirmed in two views at right angles to each other (usually the posterior and one of the lateral views). With these provisions, the opportunity for accurately detecting a subtentorial tumor is 90 per cent or better.[21]

The astrocytoma may be exhibited in the midline or off in one hemisphere, with the amount of uptake of the radiopharmaceutical agent depending upon the grade and location of such a tumor. A medulloblastoma is usually characterized by marked tumor uptake of radiopharmaceutical in the midline of the posterior fossa, seen especially in the delayed images (Fig. 85–3). Ependymomas of the fourth ventricle are also readily detected, and tend to be associated with abnormal radioactivity ventrally in the posterior fossa, adjacent to the radioactivity of the skull base.

Air Ventriculography

Air ventriculography offers both diagnostic and therapeutic possibilities. Intracra-

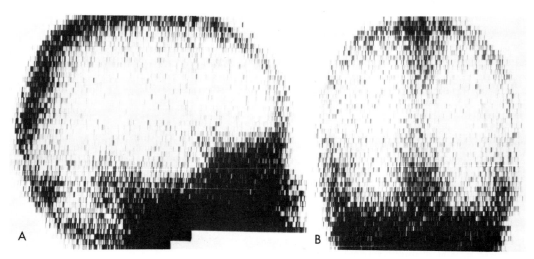

Figure 85–3 ^{99m}Technetium pertechnetate brain scan in a child with fourth ventricular medulloblastoma. *A*. Lateral view shows isolated accumulation of radiopharmaceutical beneath the tentorium and extending toward the clivus. *B*. Posterior view. The head is well flexed so that the midline radiotracer accumulation lies beneath the torcular.

nial hypertension due to hydrocephalus may be lessened immediately with the passage of a ventricular needle or catheter and removal of cerebrospinal fluid. This maneuver momentarily relieves the distressing symptoms and permits the introduction of air into the dilated ventricular system. By manipulating the head so as to get air into all four or even the first three cerebral ventricles, it is possible to assess the degree of hydrocephalus, location of the block, outline (at least partial) of the tumor, and displacements of the third and fourth ventricles and connecting aqueduct.[23]

An axial mass lesion may displace the aqueduct and fourth ventricle anteriorly if it is high in the vermis or displace the ventricle superiorly and kink the aqueduct in "dog's leg" fashion if it is positioned in the lower vermis. Hemispheric tumors will displace and rotate the aqueduct to the opposite side, and in either instance, the mass may extend into the cavity of the fourth ventricle, which expands to compensate for the tumor bulk. As air rolls along its surface, the character of the tumor, usually smooth, can be assessed (Fig. 85–4).

At operation, the surgeon is apt to work

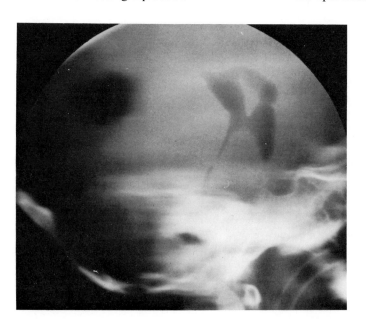

Figure 85–4 Midline tomogram, air ventriculography, lateral view. Large cystic cerebellar glioma obliterates the fourth ventricle, straightens and narrows the aqueduct, and transgresses the tentorial hiatus, indenting the posterior third ventricle.

from solid tissues to spaces—that is, from cerebellum and tumor to fourth ventricle. The ventriculogram satisfactorily outlines most of these features. The tumor size often is calculated by extrapolation, however, and the caudal limits of tumor and fourth ventricle may not be apparent.

Posterior Fossa Angiography

Vertebral angiography, particularly with subtraction views, provides artistic details of posterior fossa vasculature, but usually it adds little to the operative and prognostic management of a child's posterior fossa tumor. Angiography will outline cerebellar tonsillar herniation, and perhaps the fine vascular "blush" of an ependymoma or medulloblastoma, or the solid nodule of a cerebellar astrocytoma. Occasionally, alterations of the deep venous system noted on cerebral arteriography indicate upward herniation of tumor through the tentorial hiatus. Except for choroid plexus papilloma, there is no subtentorial tumor for which the surgeon must have a precise knowledge of its blood supply preoperatively. Hence, vertebral angiography is not the procedure of choice to investigate subtentorial tumors.

Computed Tomography

Virtually all neurosurgeons have experienced the impact of computed tomography (CT) on their treatment programs for a variety of central nervous sytem disorders. In a practical sense, at least, this procedure, by virtue of its simplicity and accuracy, renders obsolete all other traditional methods of investigation for the child with a posterior fossa tumor.

Almost any child presenting with symptoms characteristic of a posterior fossa tumor may undergo computed tomography quickly, painlessly, and usually without need for general anesthesia. The speculative discussions with parents, formerly required prior to ventriculography or angiography, are circumvented. Instead, the clinician can engage in an intelligent dialogue with relatives and provide details of the tumor's location and the probabilities as to its type. The treatment program can be staged, and the surgeon can decide on whether further investigations are required. It is anticipated that in the future more surgeons will operate solely on the basis of information provided by the CT scan.

As with radionuclide studies of the posterior fossa, a well-flexed head and low first CT section are vital to visualization of con-

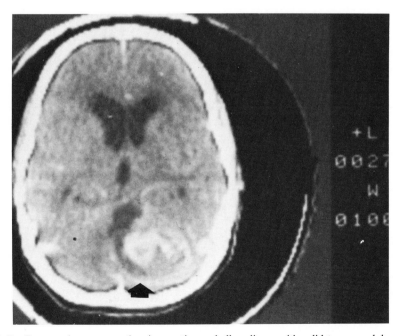

Figure 85–5 Computed tomogram showing cystic cerebellar glioma with solid tumor nodule medial and superior, capsule outline (*arrow*), and proximal hydrocephalus.

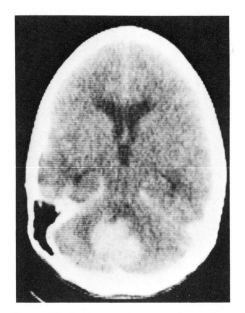

Figure 85–6 Computed tomography, enhanced view of fourth ventricular medulloblastoma.

tents in this region.[23] The unenhanced views of the cystic cerebellar glioma will show the cyst cavity with relatively low absorption factors as well as the nodule and associated perinodular edema (Fig. 85–5). Contrast enhancement more clearly details

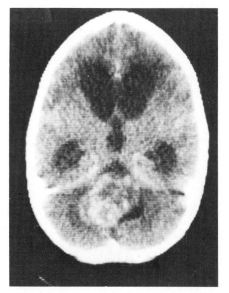

Figure 85–7 Computed tomography, enhanced view of fourth ventricular ependymoma. (Same child as shown in Figure 85–2.)

the nodular and cystic outlines. The appearance of a medulloblastoma on standard computed tomography may be disappointingly nonspecific, but the addition of contrast allows definition of the tumor because of a moderate increase in absorption factors (Fig. 85–6). Similarly, fourth ventricular ependymomas are well enhanced by contrast (Fig. 85–7).

The surgeon cannot distinguish the foregoing tumors one from another, as all may occur essentially in the axial line or all may spread from the midline laterally into one cerebellar hemisphere. The presence of the tumor and its geography are confirmed, and also the size and involvement of the fourth ventricle, proximal hydrocephalus, and associated tumor features such as edema, calcification, and hemorrhage are illustrated.

TREATMENT

Almost without exception, the posterior fossa tumor manifests itself in intracranial hypertension or an altered focal neurological state or both. In many circumstances the child is obviously or even critically ill by the time the clinical diagnosis is established. Seldom, therefore, is there any question concerning the necessity for operative treatment to relieve intracranial pressure and altered neurological function.

The immediate relief of intracranial hypertension can be achieved by decompression of the obstructed cerebrospinal fluid pathways. This is accomplished directly by tumor removal or indirectly by a diversionary shunting device. At whatever stage the operation proceeds, the acknowledged aims of tumor exploration are to identify its site, extent, and tissue type. The amazing resolution of computed tomography provides astonishing architectural details of tumor location, components, and relation to the ventricular system. Operative exploration will detail the geography further by revealing the tumor's relationship to upper cervical and lower cranial nerves, posterior inferior cerebellar arteries, and cervicomedullary junction, and most of all the insidious infiltration by tumor of the cerebellar peduncles and floor of the fourth ventricle. With this knowledge, the surgeon can then plan the extent of tumor removal to be accomplished.

Preliminary Cerebrospinal Fluid Shunting

Usually the child with a posterior fossa tumor is acutely ill and miserable with headache and vomiting. Often he presents at an awkward hour. The neurological interrogation and examination, and confirmatory computed tomography will provide an answer within a few hours of hospital admission. The surgeon's decision at this stage is whether to proceed with posterior fossa exploration immediately, temporize for a brief interval before semiurgent tumor operation, or institute an immediate effective procedure to decompress the obstructed cerebrospinal fluid pathways. The last is highly recommended as a first step in the care of a child with a posterior fossa mass.

The cerebrospinal fluid diversion can be achieved by means of an external drainage system. Because of technical and bacteriological considerations, however, it is of temporary value only. Consequently, the internal ventriculoperitoneal shunt is recommended for the following reasons: (1) It provides *immediate* and *controlled* relief of intracranial hypertension and its distressing symptoms. The disappearance of headache and vomiting can be dramatic, much to the pleasure of the child and his relatives. (2) It substantially (though not totally) improves the trunk and gait ataxia. (3) It provides relief from anorexia and permits improved nutrition prior to major operation to remove the tumor. (4) It converts an urgent tumor operation to a planned elective procedure. During the interval, appropriate drug and other support therapy can be instituted, and the family can be counseled at leisure. (5) It insures relaxation of the posterior fossa structures at the time of tumor operation, thereby permitting innocuous retraction of normal cerebellar tissue. (6) It provides a "margin of safety" during the first several postoperative days, protecting the patient from obstructive hydrocephalus related to swelling in the tumor bed or adjacent cerebellum.

There has been recent confirmation that pre–tumor removal shunting improves patient care. The report by Albright and Reigel convincingly states that treatment of the associated hydrocephalus by means of ventriculoperitoneal shunting significantly lowers the morbidity and mortality rates associated with the subsequent tumor removal.[1] Critics of the procedure have worried that shunting might promote the metastatic spread of tumor. This certainly is an argument against placing the distal end of the shunt system within the heart. But the risk of tumor dissemination is still small and can be lessened further by the addition of a tiny Millipore filtering chamber.[25]

An alternative choice of shunt, the ventriculocisternal shunt, is not appropriate for patients with fourth ventricular tumors. Apart from the technical inconvenience of having shunt tubing passing over or by the tumor, the shunt directs cerebrospinal fluid to a region where it had best not gather. That is, the patency of the lower end of the system (even if placed within the cervical subarachnoid canal) cannot be assured following operation, irradiation, or further tumor growth. Furthermore, cerebrospinal fluid is rerouted to the region of the suboccipital wound, potentially threatening its healing.

Interval Adjuncts of Therapy

The protection provided by the insertion of a bypass shunt allows a 5- to 14-day interval before the electively scheduled posterior fossa tumor operation. Obviously, the child whose tumor is unaccompanied by hydrocephalus can be operated upon at an earlier time. But the waiting period for children who have the shunt offers time to reconcile certain problems so that the child and family are properly prepared for operation.

Well-Being and Nutrition

After a shunt has been placed, the improvement in vomiting and headache promotes the child's sense of well-being. Though somewhat tender at the shunt wound site, the child is able to satisfy his appetite without upset and to become mobile again and assume surety of gait. He recognizes that, in addition to his parents, an increasingly familiar medical team is concerned about his problem. Because of this support, the child is not necessarily disappointed by the news of a second and more serious operative procedure.

Corticosteroid Therapy

While dexamethasone is more effective against the cerebral edema associated with metastatic tumors or glioblastoma, it is also of value in treatment of more benign tumors and those of the posterior fossa.[49] Its action is complex. As corticosteroids interfere with the chain reaction of cellular destruction by stablizing cell membranes, there is ultimately less leakage of fluids, electrolytes, and protein into ground-substance,[17] As it does not just act "after the fact," corticosteroid protection is offered preoperatively to all the author's patients undergoing posterior fossa tumor operation. Dexamethasone therapy begins 48 hours prior to operation and continues for approximately seven days postoperatively in doses of 4 mg every six hours. Simultaneous administration of an antacid minimizes the potential for gastric ulceration.

Family Counseling

The news of a child's brain tumor diagnosis is never easy for the parents to accept. A paramedical support team aids immeasurably in dealing with the distressed family in these trying moments. A social worker and senior neurosurgical nurse, present with the surgeon during the preoperative discussions with the family and then again immediately after the operation, can reinforce the surgeon's words and advice. The neurosurgical nurse will better understand the parents' problems and reactions to illness and, because of the team concept, will be more confident in speaking to them and answering their questions. The parents in turn are strengthened and respond by trusting the nursing staff. The social worker's intrinsic function is to deal closely with the parents and to listen to their concerns at a time when basic emotions are expressed. Since other team members have been present at all discussions, the surgeon and resident staff are not the only persons who understand the situation, and they will have less need to devote time to repeated family demands. In using this type of team approach the surgeon is not abdicating his responsibility in these matters but, rather, disseminating information so that answers to the myriad questions (many of them repetitive) are more readily available. Parents gain the most from this approach, as they are supported by many people who are interested in them and their family problems. Communication between physician and parent ultimately is clearer.

Anesthesia for Posterior Fossa Tumor Operation

A skilled anesthetist adds immeasurably to the safe conduct of the posterior fossa operation. He provides smooth anesthetic induction, placement of monitoring lines, controlled ventilation, propitious blood administration, vital sign assessments, and rapid extubation upon completion of the operation to permit early bedside evaluation of the patient.

Atropine sulfate (0.02 mg per kilogram) is administered simultaneously with induction with intravenous thiopental (4.5 mg per kilogram) and succinylcholine (1 mg per kilogram) before nasotracheal intubation. Operation is performed with the child prone, positioned on a metal support frame that permits free excursion of the abdomen (Fig. 85–8).[28] The cranium is immobilized in a Mayfield or Gardner headholder. Patients are monitored with an endoesophageal stethoscope, blood pressure cuff, radial artery Doppler ultrasonic flow detector with electrocardiograph, and rectal thermistor. Prior to transfer from the anesthetic stretcher to the operating table, the patient's eyes are treated with sterile ointment and taped shut, and the whole face is covered with a piece of adhesive foam rubber padding. A urinary catheter may be inserted if mannitol is to be administered, though hyperosmotic therapy is not usually required during a tumor operation if a shunt system has been placed previously.

While spontaneous respiration may be employed throughout the operation, controlled ventilation with nitrous oxide (66 per cent) and halothane (0.5 per cent) anesthesia is safe and offers many advantages. It promotes venous return and diminishes ventricular cerebrospinal fluid pressure, thereby decreasing both Pa_{CO_2} and Pco_2 in tissue and cerebrospinal fluid.[41] In addition blood loss tends to be lessened. The surgeon, dissecting along the floor of the fourth ventricle, need not regret the loss of monitoring of the spontaneous respiratory pattern when the patient is mechanically venti-

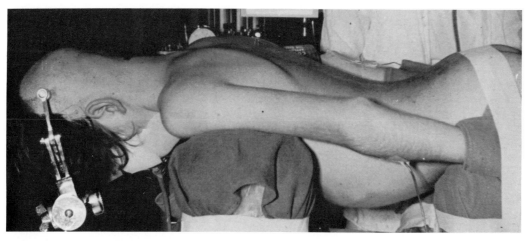

Figure 85–8   Prone positioning on four-support frame for operation on the posterior cranial fossa. Abdomen must lie free. (From Humphreys, R. P., Creighton, R. E., Hendrick, E. B., and Hoffman, H. J.: Advantages of the prone position for neurosurgical procedures on the upper cervical spine and posterior cranial fossa in children. Child's Brain, *1*:325–336, 1975. Reprinted by permission.)

lated. Compromise of vital centers can be detected just as early from cardiac arrhythmias on the continuous electrocardiograph.[28]

Accurate measurements of blood loss are difficult to obtain in most circumstances. The anesthetist can rely instead on systolic blood pressure monitoring, with blood given to maintain the systolic pressure at 70 mm of mercury in infants and 80 mm of mercury in older children. After the operation is completed and before muscle closure is begun, enough blood is administered to return the systolic pressure to preloss value. An additional 10 per cent of the estimated blood volume is then given during the closure.[40]

Operative Technique
for Posterior Fossa Exploration

The prone positioning of the patient for a posterior fossa operation is recommended, especially since controlled ventilation can be safely employed throughout.[28] The position is easily obtained. Once anesthetized, the patient is transferred from the anesthetic stretcher to the support frame with one simple roll. The monitoring devices are then placed. There is no fear that the child will be displaced (downward) during the operative exploration. As surface heat loss is especially critical in the neonate and small infant, intraoperative hypothermia is con-

trolled by heating pads or blankets or both. These can be applied to both the ventral and dorsal body surfaces of the prone patient. The worrisome threat of air embolism is minimized in the prone position, particularly in infants and young children with exceedingly vascular occipital bone and extensive ill-defined dural venous sinuses.

Working with the patient prone, the surgeon enjoys the same depth of field to which he is accustomed for supratentorial craniotomies. He may experience less neck, shoulder, and upper arm fatigue than he tends to when operating on the suboccipital region with the patient in a sitting position. Because of the excellent relaxation of brain and the controlled venous pressure that hyperventilation provides, venous ooze is not a major problem. Removal of spinal fluid is seldom difficult, since either the cerebrospinal fluid pathway is obstructed by the tumor and little of the fluid is present in the posterior fossa or the cerebrospinal fluid spaces have been decompressed by a bypass shunt. In some posterior fossa explorations, the operating microscope is employed. When the patient is positioned prone, both the surgeon and the assistant sit throughout the microdissection, each taking advantage of binocular eyepiece tubes and sharing equal territorial and visual rights.

With the patient rolled prone, the surgeon should assume personal responsibility for the positioning of the head and neck, and should select the right degree of neck flexion, bearing in mind airway stability and potential interference with cardiac venous return. The head and neck positioning should be such that an imaginary line drawn from the inion to the vertebra prominens would run parallel to the floor. This imaginary line marks the site, though not necessarily the extent, of the skin incision. For all but the most eccentric angle tumors, a vertical midline skin incision and axial bone removal will be sufficient to visualize and dissect the posterior fossa tumor. The suboccipital craniectomy need not be carried above the level of the transverse venous sinuses unless there is evidence the tumor passes upward through the tentorial hiatus. Similarly, more lateralized occipital bony removal will be required for cerebellar hemisphere tumors. In virtually all circumstances, the foramen magnum is removed. Whether or not it is necessary to excise the laminae of the atlas and axis is determined during operation by the presence of tumor or cerebellar tonsils or both within the upper cervical canal. This upper cervical laminectomy usually is required in patients with fourth ventricular medulloblastomas and ependymomas.

The method of dural opening is dictated by tumor location and personal preference. A limited lateral dural incision over the hemisphere may be sufficient to gain access to the cerebellar glioma; many of these tumors, however, encroach upon the midline structures at some point, and therefore visualization of this region also is desirable. Consquently, the orthodox Y-shaped dural opening is adequate in most circumstances. Because computed tomography is the best means of monitoring the postoperative course of a patient with a subtentorial tumor, and because of the streaking artifact on tomography produced by metallic hemostatic clips, the surgeon is advised to employ bipolar coagulation on the occipital and marginal venous sinuses.

At this juncture, magnified vision is of great value. The operating diploscope, however, has not proved to be as flexible as expected for posterior fossa tumor operations. Even when working at six times magnification, the surgeon easily loses sight of normal peripheral structures and may find himself working in the center of a bleeding tumor. Consequently the diploscope is re-

served for intra-axial brain stem tumor procedures in which 10 and 16 times magnification defines precise incision and biopsy. Otherwise, 3.5 or 4.5 times magnifying loupes and illumination with a fiberoptic headlight bring all the operative details (both normal and diseased) clearly into focus and allow the surgeon to move from side to side to gain dissecting advantage.

The surgeon needs to *know all details concerning the forth ventricle*. At all times, he should be aware of the position of the obex and the floor and lateral walls of the ventricle so that his tumor operation, proceeding inevitably in a centripetal direction to the ventricle, will not harm its components. Thus, if the obex has not been obliterated by tumor (usually the circumstance only with ependymomas arising from the cervicomedullary junction), it can be found, and cottonoids can then be passed along the floor of the ventricle for its further identification and protection. This maneuver also brings the posterior inferior cerebellar arteries into view, and they too can be appropriately protected. Their relationship to tumor bulk can also be studied.

The midline tumor may have burst through the cerebellar vermis or may require an incision in this structure for identification. Retraction of the cerebellum and dissection around the tumor can each be gently conducted with the Penfield dissectors or similar instruments. Bipolar coagulation is used throughout to sacrifice vessels entering tumor substance, and if suction dissection is necessary, it is efficiently handled with a combined suction and coagulating unit. The dorsal margin of an ependymoma or medulloblastoma is readily obtained; it is the deeper portions of these tumors that surreptitiously invade para–fourth ventricular structures. Quick section analysis of the tumor at this stage will distinguish between these two lesions and determine just how aggressive the subsequent operation should be. The medulloblastoma, for example, is often circumscribed and can be detached from its loose adherence to the floor of the ventricle. It may, however, be far more difficult to define its penetration of the cerebellar peduncles. At some point with either the medulloblastoma or ependymoma, internal decompression of the tumor will be required. If one has an idea of the size of the tumor sphere and its relationship to the ventricle, then one can begin working within the tumor perimeter, removing its contents by suction or a cutting loop. Bleeding will not stop until most of the tumor tissue has been removed. It can be lessened in children, though, by means of induced hypotension to systolic levels of 60 to 80 mm of mercury. Hypotension can be rapidly initiated by the administration of trimethaphan as a drip infusion. A combination of this agent and halothane 0.5 to 1.0 per cent is usually sufficient to maintain hypotension until tumor excision. A return to normal pressure levels is required before dural and wound closure. As tumor bulk diminishes, particularly in an ependymoma, the union between tumor and fourth ventricle floor becomes apparent. In such circumstances further tumor removal, if possible, must be judiciously performed.

Exploration of a brain stem glioma requires a vermian split and visualization of the whole floor of the fourth ventricle. Discoloration and loss of surface markings will guide the choice of site for aspiration and biopsy. The congenital or embryonic tumors (epidermoid, dermoid) must be kept intact while one follows the dermal sinus to the tumor and then attempts its total removal. Total removal is also the objective for cerebellar hemangioblastoma and uncomplicated choroid plexus papilloma.

While prone positioning of the child tends to minimize the problem, bleeding from torn superior cerebellar veins may be a nuisance during an operation for tumor. The cerebellar veins drain mainly into the adjacent venous sinuses, and those related to the transverse sinus are readily identified.[59] But those veins on the anterior and superior margin of the cerebellar hemisphere enter the great cerebral vein or proximal straight sinus, and are often excluded from the surgeon's view. Rupture of these veins may occur when the surgeon is working out in the hemisphere and has rapidly decompressed and mobilized hemispheral substance by either tumor removal or release of cystic fluid. Suddenly, venous blood flows down from the superior cerebellar surface. The surgeon should identify the tentorium and proceed along its undersurface to the site of maximal bleeding, which in turn is packed with gelatin sponge. In time, this maneuver provides adequate

hemostasis. One is also advised to search the lateral and anterior subdural spaces for formed clot, especially if cerebellar tissue begins to herniate into the wound.

At the completion of the tumor operation, the sylvian aqueduct and fourth ventricle have been at least partially cleared, and cerebrospinal fluid wells into the wound. Despite one's intentions, posterior fossa dural closure often proves frustrating. It should be attempted in patients whose benign tumors have been resected. In other circumstances, the dura can be left open and covered with gelatin sponge, and a meticulous closure of muscle, fascia, and skin can be made.

Postoperative Care and Complications

Before the child leaves the operating room, he should have been extubated, be breathing spontaneously, and demonstrate stability of the vital signs. These early baseline observations serve as a guide to further postoperative care and the management of certain complications related to the posterior fossa tumor operation.

Bleeding

As with tumor operation anywhere in the central nervous system, postoperative hemorrhage is possible, though less likely when the operation was performed with the surgeon's vision magnified. Magnification forces one to respect intracranial tissue and stanch even trivial sites of bleeding. A complicating clot, should it arise, announces its presence with rapid deterioration of consciousness and respiratory arrest.

Cerebral Edema

If a child recovers fully and rapidly from anesthesia, only to deteriorate quickly in the next several hours, he has suffered postoperative hemorrhage or local tissue edema. The surgeon distinguishes between the two by reopening the wound. Faced only with complicating edema, he must dedicate himself to antiedema treatment and basic life support (e.g., ventilatory) measures. With prompt treatment, he can properly expect that, as the child recovered once, he will do so again after the edema has spent itself—usually in five to seven days.

A much more difficult problem is that encountered when a child fails to recover from anesthesia following subtentorial tumor operation. While acute edema may be the explanation, it is also possible that brain stem ischemia or infarction occurred during the operation.

A more benign type of symptomatic tissue response may be seen about the fifth postoperative day, or if radiation treatment has been initiated, at a point 10 to 14 days into that program. In either circumstance, the child becomes more subdued, mildly lethargic, and experiences a return of anorexia and vomiting. The events often coincide with reduction of dexamethasone supplementation, and the symptoms are reversed by resuming full dosage of this medication for three to five days.

Compromise of Cranial Nerves and Their Connections

The patient and family should be cautioned that cranial nerve signs, most commonly abducens and facial, related to the tumor may be transiently worsened following the operation and, in any event, will not clear for a considerable time. Moreover, new signs may appear. These include difficulty in swallowing, nystagmus that is not subjectively distressing, and vertigo that is subjectively distressing. A skilled nurse or physician should be present when the child attempts to swallow fluids postoperatively. During this effort, the patient should lie with the "undamaged" side down. Care must be taken to avoid aspiration.

Aseptic Meningitis

Some children, usually at the fifth to seventh postoperative day, develop symptoms suggestive of purulent meningitis. Often these children have cerebellar astrocytomas and are without associated hydrocephalus. Fever, malaise, neck stiffness and tenderness, and bulging of the operative wound are all worrisome features.[7] The cerebrospinal fluid cell response (initially polymorphonuclear and then mononuclear cells), and lowered sugar and exaggerated protein contents further suggest meningitis, but no microorganism is identified following lumbar puncture. This aseptic leptomeningeal inflammation allegedly relates to the admixture of cerebrospinal fluid, blood, glioma cyst contents, and ooze from the raw cervical muscle bed. In its mildest form, the syndrome may reverse itself spontaneously; in other circumstances repeated lumbar punctures and increased doses of dexamethasone are recommended. About 20 per cent of these children subsequently demonstrate frank evidence of communicating hydrocephalus.[53]

Hydrocephalus

Patients who, prior to tumor removal, have received ventriculoperitoneal shunts have dual protection against *obstructive* hydrocephalus following tumor operation. Their cerebrospinal fluid pathways have been disimpacted of tumor, and presumably the shunt system still functions following the posterior fossa exploration. Under these circumstances, obstructive hydrocephalus usually is not a problem.

Communicating hydrocephalus may persist in some children who have experienced early aseptic meningitis. If lumbar punctures fail to alleviate the symptoms of the former, and wound bulging and discomfort persist, then either a ventriculoperitoneal or lumboperitoneal shunt system will be required.

CEREBELLAR ASTROCYTOMA

It is appropriate to follow Matson's dictum, "the child with increased intracranial pressure and evidence of a mass lesion below the tentorium is more likely to have a benign astrocytoma than a medulloblastoma."[35] Thus, the surgeon should be aggressive with treatment, as "the cerebellar astrocytoma offers the best prognosis for normal survival of any brain tumor in any age group."[35] The statement might be altered slightly in view of findings in the Vienna series and the Hospital for Sick Children series in which the statistical division between cerebellar astrocytoma and medulloblastoma is no better than even (Table 85–1).[31]

In 1959, William German, reviewing the Cushing glioma series, said in regard to cerebellar astrocytomas, ". . . we still think kindly of these tumors from a prog-

Table 85–1 POSTERIOR CRANIAL FOSSA TUMORS IN CHILDREN*

EXTRADURAL AND DURAL (9)

Dermoid	5
Chordoma	3
Meningioma	1

CEREBELLAR HEMISPHERE (123)

Astrocytoma: grades I and II	98
Grade III	7
Grade IV	5
Mixed glioma	2
Giant cell tumor	1
Medulloblastoma—desmoplastic	6
Ganglioglioma	1
Hemangioblastoma	1
Unverified	1
Other (metastasis)	1

VERMIS (116)

Medulloblastoma	99
Desmoplastic	4
Astrocytoma: grades I and II	1
Grade III	0
Grade IV	0
Mixed glioma	3
Dermoid	8
Unverified	1

FOURTH VENTRICLE (62)

Ependymoma	44
Ependymoblastoma	14
Choroid plexus papilloma	3
Astrocytoma: grades I and II	1

BRAIN STEM (127)

Astrocytoma: grades I and II	28
Grade III	17
Grade IV	20
Ganglioglioma	2
Unverified	60

CEREBELLOPONTINE ANGLE (8)

Schwannoma	7
Ependymoma	1

TRANSGRESSING TUMORS (6)

Mesenchymoma	2
Leptomeningeal Melanoma	3
Chordoma	1

* Twenty-five-year review (1950–1975) of all intracranial tumors at The Hospital for Sick Children, Toronto, yielded 344 supratentorial neoplasms and 451 posterior fossa tumors, which are classified here.

nostic standpoint, and hope we are not just whistling in the dark. If you occasionally share this uncertainty, the present results should supply the light and allow the whistling to continue.''[20] Two decades later, this sentiment is still applicable.

The cerebellar astrocytoma can arise in either hemisphere or the vermis, and may be entirely solid, almost entirely monocystic, or have a combination of solid and microcystic elements. The solid tumor is homogeneous in color and consistency, and if it forms a small nodule in a larger cystic tumor, the nodule is frequently located in the superior and medial quadrant of the tumor. The cyst is filled with proteinaceous golden fluid and surrounded by a wall consisting of poorly cellular, often degenerated tumor or a layer of reactive, nonneoplastic cerebellar tissue. Most cerebellar astrocytomas are classified as grade I despite a microscopic appearance that may vary from field to field. Compact areas of polar or fusiform fibrillated cells may alternate with microcystic regions composed of stellate astrocytes. While certain vascular endothelial changes may imply a higher grading, there is almost complete absence of mitotic figures.[50] Frankly malignant forms, fulfilling the criteria for glioblastoma multiforme, have been encountered in the cerebellum in the present series and in others.[18,35]

The lateralizing tendency (location of the tumor in one hemisphere) is accompanied by classic ipsilateral cerebellar disturbances of long standing. After the diagnosis has been all but confirmed with computed tomography, the surgeon should attempt total excision by suboccipital craniectomy, which is the treatment of choice for this neoplasm. When the dura is opened, the involved hemisphere is noted to be swollen, with compressed, pale folia despite prior use of a shunt, dexamethasone, and controlled ventilation. There will be no relief of the local tension until an aspirating needle is passed into the cyst and the yellow fluid is partially released. Following a cortical incision, the surgeon can identify the cyst wall, which is still distended by the remaining fluid, and begin to work around its perimeter in the softened layer of reactive cerebellar tissue. While it is ideal to remove the tumor intact, there are fragile sites in the tumor wall and sometimes it shreds and the cyst contents leak. If the nodule can be located, further effort should then be concentrated on its total removal (Fig. 85–9). If the tumor is entirely solid, the principles of operation are those established for removal of solid fourth ventricular tumors. There is no requirement for radiation therapy after radical operation for cerebellar astrocytoma of grades I or II.[35,50] In the Cushing era, 78 per cent of patients with cerebellar astrocytomas survived at least five years, and more recently this success rate has been bettered to 85 per cent.[20,31,36] If symptoms and signs return years after the original tumor diagnosis and treatment, it may be necessary to re-explore the lesion for drainage of the cyst.

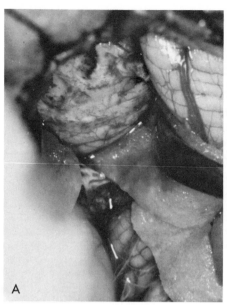
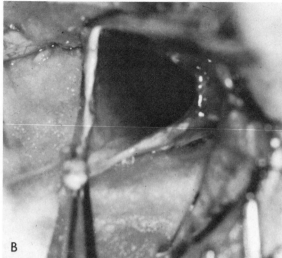

Figure 85-9 Cystic cerebellar glioma arising within the vermis. *A*. Cyst contents have been partially aspirated before excision of capsule begins. *B*. Cyst cavity has been entered and drained to facilitate identification of mural nodule and total tumor excision.

MEDULLOBLASTOMA

The dismal reputation of the cerebellar medulloblastoma as the most malignant of all brain neoplasms is deserved. As an embryonic tumor, its biological aggressiveness is associated with abbreviated clinical phenomena. But its radiosensitivity, particularly when programs of homogeneous central nervous system axis irradiation are administered, results in less gloomy patient survival rates than those originally quoted.[36,44] The treatment protocols elaborated by the current Children's Cancer Study Group may further influence medulloblastoma treatment and improve survival figures even more.

As there is no identifiable "medulloblast" cell, the tumor must originate instead from primitive cells in the neuroepithelial roof of the fourth ventricle. Such cells are destined to migrate laterally, ultimately constituting a portion of the external granular layer of the cerebellar cortex. This thesis logically explains the preponderant location of the childhood medulloblastoma within the cerebellar midline, as opposed to the less common adult tumor often located laterally over the hemisphere.[50] Tumor growth begins within the inferior medullary velum, and its sphere takes advantage of the adjacent cavity of the fourth ventricle, which it may occupy. The grayish-purple tumor substance can entirely fill this chamber, dilating it simultaneously, and because of the mechanical obstruction to the flow of cerebrospinal fluid within this ventricle and the coincident aqueduct distortion, produce hydrocephalus. Tongues of neoplastic tissue may extend up the sylvian aqueduct and laterally into the cerebellopontine recesses via the foramina of Luschka or spill from the obex dorsally over the cervicomedullary junction. This neoplasm does not usually directly invade the floor of the fourth ventricle, though it may caress its surface, from which it can often be separated by operative microdissection. There may, however, be insidious infiltration of the floor structures via one or more of the cerebellar peduncles. Definition of the tumor within these structures and the degree of indirect involvement of the brain stem provide the most taxing moments during its removal. The tumor usually thins out and broadens the vermis, and splays apart the cerebellar hemispheres. With this potential for rapid and extensive centrifugal growth, the medulloblastoma may be immediately apparent upon dural incision and reflection. If not, it comes into view with elevation or incision of the vermis. The surface is often crisscrossed with vascular strands, many of which enter the tumor directly and can be sacrificed. Consistency varies from one tumor to another and, occasionally, within any single tumor. Most have a moist granular texture described appropriately as "thick cream of wheat."[31] But other variations include tough, leathery, homogeneous tissue, cavities with old hemorrhage, or even areas of microcystic degeneration. Most tumors are quite vascular.

A medulloblastoma is composed of a monotony of irregularly arranged sheets of small round to oval cells. These cells possess the unique ability to spread with ease throughout the subarachnoid space of the cranium and spinal canal, where they may form metastases and coalesce into diffuse sheets of subarachnoid tumor. More than any other primary intracranial neoplasm, the medulloblastoma has gained the reputation for dissemination beyond the neural axis, to skeleton and other system cavities or viscera. In a minority of instances this dissemination has allegedly been promoted by the implanted bypass cerebrospinal fluid shunt.[25,30,34] Cerebellar sarcoma is not regarded as a distinct histological entity. The term refers to a medulloblastoma, usually present over one cerebellar hemisphere, with leptomeningeal involvement and microscopic features of reticulin-free islands and lobules, and has therefore been called a desmoplastic variant.[50]

The child with a medulloblastoma is more apt to be a boy between the ages of 5 and 8 years. Otherwise the general features of the "axial syndrome" are present. The biological aggressiveness of the tumor is characterized by a short history; in some instances the symptoms have been present only for four to six weeks. The clinical features are those of truncal ataxia without appendicular ataxia. The neck may be stiff on forward flexion.

The treatment of cerebellar medulloblastoma consists of operative removal of tumor tissue followed by postoperative radiation therapy. Operative exploration offers many solutions. Even with enhanced computed tomography, the distinction cannot be made between a midline cerebellar medulloblastoma and an ependymoma or solid cerebellar glioma. Posterior cranial fossa exploration therefore provides histological confirmation of neoplasm type and assists in ultimate tumor staging in terms of the lesion's size and the nature of local metastasis.[9] Radical removal of tumor bulk decreases intracranial hypertension, promotes reopening of cerebrospinal fluid pathways, lessens compression of adjacent cerebellar structures, and assists in the subsequent radiation program directed at the tumor that remains.[60] While most surgeons would favor radical removal of the tumor, it may not be possible if the tumor is spread diffusely throughout the subarachnoid space of the posterior fossa or invades the ventricular floor. The operative mortality rate (death in the first month following operation) varies from 10 to 33 per cent.[15,31] Some argue that this mortality rate is inversely proportional to the amount of tumor tissue that is removed, whereas others state that "radical or subtotal resection of the tumor or simple biopsy had no significant association with the surgical mortality."[39,44,60]

The postoperative radiation program for cerebellar medulloblastoma has been changing constantly since its inception in 1919. Understandably, small doses of radiation directed at the tumor site were used initially. With the passage of time, radiation dosage has increased to the extent that now children who have fared the best may have received doses approaching 5000 rads to the brain and 4000 rads to the spinal axis.[39] Radiation programs have become more homogeneous to take into account the propensity of a medulloblastoma to seed throughout the central nervous system axis. Currently, the brain, spinal axis, and posterior cranial fossa are irradiated; for example, the regimen under study by the Children's Cancer Study Group advocates 3500 to 4000 rads to the entire axis, and 1000 to 1500 rads to the posterior cranial fossa. Adjuvant chemotherapy has for the most part been reserved for patients with recurrent disease. Controlled studies are at present examining the value of vincristine, CCNU, procarbazine, and prednisone as part of the *initial* treatment plan.

Matson's original prediction that most children with medulloblastoma "die within two years of diagnosis" can now be altered because of improved wide radiation treatment programs.[36] A five-year survival of 40 to 77 per cent of patients treated has been reported.[5,9,27,39] To be cautious, one could predict that 50 per cent of children with medulloblastoma treated by contemporary techniques may be expected to survive the first three postoperative years at least. Whether chemotherapy can enhance this rate remains to be seen. As medulloblastoma is regarded as an embryonic tumor, the survival figures have been subjected to the predictions of Collins' law.[12] A patient with such a tumor is "at risk" during a period of time equivalent to his age at the time of diagnosis plus nine months. In 1969, McFarland and co-workers, conducting a literature review of cerebellar medulloblastoma, claimed that the cure rate for this tumor is 25 per cent if Collins' law applies.[38] Furthermore, one might expect a corollary of the law to state that the younger the patient, the worse the prognosis. Study of this thesis suggests that the clinician can expect a patient over the age of 10 years at the time of diagnosis to survive at least twice as long as one under that age.[10,42]

The problem of tumor recurrence at the primary site has in the past been clouded by the possibility that recurrence of symptoms might in fact be due to postoperative hydrocephalus or irradiation change. Now, it can be anticipated that a patient presenting with signs and symptoms similar to those encountered originally will have confirmation of tumor recurrence by computed tomography. The treatment program for recurrence within 12 months of first diagnosis may be restricted to adjuvant chemotherapy. If recurrence appears at the original site 12 months or more after completion of initial irradiation, the posterior fossa could be irradiated again up to a dose of 3000 R in 15 to 18 fractions. The radiotherapist and surgeon will have to decide about the wisdom of further operative removal of tumor bulk that might enhance the effectiveness of radiotherapy. A supratentorial recurrence at a single site after 12 or more months, when the primary location within the posterior fossa remains normal, requires operative extirpation and reirradiation to a dose of 4000 R. Spinal cord relapse 12 or more months after initial irradiation can also be treated with reirradiation to a dose of 4000 R. It is a moot point whether prior myelography or laminectomy adds significantly to the diagnosis and posttherapeutic recovery.

In summary, the suffering experienced by a child with cerebellar medulloblastoma can be immediately and effectively relieved by a cerebrospinal fluid bypass shunt. Radi-

cal tumor removal with modern operative aids carries a mortality rate of approximately 10 per cent, and when followed by homogeneous central nervous system axis irradiation should provide a three-year quality survival rate of 50 per cent and a five-year survival rate of approximately 40 per cent. Nonetheless, one should still be cautious about predicting that a patient is cured of this disease.

EPENDYMOMA

The fourth ventricle is the most common site of origin for an intracranial ependymoma.[13,14,16,31] Fifty-eight of seventy-four intracranial ependymomas in the present series were located in the fourth ventricle. This tumor tends to originate from the floor of the ventricle immediately rostral to the obex and from the region of the hypoglossal and vagal trigones. Consequently, if there is any clinical feature that distinguishes this tumor from the others occurring in this general area, it is vomiting, which can precede the other classic features of the "axial syndrome" by months. With progression of the disease, dysarthria and abnormalities of deglutition specify the exact area of brain stem involvement. Originating at the cervicomedullary junction, the fourth ventricular ependymoma can spread in all directions. Presence of tumor in the subarachnoid space below the level of the foramen magnum provokes painful stiffness of the neck.

The gross appearance of the ependymoma often resembles a placenta or cauliflower, and the tumor tends to adopt the shape of the spaces and surfaces that it occupies.[31] Therefore the tumor is usually apparent when the posterior fossa dura is opened, as it fills the cisterna magna and flows down over the cervical cord. The spurious appearance of the tumor suggests that it can be lifted from the fourth ventricle after it has been freed from the posterior inferior cerebellar arteries and adjacent cranial and cervical nerve rootlets. The same impression is gained when dissecting around rostral portions of the tumor, until finally the surgeon encounters direct invasion of the ventricle floor by the neoplasm. In 1961, Courville and Broussalian drew attention to an unusual ependymoma variant that originated in the lateral recesses of the fourth ventricle and then filled the subarachnoid space, resembling a plaster cast.[14] The extracerebellar portion of the growth differs from the usual irregular or warty ependymal tumors, as this "plastic ependymoma" has a smooth surface and grayish color.

A variety of histological patterns have been described—cellular, papillary-myxopapillary, subependymomal, and epithelioid. The Kernohan grading system has been applied to ependymomas, of which the majority are grade I type. Rubinstein has also described the features of a rare type of primitive ependymal tumor, the ependymoblastoma. It is characterized by embryonal cell forms, is highly malignant, and shows a tendency to local invasion, recurrence, and diffuse spread. But it is not unreasonable to regard even the benign form as "malignant" because of its location and its ability to seed through the subarachnoid space and implant itself on the spinal cord.[50]

The extent of the operative care for the child with a fourth ventricular ependymoma is determined during the operation when the intimacy between tumor and ventricular floor is ascertained. Those lesions that arise from the ventricular roof may be totally extirpated if they have no involvement with the floor. Many ependymomas, however, disturb the brain stem architecture so that the surgeon is unable to distinguish tumor from obex, trigones, clava, and cuneate tubercle. In this situation, it is not safe to attempt complete removal of the tumor.

It is perhaps illogical that irradiation should be employed against a tumor that in many instances is histologically benign and in most circumstances is partially buried in the brain stem. But radiotherapy programs have long been recommended. A number of factors influence survival following treatment, and interpretation of results is hampered by reports that consider supratentorial and infratentorial tumors together and blend experience with children with experience with adults. Age is of prognostic importance: the younger the child, the worse the prognosis.[13,46] In general terms, the administration of radiation therapy favorably influences survival, though chances of long life in children are still dismal, with

recently reported three-year and five-year survival rates of 17.2 per cent and 13.7 per cent respectively.*

BRAIN STEM GLIOMAS

Few pediatric neurosurgical problems are as exasperating for the clinician as the management of a child with a brain stem glioma. The clinical presentation is insidious, the tumor extension inexorable, and the prognosis almost hopeless. The pathetic neurological destruction of the child is apparent to all; moreover, the sad diplegic face must be a window to the soul, for these children quickly lose their sparkle and become lethargic, apathetic, almost immobile creatures who seem to sense their inevitable doom. Regrettably, as Villani and coworkers state, "during these 30 years no important progress has been achieved in this field."[57]

Compromise of the concentrated brain stem anatomy causes a variety of symptoms and signs that signal the presence of an intrinsic brain stem tumor. The tightly packaged long and short ascending and descending pathways, cranial nerve and other special nuclei, and the ubiquitous reticular formation can be involved in varying combinations. Remarkably, the cerebrospinal fluid pathways—sylvian aqueduct and fourth ventricle—so susceptible to distortion by more remote, extra-axial masses, remain free of insult until the final stages of the disease.

The brain stem glioma characteristically found in the pontine and medullary segments may initially be confined to just one stem segment or one side, but eventually infiltrates throughout this entire structure. Indeed, histopathologically, the tumor can vary from region to region, with classic polar spongioblastic features in some areas and evidence of marked malignancy in others. The question of tumor homogenicity is thus raised and is particularly apt at the time of biopsy.[22] Usually the neoplasm gently elevates the floor of the fourth ventricle in a smooth, rounded fashion, obliterating the topographic colliculi, sulci, and medullary striae. Tumor substance varies

---

* See references 3, 13, 16, 31, 46.

from gray through dirty white to yellow in color and has a waxy texture. Spontaneous hemorrhage may cause the clinical picture of a stroke. If the tumor clot is evacuated, neoplastic cells can be recovered from the lining bed.

Very few tumors in the brain cause such specific symptoms and signs. Still apt is Matson's description of the brain stem glioma occurring "only in children between 5 and 9 years of age who have bilateral, multiple cranial nerve signs, ataxia, upper motor neuron abnormality, [and] no evidence of increased intracranial pressure."[36] The presence of such a tumor is often shown by the child's face, where abnormalities of abducens and facial nerve function and central nystagmus are immediately apparent, along with altered deglutition and phonation. Facial paresis of the lower motor neuron type contrasts with the upper motor neuron deficits occurring in the limb distributions of one or both pyramidal systems. Interference with the connections of the input and outflow of the middle and superior cerebellar peduncles respectively induces truncal and gait ataxia. Personality is peculiarly altered—usually toward the apathetic, occasionally toward the manic. Yet consciousness is preserved, cerebrospinal fluid flow is unaltered in the early phases, and papilledema usually is absent.

Formerly, these clinical features were sufficient to convince clinicians of the diagnosis; no further confirmation was deemed necessary. Reliance on clinical diagnosis, however, may account for the occasional reported "cure" of a brain stem tumor in cases in which the signs and symptoms were related instead to a nonneoplastic lesion such as encephalitis of the brain stem.[62]

Radiographic examination of the child with a suspected brain stem tumor is mandatory, and the pneumoencephalogram is the investigation of choice. A broadened brain stem with backward convexity of the fourth ventricular floor is indicative of a mass within the brain stem. The anteroposterior tomograms outline the widened fourth ventricle, which straddles the mass yet preserves its own symmetry and angles. Certain large brain stem tumors may contain cysts, a feature not shown by any conventional investigative techniques except computed tomography. The ability of this study to outline a large tumor cyst may aid a small percentage of patients whose tumors should then be operatively explored. Otherwise, the CT scan delineates an ill-defined region of low absorption factors in the brain stem, and contrast enhancement may be of little or no assistance.

In the past it has been argued that a glioma of the brain stem is "malignant" by its location, that it cannot be operatively removed, and that even biopsy is hazardous. More recently a groundswell of support for exploration of these tumors has developed.[32,47,61] Exploration of the large tumors may uncover a tumor cyst whose evacuation improves the patient's survival. As microscopic examination of the fourth ventricle and brain stem is quite possible, it should be considered in the child with a large tumor that perhaps harbors a cyst, or in the child whose clinical signs are either atypical or of more than a year's duration, or whose tumor appears on pneumoencephalography to be partly extra-axial. The operation may also permit passage of an interventricular catheter along the aqueduct to facilitate cerebrospinal fluid drainage toward the cervical subarachnoid space. Alternatively, a ventriculoperitoneal shunt may be inserted to provide relief from obstructive hydrocephalus, which may be a problem, especially in the last few weeks of the patient's life.

Otherwise, radiation therapy must be relied upon to at least delay the tumor's relentless progression. ^{60}Cobalt programs varying from 3500 to 6000 R have been recommended.* Improvement in clinical symptoms usually follows radiation treatment, and the mean survival time in those patients so treated is longer.[33,45,57] But even the survival figures for treated patients are discrepant and vary from an average of 15.1 months to 47.2 months.[33,45] A one-year survival of 45 per cent of patients who have been irradiated can be expected. Caution should be exercised in interpreting the encouraging five-year survival statistics, particularly in the patient whose tumor has not been subjected to neuroradiological or histological confirmation. The tumor usually causes death within 18 months of diagnosis.[36]

---

* See references 6, 33, 45, 57, 58.

MISCELLANEOUS SUBTENTORIAL TUMORS

Epidermoid and Dermoid Cysts

Two of the "embryonic tumors"—the epidermoid and dermoid cysts—showing their classic gross and microscopic differentiation, may reside within the posterior fossa. In children these tumors are situated in the midline, and there is often a clue to their presence. They may be diagnosed because of the cutaneous hallmark of a midline occipital dimple, which expands into a dermal stalk that in turn proceeds in a caudal direction, plunging into deeper tissues. Alternatively, a midline occipital bony defect with sclerotic margins may be recognized in the Towne's view of a skull radiograph obtained for an unrelated reason (Fig. 85–10). The dermal stalk passes through this defect. Finally, a subtentorial embryonic tumor may be diagnosed following an episode of "chemical" or aseptic meningitis due to cyst rupture, or purulent meningitis related to the anatomical defect connecting skin surface with the subarachnoid space. In the latter circumstance, the microorganism that is recovered from cerebrospinal fluid is not the type that is expected. In the child who is older than 3 months, it is usually a gram-negative bacillus.[37,54]

Theoretically, the dermal lesion may reside in any one of several tissue layers. The dermal stalk may abort on the dural surface or probe deeper to penetrate and split the superior sagittal sinus at the level of the torcular. Or the tumor may lie within the dural component. As such it may be confined to the cisterna magna, within cerebellar tissue, or entirely within the cavity of the fourth ventricle. Radiologically, these tumors have a smooth or lobulated avascular appearance.

A subtentorial dermoid tumor should be

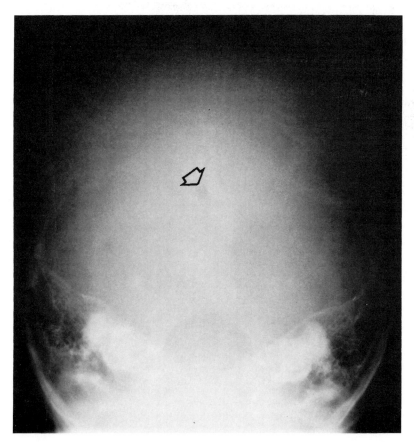

Figure 85–10 Occipital defect from dermoid track penetrating the skull just below the torcular to end in a cerebellar dermoid cyst.

excised before it produces infection or symptoms of a cerebellar–fourth ventricular space-taking mass. Obviously, the surgeon who excises a suboccipital dermal sinus must be prepared to enter the dura and evacuate the intradural stalk-cyst component.

Choroid Plexus Papilloma

The fourth ventricular choroid plexus papilloma is an uncommon tumor, especially in younger children. Its symptoms are those of hydrocephalus—which in this location is produced by at least two of the classic mechanisms, cerebrospinal fluid overproduction and fourth ventricular obstruction.[43] The clinical signs are either those of hydrocephalus developing in a previously well younger child or the features of the "axial syndrome." In 20 per cent of patients the tumor will contain calcification that is visible on plain skull films.[23] The uptake of radiopharmaceutical by the tumor in the radionuclide angiogram and the immediate blood pool images of the brain scan is striking. The anatomy of the inevitably involved choroidal arteries and the diffuse blush of the tumor are demonstrated on vertebral anteriography.

The associated hydrocephalus should be treated first, and the tumor then approached by the standard suboccipital route with the intention of total excision. Frequently the lesion fills the fourth ventricle. It may spill through the foramina of Magendie or Luschka, and occasionally exhibits malignant characteristics with invasion of the walls of the fourth ventricle or cerebellum. It is a moot question whether preoperative irradiation is of any value (especially in benign lesions) and whether it should even be recommended.[8]

Ganglioglioma

Ganglioglioma is an uncommon central nervous system tumor. This neoplasm shows a mixture of astrocytic and neuronal components, exhibiting predominance of one or other. Total tumor excision usually is not possible.

Chordoma

The chordoma, an extremely rare intracranial tumor in children, arises from intraosseous notochordal remnants of the basisphenoid.[4] Although it is benign by histological classification, this slow-growing extradural tumor on the clivus can metastasize widely. The tumor expands, progressively destroying bone anteriorly, to present as a nasopharyngeal mass, and simultaneously distorting the brain stem backward. While operative removal is indicated, it rarely is possible to excise the tumor totally through conventional or even more ingenious approaches. Characteristically, the lesion does not respond to radiation therapy.

Capillary Hemangioblastoma

Capillary hemangioblastomas of the cerebellum, denoted in the complete syndrome by the eponym von Hippel-Lindau disease, usually are well circumscribed. These tumors may be confined to a cerebellar hemisphere or be located in the midline between the cerebellar tonsils and obstruct the fourth ventricle. They have an admixture of solid and cystic components. In some instances the cystic cavities are of substantial size. In the largely cystic tumors, the associated vascular nodule may be quite discrete and resemble a cut strawberry. On vertebral angiography, it presents as a discrete vascular blush with the supplying vessels outlined (Fig. 85–11). Biologically benign, the tumor expands into neighboring structures and may hemorrhage into the cerebrospinal fluid spaces.

The ideal treatment is complete excision of cystic and solid elements. This achievement is seldom obtainable except with the lesion of the cerebellar hemisphere.

Summary

There is a safe predictability as to the nature of a posterior fossa tumor in a child. Essentially, four common neoplasms are encountered, of which one, the brain stem glioma, can be readily distinguished from the other three by clinical and radiological

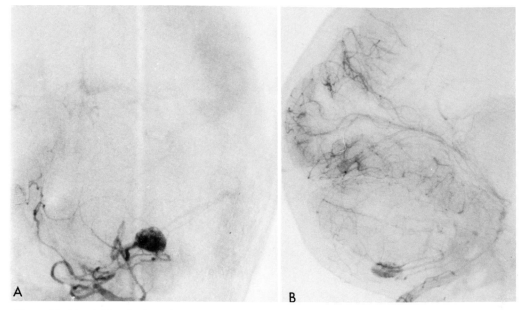

Figure 85–11 *A*. Vertebral arteriogram of capillary hemangioblastoma. A small vascular nodule just above the skull base is fed by the posterior inferior cerebellar artery. Vermian arteries and veins are shifted across the midline; hemisphere arteries are stretched on the right side. *B*. Lateral view of capillary hemangioblastoma.

evidence. The less common neoplasms are notably less frequent. Fortunately, preoperative computed tomography will diminish further the number of operative surprises for the surgeon who chances upon one of these unusual tumors.

TRANSGRESSING TUMORS

Certain neoplasms may violate the anatomical confines of the posterior cranial fossa by extension through the tentorial hiatus. Exclusive of infiltrating intra-axial gliomas, a few other lesions arising within the supratentorial compartment may extend downward to rest and perhaps produce first symptoms within the posterior fossa. The most common of these lesions is the *craniopharyngioma*, a variable portion of the capsule and contents of which may slip down over the dorsum sellae. In most instances, the standard subfrontal approach will allow the surgeon to tease that portion of the craniopharyngioma up from the posterior fossa, but on occasion a middle fossa subtemporal route is required to provide access to both faces of the tentorium.

Pineal region tumors lie at the gateway to the posterior fossa, and it is not surprising that a variety of operative approaches to this region have been advocated. Since at least a portion of the tumor lies anterior to and extends upward from the rostral cerebellum, the infratentorial supracerebellar exposure of this tumor may be used.[52]

Any of the usual infratentorial tumors, particularly the medulloblastoma and cystic cerebellar glioma, may cross the supratentorial-infratentorial border. The *medulloblastoma*, once it has invaded the subarachnoid space, may place metastatic nodules on the undersurface of the tentorium and its free edge. Alternatively, solid tumor may escape from the superior vermis and extend upward through the tentorial hiatus to involve the posterior third ventricular structures.

The cystic component of *cerebellar astrocytoma* can insinuate itself through the incisura to attach itself to the deep venous complex about the posterior end of the third ventricle. Fortunately, drainage of the tumor cyst via the suboccipital approach and retraction of the tentorium upward allow the surgeon to withdraw the tumor cyst wall back gently into the posterior fossa and to excise it.

SURVIVAL AND RECURRENCE

It is axiomatic that the words "brevity" and "chronicity" apply to all phases of malignant and benign posterior fossa tumors respectively. The child presenting with symptoms of short duration due to a malignant subtentorial tumor often experiences a rapid recovery following an uneventful tumor operation. The intense symptoms of headache and vomiting are dramatically relieved, and the truncal ataxia yields to mobility. Mildly disquieting symptoms may appear during the radiation treatment program, but at a point three months following operation and radiation, normal childhood exuberance usually has been regained. The symptom-free interval may be brief, however, especially in children with fourth ventricular tumors burrowing into the brain stem. Return of headache and vomiting several months after initial treatment may signal tumor recurrence. In the absence of recurrence or hydrocephalus, the symptom reappearances defy explanation.

Conversely, the child with a benign cerebellar tumor has often presented with chronic symptoms that resolve slowly. Although the "complete" removal of a benign tumor should insure immediate disappearance of all symptoms, such is often not the case. Morning nausea, occasional vomiting, and neck pain and stiffness may persist for weeks or months following treatment. Throughout that same time, parents may comment on the persistence of ataxic features that become obvious when the child is fatigued. The surgeon is able to document residual dysmetria and dysdiadochokinesia. Eventually the complaints and altered features subside, and a prolonged quiescent interval ensues.

Parents always have at least a degree of anxiety regarding tumor recurrence, even for confirmed benign lesions. Consequently every legitimate but ordinary headache that the child suffers is apt to require the surgeon's assessment and reassurance. When genuine symptoms related to tumor recurrence appear, they tend to do so in exactly the same form as originally. With exacerbation of the neurological signs, reinvestigation should be planned. Fortunately it is now a much easier task with radionuclide brain scanning and computed tomography. Upon confirmation of tumor recurrence,

the surgeon must make a decision concerning re-exploration, bypass cerebrospinal fluid shunting, further radiation, chemotherapy, a combination of these, or no treatment. In making the decision, there should be consideration of the latency from first treatment to confirmed recurrence, the initial quality of survival, the tumor location and histological type, and the wishes of the child and family. For example, it is advisable to treat a recurrent medulloblastoma aggressively after four years of symptom-free life, but to offer comfort only for a child in difficulty with a brain stem glioma just a few months after initial diagnosis. Whatever his decision, the surgeon can be certain that the second latent interval will be much briefer than the first, especially for malignant tumors.

When the child's tumor recurrence is confirmed, the family should be counseled again and they should make their wishes clear. Many families, faced with the child's terminal illness, would prefer to have the child at home where parents and siblings can rally around providing security and peace in the last weeks. Despite lack of medical training, many family members display imagination and confidence in their care for the dying child.

REFERENCES

1. Albright, L., and Reigel, D. H.: Management of hydrocephalus secondary to posterior fossa tumors. J. Neurosurg., *46*:52–55, 1977.
2. Amici, R., Avanzini, G., and Pacini, L.: Cerebellar Tumors. Clinical Analysis and Physiopathologic Correlations. Monographs in Neural Sciences, Vol. 4. Basel, S. Karger, 1976, pp. 80–81.
3. Barone, B. M., and Elvidge, A. R.: Ependymomas. A clinical survey. J. Neurosurg., *33*:428–438, 1970.
4. Becker, L. E., Yates, A. J., Hoffman, H. J., and Norman, M. G.: Intracranial chordoma in infancy. Case report. J. Neurosurg., *42*:349–352, 1975.
5. Bloom, H. J. G., Wallace, E. N. K., and Henk, J. M.: The treatment and prognosis of medulloblastomas in children. A study of 82 verified cases. Amer. J. Roentgen., *105*:43–62, 1969.
6. Bray, P. F., Carter, S., and Taveras, J. M.: Brain-stem tumors in children. Neurology (Minneap.), *8*:1–7, 1958.
7. Carmel, P. W., Fraser, R. A. R., and Stein, B. M.: Aseptic meningitis following posterior fossa surgery in children. J. Neurosurg., *41*:44–48, 1974.
8. Carrea, R., and Polak, M.: Preoperative radiotherapy in the management of posterior fossa

choroid plexus papillomas. Child's Brain, *3*:12–24, 1977.

9. Chang, C. H., Housepian, E. M., and Herbert, C., Jr.: Operative staging system and megavoltage radiotherapeutic technic for cerebellar medulloblastomas. Radiology *93*:1351–1359, 1969.

10. Chatty, E. M., and Earle, K. M.: Medulloblastoma. A report of 201 cases with emphasis on the relationship of histologic variants to survival. Cancer, *28*:977–983, 1971.

11. Cogan, D. G.: Neurology of the Ocular Muscles. 2nd Ed. Springfield, Ill., Charles C Thomas, 1966.

12. Collins, V. P.: Wilms' tumor: Its behavior and prognosis. J. Louisiana Med. Soc., *107*:474–480, 1955.

13. Coulon, R. A., and Till, K.: Intracranial ependymomas in children. A review of 43 cases. Child's Brain, *3*:154–168, 1977.

14. Courville, C. B., and Broussalian, S. L.: Plastic ependymomas of the lateral recess. Report of eight verified cases. J. Neurosurg., *18*:792–799, 1961.

15. Cushing, H.: Experiences with cerebellar medulloblastoma: A critical review. Acta Path. Microbiol. Scand., 7:1–86, 1930.

16. Dohrmann, G. J., Ependymomas and ependymoblastomas in children. J. Neurosurg., *45*:273–282, 1976.

17. Dougherty, T. F., and Schneebeli, G. L.: Action of steroids on reduction of edema. Clin. Neurosurg., *18*:414–425, 1971.

18. Fresh, C. B., Takei, Y., and O'Brien, M. S.: Cerebellar glioblastoma in childhood. Case report. J. Neurosurg., *45*:705–708, 1976.

19. Gay, A. J., Newman, N M., Keltner, J. L., and Stroud, M. H.: Eye Movement Disorders. St. Louis, The C. V. Mosby Co., 1974.

20. German, W. J.: The gliomas: A follow-up study. Clin. Neurosurg., 7:1–20, 1961.

21. Gilday, D. L.: Pediatric neuronuclear medicine. *In* Harwood-Nash, D. C., and Fitz, C. R., eds.: Neuroradiology in Infants and Children. St. Louis, The C. V. Mosby Co., 1976, Vol. 2, pp. 505–608.

22. Golden, G. S., Ghatak, N. R., Hirano, A., and French, J. H.: Malignant glioma of the brainstem. J. Neurol., Neurosurg. Psychiat.,*35*:732–738, 1972.

23. Harwood-Nash, D. C., and Fitz, C. R., eds.: Neuroradiology in Infants and Children. St. Louis, The C. V. Mosby Co., 1976, Vol. 2, pp. 461–504, 668–788.

24. Heiskanen, O.: Intracranial tumors of children. Child's Brain, *3*:69–78, 1977.

25. Hoffman, H. J., Hendrick, E. B., and Humphreys, R. P.: Metastasis via ventriculo-peritoneal shunt in patients with medulloblastoma. J. Neurosurg., *44*:562–566, 1976.

26. Hooper, R.: Intracranial tumors in childhood. Child's Brain, *1*:136–140, 1975.

27. Hope-Stone, H. F.: Results of treatment of medulloblastomas. J. Neurosurg., *32*:83–88, 1970.

28. Humphreys, R. P., Creighton, R. E., Hendrick, E. B., and Hoffman, H. J.: Advantages of the prone position for neurosurgical procedures on the upper cervical spine and posterior cranial fossa in children. Child's Brain, *1*:325–336, 1975.

29. Kahn, E. A., Crosby, E. C., Schneider, R. C., and

Taren, J. A.: Correlative Neurosurgery. 2nd Ed. Springfield, Ill., Charles C Thomas, 1969, pp. 173–174.

30. Kessler, L. A., Dugan, P., and Concannon, J. P.: Systemic metastases of medulloblastoma promoted by shunting. Surg. Neurol., *3*:147–152, 1975.

31. Koos, W. T., and Miller, M. H.: Intracranial Tumors of Infants and Children. St. Louis, C. V. Mosby Co., 1971.

32. Lassiter, K. R. L., Alexander, E., Jr., Davis, C. H., Jr., and Kelly, D. L., Jr.: Surgical treatment of brain stem gliomas. J. Neurosurg., *34*:719–725, 1971.

33. Lassman, L. P., and Arjona, V. E.: Pontine gliomas of childhood. Lancet, *1*:913–915, 1967.

34. Makeever, L. C., and King, J. D.: Medulloblastoma with extracranial metastasis through a ventriculovenous shunt. Report of a case and review of the literature. Amer. J. Clin. Path., *46*:245–249, 1966.

35. Matson, D. D.: Surgery of posterior fossa tumors in childhood. Clin. Neurosurg., *15*:247–264, 1968.

36. Matson, D. D.: Neurosurgery of Infancy and Childhood. 2nd Ed. Springfield, Ill., Charles C Thomas, 1969, pp. 403–479.

37. Matson, D. D., and Jerva, M. J.: Recurrent meningitis associated with congenital lumbo-sacral dermal sinus tract. J. Neurosurg., *25*:288–297, 1966.

38. McFarland, D. R., Horwitz, H., Saenger, E. L., and Bahr, G. K.: Medulloblastoma—a review of prognosis and survival. Brit. J. Radiol., *42*:198–214, 1969.

39. Mealey, J., Jr., and Hall, P. V.: Medulloblastoma in children. Survival and treatment. J. Neurosurg., *46*:56–64, 1977.

40. Meridy, H. W., Creighton, R. E., and Humphreys, R. P.: Complications during the prone position in children. Canad. Anaesth. Soc. J. *21*:445–453, 1974.

41. Michenfelder, J. D., Gronert, G. A., and Rehder, K.: Neuroanesthesia. Anesthesiology, *30*:65–100, 1969.

42. Miles, J., and Bhandari, Y. S.: Cerebellar medulloblastomata in adults: Review of 18 cases. J. Neurol. Neurosurg. Psychiat., *33*:208–211, 1970.

43. Milhorat, T. H., Hammock, M. K., Davis, D. A., and Fenstermacher, J. D.: Choroid plexus papilloma. I. Proof of cerebrospinal fluid overproduction. Child's Brain, *2*:273–289, 1976.

44. Northfield, D. W. C.: The Surgery of the Central Nervous System. A Textbook for Postgraduate Students. Oxford, Blackwell Scientific Publications, 1973, pp. 138–196.

45. Panitch, H. S., and Berg. B. O.: Brain stem tumors of childhood and adolescence. Amer. J. Dis. Child., *119*:465–472, 1970.

46. Phillips, T. L., Sheline, G. E., and Boldrey, E.: Therapeutic considerations in tumors affecting the central nervous system: Ependymomas. Radiology,*83*:98–105, 1964.

47. Pool, J. L.: Gliomas in the region of the brain stem. J. Neurosurg., *29*:164–167, 1968.

48. Raimondi, A. J., Yashon, D., Matsumoto, S., and Reyes, C. A.: Increased intracranial pressure without lateralizing signs. The midline syn-

drome. Neurochirurgia (Stuttgart), *10*:197–209, 1967.

49. Reulen, H. J., Hadjidimos, A., and Hase, U.: Steroids in the treatment of brain edema. Advances Neurosurg., *1*:92–105, 1973.

50. Rubinstein, L. J.: Tumors of the Central Nervous System. Washington, D. C., Armed Forces Institute of Pathology, 1970.

51. Sayers, M. P., and Hunt, W. E.: Posterior fossa tumors. *In* Youmans, J. R., ed.: Neurological Surgery. Philadelphia, W. B. Saunders Co., 1973, Vol. 3, pp. 1466–1489.

52. Stein, B. M.: The infratentorial supracerebellar approach to pineal lesions. J. Neurosurg., *35*:197–202, 1971.

53. Stein, B. M., Tenner, M. S., and Fraser, R. A. R.: Hydrocephalus following removal of cerebellar astrocytomas in children. J. Neurosurg., *36*:763 –768, 1972.

54. Swartz, M. N., and Dodge, P. R.: Bacterial meningitis—a review of selected aspects. I. General clinical features, special problems and unusual meningeal reactions mimicking bacterial meningitis (continued). New Eng. J. Med., *272*:842– 848, 1965.

55. Till, K.: Pediatric Neurosurgery. Oxford, Blackwell Scientific Publications, 1975, pp. 1–57.

56. Troupp, H.: Arteriovenous malformations of the brain: What are the indications for operation? *In* Morley, T. P., ed.: Current Controversies in Neurosurgery. Philadelphia, W. B. Saunders, Co., 1976, pp. 210–216.

57. Villani, R., Gaini, S. M., and Tomei, G.: Follow-up study of brain stem tumors in children. Child's Brain, *1*:126–135, 1975.

58. Whyte, T. R., Colby, M. Y., Jr., and Layton, D. D.: Radiation therapy of brain-stem tumors. Radiology, *93*:413–416, 1969.

59. Williams, P. L., and Warwick, R.: Functional Neuroanatomy of Man. Philadelphia, W. B. Saunders Co., 1975.

60. Wilson, C. B.: Medulloblastoma. Current views regarding the tumor and its treatment. Oncology, *24*:273–290, 1970.

61. Wilson, C. B.: Diagnosis and surgical treatment of childhood brain tumors. Cancer, *35*:950–956, 1975.

62. Yalaz, K., and Tinaztepe, K.: Brain stem encephalitis. Acta. Paediat. Scand., *63*:235–240, 1974.

GLIAL AND NEURONAL TUMORS OF THE BRAIN IN ADULTS

Neurological surgery's development as a specialty was intimately related to the early knowledge of brain tumors and beginning attempts at their treatment. Except for ritualistic procedures performed in ancient times and occasional attempts to treat head injuries, the first intracranial operations were performed for suspected brain tumors. Initially, the tumors were diagnosed and localized by observation of focal seizures or paresis. Later, diagnostic radiographic techniques and advances in operative techniques and general anesthesia allowed surgeons to operate with acceptable morbidity and low mortality rates. As a result of these developments, a large body of knowledge of the pathological, neurological, diagnostic, therapeutic, and prognostic aspects of brain tumors has accumulated.

CLASSIFICATION

The development of neuropathology as a specialty was stimulated by the emergence of neurological surgery as a treatment for intracranial tumors. Organization was brought to the field by Cajal and Hortega, whose metal stains allowed the separation of normal brain elements into distinct cell types. Utilizing this classification of normal elements, Bailey and Cushing separated a large series of intracranial tumors into subtypes.[22] Their classification, developed by clinicians, was particularly useful because the brain tumor types not only were grouped according to uniform histological appearance but also were clinically distinct.

The classification of Bailey and Cushing was based on the cells in the normal nervous system and their embryonic precursors. Because the embryonic derivation of mature central nervous system cells (the histogenetic line) had been traced incompletely and was in part hypothetical, Bailey and Cushing recognized that the classification was preliminary. They noted that any classification is arbitrary, since individual cellular stages are "abstractions from a continuous development."[22] In 1932, Bailey revised the original classification, subdividing glial tumors into 10 types (Table 86–1).[18]

The original classification by Bailey and Cushing and the modification by Bailey served as the foundation for further refinements by a number of authors.[207,370,461] The nomenclature in these classifications suggests that each primary brain tumor arises from a separate type of cell and that each cell type has a corresponding type of neoplasm. This assumption is inherent in the original title of Bailey and Cushing's monograph, *A Classification of Tumors of the Glioma Group on a Histogenetic Basis with a Correlated Study of Prognosis.*[22]

It is common to find a variety of glioma subtypes in different parts of the same neoplasm.[83,364] This is particularly true in experimentally produced tumors. Chemical carcinogens implanted adjacent to ependyma tend to induce neoplasms that resem-

C. A. COBB and J. R. YOUMANS

TABLE 86–1   CLASSIFICATION OF BRAIN TUMORS*

Medulloblastoma
Neuroepithelioma
Glioblastoma multiforme
Pinealoma
Spongioblastoma
Astroblastoma
Astrocytoma
Ganglioneuroma
Ependymoma
Oligodendroglioma

* As revised in 1932 by Bailey from the original 1926 classification of Bailey and Cushing.

ble ependymoma or ependymoblastoma. Subcortical parietal implantation produces glioblastoma multiforme or occasionally astrocytoma, while frontal lobe subcortical implantation often produces oligodendroglioma, and cerebellar implantation produces medulloblastoma. In spite of this tendency, however, most neoplasms are composed of several different cell types that sometimes can be separated by subculture.[454] For example, in tissue culture, a glioblastomatous portion of a tumor might continue to produce glioblastomatous cells while an oligodendrogliomatous portion continued to produce oligodendrogliomatous cells.

The field theory of tumor growth can explain the variety of cell types in a single tumor.[444] This theory suggests that neoplasms enlarge not only by cellular proliferation but also by anaplastic change in adjacent normal cellular elements. The potentially neoplastic field may be much greater in size than the microscopic or macroscopic neoplasm. This "field theory" would explain the findings of mixed tumors and would also explain the difficulty of curing anaplastic neoplasms, even by apparently total removal of all microscopic tumor.

Although subject to criticism because of its histogenetic nomenclature, the separation of primary brain tumors into different types on the basis of the predominating cell sets apart clinically distinct groups of neoplasms. In some neoplasms, it may not be possible to identify a predominant cell type, and in such circumstances, a composite label such as "oligoastrocytoma" may be required. As noted by Rubinstein, the "convenience of naming the tumor by its prevalent cell type is maintained despite the recognition of its cellular diversity."[358]

A more detailed discussion of the classification of brain tumors is given in Chapter 83.

Grading of Malignancy

Studies of separate series of primary brain tumors have shown gradual transition from well-differentiated astrocytomas, which were difficult to distinguish from gliotic brain, to anaplastic astrocytomas or glioblastomas.[208,347,409] Kernohan and associates developed a system of grading that divided primary brain tumors into four grades of progressively increasing anaplasia. The tumors that were histologically more anaplastic were found to correspond to shorter survival, a relationship that has been confirmed by subsequent investigators.[372,425] This classification has the advantages of simplicity, ease of use, and an emphasis on correlation between histological anaplasia and clinical behavior. It should be noted, however, that the histological structure of a small biopsy may not be characteristic of the entire tumor. Neoplasms that are histologically similar may have markedly different natural histories. As a result, grading oversimplifies the pathological interpretation and suggests a more precise prognosis than can be given. Proponents of grading have emphasized that it is the responsibility of the pathologist to report the microscopic structure and of the surgeon to decide the appropriate treatment.[374]

World Health Organization Classification

As different nomenclatures and tumor classifications have become prevalent, it has become difficult to compare one brain tumor series with another or to combine data for large groups of patients reported from different institutions. Each of the current classifications has its proponents. The one most popular in the United States is that devised by Russell and Rubinstein.[370] Definition of an internationally acceptable classification that could replace the myriad current classifications has been undertaken by the World Health Organization. The result closely resembles the most recent revision of Russell and Rubinstein's classification. In an effort to promote an international classification, the remainder of this chapter is based on the World Health Organization schema.[397] It is outlined in Table 86–2.

Particular types of brain tumors from series classified by other nomenclatures are discussed in terms of the analogous tumor in the World Health Organization classification. In some cases, tumor types are not analogous because of differences in classification, which in turn introduces an inaccuracy in statistical analysis.[459]

INCIDENCE OF BRAIN TUMORS

Since some of them are asymptomatic and are discovered only at autopsy, the incidence of brain tumors is unknown.

The clinically diagnosed neoplasms ac-

TABLE 86–2 WORLD HEALTH ORGANIZATION BRAIN TUMOR CLASSIFICATION

TUMORS OF NEUROEPITHELIAL TISSUE

Astrocytic tumors
  Astrocytoma
    Fibrillary
    Protoplasmic
    Gemistocytic
  Pilocytic astrocytoma
  Subependymal giant cell astrocytoma (ventricular tumor of tuberous sclerosis)
  Astroblastoma
  Anaplastic astrocytoma
Oligodendroglial tumors
  Oligodendroglioma
  Mixed oligoastrocytoma
  Anaplastic oligodendroglioma
Ependymal and choroid plexus tumors
  Ependymoma
    Variants
      Myxopapillary ependymoma
      Papillary ependymoma
      Subependymoma
  Anaplastic ependymoma
  Choroid plexus papilloma
  Anaplastic choroid plexus papilloma
Pineal cell tumors
  Pineocytoma
  Pineoblastoma
Neuronal tumors
  Gangliocytoma
  Ganglioglioma
  Ganglioneuroblastoma
  Anaplastic gangliocytoma and ganglioglioma
  Neuroblastoma
Poorly differentiated and embryonal tumors
  Glioblastoma
    Variants
      Glioblastoma with sarcomatous component
      Giant cell glioblastoma
  Medulloblastoma
    Variants
      Desmoplastic
      Medullomyoblastoma
  Medulloepithelioma
  Primitive polar spongioblastoma
  Gliomatosis cerebri

TUMORS OF NERVE SHEATH CELLS

Neurilemmoma
Anaplastic neurilemmoma
Neurofibroma
Anaplastic neurofibroma

TUMORS OF MENINGEAL AND RELATED TISSUES

Meningioma
Meningeal sarcoma
Xanthomatous tumors
Primary melanotic tumors
Others

PRIMARY MALIGNANT LYMPHOMAS

TUMORS OF BLOOD VESSEL ORIGIN

Hemangioblastoma
Monstrocellular sarcoma

GERM CELL TUMORS

Germinoma
Embryonal carcinoma
Choriocarcinoma
Teratoma

OTHER MALFORMATIVE TUMORS AND TUMORLIKE LESIONS

Craniopharyngioma
Rathke's cleft cyst
Epidermoid cyst
Dermoid cyst
Colloid cyst of the third ventricle
Enterogenous cyst
Other cysts
Lipoma
Choristoma
Hypothalamic neuronal hamartoma
Nasal glial heterotopia

VASCULAR MALFORMATIONS

Capillary telangiectasia
Cavernous angioma
Arterio-venous malformation
Venous malformation
Sturge-Weber disease

TUMORS OF THE ANTERIOR PITUITARY

Pituitary adenomas
Pituitary adenocarcinoma

LOCAL EXTENSION FROM REGIONAL TUMORS

Glomus jugulare tumors
Chordoma
Chondroma
Chondrosarcoma
Olfactory neuroblastoma
Adenoid cystic carcinoma
Other

METASTATIC TUMOR

UNCLASSIFIED TUMORS

count for only approximately half of those found in populations in which many autopsies of the central nervous system are performed.[159] Clinical and death certificate reviews report approximately five brain tumors per year per 100,000 population.[392] In studies that have more accurate data, however, approximately 10 new brain tumors are found per year per 100,000 population.[48,159,226] The rate is higher in older patients and rises to about 37 new brain tumors per year per 100,000 population in patients over 80 years of age. Age-adjusted annual incidence rates are higher for males than for females and are rising for both groups.[416] The death rate is nearly as high as the incidence rate, with 9.4 deaths per 100,000 in the same population that has an incidence rate of 10.6 per 100,000.[159] If data are extrapolated from patients with cancer, there should be more than 10 brain tumors per 100,000 of population. Approximately 18 per cent of patients who die of cancer have metastases in the central nervous system.[330] About three quarters of them have intracerebral metastases, most of which are symptomatic, while one quarter have meningeal seeding. These data indicate that metastases to the brain are underreported.

There are marked regional differences in the incidence of various types of brain tumors. These differences may have a cultural or a genetic basis.[239] For example, granulomas are comparatively rare in the United States, but they constitute approximately 20 per cent of the intracranial tumors in India.[337] In recent years, the relative incidence of granulomas in comparison with other brain tumors seems to be decreasing in India and other Asian countries.[337,438] It may, however, increase in the more economically advanced nations as travel and migration expand throughout the world.

Brain tumors are only slightly more common in patients in psychiatric hospitals than in the normal population. In a series of 5862 autopsies of mental hospital patients, brain tumors were found in only 3 per cent. Of these neoplasms, 39 per cent were gliomas, 22 per cent were metastases, and 15 per cent were meningiomas. Of the gliomas, 61 per cent were anaplastic. Fifty-seven per cent of the patients with primary brain tumors had been in the hospital less than six months, but seventy-four per cent of those with metastatic brain neoplasms had been in the hospital for six months or less.[8] The distribution of brain tumors in hospitalized psychiatric patients is no different than in the normal population. This information suggests that, although patients are occasionally admitted to psychiatric hospitals for symptoms caused by unrecognized brain tumors, it is infrequent. A brain tumor that occurs in a patient who is already hospitalized in a psychiatric hospital, however, is usually undiagnosed or diagnosed later than would be expected in the normal population. Undoubtedly many symptoms caused by the tumor are blamed on psychiatric disease in patients who carry that diagnosis.

Brain tumors commonly are misdiagnosed in patients who are thought to have vascular disease.[441] Indeed, more than one third of patients with brain tumors who were admitted to a pair of university hospitals were admitted with a diagnosis of "cerebrovascular accident."[162] One of the sources of this misdiagnosis of vascular accident is the occasional hemorrhage into a tumor. Hematomas greater than 4 cm in diameter occur in approximately 1 per cent of all patients with brain tumor, and neoplasms are found in up to 10 per cent of patients with spontaneous intracerebral hematomas.[386] Metastatic neoplasms account for most of the cases with hemorrhage. According to Yaşargil, 1 to 2 per cent of patients with spontaneous subarachnoid hemorrhage have brain tumors.[452]

SYMPTOMS DUE TO BRAIN TUMORS

Symptoms due to brain tumors can be divided into four groups: headache, seizures, focal neurological deficits, and generalized cerebral dysfunction. The symptoms accompanying specific tumors are discussed with their respective neoplasms.

Headache

Headaches in patients with brain tumors usually are not severe. Typically, the headache is mild and throbbing, usually worse in the morning and subsiding during the day. Coughing or straining tends to increase the discomfort, as does placing the head in a dependent position. If the headache is unilateral, it is usually on the same side as the mass. Indeed, if the intracranial pressure is normal and the headache is focal, it will denote the location of the tumor in most instances. Patients with elevated intracranial pressure may have generalized or focal headaches. With increased intracranial pressure the focal headache may be at the tumor or elsewhere. Presumably, the pain at distant sites is due to the stretching of dura or vessels by the increased pressure and the displacement of the intracranial contents. Supratentorial masses usually produce frontal or unlocalized headache, while posterior fossa masses produce occipital or suboccipital or generalized headache. Severe suboccipital headache that increases markedly with coughing or straining, in a patient with a brain neoplasm, should raise the question of stretching of upper cervical sensory rootlets by herniated cerebellar tonsils. Patients with brain tumors usually have headache; however, patients investigated because of headache without other symptoms or signs rarely have brain tumors.

Seizures

Seizures occur with 60 to 90 per cent of slow-growing and approximately 30 per cent of rapidly growing neoplasms.[318] Almost any type of seizure may occur with a brain tumor. Focal seizures (with or without secondary generalization) and temporal lobe seizures (especially those with a gustatory or olfactory aura) are most common.[341]

Focal Deficit

Neoplasms can interfere with brain function through many mechanisms, among them replacement of brain parenchyma, edema in surrounding tissue, compression of the microcirculation, production of herniation syndromes, and rarely the occlusion of major cerebral arteries. Any of these mechanisms can lead to localized dysfunction of brain. Usually, the dysfunction can be identified by careful neurological examination, and often it indicates the site of the neoplasm.

Caudal displacement of the brain can interfere with function of the sixth nerve. In this circumstance, sixth nerve dysfunction does not imply tumor in the sixth nerve nucleus or in the nerve itself and thus is a "false localizing sign." Other cranial nerves can be stretched or distorted, producing a variety of false localizing signs.

Generalized Dysfunction

Generalized abnormality of function of the cerebrum may range from mere impairment of intellectual functions to coma. The most common causes of generalzied cerebral dysfunction in patients with brain neoplasm are increased intracranial pressure and brain shift. These usually are due to the bulk of the neoplasm and surrounding cerebral edema. Also, hydrocephalus may contribute to the increased pressure. The degree of cerebral dysfunction may fluctuate during the day along with changes in intracranial pressure. Further, plateau waves may be accompanied by deterioration in alertness and arousal (see Chapter 24).

Generalized dysfunction may be due to metabolic or endocrine derangements. For example, the syndrome of inappropriate antidiuretic hormone secretion can lead to water intoxication, metastasis to bone can produce hypercalcemia, and metastasis to liver can produce hepatic encephalopathy.

INVESTIGATION

A detailed history and physical examination are the most important single investigative aids in evaluating a patient who may have an intracranial neoplasm. Often it is necessary to interview the family, since the patient may be demented or have memory deficits. A careful history of the onset of disease, the changes that have occurred over its duration, the time of the earliest focal neurological deficits, the impressions of other physicians, and the patient's response to treatment as well as any associated diseases in the patient or his family are important. The physical examination should be complete and include a general as well as a neurological examination. A chest x-ray is advisable and is essential if carcinoma of the lung metastatic to the brain is a reasonable possibility.

Careful inspection of skull x-rays will show an abnormality in a high percentage of patients who have a brain tumor. If calcification is shown in the tumor or if there is bony erosion, the plain skull film may give the location of the tumor. Usually the abnormality is displacement of a calcified pineal gland or erosion of the sella as a result of increased intracranial pressure. In addition to giving information concerning the tumor, skull x-rays are helpful in identifying the shape and size of the paranasal sinuses, which may be useful in planning a craniotomy. Echoencephalography is helpful in identifying shifts of the midline; however, the absence of a midline shift is not sufficient evidence to discontinue the evaluation of the patient with a history suggestive of brain tumor. Often, the electroencephalogram is abnormal with an anaplastic neoplasm and may indicate its location.[130] In patients who have a history or findings suggestive of a tumor, however, these tests usually are not cost effective because they do not add definitive information and, regardless of the findings with them, other studies must be done. In patients with temporal lobe epilepsy, the electroencephalogram may be of more importance than usual and help to establish the side of the neoplasm.[341] It is not reliable enough, though, to warrant operative treatment on its basis alone.

Undoubtedly, the most valuable study in a patient with a possible intracranial neoplasm is computed tomography. It shows the neoplasm and its effect on the adjacent structures. In some cases, the cell type can be predicted with reasonable accuracy. In addition to being the most informative study, computed tomography also has the advantage of being painless and safe.

The radioisotope scan is nearly as accurate as the CT scan at identifying the larger anaplastic gliomas, meningiomas, and schwannomas.[179] It may not however, demonstrate small lesions, deep or basal lesions, and well-differentiated astrocytomas.

Angiography identifies and localizes intracranial masses and can identify tumor type in some cases. It may be helpful in planning the operation, since vessels on the surface of the brain can be correlated with an angiogram to give an accurate localization of the portion of brain being seen in the operative field. The interpretation of angiograms may be subtle, and errors are easily made.

Occasionally, air encephalography is a valuable adjunct in diagnosing a brain tumor. Air may be injected either by lumbar puncture or through trephine openings in the skull. Injection of air through the lumbar route is particularly useful when the tumor is in the brain stem, around the sella turcica, or in the basal cisterns, and does not produce hydrocephalus. If hydrocephalus is present, injection of air into the ventricles through skull trephine openings may be preferable. If a good-quality study cannot be obtained with air as a contrast medium, injection of radiopaque materials into the ventricles may be necessary. Instillation of these materials in the lumbar subarachnoid space and their manipulation into the posterior fossa is useful for small masses along the clivus and in the cerebellopontine angle. CT scanning after injection of small volumes of subarachnoid air as a contrast medium is a very sensitive technique for the diagnosis of cerebellopontine angle masses.

OPERATIVE TREATMENT

Preoperative assessment, anesthetic management, operative technique, and postoperative care in general are discussed in Chapters 29, 30, and 31. Specific details relating to brain tumors are given in this discussion.

When intracranial pressure is elevated, the operating surgeon must be aware of the risk of cerebral herniation during induction of anesthesia. A careful induction without opportunity for carbon dioxide retention and with adequate analgesia as well as unconsciousness will reduce the likelihood of an episode of high intracranial pressure. Preoperative administration of steroids also may protect against episodes of increased intracranial pressure during induction, and in selected cases, intravenous mannitol given 15 to 30 minutes before induction may be useful.

In patients with malignant tumor, the goal of the operation is to obtain a diagnosis and achieve an "internal decompression." Since the dehydrating agents cannot be used permanently, it is best to avoid them when making the decompression. If the mass is decompressed by shrinking the brain with dehydrating agents, it may be difficult to determine how much tumor or silent cerebral tissue should be removed to insure a long-lasting decompression, but a decompression that is generous with normal hydration and normal carbon dioxide tension should be adequate postoperatively. If the patient is thought to have a benign tumor such as a meningioma, dehydrating agents should be used to achieve maximum decompression while he is being anesthetized and relaxation of the brain during the operative procedure.

Correct positioning of the patient is important. He should be positioned so that he would be comfortable if he were awake. The head should be slightly elevated and in the position that allows gravity to perform as much of the brain retraction as possible. The neck should be kept nearly straight so that venous return from the brain is unimpaired. Extreme rotation of the neck may obstruct arterial flow in the contralateral vessels.

A urethral catheter should be placed in all patients. The legs usually should be wrapped with an elastic wrap, or support hose should be applied. A pin headrest provides more solid fixation than a soft headrest. It keeps the head from moving as the skull is opened and holds it in exactly the position that the surgeon remembers it in before the drapes were applied.

The scalp incision should be fashioned so as to preserve at least one major feeding artery to the scalp flap. Incisions that extend anterior to the ear should be within 1 cm of the tragus and, in order to preserve the frontal branch of the facial nerve, should not cross the zygomatic arch. An osteoplastic craniotomy is preferable to a free bone flap. If craniotomies and dural openings are small, there will be minimal disturbance of the brain. Bipolar coagulation is particularly useful in the brain but also is useful on the dura, since it causes less dural retraction than unipolar coagulation. Whenever possible, the brain surface should be kept covered. The ideal covering agent is dura, but if a flap of dura cannot be left, wet Telfa or Biocol can be used to cover it. These materials are also useful under retractors to protect the cortex.

Bone bleeding should be controlled with bone wax. Significant bleeding from vessels of the brain or dura should be controlled by cautery. If cautery is unsuccessful or unsafe, hemostatic agents such as Gelfoam may be useful. Sometimes, in tumor cavities, cotton balls soaked with saline or hy-

drogen peroxide are required to obtain hemostasis. Oxidized cellulose mesh (Surgicel) is also useful as a hemostatic agent.

If, with normal ventilation, the brain swells during the operation, any treatable cause of brain swelling such as a kinked endotracheal tube, a pneumothorax, overhydration, or the like should be identified and corrected. Further removal of tumor or brain parenchyma may also be necessary.

The postoperative management of patients with brain tumors can be facilitated by the use of intracranial pressure monitoring. If operations last a long time, antibiotics given intravenously during the operative procedure may reduce the risks of infection.

Efficacious nonoperative treatment varies considerably from one tumor type to another. Radiotherapy and chemotherapy both are useful in some of the anaplastic lesions (see Chapters 96 and 97). Their role in most of the well-differentiated neoplasms is controversial.

ASTROCYTOMA

Astrocytomas were described by Virchow as early as the 1860's, but it was not until 1926 that Bailey and Cushing separated them into subtypes and established their relationship to other brain tumors.[22,125] Elvidge and co-workers divided astrocytomas into piloid, gemistocytic, and diffuse types.[116] The most popular grading system has not differentiated between subtypes of astrocytomas, grouping all of them into grades I through IV. The tumors that Kernohan and associates called grades III and IV can also be called anaplastic astrocytoma or glioblastoma, depending on the degree of anaplasia (see Anaplastic Astrocytoma and Glioblastoma).[409]

The World Health Organization classification subdivides the astrocytic tumors into astrocytoma with fibrillary, protoplasmic, and gemistocytic subtypes, and pilocytic astrocytoma, subependymal giant cell astrocytoma, astroblastoma, and anaplastic types (cf. Table 86–2).[397]

Incidence

Astrocytomas are the second most common primary tumors of the central nervous system, being surpassed in frequency only by glioblastomas. They constitute 17 to 30 per cent of all gliomas and 11 to 13 per cent of all brain tumors.[95,119,461] The fibrillary ones are the most common subtype.

Although 28 per cent of astrocytic tumors described by Bailey and Cushing in 1926 and 7 per cent of those described by Davis and associates in 1950 were identified as being protoplasmic, they are rare, and some recent series do not mention them.[22,95,370,455] Areas containing protoplasmic cells are seen frequently in other types of astrocytomas, but if the classification is restricted to those tumors in which protoplasmic astrocytes predominate throughout (as is true in modern series), the incidence is extremely low.

There may be a racial difference in the incidence of gliomas.[111] Among Caucasians they account for 50 per cent of primary central nervous system tumors in females and 65 per cent of those in males, but among Negroes, for only 36 per cent of those in females and 47 per cent of those in males. Despite an apparently lower incidence in blacks, there does not seem to be any change in the distribution of subtypes of glioma, suggesting that chronicity of disease is not biasing the diagnosis.[119]

Cerebral astrocytomas can occur at any age.[144,461] Average ages are 35 to 40 years.[111,298,409] There is a tendency for well-differentiated astrocytomas to occur in younger patients, while the more anaplastic ones are more frequent in the middle-aged. In adulthood they tend to be more common in men than in women. This difference in incidences in the sexes is particularly true of the less well-differentiated astrocytomas.

Pathogenesis

As is true of other gliomas, the cause of astrocytoma is unknown. A protoplasmic one has been reported around a metallic fragment that had penetrated the skull nine years previously.[123] In animal models, implantation of carcinogenic materials produces varying types of gliomas, depending on the location of the implanted material.[454] These findings suggest that gliomas can be produced by noxious materials. If the noxious substance predominantly affects deep white matter a fibrillary astrocytoma might

result, whereas if the ependymal region were affected an ependymoma might result. Cigarette smoking has been shown not to be a causative factor in production of these tumors.[75]

There can be little doubt that genetic factors have some influence in the development of a glioma. This influence is suggested by the neurocutaneous syndromes such as von Recklinghausen's disease and tuberous sclerosis, racial differences in tumor types, and rare familial occurrence of astrocytic tumors.[119,382] There does not appear to be a correlation between the occurence of brain tumors and the occurrence of genetic markers such as spina bifida, trisomy 21, or blood type.[75,101]

Bailey and Cushing recognized that different brain tumors might originate through different mechanisms. They suggested that some astrocytomas might be heterotopias.[22] Tissue culture of neoplastic astrocytes reveals a simplified structure that does not resemble the embryonic pattern of development, as would be expected if they arose from cell rests. Rather the tissue culture is more suggestive of anaplasia of adult tissues.[209]

Pathology

Macroscopic Changes

Fibrillary astrocytomas are diffuse, firm, gray or white neoplasms that widely infiltrate the brain and obliterate normal gray-white junctions (Fig. 86–1).[22,114] Frequently small cysts are present. They tend to affect the cerebral hemispheres in adults and the brain stem in children.

When fibrillary astrocytoma involves the brain stem it invades wide areas, parts of which may continue to function even though infiltrated by tumor. Similarly, it may extend into the basal ganglia under the motor strip or into speech areas without causing neurological signs referable to these areas.[96,380] There is probably little tendency to produce cerebrospinal fluid metastases. In two series of gliomas that did produce cerebrospinal fluid metastases, only 1 of a total of 77 was a fibrillary astrocytoma.[139,325] In a study of 16 posterior fossa astrocytomas (some of which may have been anaplastic), however, 3 were found that had produced meningeal seed-

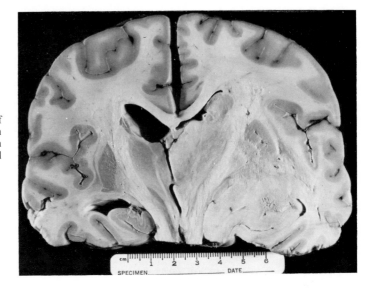

Figure 86–1 Coronal section of a fibrillary astrocytoma (Kernohan grade II) demonstrates expansion of the involved thalamus and basal ganglia.

ing. One had produced clinical symptoms before death.[372]

Penfield and associates divided a normal cerebral hemisphere into its component lobes and found that the occipital lobe occupies 50 cc, the temporal lobe 150 cc, the parietal lobe 170 cc, and the frontal lobe 175 cc.[319] They found that tumors occur with approximately equal frequency in all lobes of the hemisphere if the bulk of the lobe is taken into account. Approximately 80 per cent of the tumors of the brain stem are fibrillary astrocytomas of varying degrees of anaplasia, the remaining 20 per cent being made up primarily of pilocytic astrocytomas.[266] Approximately one fourth of tumors adjacent to or in the fourth ventricle are astrocytomas.[84]

Protoplasmic astrocytomas have a tendency to occur in the cortex. Bailey and Cushing believed them to be more malignant than fibrillary astrocytomas but less malignant than glioblastomas.[22] Owing to varying classifications, the natural history, clinical findings, optimal treatment, and prognosis still are not well defined.

Microscopic Changes

Astrocytes forming a fibrillary astrocytoma appear as a uniform field of scattered small cells with neuroglial fibers forming a background between the cell bodies (Fig. 86–2).[22] Mitoses are absent, and the nuclei are quite uniform in their shape and chromatin content, although they may vary somewhat in size.[370] The architecture of infiltrated tissues is preserved, although the normal structures may be separated from one another by expanded normal anatomical components.[379] Cystic degeneration may occur, and calcium salt deposits occasionally develop in the walls of capillaries.[370]

Differentiation between gliotic brain and the most slowly growing fibrillary astrocytomas can be difficult. The latter tend to have a cellular density that is at least slightly greater than that of normal brain. The nuclei are slightly larger and more irregular than normal and may be mildly hyperchromatic. Also, the cellular density varies in different areas of an astrocytoma. Capillary blood vessels may be slightly more prominent than in normal brain (Fig. 86–3).[111,362,409]

Scherer has described changes that he calls secondary structures.[380] These are configurations that are forced on the tumor by the brain that is being invaded. Secondary structures account for subpial and subependymal accumulation of tumor cells, and they also include concentrations of tumor cells around neurons and at the margins of the brain that is infiltrated. As fibrillary astrocytomas infiltrate fiber tracts in the nervous system, the tumor cells tend to line up and orient themselves in the direction of the fiber tract. This produces the appearance of elongated bipolar cells, a so-called pilocytic feature. This conformation is particularly well seen in the corpus callosum and the pons.

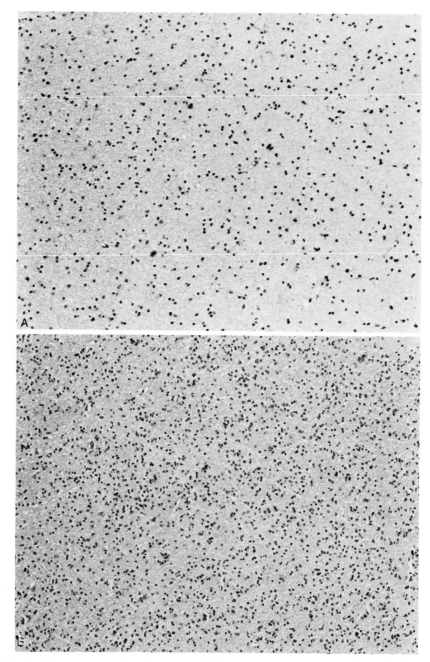

Figure 86–2   Microscopic pathological changes of fibrillary astrocytoma. *A*. Appearance of a Kernohan grade I tumor is similar to normal brain with only subtle changes in cell density, distribution, and vascularity. *B*. A Kernohan grade II tumor demonstrates increased cell density. 100 ×.

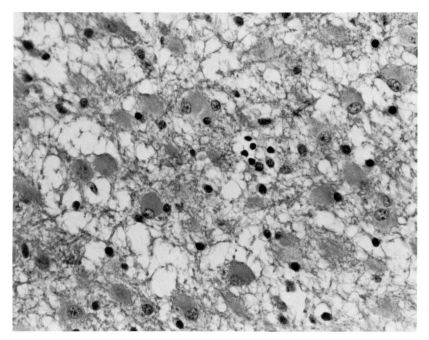

Figure 86–3 Microscopic pathological changes of gemistocytic astrocytoma include large, swollen astrocytes. 350×.

Electron microscopy reveals loosely arranged cells surrounded by fluid-filled interstitial space. The margins of these cells extend into thin processes enmeshed with other processes and containing neurofibrils.[252]

Calcification is present in approximately 15 per cent of astrocytomas when they are examined histologically, but is identified earlier by radiographs in only approximately 8 per cent. Calcified and noncalcified astrocytomas do not differ in age distribution, the preoperative duration of symptoms, the incidence of prior radiotherapy, or survival.[268]

Tissue culture of these cells reveals that they move slowly without changes in the shape of their long stiff processes. In contrast, oligodendroglial cells move more rapidly and have a rhythmic pulsation.[67] The slowness of their migration and the complex interlacing network of the astrocytic processes may prevent astrocytes from becoming detached from astrocytomas and may account for the rarity of cerebrospinal fluid metastases.

Gemistocytic Astrocytomas

Some astrocytomas contain a large number of gemistocytic astrocytes that are large and round or oval in shape, as shown in Figure 86–3. The term implies a fed or fattened cell and is derived from the German word "Gemästete."[184]

Since these tumors behave as anaplastic astrocytomas, it could be assumed that the gemistocyte is an anaplastic variant of an astrocyte. Information from experimental studies combined with the observation that gemistocytes lie near areas of necrosis suggests that they derive from astrocytes when nutrients are insufficient for cell growth. Thus, the presence of gemistocytes reflects the intense proliferative activity of adjacent cells and their rapid utilization of the available nutrients.[184]

Irradiation produces an increase in the number of undifferentiated multinucleated giant cells, extent of necrosis, thickening of the intima of blood vessels, hyaline changes in blood vessels, and small intimal hemorrhages.[131]

Grading of Astrocytomas

In an effort to simplify the classification of gliomas, Kernohan and associates categorized them on the basis of increasing pleomorphism and anaplastic characteristics.[208] Astrocytomas were grouped into grades I through IV on the basis of increasing anaplasia.[409] Grades III and IV are discussed later in the section on anaplastic astrocytomas and glioblastomas.

In grade I astrocytomas, the astrocytes have a nearly normal appearance, but the architecture of the brain is obscured. There is no pleomorphism of either cytoplasm or nucleus, and no obvious hyperchromatism or mitotic figures (see Fig. 86–2).

In grade II the cellularity, degree of fibrillary development, vascularity, and perivascular arrangement are approximately the same as in grade I for the majority of cells. Occasional cells show slight to moderate pleomorphism of cytoplasm and nucleus, and there may be hyperchromatism in some of the nuclei. They have no mitotic figures. There may be minimal adventitial or endothelial changes in vessels. In grade III, half to three quarters of the astrocytes are normal, the remainder being abnormal.

Although grading may not be applicable to some gliomas, such as pilocytic astrocytomas, it applies well to fibrillary astrocytomas.[208] For the purpose of grading, the most anaplastic area of the neoplasm will determine the natural history and therefore determines the grade. Svien and co-workers graded 161 cerebral astrocytomas, the majority of them in adults. Since in adults they usually are fibrillary, the majority of these 161 cases must have been that type. Of these 161 patients, 32 had grade I tumors and 38 had grade II tumors. The average age of the former was 34 years; of the latter, 38 years. The average ages with grades III and IV were 40 years and 43 years respectively. Preoperative duration of symptoms was longest with the low-grade tumors, being 21 months and 11 months for grades I and II.[409] Larger series have suggested that tumors of grade II are approximately twice as frequent as those of grade I.[144]

Pathological Changes in Deep-Seated Gliomas

Approximately 1 per cent of intracranial neoplasms are in the thalamus.[73,280] Two thirds of them are anaplastic and are called glioblastomas or "malignant astrocytomas."[177,280] The low-grade astrocytomas are more likely to occur at an early age, and the thalamic astrocytomas in adults are very likely to be anaplastic gliomas.[73,177,280]

Pontine and medullary tumors in children and young adults are often fibrillary astro-

cytomas with secondary structures producing a piloid pattern.[362] In a series of 25 autopsies of patients with gliomas of the brain stem, 20 per cent of the tumors were pilocytic astrocytomas, the other 80 per cent presumably being fibrillary astrocytomas (Fig. 86–4).[266]

Gliomas of the brain stem and thalamus contain a variety of cell types and have varying natural histories. Neoplasms that were anaplastic gliomas at death (and may have been less anaplastic at the time symptoms began) permit average survivals of 17 months from the time of diagnosis, while nonanaplastic fibrillary astrocytomas allow much longer survivals (in two cases of nonanaplastic fibrillary astrocytoma, average survival was 39 months from the time of diagnosis).[284] In two series of autopsies, 7 of 10 and 7 of 9 brain stem astrocytomas were anaplastic.[155,284] Cystic astrocytomas of the brain stem may have natural histories similar to those of cystic astrocytomas of the cerebellum. Milhorat has reported a patient who survived 11 years after diagnosis.[284]

The findings of the foregoing studies may be slightly biased toward the more anaplastic lesions, since these are autopsy studies and less anaplastic tumors may not have come to pathological examination. Lassiter and associates have reviewed 37 of the brain stem gliomas of which operative biopsies from 19 patients were examined histologically. Thirteen were astrocytomas and six were glioblastomas. Cysts with volumes greater than 12 cc were encountered in five patients. One of the cysts had a volume of 30 cc, which is equal to that of the normal brain stem.[229]

Anaplasia in Astrocytomas

Astrocytomas with cystic degeneration, firm consistency, and little cellularity tend to have a favorable prognosis.[125] Unfortunately, the majority of them do not have these characteristics and do undergo anaplasia.[379,449] In one reported series, of 72 patients who had regrowth of the mass after treatment of a grade I astrocytoma, 55 per cent had grade II astrocytomas at reoperation and 30 per cent had glioblastomas. Also included in this study were 65 patients who had grade II astrocytoma initially; on reoperation for regrowth of the tumor, 45 per cent had glioblastomas.[298] In spite of

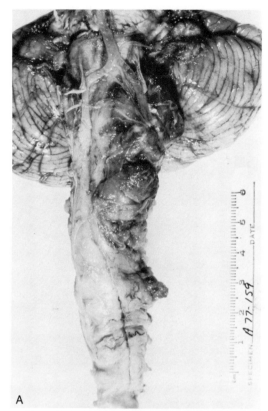

Figure 86–4 Astrocytoma of the cervico-medullary junction. *A*. Six years of slowly progressive tetraparesis was followed by rapid deterioration. Autopsy revealed anaplastic changes in a partially calcified fibrillary astrocytoma that had replaced most of the caudal medulla. *B*. Black arrow indicates the residual crescent of brain and white arrow indicates calcification.

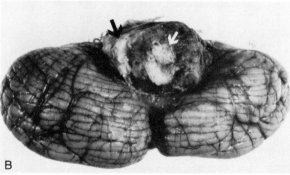

this tendency, however, some of these tumors recur more than once without histological change.[88]

Anaplasia can be suspected on gross examination if there is increased granularity, vascularity, friability, or hemorrhage and necrosis. One of these features alone is not sufficient to label an astrocytoma as anaplastic.[96] If more than one or two mitotic figures per high-power field are present, however, it is highly anaplastic. Previous operation may have induced foreign body giant cells, which makes microscopic diagnosis more difficult.

Mixed Gliomas

Although a tumor is labeled for its predominant cell type, most astrocytomas have a scattering of other recognizable cell types, some of which may be surrounded by the tumor as it extends into previously uninvolved brain, and some of which seem neoplastic. At times, this diversity of cell type is so great that it is impossible to determine a predominant cell. Such unusual tumors are appropriately called mixed tumors, particularly those combining astrocytes and oligodendroglial cells (Fig. 86–5).

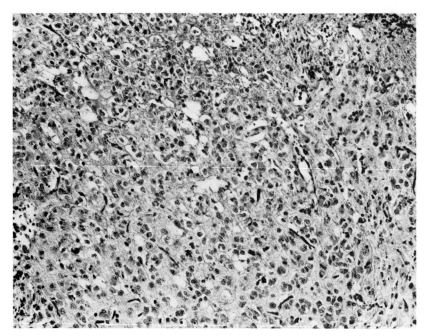

Figure 86–5 Microscopic pathological changes of oligoastrocytoma. The tumor contains a mixture of neoplastic astrocytes and oligodendroglial cells, 120 ×.

Clinical Presentation

Duration of symptoms in patients with astrocytomas is approximately 21 months with grade I, and 11 months with grade II tumors.[409] Gonzales and Elvidge reported a patient with a 30-year history of seizures who subsequently was found to have an astrocytoma.[147] Gol noted a median length of history of 10 months, and Elvidge and Martinez-Coll reported a duration of symptoms of 27 months.[115,144]

Headache and Vomiting

Although headache and vomiting are not the most frequent presenting complaints, headache is the most frequent symptom in astrocytomas of the cerebrum and occurs in approximately 72 per cent of patients. In approximately 11 per cent the headache is more marked on one side, and of these, about 75 per cent have it on the side of the neoplasm.[144] Vomiting occurs in approximately 31 per cent of patients with cerebral astrocytomas.

Seizures

The most frequent initial symptom with astrocytomas is epilepsy. It has been reported in 40 to 75 per cent of patients.[144,147,319] Its incidence varies little between various subtypes, since development is more related to the chronicity of parenchymal tumors than to the tissue type.[113,341] Lesions adjacent to the cortex are more likely to be associated with epilepsy than those deep to the cortex. Tumors near the motor strip are more likely to cause it than those in the temporal or frontal lobe, and those in the occipital lobe are least likely (Fig. 86–6).[319]

Astrocytomas may produce either generalized or focal seizures. Among Gol's patients, 46 per cent had generalized seizures and 28 per cent had "minor" seizures.[144] The seizures tend to be focal with centroparietal tumors, generalized with frontal tumors, and "temporal lobe"–type with temporal lobe tumors.[42] They may have their origin one to several centimeters from the boundary of a tumor, suggesting that "insufficiency of transient blood supply may set off the abnormal, excessive electrical discharge for the seizure."[147] Approximately 20 per cent of patients who undergo operations for seizures are found to have brain tumors.[341] In many of these patients, a tumor has been suspected before operation; however, in about 10 per cent it is not

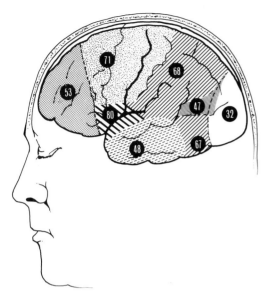

Figure 86–6 Likelihood of seizures (per cent) with tumors in various locations. (Modified from Penfield, W., Erickson, T. C., and Tarlov, I.: Relation of intracranial tumors and symptomatic epilepsy. Arch. Neurol. Psychiat., *44*:300–315, 1940.)

suspected until disclosed by the operation. An initial olfactory or gustatory aura suggests a neoplasm in the sylvian region.

It has been estimated that intracranial tumors are present in 5 to 10 per cent of patients being treated for seizures in large general hospital clinics, an incidence confirmed by CT scan.[136,443] Wyke has identified brain tumors in 30 per cent of 1661 patients with seizures who were selected for study for possible presence of an operatively treatable lesion.[451] In patients who undergo operations for excision of seizure foci, slowly growing gliomas, most of which are astrocytomas, constitute 65 per cent of the neoplasms.[341] The presence of cysts in the tumor does not influence the likelihood of seizures.[95] Preoperative duration of symptoms in patients who undergo operation for seizures and are found to have gliomas range from a few months to 31 years, the median interval being 3 years.[341]

Focal Deficits

Focal neurological deficits are common. Although only 19 per cent of patients complain of paresis or paralysis, facial paresis can be detected in approximately 55 per cent and limb paresis in 41 per cent. Other symptoms such as impaired vision, dyspha-

sia, diplopia, and vertigo, and neurological findings such as homonymous hemianopia and sensory abnormalities occur in 15 to 20 per cent of patients. Approximately 13 per cent have unequal pupils, and when pupillary inequality is present, the smaller pupil is on the side of the lesion in 80 per cent of cases.[144]

Mental Changes and Generalized Dysfunction

Approximately one third of patients with cerebral astrocytomas have mental impairment, and drowsiness occurs in about one fifth of them.[144] Often the mental changes are due to direct involvement of the limbic system by the tumor. Tumors of the third ventricle, of glial origin or otherwise, are most likely to produce these symptoms, and frontal lobe tumors produce them nearly as frequently. They are less likely with parietal lobe tumors. Their high incidence in third ventricular tumors may not be due to hydrocephalus, since posterior fossa tumors, which often produce hydrocephalus, seldom cause them. Of nine temporal lobe masses in patients in whom psychiatric disease was diagnosed initially (schizophrenia in four, depression in four, anxiety state in one), three were astrocytomas and a fourth was a ganglioglioma of the temporal lobe.[261]

On examination, the most frequent finding is papilledema, which is present in approximately 60 per cent of patients.[144] If spontaneous pulsations are present in the retinal veins, intracranial pressure can be predicted to be less than 190 mm of water.[235]

Symptoms of Deep-Seated Tumors

Thalamic Astrocytoma

Thalamic tumors usually produce symptoms of increased intracranial pressure, apathy or dulling of intellect, visual abnormalities, and paresis.[280] Nystagmus, which usually is thought to arise from the posterior fossa, is common. Approximately one third of the patients have a small pupil on the side of the tumor. It is of interest that despite the location of thalamic tumors in a major sensory relay system, the most common neurological finding is hemiparesis, which accompanies three fourths of them.[73] Sensory findings are present in only 37 per cent of these patients. Ten to twenty per cent of patients with thalamic neoplasms have dysphasia.[73,280]

Brain Stem Astrocytoma

Headache occurs in approximately 55 per cent of these patients.[155,229] Half to three quarters of them have difficulty with gait, and approximately half have nausea. Limb paresis is also present in approximately 50 per cent of cases, and cranial nerve deficits in about 80 per cent. The seventh nerve is involved in 70 per cent, the sixth nerve in 60 per cent, and the fifth nerve in 50 per cent. The third nerve also is frequently affected.

When cranial nerve paralyses are considered, neoplasms account for approximately 18 per cent of the third, 8 per cent of the fourth, and 31 per cent of the sixth cranial nerve involvement.[368] Interestingly, cases of sixth nerve palsy due to neoplasm, only 11 per cent are due to a supratentorial tumor, 9 per cent to a parasellar tumor, and 80 per cent to an infratentorial tumor. Glioma of the pons causes 36 per cent of sixth palsy due to neoplasm. The nerves most commonly affected by pontomedullary tumors are the sixth and seventh cranial nerves, the next most common being the fifth and tenth cranial nerves.[232] Brain stem gliomas occur much less frequently after the fifth decade than in earlier decades, and patients over 50 who present with clinical and radiographic evidence of a brain stem tumor should be suspected of having metastasis to the brain stem.

Investigation

Plain Roentgenography

Routine x-rays of the skull are abnormal in approximately 50 per cent of patients with astrocytomas of the cerebral hemispheres.[144] The most common abnormality is erosion of the sella turcica (Fig. 86–7).[424] Frontal lobe tumors are more likely than parietal or temporal lobe tumors to produce this change, probably because the former tend to be discovered later after more long-standing elevation of intracranial pressure. Radiographically visible calcification is present in only 8 to 12 per cent of astrocytomas.[95,268]

Electroencephalography

The electroencephalogram, often abnormal with astrocytomas of the cerebral hemispheres, is localizing in approximately 45 per cent of patients and lateralizing in another 30 per cent.[144,341] In only approximately one third is it particularly helpful in making the diagnosis. A wide variety of

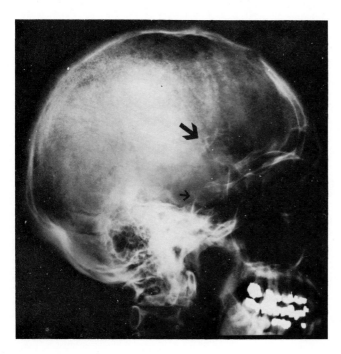

Figure 86–7 Skull x-ray of an astrocytoma reveals tumor calcification (*large arrow*) and erosion of the dorsum sellae from chronic increased intracranial pressure (*small arrow*). (Courtesy of Arthur B. Dublin, University of California, Davis.)

patterns can be present, including centrencephalic and three-per-second spike and wave activity.[147,423]

Abnormal electroencephalograms are found in approximately 85 per cent of patients with seizures due to astrocytomas. These changes may be subtle and tend to be of minor degree in comparison with those seen with the more anaplastic tumors.

Isotope Scanning

Because of the variety of histological classifications that have been used, the accuracy of isotope scans is difficult to determine. Holman reported 67 per cent accuracy in diagnosing grade I and II astrocytomas, while Fulghum and associates have noted that 50 per cent of such patients have positive scans.[135,179] In other series, low-grade astrocytomas have been demonstrated in even lower percentages.[59] Although Altenburg and Schmidt reported that 73 per cent of patients with astrocytomas had positive radioisotope scans, all the positive scans were of neoplasms with anaplastic features.[5] In one series of 813 patients with low- to intermediate-grade astrocytomas, none had abnormal radioisotope scans.[125] Grade II astrocytomas are more likely than those of grade I to yield a positive scan.[294]

Computed Tomography

Computed tomography has revolutionized the diagnosis of astrocytomas. Accuracy up to 100 per cent has been cited for identification of supratentorial lesions (including both anaplastic and nonanaplastic).[6] Ninety-eight per cent of those in grade I show decreased density on CT scan.[405] These tumors are not enhanced with contrast and have little or no edema around them (Fig. 86–8). Calcification can sometimes be seen in low-grade gliomas (Fig. 86–9).

The grade II astrocytomas are less dense than surrounding brain in approximately 40 per cent of patients, and are isodense or of increased density in the remainder.[405] Approximately 70 per cent of grade II tumors have edema around them, and 90 per cent are enhanced after contrast infusion. The accuracy of CT scanning is considerably improved by using larger volumes of contrast material and more sophisticated scanners.[6]

Computed tomography is useful in evaluating the effect of treatment. Changes in tumor size and ventricular size can be noted. Also, delayed radiation necrosis can be identified, although it cannot always be distinguished from neoplasm.[315]

Angiography

Prior to the introduction of computed tomography, angiography was the standard definitive study in most patients with astrocytomas. It is normal in only approximately 10 per cent of patients with grade I or II astrocytomas.[125] Abnormal circulation was seen in approximately 15 per cent of fibrillary astrocytomas in one series, although others have suggested that a blush on angiography implies anaplasia in the neoplasm.[99,221,399]

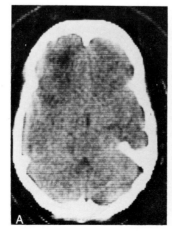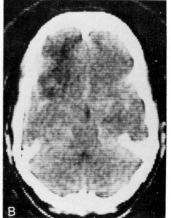

Figure 86–8 *A*. CT scan of a left frontal fibrillary astrocytoma reveals a low-density lesion. *B*. The tumor is not enhanced after intravenous administration of meglumine iothalamate.

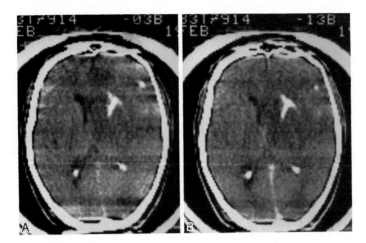

Figure 86–9 *A*. CT scan of a right frontal oligoastrocytoma shows calcification and midline shift. *B*. Contrast enhancement does not affect the appearance of the tumor. The patient was a 51-year-old man with a 13-year history of seizures.

Encephalography

Until angiography became popular in the late 1950's, pneumoencephalography and ventriculography were the definitive studies for evaluation of brain tumors. Encephalography is highly accurate in lateralizing astrocytomas and shows the location of the lesion in approximately 90 per cent of patients.[144] There are a variety of encephalographic changes that may be seen, including compression or displacement of the ventricles. In patients with brain stem tumors, encephalography may still be required for diagnosis.

Investigation of Deep-Seated Tumors

Thalamic Astrocytoma

Pneumoencephalography, ventriculography, and arteriography are of nearly equal diagnostic value in patients with thalamic neoplasms.[232] Characteristic encephalographic findings include elevation of the floor of the body of the lateral ventricle (present in 96 per cent), displacement and bowing of the third ventricle (present in approximately 90 per cent), partial obstruction of the posterior portion of the third ventricle, ventricular enlargement, and compression of the ambient cistern.[73] These same findings would be expected to be identified by CT scanning.

Analysis of ventricular fluid and lumbar spinal fluid reveals increased protein in approximately 50 per cent of patients. Occasionally the cell counts are increased.[73]

Brain Stem Astrocytoma

Radiographic diagnosis of brain stem tumors can be confusing and difficult. Intraventricular masses, cerebellar masses, and extra-axial masses can masquerade as tumors in the brain stem. Encephalitis can produce enlargement of the brain stem, and metastasis to the brain stem can produce the same clinical and investigative findings as primary tumors.[100,375]

The radioisotope brain scan is abnormal in only approximately 5 per cent of patients with brain stem gliomas.[120] The encephalogram is abnormal in 84 to 100 per cent.[232]

Treatment and Results

Hemispheric Astrocytoma

Management of patients with astrocytomas is directed toward establishing a histological diagnosis and inferring a prognosis, relief of symptoms, and prolongation of useful life. With neoplasms located in areas of the brain that are silent, such as the frontal lobe of the nondominant hemisphere, aggressive operative resection including lobectomy may be appropriate. In more critical areas, such as the motor strip, only biopsy may be indicated. In extremely sensitive areas, such as the brain stem, confident neuroradiological diagnosis may be sufficient.

The operative mortality rate depends on the condition of the patients prior to operation and on whether steroids are used. Some authors have reported death rates of zero to 8 per cent with cerebral hemisphere astrocytomas.[233,258] In one series of 206 patients who had neoplasms and were operated on because of seizures, the operative mortality rate was only 3 per cent.[341]

The operative death rate is also influenced by the aggressiveness of the resection. Gol reported the death of 16 per cent of patients who underwent partial resection and internal decompression, whereas after biopsy alone the rate was 37 per cent.[144] These numbers are biased because surgeons tend to perform biopsy in patients who have more dangerously placed tumors or who are in poor neurological condition. If patients are premedicated with steroids, the mortality rate of biopsy may be as low as 3 per cent even with anaplastic astrocytomas.[267]

To a large extent, neurological function after operation depends on the condition of the patient before operation. For those who are in good neurological condition, a good result usually follows operation. With severe neurological deficits preoperatively, continuing neurological problems can be expected. Between 20 and 40 per cent of patients are able to work after operation for astrocytoma; however, a large number are severely disabled.[125,144]

The natural history of fibrillary astrocytoma is one of progressive growth, with anaplasia developing in two thirds of cases and eventually leading to death.[298] Operative decompression postpones death. The effect of radiotherapy in fibrillary astrocytoma is less clear. There are pathological changes that follow radiotherapy, and most authors have found that groups of patients who are treated with operation followed by radiotherapy survive longer than those who are treated with operation alone (Table 86–3). Unfortunately, there are no randomized prospective studies of the usefulness of radiotherapy in nonanaplastic astrocytomas. There is general agreement, however, that between 35 and 50 per cent of patients survive for five years if operative treatment and radiotherapy are combined. There is considerable disparity between the five-year survivals in different series in which radiotherapy was not used. Many of these series included a mixture of tumor types such as cerebellar astrocytomas, gemistocytic astrocytomas, and third ventricular tumors. The natural histories of these vari-

TABLE 86–3 FIVE-YEAR SURVIVAL OF ASTROCYTOMA

SERIES	WITH RADIOTHERAPY (PER CENT)	WITHOUT RADIOTHERAPY (PER CENT)
Bloom et al.*	49	26
Leibel et al.†	35	23
Levy and Elvidge‡	36	26
Uihlein et al.§	54	65

* The treatment and prognosis of medulloblastoma in children: A study of 82 verified cases. Amer. J. Roentgen. *105*:43–62, 1969.
† The role of radiation therapy in the treatment of astrocytomas. Cancer, *35*:1551–1557, 1975.
‡ Astrocytoma of brain and spinal cord: Review of 176 cases, 1940–1949. J. Neurosurg., *13*:413–443, 1956.
§ Comparison of surgery and surgery plus irradiation in the treatment of supratentorial gliomas. Acta. Radiol. [Ther.] (Stockholm), *5*:67–78, 1966.

ous lesions differ from one another, and all these factors make interpretation of results difficult. If surgeons recommend radiotherapy for patients in good neurological condition, and do not recommend it for patients who are in poor neurological condition, selection bias would be expected to produce better survival in the irradiated group.

Clinical improvement following radiotherapy has been noted in up to 90 per cent of patients who survived three months or more.[426] Again, it is not known whether this improvement is due to the radiotherapy, to the operative treatment, or to the resolution of edema produced by treatment modalities.

If radiotherapy is to be undertaken, large doses must be given. Whole brain irradiation with 4500 rads with an additional 1000 rads to the tumor has been recommended. In patients with posterior fossa tumors, Millipore filter analysis of ventricular or spinal fluid may allow detection of neoplastic cells in spinal fluid and indicate a need for craniospinal irradiation.[372] If this is to be done, one must remember that lumbar puncture and cerebrospinal fluid aspiration may be risky in patients with tumors.

Use of radiotherapy is not without risk (see Chapter 97). It delays wound healing and makes postoperative wound infection more likely. Also, radionecrosis may occur and be clinically indistinguishable from tumor recurrence. In some patients who develop radionecrosis, there is no further evidence of tumor; more commonly, however, the astrocytoma persists.[243] Radionecrosis tends to develop late after radiotherapy.[458] Computed tomography reveals mass effect with a mottled lucency.[315] Contrast enhancement of a recurrent mass, although it is possible in areas of radiation necrosis, more likely indicates recurrent tumor.

Other radiation effects on the brain may occur. Symmetrical enlargement of the ventricles is seen three to six months after treatment in approximately 50 per cent of patients receiving 3000 to 6000 rads to the entire brain. This change can be the result of operation; it can, however, also result from diffuse cerebral damage due to whole brain radiotherapy. As yet, there is no known clinical correlate to this ventricular enlargement.[315]

Grading of astrocytomas correlates with survival.[111,298] In the original series of Svein and associates, the three-year survival rates were 62.5 per cent with grade I and 16.8 per cent with grade II neoplasms. The degree of anaplasia of the astrocytic element also influences the survival of patients with mixed gliomas; a mixed glioma with a grade II astrocytic component has the natural history of a grade II astrocytoma.

One of the most important factors affecting survival is the age of the patient. The five-year rate for patients less than 30 years of age was 81 per cent, whereas that for patients older than 30 years was only 15 per cent.[372] In part, this effect of age may reflect the inclusion of tumors of different cell types such as cerebellar astrocytomas and hypothalamic gliomas with the low-grade astrocytomas of children. These more slowly growing cell types are quite uncommon in the older age groups.

Length of survival with gemistocytic astrocytoma is variable. In one series the average time was three years and eight months.[115] In another, 10 per cent of the patients were living at five years.[223] Eventually, most gemistocytic astrocytomas evolve into glioblastomas.[370]

Patients with extensive tumor resections survive longer than patients with less extensive resections. With external decompression alone, no patient in Davidoff's series lived five years.[90] Survival after subtotal removal is almost twice that after biopsy or partial removal, and after gross total removal approximately 40 per cent of patients are alive at five years compared with 13 per cent after subtotal removal.

If seizures are a primary manifestation of the neoplasm, intraoperative electrocorticography may make it possible to control them after operation or even to make the patient seizure-free.[34] This technique requires that skin and bone flaps include the rolandic fissure so that the motor cortex can be identified by electrical stimulation. Removal of tumor from under the white matter beneath the insula should be avoided in order to lessen the risk of postoperative paresis or paralysis. Where tumor is adjacent to important white matter fiber tracts, the tumor should be divided sharply with as little manipulation as possible to minimize the disturbance of the fiber tract. If these techniques are utilized, the majority of patients have less tendency to seizures or become seizure-free, and there is little morbidity.[147,341]

Cushing advocated an aggressive approach to recurrent tumors.[88] Few other authors have addressed this problem. Lorenz found that recurrent astrocytomas were larger, more diffuse, and more difficult to resect than those encountered at the original operation.[247] Others have recommended that repeat operation not be performed for most recurrent astrocytomas.[125] Despite these discouraging comments, reoperation for recurrent astrocytoma sometimes gives gratifying results and adds years to the patient's life. If the neoplasm has become anaplastic, treatment with radiotherapy and possibly chemotherapy may be advisable. If it remains nonanaplastic and slow-growing, and if a significant bulk of it can be resected, reoperation probably will be worthwhile. In particular, a cystic lesion shown on CT scan is a prime candidate for reoperation.

If radiotherapy has not been used as part of the initial treatment, the recurrence can be treated with irradiation. In Bouchard's series all patients who underwent irradiation for recurrent astrocytomas improved clinically either during or subsequent to treatment.[44]

Thalamic Astrocytoma

Decisions concerning treatment of thalamic astrocytomas are difficult. Failure to obtain tissue for histological diagnosis can lead to inappropriate treatment of a potentially curable lesion such as an abscess.[231] If the diagnosis of neoplasm can be made with confidence on the basis of angiography and computed tomography, however, biopsy may be unwise. If there is any question of the nature of the mass, biopsy is necessary, but in some circumstances it is judicious to wait for the nature of the disease process to declare itself.

Needle biopsy of the thalamus can cause significant morbidity and death. In two series, 6 of 17 and 2 of 18 patients developed transtentorial herniation after needle biopsy.[73,177] Intensive corticosteroid premedication and stereotaxic control may, however, allow it to be done with relative safety.[267,389]

Extensive resection of thalamic tumors is not appropriate. If symptoms are produced by obstruction of flow of cerebrospinal fluid, ventricular shunting is indicated. Torkildsen has recommended ventricular shunting and radiotherapy for all tumors in this region, regardless of their histological nature (although radiotherapy is inappropriate for some of these masses).[420] Approximately half the patients with thalamic neoplasms improve with external radiotherapy.[232] Interstitial radiotherapy has also been suggested, but it remains experimental.[299] Some of this improvement may be due to concurrent ventricular shunting, steroids, and other medications.

As would be expected from the variety of neoplasms that occur in the thalamus, survival statistics vary considerably. Most series report three-year survivals of 40 to 60 per cent.[155,232]

Brain Stem Astrocytoma

Approximately 20 per cent of "brain stem gliomas" are pilocytic rather than fibrillary astrocytomas.[266] This figure explains the 20 per cent five-year survival rate after radiotherapy. These tumors occur infrequently after the fifth decade. Patients over 50 who present with clinical and radiographic evidence of a brain stem tumor should be suspected of having a metastasis.[100]

Even in brain stem glioma, operative treatment may occasionally result in improvement. This is particularly true in children who may have cystic tumors. Lassiter and co-workers discovered cystic tumors in 5 of 34 patients who underwent operative exploration for brain stem gliomas. The cysts varied from 12 to 30 cc in volume.[229] With computed tomography, cystic lesions

of the brain stem may be detectable prior to operation. If a large cyst is present, if there is doubt regarding the tumor type, or if knowledge of its histological nature may affect treatment, an operation may be advisable. If operative treatment is undertaken, biopsy should include only visibly abnormal tissue. Most patients with this tumor will not require operative treatment.

Fifteen to thirty per cent of patients with brain stem tumors survive for five years, and occasional patients survive for long periods.[44,266,326] Astrocytomas of the brain stem may extend into the cerebellum, the internal capsule, or the basal ganglia. For this reason, when radiotherapy is used, the treatment fields should be large.[232]

PILOCYTIC ASTROCYTOMA

The pilocytic astrocytoma is the subject of more controversy than any of the other common primary gliomas. Originally termed spongioblastoma unipolare, it has also been called juvenile pilocytic astrocytoma and has been referred to by names designating the location of the mass such as hypothalamic glioma or cerebellar astrocytoma.[22,370]

The original spongioblastoma unipolare seen in young patients was commonly adjacent to the third ventricle or in the cerebellum and rarely in the cerebral hemisphere.[22] It was called spongioblastoma by Zülch, but he also included brain stem gliomas and optic nerve gliomas in the subgroup.[461] These tumors are grouped together on the basis of similar biological characteristics. The pathological changes are also similar in several of these groups, and Rosenthal fibers (which can also occur in a wide variety of other pathological conditions) are present in each of them. They are biologically indolent and, in this respect, differ from the fibrillary astrocytomas of adulthood. Examples are the optic nerve, hypothalamic, and cerebellar tumors that grow very slowly. Most pontine gliomas have a more aggressive natural history than the hypothalamic gliomas.

There are differences in histological appearance between cerebellar tumors and those in the hypothalamic and chiasmal areas, but these differences may result from the local environment. The compact optic nerve may produce a pilocytic lesion, and the less confining cerebellum, a spongy tumor. The brain stem glioma is usually a fibrillary astrocytoma. Twenty per cent of brain stem gliomas have the histological characteristics of hypothalamic glioma and a reasonably benign natural history.[266]

A compromise between these divergent views has been adopted by Davis and is also used in the World Health Organization Brain Tumor Classification.[96,397] The specific pathological changes usually found in astrocytomas adjacent to the third ventricle, in the cerebellum, in the optic nerve or chiasm, and occasionally in the brain stem, determine the name of the tumor. Davis calls these neoplasms juvenile astrocytomas.[96] They are called pilocytic astrocytomas in the World Health Organization classification, and they include the juvenile pilocytic astrocytomas of Russell and Rubinstein as well as most cerebellar astrocytomas.

Hypothalamic-Chiasmal Glioma

Gliomas of the chiasm, hypothalamus, and third ventricular region present differently to different medical specialists. Ophthalmologists see patients whose complaints are primarily visual. Neurological surgeons see those whose symptoms and signs are referable to the hypothalamic or third ventricular areas.[351] These tumors usually occur in childhood, the average age being 4 years and the peak incidence lying between 3 and 7 years.[140,287,461] Older persons can be affected, and patients 67 and 79 years old have been reported.[81,287] Women are more likely than men to be affected.[78,259,310]

The incidence of optic nerve or chiasmal gliomas is approximately 1 per cent of gliomas of the nervous system, and they account for 3 to 4 per cent of all orbital tumors.[295] Chiasmal tumors have a tendency to project into the third ventricle and to have a looser architecture adjacent to the ventricle and to be more compact in the more distal portions of the optic nerve.[78]

On histological examination, pilocytic areas alternate with more loosely organized areas. The cell types are a mixture of fibrillary and "protoplasmic" astrocytes, the latter predominating in the less compact portions of the tumor. Rosenthal fibers are common. When the tumor extends into the optic nerves it may elicit neoplastic proliferation of the meninges.[78] Variable numbers of oligodendroglial cells occur. Electron microscopy reveals a predominance of astrocytes with secretory activity, as shown by increased endoplasmic reticulum and Golgi apparatus.[7] The increase in secretory activity may account for the accumulation of extracellular myxoid material seen in these tumors.

The natural history of these lesions is variable. Some tumors inexorably enlarge at a slow rate, while others do not change. The enlargement may occur not only by proliferation of tumor cells but also by hyperplasia of surrounding tissues or by accumulation of secretory products within the tumor.[7] Verhoeff has suggested that the original glioma enlarges by producing anaplasia in adjacent normal or reactive astrocytes.[429]

Clinical Presentation

The clinical findings of hypothalamic, chiasmal, and optic nerve gliomas depend on the site of involvement. Gliomas of the optic nerve may be large without producing profound visual deficits.[150] (Optic nerve tumors are discussed in greater detail in Chapter 95.) Approximately 75 per cent of optic nerve gliomas involve the optic chiasm, and two thirds of the tumors that involve the optic chiasm also involve the hypothalamus.[287]

Chiasmal involvement produces visual field loss. Hypothalamic involvement produces precocious puberty in approximately 20 per cent, diencephalic syndrome in approximately 20 per cent, diabetes insipidus in approximately 10 per cent, and obesity or failure of development of secondary sex characteristics in other patients.[351] Headache is present in approximately 10 per cent in ophthalmological series, but in about 33 per cent of patients in neurosurgical series.[259,287,310] Dodge and co-workers noted loss of vision in 91 per cent of patients with chiasmal gliomas, optic atrophy in 62 per cent, headache in 47 per cent, papilledema in 32 per cent, metabolic disturbances in 26 per cent, proptosis in 18 per cent, motor symptoms in 12 per cent, and convulsions in 9 per cent.[106] Between 10 and 50 per cent of patients with optic nerve gliomas have the stigmata of von Recklinghausen's syndrome.[78]

Investigation

Routine radiographs of the skull are abnormal in approximately 50 per cent of patients, the abnormalities often being due to increased intracranial pressure. Enlargement of the chiasmatic sulcus can be identified in approximately 25 per cent of patients.[384] If the tumor extends through the optic canal, the canal will be eroded. An optic canal more than 7 mm in diameter or with one side more than 20 per cent larger than the other suggests an expanding lesion in the canal, although it does not assure that the mass is a glioma.[118,142] Calcification is seen with approximately 20 per cent of chiasmatic and hypothalamic gliomas and, when seen, consists of a small nodule of calcium or granules of calcium. It is seen only in the very large tumors.[384]

In the past, encephalography and ventriculography have been the studies used to diagnose these neoplasms. When tumors are less than 1 cm in diameter, the only findings may be an enlarged optic nerve outlined by air, or slight separation of chiasmatic and infundibular recesses of the third ventricle. In tumors 1 to 2 cm in diameter, the anterior recesses of the third ventricle are displaced superiorly and posteriorly, and a filling defect is seen in the chiasmatic cistern. On occasion, the cistern may be completely obliterated. With tumors larger than 2 cm in diameter, there usually is hydrocephalus due to obstruction of the foramen of Monro.[384] At present, the diagnosis is made more secure by the addition of computed tomography (Fig. 86–10). This procedure also permits estimation of the intracranial extent of optic nerve glioma and allows it to be followed over long periods, for intermittent assessment of size.

Diagnosis can be particularly difficult in anterior third ventricular neoplasms. Of 16 patients with confirmed tumors of the third ventricle, 11 had infiltrating astrocytomas, 2 had hematomas, 1 had a malignant neoplasm, 1 had a cyst, and 1 had a teratoma.[403]

Treatment and Results

Treatment of gliomas of the chiasm and hypothalamus has been directed toward histological diagnosis and relief of hydrocephalus. In the young patient, particularly if von Recklinghausen's disease coexists, there is usually little difficulty in establishing the diagnosis on the basis of clinical and radiological criteria. Confusion can arise in the older patient. In a series of 51 patients with optic gliomas, 14 of 29 (48 per cent) with chiasmal gliomas and 3 of 11 (27 per cent) with optic nerve gliomas were more than 15 years of age.[287] A diagnosis of optic nerve glioma was made in two patients following biopsy, but subsequently, one of them, a 43-year-old man, was found to have Hodgkin's disease; and the other, a 19-year-old woman, had reticulum cell sarcoma. An arachnoid cyst has also been reported in the optic nerve and chiasm.

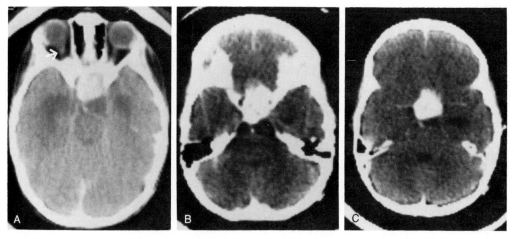

Figure 86–10 CT scan of a chiasmal glioma. *A*. Tumor thickens the left optic nerve (*arrow*) and lies between the anterior clinoid processes. *B*. Tumor extends superiorly to the region of the optic chiasm. *C*. Contrast enhancement of tumor in the hypothalamus.

Drainage of this cyst has resulted in improvement in vision.[76]

Recommendations for treatment of the hydrocephalus vary. Torkildsen advised ventriculocisternal shunting in all patients who have obstructive third ventricular tumors.[420] Ventriculoperitoneal shunts are probably preferable, however, since they are easier to place and function more reliably. Roberson and Till recommend subtotal excision of the tumor if this appears feasible on preoperative radiographic investigation and at the time of operation—if the patient is in sufficiently good condition to survive for six months.[351]

In many patients, operation will be necessary for diagnosis or for relief of hydrocephalus. Most authors recommend radiotherapy for chiasmal and hypothalamic gliomas.[44,259,266,351] Miller and co-workers agree that radiotherapy may be useful for hypothalamic gliomas, but they advocate withholding this treatment in gliomas limited to the chiasm.[287] Glaser and colleagues believe that radiotherapy does not offer any better result than no treatment.[140] Since patients with hypothalamic gliomas commonly have endocrine derangements, hormonal support also may be needed.[218]

The outcome of treatment depends on the preoperative condition of the patients. If they are in poor neurological condition on admission, the results do not warrant further treatment. An exception to this rule might be the one with the diencephalic syndrome.[351]

Part of the problem in determining the efficacy of radiotherapy is the quite variable natural history of hypothalamic gliomas. MacCarty and associates noted progressive visual deterioration in approximately one third of patients with chiasmal gliomas.[259] Among Roberson and Till's 18 patients for whom survival information is available, 5 died, 2 as a result of operative intervention and 1 a year after biopsy and radiotherapy. The rest were alive at follow-up, up to 13 years later.[351] In another series, of five patients who survived operation and later died of tumor, two succumbed between 1 and 5 years after operation, one less than 10 years after operation, and two between 16 and 20 years after operation.[287] Unless the patients are followed for many decades, the result of treatment and the natural history of the disease cannot be known.

One of the arguments against biopsy of hypothalamic and chiasmal gliomas is the risk of operative death with a relatively benign tumor. This mortality rate is much higher among patients who are in poor condition prior to operation or who have extensive tumors. In the series reported by Miller and associates, 11 patients died in the immediate postoperative period.[287] All deaths were prior to 1962, and in the 14 operations since 1963 there were no deaths. In two other recent series there were no operative deaths.[259,310]

Hoyt and Baghdassarian have assessed the effect of radiotherapy on visual acuity in patients with chiasmal gliomas. Deterioration occurred in 11 of 38 eyes. There was no difference in acuity changes between those with irradiated tumors and those with nonirradiated tumors.[185] Actually, acuity may improve spontaneously and proptosis may decrease even without radiotherapy.[140] Others have suggested that radiotherapy may be advantageous, since on long-term follow-up, three of four patients without it had died, whereas only two of seven patients with it had died.[287]

In summary, it is unclear whether radiotherapy is beneficial with chiasmal gliomas. It would appear to be prudent to use it for large hypothalamic gliomas, since they have an unfavorable prognosis. With small hypothalamic gliomas in patients who are in good condition, there is controversy regarding its use. The same is true for patients with neoplasm restricted to the chiasm. The role of biopsy has yet to be determined.

Cerebellar Pilocytic Astrocytoma

Cerebellar astrocytomas make up approximately 4 per cent of intracranial tumors and 8 per cent of gliomas.[306,461] They constitute approximately 20 per cent of cerebellar and fourth ventricular tumors.[306] The average age of the patients varies widely; it was 9 years and 20 years in two large series, but most authors have found it to be between 10 and 15 years.[87,115,138,306,461] Approximately one third of patients are older than 15 years, with the ages ranging up to 60 years.[145,306] Males and females are approximately equally affected.

Pathology

Pilocytic cerebellar astrocytomas occur in the midline in one third to two thirds of patients, the more lateral tumors tending to occur in older patients.[115,145,306] Penfield is reported to have believed that the tumor produced a transudate that collected outside the tumor, forming a cyst in which the tumor lay as a mural nodule.[115] The cyst may be many times as large as the neoplasm, which is a nodule in the wall of the cyst in approximately 47 per cent of cases and constitutes most of the wall in approximately 45 per cent.[145] Approximately 8 per cent of patients have more than one cyst.

The neoplastic tissue is firm to tough and well demarcated from cerebellum. Occasionally, it is softer as a result of mucoid degeneration. In approximately 15 per cent the neoplasm is a typical "diffuse" astrocytoma of adulthood.[370]

Leviton and co-workers have derived a discriminate function to predict survival in cerebellar astrocytomas in children. Histological factors that are favorable include microcysts, foci of oligodendroglial cells, low cell density, endothelial proliferation, and perivascular desmoplasia.[238] High cell density is unfavorable. Two thirds of cerebellar astrocytomas in children have favorable histological characteristics (Fig. 86–11).[447]

Clinical Presentation

The average duration of symptoms is one to two years.[95,115] All patients develop headache, and it is the initial symptom in 90 to 95 per cent.[138,306,447] A typical history consists of morning headache and vomiting in an otherwise apparently well person. Papilledema is present in approximately 90 per cent of patients, and gait disturbance, ataxia, cranial nerve palsy, nystagmus, and lethargy are common.[145] In earlier years, blindness due to papilledema was common also, but in recent years earlier diagnosis and treatment have made this unusual.

Investigation

Plain skull films often show evidence of hydrocephalus or, in children, may show spreading of the cranial sutures. Only approximately 4 per cent of patients with cerebellar astrocytomas have radiographically identifiable calcium salts in their tumor.[268] The isotope brain scan is highly accurate in identifying these neoplasms.[138] Computed tomography also is highly reliable (Fig. 86–12). Contrast enhancement may result in layering of contrast material in the dependent portion of the cyst.[212] Angiography reveals hydrocephalus, rules out a vascular lesion of the cerebellum, and in many cases is able to identify the tumor. Ventriculography identifies the mass effect of the tumor in approximately 90 per cent of patients.[138,145]

Treatment and Results

Although most patients have had the tumor removed, there are a few who had no operation or in whom only a cyst decompression or biopsy has been done. Hausman and Stevenson have reported a patient with a cerebellar astrocytoma who had no operation and who survived 45 years after the onset of symptoms before he died of his neoplasm.[171] Bucy reported a patient who was asymptomatic for 15 years after drainage of the cyst.[56] Geissinger and Bucy had a patient who underwent suboccipital craniectomy and biopsy of the tumor and was subsequently asymptomatic for 30 years before she developed diplopia and headaches.[138] At a second operation, a large fluid-filled cyst was found, but no evidence of tumor either grossly or in several biopsy specimens.

Despite the rare occurrence of spontaneous regression or effective treatment by cyst decompression, the optimal treatment is removal of the tumor. Preoperative shunting may lessen the cerebellar symptoms and the symptoms of hydrocephalus and decrease the operative morbidity and the number of deaths.[2] If cerebrospinal fluid pathways are unequivocally patent, as determined by a normal postoperative cisternogram, the cerebrospinal fluid shunt can be occluded.[3] Successful removal of the tumor may not, however, obviate the need for ventricular shunting because adhesive arachnoiditis may develop and obstruct cerebrospinal fluid circulation. The hydrocephalus occurring after posterior fossa operation is of a communicating type rather than the noncommunicating hydrocephalus produced by tumors.[62,281]

Anaplasia in cerebellar astrocytomas is

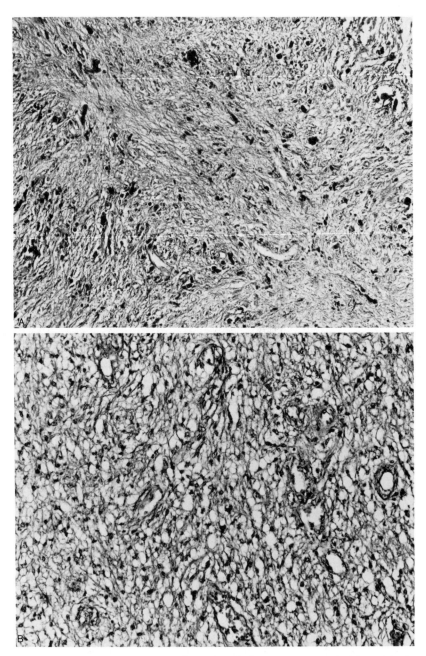

Figure 86–11   Microscopic pathological changes of cerebellar astrocytoma. Staining with phosphotungstic acid-hematoxylin reveals Rosenthal fibers in *A* and both compact and loose architecture. *A*, 140 ×; *B*, 170 ×.

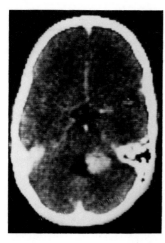

Figure 86–12 CT scan of cerebellar astrocytoma reveals a contrast-enhanced mass adjacent to a cyst.

quite unusual. Bernell and associates have reported two patients whose cerebellar astrocytomas recurred 20 and 23 years after gross total excision, and Budka reported a recurrence after 28 years.[35,58] Anaplasia was present at recurrence in each of these neoplasms. Cerebellar astrocytoma has metastasized through a ventriculoperitoneal shunt to cause widespread systemic disease.[54]

The extent of tumor resection determines survival. Of patients followed up for five years or longer, 1 of 6 who underwent biopsy alone was alive, while 2 of 5 with partial resections, 11 of 20 with subtotal resections, and 22 of 29 with gross total removal were alive.[90] Altered consciousness is also an important factor more closely related to survival than are histological criteria.

Long-term survival of patients who undergo successful gross total excision of cerebellar astrocytomas is nearly 100 per cent.[138,461] Of 12 patients followed for long periods, 9 were alive an average of 31.4 years after operation, 2 had died of recurrence of tumor, and 1 had committed suicide 30 years after operation.[113] Twelve other patients with long-term follow-up were all living an average of 36.3 years after operation. Four of these patients had initially undergone an incomplete removal and one had undergone only biopsy and cyst aspiration.[138]

The risks of operative treatment are quite small. In a series of 12 patients with cerebellar astrocytomas, there was only one postoperative death, which was due to an anesthetic accident.[259] A 3.8 per cent operative mortality rate has been reported in patients operated on since 1938.[138] Gol and McKissock found postoperative mortality rates of 14 per cent if hydrocephalus was not severe but of 58 per cent in the presence of severe hydrocephalus.[145] Leviton and co-workers have reported no operative deaths in 76 consecutive operations for cerebellar astrocytoma.[238]

The most common complication of operative treatment is pseudomeningocele, which occurs in approximately 12 per cent of patients. Geissinger and Bucy found only 1 of 22 patients who had such severe neurological dysfunction as to "curtail a normal independent existence," although 5 of the 22 (23 per cent) had "significant neurologic deficit," which consisted of decreased visual acuity in 4 and a wide-based gait in the fifth.[138] In Gol and McKissock's series, 88 per cent of patients who survived operation were able to "earn their living or continue with their education in a fairly normal fashion."[145]

The evidence is unclear whether radiotherapy is or is not of benefit for cerebellar astrocytomas. Of seven patients in a series surviving 12 to 39 years after incomplete removal of the tumor, none received radiotherapy.[138] Davis and co-workers reported 14 patients who received postoperative irradiation and 11 patients who did not receive irradiation. Seven patients were alive in each group at the time of the report.[95]

There is a marked difference in survival between patients with cystic and those with noncystic cerebellar astrocytomas. Some noncystic tumors undoubtedly are fibrillary as opposed to pilocytic. For five patients with noncystic tumors, the average postoperative survival was 6.5 years, with only one patient still alive, while of nine with cystic tumors, seven were alive for an average of 29.1 years after operation.[113] Of four patients who received radiotherapy after operation, one had a "diffuse astrocytoma" and died of disease at six months. The other three were living and well 21 to 118 months after treatment.[266]

Cerebellar astrocytomas should be operatively removed if it can be done with reasonable safety. Tumor attached to the brain stem or floor of the fourth ventricle should not be resected. If it is fibrillary rather than pilocytic in cell type, radiotherapy may be useful. It would also be reasonable to follow patients postoperatively with CT scanning, and if neoplastic growth is identified, reoperation or radiotherapy could be used.

Macrocystic Cerebral Pilocytic Astrocytoma

Macrocystic pilocytic astrocytomas may occur in the cerebrum and, in this location, have the same good prognosis as they do when they occur in the cerebellum.[18] They tend to affect young adults.[115,173] Most authors have included them with other types of cerebral astrocytomas and have not commented on any unusual pathological or clinical characteristics.[45,111,409,440,455]

Cysts occur in 25 to 50 per cent of all cerebral astrocytomas.[95,144] A macrocystic form occurs in approximately 10 per cent.[95] Ringertz has stated that 11 per cent have a structure similar to cerebellar astrocytomas, although some other authors believe the incidence to be lower.[144,173,347]

Pathologically, the cerebral lesion consists of a tumor nodule in the wall of a large cyst exactly as it does in the cerebellum (Fig. 86–13).[95] Although the tumor appears macroscopically to be a very well-defined entity, the microscopic pattern varies. It may be reported as a piloid astrocytoma, a fibrillary astrocytoma, or a giant cell astrocytoma.[144] There has been insufficient description of the microscopic details of this neoplasm to allow more precise histological delineation.

The literature contains several reports referring to long survival of patients with macrocystic astrocytomas. Elvidge and Martinez-Coll have reported eight cases of cystic piloid astrocytoma of the cerebral hemisphere in which average survival was 11.9 years and in which four of the patients were still living at the time of the report.[115] These patients were again reported in 1968 and continued to survive 28, 29, 33, and 38 years respectively after the initial operation.[113] Davidoff reported that while only 29 per cent of cerebral astrocytomas were cystic, 56 per cent of his patients who survived longer than eight years had cystic lesions. One physician with a macrocystic astrocytoma was alive and well 26 years after subtotal removal of his tumor.[90] Leibel and associates described three patients with macrocystic cerebral astrocytomas that were thought to have been totally resected. Two patients survived 8 years and 12 years after operation; a third patient died of congestive heart failure without evidence of tumor recurrence 12 years after operation.[233]

SUBEPENDYMAL GIANT CELL ASTROCYTOMA

This descriptive name is applied to a tumor that occurs in approximately 15 per cent of patients with tuberous sclerosis. It may occur without evidence of tuberous sclerosis or with an incomplete form of it.[129,203] The tumor is usually encountered in children, but adults may be affected.

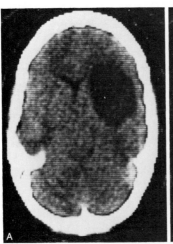 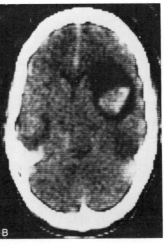

Figure 86–13 *A.* CT scan of cerebral macrocystic pilocytic astrocytoma reveals a large cyst with no obvious tumor in a 26-year-old woman with headache and seizures. *B.* Contrast enhancement demonstrates a mural nodule.

Pathology

Since this tumor is so intimately associated with tuberous sclerosis, the pathological changes of the latter are important. There are three pathologically distinct intracranial lesions with tuberous sclerosis. One is a cortical tuber, a pale whitish nodule that arises in a gyrus and is firm and rubbery. Microscopic examination reveals a gradual transition from normal cortex to abnormal tissue. Within the tuber the cortical laminations are disordered, there is an increased number of astrocytes, and giant cells are found.[203] A second type is the small subependymal nodule that resembles wax dripping along a candle. For this reason, these lesions have been called "candle gutterings." They consist of small circumscribed masses of elongated astrocytes in association with gemistocytic astrocytes and are covered by an intact layer of ependymal cells. The third lesion is the subependymal giant cell astrocytoma (Fig. 86–14). It is an intraventricular neoplasm arising from the lateral ventricle or the anterior part of the third ventricle and often produces ventricular obstruction. It has a combination of two cell types. In some areas there are predominantly elongated astrocytes, while in other areas giant cells predominate. The giant cells are thought to be gemistocytic astrocytes.[370] In tissue culture, they have been identified as monstrous astrocytes with ballooning cytoplasm and many processes.[209] Vascularity may be greatly increased.[175,362]

Clinical Presentation

Patients with tuberous sclerosis typically have a triad of mental retardation, seizures, and facial adenoma sebaceum. The presence of subependymal giant cell astrocytoma is announced by symptoms and signs of hydrocephalus.

Investigation

Calcification is seen on plain x-ray in approximately two thirds of subependymal giant cell astrocytomas.[129,203] Isotope scan is highly reliable, and CT scan also accurately identifies the tumor, which tends to be vascular and to be enhanced by contrast (Fig. 86–15). Since the neoplasms project into the low-density ventricular compartment, they should be easily distinguished from the surrounding low-density fluid. Angiography reveals hypervascularity, par-

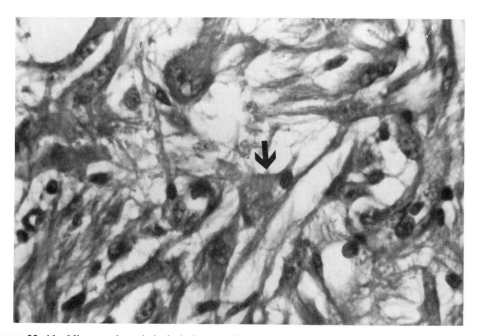

Figure 86–14 Microscopic pathological changes of subependymal giant cell astrocytoma. Giant astrocytes (*arrow*) are demonstrated. 440 ×. (Courtesy of Surl L. Nielson, M.D., University of California, Davis.)

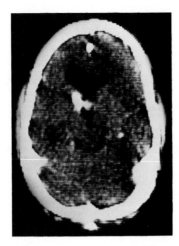

Figure 86–15 CT scan of a subependymal giant cell astrocytoma shows an enhanced subependymal mass that projects into the left ventricle at the site of the foramen of Monro and has produced unilateral hydrocephalus. (Courtesy of Arthur B. Dublin, M.D., University of California, Davis.)

ticularly in the late arterial phase, with contrast material pooling in small rounded collections.[175] Early venous drainage is not a prominent feature.

Treatment and Results

Treatment of subependymal giant cell astrocytoma is directed toward decompression of the obstructed ventricular system and removal of the intraventricular tumor. Both goals usually can be accomplished by removal of the tumor.[203] Shunting of the ventricular fluid may be required. If so, a ventriculoatrial or ventriculoperitoneal shunt is preferable. If the tumor appears to have been resected, recurrence is quite unlikely.

Even if management of the tumor is uncomplicated, other stigmata of tuberous sclerosis such as seizures and mental retardation will usually interfere with the quality of the patient's life.

ASTROBLASTOMA

Astroblastomas make up 2 to 5 per cent of all gliomas.[22,116,455] Although they can occur in the cerebellum, they usually arise in the cerebral hemispheres of young adults.[20,370] Large cysts are frequent. The prognosis is intermediate between those of astrocytoma and glioblastoma.[370] The diagnosis should not be made unless the entirety of a neoplasm has been sampled for histological study.

ANAPLASTIC ASTROCYTOMA

When an astrocytoma develops areas of anaplasia, it is called an anaplastic astrocytoma. Histological signs of anaplasia include cellular and nuclear pleomorphism, mitoses, endothelial proliferation, hemorrhage, and necrosis. At least two of these features must be present in order to qualify an astrocytic neoplasm as anaplastic.[96] Extreme degrees of anaplasia produce the histological pattern of glioblastoma, as is discussed later. Some authors have considered the glioblastoma to correspond with grade IV astrocytoma, and anaplastic astrocytoma to correspond with grade III astrocytoma in the Kernohan classification. Other authors have considered "glioblastoma" to be a term applying to evidence of anaplasia in any of the glial neoplasms and have not used the term "anaplastic astrocytoma." This differentiation is discussed further in the section on glioblastomas.

Each of the common well-differentiated glial neoplasms has an anaplastic variant. Examples are anaplastic astrocytoma, anaplastic oligodendroglioma, and anaplastic ependymoma. In these variants, the cell of origin can still be identified. Since the cell line of origin may not be apparent in a glioblastoma, glioblastomas must be considered as a separate entity. Unfortunately, clinical studies have so mixed and confused the differentiation between glioblastoma and anaplastic astrocytoma that clinical differences between these two pathological groups cannot be isolated. For this reason, anaplastic astrocytomas are discussed with glioblastoma. It should be understood that anaplastic astrocytomas tend to be less anaplastic than glioblastomas and, therefore, have a slightly better prognosis. Also it should be understood that not all glioblastomas are of the astrocytic series, some being derived from oligodendroglial or ependymal tumors, although all anaplastic astrocytomas are of the astrocytic series.

OLIGODENDROGLIOMA

An oligodendroglioma arises from the neoplastic proliferation of oligodendroglial cells. These cells were not recognized as a discrete entity until 1900, when Robertson, while studying platinum stains of brain, identified a cell he called a "mesoglial cell."[353] In 1921 Hortega, noting its paucity of dendrites, coined the term "oligodendroglial."[182] Although the occurrence of tumors of this cell line was predicted by Bailey and Hiller, they were not recognized until 1926 when Bailey and Cushing reported nine cases.[22,23] In 1929 Bailey and Bucy reported four cases and presented a thorough clinical and pathological discussion of the neoplasm.[19]

Incidence

Oligodendrogliomas make up about 4 per cent of all gliomas. Approximately 60 per cent of the patients are men, and their average age is 40 years. Although this tumor is rare in children, it does occur and has been reported as early as six weeks of age. Patients with tumors near the midline are, on the average, 12 years younger than those with hemispheric tumors.*

Pathogenesis

The cause of oligodendrogliomas is unknown. Interestingly, they have been reported to occur in the frontal lobes of each of twins.[314] Also, one has developed in a glial scar following a head injury.[104] They are the most common tumors induced by the nitrosoureas in experimental animals.[213]

Pathology

At least 90 per cent of oligodendrogliomas are above the tentorium.[112,181,264] Of the supratentorial oligodendrogliomas, 10 to 20 per cent occur in either the third ventricle or the lateral ventricle, or arise from the thalamus and project into a ventricle.[112,181] The remaining 80 to 90 per cent

are located in the cerebral hemispheres. At least half of these hemispheric tumors are in the frontal lobe.[345,388,448]

Macroscopically, these tumors are pinkish-red, friable masses. There may be a false plane of demarcation between what is obviously tumor and what appears to be uninvaded brain. One fifth of those in the hemisphere are cystic.[112,156,352] Some of the hemispheric tumors are surface lesions that may appear initially to grow from dura and to indent brain.[388] As dissection proceeds, however, these are found to be exophytic lesions from brain that have become attached to dura. They may also grow into the ventricular space and diffusely along the ventricular wall to cover the wall with a carpet of neoplastic cells.[56]

A typical oligodendroglioma is a uniform cellular neoplasm that resembles a honeycomb at low magnification (Fig. 86–16).[19] The nuclei are round and equal in size with diffusely scattered chromatin. Mitoses may be absent or occur occasionally. Vascularity also varies and may be increased significantly in some.[95] If a biopsy is allowed to stand for several hours before fixation and staining, the cells alter and develop a perinuclear halo referred to as "acute swelling" by Penfield and Cone.[317] Metallic impregnation may further identify the cell type.[65]

Approximately one third of tumors that are eventually labeled oligodendroglioma have a significant component of neoplastic astrocytes or neoplastic ependymal cells.[181,206,448] Some of these astrocytes are nonneoplastic but are engulfed by the invading oligodendroglioma. Others are neoplastic and coexist with neoplastic oligodendroglia. In this circumstance, the predominant cell type is not clear and the neoplasm is termed an oligoastrocytoma.[358]

Calcium salts are found by histological examination in approximately 70 per cent of oligodendrogliomas.[112,352] They are much less frequent in subtentorial tumors.[264] Usually they occur in or adjacent to vessel walls, but they may also occur in the tumor parenchyma.[206] Necrotic areas develop in these tumors, particularly in the portions with endothelial proliferation. Degenerative changes may result in the deposition of fat in the cytoplasm of the cell.[19]

Oligodendrogliomas account for approximately 10 per cent of tumors with menin-

---

* See references 22, 95, 112, 154, 156, 181, 264, 345, 352, 388, 441, 448, 455.

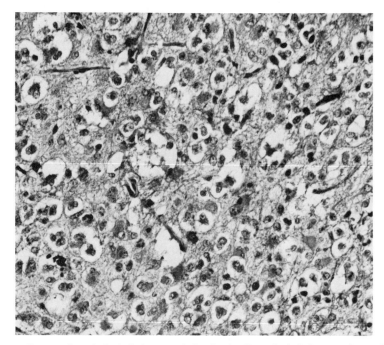

Figure 86–16   Microscopic pathological changes of oligodendroglioma include increased vascularity and a uniform pattern of cells with perinuclear halos. 220 ×.

geal gliomatosis.[325] Also, approximately 10 per cent of oligodendrogliomas metastasize through the ventricular system.[112] They gain access to the cerebrospinal fluid through the ventricular wall. The likelihood of spread by way of the cerebrospinal fluid is unrelated to the histological features of the tumor. These metastases are unusual if tumor invades the subarachnoid space rather than the ventricle.[206] Dissemination outside the central nervous system is unusual, and when it does occur, operative treatment has preceded it. Extracranial metastasis may take place via either lymphatic channels or hematogenous routes.[192,398]

Anaplastic Oligodendroglioma

As many as one fourth of oligodendrogliomas may be anaplastic.[448,460] The honeycomb pattern of the usual oligodendroglioma is distorted in the anaplastic variant.[112] Duration of symptoms is shorter preoperatively than with nonanaplastic ones, and survival is shortened.[345]

There is disagreement about the relation between oligodendrogliomas and glioblastomas. In rare situations, oligodendrogliomas have been documented to dedifferentiate to glioblastomas.[95,206] It is not known whether the glioblastoma element arises from anaplasia of oligodendroglial cells or from an astrocytic component of an oligodendroglioma.[26,460]

Clinical Presentation

Typically patients harboring oligodendrogliomas have a long history of symptoms averaging seven to eight years.[95,352,439] The preoperative history can extend to 21 years.[112] With tumors near the midline, however, it is much shorter, averaging about eight months. The midline tumors tend to cause increased intracranial pressure early in the course, and one third of midline tumors reported in one series presented with attacks of decerebrate rigidity.[388]

The initial symptom is seizures in approximately 50 per cent of cases.[264,387,439] Headache is also a common early symptom. By the time the tumor is diagnosed, 70 to 90 per cent of patients have seizures.[318] Ten per cent of those with seizures caused by neoplasm will be found to have oligodendroglioma. Only the common neoplasms such as glioblastoma, metastatic tumor, or meningioma are more likely to be found in a patient evaluated for seizures.[164] Papilledema and focal neurological deficits are each present in approximately one third to one half of patients.[181,264,439] Rarely, spontaneous hemorrhage may occur and can lead to sudden coma or death.[206]

Investigation

Radiographically identifiable tumor calcification is present in 40 to 60 per cent of oligodendrogliomas.[112,345,439] Its incidence is unrelated to the age of the patient.[112] The appearance of the calcium has been described as "blotchy or wavy, irregular shadows."[19] It can also appear as rounded patches of radio-opaque material, and it may not be at the center of the tumor but may be restricted to only one portion of its periphery.

Spinal fluid findings usually are not helpful. Occasionally, pleocytosis occurs and has included up to 500 cells that appear to be lymphocytes.[398] The electroencephalogram usually is abnormal, but the abnormality may be nonfocal and may even suggest an atrophic process.[263,439]

Oligodendrogliomas may be identified by isotope brain scans.[439] CT scanning demonstrates calcification in 90 per cent and approximately 66 per cent show enhancement (Fig. 86–17).[431] Angiography reveals an avascular mass. Draining veins, which are in their normal location, may be enlarged.[430,448]

Treatment and Results

The standard treatment for oligodendroglioma has been resection. Aggressive operation with excision of considerable bulk of tumor leads to longer survival than more restricted resection.[112,181,439] Tumors located in the occipital lobe have a somewhat better prognosis than those at other sites because occipital tumors can be removed by generous occipital lobectomy. Frontal and temporal tumors tend to invade the basal ganglia or corpus callosum before they are identified and thus have a worse prognosis. There is disagreement regarding the effectiveness of radiotherapy for these lesions. It has been recommended on the basis of a study of one group of patients, some of whom were treated by operation alone and some of whom were treated by operation followed by radiotherapy. Only 31 per cent of the unirradiated group survived five years, in comparison with 85 per cent of those who underwent radiotherapy. Unfortunately the data were biased by the inclusion in the unirradiated group of at least two patients who died shortly after operation but not within the 30-day period allotted for operative death.[387] Weir and Elvidge reported the average survival for patients who underwent operation and radiotherapy to be 4 years as compared with 6.4 years for patients who underwent operative treatment only.[439] Other authors have found no effect or only a slight prolongation of life with added radiotherapy.[264,352] Long survivals occur occasionally—for 20 years in an estimated 6 per cent.[352] Indeed, survivals of 20 to 40 years have been reported.[95,181] Patients who live for many years often have had multiple operations. Kernohan has reported one who has undergone eight operations over a span of 41 years and is still living.[206]

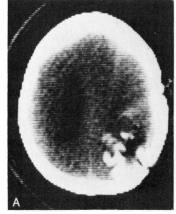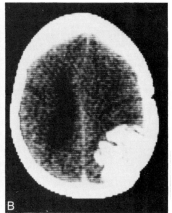

Figure 86–17 CT scan of oligodendroglioma. *A*. Unenhanced scan shows tumor calcification and hydrocephalus (due to brain shift not demonstrated in this illustration). *B*. Intravenous contrast agent densely enhances the tumor. (Courtesy of Arthur B. Dublin, M.D., University of California, Davis.)

The operative mortality rate was 15 per cent in Cushing's series published in 1932.[88] With current techniques for control of intracranial pressure and modern postoperative management, the expected operative mortality rate is approximately 5 per cent.[264,439] Postoperative seizures are quite common, occurring in approximately 80 per cent of patients.[388]

EPENDYMOMA

Ependymomas were first set apart as a single group by Bailey.[16] They are glial neoplasms composed predominantly of ependymal cells and constitute approximately 5 per cent of gliomas.* The incidence varies widely among different series; it is higher in those with a large proportion of young patients and those that include choroid plexus papillomas as a type of ependymoma.[410] In addition there seems to be a higher incidence in Asia and Japan.[390] The average age of patients is approximately 20 years.[223,256] Patients have been reported as young as 1 week of age, however, and the authors have treated a 72-year-old man.[371] There is a slight male preponderance. Approximately two thirds of all ependymomas occur in the infratentorial compartment, and ependymomas account for approximately 25 per cent of tumors in and around the fourth ventricle.[84,390,410] Most series show childhood tumors to be predominantly infratentorial, whereas adults may develop either supratentorial or infratentorial ependymomas.[108,127]

Pathology

The gross appearance of an ependymoma is that of a soft, pale, and sometimes nodular mass. It may be predominantly intraventricular, in which case it conforms to the shape of its enclosure, or it may burrow into the cerebral white matter (Fig. 86–18). Approximately half of those occurring in the fourth ventricle arise from the lateral recess. The remaining tumors arise from the floor of the fourth ventricle or rarely from the posterior medullary velum or obex.[322,391] Half of those in the fourth ventricle extend into the subarachnoid space.[349] When this extension occurs, the tumor tends to encase the medulla or upper cervical spinal cord (it is described as "plastic ependymoma") in a pattern thought to be due to its growth within the confines of the arachnoid around the medulla.[82] The tendency for ependymomas to grow through the foramina of Luschka accounts for 80 per cent of gliomas in the cerebellopontine angle.[450] Those in the fourth ventricle occasionally extend into the central canal or through the aqueduct of Sylvius.[223]

Approximately 50 per cent of supratentorial ependymomas are primarily intraventricular or arise in the ventricle and grow into the cerebral white matter. The other approximately 50 per cent are separate from the ependymal surface of the ventricle.[127,349] They must arise from rests of cells adjacent to but not contiguous with the ventricular surface.[410] Approximately 25 per cent of the intraventricular tumors occur in the third ventricle, and the other 75 per cent occur either in or near the lateral ventricles.[223] The various portions of the lateral ventricles are affected almost equally. These tumors may erode through the cerebral substance and invade dura and skull.[52] About 40 per cent of supratentorial ependymomas are cystic.[410] Those in the posterior fossa are less likely to be cystic.

Ependymomas can be classified in several ways. Previously, cellular, mixed, papillary, and epithelioid histological types have been identified.[127] Since these histological variations do not seem to correlate with differences in prognosis, however, they seem unnecessary.[205,390] A category of ependymoblastoma has been included by some, but it seems desirable to avoid use of this term, which is surrounded by disagreement.[22,127,205,360,390] Although Kernohan has advocated the separation of ependymomas into four grades of increasing histological anaplasia, this also seems unnecessary, since most of them behave either as hamartomas (subependymomas), which are very slowly growing, as well-differentiated neoplasms (papillary type), or as more rapidly growing neoplasms (anaplastic type).[256] Each of these types has distinct histological features, and it seems preferable to separate ependymomas into histological types rather than grades. The World Health Organization classification divides them into

---

* See references 10, 18, 349, 410, 455, 461.

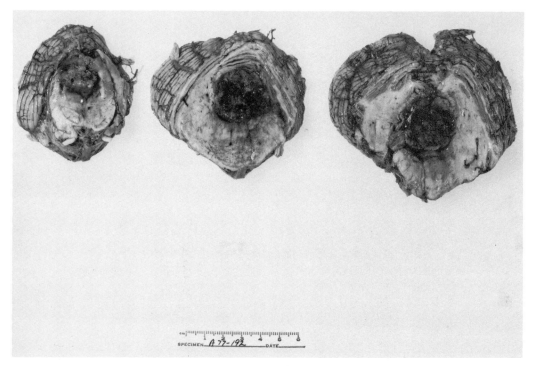

Figure 86–18   Ependymoma of the fourth ventricle in a 36-year-old man with a 10-year history of hydrocephalus treated by ventricular shunting. The tumor fills the entire fourth ventricle and extends into the cerebral aqueduct.

myxopapillary, papillary, and subependymoma types of nonanaplastic ependymoma and anaplastic ones. The majority of clinically symptomatic ependymomas fall into the groups designated as papillary and anaplastic. The myxopapillary variety occur in the cauda equina and are not included in this discussion. The subependymomal ones are covered in a separate section of this chapter.

The pathology of these tumors is complex. Neoplastic astrocytes have been found coexisting with neoplastic ependymal cells.[253] Tissue culture has confirmed that many ependymomas contain both an ependymal cell line and astrocytic cell line (particularly those tumors that occur in the spinal cord).[209]

The tumors are composed of polygonal or tapered cells containing moderately large vesicular nuclei with scattered chromatin.[16,18] Blepharoplasts, small granules seen by light microscopy and representing the basal portion of cilia, are sometimes seen in the cytoplasm of ependymal cells, especially with phosphotungstic acid–hematoxylin stains. Blepharoplasts tend to occur adjacent to the cell surface that abuts on the

ventricular cavity or to a false central canal that a neoplasm is attempting to form. Histological evidence of calcium is present in approximately one third and, when present in a supratentorial one, may betoken a better prognosis.[268,410] There is a tendency for cells in an ependymoma to arrange themselves in a radial pattern around blood vessels with their thin, tapering processes directed toward the vessel (a gliovascular complex) (Fig. 86–19). Occasionally, they arrange themselves in a radial pattern around a lumen resembling a central canal (a Flexner-Wintersteiner rosette) (Fig. 86–20).[16]

Most patients with cerebrospinal fluid metastases of ependymomas have had tumors in the fourth ventricle with a tongue of tumor projecting through the foramen magnum. It has been suggested that movement of the head might manipulate a tongue of tumor projecting across the cervicomedullary junction and be capable of dislodging tumor cells into the spinal fluid.[410] Approximately half of those that have metastasized have been anaplastic ependymomas.[391] Papillary ependymomas can metastasize, and one arising in the cauda equina has me-

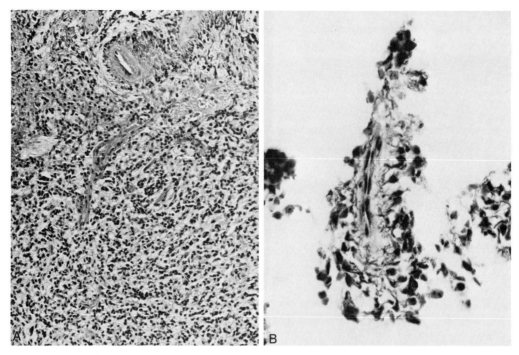

Figure 86–19 *A*. Microscopic pathological changes of anaplastic ependymoma. 100 ×. *B*. Touch preparation of the same tumor shows cells attached to a vessel by thick processes. 300 ×.

tastasized to the fourth ventricle.[360] The frequency of spread via the cerebrospinal fluid is in doubt, however. Ependymomas account for only approximately 12 per cent of neoplasms that metastasize by this route.[55] Spinal fluid metastases seem to be common in some series, occurring in as many as one third of patients, while being uncommon in other series.[223,321,410] Dissemination outside the central nervous system

has been reported after operation but is quite rare.[255]

Clinical Presentation

The duration of symptoms is variable. The average with intracranial lesions is 16 months.[256] Thirty-six per cent of patients have symptoms for less than three

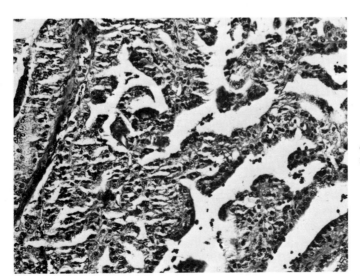

Figure 86–20 Microscopic pathological changes of papillary ependymoma. 140 ×.

months.[321] Those with infratentorial tumors have symptoms for longer than those with lateral ventricle lesions. Also, tumors that are discrete and easily separated from the tumor bed cause symptoms for longer periods than those that are more invasive.[223] Undoubtedly, these tumors are present for longer than their symptoms would suggest. Their intraventricular location makes them clinically silent until they become large.[22]

Almost 90 per cent of patients with ependymomas have papilledema, and 80 per cent complain of headache. Nausea and vomiting are present in approximately 75 per cent. Approximately 60 per cent have ataxia or vertigo.[321] Seizures are present with only one third of supratentorial lesions, and patients with this type of tumor constitute only approximately 1 per cent of those with seizures due to brain tumors.[164,319] The presenting symptoms of fourth ventricular tumors are headache and vomiting, while those of lateral ventricle tumors are more likely to be focal neurological deficits.

Investigation

Skull x-rays usually reveal evidence of increased intracranial pressure, and in approximately 20 per cent of patients with supratentorial ependymomas, calcification can be identified.[268,321,410] Radiographically visible calcification is less common in infratentorial tumors.[321,410] Radioisotope scanning is abnormal in 90 per cent.[179]

The standard diagnostic technique for demonstration of fourth ventricular ependymomas has been ventriculography, often with supplemental subarachnoid placement of air. Vertebral angiography is also a reliable method. Computed tomography has, however, largely replaced these techniques (Figs. 86–21 and 86–22). Even with good radiography, the differentiation between tumors of the brain stem and tumors of the fourth ventricle may be difficult. If an intraventricular ependymoma is mistakenly identified as a brain stem tumor, the patient may be treated with radiotherapy without opportunity to benefit from operative decompression.[321]

Detection of cerebrospinal fluid metastases may require myelography. Their occurrence can be anticipated if neoplastic cells are demonstrated in the cerebrospinal fluid.[346,371]

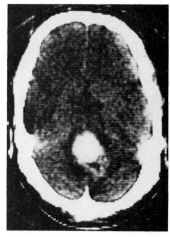

Figure 86–21 CT scan of ependymoma of the fourth ventricle (same patient as Figure 86–18).

Treatment and Results

Because fourth ventricular ependymomas may arise from or encase the brain stem, and because the supratentorial ones are often quite large and may be invasive, their complete removal at operation is uncommon. In a series of 65 patients, complete excision was not possible in any case.[223] Operative decompression does allow diagnosis and determination of the degree of anaplasia, and it confirms the presence of a neoplasm that is likely to be sensitive to radiotherapy. Further, it may allow relief of obstruction of the ventricles and reduction in compression of surrounding brain.

Posterior fossa ependymomas are approached through a midline suboccipital craniectomy. If a cuff of muscle is left attached to the occipital bone, the wound can be closed more securely and the likelihood of cerebrospinal fluid leak will be lessened. Laminectomies at C1 and often at C2 should be performed to allow decompression of the foramen magnum. Removal of the C1 arch should extend laterally to the groove in the superior aspect of C1. This groove is formed by the vertebral artery, and removal of bone more laterally is hazardous. The dura is opened with a Y- or a question mark–shaped incision so that the midline and the dorsal lateral aspect of the medulla on each side are exposed. The vallecula is then entered, and the cerebellar tonsils are separated. Usually the tumor presents in the vallecula (Fig. 86–23). Often it has escaped the vallecula and lies

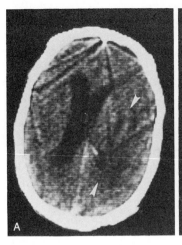
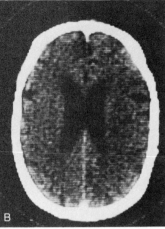

Figure 86–22 *A*. CT scan of anaplastic ependymoma demonstrates a low-density mass with no contrast enhancement. *B*. Repeat enhanced scan five months after radiotherapy shows resolution of the mass. This 71-year-old man with confusion became neurologically normal after radiotherapy, but later died of neoplasm regrowth.

in the subarachnoid space around the medulla. If the tumor is small, total excision of all visible tumor may be possible. In the majority of patients, however, the goal of operative treatment should be decompression by removal of as much tumor as can be accomplished without undue risk of neurological deficit. If tumor appears to extend through the foramen of Luschka, it is helpful to inspect the cerebellopontine angle. Removal of tumor lying between the cranial nerves or encasing the anterior and lateral aspects of the medulla is unwise. In most circumstances, the dura should be left open or a dural graft should be used to in-

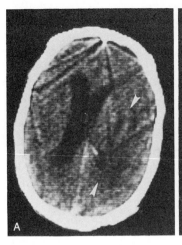

Figure 86–23 Ependymoma of the fourth ventricle. The tumor presents in the vallecula and displaces the cerebellar tonsil (*arrow*). (Courtesy of Barry N. French, M.D., University of California, Davis.)

sure that postoperative tumor swelling does not compress the brain stem. If a dural graft is used, the likelihood of postoperative chemical meningitis from blood and muscle transudates from the subarachnoid space is lessened, as may also be the likelihood of postoperative communicating hydrocephalus. In patients who have symptoms from obstructive hydrocephalus, preoperative ventriculoperitoneal shunting or ventricular drainage improves the postoperative course.

Supratentorial ependymomas are approached in the same way as other tumors in the hemisphere. Removal should not be so aggressive as to produce unnecessary neurological deficit. The rare supratentorial neoplasm that occurs in the third ventricle should be approached in the same way as a colloid cyst in the same location (see Chapter 91). An alternative method for management of third ventricular tumors is preoperative ventriculoperitoneal shunting from one or both ventricles followed by biopsy through a ventriculoscope or by stereotaxic needle biopsy, and radiotherapy.

Of all intracranial tumors, ependymomas rank second only to medulloblastomas in their radiosensitivity.[383] Radiotherapy followed by excision has revealed necrosis of tumor, and patients treated by radiotherapy without operation have had remission of symptoms.[321] Computed tomography can demonstrate reduction in tumor size after radiotherapy (cf. Fig. 86–22). There does not seem to be any correlation between the histological appearance of a tumor and its radiosensitivity. Symptoms of elevated intracranial pressure may become more severe during radiotherapy, and some radiotherapists have recommended starting with small doses of radiation and gradually increasing them until a full daily dose is reached.[223] At least 4500 rads should be given, and if recurrence occurs, retreatment with 1500 to 2000 rads may be helpful.[321,391]

Because of the infrequency of symptomatic metastases there is disagreement regarding the advisability of neuraxis radiation.[322] Not only are cerebrospinal fluid metastases uncommon, but radiation of the neuraxis is not always effective in preventing them.[223] It is, however, reasonable to use it for patients with tumors of the fourth ventricle that project through the foramen magnum and histologically are anaplastic. For other patients, Nuclepore filtration can be used to detect potential for metastases in the cerebrospinal fluid.[346] If Nuclepore filtration fails to reveal neoplastic cells, then neuraxis radiation can be withheld.

In common with the prognosis for most primary brain tumors, the likelihood of cure of an intracranial ependymoma is slight.[391] Operative decompression and subsequent radiotherapy can, however, add months or years to the patient's life. Operative risks in the supratentorial ependymomas are similar to those with other supratentorial neoplasms. The mortality rates in earlier series varied from 20 to 50 per cent, but current rates should be in the range of 5 to 8 per cent. Fourth ventricular tumors pose greater operative risks than supratentorial ones.[349] Even in early series and without radiotherapy, five-year survival rates with infratentorial tumors were as high as 35 per cent. Survival can be increased by adding postoperative radiotherapy, and with it the chances of the patient's living for five years are 80 per cent with supratentorial tumors and 90 per cent with infratentorial ones.[321] Even an apparently long survival without symptoms does not rule out the possibility of late recurrence. Patients have been reported to live for more than 10 years and later die of a recurrence.[223]

Morbidity in patients who have survived removal of an infratentorial ependymoma usually is mild. Presumably, if the surgeon was so aggressive as to endanger the brain stem, the patient did not survive, while if the surgeon was more cautious, the likelihood of a new neurological deficit was not great. These statements may no longer be true with prolonged, intensive, postoperative care available and the frequent use of continuous intracranial pressure monitoring, pulmonary therapy, tracheostomy, steroids and dehydrating agents, and better control of electrolyte abnormalities.

Morbidity is greater with supratentorial than with infratentorial ependymomas. Approximately 50 per cent of patients are in good or excellent condition after operation for supratentorial ependymomas.[223] With prudent operative procedures and aggressive radiotherapy, it may be possible to reduce this operative morbidity below 50 per cent.

Since supratentorial lesions are more likely to be anaplastic, they are likely to recur sooner than the infratentorial ones.[349,390,410] Even those that are well differentiated may become anaplastic. One report describes a tumor that was an ependymoma at the initial operation but had developed into a glioblastoma by the time of death 26 months later.[127]

SUBEPENDYMOMA

A subependymoma is a well-demarcated expansive growth arising from the neuroglia along the ventricular surface. First described as a separate entity by Scheinker, it usually has been an incidental finding at autopsy, most often in the fourth ventricle of middle-aged or elderly patients.[46,143,377] Some of them may be more nearly malformations than neoplasms. The tumor is composed of mature fibrillary astrocytes with large numbers of glial fibers intermixed with ependymal cells (Fig. 86–24). It mimics the architecture of the normal embryonic subependymal glia.[141] Similar tumors have also been reported in the septum pellucidum.[132] Approximately one third of them contain calcification at histological examination.

Although subependymomas have been reported to follow streptococcal meningitis, most of them are presumed to arise from rests of the subependymal cell plate.[141,362] Areas of apparent subependymoma have been described in an otherwise typical fourth ventricular ependymoma.[134] When a neoplasm of this nature is identified, it should be named for the more anaplastic portion. This course is justified because the

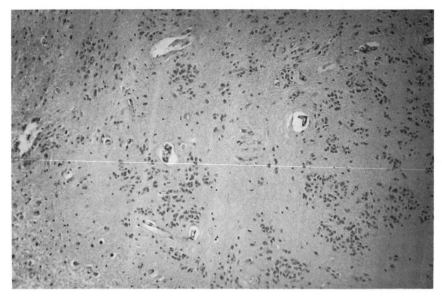

Figure 86–24 Microscopic pathological changes of subependymoma. Nests of cells are scattered over a fibrillary background. 100 ×. (Courtesy of Surl L. Nielson, M.D., University of California, Davis.)

ependymoma portion will determine the patient's course.

CHOROID PLEXUS PAPILLOMA

Embryologically, the cells of the choroid plexus derive from the ependymal lining of the neural tube. Tumors of the choroid plexus were first reported by Guerard in 1833.[160] A successful removal with survival of the patient was not accomplished until 1919.[320]

This neoplasm accounts for about 0.5 per cent of all intracranial tumors but for about 4 per cent of intracranial tumors in patients less than 12 years of age.* Its incidence is also increased in patients with von Recklinghausen's disease. Indeed, a hypertrophied, calcified choroid plexus has been suggested as a radiographic sign of von Recklinghausen's disease (although this is usually due to a meningioma rather than a choroid plexus papilloma).[453] The tumors may develop at any age, including infancy.[47,109] Thirty-five to forty-five per cent of them occur in patients less than 20 years of age.[13,41,174] The oldest patient reported was 74 years old.[428] They occur with the

same frequency in males and females. Approximately 50 per cent of them are in the fourth ventricle.[301,349] The third and fourth ventricles are particularly likely to be involved in adults, but the lateral ventricles are more likely to be affected in children.[274,349] About 20 per cent arise from tufts of the choroid plexus that extend into or through the foramina of Luschka. Some 50 per cent of third ventricular tumors extend into another ventricle.

Most series show a preponderance of lesions in the left rather than the right ventricle.[13,216,274] The clinical signs suggesting right ventricular lesions may not have been appreciated in the early experience with intracranial tumors; therefore, such patients may not have been referred to neurosurgeons. This interpretation would explain why no such left-sided preponderance appears in recent series as was reported in the 1930's, when as many as 93 per cent of supratentorial papillomas were found to occur on the left side.[428] The finding of choroid plexus papillomas in siblings may be accounted for by the presence of von Recklinghausen's disease.[214]

Pathology

On macroscopic examination, these tumors are soft, quite vascular, and irregu-

---

* See references 13, 41, 93, 174, 248, 274, 349, 401, 461.

lar, with an appearance somewhat like a purplish to gray cauliflower. They tend to conform to the contours of the ventricle in which they lie and may extend through foramina to adjacent ventricles or to the subarachnoid space.[93,349] They may be forced into the brain tissue but do not invade the brain.[216] Lateral ventricular tumors may obstruct drainage from the temporal horn, the result being a large encysted temporal horn. Tumor secretions may be trapped by the adjacent ventricular walls and produce smaller cysts in or close to the tumor.

Their histological appearance closely resembles the architecture of a normal choroid plexus. They have a connective tissue stroma and an epithelium of cuboid or columnar cells with abundant mitochondria and no blepharoplasts or cilia (Fig. 86–25).[93] Electron microscopy reveals cilia and blepharoplasts in an occasional cell, but they are much less frequent than in ependymomas.[252] By light microscopy, hyaline or mucoid degeneration of the stroma is seen to be present in some cases.[216] A rare histological variant composed of mucus-secreting cells has been described and labeled "acinar choroid plexus adenoma."[97]

Malignant choroid plexus tumors are rare.[241,370] Anaplastic features include invasion of surrounding neural structures with loss of papillary architecture and pleomorphism of cells and nuclei. Mitoses may be numerous, and foci of necrosis may occur. Histological evidence of anaplasia does not always indicate a short postoperative survival.[445] Metastasis from carcinoma outside the central nervous system encroaching on the third ventricle or metastasis to the choroid plexus is a source of tumor that can be mistaken for carcinoma arising primarily in the choroid plexus.[349]

Metastases of choroid plexus papillomas are found in up to 20 per cent of patients at postmortem examination.[174] They occur through the cerebrospinal fluid. Lateral ventricular papillomas in children are more anaplastic and metastasize more frequently than fourth ventricular tumors in adults.[41] Spread outside the central nervous system is rare.[432]

Hydrocephalus is a common but not invariable accompaniment of choroid plexus papillomas and has been thought to be due to oversecretion of cerebrospinal fluid.[92,396,430] Production of this fluid has been measured at rates as high as 1656 ml per day.[285] Russell has attributed the hydrocephalus to recurrent episodes of hemorrhage from the tumor that cause obstruction of the cerebrospinal fluid pathways.[369] Removal of the tumor is not always followed by resolution of the hydrocephalus,

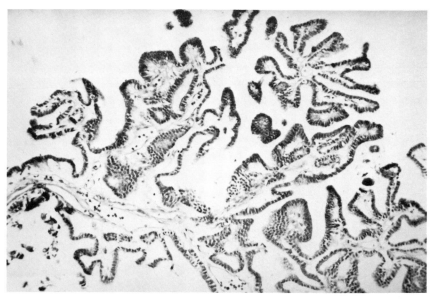

Figure 86–25 Microscopic pathological changes of choroid plexus papilloma mimic the normal choroid plexus. A connective tissue nourishes the fronds of tumor. 80 ×. (Courtesy of Surl L. Nielson, M.D., University of California, Davis.)

which suggests that either overproduction or poor reabsorption may cause ventricular enlargement.

Clinical Presentation

The characteristic presenting symptoms of choroid plexus papillomas suggest only an increase in intracranial pressure, usually without focal signs.[274,329] Although the onset may be relatively rapid in childhood, in adults the history commonly is one to two years in length.[13,301,349] Adults usually complain of headache, nausea, and vomiting. Examination reveals papilledema or other evidence of increased intracranial pressure. With fourth ventricular tumors, nystagmus and ataxia are common. Occasionally, patients present with intraventricular hemorrhage caused by the tumor.[1,117,275]

Investigation

Skull x-rays usually reveal evidence of increased pressure. Tumor calcification is present in approximately 13 per cent.[13] In fact, 15 of Matson and Crofton's 16 patients with this type of tumor had such a finding.[274] Angiography reveals hydrocephalus and occasionally demonstrates the associated tumor blush.[25,41,216] The isotope brain scan is abnormal in more than 50 per cent of patients.[312] Potassium perchlorate is able to suppress isotope concentration in some of them.[202]

In the past, the definitive study has been ventriculography. Characteristically, it reveals either a fourth ventricular tumor with noncommunicating hydrocephalus or a lateral ventricular tumor with communicating hydrocephalus. The cerebrospinal fluid is usually under increased pressure.[174] The spinal fluid protein may be either normal or increased, and the level may be as high as 2000 mg per 100 ml.[248] Crenated red blood cells or xanthochromia often is present.[41,301] If there is a tumor in the lateral ventricle, there should be a shift of the midline structures away from the side of the tumor. Progressive hydrocephalus beginning long after tumor resection may signal tumor recurrence. Computed tomography is exceedingly accurate (Fig. 86–26). These tumors do not have a blood-brain

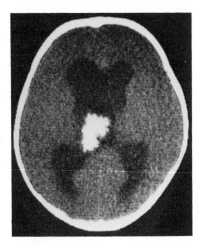

Figure 86–26   CT scan of choroid plexus papilloma shows a calcified tumor in the left lateral ventricle producing communicating hydrocephalus involving the left lateral ventricle more than the right one. (Courtesy of Frank A. Brown, M.D., Sutter Community Hospitals, Sacramento, California.)

barrier and should be enhanced by contrast, may contain calcium, and usually are accompanied by changes in the ventricles.

Treatment and Results

The treatment for choroid plexus papilloma is operative removal. If the tumor is in the fourth ventricle, a standard midline suboccipital craniectomy is performed. If upward herniation through the tentorium seems imminent, preoperative ventriculoperitoneal shunting and tentorial section may reduce the risk of subsequent excision.[69] Obstruction of the arterial supply to the tumor as the initial step in tumor removal greatly facilitates the remainder of the operation. The tumor may exit the foramina of Luschka or be embedded in the floor of the fourth ventricle, precluding total removal.[216]

The usual approach to third ventricular tumors has been through the lateral ventricle and foramen of Monro.[301] Transcallosal exposure also is feasible.

Tumors of the lateral ventricles usually occur at the atrium. They may be approached through the posterior cortex or through the dilated temporal horn. The tumor may be attached to the ependyma by light adhesions, but its vascular supply will come from the glomus of the choroid plexus.[274] It should be mobilized, and the vascular pedicle should then be divided. Once the vascular supply has been obliterated, the tumor shrinks greatly in size and can often be removed intact. If it is entered before the pedicle is divided, however, vigorous bleeding may occur.

Radiotherapy is not of much value with choroid plexus papillomas.[274,301] Some authors have suggested that, although radiotherapy does not reduce the bulk of the tumor, it may reduce vascularity.[69] This hypothesis still remains in question. Radiotherapy should not be given to patients with fourth or lateral ventricle tumors that can be resected. In patients with anaplastic neoplasms, particularly if their growths occur in the lateral ventricles, postoperative radiotherapy may be advisable.[13,274]

Operative mortality rates vary from 18 per cent in a recent series to more than 30 per cent in series that include patients operated on before 1945.* Adults tend to fare better than children, and fourth ventricular neoplasms have a better prognosis than lateral ventricular neoplasms. The morbidity is related not only to nervous system injury at the time of operation but also to the degree and duration of hydrocephalus. Morbidity tends to be less with third and fourth ventricular tumors (25 per cent of patients have severe or mild deficits). If hydrocephalus has not been longstanding or severe, and if the neoplasm can be successfully removed, the result usually is gratifying.[216] Of 17 patients with fourth ventricular tumors reported by Herren, 13 "recovered." Of 4 with third ventricular tumors, only 1 "recovered," and of 14 with lateral ventricular tumors, 9 "recovered."[174] Clinical relapse due to regrowth of the tumor can occur as late as 19 years after its removal.[13]

Hydrocephalus is usually relieved by tumor removal. Shunting without removal of tumor has been shown to be ineffective in at least one patient.[342]

NEURONAL TUMORS

There is considerable controversy regarding the classification and nomenclature of neuronal tumors.[166] The World Health Organization subdivides them into five types: gangliocytoma, ganglioglioma, gan-

glioneuroblastoma, anaplastic ganglioglioma, and neuroblastoma.[397] A gangliocytoma has abnormal ganglion cells with non-neoplastic glia. If glia are also neoplastic, it is called a ganglioglioma. Anaplastic forms are postulated to exist for gangliocytoma and have been documented for ganglioglioma.[358] If the neoplasm includes a spectrum of cells from mature ganglion cells to immature neuroblasts, it is considered a ganglioneuroblastoma, while if only the immature neuroblasts are present, it is a neuroblastoma.

A gangliocytoma may be a hamartoma consisting of ectopic autonomic neural tissue and not be strictly neoplastic.[358,362] Whatever the exact origin of the ganglion cells in neuronal tumors, the consensus is that they have their origin early in the development of the central nervous system.[77]

Neuronal tumors are rare, accounting for approximately 0.5 to 2 per cent of tumors.[18,77] Gangliogliomas occur at all ages but are most common between the ages of 10 and 30 years. In contrast, cerebral neuroblastomas are almost exclusively tumors of childhood.[183,313]

Pathology

Gangliogliomas are encapsulated tumors that may be cystic. They can occur in almost any part of the central nervous system but are most common in the region of the third ventricle.[207] In a series of 25 of these neoplasms, 36 per cent were in the body and frontal horn of the lateral ventricle, 20 per cent were in the wall of the third ventricle, 20 per cent were in the temporal horn of the lateral ventricle, and 24 per cent were in the fourth ventricle.[77] Neuronal, glial, and mesenchymal cells all participate in the ganglioglioma and are intermingled.[362] The ganglion cells may be multinucleated but appear mature. The relative proportion of glial and ganglion cells varies from one location to another in a single tumor and from one tumor to another. Rosenthal fibers may be seen, and calcium salts may be deposited in and around ganglion cells and glial cells.[361] Vascularity may be moderate, but there are usually no mitoses. Recognition of gangliocytoma and ganglioglioma may be difficult, since the neuronal characteristics may be lost or overshadowed by anaplastic glia.[358] An astrocytoma may be mistaken

---

* See references 13, 41, 174, 274, 301, 349.

for a ganglioglioma if the tumor is sampled at its edges where it is invading and has included prexisting normal neurons.[207]

Anaplasia can occur in gangliogliomas. Usually it is the glial element that becomes anaplastic.[358] Kernohan and Sayre believe that these tumors have the same natural history as an astrocytoma of comparable anaplasia.[207]

Treatment and Results

These tumors should be treated as well-differentiated astrocytomas unless anaplasia is present. They are often slow growing, but are capable of undergoing anaplasia to become glioblastomas.[419] A patient has been reported who survived 23 years after operation for ganglioglioma and later died of anaplastic astrocytoma.[370]

GLIOBLASTOMA

The criteria differentiating glioblastoma from anaplastic astrocytoma vary from one author to another. According to one set of definitions, a neoplasm is considered to be an anaplastic astrocytoma if an astrocytic origin can be identified and a glioblastoma if no recognizable precursors can be found.[110] Other authors separate anaplastic astrocytoma from glioblastoma on the basis of degree of anaplasia.[184] These traits tend to accompany one another, so those tumors without definable astrocytic ancestry (or less commonly oligodendroglial or ependymal ancestry) tend to be more anaplastic histologically than those in which an astrocytic heritage can be identified. Usually it is possible to identify recognizable astrocytes from neoplasms with moderate cellular pleomorphism, numbers of mitoses, and endothelial changes. Less frequently, it is possible to identify the cellular origin of neoplasms that have marked hypercellularity, extreme pleomorphism of cells and nuclei, cells that do not appear to be glial, prominent endothelial proliferation, and necrosis. The histological variability of neoplasms with this latter microscopic appearance prompted the original name of glioblastoma multiforme.[17] The World Health Organization classification differentiates anaplastic astrocytoma from glioblastoma on the basis of degree of anaplasia and microscopic variability. As a result of these diverse standards, it should be noted, the name given to a particular tumor is a subjective decision.

In most reports, it is not possible to distinguish between anaplastic astrocytomas and glioblastomas. Often they include such phrases as "glioblastomatous areas of an astrocytoma" and other confusing pathological descriptions. Because of this difficulty with classification and nomenclature, this discussion deals with anaplastic astrocytomas and glioblastomas together in the clinical descriptions with comments pertinent to the differing degrees of anaplasia where appropriate.

Glioblastoma was originally termed spongioblastoma multiforme by Bailey and Cushing following the common usage of that day.[22] At the time of their original report, they commented that this was not an ideal name for these tumors, since the majority of cells did not look like spongioblasts. Shortly after the original report, Bailey recommended the term "glioblastoma multiforme."[17] Common usage has shortened it to "glioblastoma." Although the glioblast is a theoretical cell and has not been identified, this name has remained in the literature. The only arguments against it have come from authors such as Kernohan and his associates who prefer to consider astrocytomas as a continuum in which glioblastoma represents the extreme in grading of anaplasia and in which numerical grades might be preferable.[208]

Incidence

Glioblastomas constitute approximately one fourth of intracranial tumors in neurosurgical and neuropathological series and approximately half of all gliomas.[22,94,111,436,456]

The greatest number of them occur between the ages of 40 and 60, but the incidence of all brain neoplasms probably is underestimated, particularly in older patients. If age-adjusted rates are applied to Kurland's series the incidence of primary brain tumors increases with increasing age.[226] In a series of 100 patients who had brain tumors after 60 years of age, one third had glioblastomas.[289] The average age of the 77 patients reported by Bailey and Cushing was 41 years.[22] More recent series have contained higher proportions of older patients, and nearly one fourth in one series were between the ages of 60 and 70.[111,158,311] Of the 162 patients reported by Jelsma and Bucy, 85 per cent were between the ages of 40 and 70 years.[193] Glioblastomas are rare in childhood. A congenital example in the right basal ganglia of a stillborn infant has been reported.[362] Among 32 children with them, however, only one was less than 1 year of age.[216] There is some tendency for patients who survive longer, and who probably have less aggressive neoplasms, to have the onset of symptoms at a younger age.[61] Anaplastic astrocytomas are much more common in younger persons than are glioblastomas, with 15 per cent of them occurring before the age of 10, while only 2 per cent of glioblastomas occur before that age. Males are affected more frequently than females, 55 to 65 per cent of patients in most series being male.[111,130,308]

Pathogenesis

The cause of glioblastoma and anaplastic astrocytoma is unknown. It is known, however, that a well-differentiated astrocytoma may gradually become more anaplastic as it evolves and eventually dedifferentiate to glioblastoma. This type of change also may occur in gliomas with other cell types. Various authors have postulated toxic, traumatic, viral, and other causes for tumors of the astrocytic series. There is little experimental work to prove that these factors are causative. Gliomas have been produced by hematogenous or intracerebral injection of carcinogens or viruses.[412] Haymaker and associates found that 3 of 10 monkeys surviving 3 to 5 years after 600 or 800 rads of 55 mev protons developed glioblastoma.[172]

Monson and co-workers reported that deaths due to brain neoplasms are four times as common as expected in workers exposed to vinyl chloride.[291] It should, however, be noted that the analysis of their data is open to question. For example, the expected number of brain tumors in the population studied was 1.2, and they discovered 5, of which 3 were glioblastoma. When the probable underreporting of brain tumors is taken into consideration, these figures may not be significant. Another example of possible misinterpretation of a relation between exposure to vinyl chloride and development of brain tumors is shown

by a patient who was reported to have a glioblastoma and survived 15 years after the diagnosis was made.[303] The length of survival brings the diagnosis into question.

In a study of brain tumors in Kentucky, Brooks noted that there were seven counties in which there were 4.4 times as many brain tumors as expected. Six of the seven high-incidence counties were within one area in the eastern central part of the state. The origin of this regional concentration is not clear, but environmental factors were suggested.[50] There may also be a greater incidence of brain tumors in farm workers.[74] There does not appear to be any correlation between genetic markers such as spina bifida or trisomy 21 and brain tumors or an increased risk of glioblastoma or other neoplasms in relatives of patients with glioblastoma.[101,170] Rare patients with glioblastoma have had trauma as the apparent inciting event.[265]

Pathology

Macroscopic Changes

Glioblastoma may occur as either a circumscribed mass or a diffusely infiltrating neoplasm. At operation, it has a variety of appearances, depending on the presence of necrosis, cystic degeneration, or hemorrhage. Approximately one fifth of the tumors are well circumscribed.[379] Approximately 60 per cent are solid, and the others are cystic.[130] Necrosis is present in approximately half of them. Small areas of hemorrhage are seen in about 40 per cent, and massive hemorrhage in 2 per cent (Fig. 86–27).

The cut surface of glioblastoma alternates between areas of moderately firm tumor that may be grayish or pinkish, areas of creamy yellow necrosis, and areas of recent or old hemorrhage that may be red or brown. The ends of a larger vessel may be visible, and cysts may be present. When neoplastic cysts are present, pleocytosis can be identified in at least 80 per cent of samples of cyst fluid, and these cells are often neoplastic.[60]

The frontal and temporal lobes are most commonly affected by glioblastoma; there is, however, no area containing glial tissue that is exempt from it.[257] Even the optic nerve may be involved.

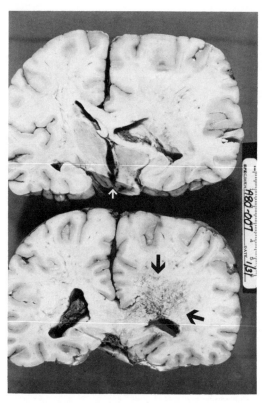

Figure 86–27 Coronal section of glioblastoma demonstrates tumor above the right occipital horn (*black arrows*) and brain stem hemorrhages that have resulted from transtentorial herniation (*white arrow*).

Anaplastic astrocytomas of the brain stem usually are unilateral, at least at their onset. As they extend into the proximal portions of cranial nerves they tend to expand the brain stem in a lobulated fashion. Lobules of tumor may even surround the basilar artery. The neoplasm may protrude into the subarachnoid space, particularly in the cerebellopontine angle. They are inclined to infiltrate along fiber tracts in the brain stem.[146] Most of these tumors occur in the pons, but they occasionally arise in the medulla oblongata and other portions of the brain stem.[297,332]

A wide variety of neoplasms may occur in the thalamus. In most series, approximately half of them are either glioblastomas or anaplastic astrocytomas.[73,117,280] The more rapidly growing tumors are most likely to be found in older patients.[73] Glioblastomas of the cerebellum are exceedingly rare, and only five well-documented cases could be identified in a recent review.[107]

Examination of the cut surface of a glioblastoma reveals obvious areas of abnormality in most cases. The portion that is most easily identified is the degenerated portion. In the absence of degeneration or hemorrhage, an astrocytic neoplasm may appear as a diffuse increase in volume of the brain. The cortex is usually more translucent than normal and may be somewhat yellow. It is also enlarged, and the boundary line between gray and white matter is less distinct than usual. In the white matter, an astrocytoma appears as more transparent, slightly grayish, and homogenous and may be either more or less firm than normal brain. There is no correlation between the presence of fibrillary processes on microscopic examination and the firmness of the neoplasm.[379]

Growth of the neoplasm may be by infiltration of its cells between normal cells or by expansive growth in which the normal tissue is displaced.[379] If the zone of infiltration is narrow, it may be possible to excise a tumor completely even though it is malignant. For instance, the narrow zone of infiltration is a major difference between the curable cystic cerebellar astrocytoma and the diffusely infiltrating astrocytoma that is unresectable. Scherer's autopsy series reveals, however, that although 20 per cent of glioblastomas have a narrow zone of infiltration, only 3 per cent appear to be poten-

In comparison with other portions of the cerebral hemispheres, the occipital lobe is an uncommon site for glioblastoma. Anaplastic astrocytomas arising from pre-existing fibrillary astrocytomas are relatively frequent in the pons and occur in the remainder of the brain stem as well. Glioblastomas without evidence of origin from a more differentiated astrocytic tumor are rare in the posterior fossa.

In the frontal lobe these tumors tend to invade the corpus callosum and extend to the opposite side. If this spread is obvious, it assumes a "butterfly" pattern with both frontal lobes and the corpus callosum involved. Those in the more inferior aspects of the frontal lobe may follow the uncinate fasciculus into the temporal lobe. The more medial and posterior frontal ones tend to extend into the basal ganglia, as do temporal lobe glioblastomas also. Those in medial parietal or occipital lobes tend to extend across the corpus callosum to involve the opposite hemisphere (Fig. 86–28).

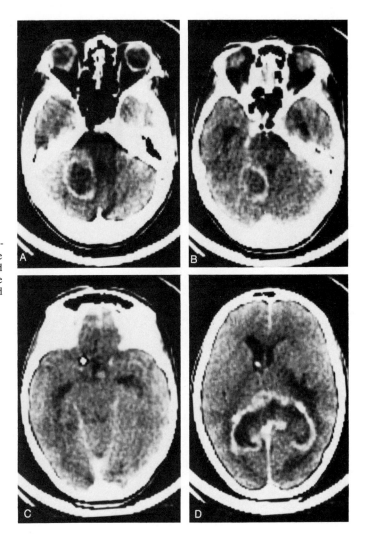

Figure 86–28 CT scan of glioblastoma shows apparently separate tumor foci in posterior fossa, *A* and *B*, and corpus callosum, *D*. These are separated by apparently involved brain, *C*.

tially resectable.[380] Jelsma and Bucy report that tumors that appear to be circumscribed have a more favorable prognosis.[193]

Infiltrative growth with preservation of the pre-existing parenchyma is a prominent characteristic of astrocytic tumors of all types. When infiltration is extreme, astrocytoma may involve an entire hemisphere or possibly even both hemispheres. This extreme degree of infiltration has been named gliomatosis cerebri.[153]

Differentiation between multicentric origin and regional metastasis or spread along narrow pathways is difficult. Approximately 20 per cent of glioblastomas appear as multiple foci (see Fig. 86–28).[29,290,380] Undoubtedly, however, not all of these foci are separate independent neoplasms. Extensive serial sectioning of brain and histological examination demonstrate that separate primaries are present in 5 to 10 per cent.[380] If only widely separated foci are accepted as discrete primary neoplasms, then only approximately 2 per cent are of multicentric origin.[29,370]

Symptomatic metastasis of glioblastoma through cerebrospinal fluid pathways is relatively rare. It occurs more frequently with tumors that are extremely anaplastic and those that reach the ventricular ependyma.[63,364] When it does occur, the spread may be along the ependymal surface as a carpet in the ventricle, or to the spine or the leptomeninges along the base of the brain.[257] Distant metastases through cerebrospinal fluid are more common from such tumors as oligodendrogliomas, whose cells are easily dispersed.[28,110] Possibly these cells are more likely to be detached, since they are less firmly fixed by numerous processes. Although extension of the tumor through the hemisphere into the subarachnoid space is not uncommon, it is less likely to produce cerebrospinal fluid metastasis.

Cytological studies of the cerebrospinal fluid show tumor cells in approximately 10 to 40 per cent of patients with deeply situated glioblastomas.[346,433] In contrast, only 5 per cent of patients with grade III and grade IV astrocytomas have cerebrospinal fluid metastases.[372] As many as 60 per cent of cerebrospinal fluid metastases due to primary brain tumors arise from glioblastomas.[55] Many of them are too small to be seen without a microscope.

Glioblastomas in the posterior fossa may be more likely to metastasize than those in other locations. In one such series, four of six spread to the spine and produced symptoms.[372]

In the absence of a previous operation, dissemination outside the central nervous system is rare. Several explanations for this fact have been offered. Among them are that growth of the primary neoplasm is so rapid that there is not time for a metastatic lesion to become apparent, that there are no lymphatics in the central nervous system, that there are no easily detached clumps of cells in intracerebral veins, that veins are compressed by neoplasm outside the vessel, and that the immune system is active outside but relatively ineffective inside the central nervous system.[385] The scarcity of systemic metastases in patients with glioblastoma cannot be entirely attributed to a hostile systemic environment, however, since the tumor can be transplanted into subcutaneous tissue and may metastasize through ventricular shunts.[152,225,435] Although they commonly invade vessels, the number of cells that are available to spread through a vein probably is insufficient.[225] A clump of cells rather than a single cell may be required for an intravascular metastasis that will survive. Once the cells reach the lymphatic channels, they can be disseminated by this route.[163] Metastases following operations occur with approximately equal frequency to the lungs and lymph nodes.

The frequency of metastases outside the neuraxis is difficult to determine. Only 0.4 per cent of neuroectodermal neoplasms metastasize outside the nervous system. Of those that do, however, 66 per cent are glioblastomas.[395] Of all intracranial tumors

with proved distant metastases, approximately 30 per cent are glioblastomas.[139] Approximately 50 per cent of these are in lung, 40 per cent in lumph nodes, and 35 per cent in bones. The liver is also involved in some patients.

The fact that metastases of glioblastoma follow operations or shunting procedures, but occur spontaneously only if they gain access to large veins, suggests that it is the anatomical location of the tumor that determines the rarity of systemic dissemination. The reason for the dearth of lymphatic metastases is obvious, since most glioblastomas do not have access to lymphatics. The mechanisms by which hematogenous spread is inhibited remain in question.

Systemic metastases in the absence of operative treatment occur in neoplasms that invade the vessels to an unusual degree.[9,187,361] Although glioblastoma erodes the inner aspect of the dura relatively frequently, it is rare for it to penetrate the outer layer; thus entry into the extracranial circulation is prevented.[204] Occasionally, however, it breaks through the floor of the anterior or middle fossa and may present in the middle ear or paranasal sinuses.[300] Theoretically, invasion via this route could provide access to the extracranial circulation.

Microscopic Changes

Glioblastomas are characterized by microscopic variability. Hypercellularity, pleomorphism of cells and nuclei, mitoses, capillary endothelial proliferation, and necrosis are seen (Fig. 86–29).[184] Calcium salts are present in 3 per cent. Electron microscopy reveals large numbers of mitochondria and ribosomes, and extensive cellular space, and nuclear pleomorphism.[253,336] The neoplastic cells may be so undifferentiated that an astrocytic origin is unrecognizable.[362]

There is a tendency for cells to cluster around areas of necrosis. This pattern has been described as a "pseudopalisade." Pseudopalisading occurs in approximately 80 per cent of the tumors and, if seen, is highly suggestive of the diagnosis.[370] Vascular changes include increased numbers of capillaries as well as proliferation of their endothelium. Endothelial cells may be enlarged and may contain mitotic figures. If the hyperplasia is marked, thrombosis may result.

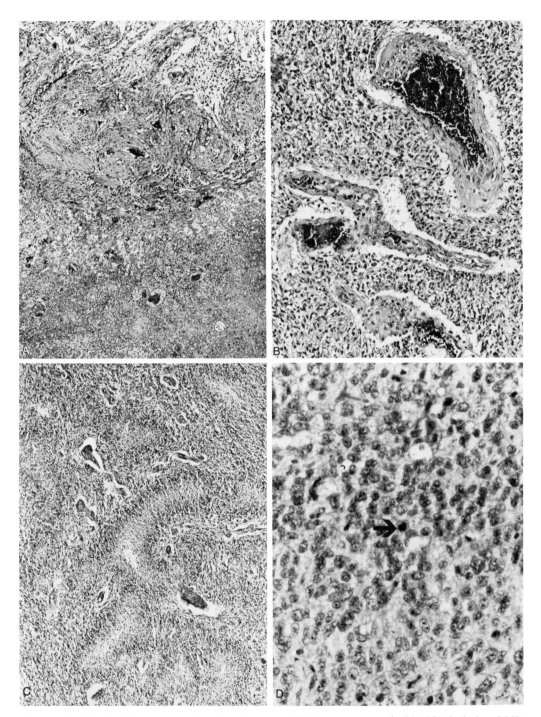

Figure 86–29 *A*. Microscopic pathological changes of glioblastoma are marked by histological variability. 50 ×. *B*. Endothelial hyperplasia may be intense. 100 ×. *C*. Bands of necrosis may be present. 30 ×. *D*. Mitoses can be found (*arrow*). 200 ×.

Astroblastic foci may be seen in anaplastic astrocytomas. These foci consist of perivascular anaplastic cells with thick processes directed toward the vessel. They occur in approximately 17 per cent of glioblastomas, 38 per cent of anaplastic astrocytomas, and 54 per cent of gemistocytic astrocytomas. Their presence in a glioblastoma may suggest an origin from gemistocytic astrocytoma.[370]

The inherent histological characteristics of glioblastoma are independent of its location in the brain and have been termed "primary" by Scherer. The form and structure of the neoplasms may also be affected by the invaded brain, the result being "secondary structures" whose histological patterns are determined by the tissue they invade. Some of these secondary structures are visible without the aid of magnification, as, for example, glioblastomas may stop growing at gray-white junctions without invasion of the deep nuclei and the cortex. Other secondary structures are microscopic. For instance, neoplastic cells tend to follow white matter tracts and to orient themselves along them. As they reach the pial surface of the brain they tend to spread in the subpial layer, and likewise when they reach the ventricular surface they tend to spread in the subependymal layer.[378]

As a neoplasm invades dura, fibrous connective tissue proliferates. This proliferation may produce hyperplastic dura that resembles a meningioma. Deep to this tissue is a gradual transition to a typical glioblastoma. Biopsy of the superficial portion of such a tumor may be confusing and may suggest a diagnosis of fibrosarcoma. Another source of connective tissue in glioblastomas is the response to necrosis. Initially there is a microglial infiltration of areas of degeneration and necrosis. Later it is replaced by organization and neovascularization.

Histological examination of glioblastoma after irradiation may be confusing. Radiotherapy produces an increase in the number of giant cells and cells with bizarre nuclei. There is also an increase in the areas of necrosis and degeneration and, possibly, in the number of hemorrhages. Blood vessel walls may be necrotic, and there may be thromboses. These changes are not noted in all neoplasms undergoing radiotherapy. In fact, some are unchanged.[94]

Although anaplasia and variability are characteristic of glioblastomas, more-differentiated normal appearing cells may also occur. These more-differentiated areas may be sufficient in number to demonstrate the cell of origin. If the tumor type from which it arises can be identified, the glioblastoma is referred to as a secondary glioblastoma; if no tumor of origin can be identified, it is referred to as a primary glioblastoma. An apparent primary glioblastoma is more common than the secondary type; this does not, however, mean that an astrocytic precursor was not initially present. It may be that in most "primary glioblastomas" a pre-existing astrocytoma developed anaplasia throughout so that no evidence of the initial tumor remained. Some authors believe that glioblastoma may arise de novo without transition through a more differentiated neoplasm.[347,380,462]

Giant Cell Glioblastoma

The same factors that produce gemistocytic astrocytes in astrocytomas are capable of producing giant cells in glioblastomas.[184] Giant cells are a frequent sequela of radiotherapy and, in this circumstance, may arise not because of inadequate nutrition but because of a basic change in the cell itself.

Giant cell glioblastomas usually are well demarcated and firm. Cysts may be present, however. The giant cells may be as large as 200 to 300 microns in diameter and may be seen without magnification.[36,53] Although the presence of reticulin has suggested that they have a sarcomatous origin, the results of ultrastructural study have been more consistent with an astrocytic origin.[53,254] Typical glioblastomas or gemistocytic astrocytomas have been found adjacent to areas of giant cell glioblastoma.[30]

Gliosarcoma

In 1895 Stroebe recognized that malignant glial elements can coexist with sarcomatous elements.[407] The resulting neoplasm is called a gliosarcoma. Considerable controversy has surrounded this neoplasm, which can develop from a sarcomatous tumor that incites a gliomatous reaction or from a glioblastoma that produces sarcomatous change in invaded dura or in the vessels within the tumor.

Gliosarcoma occurs in approximately 2

per cent of patients with gliomas. At macroscopic examination, the area of sarcoma is denser and whiter than the usual glioblastoma.[121] The histological characteristics are best seen with reticulin stains. These stains identify a transition between endothelial proliferation and sarcomatous change in vessels.[370]

Glioblastomas may infiltrate the leptomeninges. This invasion is soon followed by attachment of the tumor to the dura mater. The pattern of attachment may simulate a meningioma, and biopsy of the surface may be confusing. Biopsy of the depths of the tumor, however, will reveal characteristic glioblastoma. Approximately 47 per cent of cortical neoplasms that invade the dura mater are malignant gliomas; another 33 per cent are metastases of other types of tumor.[4] Since approximately 50 per cent of cerebellar astrocytomas invade the subarachnoid space, invasion of the leptomeninges does not always imply anaplasia.[370]

Clinical Presentation

Glioblastomas, depending on their location, present with a wide variety of symptoms that have usually persisted for a few months. Since they may arise secondarily from a pre-existing well-differentiated astrocytoma, however, there may have been a long period of symptoms related to the astrocytoma.

The approximate duration of symptoms is less than one month in 30 per cent, three months in 60 per cent, six months in 70 per cent, and longer than two years in only 7 per cent.[61,130,158] Onset is apoplectic in approximately 4 per cent. Anaplastic astrocytomas cause symptoms for longer than glioblastomas, for more than one year in approximately 34 per cent of patients.[370]

Headache is the most common symptom with glioblastoma. It is present in over 70 per cent and is the initial symptom in 40 per cent of patients.[130,193] In 25 per cent of patients, it is unilateral, and on the same side as the tumor in over 90 per cent of those. Although motor disorders are the initial symptom in only about 3 per cent, approximately 43 per cent of patients complain of them by the time of diagnosis.[130,193] Mental changes are noted in 45 per cent and are the initial symptom in approximately 7 per cent of patients. Seizures occur in about 33 per cent of patients and are the initial symptom in 15 per cent.[319]

The neurological examination usually reveals obvious abnormalities. Their percentages are approximately as follows: Abnormal reflexes, 83 per cent; confusion or disorientation, 50 per cent; papilledema, 45 per cent, drowsiness or lethargy, 28 per cent, visual field abnormalities, 25 per cent; parietal lobe signs, 26 per cent; hypesthesia or hypalgesia, 19 per cent; stupor or coma, 19 per cent; and third or sixth nerve palsy, 5 per cent.[193]

Patients with glioblastoma of the optic nerve develop signs and symptoms mimicking optic neuritis and may progress to total blindness within two months and to death within a few months.[165,186,276] Nearly all glioblastoma of the brain stem arises as a result of anaplasia of a previous astrocytoma. The signs are the same as those of astrocytoma, but the course is more rapid. Glioblastoma of the thalamus presents with the same signs and symptoms as astrocytoma of the thalamus, although with more rapid progression. Glioblastoma of the hemisphere presents with focal neurological deficit related to the location of tumor and in most cases accompanied by changes in mentation and elevated intracranial pressure.

Glioblastomas may cause symptoms by generalized increased intracranial pressure, either from tumor mass or obstruction of cerebrospinal fluid pathways. Focal neurological deficits may be due to displacement and distortion of fiber tracts by localized masses, to replacement of brain by tumor, or to edema interfering with brain function. Cysts can develop, especially in previously treated lesions, and may be the primary cause of symptoms.[323] Involvement of vessels by neoplasm is a less common cause of symptoms. Vascular involvement can cause either ischemic or hemorrhagic symptoms.[168,230,402]

The hemorrhage that occurs in glioblastoma is usually the result of rupture of small vessels in areas of necrosis.[354] Approximately 50 per cent of patients with brain tumor who present with subarachnoid hemorrhage have primary gliomas, and 30 per cent have anaplastic gliomas. A rarer mechanism for bleeding consists of invasion of a cerebral artery by glioma with secondary rupture of the artery. A patient in whom rupture of the middle cerebral artery led to death has been reported.[168]

Investigation

The investigation of patients with glioblastoma has been revolutionized by computed tomography. In spite of the advances in diagnosis with this device, however, other investigational techniques often are helpful. In centers in which computed tomography is not available, the sequence of investigative studies used in earlier years may be necessary.

Plain x-rays of the skull are abnormal in approximately 60 per cent of these patients.[130,157] A calcified pineal gland is shifted in 33 per cent, there is evidence of increased intracranial pressure in 25 per cent, and abnormal calcification is present in approximately 2 per cent.[130]

The electroencephalogram is abnormal in 92 per cent and is localizing in 75 per cent of patients with glioblastomas.[130,311] Sometimes, however, it is localizing to the wrong lobe of the brain and, in rare cases, to the wrong hemisphere.[130] Markedly abnormal recordings with a tumor suggest an anaplastic lesion, while a normal or nearly normal one suggests a well-differentiated tumor.[151]

Deep-lying neoplasms cause abnormalities in 90 per cent of cases if the intracranial pressure is elevated, but in only 33 per cent if this pressure is normal.[73]

Radioisotope uptake is abnormal in 90 per cent of the patients (Fig. 86–30).[135,294,311] The concentration gradient between tumor and surrounding brain is approximately 8 to 1 for technetium pertechnetate, which accounts for the requirement that lesions be 1.5 to 2 cm in diameter to allow detection.[179] The scan may change dramatically over short periods of time.[334] If an initial evaluation fails to reveal the neoplasm, repeat scanning after a few weeks may detect it. Tracers such as xenon are less accurate than technetium.[167] It is not possible to make a specific diagnosis of glioblastoma from the radioisotope scan. Occasionally, a multifocal glioblastoma will show apparently separate lesions that suggest metastatic disease.[331] A "doughnut" sign may be produced that is easily misinterpreted as an abscess.[200] When the tumor is attached to the dura, the usefulness of the scan is reduced, and the mass may be incorrectly diagnosed as either a meningioma or a metastasis.[4,393] Cerebrospinal fluid metastases from this tumor can produce a carpet of glioblastoma throughout the basal meninges, a distribu-

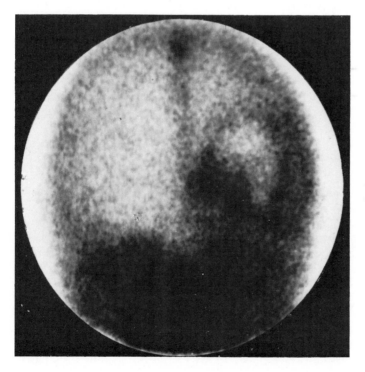

Figure 86–30 Uptake of isotope in a ring in the left hemisphere demonstrates a glioblastoma.

tion that is referred to as "meningeal glio-mastosis." In this circumstance, the radio-isotope brain scan may reveal uptake throughout the basal cisterns, a pattern that looks much like an isotope cisternogram.[227]

The current diagnostic procedure of choice for glioblastoma is the CT scan enhanced with water-soluble iodinated contrast material.[6] Indeed, the method is so accurate that false negative scans have been published as case reports.[415] The appearance on the scan of nonanaplastic gliomas usually is as a low-density lesion that is well defined and regular in shape. There is little edema around the neoplasm.[414] In the anaplastic lesions such as the glioblastomas, the area of low density is irregular and poorly defined. There may be "fingers" of edema extending into the adjacent white matter (Fig. 86–31). The density may be increased in glioblastomas or low-grade gliomas. In the latter, it may correspond to calcification within the tumor. If increased density is present in a glioblastoma, hemorrhage into the tumor should be considered. In contrast to glioblastomas, which are enhanced more than 90 per cent of the time, low-grade gliomas usually cannot be enhanced.[404,414] The contrast enhancement of glioblastoma usually is heterogeneous but may have a ringlike pattern. The margins of the ring often are unequal in thickness. The mass effect tends to be greater with glio-blastomas than with less anaplastic astrocytomas. Contrast enhancement always occurs in tumors in which angiographic evidence of vascularity is present; it may, however, occur without evidence of abnormal vessels.

Slightly more than 50 per cent of these tumors have a central lucent area on CT scan, and clinical deterioration correlates with an increase in the size of that area in 80 per cent of them (cf. Fig. 86–31). Edema tends to be more marked in patients who deteriorate.[304] The CT scan is at least as useful as radioisotope scanning in assessing progression of the tumor and is more helpful with regard to development of cysts or hemorrhage within it.[68,222,323]

Lumbar puncture should not be performed in patients suspected of having glioblastomas. The information obtained usually is nonspecific and does not justify the significant risk that accompanies the procedure. Among 122 patients reported by Frankel and German who underwent lumbar puncture and who had the tumor, there were two fatalities "directly attributable to the lumbar puncture."[130] Spinal fluid pressure was elevated above 190 mm of water in 80 per cent of the cases, and the protein was increased about 45 mg per 100 ml in 76 per cent of them. Increased numbers of white cells (more than five white cells per cubic centimeter) were present in 23 of 96

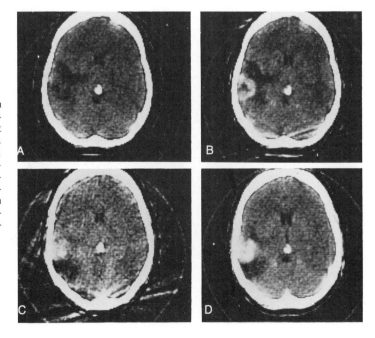

Figure 86–31 *A*. CT scan shows decreased density of glioblastoma. *B*. Intravenous contrast agent reveals an enhanced mass with a central area of lucency and surrounding edema. *C*. Repeat enhanced scan four months after beginning radiotherapy and chemotherapy demonstrates reduction in the mass. *D*. Clinical deterioration one month later is accompanied by enlargement of the mass.

patients. Glioblastomas routinely elevate polyamine content in cerebrospinal fluid.[270] Abnormal adenylate kynase activity can also be demonstrated in patients with anaplastic gliomas.[355] Low cerebrospinal fluid sugar levels have been reported with glioblastomas, in one case as low as zero.[79,105] All these findings are of interest but are not of definitive help in the diagnosis or management of the tumors.

In past decades, ventriculography was the diagnostic procedure of choice in evaluating patients with brain tumors. Ventriculography in 131 patients with glioblastoma was localizing in 77 per cent, demonstrated inadequate filling of the ventricles in 11 per cent, was lateralized but without localization in 5 per cent, and was falsely localizing in 12 per cent.[130] Pneumoencephalography was less useful, since there is approximately a 50 per cent likelihood of inadequate filling of the ventricles in patients with glioblastoma. Currently, ventriculography is rarely necessary. Although spinal fluid analysis may or may not be diagnostic in patients with glioblastoma, cyst fluid usually reveals neoplastic cells, and pleocytosis may be marked.[60] The cyst fluid also has increased beta-lipoproteins and decreased albumin in patients with glioblastomas in comparison with patients who have less anaplastic gliomas.[60]

In the 1940's and 1950's, angiographic studies frequently were not helpful in the assessment of patients with glioblastoma. By 1963 Busch found abnormal vessels or a tumor blush in 58 per cent and an avascular area in another 4 per cent.[61] In 1964, Paillas and Combalbert reported angiograms to be abnormal in 90 per cent of patients with glioblastoma. Current techniques are more likely to show the tumors (Fig. 86–32). All 335 patients reported in a recent series had abnormal angiograms.[158]

A central nervous system mass in a patient with a neoplasm outside the central nervous system does not always herald central nervous system metastasis. Raskind and Weiss reported eight patients with primary malignant neoplasms outside the central nervous system who also had evidence of an intracranial mass. In these eight, they found two meningiomas, two chronic subdural hematomas, one astrocytoma, one glioblastoma, one intracerebral hematoma, and one enchondroma.[340]

Treatment and Results

The traditional treatment of glioblastoma is by operation. Often radiotherapy is used, and recently chemotherapy has been added (see Chapters 96 and 97).

As early as the monograph by Bailey and Cushing, it was recognized that radical operations and radiotherapy were not curative.[22] Even hemispherectomy has been

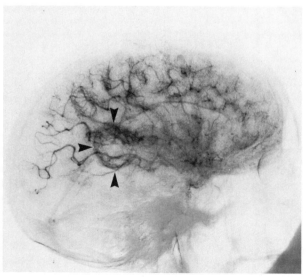
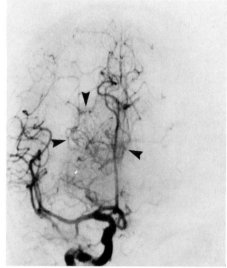

Figure 86–32 Angiography of glioblastoma reveals a tumor blush (*arrows*) and early filling of the straight sinus.

tried in a futile attempt at cure.[394] Although the tumor appears well demarcated from the surrounding brain in some areas, in other areas glioblastoma merges with normal tissue. If the tumor is large, it is likely that it invades the corpus callosum or basal ganglia and crosses to the opposite side of the brain or to the brain stem. Of course, there is little value in removing the hemisphere if tumor is left in the corpus callosum or in the opposite hemisphere or brain stem.

A variety of types of operative treatment have been utilized. Biopsy with external decompression was found unacceptable, since it was accompanied by high rates of mortality and morbidity. Many patients had severe focal neurological deficits such as aphasia and hemiplegia, and lingered for weeks or months in a demented or stuporous condition.[61,188] A few authors have recommended radiotherapy without a tissue diagnosis or no treatment when glioblastoma has been confidently diagnosed on clinical and radiological criteria.[33] Recently, the high operative risk of biopsy alone has been reduced by careful preoperative and postoperative medication with glucocorticoids and stereotaxic needle positioning.[267,389] If these techniques are used, a histological diagnosis can be obtained in approximately 90 per cent of patients with a 2 per cent mortality rate and 4 per cent neurological morbidity.[389] In spite of the reduced risk of biopsy, some neoplasms are still best treated without tissue diagnosis. This is particularly true of those in the brain stem and some of those in the thalamus.

In patients who undergo biopsy alone, the surgeon still may need to treat the elevated intracranial pressure. It must be remembered that intracranial pressure can be elevated not only by the presence of a focal mass but also by cerebral edema or trapped cerebrospinal fluid. The appropriate method for lowering intracranial pressure will depend on the relative contributions of each of these components to the elevated pressure. Glucocorticoids may be helpful in lowering intracranial pressure in patients with supratentorial tumors.[33,286] They are also reported to reduce increased intracranial pressure due to hydrocephalus in patients with posterior fossa tumors.[49]

If operative treatment is undertaken, it is advisable to remove as much of the tumor as possible.[178] If the tumor *displaces* brain it may be possible to remove tumor—even from areas that would appear to be important—without increasing neurological deficit. Tumor displacing brain usually is necrotic or hemorrhagic and, therefore, of a different color than normal brain. Tumor that *infiltrates* brain tends to be more the appearance and color of normal brain. Removal of infiltrating tumor in areas of important fiber tracts such as the internal capsule or areas with specific function such as the motor cortex is unwise. Despite the infiltration of the tumor, the brain may be functional, and resection could produce a serious deficit.

Aggressive resection of this tumor gives longer survivals than limited resection. Three-year survival rates of as high as 20 per cent and five-year survival rates of 12 per cent have been reported after extensive resection and radiotherapy.[39,308] It is possible that aggressive resection may be necessary to reduce the "tumor burden" and allow maximum effectiveness of irradiation and chemotherapy.[442] Resection also may improve effectiveness of radiotherapy by removing anoxic neoplastic cells that are radioresistant.[196] Jelsma and Bucy found that after extensive resection, the six-month survival rate was twice as high as after partial resection. They also found postoperative improvement in 89 per cent of patients who underwent extensive resection, whereas only 30 per cent with partial resection and 10 per cent with external decompression were improved. The external decompression consisted of removal of a bone flap and sometimes opening of the dura, but without resection of tumor.[193] It is obvious that the potential for the relief of neurological deficit depends on the cause of the deficit. If symptoms are caused by increased intracranial pressure and by brain shift, they are more amenable to operative treatment than deficit caused by infiltration of tumor into sensitive areas of the brain such as the internal capsule.

Younger patients tend to survive longer than those who are older. In one series of patients with grade III and grade IV astrocytomas, 76 per cent of those who were 30 years old or younger were alive one year after operation in contrast to only 50 per cent of those older than 30 years of age.[372] At five years, 25 per cent of the younger patients were alive in contrast to 3 per cent of the older patients.

Operative Deaths

The operative mortality rate has improved over the decades. It was 48 per cent between 1945 and 1959, and 2.9 per cent between 1962 and 1964 in a series reported by Jelsma and Bucy.[193] This marked improvement was due to a number of factors, which included earlier diagnosis, improved anesthesia, better control of hemorrhage at operation, the use of glucocorticoids, and removal of larger amounts of tumor tissue to effect internal decompression. The overall mortality rate reported in most series in the 1960's was 10 to 30 per cent.[158,425] The current rate is approximately 5 to 10 per cent.

Glucocorticoids are quite helpful in the operative treatment of glioblastoma. They not only reduce the number of operative deaths but also reduce intracranial pressure and may relieve symptoms temporarily. Improvement is usually apparent within 12 to 18 hours after treatment is begun and reaches a maximum in three to four days.[133] If the more usual doses of steroids are not effective, very large ones may be. Daily doses of as much as 96 mg of dexamethasone or 2000 mg of methylprednisolone have been demonstrated to be useful.[242,344] Both dexamethasone and methylprednisolone inhibit the growth of glioblastoma in tissue culture and may provide some long-term improvement. Inhibition of growth is dose dependent.[283] The mechanism of this chemotherapeutic effect of glucocorticoids is unknown.

Operative Technique

The head should be positioned so that the brain falls away from the area of dissection. Only the portion of brain to be dissected should be exposed. The remainder should have its dural covering left intact or should be protected by moist plastic-covered cotton (Telfa) or collagen sponge (Biocol). The dura should not be opened widely if intracranial pressure is high. Under these circumstances, if a cyst is present, a needle should be passed through a small hole in the dura to aspirate it. If no cyst is present, hyperventilation should be performed. The surgeon should insure that venous drainage from the head is not obstructed by poor positioning, that the head is elevated above the heart, that the endotracheal tube is not kinked and no interference with ventilation (such as pneumothorax) is present, and that arterial blood gas levels are adequate.

After the dura has been opened the next task is to locate the tumor. If large cortical veins are easily identifiable on the preoperative angiogram, it may be possible to correlate them with veins seen in the operative field and use them to locate the tumor.

Often the moistened palpating finger can identify a different consistency in an area of neoplasm. It may feel either more or less firm than normal brain. An open-ended blunt biopsy needle may also be used to take a core of tissue in the region of suspected tumor. This technique is less traumatic than biopsy by a cortical incision. Fluorescein and ultraviolet light or intravenously injected radioisotope and a probe sensitive to it have been used to localize tumor and detect residual neoplasm in the bed of the tumor cavity in the past.

Once the neoplasm has been identified, an internal decompression can be performed with suction and biopsy forceps. If it is in the temporal, occipital, or frontal pole, a lobectomy usually may be used without increasing the neurological deficit. Hemostasis can be obtained with unipolar or bipolar coagulation, with Gelfoam, or with bits of oxidized cellulose mesh (Surgicel). Sometimes troublesome bleeding can be controlled most easily with the combined use of a Frazer sucker and a Greenwood suction bipolar forceps. The sucker is used to keep the bleeding vessel exposed while it is coagulated. Placing cotton balls soaked with saline or hydrogen peroxide in the tumor bed will help control bleeding. A tempting but serious error is continued resection of tumor after the operative field becomes obscured by bleeding. In such circumstances, it is not advisable to complete the removal of tumor in hopes that the bleeding will stop once the tumor has been removed. Hemostasis should be obtained prior to further dissection so that the operation is always a controlled procedure.

The motor strip and other important landmarks may be displaced up to 2 cm by tumor.[327] If the tumor is in the region of the motor strip, localization of the strip by electrical stimulation may be helpful. Bipolar electrodes 2 mm apart stimulated with square waves of 2 msec duration and 60 Hz with a voltage of approximately 2 should be sufficient.[296] Stimulation identifies the motor strip in patients under general anesthesia as long as muscle relaxants are not used. The sensory strip also can be localized with an averaging computer if appropriate equipment is available.

Retraction by metal retractors should be minimized. Whenever possible, retraction should be applied to tumor rather than to brain by pulling the tumor away from the brain. Finger dissection rarely is indicated, but the palpating finger is useful to identify remnants of tumor in the depths of a tumor cavity and to identify retained cotton balls or cotton patties prior to closure of the wound. Postoperative intracranial pressure monitoring and liberal use of computed tomography are appropriate when there is a possibility of increased intracranial pressure or a focal mass after operation. Further details of operative management are found in Chapters 31 and 32.

In some cases an internal decompression is needless or would produce excessive morbidity. In these patients, a needle biopsy through a burr hole can be guided by CT scan. This technique permits an accurate and safe biopsy with minimal brain manipulation. A burr hole is made over the lesion at a site that will allow a single slice of the scan to pass through both the burr hole and the lesion. A biopsy needle is placed in the cortex to approximately half the depth that will be required to reach the lesion. The patient is scanned and the required correction in direction is made. Repeat scanning makes it possible to aim the needle perfectly. The needle is then advanced and a biopsy is taken. This procedure requires a body scanner with a large gantry opening.

Radiotherapy

Radiotherapy has been demonstrated to be beneficial to patients with glioblastoma.[24] Unfortunately, the dosage required for the benefit may cause radiation necrosis. There have been a few patients who died of this complication in whom no residual tumor was found at autopsy.[14,243] The technique of radiotherapy remains a matter of disagreement. Some authors recommend irradiating limited fields with high dosages, while others recommend whole brain irradiation so that no portion of the neoplasm escapes treatment.[80,338] Patients who receive large radiation doses over extensive fields tend to survive longer than those who receive smaller doses over smaller areas.

In most failures of radiotherapy, however, there is regrowth of tumor within the area that was irradiated, although some recurrences are in unirradiated areas.[338,372]

Radiation doses of more than 3500 rads are significantly more effective than lesser doses in treating both grade III and grade IV astrocytomas.[425] Various attempts have been made to enhance the effect of radiotherapy. Hypothermia enhances it, but the mortality rate is high as a result of pulmonary infection.[38] In a preliminary study, metronidazole appears to have increased its effectiveness.[427]

Irradiation of the entire neuraxis usually has not been used to treat glioblastoma. Perhaps glioblastomas and anaplastic astrocytomas of the posterior fossa should receive it because cerebrospinal fluid metastases are more likely with them. Millipore filtration of cerebrospinal fluid has been recommended for cytological study in patients with posterior fossa glioblastomas.[372] If malignant cells are found, radiotherapy of the neuraxis would be appropriate. Nevertheless, its potential for interfering with the ability of the bone marrow to resist chemotherapy must be kept in mind.

The sequelae of radiotherapy are discussed in Chapter 97. The incidence of postirradiation injury has been low, in part because the majority of patients do not survive sufficiently long to develop radiation necrosis.[383] There are several types of radiation injury. The first is edema that occurs during treatment or shortly after its completion. This effect is self-limited and usually is well controlled by glucocorticoids. The second type of radiation injury probably is due to demyelination and produces symptoms several weeks or a few months after radiotherapy is completed.[228] Demyelination is transient, and the symptoms resolve spontaneously.[383] The third clinical pattern of radiation injury is radiation necrosis.[38,91] The incidence of the necrosis reaches its peak 1 to 3 years after treatment, but it may occur as soon as a few months and has been reported as late as 12 years.[219,228] It regularly occurs in monkeys irradiated with 6000 rads over six weeks.[70] The symptoms are the same as those of recurrent tumor, and the two cannot be distinguished with confidence by radiological studies.[128,269] Since few patients undergo repeat craniotomy, and since autopsy rates are low in patients with glioblastomas, the incidence of radiation necrosis is not well known.

Nearly 50 per cent of patients who undergo operation followed by radiotherapy and chemotherapy for malignant gliomas develop ventricular enlargement.[304] In some, this enlargement can be attributed to obstruction of cerebrospinal fluid flow by neoplasm or communicating hydrocephalus due to blood in the subarachnoid spaces as a result of operative treatment. In others, it may result from brain atrophy following radiotherapy.

Radiotherapy apparently can cause malignancy. Haymaker and co-workers noted a 30 per cent incidence of glioblastoma after irradiation of monkeys with 600 to 800 rads of protons. In addition, mesodermal tumors have been reported in humans after radiotherapy. Two patients have developed meningiomas 15 and 25 years after irradiation for glioma.[305] A series of sarcomas following radiotherapy for pituitary tumors has been reported.[437]

Results

Results of treatment by operative decompression and radiotherapy usually have been evaluated by length of survival. It is also possible to observe whether the tumor decreases in size or has a stable size before resuming growth. This assessment can be done either by serial radioisotope brain scans or by CT scans. A craniotomy flap alters the radioisotope brain scan for up to four or five years, but the scans are still accurate in predicting recurrence of neoplasm.[126,189,234] Changes in vasculature of the tumor as judged by angiography do not correlate with the clinical response to treatment.[215]

Many factors correlate with survival in patients with anaplastic astrocytomas. Gehan and Walker analyzed 225 patients entered in a brain tumor study. Characteristics that were associated with improved survival were treatment with radiotherapy, young age, clinical presentation with seizures, cranial nerve palsies, treatment with chemotherapy, encapsulated neoplasm, and tumor not in the parietal lobe. Other factors were not statistically significant.[137] Tumors containing calcium also have a more favorable prognosis than those without calcification.[413] Grade IV neoplasms are linked to a shorter survival than those in grade III.[208,372,425] Patients with astrocytomas with "areas of glioblastoma" live longer than those with glioblastoma without obvious astrocytic origin. Of the 162 patients reported by Jelsma and Bucy, only 10 survived two years or longer. All 10 of these patients had anaplasia in a pre-existing astrocytoma, and 3 had had previous operations for astrocytomas. Russel and Rubinstein reported only 2 of 74 patients with glioblastomas without apparent astrocytic ancestry who survived three or more years, while 8 of 32 patients with glioblastomatous areas in astrocytomas lived three years or longer.[370]

With tumors in the frontal region the outlook is more favorable than with those in other lobes of the brain.[130,338] Right hemisphere lesions have a slightly better prognosis than those in the left hemisphere, and deep-lying or bilateral ones have a more ominous prognosis than those restricted to one side of the brain. The differences in survival of patients with neoplasms in these several locations may be, to some extent, the result of different degrees of resection, the most extensive resection being performed in right frontal tumors and the most restricted resection in glioblastomas in the midline or the dominant hemisphere. The radiation dose also affects survival time, with longer survivals in patients who receive larger doses.[308]

Survival with this tumor is longer in young adults than in older adults. The five-year survival rate in young adults is as high as 20 per cent but is only 6 per cent in those older than 36 years of age.[308] There is also a more favorable prognosis for patients with long histories of preoperative symptoms than for patients with short histories. It is probable that the majority of these younger adults with long histories have anaplastic astrocytomas, accounting for their longer survival, and that the older adults have glioblastoma without areas of more differentiated astrocytic neoplasm.[61]

Although most patients with glioblastomas do not live long, some live for many years. Elvidge and Barone have reported a woman who was asymptomatic 20 years after radical removal of a right hemisphere glioblastoma not treated with radiotherapy. They have also reported a 17-year survival after radical removal of a left parieto-occipital glioblastoma. This second patient was treated with a tumor dose of 4876 rads. It was suggested that failure of a glioblastoma to recur may be based on immunity acquired by the host against the tumor.[114] In some patients with an initial pathological diagnosis of glioblastoma who survive unusually long, the initial pathological diagnosis may have been incorrect. This explanation does not, however, seem to apply to all long survivals.[114,161]

Anaplastic gliomas of the optic nerve have a particularly poor prognosis. Of a total of 15 cases in one series, only two patients survived more than two years from the onset of symptoms.[186] Death usually occurs six to nine months after symptoms start, and sudden death is not uncommon, particularly in the immediate postoperative period. Fortunately, these tumors are quite rare.

Immunotherapy

Cell-mediated immunity is depressed in patients with anaplastic gliomas and, to a lesser extent, in those with schwannomas and meningiomas.[417] There is further depression of immunity in the immediate postoperative period.[51,245] The significance of these findings is unknown.

Access of brain antigens to the immune system has been documented by the finding of "antiglioma antibodies" in 82 per cent of patients with astrocytomas and by immune responses in tissue culture.[217] Immune surveillance depends not only on access of the pathological cells to the immune system but also on a surface made unique by a particular set of antigens. Astrocytic cells have a particularly large surface area and require approximately 10 times as much antibody to saturate all the antigenic sites as is required by rat lymphoma cells.[98]

The efferent limb of the cellular immune system should have access to the central nervous system by way of circulating cells. At least in multiple sclerosis, the humoral immune system has access to the central nervous system, as demonstrated by the production of immunoglobulins from cells in the cerebrospinal fluid.[373]

Circulating factors that are incapable of crossing the blood-brain barrier may not have access to the rapidly growing portion of tumor, since the rapidly growing cells are at the periphery of the tumor, beyond the limits of its neovascular supply, and are nourished by the vascular system of the in-

vaded brain.[237] The effect of the humoral and cellular immune systems in central nervous system neoplasms is unknown.

A prospective randomized clinical trial has been performed in an effort to assess the effect of specific active immunotherapy.[39] Immunotherapy was not found to be beneficial in this trial, but irradiated tumor cells were used and may not have provided a sufficient antigenic stimulus. Also, the immunotherapy was delivered during the period of immunosuppression produced by radiotherapy.[277] It has been suggested that immunotherapy may be beneficial in the treatment of these tumors, but its value is not proved.[442] Furthermore, manipulation of the immune system may interfere with natural immunological defenses.[148] Gliomas have some antigens in common with normal brain, and active specific immunotherapy directed against brain antigens can produce encephalitis in experimental animals. There are other antigens that occur in a variety of glioblastomas but do not occur in normal brain. These have been postulated either to be embryonic antigens or to reflect a common viral etiology for a variety of central nervous system neoplasms.[434] Perhaps active immunotherapy specific for these antigens will be useful.

MEDULLOBLASTOMA

Medulloblastoma is a primary brain tumor occuring in the cerebellum. It is composed of uniform small cells with frequent mitoses, and was definitively described by Bailey and Cushing.[21] Initially they intended to name it spongioblastoma cerebelli. When it was realized, however, that this term conflicted with the spongioblastoma of the cerebral hemisphere named by Globus and Strauss, it was renamed medulloblastoma. Bailey and Cushing recognized that this tumor frequently was called a neuroblastoma or sarcoma, but believed both of these names inappropriate for histogenetic reasons and preferred a name that implied an origin from multipotential cells.

The cell type of origin of medulloblastoma continues to be controversial.[361] Bailey and Cushing believed the undifferentiated cells described by Schaper were the source of medulloblastoma.[21,376] These undifferentiated cells migrate from the midline over the surface of the cerebellum during early life. They were thought by Schaper to be capable of either neuroblastic or spongioblastic differentiation. This multipotentiality may account for the finding of areas of spongioblastic differentiation with neuroglial fibrillae and smaller, more heavily stained nuclei as well as other areas of neuroblastic differentiation characterized by larger nuclei with a single large nucleolus.[21] The predominance of medulloblastoma in early life and the relative lack of differentiation of the cells were also compatible with origin from embryonic nests of a primitive cell.[86]

Cajal believed that the external granular cells were destined for neuroblastic differentiation. In line with Cajal's suggestion, Stevenson and Echlin thought that a neoplasm of these cells should be called a neuroblastoma or even more specifically, a granuloblastoma.[64,406] The external granular layer of the cerebellum arises from cells that migrate from the posterior medullary velum. The germinal bud in this area normally disappears early in life, although in some patients scattered collections of cells remain. The cells that have arisen in this region and that migrate over the surface of the cerebellum remain as the external granular layer for the first 18 to 20 months.[335] The origin of medulloblastoma from the external granular layer is supported by the findings in a patient in whom diffuse neoplasia of the external granular layer merged with a focus of medulloblastoma.[367] There is also cytological similarity between external granular cells and medulloblastoma cells.[197]

Origin from neurons in the granular layer has been suggested by Zimmerman. He found that implantation of carcinogens in the cerebellum of some experimental animals resulted in medulloblastomas.[455] This implies that medulloblastoma can be a neoplasm of mature cells that are normally present.

The finding of striated muscle in medulloblastomas has produced considerable confusion. Neoplastic muscle would require precursors of mesenchymal origin, while the medulloblastoma presumably arises from precursors of neuroepithelial origin. If mixed mesenchymal and neuroepithelial heritage is present for a medullomyoblastoma, the tumor would, by definition, be a teratoma.

Incidence

Medulloblastomas constitute approximately 8 per cent of gliomas and 33 per cent of tumors in and around the fourth ventricle.* Although it is thought of as a childhood tumor, approximately one third occur in adults. In the adult, women appear to be affected as commonly as men. Approximately half of the laterally placed medulloblastomas occur in adults, whereas midline ones are much more likely to occur in childhood. As a corollary of this, the average age of patients with laterally placed tumors is approximately 17 years, while the average age of all those with medulloblastomas is only about 14 years.

Although medulloblastoma occurs with a higher than normal frequency in children with the nevoid basal cell carcinoma syndrome, adults with this syndrome have not been shown to develop them.[302] The possibility of greater incidence in siblings has been raised by intriguing cases such as the occurrence of medulloblastomas in newborn twin sisters.[32]

Pathology

Macroscopic Changes

Medulloblastoma usually arises in the region of the roof of the fourth ventricle and is a well-circumscribed lesion.[21] Like other fourth ventricular tumors, it tends to present between the cerebellar tonsils and may extend through the foramen magnum. The fourth ventricle is expanded by tumor, and occasionally tumor projects through the aqueduct of Sylvius.[21,350] Midline lesions are adherent to the floor of the fourth ventricle in approximately 50 per cent of cases. It has been reported to have invaded the anterior vermis and covered the corpora quadrigemina.[350] It is not clear whether the tumors in this location have their origin from the pineal region and have extended caudally or whether this is an unusual extension of a medulloblastoma.

Tumors apparently identical with medulloblastoma have been observed in the cerebral hemispheres, but they are quite un-

---

* See references 21, 34, 72, 84, 86, 111, 154, 159, 350, 363, 400.

common. Bailey and Cushing initially found 11 such cases; however, on re-examination by Cushing, all but two were reclassified as other types of tumors. Cushing suggested that even these two remaining ones might properly be reclassified.[86] Ringertz and Tola reviewed a large series of gliomas without finding any evidence of cerebral medulloblastoma.[350]

Medulloblastomas are particularly likely to metastasize to the subarachnoid space and may develop subarachnoid implants over the surface of the cerebellum.[21] The frequency with which they spread via the cerebrospinal fluid may be, in part, due to the ease of dispersion of tumor cells.[28] Cerebrospinal fluid metastases may produce a diffuse opacity of the arachnoid or "buttonlike" nodules of tumor, or may occur in the spinal region or in the floor of the third ventricle.[350] At operation, local subarachnoid metastases can be recognized in approximately 10 per cent, and on pathological examination, metastases can be identified in more than half the cases.[102,367] Because of the infrequency of medulloblastoma, it constitutes only 10 to 50 per cent of neuroepithelial tumors that metastasize in cerebrospinal fluid.[55,325]

Typically this neoplasm is soft. Occasionally it is firmer owing to proliferation of fibrous tissue. This collagenous reaction is found in a variant called desmoplastic medulloblastoma in which meningeal reactive changes are quite prominent.[367] It is particularly likely to occur in the cerebellar hemisphere rather than in the vermis (probably because hemispheric tumors are more likely to invade the meninges).

Extracranial metastases may also arise from medulloblastoma and are particularly likely to involve bone.[37] There are rare cases of extracranial metastases in the absence of previous operative treatment; most, however, have followed craniotomy or cerebrospinal fluid shunting for hydrocephalus.[260,356] As many as one fourth of systemic metastases from neuroectodermal tumors arise from medulloblastoma.[395]

Microscopic Changes

Under the microscope, medulloblastoma appears as a mass of cells that are "rounded or pear-shaped, sometimes spindle-shaped, with scanty cytoplasm and big oval nuclei containing an abundant network of chromatin" (Fig. 86–33).[21] The ultrastructure of these cells is very primitive, with the glial or neuronal differentia-

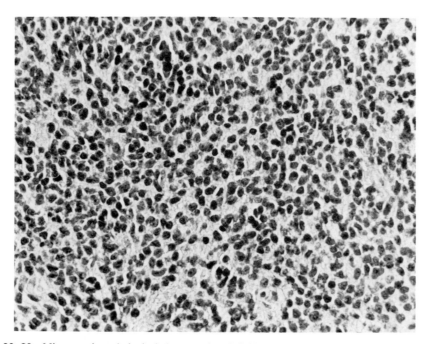

Figure 86–33 Microscopic pathological changes of medulloblastoma. A densely packed field of uniform cells is shown. 250 ×.

tion that would be expected of an embryonic tissue.[272] They may be densely packed in a sheet without any obvious architecture or may lie in strands, pallisade around irregular spaces, or form "pseudorosettes."[21] A pseudorosette is a circular arrangement of cells clustering around a nuclear free center. This type of rosette is thought to be typical of neuroblastic differentiation.

Microscopic fields that resemble oligodendroglioma may occur in medulloblastomas. Ringertz and Tola attributed this appearance to fixation artifact.[350] Rubinstein and Northfield have suggested that they are oligodendroglial cells and that they illustrate the greater variation and possibilities for differentiation inherent in the multipotential cell of origin of medulloblastoma. Oligodendroglial cells exemplify glial differentiation in medulloblastomas. Phosphotungstic acid–hematoxylin staining reveals polar cells . with fine fibrillary processes suggesting spongioblastic differentiation.[367]

Gangliogliomatous maturation has been documented in three medulloblastomas. Although medulloblastomas are more common in men, the three patients in whom these changes were observed were women.[201] There may be a humoral factor in the female that augments this type of cell differentiation.

Striated muscle fibers have been identified in medulloblastoma.[288] Since neuroglial cells have also been proved to be present, the tumor cannot be regarded as a sarcoma but must be a variant of a teratoma in which neuroepithelial differentiation gives rise to medulloblastoma and mesenchymal components give rise to striated muscle.[15,288]

Proliferation of vascular walls occurs in approximately one fourth of patients with medulloblastoma but does not lead to extensive thrombosis and necrosis.[350] Calcification is present in approximately 6 per cent.[268]

A great increase in interstitial tissue may occur and add to the firmness of a medulloblastoma.[86] This is particularly likely if the neoplasm is superficial and has extensive distribution in the meninges. In this circumstance, tumor may be identifiable only as nests of cells in a network of connective tissue (Fig. 86–34).[350] If portions of the tumor that infiltrate brain tissue are examined, more typical cells can be perceived.

This connective tissue reaction has been named desmoplasia, and the tumor, desmoplastic medulloblastoma. Rubinstein and Northfield have suggested that some of them may stimulate a more intense connec-

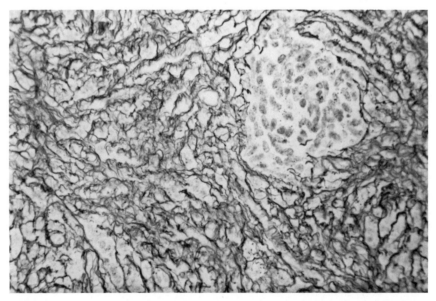

Figure 86–34 Microscopic pathological changes of desmoplastic medulloblastoma. Nests of cells are embedded in a connective tissue background (reticulin stain). 250 ×. (Courtesy of Surl L. Nielson, M.D., University of California, Davis.)

tive tissue reaction than others because of an intrinsic property of the tumor. The resulting meningeal reaction may seal off the subarachnoid space around a medulloblastoma and restrict further invasion by the tumor.[367]

Radiotherapy of medulloblastomas results in widespread necrosis, cellular pleomorphism, and the formation of giant cells. Oppenheimer has suggested that after irradiation the pleomorphic areas and giant cells are incapable of reproduction but that cells that escape this radiotherapeutic change can reproduce the original tissue.[309] This theory agrees with the findings in astrocytomas in which gemistocytes and giant cells may indicate a nondividing cell.[184] Irradiated medulloblastoma may resemble glioblastoma.[363]

Clinical Presentation

The average duration of symptoms prior to operation in patients with medulloblastomas is four or five months.[350,400] Symptoms progress rapidly after their onset.

In 75 to 80 per cent of adults, the first symptoms indicate only increased intracranial pressure.[21,244] Common presenting symptoms are headache, nausea, and vomiting as well as visual changes.[400] Usually there is a history of difficulty with gait, and cerebellar signs can be identified. Brain stem abnormalities such as abducens nerve palsy are common.

Although it is possible for the symptoms of medulloblastoma to have a sudden onset due to hemorrhage in the tumor, this is uncommon.[278] They can also present with

paroxysms of arterial hypertension suggestive of pheochromocytoma.[66] Metastases to the spine, just like other intradural extramedullary masses, manifest themselves with spinal cord compression.

Investigation

Ventriculography has been the procedure of choice in the past. With a very large lesion it may be interpreted as demonstrating a posterior third ventricular tumor.[34] Currently the diagnostic procedure of choice is computed tomography (Fig. 86–35). It may reveal not only the tumor but also associated hydrocephalus. Other contrast studies usually add little to the information gained from CT scanning.[339] Diagnosis may be aided by cytological examination of cerebrospinal fluid. Approximately half the patients have abnormal cells that can be isolated by Nuclepore filtration.[346] Distant metastases to bone may produce either osteoplastic or osteolytic lesions.[37] Cerebrospinal fluid metastases may require myelography for identification.

Treatment and Results

At the time of their initial report, Bailey and Cushing recommended limited decompression and subsequent radiotherapy.[21] Further experience led to the recommendation that tumor removal should be sufficiently extensive to open cerebrospinal fluid pathways.[86] Radiotherapists have also recommended sufficiently aggressive removal to re-establish cerebrospinal fluid

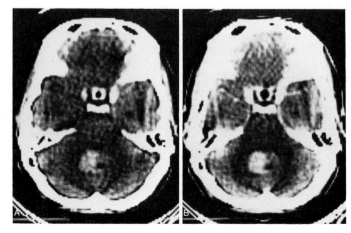

Figure 86–35 *A*. Unenhanced CT scan of a medulloblastoma shows a cerebellar mass. *B*. Infusion of iodinated contrast material enhances the tumor density.

circulation.[220] If cerebrospinal fluid circulation is to be restored, the tumor must be withdrawn from the aqueduct of Sylvius and most of it removed from the fourth ventricle. Often this effect can be accomplished by using suction dissection.[86] If the patient is in the sitting position, a gush of cerebrospinal fluid through the aqueduct signals its being unblocked. During tumor dissection, the subarachnoid space should be covered with cottonoid or another material that will prevent its contamination with tumor fragments.[319]

There is disagreement regarding the relationship between extent of resection and duration of survival. Some authors believe that moderate tumor removal sufficient to restore cerebrospinal fluid circulation is not as effective as radical tumor removal, which is associated with fewer operative deaths, less postoperative morbidity, and a longer survival after radiotherapy.[211,446] One series reported the survival of 44 per cent of patients with "complete" excisions, as opposed to only 22 per cent of those with "partial" excisions.[40] Berger and Elvidge, however, found no difference in average duration of survival of patients who underwent biopsy and irradiation and those who underwent decompressive operation and irradiation.[34]

The operative death rate has been approximately 20 per cent in most series.[34,86,350] In recent series this rate has been reduced to nearly 10 per cent.[283]

Radiotherapy greatly increases the survival time.[21] Without it the tumor can grow rapidly and prove fatal only a few months after extensive resection.[418] Radiotherapy should not be substituted for combined operative and radiotherapeutic management because other lesions, such as astrocytoma and hemangioglioblastoma, may mimic medulloblastoma but require operative removal. As noted by Cushing, radiotherapy should encompass the entire neuraxis.[86] Most radiotherapists recommend approximately 5500 rads of radiation to the posterior fossa and 4000 to 4500 rads to the remainder of the neuraxis.[211,220] The junction between fields should vary from one treatment to the next so that one area of the spinal cord does not receive either no radiation or a very large dose. During the course of treatment, bone marrow activity should be monitored, since leukopenia may be sufficiently severe to require a change in

schedule. If tumor recurs, a second course may be useful. Even with aggressive operative excision and radiotherapy, residual tumor usually remains in the posterior fossa, identifiable on CT scan and at autopsy.[11,40,222]

Chemotherapy has demonstrated benefit in patients with medulloblastoma. The risks of intrathecal chemotherapy are significant.[442] Further details are given in Chapter 96.

Survival for five years has been reported for up to 58 per cent of small groups of patients, but most authors report survival of only approximately 40 per cent for that length of time.[34,102,180,282]

Larger radiation doses also prolong survival.[282] Inadequate irradiation accounts for the poorer results in some early series.[350] Patients with desmoplastic lesions live slightly longer than those with typical ones.[72,102,367] The better prognosis may be due to a lesser tendency to invade the fourth ventricle and produce cerebrospinal fluid metastases as well as to the lateral and superficial localization of desmoplastic lesions, which allows more complete removal.[367]

The morbidity of aggressive treatment has been great, particularly in children. In one series, only 6 of 10 children alive three or more years after treatment were making satisfactory progress in school, and 1 of these 6 was blind.[40]

Initially these tumors were thought to be uniformly and rapidly fatal. Age and the aggressiveness of treatment have, however, been found to influence the prognosis. The natural history of the tumor has a longer course in adults than in children, but in contrast, aggressive treatment seems to influence the tumor more in children and they survive longer than when the same treatment is given to adults. Bloom and colleagues have reported that 26 per cent of children survive for 10 years, and Quest and co-workers have reported that 23 per cent live beyond the age of diagnosis plus nine years.[40,333]

Collin's law states that in a patient with a congenital neoplasm, if survival after treatment equals the patient's age at diagnosis plus nine months, then the patient should be cured. This rule has been applied to medulloblastomas; of 24 patients reported by King and Sagerman, however, 3 survived long enough to be considered cured according to Collin's law, and 2 of these 3 later died of the neoplasm.[211] Other authors have also reported patients who violate Collin's law.[15,220]

MEDULLOEPITHELIOMA

Medulloepithelioma is a rare primitive neoplasm that occurs in young children. On microscopic examination, the tissue consists of cells lining up in pallisades around a central cell-free zone. It is quite anaplastic, but there is insufficient experience available to make firm statements about natural history or recommended treatment.[362]

PRIMITIVE POLAR SPONGIOBLASTOMA

This tumor is listed in the World Health Organization outline, but fewer than 10 cases have been reported in the world's literature.[357,361] It is a rare neoplasm of childhood that grows rapidly. It has primitive cells that resemble the migrating spongioblasts that are seen during embryogenesis. The cells are tapered, and the nuclei align in rows.

GLIOMATOSIS CEREBRI

"Gliomatosis cerebri" is a term that refers to the extremely widespread distribution of astrocytoma, a condition that is most common in anaplastic astrocytoma. The lesion has the natural history of anaplastic glioma.[153] Diagnosis may be difficult if no focal mass effect is present. Treatment consists of biopsy to establish diagnosis and subsequent radiotherapy and chemotherapy.

REFERENCES

1. Abbott, K. H., Rollas, Z. H., and Meagher, J. N.: Choroid plexus papilloma causing spontaneous subarachnoid hemorrhage: Report of case and review of literature. J. Neurosurg. *14*:566–570, 1957.
2. Abraham, J., and Chandy, J.: Ventriculo-atrial shunt in the management of posterior-fossa tumours: Preliminary report. J. Neurosurg., *20*:252–253, 1963.
3. Albright, L., and Reigel, D. H.: Management of hydrocephalus secondary to posterior fossa tumors. J. Neurosurg., *46*:52–55, 1977.
4. Alliez, B., Paillas, J. E., Vigouroux, M., Pelissier, J-F., and Debaene, A.: Tumeurs cérébrales envahissant la dure-mère: Etude anatomique, clinique et radiologique. Neurochirurgie, *18*:453–469, 1972.
5. Altenburg, H., and Schmidt, H.: Vergleichende Untersuchungen zwischen szintigraphischen, angiographischen und histologischen Befunden beim Astrocytom. Proc. German Society for Neurosurgery, Dusseldorf, 1971. Amsterdam, Excerpta Medica, 1973.
6. Ambrose, J., Gooding, M. R., and Richardson, A. E.: Sodium iothalamate as an aid to diagnosis of intracranial lesions by computerized transverse axial scanning. Lancet, *2*:669–674, 1975.
7. Anderson, D. R., and Spencer, W. H.: Ultrastructural and histochemical observations of optic nerve gliomas. Arch. Ophthal. (Chicago), *83*:324–335, 1970.
8. Andersson, P. G.: Intracranial tumors in a psychiatric autopsy material. Acta Psychiat. Scand., 46:213–224, 1970.
9. Anzil, A. P.: Glioblastoma multiforme with extracranial metastases in the absence of previous craniotomy: Case report. J. Neurosurg., *33*:88–94, 1970.
10. Arendt, A.: Ependymomas. *In* Vinken, P. J., and Bruyn, G. W., eds.: Handbook of Clinical Neurology. Vol. 18, Tumours of the Brain and Skull, Part IV. Amsterdam, North-Holland Publishing Co., 1975. pp. 105–150.
11. Aron, B. S.: Twenty years' experience with radiation therapy of medulloblastoma. Amer. J. Roentgen., *105*:37–42, 1969.
12. Aronson, S. M., Garcia, J. H., and Aronson, B. E.: Metastatic neoplasms of the brain: Their frequency in relation to age. Cancer, *17*:558–563, 1964.
13. Arseni, C., Constantinescu, A., Danaila, L., and Istrate, C.: The choroid plexus papillomas. Neurochirurgia (Stuttgart), *17*:121–129, 1974.
14. Asbury, A. K., Ojemann, R. G., Nielsen, S. L., and Sweet, W. H.: Neuropathologic study of fourteen cases of malignant brain tumor treated by boron-10 slow neutron capture radiation. J. Neuropath. Exp. Neurol., *31*:278–303, 1972.
15. Bailey, O. T.: Medulloblastoma. *In* Minckler, J., ed.: Pathology of the Nervous System. New York, McGraw-Hill Book Co., 1971, pp. 2071–2081.
16. Bailey, P.: A study of tumors arising from ependymal cells. Arch. Neurol. Psychiat., *11*:1–27, 1924.
17. Bailey, P.: Further remarks concerning tumors of the glioma group. Bull. Johns Hopkins Hosp., *40*:354–389, 1927.
18. Bailey, P.: Cellular types in primary tumors of the brain. *In* Penfield, W., ed.: Cytology and Cellular Pathology of the Nervous System. 1932. Reprinted, New York, Hafner Publishing Co., 1965, pp. 905–951.
19. Bailey, P., and Bucy, P. C.: Oligodendrogliomas of the brain. J. Path. Bact., *32*:735–751, 1929.
20. Bailey, P., and Bucy, P. C.: Astroblastomas of the brain. Acta Psychiat. Neurol. Scand., *5*:439–461, 1930.

21. Bailey, P., and Cushing, H.: Medulloblastoma cerebelli: A common type of midcerebellar glioma of childhood. Arch. Neurol. Psychiat., *14*:192–224, 1925.
22. Bailey, P., and Cushing, H.: A Classification of the Tumors of the Glioma Group on a Histogenetic Basis with a Correlated Study of Prognosis. Philadelphia, J. B. Lippincott Co., 1926; Reprinted, New York, Argosy-Antiquarian Ltd., 1971.
23. Bailey, P., and Hiller, G.: The interstitial tissues of the central nervous system: A review. J. Nerv. Ment. Dis., *59*:337–361, 1924.
24. Bailey, P., Sosman, M. C., and Dessel, A. V.: Roentgen therapy of gliomas of the brain. Amer. J. Roentgen., *19*:203–264, 1928.
25. Banna, M.: Angiography of malignant choroid plexus papilloma. Brit. J. Radiol., *44*:412–415, 1971.
26. Barnard, R. O.: The development of malignancy in oligodendrogliomas. J. Path. Bact., *96*:113–123, 1968.
27. Bartal, A. D., Hielbronn, Y. D., and Schiffer, J.: Extensive resection of primary malignant tumors of the left cerebral hemisphere. Surg. Neurol., *1*:337–342, 1973.
28. Batzdorf, U., and Gold, V.: Dispersion of central nervous system tumors: Correlation between clinical aspects and tissue culture studies. J. Neurosurg., *41*:691–698, 1974.
29. Batzdorf, U., and Malamud, N.: The problem of multicentric gliomas. J. Neurosurg., *20*:122–136, 1963.
30. Becker, D. P., Benyo, R., and Roessmann, U.: Glial origin of monstrocellular tumor: Case report of prolonged survival. J. Neurosurg., *26*:72–77, 1967.
31. Beks, J. W. F., Doorenbos, H., and Walstra, G. J. M.: Clinical experiences with steroids in neurosurgical patients. *In* Reulen, H. J., and Schürmann, K., eds.: Steroids and Brain Edema. New York, Springer-Verlag, 1972, pp. 233–238.
32. Belamaric, J., and Chau, A. S.: Medulloblastoma in newborn sisters: Report of two cases. J. Neurosurg., *30*:76–79, 1969.
33. Bender, M. B., and Elizan, T.: The non-surgical management of brain tumor. Trans. Amer. Neurol. Ass., 87:20–24, 1961.
34. Berger, E. C., and Elvidge, A. R.: Medulloblastomas and cerebellar sarcomas: A clinical survey. J. Neurosurg., *20*:139–144, 1963.
35. Bernell, W. R., Kepes, J. J., and Seitz, E. P.: Late malignant recurrence of childhood cerebellar astrocytoma: Report of two cases. J. Neurosurg., *37*:470–474, 1972.
36. Bingas, B.: On the primary sarcomas of the brain. Acta Neurochir. (Wien), suppl. *10*:186–189, 1964.
37. Black, S. P. W., and Keats, T. E.: Generalized osteosclerosis secondary to metastatic medulloblastoma of the cerebellum. Radiology, *82*:395–400, 1964.
38. Bloch, M., Bloom, H. J. G., Penman, J., and Walsh, L.: Observations on patients with cerebral astrocytoma (glioblastoma multiforme) treated by irradiation under whole-body hypothermia. Brit. J. Cancer, *20*:722–728, 1966.
39. Bloom, H. J. G.: Combined modality therapy for intracranial tumors. Cancer, *35*:111–120, 1975.
40. Bloom, H. J. G., Wallace, E. N. K., and Henk, J. M.: The treatment and prognosis of medulloblastoma in children: A study of 82 verified cases. Amer. J. Roentgen., *105*:43–62, 1969.
41. Bohm, E., and Strang, R.: Choroid plexus papillomas. J. Neurosurg., *18*:493–500, 1961.
42. Bormann, H., and Schiefer, W.: Krampfanfälle bei Tumoren des Groshirns. Deutsch. Z. Nervenheilk., *166*:1–16, 1951.
43. Bouchard, J.: Radiation therapy of intracranial tumors: Long-term results. Acta Radiol. [Ther.] (Stockholm), *5*:11–16, 1966.
44. Bouchard, J.: Radiation Therapy of Tumors and Diseases of the Nervous System. Philadelphia, Lea & Febiger, 1966.
45. Bouchard, J., and Peirce, C. B.: Radiation therapy in the management of neoplasms of the central nervous system, with a special note in regard to children: Twenty years' experience, 1939–1958. Amer. J. Roentgen., *84*:610–628, 1960.
46. Boykin, F. C., Cowen, D., Iannucci, C. A. J., and Wolf, A.: Subependymal glomerate astrocytomas. J. Neuropath. Exp. Neurol., *13*:30–49, 1954.
47. Braunstein, H., and Martin, F.: Congenital papilloma of choroid plexus: Report of a case, with observations on pathogenesis of associated hydrocephalus. Arch. Neurol. Psychiat., *68*:475–480, 1952.
48. Brewis, M., Poskanzer, D. C., Rolland, C., and Miller, H.: Neurological disease in an English city. Acta Neurol. Scand., *42*: Suppl. 24:1–89, 1966.
49. Brock, M., Zillig, C., Wiegand, H., Zywietz, C., and Mock, P.: The influence of dexamethasone therapy in ICP in patients with tumors of the posterior fossa. *In* Beks, J. W. F., Bosch, D. A., and Brock, M., eds.: Intracranial Pressure III. Berlin, Springer-Verlag. 1976. pp. 236–246.
50. Brooks, W. H.: Geographic clustering of brain tumors in Kentucky. Cancer, *30*:923–926, 1972.
51. Brooks, W. H., Caldwell, H. D., and Mortara, R. H.: Immune responses in patients with gliomas. Surg. Neurol., *2*:419–423, 1974.
52. Broussalian, S. L.: Intracranial ependymo-choroidal tumors: An analysis of fifty-three cases. Bull. Los Angeles Neurol. Soc., *23*:119–128, 1958.
53. Brucher, J. M.: The classification and diagnosis of intracranial sarcomas. Acta Neurochir. (Wien), suppl. *10*:190–200, 1964.
54. Brust, J. C. M., Moiel, R. H., and Rosenberg, R. N.: Glial tumor metastases through a ventriculo-pleural shunt: Resultant massive pleural effusion. Arch. Neurol. (Chicago), *18*:649–653, 1968.
55. Bryan, P.: CSF seeding of intra-cranial tumours: A study of 96 cases. Clin. Radiol., *25*:355–360, 1974.
56. Bucy, P. C.: Intrinsic tumors of the cerebellum and brain stem. *In* Bancroft, F. W., and Pilcher, C., eds.: Surgical Treatment of the Nervous System. Philadelphia, J. B. Lippincott Co., 1946, pp. 204–238.
57. Bucy, P. C., and Gustafson, W. A.: Structure, nature and classification of cerebellar astrocytomas. Amer. J. Cancer, *35*:327–353, 1939.

58. Budka, H.: Partially resected and irradiated cerebellar astrocytoma of childhood: Malignant evolution after 28 years. Acta Neurochir. (Wien), *32*:139–146, 1975.

59. Bull, J.: Localization of cerebral lesions by radioactive isotopes and ultra sound. Proc. Roy. Soc. Med., *58*:1051–1053, 1965.

60. Burgman, G. P., and Lobkova, T. N.: Fluid composition in cerebral cysts of different histological origin. Vop. Neirokhir., *34*:47–50, 1970.

61. Busch, E. A. V.: Indications for surgery in glioblastomas. Clin. Neurosurg., *9*:1–17, 1963.

62. Cabanes, J., Vazquez, R., and Rivas, A.: Hydrocephalus after posterior fossa operations. Surg. Neurol., *9*:42–46, 1978.

63. Cairns, H., and Russell, D. S.: Intracranial and spinal metastases in gliomas of the brain. Brain, *54*:377–420, 1931.

64. Cajal, S. R.: Histologie du Système Nerveux de l' Homme et des Vertébrés. Vol. 2. Paris, A. Maloine, 1909.

65. Calvo, W.: Observations on the metallic impregnations of brain tumours. Acta Neurochir. (Wien), Suppl *10*:85–97, 1964.

66. Cameron, S. J., and Doig, A.: Cerebellar tumours presenting with clinical features of phaeochromocytoma. Lancet, *2*:492–494, 1970.

67. Canti, R. G., Bland, J. O. W., and Russell, D. S.: Tissue culture of gliomata. Ass. Res. Nerv. Ment. Dis. Proc., *16*:1–24, 1937.

68. Carella, R. J., Pay, N., Newall, J., Farina, A. T., Kricheff, I. I., and Cooper, J. S.: Computerized (axial) tomography in the serial study of cerebral tumors treated by radiation: A preliminary report. Cancer, *37*:2719–2728, 1976.

69. Carrea, R., and Polak, M.: Preoperative radiotherapy in the management of posterior fossa choroid plexus papillomas. Child's Brain, *3*:12–24, 1977.

70. Caveness, W. F.: Pathology of radiation damage to the normal brain of the monkey. Nat. Cancer Inst. Monogr., *46*:57–76, 1977.

71. Chassard, J. L., Dutou, L., Gérard, J. P., and Papillon, J.: La radiothérapie post-opératoire des gliomes hémisphériques de l' adulte: A propos d'une statistique de 134 observations. J. Radiol. Elect., *57*:391–398, 1976.

72. Chatty, E. M., and Earle, K. M.: Medulloblastoma: A report of 201 cases with emphasis on the relationship of histologic variants to survival. Cancer, *28*:977–983, 1971.

73. Cheek, W. R., and Taveras, J. M.: Thalamic tumors. J. Neurosurg., *24*:505–513, 1966.

74. Choi, N. W., Schuman, L. M., and Gullen, W. H.: Epidemiology of primary central nervous system neoplasms: I. Mortality from primary central nervous system neoplasms in Minnesota. Amer. J. Epidem., *91*:238–259, 1970.

75. Choi, N. W. Schuman, L. M., and Gullen, W. H.: Epidemiology of primary central nervous system neoplasms: II. Case-control study. Amer. J. Epidem., *91*:467–485, 1970.

76. Chowdhury, A. M.: Cyst within the parenchyma of the optic chiasm. Brit. J. Ophthal., *60*:581–582, 1976.

77. Christensen, E.: Nerve cell tumors: Central and peripheral. *In* Minckler, J., ed.: Pathology of the Nervous System. New York, McGraw-Hill Book Co., 1971. pp. 2081–2093.

78. Cogan, D. G.: Tumors of the optic nerve. *In* Vincken, P. J., and Bruyn, G. W., ed.: Handbook of Clinical Neurology. Vol. 17. Amsterdam, North-Holland Publishing Co., 1974, pp. 350–374.

79. Cole, M., Gordy, P. D., and Brondos, G. A.: Low cerebro-spinal fluid sugar associated with malignant glioma. Surg. Neurol., *2*:399–402, 1974.

80. Concannon, J. P., Kramer, S., and Berry, R.: The extent of intracranial gliomata at autopsy and its relationship to techniques used in radiation therapy of brain tumors. Amer. J. Roentgen., *84*:99–107, 1960.

81. Condon, J. R., and Rose F. C.: Optic nerve glioma., Brit. J. Ophthal., *51*:703–706, 1967.

82. Courville, C. B., and Broussalian, S. L.: Plastic ependymomas of the lateral recess: Report of eight verified cases. J. Neurosurg., *18*:792–799, 1961.

83. Cox, L. B.: The cytology of the glioma group; with special reference to the inclusion of cells derived from the invaded tissue. Amer. J. Path., *9*:839–898, 1933.

84. Craig, W. M., and Kernohan, J. W.: Tumors of the fourth ventricle. JAMA, *111*:2370–2377, 1938.

85. Cronqvist, S., and Agee, F.: Regional cerebral blood flow in intracranial tumours. Acta. Radiol. [Diagn.] (Stockholm), *7*:393–404, 1968.

86. Cushing, H.: Experiences with the cerebellar medulloblastomas. A critical review. Acta Pathol. Scand., *7*:1–86, 1930.

87. Cushing, H.: Experiences with the cerebellar astrocytomas: A critical review of seventy-six cases. Surg. Gynec. Obstet., *52*:129–204, 1931.

88. Cushing, H.: Intracranial Tumors: Notes upon a Series of Two Thousand Verified with Surgical-Mortality Percentages Pertaining Thereto. Springfield, Ill., Charles C Thomas, 1932.

89. Dastur, H. M., and Desai, H. D.: A comparative study of brain tuberculomas and gliomas based upon 107 case records of each. Brain, *88*:375–396, 1965.

90. Davidoff, L. M.: Some random thoughts on the astrocytomas. Bull. NY Acad. Med., *42*:85–99, 1966.

91. Davidoff, L. M., Dyke, C. G., Elsberg, C. A., and Tarlov, I. M.: The effect of radiation applied directly to the brain and spinal cord. Radiology, *31*:451–463, 1938.

92. Davis, L. E.: A physio-pathologic study of the choroid plexus with the report of a case of villous hypertrophy. J. Med. Res., *44*:521–534, 1924.

93. Davis, L. E., and Cushing, H.: Papillomas of the choroid plexus: With the report of six cases. Arch. Neurol. Psychiat., *13*:681–710, 1925.

94. Davis, L., Martin, J., Goldstein, S. L., and Ashkenazy, M.: A study of 211 patients with verified glioblastoma multiforme. J. Neurosurg., *6*:33–44, 1949.

95. Davis, L., Martin, J., Padberg, F., and Anderson, R. K.: A study of 182 patients with verified astrocytoma, astroblastoma and oligodendroglioma of the brain. J. Neurosurg., *7*:299–312, 1950.

96. Davis, R. L.: Astrocytomas. *In* Minckler, J., ed.: Pathology of Diseases of the Nervous System.

New York, McGraw-Hill Book Co., 1971, pp. 2007–2026.

97. Davis, R. L., and Fox, G. E.: Acinar choroid plexus adenoma: Case report. J. Neurosurg., *33*:587–590, 1970.

98. Day, E. D., and Bigner, D. D.: Specificity, cross-reactivity, and affinity of ^{125}I-labeled antiglioma antibodies for monolayers of cultured glioma cells. Cancer Res., *33*:2362–2372, 1973.

99. Decker, K.: Klinische Neuroradiologie. Stuttgart, G. Thieme, 1960, pp. 226–246.

100. Derby, B. M., and Guiang, R. L.: Spectrum of symptomatic brain-stem metastases. J. Neurol. Neurosurg. Psychiat., *38*:888–895, 1975.

101. DeWeerdt, C. J., and Schut, T.: Some aspects of heredity of brain tumours. Psychiat. Neurol. Neurochir. (Amst.), *75*:293–298, 1972.

102. Dexter, D., and Howell, D. A.: Medulloblastomas and arachnoidal sarcomas. Brain, *88*:367–374, 1965.

103. DiChiro, G.: Relative value of air studies, angiography and radioisotope scanning in the diagnosis of glial intracranial tumors. Progr. Neurol. Surg., *2*:292–317, 1968.

104. Diezel, P.: gliom nach Trauma. Frankf. Z. Path., *60*:316–326, 1949.

105. Dodge, H. W., Sayre, G. P., and Svien, H. J.: Sugar content of the cerebrospinal fluid in diffuse neoplastic involvement of the meninges. Mayo Clin. Proc., *27*:259–266, 1952.

106. Dodge, H. E., Love, J. G., Craig, W. M., Dockerty, M. B., Kearns, T. P., Holman, C. B., and Hayles, A. B.: Gliomas of the optic nerves. Arch. Neurol. Psychiat., *79*:607–621, 1958.

107. Dohrmann, G. J., and Dunsmore, R. H.: Glioblastoma multiforme of the cerebellum. Surg. Neurol., *3*:219–223, 1975.

108. Dohrmann, G. J., Farwell, J. R., and Flannery, J. I.: Ependymomas and ependymoblastomas in children. J. Neurosurg., *45*:273–283, 1976.

109. Drucker, G. A.: Papillary tumor of the choroid plexus in a newborn infant. Arch. Path. (Chicago), *28*:390–395, 1939.

110. Eade, O. E., and Urich, H.: Metastasising gliomas in young subjects. J. Path., *103*:245–256, 1971.

111. Earle, K. M., Rentschler, E. H., and Snodgrass, S. R.: Primary intracranial neoplasms: Prognosis and classification of 513 verified cases. J. Neuropath. Exp. Neurol., *16*:321–331, 1957.

112. Earnest, F., Kernohan, J. W., and Craig, W. M.: Oligodendrogliomas: A review of two hundred cases. Arch. Neurol. Psychiat., *63*:964–976, 1950.

113. Elvidge, A. R.: Long-term survival in the astrocytoma series. J. Neurosurg., *28*:399–404, 1968.

114. Elvidge, A. R., and Barone, B. M.: Long-term postoperative survival in two cases of glioblastoma multiforme. J. Neurosurg., *22*:382–386, 1965.

115. Elvidge, A. R., and Martinez-Coll, A.: Long-term follow-up of 106 cases of astrocytoma, 1928–1939, J. Neurosurg., *13*:318–331, 1956.

116. Elvidge, A., Penfield, W., and Cone, W.: The gliomas of the central nervous system: A study of two hundred and ten verified cases. Asso. Res. Nerv. Ment. Dis. Proc., *16*:107–181, 1937.

117. Ernsting, J.: Choroid plexus papilloma causing spontaneous subarachnoid haemorrhage. J. Neurol. Neurosurg. Psychiat., *18*:134–136, 1955.

118. Evans, R. A., Schwartz, J. F., and Chutorian, A. M.: Radiologic diagnosis in pediatric ophthalmology. Radiol. Clin. N. Amer., *1*:459–495, 1963.

119. Fan, K.-J., Kovi, J., and Earle, K. M.: The ethnic distribution of primary central nervous system tumors: AFIP, 1958 to 1970. J. Neuropath. Exp. Neurol., *36*:41–49, 1977.

120. Feigin, D. S., Welch, D. M., Siegel, B. A., and James, E. A.: The efficacy of the brain scan in diagnosis of brainstem gliomas. Radiology, *116*:117–120, 1975.

121. Feigin, I., Allen, L. B., Lipkin, L., and Gross, S. W.: The endothelial hyperplasia of the cerebral blood vessels with brain tumors, and its sarcomatous transformation. Cancer, *11*:264–277, 1958.

122. Fewer, D., Wilson, C. B., Boldrey, E. B., Enot, K. J., and Malcolm, R. P.: The chemotherapy of brain tumors: Clinical experience with carmustine (BCNU) and vincristine. JAMA, *222*:549–552, 1972.

123. Finkemeyer, H., and Behrend, R. C.: Hirntrauma und Gliomentstehung. Zbl. Neurochir., *16*:318–324, 1956.

124. Finkemeyer, H., Krämer, W., Pfingst, E., and Tzonos, T.: Malignität und Rezidiv bei den hirneigenen Tumoren. Zbl. Neurochir., *25*:281–299, 1965.

125. Finkemeyer, H., Pfingst, E., and Zülch, K. J.: The astrocytomas of the cerebral hemispheres. *In* Vinken, P. J., and Bruyn, G. W., eds.: Handbook of Clinical Neurology. Amsterdam, North-Holland Publishing Co. 1975, pp. 1–47.

126. Flipse, R. C., Vuksanovic, M., and Fonts, E. A.: Sequential brain scanning in radiation therapy of malignant tumors of the brain. Amer. J. Roentgen., *102*:93–96, 1968.

127. Fokes, E. C., and Earle, K. M.: Ependymomas: Clinical and pathological aspects. J. Neurosurg., *30*:585–594, 1969.

128. Foltz, E. L., Holyoke, J. B., and Heyl, H. L.: Brain necrosis following x-ray therapy, J. Neurosurg, *10*:423–429, 1953.

129. Fowler, G. W., and Williams, J. P.: Technetium brain scans in tuberous sclerosis. J. Nucl. Med., *14*:215–218, 1973.

130. Frankel, S. A., and German, W. J.: Glioblastoma multiforme: Review of 219 cases with regard to natural history, pathology, diagnostic methods, and treatment. J. Neurosurg., *15*:489–503, 1958.

131. Frazier, C. H., and Alpers, B. J.: Effect of irradiation on the gliomas. Ass. Rev. Nerv. Ment. Dis. Proc., *16*:68–106, 1937.

132. French, J. D., and Bucy, P. C.: Tumors of the septum pellucidum. J. Neurosurg., *5*:433–449, 1948.

133. French, L. A., and Galicich, J. H.: The use of steroids for control of cerebral edema. Clin. Neurosurg., *10*:212–223, 1964.

134. Fu, Y. S., Chen, A. T. L., Kay, S., and Young, H. F.: Is subependymoma (subependymal glomerate astrocytoma) an astrocytoma or ependymoma? Cancer, *34*:1992–2008, 1974.

135. Fulghum, J. S., Adcock, D. F., Guinto, F. C.,

Krigman, M. R., and Radcliffe, W. B.: Radionuclide imaging and tumor vascularity in supratentorial gliomas. Invest. Radiol., *6*: 388–391, 1971.

136. Gall, M. V., Becker, H., and Hacker, H.: Computer tomography (CT scan) in the diagnosis of epilepsy. Nervenarzt, *48*:72–76, 1977.

137. Gehan, E. A., and Walker, M. D.: Prognostic factors for patients with brain tumors. Nat. Cancer Inst. Monogr., *46*:189–195, 1977.

138. Geissinger, J. D., and Bucy, P. C.: Astrocytomas of the cerebellum in children: Long-term study. Arch. Neurol. (Chicago), *24*:125–135, 1971.

139. Glasauer, F. E., and Yuan, R. H. P.: Intracranial tumors with extracranial metastases: Case report and review of the literature. J. Neurosurg., *20*:474–493, 1963.

140. Glaser, J. S., Hoyt, W. F., and Corbett, J.: Visual morbidity with chiasmal glioma. Arch. Ophthal. (Chicago), *85*:3–12, 1971.

141. Globus, J. H., and Kuhlenbeck, H.: The subependymal cell plate (matrix) and its relationship to brain tumors of the ependymal type. J. Neuropath. Exp. Neurol., *3*:1–35, 1944.

142. Goalwin, H. A.: One thousand optic canals. JAMA, *89*:1745–1748, 1927.

143. Godwin, J. T.: Subependymal glomerate astrocytoma: Report of two cases. J. Neurosurg., *16*:385–389, 1959.

144. Gol, A.: The relatively benign astrocytomas of the cerebrum: A clinical study of 194 verified cases. J. Neurosurg., *18*:501–506, 1961.

145. Gol, A., and McKissock, W.: the cerebellar astrocytomas: A report on 98 verified cases. J. Neurosurg., *16*:287–296, 1959.

146. Golden, G. S., Ghatak, N. R., Hirano, A., and French, J. H.: Malignant glioma of the brainstem: A clinicopathological analysis of 13 cases. J. Neurol. Neurosurg. Psychiat., *35*: 732–738, 1972.

147. Gonzales, D., and Elvidge, A. R.: On the occurrence of epilepsy caused by astrocytoma of the cerebral hemispheres. J. Neurosurg., *19*:470–482, 1962.

148. Good, R. A.: Harnessing the immunity system: From potential to reality. CA, *25*:178–186, 1975.

149. Goodhart, G. W.: Adenoma of the choroid plexus. Guy's Hosp. Rep., *69*:217–222, 1918.

150. Goodman, S. J., Rosenbaum, A. L., Hasso, A., and Itabashi, H.: Large optic nerve glioma with normal vision. Arch. Ophthal. (Chicago), *93*:991–995, 1975.

151. Götze, W., and Kubicki, S.: Zur Artdiagnose der Hirngeschwülste. Acta Neurochir. (Wien), *5*:512–528, 1957.

152. Grace, J. T., Perese, D. M., Metzgar, R. S., Sasabe, T., and Holdridge, B.: Tumor autograft responses in patients with glioblastoma multiforme. J. Neurosurg., *18*:159–167, 1961.

153. Grant, N.: Diffuse glioblastosis. *In* Vinken, P. J., and Bruyn, G. W., eds.: Handbook of Clinical Neurology. Amsterdam, North-Holland Publishing Co., 1975, Vol. 18. pp. 73–79.

154. Green, J. R., Waggener, J. D., and Kriegsfeld, B. A.: Classification and incidence of neoplasms of the central nervous system. Advances Neurol., *15*:51–55, 1976.

155. Greenberger, J. S., Cassady, J. R., and Levene, M. B.: Radiation therapy of thalamic, midbrain and brain stem gliomas. Radiology, *122*:463–468, 1977.

156. Greenfield, J. G., and Robertson, E. G.: Cystic oligodendrogliomas of the cerebral hemispheres and ventricular oligodendrogliomas. Brain, *56*:247–264, 1933.

157. Griffiths, T.: Observations on cranial radiography in a series of intracranial tumours. Brit. J. Radiol., *30*:57–69, 1957.

158. Grunert, V., Jellinger, K., Sunder-Plassmann, M., and Wöber, G.: Glioblastoma multiforme: a preliminary follow-up study. Mod. Aspects. Neurosurg., *3*:108–115, 1973.

159. Gudmundsson, K. R.: A survey of tumours of the central nervous system in Iceland during the 10-year period 1954–1963. Acta Neurol. Scand., *46*:538–552, 1970.

160. Guerard: Tumeur fongueuse dans le ventricule droit du cerveau chez une petite fille de 3 ans. Bull. Soc. Anat. Paris, *8*:211–214, 1833.

161. Gullotta, F., and Bettag, W.: Zur Frage der längeren Überlebenszeit bei glioblastomen. Acta Neurochir. (Wien), 16:122–128, 1967.

162. Gupta, S., Boop, W. C., and Flanigan, S.: Brain tumor or cerebrovascular accident? J. Arkansas Med. Soc., *69*:388–391, 1973.

163. Gyepes, M. T., and D'Angio, G. J.: Extracranial metastases from central nervous system tumors in children and adolescents. Radiology, *87*:55–63, 1966.

164. Haller, P., and Patzold, U.: Diagnostic value of epileptic seizures for location and morphology of brain tumors: Contribution to preferred localization of cerebral neoplasms. Z. Neurol., *203*:311–336, 1973.

165. Hamilton, A. M., Garner, A., Tripathi, R. C., and Sanders, M. D.: Malignant optic nerve glioma: Report of a case with electron microscope study. Brit. J. Ophthal., *57*:253–264, 1973.

166. Hamperl, H.: The nomenclature of tumours of the nervous system. Acta Neurochir. (Wien) suppl., *10*:5–23, 1964.

167. Handa, J., Handa, H., Torizuka, K., Hamamoto, K., and Kousaka, T.: Serial brain scanning with radioactive xenon and scintillation camera. Amer. J. Roentgen., *109*:701–706, 1970.

168. Hart, M. N., and Byer, J. A.: Rupture of middle cerebral artery branches by invasive astrocytoma. Neurology (Minneap.), *24*:1171–1174, 1974.

169. Hart, M. N., Petito, C. K., and Earle, K. M.: Mixed gliomas. Cancer, *33*:134–140, 1974.

170. Harvald, B. H., and Hauge, M.: On the heredity of glioblastoma. J. Nat. Cancer Inst., *17*:289–296, 1956.

171. Hausman, L., and Stevenson, L.: Astrocytoma of the cerebellum: Survival of forty-five years without operation. Arch. Neurol. Psychiat., *30*:1100–1110, 1933.

172. Haymaker, W., Rubinstein, L. J., and Miquel, J.: Brain tumors in irradiated monkeys. Acta Neuropath. (Berlin), *20*:267–277, 1972.

173. Hensell, V.: A special group of astrocytomas: The so-called "Bergstrand tumours." Mod. Aspects Neurosurg., *3*:137–138, 1973.

174. Herren, R. Y.: Papilloma of the choroid plexus. Arch. Surg. (Chicago), *42*:758–774, 1941.

175. Herz, D. A., Liebeskind, A., Rosenthal, A., and

Schechter, M. M.: Cerebral angiographic changes associated with tuberous sclerosis. Radiology, *115*:647–649, 1975.

176. Hirano, A., and Matsui, T.: Vascular structures in brain tumors. Hum. Path., *6*:611–621, 1975.

177. Hirose, G., Lombroso, C. T., and Eisenberg, H.: Thalamic tumors in childhood: Clinical, laboratory, and therapeutic considerations. Arch. Neurol. (Chicago), *32*:740–744, 1975.

178. Hitchcock, E., and Sato, F.: Treatment of malignant gliomata, J. Neurosurg., *21*:497–505, 1964.

179. Holman, B. L.: The brain scan. Postgrad. Med., *54*:143–149, 1973.

180. Hope-Stone, H. F.: Results of treatment of medulloblastomas. J. Neurosurg., *32*:83–88, 1970.

181. Horrax, G., and Wu, W. Q.: Postoperative survival of patients with intracranial oligodendroglioma with special reference to radical tumor removal: A study of 26 patients. J. Neurosurg., *8*:473–497, 1951.

182. Hortega, P. DelR.: Estudios sobre la neuroglia: La glia de escasas radiaciones (oligodendroglia). Bol. Real. Soc. Espan. Hist. Nat., *21*:63–92, 1921.

183. Horten, B. C., and Rubinstein, L. J.: Primary cerebral neuroblastoma: A clinicopathological study of 35 cases. Brain, *99*:735–756, 1976.

184. Hoshino, T., Wilson, C. B., and Ellis, W. G.: Gemistocytic astrocytes in gliomas: An autoradiographic study. J. Neuropath. Exp. Neurol., *34*:263–281, 1975.

185. Hoyt, W. F., and Baghdassarian, S. A.: Optic glioma of childhood: Natural history and rationale for conservative management. Brit. J. Ophthal., *53*:793–798, 1969.

186. Hoyt, W. F., Meshel, L. G., Lessell, S., Schatz, N. J., and Suckling, R. D.: Malignant optic glioma of adulthood. Brain, *96*:121–132, 1973.

187. Hulbanni, S., and Goodman, P. A.: Glioblastoma multiforme with extraneural metastases in the absence of previous surgery. Cancer, *37*:1577–1583, 1976.

188. Hunt, W. E.: Surgical treatment of adult brain tumors. Progr. Exp. Tumor Res., *17*:400–407, 1972.

189. Hurley, P. J.: Effect of craniotomy on the brain scan related to time elapsed after surgery. J. Nucl. Med., *13*:156–158, 1972.

190. Hyman, R. A., Loring, M. F., Liebeskind, A. L., Naidich, J. B., and Stein, H. L.: Computed tomographic evaluation of therapeutically induced changes in primary and secondary brain tumors. Neuroradiology, *14*:213–218, 1978.

191. Jachuck, S. J., Ramani, P. S., Clark, F., and Kalbag, R. M.: Electrocardiographic abnormalities associated with raised intracranial pressure. Brit. Med. J., *1*:242–244, 1975.

192. James, T. G. I., and Pagel, W.: Oligodendroglioma with extracranial metastases. Brit. J. Surg., *39*:56–65, 1951.

193. Jelsma, R., and Bucy, P. C.: The treatment of glioblastoma multiforme of the brain. J. Neurosurg., *27*:388–400, 1967.

194. Jennett, W. B., McDowall, D. G., and Barker, J.: The effect of halothane on intracranial pressure in cerebral tumors: Report of two cases, J. Neurosurg., *26*:270–274, 1967.

195. Jennett, W. B., Barker, J., Fitch, W., and McDowall, D. G.: Effect of anaesthesia on intracranial pressure in patients with space-occupying lesions. Lancet, *1*:61–64, 1969.

196. Jones, A.: Radiotherapy of gliomata: Clinical and biological factors. Proc. Roy. Soc. Med., *56*:673–680, 1963.

197. Kadin, M. E., Rubinstein, L. J., and Nelson, J. S.: Neonatal cerebellar medulloblastoma originating from the fetal external granular layer. J. Neuropath. Exp. Neurol., *29*:583–600, 1970.

198. Kahn, E. A., and Luros, J. T.: Hydrocephalus from overproduction of cerebrospinal fluid (and experiences with other papillomas of the choroid plexus). J. Neurosurg., *9*:59–67, 1952.

199. Kalyanaraman, K., Smith, B. H., and Alker, G. J.: Intracranial tumors of apoplectiform onset. New York J. Med., *73*:2133–2139, 1973.

200. Kamata, K., Harano, H., Hori, S., Shinohara, T., Toyama, K., Nakayama, K., Nemoto, H., Nakamichi, G., Iwasaki, N., and Sakamoto, S.: Doughnut sign in brain scanning. Neurol. Surg. (Tokyo), *2*:757–762, 1974.

201. Kane, W., and Aronson, S. M.: Gangliogliomatous maturation in cerebellar medulloblastoma. Acta Neuropath. (Berlin), *9*:273–279, 1967.

202. Kaplan, W. D., McComb, J. G. Strand, R. D., and Treves, S. Suppression of ^{99m}Tc-Pertechnetate uptake in a choroid plexus papilloma. Radiology, *109*:395–396, 1973.

203. Kapp, J. P., Paulson, G. W., and Odom, G. L.: Brain tumors with tuberous sclerosis. J. Neurosurg., *26*:191–202, 1967.

204. Kawano, N., Yada, K., Ogawa, Y., and Sasaki, K. Spontaneous transdural extension of malignant astrocytoma: Case report. J. Neurosurg., *47*:766–770, 1977.

205. Kernohan, J. W.: Ependymomas. *In* Minckler, J., ed.: Pathology of the Nervous System. New York, McGraw-Hill Book Co., 1971, pp. 1976–1993.

206. Kernohan, J. W.: Oligodendrogliomas. *In* Minckler, J., ed.: Pathology of the Nervous System. New York, McGraw-Hill Book Co., 1971, pp. 1993–2007.

207. Kernohan, J. W., and Sayre, G. P.: Tumors of the Central Nervous System. Atlas of Tumor Pathology. Fascicle 35. Washington, D.C., Armed Forces Institute of Pathology, 1952.

208. Kernohan, J. W., Mabon, R. F., Svien, H. J., and Adson, A. W.: A simplified classification of the gliomas. Mayo Clin. Proc., *24*:71–75, 1949.

209. Kersting, G.: Tissue culture of human gliomas. Progr. Neurol. Surg., *2*:165–202, 1968.

210. Kersting, G.: Tissue culture of recurrent gliomas. Mod. Aspects Neurosurg., *3*:122–124, 1973.

211. King, G. A., and Sagerman, R. H.: Late recurrence in medulloblastoma. Amer. J. Roentgen., *123*:7–12, 1975.

212. Kingsley, D., and Kendall, B. E.: Dependent layering of contrast medium in cystic astrocytomas. Neuroradiology, *14*:107–110, 1977.

213. Koestner, A., Swenberg, J. A., and Wechsler, W.: Experimental tumors of the nervous system induced by resorptive N-nitrosourea compounds. Progr. Exp. Tumor Res., *17*:9–30, 1972.

214. Komminoth, R., Woringer, E., Baumgartner, J., Braun, J. P., and LeMaistre, D.: Papillome intraventriculaire familial. Neurochirurgie, *11*:267–272, 1965.

215. Koo, A. H., Fewer, D., Wilson, C. B., and Newton, T. H.: Lack of correlation between clinical and angiographic findings in patients with brain tumors under BCNU chemotherapy. J. Neurosurg., *37*:9–14, 1972.

216. Koos, W. T., and Miller, M. H.: Intracranial Tumors of Infants and Children. Stuttgart, Georg Thieme Verlag, 1971.

217. Kornblith, P. L., Dohan, F. C., Wood, W. C., and Whitman, B. O.: Human astrocytoma: Serum-mediated immunologic response. Cancer, *33*:1512–1519, 1974.

218. Korsgaard, O., Lindholm, J., and Rasmussen, P.: Endocrine function in patients with suprasellar and hypothalamic tumours. Acta Endoc. (Kobenhavn), *83*:1–8, 1976.

219. Kramer, S.: The hazards of therapeutic irradiation of the central nervous system. Clin. Neurosurg., *15*:301–318, 1967.

220. Kramer, S.: Radiation therapy in the management of brain tumors in children. Ann. N.Y. Acad. Sci., *159*:571–584, 1969.

221. Krayenbuhl, H. A., and Yasargil, M. G.: Cerebral Angiography. Philadelphia, J. B. Lippincott Co., 1968.

222. Kretzschmar, K., Aulich, A., Schindler, E., Lange, S., Grumme, T., and Meese, W.: The diagnostic value of CT for radiotherapy of cerebral tumors. Neuroradiology, *14*:245–250, 1978.

223. Kricheff, I. I., Becker, M., Schneck, S. A., and Taveras, J. M.: Intracranial ependymomas: A study of survival in 65 cases treated by surgery and irradiation. Amer. J. Roentgen., *91*:167–175, 1964.

224. Kullberg, G., and West, K. A.: Influence of corticosteroids on the ventricular fluid pressure. Acta Neurol. Scand., *41*: suppl. 13:445–452, 1965.

225. Kung, P. C., Lee, J. C., and Bakay, L.: Vascular invasion by glioma cells in man: An electron microscopic study. J. Neurosurg., *31*:339–345, 1969.

226. Kurland, L. T.: The frequency of intracranial and intraspinal neoplasms in the resident population of Rochester, Minnesota. J. Neurosurg, *15*:627–641, 1958.

227. Lake, P., Friedenberg, M. J., and McCammon, C. J.: Diagnosis of basal meningeal gliomatosis by brain scan: Significance of basal cistern sign. J. Neurosurg., *37*:100–102, 1972.

228. Lampert, P. W., and Davis, R. L.: Delayed effects of radiation on the human central nervous system: "Early" and "late" delayed reactions. Neurology (Minneap.), *14*:912–917, 1964.

229. Lassiter, K. R. L., Alexander, E., Davis, C. H., Jr., and Kelly, D. L.: Surgical treatment of brain stem gliomas. J. Neurosurg., *34*:719–725, 1971.

230. Launay, M., Fredy, D., Merland, J. J., and Bories, J.: Narrowing and occlusion of arteries by intracranial tumors. Neuroradiology, *14*:117–126, 1977.

231. Law, J. D., Lehman, R. A. W., Kirsch, W. M.,

and Ehni, G.: Diagnosis and treatment of abscess of the central ganglia. J. Neurosurg., *44*:226–232, 1976.

232. Lee, F.: Radiation of infratentorial and supratentorial brain-stem tumors. J. Neurosurg., *43*: 65–68, 1975.

233. Leibel, S. A., Sheline, G. E., Wara, W. M., Boldrey, E. B., and Nielson, S. L.: The role of radiation therapy in the treatment of astrocytomas. Cancer, *35*:1551–1557, 1975.

234. Leonard, J. R., Witherspoon, L. R., Mahaley, M. S., and Goodrich, J. K.: Value of sequential postoperative brain scans in patients with anaplastic gliomas. J. Neurosurg., *42*:551–556, 1975.

235. Levin, B. E.: The clinical significance of spontaneous pulsations of the retinal vein. Arch. Neurol. (Chicago), *35*:37–40, 1978.

236. Levin, V. A, Crafts, D. C., Norman, D. M., Hoffer, P. B., Spire, J.-P., and Wilson, C. B.: Criteria for evaluating patients undergoing chemotherapy for malignant brain tumors. J. Neurosurg., *47*:329–335, 1977.

237. Levin, V. A., Freeman-Dove, M., and Landahl, H. D.: Permeability characteristics of brain adjacent to tumors in rats. Arch. Neurol. (Chicago), *32*:785–791, 1975.

238. Leviton, A., Fulchiero, A., Gilles, F. H., and Winston, K.: Survival status of children with cerebellar gliomas. J. Neurosurg., *48*:29–33, 1978.

239. Levy, L. F., and Auchterlonie, W. C.: Primary cerebral neoplasia in Rhodesia. Int. Surg., *60*:286–292, 1975.

240. Levy, L. F., and Elvidge, A. R.: Astrocytoma of brain and spinal cord: Review of 176 cases, 1940–1949. J. Neurosurg., *13*:413–443, 1956.

241. Lewis, P.: Carcinoma of the choroid plexus. Brain, *90*:177–186, 1967.

242. Lieberman, A., Lebrun, Y., Glass, P., Goodgold, A., Lux, W., Wise, A., and Ransohoff, J.: Use of high dose corticosteroids in patients with inoperable brain tumours. J. Neurol. Neurosurg. Psychiat., *40*:678–682, 1977.

243. Lindgren, M.: On tolerance of brain tissue and sensitivity of brain tumours to irradiation. Acta Radiol. (Stockholm), suppl. 170:1–73, 1958.

244. Lins, E.: Medulloblastoma in the adult (das Medulloblastom des Erwachsenen). Acta Neurochir. (Wien), *31*:67–72, 1974.

245. Liske, R.: A comparative study of the action of cyclophosphamide and procarbazine on the antibody production in mice. Clin. Exp. Immun., *15*:271–280, 1973.

246. Little, J. B.: Cellular effects of ionizing radiation. New Eng. J. Med., *278*:308–315, 1968.

247. Lorenz, R.: Zur Frage der Rezidivoperationen bei Gliomen. Zbl. Neurochir., *28*:27–34, 1967.

248. Low, N. L., Correll, J. W., and Hammill, J. F.: Tumors of the cerebral hemispheres in children. Arch. Neurol. (Chicago), *13*:547–554, 1965.

249. Löwenberg, K., and Waggoner, R. W.: Gross pathology of the oligodendrogliomas. Arch,. Neurol. Psychiat., *42*:842–861, 1939.

250. Lumsden, C. E., and Pomerat, C. M.: Normal oligodendrocytes in tissue culture: A preliminary report on the pulsatile glial cells in tissue cultures from the corpus callosum of the nor-

mal adult rat brain. Exp. Cell Res., *2*:103–114, 1951.

251. Lund, M.: Epilepsy in association with intracranial tumor. Acta Psychiat. Scand., suppl. 81: 1–149, 1952.

252. Luse, S. A.: Electron microscopic studies of brain tumors. Neurology (Minneap.), *10*:881–905, 1960.

253. Luse, S. A.: Electron microscopy of brain tumors. *In* Fields, W. S., and Sharkey, P. C., eds.: The Biology and Treatment of Intracranial Tumors. Springfield, Ill., Charles C Thomas, 1962, pp. 75–103.

254. Lynn, J. A., Panopio, I. T., Martin, J. H., Shaw, M. L., and Rice, G. J.: Ultrastructural evidence for astroglial histogenesis of the monstrocellular astrocytoma (so-called monstrocellular sarcoma of brain). Cancer, *22*: 356–366, 1968.

255. Maass, L.: Occipital ependymoma with extracranial metastases. J. Neurosurg., *11*:413–421, 1954.

256. Mabon, R. F., Svien, H. J., Kernohan, J. W., and Craig, W. M.: Ependymomas. Mayo Clin. Proc., *24*:65–70, 1949.

257. MacCabe, J. J.: Glioblastoma. *In* Vinken, P. J., and Bruyn, G. W., eds.: Handbook of Clinical Neurology. Vol. 18. Amsterdam, North-Holland Publishing Co. 1975, pp. 49–71.

258. MacCarty, C. S.: Results of the surgical management of glial tumors of the brain. *In* Fields, W. S., and Sharkey, P. C., eds.: The Biology and Treatment of Intracranial Tumors. Springfield, Ill., Charles C Thomas, 1962, pp. 434–456.

259. MacCarty, C. S., Boyd, A. S., and Childs, D. S.: Tumors of the optic nerve and optic chiasm. J. Neurosurg., *33*:439–444, 1970.

260. Makeever, L. C., and King, J. D.: Medulloblastoma with extracranial metastasis through a ventriculovenous shunt: Report of a case and review of the literature. Amer. J. Clin. Path., *46*:245–249, 1966.

261. Malamud, N.: Psychiatric disorder with intracranial tumors of limbic system. Arch. Neurol. (Chicago), *17*:113–123, 1967.

262. Manganiello, L. O. J.: Massive spontaneous hemorrhage in gliomas (a report of seven verified cases). J. Nerv. Ment. Dis., *110*:277–298, 1949.

263. Mansuy, L., Thierry, A., and Tommasi, M.: Oligodendroglioma. *In* Vinken, P. J., and Bruyn, G. W., eds.: Handbook of Clinical Neurology. Vol. 18. Amsterdam, North-Holland Publishing Co., 1975, pp. 81–103.

264. Mansuy, L., Allègre, G., Courjon, J., and Thierry, A.: Analyse d'une série opératoire de 49 oligodendrogliomes: Avec 3 localizations infra-tentorielles. Neurochirurgie, *13*:679–700, 1967.

265. Manuelidis, E. E.: Glioma in trauma. *In* Minckler, J.: Pathology of the Nervous System. New York, McGraw-Hill Book Co., 1971, pp. 2237–2240.

266. Marsa, G. W., Probert, J. C., Rubinstein, L. J., and Bagshaw, M. A.: Radiation therapy in the treatment of childhood astrocytic gliomas. Cancer, *32*:646–655, 1973.

267. Marshall, L. F., Jennett, B., and Langfitt, T. W.: Needle biopsy for the diagnosis of malignant glioma. JAMA, *228*:1417–1418, 1974.

268. Martin, F., and Lemmen, L. J.: Calcification in intracranial neoplasms. Amer. J. Path., *28*:1107–1131, 1952.

269. Martins, A. N., Johnston, J. S., Henry, J. M., Stoffel, T. J., and DiChiro, G.: Delayed radiation necrosis of the brain. J. Neurosurg., *47*:336–345, 1977.

270. Marton, L. J., Heby, O., and Wilson, C. B.: Increased polyamine concentrations in the cerebrospinal fluid of patients with brain tumors. Int. J. Cancer, *14*:731–735, 1974.

271. Maspes, P. E., and Paoletti, P.: Recent advances in chemical composition and metabolism of brain tumors. Progr. Neurol. Surg., *2*:203–266, 1968.

272. Matakas, F., and Cervós-Navarro, J.: The ultrastructure of medulloblastomas. Acta Neuropath. (Berlin), *16*:271–284, 1970.

273. Matson, D. D.: Hydrocephalus in premature infant caused by papilloma of the choroid plexus: With report of surgical treatment. J. Neurosurg., *10*:416–420, 1953.

274. Matson, D. D., and Crofton, F. D. L.: Papilloma of the choroid plexus in childhood. J. Neurosurg., *17*:1002–1027, 1960.

275. Matsushima, M., Yamamoto, T., Motomochi, M., and Ando, K.: Papilloma and venous angioma of the choroid plexus causing primary intraventricular hemorrhage: Report of two cases. J. Neurosurg., *39*:666–670, 1973.

276. Mattson, R. H., and Peterson, E. W.: Glioblastoma multiforme of the optic nerve: Report of a case. JAMA, *196*:119–120, 1966.

277. Mavligit, G. M., Gutterman, J. U., and Hersh, E. M.: Primary brain tumors: Tumor immunity and immunocompetence. Surg. Neurol., *1*: 261–263, 1973.

278. McCormick, W. F., and Ugajin, K.: Fatal hemorrhage into a medulloblastoma. J. Neurosurg., *26*:78–81, 1967.

279. McDonald, J. V.: Persistent hydrocephalus following the removal of papillomas of the choroid plexus of the lateral ventricles. J. Neurosurg., *30*:736–640, 1969.

280. McKissock, W., and Paine, K. W. E.: Primary tumours of the thalamus. Brain, *81*:41–63, 1958.

281. McLaurin, R. L., and Ford, L. E.: Obstruction following posterior fossa surgery: The postoperative Dandy-Walker syndrome. Johns Hopkins Med. J., *122*:309–318, 1968.

282. Mealey, J., and Hall, P. V.: Medulloblastoma in children: Survival and treatment. J. Neurosurg., *46*:56–64, 1977.

283. Mealey, J., Chen, T. T., and Schanz, G. P.: Effects of dexamethasone and methylprednisolone on cell cultures of human glioblastomas. J. Neurosurg., *34*:324–334, 1971.

284. Milhorat, T. H.: Pontine glioma. JAMA, *232*: 595–596, 1975.

285. Milhorat, T. H., Hammock, M. K., Davis, D. A., and Fenstermacker, J. D.: Choroid plexus papilloma: I. Proof of cerebrospinal fluid overproduction. Child's Brain, *2*:273–289, 1976.

286. Miller, J. D., Sakalas, R., Ward, J. D., Young, H. F., Adams, W. E., Vries, J. K., and Becker, D. B.: Methylprednisolone treatment in patients with brain tumors. Neurosurgery, *1*:114–117, 1977.

287. Miller, N. R., Iliff, W. J., and Green, W. R.:

Evaluation and management of gliomas of the anterior visual pathways. Brain, 97:743–754, 1974.

288. Misugi, K., and Liss, L.: Medulloblastoma with cross-striated muscle: A fine structural study. Cancer, 25:1279–1285, 1970.

289. Moersch, F. P., Craig, W. M., and Kernohan, J. W.: Tumors of the brain in aged persons. Arch. Neurol. Psychiat., 45:235–245, 1941.

290. Moertel, C. G., Dockerty, M. B., and Baggenstoss, A. H.: Multiple primary malignant neoplasms: III. Tumors of multicentric origin. Cancer, 14:238–248, 1961.

291. Monson, R. R., and Peters, J. M., and Johnson, M. N.: Proportional mortality among vinylchloride workers. Lancet, 2:397–398, 1974.

292. Moore, G. E., Peyton, W. T., French, L. A., and Walker, W. W.: The clinical use of fluorescein in neurosurgery. J. Neurosurg., 5:392–398, 1948.

293. Moore, M. T., and Stern, K.: Vascular lesions in the brain-stem and occipital lobe occurring in association with brain tumours. Brain, 61:70–98, 1938.

294. Moreno, J. B., and Deland, F. H.: Brain scanning in the diagnosis of astrocytomas of the brain. J. Nucl. Med., 12:107–111, 1971.

295. Moss, H. M.; Expanding lesions of the orbit: A clinical study of 230 consecutive cases. Amer. J. Ophthal., 54:761–770, 1962.

296. Mullan, S.: Surgery of brain tumors. In Vinken, P. J., and Bruyn, G. W., eds.: Handbook of Clinical Neurology. Vol. 18. Amsterdam, North-Holland Publishing Co., 1975, pp. 471–480.

297. Müller, W.: Über das Vorkommen von glioblastomen im kaudalen Hirnstamm. Acta Neurochir. (Wien), 28:65–80, 1973.

298. Müller, W., Afra, D., and Schroder, R.: Supratentorial recurrences of gliomas: Morphological studies in relation to time intervals with astrocytomas. Acta Neurochir. (Wein), 37:75–91, 1977.

299. Mundinger, F., and Metzel, E.: Interstitial radioisotope therapy of intractable diencephalic tumors by the stereotaxic permanent implantation of iridium^{192}, including bioptic control. Confin. Neurol., 32:195–202, 1970.

300. Nager, G. T.: Gliomas involving the temporal bone: Clinical and pathological aspects. Laryngoscope, 77:454–488, 1967.

301. Nasser, S. I., and Mont, L. A.: Papillomas of the choroid plexus. J. Neurosurg., 29:73–77, 1968.

302. Neblett, C. R., Waltz, T. A., and Anderson, D. E.: Neurological involvement in the nevoid basal cell carcinoma syndrome. J. Neurosurg., 35:577–584, 1971.

303. Nicholson, W. J., Hammond, E. C., Seidman, H., and Selikoff, I. J.: Mortality experience of a cohort of vinyl chloride-polyvinyl chloride workers. Ann. N.Y. Acad. Sci., 296:225–230, 1975.

304. Norman, D., Enzmann, D. R., Levin, V. A., Wilson, C. B., and Newton, T. H.: Computed tomography in the evaluation of malignant glioma before and after therapy. Radiology, 121:85–88, 1976.

305. Norwood, C. W., Kelly, D. L., Davis, C. H., and Alexander, E.: Irradiation-induced meso-

dermal tumors of the central nervous system: Report of two meningiomas following x-ray treatment for gliomas. Surg. Neurol., 2:161–164, 1974.

306. Obrador, S., and Blazquez, M. G.: Benign cystic tumours of the cerebellum. Acta Neurochir. (Wien), 32:55–68, 1975.

307. Olivecrona, H.: The surgical treatment of intracranial tumors. In Olivecrona, H., and Tönnis, W.: Handbuch der Neurochirurgie. Vol. 4. New York, Springer-Verlag, 1967.

308. Onoyama, Y., Abe, M., Sakamoto, T., Nishidai, T., and Suyama, S.: Radiation therapy in treatment of glioblastoma. Amer. J. Roentgen., 126:481–492, 1976.

309. Oppenheimer, D. R.: The effect of irradiation on a medulloblastoma. J. Neurol. Neurosurg. Psychiat., 32:94–98, 1969.

310. Oxenhandler, D. C., and Sayers, M. P.: The dilemma of childhood optic gliomas. J. Neurosurg., 48:35–41, 1978.

311. Paillas, J. E., and Combalbert, A.: Évolution comparée des gliomes du cerveau. A propos d'une statistique opératoire de 333 cas observés avec les mêmes méthodes durant une même décennie. Rev. Neurol. (Paris), 111:43–60, 1964.

312. Palacios, E., and Lawson, R. C.: Choroid plexus papillomas of the lateral ventricles. Amer. J. Roentgen., 115:113–119, 1972.

313. Parker, J. C., Mortara, R. H., and McCloskey, J. J.: Biological behavior of the primitive neuroectodermal tumors: Significant supratentorial childhood gliomas. Surg. Neurol., 4:383–388, 1975.

314. Parkinson, D., and Hall, C. W.: Oligodendrogliomas: Simultaneous appearance in frontal lobes of siblings. J. Neurosurg., 19:424–426, 1962.

315. Pay, N. T., Carella, R. J., Lin, J. P., and Kricheff, I. I.: The usefulness of computed tomography during and after radiation therapy in patients with brain tumors. Radiology, 121:79–83, 1976.

316. Pendergrass, H. P., McKusick, K. A., New, P. F. J., and Potsaid, M. S.: Relative efficacy of radionuclide imaging and computed tomography of the brain. Radiology, 116:363–365, 1975.

317. Penfield, W., and Cone, W.: Acute swelling of oligodendroglioma: A specific type of neuroglia change. Arch. Neurol. Psychiat., 16:131–153, 1926.

318. Penfield, W., and Feindel, W.: Medulloblastoma of the cerebellum with survival for seventeen years. Arch. Neurol. Psychiat., 57:481–484, 1947.

319. Penfield, W., Erickson, T. C., and Tarlov, I.: Relation of intracranial tumors and symptomatic epilepsy. Arch. Neurol. Psychiat., 44:300–315, 1940.

320. Perthes: Glückliche Entfernung eines Tumors des Plexus chorioides aus dem Seitenventrikel des Cerebrum. München Med. Wschr., 66:677–678, 1919.

321. Phillips, T. L., Sheline, G. E., and Boldrey, E.: Therapeutic considerations in tumors affecting the central nervous system: Ependymomas. Radiology, 83:98–105, 1964.

322. Pierluca, P.: Ependymomas of the posterior

fossa. Neurochirurgie, *23*:suppl. 1:111–147, 1977.

323. Poisson, M., Philippon, J., van Effenterre, R., Racadot, J., and Sichez, J. P.: Cerebral pseudocysts following chemotherapy of glioblastomas. Acta Neurochir. (Wien), *39*:143–149, 1977.

324. Polak, M.: On the true nature of the so-called medulloblastoma. Acta Neuropath. (Berlin), *8*: 84–95, 1967.

325. Polmeteer, F. E., and Kernohan, J. W.: Meningeal gliomatosis: A study of forty-two cases. Arch. Neurol. Psychiat., *57*:593–616, 1947.

326. Pool, J. L.: Gliomas in the region of the brain stem. J. Neurosurg., *29*:164–167, 1968.

327. Pool, J. L., and Kamrin, R. P.: The treatment of intracranial gliomas by surgery and radiation. Progr. Neurol. Surg., *1*:258–299, 1966.

328. Pool, J. L., Ransohoff, J., and Correll, J. W.: The treatment of malignant brain tumors, primary and metastatic. New York J. Med., *57*:3983–3988, 1957.

329. Posey, L. C.: Papilloma of the choroid plexus: Report of a case and summary of recorded cases. Arch. Path. (Chicago), *34*:911–916, 1942.

330. Posner, J. S., and Shapiro, W. R.: Brain tumor: Current status of treatment and its complications. Arch. Neurol. (Chicago), *32*:781–784, 1975.

331. Prather, J. L., Long, J. M., van Heertum, R., and Hardman, J.: Multicentric and isolated multifocal glioblastoma multiforme simulating metastatic disease. Brit. J. Radiol., *48*:10–15, 1975.

332. Queiroz, L. S., Cruz-Neto, J. N., and Faria, J. L.: Glioblastoma multiforme of the medulla oblongata: A case report. Acta Neuropath. (Berlin), *29*:355–360, 1974.

333. Quest, D. D., Brisman, R., Antunes, J. L., and Housepian, E. M.: Period of risk for recurrence in medulloblastoma. J. Neurosurg., *48*:159–163, 1978.

334. Quinn, J. L.: Serial brain scans in glioblastoma multiforme. Radiology, *101*:367–370, 1971.

335. Raaf, J., and Kernohan, J. W.: Relation of abnormal collections of cells in posterior medullary velum of cerebellum to origin of medulloblastoma. Arch. Neurol. Psychiat., *52*:163–169, 1944.

336. Raimondi, A. J.: Ultrastructure and the biology of human brain tumors. Progr. Neurol. Surg., *1*:1–63, 1966.

337. Ramamurthi, B.: Intracranial tumors in India: Incidence and variations. Int. Surg., *58*:542–547, 1973.

338. Ramsey, R. G., and Brand, W. N.: Radiotherapy of glioblastoma multiforme. J. Neurosurg., *39*:197–202, 1973.

339. Rappaport, Z. H., and Epstein, F.: Computerized axial tomography in the preoperative evaluation of posterior fossa tumors in children. Child's Brain, *4*:170–179, 1978.

340. Raskind, R., and Weiss, S. R.: Conditions simulating metastatic lesions of the brain: Report of eight cases. Int. Surg., *53*:40–43, 1970.

341. Rasmussen, T.: Surgery of epilepsy associated with brain tumors. Advances Neurol., *8*:227–239, 1975.

342. Ray, B. S., and Peck, F. C.: Papilloma of the choroid plexus of the lateral ventricles causing hydrocephalus in an infant. J. Neurosurg., *13*:405–410, 1956.

343. Redondo, A., Daumas-Duport, C., Vedrenne, C., Chodkiewicz, J. P., and Constans, J. P.: Tumeurs intra-craniennes chez les malades mentaux. Neurochirurgia (Stuttgart), *6*:217–221, 1972.

344. Renaudin, J., Fewer, D., Wilson, C. B., Boldrey, E. B., Calogero, J., and Enot, K. J.: Dose dependency of Decadron in patients with partially excised brain tumors. J. Neurosurg., *39*:302–305, 1973.

345. Reymond, A., and Ringertz, N.: L'oligodendrogliome: Étude anatomo-clinique de 74 cas. Schweiz. Arch. Neurol. Psychiatr., *65*:221–254, 1950.

346. Rich, J. R.: A survey of cerebrospinal fluid cytology. Bull. Los Angeles Neurol. Soc., *34*:115–131, 1969.

347. Ringertz, N.: "Grading" of gliomas. Acta Path. Microbiol. Scand., *27*:51–64, 1950.

348. Ringertz, N., and Nordenstam, H.: Cerebellar astrocytoma. J. Neuropath. Exp. Neurol., *10*:343–367, 1951.

349. Ringertz, N., and Reymond, A.: Ependymomas and choroid plexus papillomas. J. Neuropath. Exp. Neurol., *8*:355–380, 1949.

350. Ringertz, N., and Tola, J. H.: Medulloblastoma. J. Neuropath. Exp. Neurol., *9*:354–372, 1950.

351. Roberson, C., and Till, K.: Hypothalamic gliomas in children. J. Neurol. Neurosurg. Psychiat., *37*:1047–1052, 1974.

352. Roberts, M., and German, W. J.: A long term study of patients with olidogendrogliomas. J. Neurosurg., *24*:697–700, 1966.

353. Robertson, F.: A microscopic demonstration of the normal and pathological histology of mesoglia cells. J. Ment. Sci., *46*:724, 1900.

354. Rockswold, G. L., and Seljeskog, E. L.: Spontaneous subarachnoid hemorrhage: Initial presentation of brain tumors. Minn. Med., *55*:805–806, 1972.

355. Ronquist, G., Ericsson, P., Frithz, G., and Hugosson, R.: Malignant brain tumours associated with adenylate kinase in cerebrospinal fluid. Lancet, *1*:1284–1286, 1977.

356. Rubinstein, L. J.: Extracranial metastases in cerebellar medulloblastoma. J. Path. Bact., *78*:187–195, 1959.

357. Rubinstein, L. J.: Discussion on polar spongioblastomas. Acta Neurochir. (Wien), Suppl. 10:126–140, 1964.

358. Rubinstein, L. J.: Morphological problems of brain tumors with mixed cell population. Acta Neurochir. (Wien), suppl. 10:141–165, 1964.

359. Rubinstein, L. J.: Development of extracranial metastases from a malignant astrocytoma in the absence of previous craniotomy: Case report. J. Neurosurg., *26*:542–547, 1967.

360. Rubinstein, L. J.: The definition of the ependymoblastoma. Arch. Path. (Chicago), *90*:35–45, 1970.

361. Rubinstein, L. J.: Cytogenesis and differentiation of primitive central neuroepithelial tumors. J. Neuropath. Exp. Neurol., *31*:7–26, 1972.

362. Rubinstein, L. J.: Tumors of the Nervous System. Bathesda, Md., AFIP. 1972.

363. Rubinstein, L. J.: The cerebellar medulloblastoma: Its origin, differentiation, morphological

variance, and biological behavior. *In* Vinken, P. J., and Bruyn, G. W., eds.: Handbook of Clinical Neurology. Vol. 18. Amsterdam, North-Holland Publishing Co., 1975, pp. 167–193.

364. Rubinstein, L. J.: Current concepts in neuro-oncology. Advances Neurol., *15*:1–25, 1976.

365. Rubinstein, L. J., and Herman, M. M.: A light and electron-microscopic study of temporal-lobe ganglioglioma. J. Neurol. Sci., *16*:27–48, 1972.

366. Rubinstein, L. J., and Logan, W. J.: Extraneural metastases in ependymoma of the cauda equina. J. Neurol. Neurosurg. Psychiat., *33*:763–770, 1970.

367. Rubinstein, L. J., and Northfield, D. W. C.: The medulloblastoma and the so-called "arachnoidal cerebellar sarcoma": A critical re-examination of a nosological problem. Brain, *87*:379–412, 1964.

368. Rucker, C. W.: The causes of paralysis of the third, fourth and sixth cranial nerves. Amer. J. Ophthal., *61*:1293–1298, 1966.

369. Russell, D. S.: Hydrocephalus. Asso. Res. Nerv. Ment. Dis. Proc., *34*:160–175, 1954.

370. Russell, D. S., and Rubinstein, L. J.: Pathology of Tumours of the Nervous System. 4th Ed. Baltimore, Williams & Wilkins Co., 1977.

371. Sagerman, R. H., Bagshaw, M. A., and Hanbery, J.: Considerations in the treatment of ependymoma. Radiology, *84*:401–408, 1965.

372. Salazar, O. M., Rubin, P., McDonald, J. V., and Feldstein, M. L.: Patterns of failure in intracranial astrocytomas after irradiation: Analysis of dose and field factors. Amer. J. Roentgen., *126*:279–292, 1976.

373. Sandberg-Wollheim, M.: Immunoglobulin synthesis in vitro by cerebrospinal fluid cells in patients with multiple sclerosis. Scand. J. Immun., *3*:717–730, 1974.

374. Sayre, G. P.: The system of grading of gliomas. Acta Neurochir. (Wien), Suppl. 10:98–116, 1964.

375. Schain, R. J., and Wilson, G.: Brain stem encephalitis with radiographic evidence of medullary enlargement. Neurology (Minneap.), *21*:537–539, 1971.

376. Schaper, A.: Die frühesten Differenzirungsvorgänge im Centralnervensystem. Wilhelm Roux Arch. Enlwicklungsmechanik Organismen, *5*:81–132, 1897.

377. Scheinker, I. M.: Subependymoma: A newly recognized tumor of subependymal derivation. J. Neurosurg., *2*:232–240, 1945.

378. Scherer, H. J.: Structural development in gliomas. Amer. J. Cancer, *34*:333–351, 1938.

379. Scherer, H. J.: Cerebral astrocytomas and their derivatives. Amer. J. Cancer, *40*:159–198, 1940.

380. Scherer, H. J.: The forms of growth and their practical significance. Brain, *63*:1–35, 1940.

381. Schoenberg, B. S., and Christine, B. W.: Neoplasms of the brain and cranial meninges: A study of incidence, epidemiological trends, and survival. Neurology (Minneap.), *20*:399, 1970.

382. Schoenberg, B. S., Glista, G. G., and Reagan, T. J.: The familial occurrence of glioma. Surg. Neurol., *3*:139–145, 1975.

383. Schulz, M. D., Wang, C.-C., Zinninger, G. F., and Tefft, G. F.: Radiotherapy of intracranial

neoplasms: With a special section on the radiotherapeutic management of central nervous system tumors in children. Progr. Neurol. Surg., *2*:318–379, 1968.

384. Schuster, G., and Westberg, G.: Gliomas of the optic nerve and chiasm. Acta Radiol. [Diagn.] (Stockholm), *6*:221–232, 1967.

385. Schuster, H., Jellinger, K., Gund, A., and Regele, H.: Extracranial metastases of anaplastic cerebral gliomas. Acta Neurochir. (Wien), *35*:247–259, 1976.

386. Scott, M.: Spontaneous intracerebral hematoma caused by cerebral neoplasms. J. Neurosurg., *42*:338–342, 1975.

387. Sheline, G. E., Boldrey, E., Karlsberg, P., and Phillips, T. L.: Therapeutic considerations in tumors affecting the central nervous system: Oligodendrogliomas. Radiology, *82*:84–89, 1964.

388. Shenkin, H. A., Grant, F. C., and Drew, J. H.: Postoperative period of survival of patients with oligodendroglioma of the brain: Report of twenty-five cases. Arch. Neurol. Psychiat., *58*:710–715, 1947.

389. Shetter, A. G., Bertuccini, T. V., and Pittman, H. W.: Closed needle biopsy in the diagnosis of intracranial mass lesions. Surg. Neurol., *8*:341–345, 1977.

390. Shuangshoti, S., and Panyathanya, R.: Ependymomas: A study of forty-five cases. Dis. Nerv. Syst., *34*:307–314, 1973.

391. Shuman, R. M., Alvord, E. C., and Leech, R. W.: The biology of childhood ependymomas. Arch. Neurol. (Chicago), *32*:731–739, 1975.

392. Silverberg, E.: Cancer statistics, 1977. CA, *27*:26–41, 1977.

393. Silverberg, G. D., and Hanbery, J. W.: Meningeal invasion by gliomas. J. Neurosurg., *34*:549–554, 1971.

394. Smith, A.: Speech and other functions after left (dominant) hemispherectomy. J. Neurol. Neurosurg. Psychiat., *29*:467–471, 1966.

395. Smith, D. R., Hardman, J. M., and Earle, K. M.: Metastasizing neuroectodermal tumors of the central nervous system. J. Neurosurg., *31*:50–58, 1969.

396. Smith, J. F.: Hydrocephalus associated with choroid plexus papillomas. J. Neuropath. Exp. Neurol., *14*:442–449, 1955.

397. Sobin, L. H.: Personal communication, 1977.

398. Spataro, J., and Sacks, O.: Oligodendroglioma with remote metastases: Case report. J. Neurosurg., *28*:373–379, 1968.

399. Spettowa, S., and Kusmiderski, J.: Angiography of supratentorial astrocytomas. Acta Med. Pol., *9*:475–479, 1968.

400. Spitz, E. B., Shenkin, H. A., and Grant, F. C.: Cerebellar medulloblastoma in adults. Arch. Neurol. Psychiat., *57*:417–422, 1947.

401. Stanley, P.: Papillomas of the choroid plexus. Brit. J. Radiol., *41*:848–857, 1968.

402. Steele, J. R., Cohen, F. L., and Weber, W. R.: Middle cerebral artery occlusion within an irradiated glioblastma multiforme. Surg. Neurol., *9*:173–176, 1978.

403. Stein, B. M., Fraser, R. A. R., and Tenner, M. S.: Tumours of the third ventricle in children. J. Neurol. Neurosurg. Psychiat., *35*:776–788, 1972.

404. Steinhoff, H., Grumme, T., Kazner, E., Lange,

S., Lanksch, W., Meese, W., and Wüllenweber, R.: Axial transverse computerzied tomography in 73 glioblastomas. Acta Neurochir. (Wien), *42*:45–56, 1978.

405. Steinhoff, H., Lanksch. W., Kazner, E., Grumme, T., Meese, W., Lange, S., Aulich, A., Schinder, E., and Winde, S.: Computed tomography in the diagnosis and differential diagnosis of glioblastomas. Neuroradiology, *14*:193–200, 1977.

406. Stevenson, L., and Echlin, F.: Nature and origin of some tumors of the cerebellum: Medulloblastoma. Arch. Neurol. Psychiat., *31*:93–109, 1934.

407. Stroebe, H.: Ueber Entstehung und bau der Gehirngliome. Beitr. Path. Anat., *18*:405–437, 1895.

408. Svien, H. J., Gates, E. M., and Kernohan, J. W.: Spinal subarachnoid implantation associated with ependymoma. Arch. Neurol. Psychiat., *62*:847–856, 1949.

409. Svien, H. J., Mabon, R. F., Kernohan, J. W., and Adson, A. W.: Astrocytomas. Mayo Clin. Proc., *24*:54–64, 1949.

410. Svien, H. J., Mabon, R. F., Kernohan, J. W., and Craig, W. M.: Ependymoma of the brain: Pathologic aspects. Neurology (Minneap.) *3*:1 15, 1953.

411. Svoboda, D. J.: Oligodendroglioma in a six-week old infant. J. Neuropath. Exp. Neurol., *18*: 569–574, 1959.

412. Swenberg, J. A.: Chemical- and virus-induced brain tumors. Nat. Cancer Inst. Monogr., *46*: 3–10, 1977.

413. Takeuchi, K., and Hoshino, K.: Statistical analysis of factors affecting survival after glioblastoma multiforme. Acta Neurochir. (Wien), *37*:57–73, 1977.

414. Tchang, S., Scotti, G., Terbrugge, K., Melançon, D., Bélanger, G., Miller, C., and Ethier, R.: Computerized tomography as a possible aid to histological grading of supratentorial gliomas. J. Neurosurg., *46*:735–739, 1977.

415. Tentler, R. L., and Palacios, E.: False-negative computerized tomography in brain tumor. JAMA, *238*:339–340, 1977.

416. Teppo, L., Hakama, M., Hakulinen, T., Lehtonen, M., and Saxén, E.: Cancer in Finland 1953–1970: Incidence, mortality, prevalence. Acta Path. Microbiol. Scand. [A], suppl. 252, 1975.

417. Thomas, D. G. T., Lannigan, C. B., and Behan, P. O.: Impaired cell-mediated immunity in human brain tumours. Lancet, *1*:1389–1390, 1975.

418. Tola, J. S.: The histopathological and biological characteristics of the primary neoplasms of the cerebellum and the fourth ventricle, with some aspects of their clinical picture, diagnosis and treatment (on the basis. of 71 verified cases). Acta Chir. Scand., suppl. 164:1–112, 1951.

419. Tönnis, W., and Zülch, K. J.: Intrakranielle Ganglienzellgeschwülste. Zbl. Neurochir., *4*:273–307, 1939.

420. Torkildsen, A.: Should extirpation be attempted in cases of neoplasm in or near the third ventricle of the brain: Experiences with a palliative method. J. Neurosurg., *5*:249–275, 1948.

421. Treip, C. S.: A congenital medulloepithelioma of the midbrain. J. Path. Bact., *74*:357–363, 1957.

422. Trouillas, P., and Lapras, C.: Immunothérapie active des tumeurs cérébrales; Apropos de 20 cas. Neurochirurgie, *16*:143–170, 1970.

423. Tukel, K., and Jasper, H.: The electroencephalogram in parasagittal lesions. Electroenceph. Clin. Neurophysiol., *4*:481–494, 1952.

424. Twining, E. W.: Radiology of the third and fourth ventricles. Brit. J. Radiol., *12*:385–418, 569–598, 1939.

425. Uihlein, A., Colby, M. Y., Layton, D. D., Parsons, W. R., and Carter, T. L.: Comparison of surgery and surgery plus irradiation in the treatment of supratentorial gliomas. Acta. Radiol. [Ther.] (Stockholm), *5*:67–78, 1966.

426. Urtasun, R. C.: ^{60}Co radiation treatment of pontine gliomas. Radiology, *104*:385–387, 1972.

427. Urtasun, R. C., Band, P. R., Chapman, J. D., and Feldstein, M. L.: Radiation plus metronidazole for glioblastoma. New Eng. J. Med., *296*:757, 1977.

428. van Wagenen, W. P.: Papillomas of the choroid plexus: Report of two cases, one with removal of tumor at operation and one with "seeding" of the tumor in the ventricular system. Arch. Surg. (Chicago), *20*:199–231, 1930.

429. Verhoeff, F. H.: Tumors of the optic nerve. *In* Penfield, W., ed.: Cytology and Cellular Pathology of the Nervous System. 1932. Reprinted, New York, Hafner Publishing Co., 1965, pp. 1029–1039.

430. Vigouroux, A.: Écoulement de liquide céphalorachidien hydrocéphalie papillome des plexus choroïdes du IVe ventricule. Rev. Neurol. (Paris), *16*:281–285, 1908.

431. Vonofakos, D., Marcu, H., and Hacker, H.: Oligodendrogliomas: CT patterns with emphasis on features indicating malignancy. J. Comput. Assist. Tomogr. *3*:783–788, 1979.

432. Vraa-Jensen, G.: Papilloma of the choroid plexus with pulmonary metastases. Acta Psychiat. Neurol. Scand., *25*:299–306, 1950.

433. Wagner, J. A., Frost, J. K., and Wisotzkey, H.: Subarachnoid neoplasia: Incidence and problems of diagnosis. Southern Med. J., *53*:1503–1508, 1960.

434. Wahlström, T., Linder, E., Saksela, E., and Westermark, B.: Tumor-specific membrane antigens in established cell lines from gliomas. Cancer, *34*:274–279, 1974.

435. Wakamatsu, T., Matsuo, T., Kawano, S., Teramoto, S., and Matsumura, H.: Glioblastoma with extracranial metastasis through ventriculopleural shunt: Case report. J. Neurosurg., *34*:697–701, 1971.

436. Walker, M. D.: Malignant brain tumors—A synopsis. CA, *25*:114–120, 1975.

437. Waltz, T. A., and Brownell, B.: Sarcoma: A possible late result of effective radiation therapy for pituitary adenoma: Report of two cases. J. Neurosurg., *24*:901–907, 1966.

438. Weinman, D. F.: Incidence and behavior pattern of intracranial tumors in Ceylon. Int. Surg., *58*:548–554, 1973.

439. Weir, B., and Elvidge, A. R.: Oligodendrogliomas: An analysis of 63 cases. J. Neurosurg., *29*:500–505, 1968.

440. Weir, B., and Grace, M.: The relative signifi-

cance of factors affecting postoperative survival in astrocytomas, grades one and two. Canad. J. Neurol. Sci., *3*:47–50, 1976.

441. Weisberg, L. A., and Nice, C. N.: Intracranial tumors simulating the presentation of cerebrovascular syndromes: Early detection with cerebral computed tomography (CCT). Amer. J. Med., *63*:517–524, 1977.

442. Weiss, H. D., Gutin, P. H., and Walker, M. D.: Unresolved problem of treatment of glioma. JAMA, *229*:1284–1285, 1974.

443. White, J. C., Liu, C. T., and Mixter, W. J.: Focal epilepsy: A statistical study of its causes and the results of surgical treatment. I. Epilepsy secondary to intracranial tumors. New Eng. J. Med., *238*:891–899, 1948.

444. Willis, R. A.: Pathology of Tumours. 3rd Ed. London, Butterworth & Co., 1960.

445. Wilkins, H., Smith, R., and Halpert, B.: Neoplasm of the choroid plexus of the left lateral ventricle. J. Neurosurg., *5*:406–410, 1948.

446. Wilson, C. B.: Medulloblastoma: Current views regarding the tumor and its treatment. Oncology, *24*:273–290, 1970.

447. Winston, K., Gilles, F. H., Leviton, A., and Fulchiero, A. Cerebellar gliomas in children. J. Nat. Cancer Inst., *58*:833–838, 1977.

448. Wislawski, J.: Cerebral oligodendrogliomas. Clinical manifestations, surgical treatment and histological findings in seventy cases. Pol. Med. J., *9*:163–172, 1970.

449. Witthaut, H.: Klinische Untersuchungen zur Frage einer biologisch-prognostischen Einteilung der Astrocytome des Groshirns unter Zugrundelegung der histologischen Klassifikation nach dem Prinzip des "Grading." Aerztl. Wschr., *14*:725–730, 1959.

450. Woltman, H. W., Kernohan, J. W., and Adson, A. W.: Gliomas of the cerebellopontine angle. Mayo Clin. Proc., *24*:77–82, 1949.

451. Wyke, B. D.: The cortical control of movement: A contribution to the surgical physiology of seizures. Epilepsia, *1*:4–35, 1959.

452. Yasargil, M. G.: Die subarachnoidale blutung. Schweiz. Med. Wschr., *99*:1629–1632, 1969.

453. Zatz, I. M.: Atypical choroid plexus calcifications associated with neurofibromatosis. Radiology, *91*:1135–1139, 1968.

454. Zimmerman, H. M.: The natural history of intracranial neoplasms with special reference to the gliomas. Amer. J. Surg., *93*:913–924, 1957.

455. Zimmerman, H. M.: Brain tumors: Their incidence and classification in man and their experimental production. Ann. N.Y. Acad. Sci., *159*:337–359, 1969.

456. Zimmerman, H. M.: Introduction to tumors of the central nervous system. *In* Minckler, J., ed.: Pathology of the Nervous System. New York, McGraw-Hill Book Co., 1971, pp. 1947–1951.

457. Zimmerman, H. M.: Experimental neuroneoplasia. *In* Minckler, J., ed.: Pathology of the Nervous System. New York, McGraw-Hill Book Co., 1971, pp. 1951–1960.

458. Zülch, K. J.: Über die Strahlensensibilität der Hirngeschwülste und die sogenannte Strahlenspatnekrose des Hirns. Deutsch. Med. Wschr., *85*:293–298, 1960.

459. Zülch, K. J.: Some remarks on the spongioblastoma of the brain. Acta Neurochir. (Wien), suppl. 10:121–125, 1964.

460. Zülch, K. J.: On the definition of the polymorphous oligodendroglioma. Acta Neurochir. (Wien), suppl. 10:166–172, 1964.

461. Zülch, K. J.: Brain Tumors: Their Biology and Pathology. New York, Springer-Verlag, 1965.

462. Zülch, K. J.: Biology and morphology of glioblastoma multiforme. Acta Radiol. [Ther.] (Stockholm), *8*:65–77, 1969.

463. Zülch, K. J., and Wechsler, W.: Pathology and classification of gliomas. Progr. Neurol. Surg., *2*:1–84, 1968.

87

LYMPHOMAS OF THE
BRAIN IN ADULTS

Brain tumors may derive from any of the cellular elements normally present in the brain. Consequently, the lymphoreticular system, a constituent of the brain, is able to produce tumors. In the brain, this system is represented by lymphocytes, plasma cells, macrophages, and reticulum cells.[10] In order to simplify terminology, neoplasms of these cellular elements have been collectively referred to in the World Health Organization classification as malignant lymphomas.[59] Although there is a possibility that benign lymphomas may exist as a transitional stage between inflammatory response and malignant form, all clinically significant lymphomas are malignant. Thus, in this chapter, the shorter term "lymphoma" is used rather than "malignant lymphoma."

The histological similarity between brain neoplasms deriving from lymphatic elements and lymphomas outside the central nervous system allowed Mallory to suspect a lymphoma ancestry in a tumor referred to by Bailey as "perivascular sarcoma."[5] Despite Mallory's correct interpretation of the cell of origin, credit for identification of lymphomas of the brain is usually given to Yuile, who noted morphological similarity between "primary reticulum cell sarcomas of the brain," which he attributed to microglial origin, and tumors of histiocytic elements outside the central nervous system.[73] The 12 cases described by Abbott and Kernohan in 1943 and the seven "microgliomas" described by Russell and coworkers in 1948 established brain neoplasms arising from lymphatic elements as a nosological entity.[1,55]

The cell of origin of lymphoma of the brain has not been determined. Potential cells of origin include histiocytes in the leptomeninges or vascular adventitia, hematogenous macrophages, or microglial cells.* The precise identification of these cell types and their relation to one another are not well understood.[10,35,51,64,72] The resulting lymphoma usually contains a mixture of microglial and reticulum cell elements as well as small undifferentiated cells. It is possible that the lymphoma arises from undifferentiated cells and that the more differentiated portions represent maturation. It is also possible that the poorly differentiated areas represent dedifferentiation of more mature forms.[52] Typical "microgliomas" have been suggested to be of B-cell origin and to produce immunoglobulins.[26,65] B-cell origin is supported by the monoclonal nature of most individual tumors.

There is disagreement concerning the subclassification of lymphomas primary to the brain, although there are no features that distinguish these primary lymphomas from the "secondary" lymphomas, which have been well classified.[34,55,61,75] This disagreement is in part due to the inadequacy of information regarding the origin and life history of the lymphatic elements of the central nervous system and in part due to the rarity of this type of neoplasm.[19] Names used to denote this tumor type include "microglioma," microgliomatosis," reticulum cell sarcoma," "reticulomicrogliomatosis," "reticulomicroglial sarcoma," "reticulosarcoma," "diffuse reticulosarcomatosis" "reticuloendotheliomatosis," "reticulopathy," "retothelio sarcoma," "perithelial sarcoma," "adventitial sarcoma,"

---

* See references 4, 19, 46, 64, 66, 74.

C. A. COBB AND J. R. YOUMANS

"histiocytic sarcoma," and "malignant lymphoma."[27] Neoplasms that are histologically like Hodgkin's sarcoma may also be included in this general type of brain tumor.[61] One subclassification has separated a microglial type, a reticulum cell sarcoma type, a Hodgkin's type, and a mixed type.[9] Another subclassification divides these neoplasms into Hodgkin's granuloma and sarcoma, reticulum sarcoma, lymphosarcoma, and plasmacytoma.[74,75]

Unfortunately, a patient with multicentric central nervous system tumors of lymphatic origin can have apparently separate subtypes in different masses.[74] Furthermore, a single neoplasm may contain portions that appear to be microglioma and other portions that appear to be reticulum cell sarcoma.[52,75] Primary brain tumors with the histological features of Hodgkin's disease also contain microglial elements.[9] Thus, neoplasms in the separate lymphoma subcategories contain mixtures of cell types and differ primarily in the cell type that predominates in the area that is sampled. Because of these difficulties with subclassification and the belief that these separate subclassifications do not convey important pathological or clinical differences, the World Heath Organization classification includes all these neoplasms in the category of malignant lymphoma.[52,75]

Identification of a lymphoma as a neoplastic rather than an inflammatory process may be difficult, since in either case the same cell type may proliferate.[41,67] Known infectious agents can produce inflammation that resembles lymphoma.[35] Some cellular proliferations are described as neoplasms on the basis of the clinical progression of disease and cellular pleomorphism and anaplasia.[38,42] There may even be a gradation from reactive proliferation of cells of the lymphatic system to neoplastic proliferation. The identification of transitional cases between neoplastic and inflammatory diseases has aroused speculation that brain lymphomas may be caused by an oncogenic virus producing an inflammatory process that transforms into a neoplasm.[52,67–69]

Although the cause of malignant lymphoma has not yet been determined, diseases associated with a greater incidence of them have been identified. They occur in approximately 240 per 100,000 patients whose immune responses are suppressed and may occur more frequently after renal transplantation and with the inflammatory form of Mikulicz's syndrome and Wiskott-Aldrich syndrome.[4,43,58] A "perithelial sarcoma," which would probably be currently classified as a lymphoma, has occurred at the site of a previous head injury, which raises the question of traumatic etiology.[23]

Any mechanism postulated to account for lymphomas of the brain must not only allow for spread of tumor through Virchow-Robin spaces but should also allow for the widespread transformation of normal cells into malignant cells.[1] Immunosuppressive therapy may have an oncogenic potential by causing chromosomal breakage, depression of the host's surveillance of neoplasms, or activation of an oncogenic virus. Also the postulated increased incidence of lymphomas associated with this therapy may result from its use as a treatment for diseases in which there is repeated antigenic stimulation.[53,68] In this last circumstance, the repeated antigenic stimulation, rather than the immunosuppressive therapy, may be the activating mechanism for the lymphoma.[53]

INCIDENCE

Central nervous system lymphomas are discovered in 0.1 per cent of autopsies and account for 1 to 3 per cent of central nervous system tumors.[32,50,57,75]

Although an increased incidence of lymphomas has been suggested to follow immunosuppressive therapy, primary brain lymphomas occur in only 0.24 per cent of patients who are undergoing immunological suppression, an incidence similar to that expected for the general population.[4]

The usual age of patients with primary brain lymphomas is between 40 and 60 years; however, there is a wide spectrum of ages, with no age exempt from the disease.* Patients as young as 16 days and as old as 90 years have had lymphomas of the brain.[9,32] The incidence is the same in both sexes.

Eight per cent of all lymphomas are primary in the central nervous system.[2] Half of the patients with lymphomas of the brain have systemic lymphoma.[74,75] Intracranial lymphoma occurs in approximately 60 per cent of patients with acute lymphocytic leu-

* See references 9, 23, 32, 37, 42, 56, 57.

kemia, in 25 per cent of patients with non-Hodgkin's lymphoma, and in only 1 to 3 per cent of patients with Hodgkin's disease.[14,30,31] Some of the patients harboring lymphoma in brain as well as in extraneural sites may be manifesting multifocal origin rather than metastatic disease, and some patients may develop extraneural lymphoma as a result of spread from the central nervous system.[45,60,67]

Lymphoma of the brain can occur as a discrete mass or may consist of widespread infiltration.[1] If a discrete mass, it may be either soft or firm. Usually it is homogeneous without significant necrosis or hemorrhage and is gray-pink in color.[37,57] The absence of necrosis may be due to the intimate relationship between the neoplasm and the vascular system.[4] The tumor margins are indistinct, and the surrounding brain usually is edematous.

If the neoplasm occurs as a diffuse, unlocalized process, the brain may look relatively normal on macroscopic examination. Microscopic examination, however, reveals widespread proliferation of microglia, suggesting that much of the brain may have developed a neoplastic "field" (see Chapter 86).[3] This diffuse involvement may resemble an exudative cellular inflammatory process.

The occurrence of multiple foci and of diffuse infiltrative growth is characteristic of lymphoma. Even in patients with discrete tumor masses, infiltration and small foci of neoplasm at a distance from the larger mass occur in more than 85 per cent of cases.[2,6] Since the diffuse pattern of lymphoma is difficult to recognize, it is not possible to make an accurate estimate of its incidence. Quite probably the rates are higher than the 7 per cent identified as occurring in a diffuse pattern and the 10 per cent noted to be multifocal by Burstein and associates.[9] If a parallel can be drawn between primary central nervous system lymphomas and secondary lymphomas (those associated with systemic lymphomas), the great majority of primary lymphomas would be expected to be diffuse.[29] Since there are so few other pathological differences between primary and secondary lymphomas, it would be expected that meticulous autopsy studies would reveal previously unrecognized primary malignant lymphomas occurring without focal masses.

Lymphomas can occur in any portion of the central nervous system. Secondary lymphomas in the spinal extradural space are the ones that most frequently cause neurological involvement, and these are discussed in other chapters. Approximately half of primary central nervous system lymphomas occur in the cerebral hemispheres, and 10 to 30 per cent occur in the posterior fossa.[9,23,32] The two sides of the brain are equally affected. The frequency with which discrete masses are distributed in the various lobes of the brain corresponds to the surface area of the particular lobe. Spread along leptomeninges and periventricular surfaces is common because the neoplasm usually abuts either a meningeal or ependymal surface.[30,57] Leptomeningeal spread occurs in approximately 95 per cent of patients.[6] Even more characteristic than periventricular and meningeal spread is the occurrence of neoplasm in a perivascular pattern and in Virchow-Robin spaces. This phenomenon may be due either to the origin of the tumor from cells intimately related to blood vessels or to spread of the neoplasms to these spaces.

Lymphoma is particularly likely to involve the choroid plexus and the septum pellucidum.[9,57,75] This tendency may be related to intraventricular spread of tumor. Lymphomas frequently involve the corpus callosum and have a "butterfly" distribution. Indeed, if a brain tumor has this type of distribution, the chance that it is a lymphoma has been estimated to be as high as 10 per cent.[15,32]

MICROSCOPIC PATHOLOGY

The characteristic microscopic features of central nervous system lymphomas are extensive spread of neoplasm beyond the apparent macroscopic border, perivascular distribution of tumor (particularly in Virchow-Robin spaces), and microglial cells with varying degrees of differentiation (Fig. 87–1).[54,55] Often they are quite cellular, and the cells may be pleomorphic with frequent mitoses. Multinucleated giant cells suggesting Hodgkin's disease may occur.[61] Typical neoplastic cells are round or oval. Nuclei are distinct, have an elongated, dented or twisted shape, and contain delicate chromatin. A small cell with scant cytoplasm and a large dense nucleus may also be seen and, it has been suggested, may be a primi-

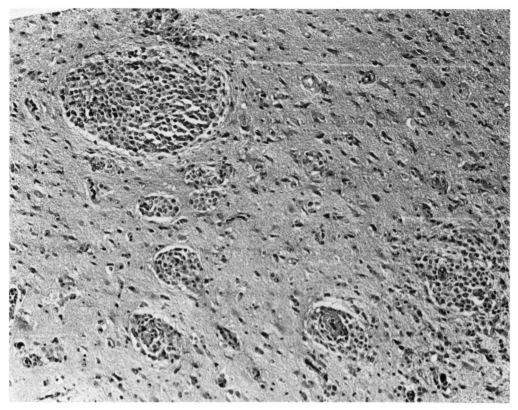

Figure 87–1 Histological examination of the margin of a malignant lymphoma shows tumor cells clustering around vessels. Nuclear variability is apparent. Hematoxylin and Eosin, 180×.

tive multipotential cell.[13] Although scattered areas of necrosis are seen occasionally, necrosis is not a pronounced feature.

Collections of neoplastic cells may arise remote from the main mass of tumor.[55] This is particularly true when these collections are related to vessels. The association of lymphoma with vessels parallels an association with reticulin, a material that is still poorly characterized.[1,11] The individual lymphoma cells occur in the walls of vessels and are surrounded by a reticulin stroma. As the neoplastic cells separate the reticulin fibers around vessels and new reticulin is formed, multiple rings of reticulin occur in a perivascular pattern with proliferating cells between the concentric rings (Fig. 87–2).[3,19]

Lymphomas may be accompanied by gliosis with increased numbers of fibrous astrocytes and glial fibers. This has been estimated to occur in 95 per cent of cases.[6,55] There can also be a reactive proliferation of microglial cells as a response to primary lymphoma of the brain, a feature that is not prominent in most non-lymphoma metastases.[6,47] A fibroblastic response also may occur.[44]

CLINICAL PRESENTATION

The presenting signs and symptoms of intracranial lymphomas may suggest an expanding intracerebral mass. In this circumstance, the clinical diagnosis usually is glioblastoma multiforme.[56,74] Lymphoma may also present with signs and symptoms suggestive of encephalitis.

The duration of symptoms with intracranial lymphoma is quite variable. In rare cases, many years elapse between the onset of symptoms and the diagnosis. In most series, the average duration of symptoms is from three to six months.[7,9,32,37,57] The course of the illness tends to be less rapid with the diffuse form of cerebral lymphoma than with localized masses of tumor.[20] This difference may be due to the more extensive cerebral edema seen with the localized tumor mass.

When the presentation suggests encepha-

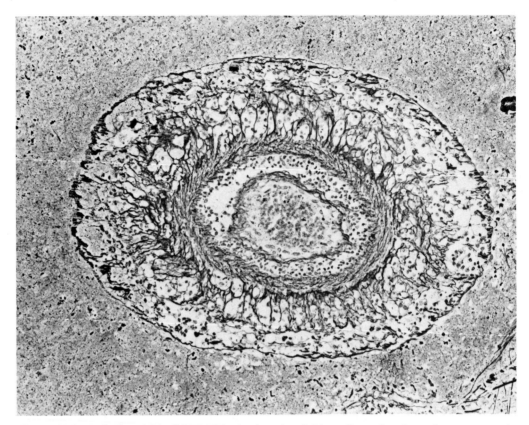

Figure 87–2   Reticulin staining of a vessel that has been invaded by malignant lymphoma demonstrates reticulin fibers surrounding tumor cells. Reticulin stain, 180×.

litis, the patients develop malaise, lethargy, anorexia, headache, and fever, sometimes with cerebellar or pseudobulbar signs. This presentation was seen in 6 of the 29 patients reported by Burstein and associates.[9]

In the more common form of presentation the lymphoma mimics a glioblastoma multiforme or a metastatic tumor. Increased intracranial pressure produces headache early in the clinical course. Mental changes are common and include changes in personality as well as confusion, irritability, drowsiness, and inattentiveness. Focal neurological signs and symptoms may or may not be present, depending on the extent and location of tumor infiltration. Localized motor deficits are present in fewer than half of the cases, and seizures are uncommon.[20,23,56]

INVESTIGATION

The cerebrospinal fluid is almost always abnormal with lymphoma of the brain.[22,39,57] Often the pressure is elevated and the pro-

tein concentration is increased in nearly all cases. The protein content may be particularly high with an encephalitic type of distribution and can reach as much as 625 mg per 100 ml. Lymphoma may cause an increase of the macroglobulins in the blood and spinal fluid (Fig. 87–3). In the future, analysis for this component may become a significant tool in the diagnosis of this tumor.[39] Routine cell counts of the cerebrospinal fluid usually are normal except in patients with an encephalitic distribution of tumor. In this group, cell counts average 55 mononuclear cells per cubic millimeter. The cerebrospinal fluid glucose level may be lowered and may reach values as low as 0 mg per 100 ml. Cytological studies reveal neoplastic cells in more than 50 per cent of patients, and this finding may be diagnostic even in the presence of a normal spinal fluid cell count and normal spinal fluid protein.[39] In 12 of 33 patients with extraneural lymphoma in whom autopsy revealed central nervous system involvement, cytological examination of cerebrospinal fluid revealed neoplastic cells in 8.[49] Although analysis of

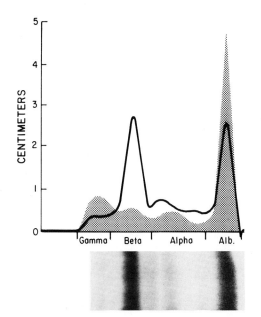

Figure 87–3 Serum protein electrophoresis demonstrates macroglobulinemia in an unusual case of malignant lymphoma primary in the brain. The normal electrophoretic pattern is shaded.

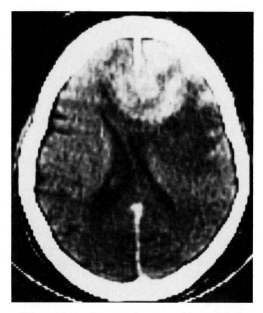

Figure 87–4 Computed tomographic scan demonstrates a bifrontal primary malignant lymphoma that has been enhanced by iodinated contrast medium.

the spinal fluid may contribute to diagnosis in patients with lymphoma, the physician must remember that lumbar puncture in patients with intracranial masses may be hazardous.

Skull x-rays are abnormal in approximately half of these patients. When abnormal they usually reveal a pineal shift. Signs of chronic increased intracranial pressure may also be present. Calcification of the tumor is not seen.[57]

Electroencephalography demonstrates abnormality in approximately 80 per cent of patients.[23,57] This abnormality may be either diffuse or focal. If the diffuse unlocalized form of lymphoma is excluded, all patients with lymphoma have abnormal electroencephalograms.

Technetium brain scans are highly accurate in identifying lymphomas.[22,57] Other radioisotope tracers such as arsenic and copper are less accurate. Isotope scans may be interpreted as demonstrating multiple lesions "diagnostic" of metastatic carcinoma. Computed tomography usually shows parenchymal tumors, but often does not show leptomeningeal tumors (Fig. 87–4).[8,16]

Angiograms are abnormal in more than 80 per cent of cases.[57] Angiographic tumor staining is rare; the usual finding is a localized intracerebral mass. Air encephalography is quite accurate. It revealed abnormal-

ity in all the patients reported by Hanbery and Dugger, and in two thirds of the patients reported by Schaumberg and associates.[23,57] Angiography and encephalography would be expected to be less reliable in the encephalitic presentation of lymphoma, and the normal studies may have been those of patients with this distribution of tumor.

TREATMENT

Central nervous system lymphoma is radiosensitive, and radiotherapy may produce a dramatic decrease in symptoms. Without operative decompression or radiotherapy, the average length of survival after diagnosis is only three weeks. Perhaps this is true because only those patients too ill for operative treatment are included in this group. If operative treatment is added, the survival time increases to approximately two months.[9] Because of the recognized advantages of radiotherapy, few series have included an unirradiated group of patients. In series in which radiotherapy is used, average survival varies from 17 months to four years.[9,32,57,75] Adams has reported a patient who underwent irradiation and at autopsy six years later was found to have only "one small nodule of neoplasm."[4] Bertelsen has reported a patient who underwent a limited operative resection and postoperative radiotherapy, and subsequently died of a pulmonary embolus. At autopsy no residual neoplasm was identified.[7] Burstein and colleagues have reported one patient who survived 10 years and another patient who was alive and well 17 years after treatment with combined operation and radiotherapy.[9] Although 47 per cent of the patients reported by Littman and Wang survived for three or more years, only one survived more than six years.[40]

Because of the efficacy of radiotherapy in malignant lymphomas, the goal of operative treatment should primarily be to obtain tissue to establish the diagnosis. In a neoplasm located in a "silent" portion of the brain, this may be performed most safely by generous operative decompression. In other circumstances, a stereotaxic biopsy through a burr hole may be advisable. Occasionally, cytological analysis of spinal fluid may be sufficient for diagnosis. Histological diagnosis should be followed by whole brain radiotherapy of approximately 4500 rads with an addition of 500 to 1000 rads directly to the tumor.[40] Radiotherapy of the spinal axis should be added if there are clinical manifestations of spinal disease, if neoplastic cells are revealed in the spinal fluid, or if the clinical presentation or investigative studies suggest disseminated lymphoma. Recurrence of tumor in the irradiated field can occur even after adequate radiotherapy.

The role of chemotherapy in the treatment of lymphoma of the brain has not been defined.[31] Glucocorticoids have produced dramatic improvement in some cases.[71] It would be expected that with restricted operative treatment combined with aggressive radiotherapy (possibly including neuraxis irradiation) and postoperative chemotherapy, the prognosis in primary central nervous system malignant lymphoma would be relatively favorable for many years of survival, and cure may be possible.

Acknowledgment. The authors wish to express their appreciation to Dr. Surl Nielsen, Section of Neuropathology, University of California, Davis, for obtaining the illustrations for this chapter.

REFERENCES

1. Abbott, K. H., and Kernohan, J. W.: Primary sarcomas of the brain: Review of the literature and report of twelve cases. Arch. Neurol. Psychiat., *50*:43–66, 1943.
2. Adams, J. H.: The classification of microgliomatosis with particular reference to diffuse microgliomatosis. Acta Neuropath. (Berlin), suppl. 6:119–123, 1975.
3. Adams, J. H., and Jackson, J. M.: Intracerebral tumours of reticular tissue: The problem of microgliomatosis and reticulo-endothelial sarcomas of the brain. J. Path. Bact., *91*:369–381, 1966.
4. Adams, R. D.: Certain notable clinical attributes of the histiocytic sarcomas of the central nervous system. Acta Neuropath. (Berlin), suppl. 6:117–180, 1975.
5. Bailey, P.: Intracranial sarcomatous tumors of leptomeningeal origin. Arch. Surg., (Chicago), *18*:1359–1402, 1929.
6. Barnard, R. O., and Scott, T.: Patterns of proliferation in cerebral lymphoreticular tumors. Acta Neuropath. (Berlin), suppl. 6:125–130, 1975.
7. Bertelsen, K.: Primary cerebral reticulosarcoma. Acta Path. Microbiol. Scand. [A], *78*:209–214, 1970.
8. Brant-Zawadzki, M., and Enzmann, D. R.: Computed tomographic brain scanning in patients with lymphoma. Radiology, *129*:67–71, 1978.
9. Burstein, S. D., Kernohan, J. W., and Uihlein, A.: Neoplasms of the reticuloendothelial system of the brain. Cancer, *16*:289–305, 1963.
10. Carr, I., Hancock, B. W., Henry, L., and Ward, A. M.: Lymphoreticular Disease. London, Blackwell Scientific Publications, 1977.
11. Cervos-Navarro, J., and Matakas, F.: The ultrastructure of reticulin. Acta Neuropath. (Berlin), suppl. 6:173–176, 1975.
12. Constantinidis, J., and Escourolle, R.: Réticulose pallido-pédonculaire bilatérale et nécrosante. Schweiz. Arch. Neurol. Neurochir. Psychiat., *106*:223–240, 1970.
13. Cravioto, H.: Human and experimental reticulum cell sarcoma (microglioma) of the nervous system. Acta Neuropath. (Berlin), suppl. 6:135–140, 1975.
14. Currie, S., and Henson, R. A.: Neurological syndromes in the reticuloses. Brain, *94*:307–320, 1971.
15. Ebels, E. J.: Reticulosarcomas of the brain presenting as butterfly tumours: Possible implications for treatment. Europ. Neurol., *8*:333–338, 1972.
16. Enzmann, D. R., Krikorian, J., Norman, D., et al.: Computed tomography in primary reticulum cell sarcoma of the brain. Radiology, *130*:165–170, 1979.
17. Frankhauser, R., Fatzer, R., and Luginbühl, H.: Reticulosis of the central nervous system (CNS) in dogs. Advances Vet. Sci., *16*:35–71, 1972.
18. Fisher, D., Mantell, B. S., and Urich, H.: The clinical diagnosis and treatment of microgliomatosis: Report of a case. J. Neurol. Neurosurg. Psychiat., *32*:474–478, 1969.
19. Fisher, E. R., Davis, E. R., and Lemmen, L. J.: Reticulum-cell sarcoma of brain (microglioma). Arch. Neurol. Psychiat., *81*:591–598, 1959.
20. Foncin, J.-F., and Faucher, J.-N.: Primary and borderline brain lymphosarcoma: A neuropathological review of nine cases. Acta Neuropath. (Berlin), suppl. 6:107–113, 1975.
21. Gazso, L., Slowik, F.: Primary lymphomas of the

central nervous system; in vitro culture observations. Acta Neuropath. (Berlin), suppl. 6: 103–106, 1975.

22. Gunderson, C. H., Henry, J., and Malamud, N.: Plasma globulin determinations in patients with microglioma: Report of five cases. J. Neurosurg., 35:406–415, 1971.

23. Hanbery, J. W., and Dugger, G. S.: Perithelial sarcoma of the brain: A clinicopathological study of thirteen cases. Arch. Neurol. Psychiat., 71:732–761, 1954.

24. Hirano, A.: A comparison of the fine structure of malignant lymphoma and other neoplasms in the brain. Acta Neuropath. (Berlin), suppl. 6:141–145, 1975.

25. Horvat, B., Pena, C., and Fisher, E. R.: Primary reticulum cell sarcoma (microglioma) of brain: An electron microscopic study. Arch. Path. (Chicago), 87:609–616, 1969.

26. Houthoff, H. J., Poppema, S., Ebels, E. J., and Elema, J. D.: Intracranial malignant lymphomas. Acta Neuropath. (Berlin), 44:203–210, 1978.

27. Hubert, J. W. A.: Tumours of the reticuloendothelial system. In Vinken, P. J., and Bruyn, G. W., eds.: Handbook of Clinical Neurology. Vol. 18. Amsterdam, North-Holland Publishing Co., 1975, pp. 233–267.

28. Ishida, W. Y.: Fine structure of primary reticulum cell sarcoma of the brain. Acta Neuropath. (Berlin), suppl. 6:147–153, 1975.

29. Jänisch, W., Gerlach, H., and Remus, I.: Neoplastic involvement of the CNS in generalized lymphomas. Acta Neuropath. (Berlin), suppl. 6:81–84, 1975.

30. Janisch, V. W., Gerlach, H., Schreiber, D., et al.: Isolated neoplastic foci in the central nervous system in generalized non-Hodgkin's-lymphoma. A prospective pathomorphological study. Zbl. Allg. Path., 122:195–203, 1978.

31. Jellinger, K., and Slowik, F.: Affection of the nervous system in leucoses and malignant lymphomas. Zbl. Allg. Path., 122:439–461, 1978.

32. Jellinger, K., Radaskiewicz, T., and Slowik, F.: Primary malignant lymphomas of the central nervous system in man. Acta Neuropath. (Berlin), suppl. 6:95–102, 1975.

33. Jernstrom, P., Crockett, H. G., and Bachhuber, R. G.: Primary lymphosarcoma of cerebral meninges. J. Neurosurg., 24:679–683, 1966.

34. Kepes, J. J., and Kepes, M.: Lymphoreticular proliferative disorders of the CNS and other organs: Analogies and differences. Acta Neuropath. (Berlin), suppl. 6:75–79, 1975.

35. Kershman, J.: Genesis of microglia in the human brain. Arch. Neurol. Psychiat., 41:24–50, 1939.

36. Kersting, G., and Neumann, J.: "Malignant lymphoma" of the brain following renal transplantation. Acta Neuropath. (Berlin), suppl. 6:131–133, 1975.

37. Kinney, T. D., and Adams, R. D.: Reticulum cell sarcoma of the brain. Arch. Neurol. Psychiat., 50:552–564, 1943.

38. Koestner, A.: Primary lymphoreticuloses of the nervous system in animals. Acta Neuropath. (Berlin), suppl. 6:85–89, 1975.

39. Kolar, O. J.: Differential diagnostic aspects in malignant lymphomas involving the central nervous system. Acta Neuropath. (Berlin), suppl. 6:181–186, 1975.

40. Littman, P., and Wang, C. C.: Reticulum cell sarcoma of the brain: A review of the literature and a study of 19 cases. Cancer, 35:1412–1420, 1975.

41. Marshall, A. H. E.: Cytology and Pathology of the Reticular Tissue, London, Oliver & Boyd, 1956.

42. Miller, A. A., and Ramsden, F.: Primary reticulosis of the central nervous system "microgliomatosis." Acta Neurochir. (Wien), 11:439–478, 1963.

43. Model, L. M.: Primary reticulum cell sarcoma of the brain in Wiskott-Aldrich syndrome: Report of a case. Arch. Neurol. (Chicago), 34:633–635, 1977.

44. Onofrio, B. M., Kernohan, J. W., and Uihlein, A.: Primary meningeal sarcomatosis: A review of the literature and report of 12 cases. Cancer, 15:1197–1208, 1962.

45. Peison, B.: Microglial glioma of brain with extracerebral involvement. Cancer, 20:983–990, 1967.

46. Peison, B., and Voris, D.: Primary sarcoma of the reticuloendothelial system of the brain: Report of a case. J. Neurosurg., 23:630–634, 1965.

47. Plafker, J., Martinez, A. J., and Rosenblum, W. I.: A neoplasm of the reticuloendothelial system involving brain (microglioma) and viscera (reticulum cell sarcoma). Southern Med. J., 65:385–389, 1972.

48. Polak, M.: Microglioma and/or reticulosarcoma of the nervous system. Acta Neuropath. (Berlin), suppl. 6:115–118, 1975.

49. Rawlinson, D. G., Billingham, M. E., Berry, P. F., and Kempson, R. L.: Cytology of the cerebrospinal fluid in patients with Hodgkin's disease or malignant lymphoma. Acta Neuropath. (Berlin), suppl. 6:187–191, 1975.

50. Reznik, M.: Pathology of primary reticulum cell sarcoma of the human central nervous system. Acta Neuropath. (Berlin), suppl. 6:91–94, 1975.

51. Rio-Hortega, P. del: Microglia. In Penfield, W., ed.: Cytology and Cellular Pathology of the Nervous System. 1932, Reissued by Hafner Publishing Company, New York, 1965, pp. 482–534.

52. Rubinstein, L. J.: Microgliomatosis. Acta Neurochir. (Wien), suppl. 10:201–207, 1963.

53. Rubinstein, L. J.: Current concepts in neuro-oncology. Advances Neurol., 15:1–25, 1976.

54. Russell, D. S., and Rubinstein, L. J.: Pathology of Tumours of the Nervous System. 4th Ed. Baltimore, Williams & Wilkins Co., 1977, pp. 101–115.

55. Russell, D. S., Marshall, A. H. E., and Smith, F. B.: Microgliomatosis: A form of reticulosis affecting the brain. Brain, 71:1–15, 1948.

56. Samuelsson, S.-M., Werner, I., Pontén, J., et al.: Reticuloendothelial (perivascular) sarcoma of the brain. Acta Neurol. Scand., 42:567–580, 1966.

57. Schaumburg, H. H., Plank, C. R., and Adams, R. D.: The reticulum cell sarcoma-microglioma group of brain tumors: A consideration of their clinical features and therapy. Brain, 95:199–212, 1972.

58. Schneck, S. A., and Penn, I.: Cerebral neoplasms associated with renal transplantation. Arch. Neurol. (Chicago), 22:226–233, 1970.

59. Sobin, L. H.: Personal communication, 1977.

60. Sorger, K.: Reticulum cell sarcoma of the central

nervous system. Canad, Med. Ass. J., *89*:503–507, 1963.

61. Sparling, H. J., and Adams, R. D.: Primary Hodgkin's sarcoma of the brain. Arch. Path. (Chicago), *42*:338–344, 1946.

62. Stensaas, L. J., and Horsley, W. W.: Production of lymphoid tissue in the rat brain by implants containing phytohemagglutinin. Acta Neuropath. (Berlin), *31*:71–84, 1975.

63. Tani, E., and Ametani, T.: Nuclear characteristics of malignant lymphoma in the brain. Acta Neuropath. (Berlin), suppl. 6:167–171, 1975.

64. Torvik, A.: The relationship between microglia and brain macrophages: Experimental investigations. Acta Neuropath. (Berlin), suppl. 6: 297–300, 1975.

65. Varadachari, C., Palutke, M., Climie, A. R. W., et al.: Immunoblastic sarcoma (histiocytic lymphoma) of the brain with B cell markers: Case report. J. Neurosurg., *49*:887–892, 1978.

66. Vuia, O.: Primary cerebral reticulosis and plasma cell differentiation. Acta Neuropath. (Berlin), suppl. 6:161–166, 1975.

67. Vuia, O., and Hager, H.: Primary cerebral blastomatous reticulosis: Clinical, pathohistological and ultrastructural study. J. Neurol. Sci., *19*:407–423, 1973.

68. Vuia, O., and Mehraein, P.: Primary reticulosis of the central nervous system. J. Neurol. Sci., *14*:469–482, 1971.

69. Wilke, G.: Über primäre reticuloendotheliosen des Gehirns. Deutsch. Z. Nervenheilk., *164*: 332–380, 1950.

70. Williams, J. L., and Peters, H. J.: Malignant reticulosis limited to the central nervous system: Case report. J. Neurosurg., *26*:532–535, 1967.

71. Williams, R. S., Crowell, R. M., Fisher, C. M., et al.: Clinical and radiologic remission in reticulum cell sarcoma of the brain. Arch. Neurol. (Chicago), *36*:206–210, 1979.

72. Wyburn-Mason, R.: The Reticulo-Endothelial System in Growth and Tumour Formation. London, Henry Klimpton, 1958.

73. Yuile, C. L.: Case of primary reticulum cell sarcoma of the brain: Relationship of microglia cells to histiocytes. Arch. Path. (Chicago), *26*:1036–1044, 1938.

74. Zimmerman, H. M.: Malignant lymphomas. *In* Minckler, J., ed.: Pathology of the Nervous System. New York, McGraw-Hill Book Co., 1971, pp. 2165–2178.

75. Zimmerman, H. M.: Malignant lymphomas of the nervous system. Acta Neuropath. (Berlin), suppl. *6*:69–74, 1975.

88

SARCOMAS AND NEOPLASMS OF BLOOD VESSELS

Intracranial neoplasms of connective tissue and blood vessels make up three overlapping groups of tumors. They are the sarcomas, the meningiomas, and the hemangiopericytomas and hemangioblastomas. The most common of these is the meningioma group, which is discussed in detail in Chapter 92. Unfortunately, meningiomas were initially described and classified by Cushing four years before the development of the histogenetic classification of glial tumors.[43] Rather than basing the meningioma group on a common cell of origin, he included tumors in this group if they were primary neoplasms of the leptomeninges. As a result of this topographic rather than histogenetic classification, a tumor that appeared to be a neoplasm of vascular endothelium might in the past have been called a hemangioblastoma if it occurred in the cerebellum or an angioblastic meningioma if it rose from supratentorial leptomeninges. This confusion has tended to blur the distinction between meningiomas and nonmeningeal connective tissue tumors.

Intracranial sarcomas are composed of anaplastic connective tissue. Since most of the intracranial connective tissue is located either in meninges or in vascular structures, most intracranial sarcomas derive originally from meningeal or vascular tissues.

The World Health Organization classification separates neoplasms of meningeal and related tissues from tumors of blood vessel origin (Table 88–1). In this chapter, vascular neoplasms are considered to include hemangioblastoma (hemangioendothelioma) and hemangiopericytoma and sarcomas include all anaplastic tumors of connective tissue origin.

In early descriptions, Bailey, Cushing, and Eisenhardt divided vascular tumors into hemangioblastomas and angioblastic meningiomas.[14] They described angioblastic meningiomas as sharing the histological features of hemangioblastoma. The elaborate meningioma classification of Cushing and Eisenhardt separated angioblastic meningiomas into three subtypes.[45] The first of these was the neoplasm that had originally been described in 1928 and has since been recognized as histologically identical with extraneural hemangiopericytoma.[14,144] The second subtype was transitional between the hemangioblastoma subtype and typical meningioma, and the third subtype resembled hemangioblastoma of the cerebellum.

When Courville and Abbott revised the classification of meningiomas in 1941, they preserved the single category of angioblastic meningioma to include all primary meningeal tumors that have prominent vascularity.[37] Bailey and Ford also recognized angioblastic meningiomas as a single entity.[8]

Unfortunately, the early series contained too few meningiomas for detailed study. Since angioblastic meningiomas make up only approximately 3 per cent of all meningiomas, large series are required for analysis of subdivisions in the angioblastic group.[14,71] At present there is general agreement that some angioblastic meningiomas resemble hemangioblastomas and others

---

C. A. COBB and J. R. YOUMANS

TABLE 88–1 WORLD HEALTH ORGANIZATION CLASSIFICATION OF TUMORS OF MENINGES, RELATED TISSUES, AND BLOOD VESSELS

TUMORS OF MENINGEAL AND RELATED TISSUES
Meningioma
  Meningotheliomatous
  Fibrous
  Transitional
  Psammomatous
  Angiomatous
  Hemangioblastic
  Hemangiopericytic
  Papillary
  Anaplastic
Meningeal sarcomas
  Fibrosarcoma
  Polymorphic cell sarcoma
  Primary meningeal sarcomatosis
Xanthomatous tumors
  Fibroxanthoma
  Xanthosarcoma
Primary melanotic tumors
  Melanoma
  Meningeal melanomatosis
Others
TUMORS OF BLOOD VESSEL ORIGIN
Hemangioblastoma
Monstrocellular sarcoma

resemble hemangiopericytomas.* A recent report states that many of these tumors are neither hemangioblastic nor hemangiopericytic variants but are the more common meningioma subtypes with unusually prominent vascularity (see Chapter 92).[71] One sixth to one third of angioblastic meningiomas are hemangiopericytomas, and an equal number are hemangioblastomas.[71,118,139]

There is disagreement regarding preservation of the term "angioblastic meningioma." Russell and Rubinstein have argued that there is a continuum from intraparenchymal cystic cerebellar hemangioblastoma to solid supratentorial hemangiopericytoma of the meninges.[132] Horten and associates found hemangioblastic areas in 2 of 34 (6 per cent) hemangiopericytomas and transitional features to ordinary meningioma in 2 of 29 (7 per cent) hemangiopericytomas.[65] If such a continuum is accepted as typical of these neoplasms, it can be suggested that both hemangioblastomas and hemangiopericytomas arise from polyblastic cells, possibly arachnoidal cells, whose differentiation is determined by the surrounding tissues in which they grow.

Several features support a distinction between hemangiopericytoma and heman-

* See references 17, 58, 71, 103, 118, 139.

gioblastoma. The original description of hemangiopericytoma stressed the normal appearance of the endothelial cells as opposed to the abnormal appearance of the neoplastic endothelial cells seen in hemangioblastoma.[144] There are also differences in the macroscopic characteristics of hemangiopericytomas and hemangioblastomas and in their electron microscopic appearances.[35,119] The failure to recognize hemangiopericytoma in a patient with Lindau's disease also argues against consideration of these as minor variations of a single tumor.

The outlook for patients with angioblastic meningioma depends on whether the tumor is of the hemangioblastic type, in which the prognosis is favorable, or the hemangiopericytic type, in which it is poor.[14,71,137]

HEMANGIOBLASTOMA

A hemangioblastoma arises from proliferation of endothelial cells that are not markedly anaplastic. A variety of names have been applied to this tumor.[14,83,133] They include "capillary hemangioma," "hemangioendothelioma," "angioreticuloma," "hemangioperithelioma," and "Lindau tumor." It usually occurs in the posterior fossa and often produces a large cyst. Originally it was thought to arise from a vascular anlage in the posterior medullary velum, but its occurrence above the tentorium is against this theory.[84] If an arachnoidal or pial origin is accepted, neoplasms in the cerebellar parenchyma abutting against the pial surface of the cerebellum and neoplasms of the meninges could both be accounted for.[14,132]

In 1926, Lindau exhaustively reviewed the literature and a series of cases and recognized the relationship between vascular cystic cerebellar tumors, vascular tumors of the retina (described by von Hippel in 1904), and tumors and cysts in other sites.[83,147] Lindau commented on the familial occurrence of hemangioblastoma.[84] More recent authors have suggested that a family history of retinal hemangioblastoma or cerebellar hemangioblastoma, as well as any component of the multisystem disease described by Lindau, is strongly suggestive of a diagnosis of Lindau's disease.[3,23,155] Multiple cerebellar hemangioblastomas probably also constitute confirmation of

Lindau's disease. They may, however, be overlooked or thought to be recurrence of a previously treated tumor rather than a new primary neoplasm.[24,131,155]

Incidence

These tumors make up approximately 1.5 to 2.0 per cent of all brain tumors and 7 to 12 per cent of posterior fossa tumors. About 1.5 per cent of meningiomas are, histologically, hemangioblastoma. The extremes of age at which they have been reported go from newborn to the eighth decade. Usually, they occur in young adults, the average age of patients being between 30 and 40 years in most series. Patients with Lindau's disease present at a younger age than those without it. Hemangioblastoma is slightly more frequent in males than in females; if only those in young adult men are considered, they constitute 3 per cent of brain tumors.*

In his 1926 review, Lindau noted the variety of abnormalities that may occur in these patients, including multiple hemangioblastomas, hemangioblastoma of the retina (von Hippel tumor), renal tumors, renal cysts, pancreatic cysts, and "tubular adenomata" of the epididymis.[85] In the majority of patients with the cerebellar lesion, Lindau's disease cannot be identified. There is a complicated relationship between cerebellar hemangioblastoma, retinal hemangioblastoma, and Lindau's disease. A minority of patients (approximately 20 per cent) with the cerebellar disease either have a family history of hemangioblastoma or have multiple central nervous system lesions. Retinal hemangioblastoma is unusual (6 per cent) in patients with hemangioblastoma of the cerebellum, but cerebellar hemangioblastoma occurs in 20 per cent of the patients with retinal hemangioblastoma. Even when Lindau's disease is present, only half the patients have cerebellar hemangioblastomas. Lindau's disease, when it occurs, is inherited as an autosomal dominant gene affecting males and females with equal frequency.†

Hemangioblastomas of the cerebral hemispheres are rare and account for 2 to 8 per cent of all tumors of this type.[6,103,138] They may be multiple and may be associated with retinal hemangioblastomas or other evidence of Lindau's disease.[64,67,118]

Pathology

Macroscopic Changes

Cerebellar hemangioblastomas are pinkish or yellow, usually abut the pial surface of the cerebellum, and often are associated with a cyst.[84,133] Their location may be marked by enlarged arteries and veins on the cerebellar surface near the tumor. They are sharply demarcated from the surrounding cerebellum. When a cyst is present its wall is smooth and white, and it contains yellow or clear cyst fluid. Hemorrhage can stain the cyst wall with a rusty brown pigment and may produce a brown discoloration of the cyst fluid. Protein in the fluid may exceed 5 grams per 100 ml.[136]

The mural nodule of a cystic cerebellar hemangioblastoma is found on the pial side of the cyst.[111,122,132] The tumor extends past the pia to involve the dura, usually the inferior aspect of the tentorium, in approximately 20 per cent of cases.[116,136] Dural attachment occurs in only half of supratentorial hemangioblastomas, but the cerebral tumor that appears to be subcortical may be in contact with pia in the depths of a sulcus.[65,123]

Identification of the mural nodule may be difficult. Because of this Sargent and Greenfield have suggested that a cerebellar cyst should always be presumed to have hemangioblastoma in its wall.[133] The mural nodule may be of any size, even as small as 2 mm, and its size is unrelated to the size of the cyst.

Hemangioblastoma may affect any part of the brain.[65,138] Approximately 10 per cent are supratentorial. Undoubtedly the incidence of supratentorial tumors of this type has been underestimated in the past because of classifying many of them as angioblastic meningiomas. Hemangioblastomas constitute a small proportion of fourth ventricular tumors.[40] In approximately 10 per cent of cases, the brain stem is the site of this tumor, in which case the tumor is particularly likely to be found in the area postrema.[96,132]

Cerebellar hemangioblastomas are cystic

---

* See references 18, 41, 68, 69, 72, 85, 101, 109, 111, 113, 118, 132, 136, 138, 139, 154, 157.

† See references 41, 69, 84, 85, 96, 101, 113.

in about 70 per cent of cases.[70,101,110] Even in those classified as "solid," small cystic areas are commonly found. There may be multiple cysts, or a single cyst may have a volume as large as 90 ml. Hemangioblastomas of the cerebrum and brain stem are cystic in only approximately 20 per cent of cases.[94,132,138] The tendency to develop cysts in the cerebellar lesions suggested to Lindau that the tumor produced fluid that the nervous system was unable to absorb because of the absence of a lymphatic circulation.[84] Perhaps the cerebral hemispheres are better able to absorb the fluid produced by neoplasms than the cerebellum and this in part accounts for the greater frequency of cystic hemangioblastomas and astrocytomas in the cerebellum. There is no histological subtype that is particularly likely to be associated with a cyst.[70]

Rarely cerebellar hemangioblastoma may give rise to cerebrospinal fluid metastases.[99] These metastases occur in the spinal canal and are seen only after posterior fossa craniotomy.

Microscopic Changes

Hemangioblastoma consists of a proliferation of vascular spaces and endothelial cells separated by fat-laden stromal cells. The endothelial cells proliferate in greater numbers than required to line the vascular spaces and form a multilayered envelope of cells of uniform cytological appearance. They have few or no mitoses (Fig. 88–1).[65,155] The name "hemangioblastoma" is unfortunate, since it carries the connotation of an aggressive, primitive, anaplastic neoplasm, which reflects neither the tumor's benign natural history nor the uniform cellular structure with a very low mitotic rate and little pleomorphism. The hemangioblastic variant of angioblastic meningioma has the same histological appearance as a hemangioblastoma and is considered to be one.

Reticulin stains demonstrate a network of fibers that surround the separate vessels and outline the neoplastic endothelial proliferation arising from each capillary, as shown in Figure 88–1. Calcium is rarely seen.[75,118]

Apparently solid hemangioblastomas may contain small cysts whose walls are composed of neoplastic tissue. The typical cystic one has a mural nodule of tumor in a cyst whose wall is composed of compressed cerebellum.[35,132,133] Histological examination of this wall shows only gliosis. The neoplastic tissue is not surrounded by a capsule, but the zone of infiltration is so narrow that the tumor is essentially noninvasive.[70,84,132] The histological pattern may resemble metastatic hypernephroma. Sometimes the two can be differentiated by mitotic figures and prominent nucleoli that suggest anaplastic neoplasm rather than hemangioblastoma.[136]

The stroma interspersed between capillaries was thought by Lindau to contain endothelial cells that had ingested lipids, possibly lipids that resulted from degeneration of myelin.[84] These fat-laden cells can enlarge and develop into multinucleated giant cells. Immunological studies have demonstrated an endothelial origin for the perivascular cells, but not for the stromal cells, which originate either from pericytes or from a separate cell line that replicates in parallel with the endothelial cell line.[71,74] Spence and Rubinstein have suggested that the stromal cells may be aberrant angiogenic mesenchymal precursors that are prevented from maturing into endothelial cells.[141] An alternative explanation is that the stromal cells are of pial origin.[132] Whatever the origin of cells making up hemangioblastoma, some cellular plasticity must be present, since at least 10 per cent of hemangioblastomas have areas resembling meningioma.[45,65]

There is disagreement regarding the interpretation of electron microscopy of hemangioblastoma. Some authors believe that the perivascular and stromal cells represent a single cell type.[27,31] Cytoplasmic whorled structures have been suggested to be either mast cells or areas of myelin production.[27,30]

Clinical Presentation

Headache is the first symptom of approximately 80 per cent of these tumors and is present at some time in the course of 90 to 95 per cent of patients with hemangioblastomas of the cerebellum. The headache is suboccipital and intermittent. Vomiting occurs in approximately 60 per cent of cases. Vertigo and diplopia also are common. Occasionally, hydrocephalus produces severe mental changes, and a degree of mental change marks 25 per cent of

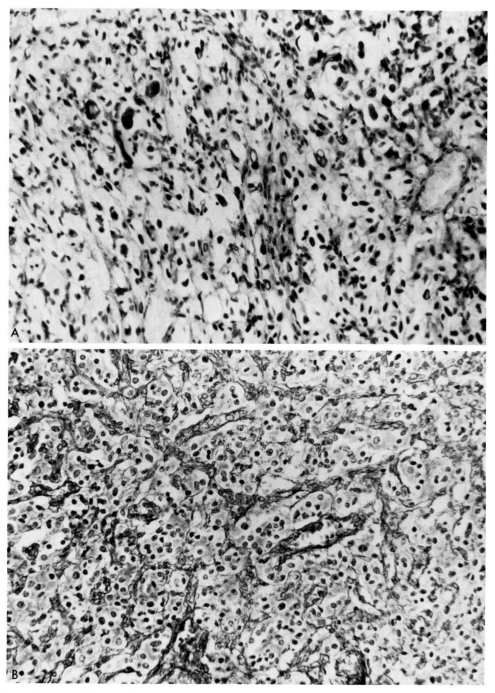

Figure 88–1   *A*. Microscopic pathological changes of hemangioblastoma. Numerous endothelium-lined vascular spaces are separated by fat-laden cells. 450 ×. *B*. Reticulin stain emphasizes the vascular nature of the tumor. 450 ×. (Courtesy of Surl L. Nielsen, M.D., University of California, Davis.)

cases. Rarely, the initial manifestation is a subarachnoid or parenchymal hemorrhage; in the case of a similar tumor of the occipital bone, it was acute epidural hematoma. In the supratentorial meninges these tumors mimic meningiomas in their clinical presentations.

Average duration of symptoms before operation is approximately seven months, although it may extend to 10 years. Tumors in the brain stem cause symptoms for one to two years, and cerebral lesions, for a median span of approximately two years. Cerebellar deficit is the initial symptom in only approximately 10 per cent, but occurs at some time in 60 per cent of patients. Nystagmus and ataxia are present in approximately 60 per cent, and papilledema is present in 70 per cent of cases. Cranial nerve paresis is noted in 30 per cent, and corticospinal tract involvement can be identified in 25 per cent of them. The sixth and seventh cranial nerves are equally likely to be affected.*

Clinical signs allow accurate localization to the cerebellum in only half the patients, and in some findings may be confusing, perhaps because of multiple masses. Occasionally, patients with cerebellar hemangioblastoma develop paralysis of upward gaze. This is particularly likely to occur when the tumor is in the roof of the fourth ventricle.[100]

Although several authors had described cases prior to von Hippel's report, hemangioblastoma of the retina is called von Hippel's disease. It appears as a reddish retinal mass peripherally situated between a dilated artery and vein.[100,147] Often there are inflammation and exudates that obscure the dilated vessels. Hemorrhage may cause retinal detachment. The end result of the hemorrhage is a painful blind eye with glaucoma, cataract, and uveitis. Even after enucleation and pathological examination the diagnosis of von Hippel's disease may be difficult because of reactive gliosis and connective tissue proliferation in the region of the tumor. Reticulin stains will outline the neoplastic elements and may be of use in making the diagnosis.[84] When ocular and cerebellar tumors coexist, visual symptoms usually precede clinical evidence of the

cerebellar lesion. In one third of patients with retinal hemangioblastoma, the eye tumors are multiple.[96]

Identification of retinal hemangioblastoma may allow preoperative diagnosis of Lindau's disease in a patient with a cerebellar tumor. Cerebellar hemangioblastomas are also associated with an increased incidence of pheochromocytoma and renal tumors.[32,106,148] The benign components of Lindau's disease (cysts of the pancreas, kidney, and liver; and tumors of the epididymis) may also be present, although they rarely are symptomatic.[51,58]

Investigation

Patients suspected of having hemangioblastoma should have a careful physical examination to insure that other components of Lindau's disease are not present. Detailed funduscopic examination of the peripheral retina should be performed and evaluation for possible hypernephroma or pheochromocytoma considered. Erythrocytosis, if present, should be carefully documented because it may be useful in following the effects of treatment on the neoplasm.[69,70]

Although skull x-rays reveal evidence of increased intracranial pressure in approximately one third of patients, tumor calcification does not occur to a sufficient extent to allow localization with plain radiographs.[69,96,113] Identification and localization of the tumor usually require computed tomography or angiography. Isotope scan demonstrates approximately 80 per cent of cerebellar hemangioblastomas, but can miss those that are predominantly cystic, even when they occur in the supratentorial space.[69,94,96]

The CT scan reveals a tumor with density similar to that of brain that is enhanced by contrast. It may or may not be associated with a cyst (Fig. 88–2).[53] The mass effect of the tumor narrows the pontine and quadrigeminal cisterns and collapses the fourth ventricle, which in turn causes enlargement of the lateral ventricles.

Angiography is particularly useful in patients with hemangioblastoma (Figure 88–3). A meshwork of small vessels or occasionally a homogeneous stain may identify the neoplasm and may allow accurate local-

---

* See references 18, 41, 46, 68–70, 91, 96, 101, 102, 109–111, 113, 118, 136, 138.

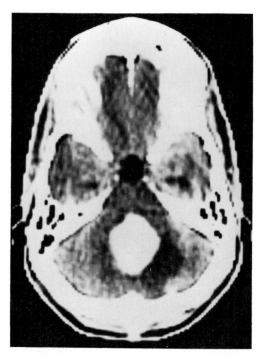

Figure 88-2 Computed tomography of a hemangioblastoma after intravenous injection of iodinated contrast material demonstrates a densely enhanced tumor of the vermis. (Courtesy of Frank A. Brown, M.D., Sutter Community Hospitals, Sacramento, California.)

ization of a tumor nodule.[86] Rarely is the angiogram normal with this tumor, and it may identify multiple neoplasms overlooked by CT scanning.[69,110,113] Occasionally angiography identifies an avascular mass without apparent neoplastic circulation.

To a large extent, ventriculography has been replaced by other studies. When performed, it demonstrates upward displacement of the posterior portion of the third ventricle as well as forward and sometimes lateral displacement of the fourth ventricle. Myelography is unwise in most cases of cerebellar tumor, but in patients with tumors of the caudal medulla, myelography, air encephalography, or possibly CT scan enhanced by subarachnoid instillation of water-soluble contrast material may demonstrate a lobulated tumor that can mimic tonsillar herniation.[22] Spinal fluid is often under increased pressure, and the protein level is raised in approximately half the patients. The protein level in the cyst contents is high, averaging 3.7 gm per 100 ml.[70,113]

Erythrocytosis occurs in 10 to 50 per cent of patients with cerebellar hemangioblastomas and has been reported with those in

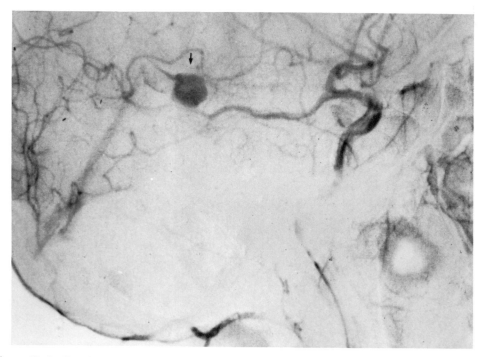

Figure 88-3 Vertebral angiography shows a small hemangioblastoma. (Courtesy of Michel Djindjian, M.D., Hôpital Henri Mondor, Paris; and Arthur B. Dublin, M.D., University of California, Davis.)

the supratentorial area.* This erythrocytosis subsides after removal of the tumor in at least half the cases, but may recur if tumor recurs.[29,148] The increase in the red cell mass is due to secretion of erythropoietin by cytoplasmic secretory granules in the tumor.[67,124,148] Both cystic and solid hemangioblastomas can cause proliferation of erythrocytres, but it is more common with the solid ones.[70,113,138] There may be a relationship between the lipid-containing stromal cells and erythropoietin, since neoplasms tend to produce erythrocytosis only if they contain cells that are swollen with lipid material.[70]

Treatment and Results

For many years, this tumor has been recognized as one of the most favorable for operative treatment.[133] If the entire tumor is removed, the morbidity usually is minimal and regrowth is unusual. Indeed, regrowth of the tumor suggests a second primary neoplasm.

The operative approach to the cerebellar lesion should allow a wide resection of the bone. If a cyst is present, the fluid should be saved for erythropoietin assay in case a mural nodule cannot be identified.[69] Decompression of the cyst is of temporary benefit. Fewer than 20 per cent of patients are helped for more than 48 hours.[35,69,110,113,133] The cyst should be opened, and a mural nodule should be identified if possible.[69,111] Even if none is found, it probably is present but has been overlooked.[35] In this circumstance, repeat vertebral angiography usually will reveal the nodule and reoperation for its excision is reasonable. If a solid tumor is identified, operative removal may be more difficult. The neoplasm tends to be vascular, and dissection is best performed through the cerebellar tissue adjacent to the tumor.[111,116]

After tumor removal, the posterior fossa dura should be left open.[113] Postoperative ventricular shunting is required in only 10 per cent of patients.[69] A superior vermis tumor may be less difficult to remove if it is approached through the tentorium.[111]

The operative mortality rate was 25 to 30 per cent in the early experience with cerebellar hemangioblastoma.[18,100] In the 1950's, death rates of 15 to 20 per cent could be expected.[111,136] Most current series report rates of approximately 15 per cent.[69,101,138] Usually, however, they include patients operated on before the development of modern antibiotics and glucocorticoids and the widespread availability of assisted ventilation in the postoperative period. Many of the deaths in the past were due to meningitis resulting from cerebrospinal fluid leakage. This is less of a problem with more deliberate wound closure and with early detection and aggressive antibiotic treatment of meningitis. Some operative death rates as low as 6 to 8 per cent have been reported.[101,113]

There is little difference in the operative mortality rates for partial and total removal of tumors, but undoubtedly the tumors that are more difficult to remove undergo partial excision, and if a more aggressive removal were attempted, the death rate for this group might be high. Patients with solid tumors are three times as likely to die in the postoperative period as are patients with cystic tumors.[69,138] This increased risk is due to greater difficulty with hemostasis and greater likelihood of involvement of the brain stem and fourth ventricle.[109] Few reports of excision of brain stem hemangioblastomas are available. Operative deaths for these lesions, even with the most modern postoperative care, amount to approximately 33 per cent.[33,138] Postoperative deaths may be due to posterior fossa hematoma, supratentorial hematoma, brain stem infarction, or systemic complications such as pulmonary emboli.[113] For the hemangioblastic type of angioblastic meningioma, the operative mortality rate is approximately the same as for cerebellar hemangioblastoma.[118]

Radiotherapy of this tumor has not been subjected to a prospective randomized trial, but clinical impressions suggest that it offers little or no benefit for those in the central nervous system.[73,113,138] It does not suppress the erythropoietic activity of the tumor and does not prevent regrowth after incomplete removal.

In patients who survive the initial operation, the approximate survival rates are 90 per cent at 5 years, 80 per cent at 10 years, and 35 per cent at 20 years. Often death is not due to the neoplasm or its treatment.[101,113,138] If only patients who have in-

---

* See references 29, 41, 70, 96, 109, 113, 117, 136, 138.

complete removal of tumor are studied, more than 50 per cent die of tumor recurrence. After apparently total excisions, recurrence of tumor occurs in 3 to 10 per cent.[69,110,113] If it does occur, reoperation may be required and can be done repeatedly.[101]

Recurrence of symptoms of cerebellar hemangioblastoma may be due to a new primary tumor, a problem that has been estimated to arise in at least 5 to 10 per cent of patients.[101,111,113] The usual time between first and second operations is five to seven years.[116]

Seventy-five to ninety per cent of patients have little neurological deficit after operation.[69,77,111] Some of the neurological dysfunction that does occur after operation may be due to causes unrelated to the cerebellar tumor, while recurrent or new neoplasm explains much of the remaining dysfunction.

HEMANGIOPERICYTOMA

In 1942 Stout and Murray described an extraneural tumor composed of a proliferation of capillary blood vessels with normal endothelial cells surrounded by neoplastic perivascular cells that were presumed to arise from pericytes.[144] The neoplasm was named hemangiopericytoma. It has subsequently been realized that this tumor is identical with the angioblastic type of meningioma reported by Bailey, Cushing, and Eisenhardt, and with the variant I of angioblastic meningioma defined by Cushing and Eisenhardt.[14,45,103] Early reports of brain tumors in which the pathological changes were correctly identified as those of hemangiopericytoma were isolated cases, but this neoplasm has become more familiar to pathologists and larger series are being reported.[65,118,139]

The spectrum of hemangiopericytoma remains undefined. A neoplasm formerly called papillarly meningioma may be a variant of hemangiopericytoma.[88] Some rare neoplasms containing both hemangiopericytic areas and areas of typical meningioma or hemangioblastoma have been reported. The authors have such a case. The rarity of this occurrence is, however, stressed by the fact that Muller and Mealey deny the existence of tumors that cross these boundaries.[65,88,103]

Incidence

Owing to the infrequency of clinical reports, the incidence of hemangiopericytoma has been difficult to determine. In 1971, Muller and Mealey were able to discover only 44 cases; many more have, however, been reported subsequently.[103] Approximately 1 per cent of meningiomas are of the hemangiopericytic variety.[72,118]

If an analogy can be made with extraneural hemangiopericytoma, the neoplasm would be expected to affect the sexes equally and to occur at all ages.[7,73] Most reports of central nervous system hemangiopericytomas have included few clinical details. The incidence may be higher in men than in women.[56] The average age of patients is in the early forties, but the tumor may occur over a wide spread of ages.

Pathology

Macroscopic Changes

Hemangiopericytomas usually present as firm vascular tumors attached to the meninges. They tend to compress and displace the brain rather than to invade it.[56] They may arise in any of the locations in which meningiomas are found, including the choroid plexus.[93] Approximately 80 per cent of them are supratentorial, but they can occur in the cerebellopontine angle, the foramen magnum, or the spine.[65] Approximately 10 per cent appear to be separate from the meninges and are found in the central nervous system parenchyma.[65,155] They may arise from pia in the depths of sulci or may have some other source that has not yet been identified.

Microscopic Changes

The histological pattern is a meshwork of capillaries lined by normal endothelial cells outside of which is found a dense collection of neoplastic rounded or elongated cells containing mitoses (Fig. 88–4).[56,143] Necrosis may be seen, as may cellular pleomorphism and binucleate or multinucleate cells. The mitotic rate usually is one to five mitoses in 10 separate high-power fields, although up to 25 to 50 mitoses per high-power field may be seen.[65] Histological identification may be aided by reticulin stains. These stains demonstrate an abun-

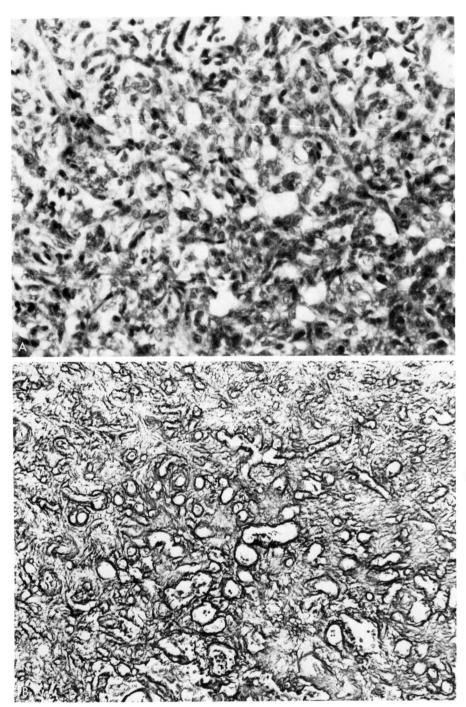

Figure 88–4   *A*. Microscopic pathological changes of hemangiopericytoma. A meshwork of capillaries lined by normal endothelial cells are surrounded by neoplastic cells. 450 ×. *B*. Reticulin stain emphasizes the vascular pattern. 250 ×.

dant reticulin stroma around most tumor cells and show the neoplastic cells to be outside the perivascular reticulin sheath. Immunological studies confirm that the neoplastic cells are not endothelial in origin.[71]

A histological pattern of dense cellularity, frequent mitoses, and foci of necrosis or hemorrhage suggests that the natural history will be more malignant than if these changes are not present and that metastases can be expected.[47,95] Only one series has been studied for the effect of anaplasia on prognosis in those of the nervous system, and a statistically significant correlation could not be identified.[56]

Electron microscopy has demonstrated the similarity between smooth muscle and the neoplastic cells of hemangiopericytoma both in the central nervous system and in extraneural sites.[16,59,114]

Clinical Presentation

Hemangiopericytomas of the meninges present with the symptoms and signs that would be expected for meningiomas in the same location.[118] The most common symptom is headache, which is noted in half the patients.[56] Paresis is present in approximately 25 per cent, and seizures occur in approximately 20 per cent of patients. Symptoms are present for a mean of eight months with the hemangiopericytic type of angioblastic meningioma as opposed to two years with the hemangioblastic type.[118]

Investigation

The laboratory findings in hemangiopericytoma are similar to those found in meningiomas. Computed tomography shows it, and it is enhanced by intravenous contrast media.

Treatment and Results

As for extraneural hemangiopericytomas, the treatment of choice for those in the central nervous system is complete excision.[7] Operative removal may be made more difficult by intraoperative hemorrhage.[56] Radiotherapy may be beneficial in

central nervous system tumor, although it does not seem to help extraneural ones.[47,52]

Symptoms of tumor regrowth occur in approximately 75 per cent of cases.[71,78,139] Since the mean survival is 7.3 years after initial operation, long-term follow-up is required.[56] Of patients who survive the postoperative period but later die of recurrence, three fourths have local recurrence and one fourth have metastases.[118] Extraneural metastases occur in 12 to 25 per cent of these patients.[56,155] As is true of other central nervous system tumors, bone and lung are the most common sites for metastases.

SARCOMAS

In the nineteenth century, the term "sarcoma" was applied to so-called fleshy tumors, and most brain tumors were placed in this category. After Bailey and Cushing demonstrated that the majority of brain tumors were of neuroglial origin, the diagnosis of sarcoma was made less often because of its restriction to tumors of proved mesodermal origin.[13,66,151] Unfortunately, the origin of the meninges was unclear, and controversy surrounded the relative contribution of neural crest and mesodermal elements.[61,62,150] Neoplasms presumed to arise from leptomeninges (e.g., meningiomas) were separated and labeled as a discrete group, and their classification was not based on histogenesis. The confusion produced by histogenetic classification with selected exceptions was lessened by the pragmatic definition of sarcoma as an anaplastic tumor composed of cells of the connective tissue type.[1,156] Perhaps the most convenient definition of sarcoma of the brain identifies it as a neoplasm resembling extraneural neoplasms that have been identified as sarcomas.[66] Thus, if an anaplastic neoplasm of muscle is called a rhabdomyosarcoma in the leg, a similar tumor in the brain would be a sarcoma.

Classification

If a sarcoma is a tumor of connective tissue elements, it should be able to occur in dura and leptomeninges, cerebral vessels, the velum of the choriodal tela, and the other sites of concentration of connective tissue.[34,48,66] Early classifications are confusing and undoubtedly included malignant lymphomas, subarachnoid metastases from medulloblastoma, and anaplastic (malignant) meningiomas as well as lesions that, in retrospect, may have been nonneoplastic.* Terms such as "perivascular sarcoma" and "perithelial sarcoma," which are based on the distribution of tumor in the brain rather than on histological characteristics, have been difficult to correlate with the more common cellular types of sarcomas such as fibrosarcoma or osteogenic sarcoma.

The World Health Organization does not list sarcomas separately but includes them in the general category of tumors of meningeal and related tissues.[140] The subdivisions of this category are outlined in Table 88–1.

Some authors list anaplastic meningiomas as sarcomas.[10,36] In the World Health Orgnization classification, neoplasms that are the result of anaplastic change in a meningioma are considered anaplastic meningiomas and are not listed as sarcomas. Differentiation between anaplastic meningioma and meningeal fibrosarcoma depends on the degree of anaplasia and brain invasion and possibly on cellular differences that can be recognized by electron microscopy. If meningothelial portions of meningiomas arise from arachnoid cells, while fibroblastic areas arise from connective tissue elements in the meninges, anaplasia of these separate elements might preserve differences between some anaplastic meningiomas and fibrosarcomas.[21] In practice, these differences are blurred. Typical meningotheliomatous meningiomas may recur as histological fibrosarcoma, and meningiomas have developed some degree of anaplasia in 12 per cent of recurrent tumors.[34,72,126] If an anaplastic tumor has areas that can be recognized as meningiomatous, it is considered to be an anaplastic meningioma unless it is markedly anaplastic, in which case it may be called a sarcoma.[129] If an anaplastic meningeal tumor contains no evidence of meningioma origin, it is considered to be a fibrosarcoma. Invasion of brain has been variously regarded as a property of fibrosarcoma and of anaplastic meningioma.[72,76,132] Some authors, however, never classify invasive tumors as anaplastic meningiomas but believe that invasion of brain is sufficient evidence to label a neoplasm as meningeal sarcoma.[157]

The neoplasm called monstrocellular sarcoma or giant cell fibrosarcoma is probably an anaplastic glioma with giant astrocytes and has been discussed in Chapter 86. Although it is included under vascular tumors in the World Health Organization classification, there is considerable doubt about the existence of a nongliomatous tumor of this type.

Circumscribed arachnoidal cerebellar sarcoma is a connective tissue mass in the posterior fossa and has been shown usually to consist of a fibrous response of the meninges to invading medulloblastoma and not to be an independent sarcoma.[130] In a similar fashion, gliomas may elicit an intense connective tissue response (cf. Chapter 84). This response may be so intense that an independent sarcoma arises.[48,127,145] The sarcomatous component probably develops from blood vessel walls.[49] A primary sarcoma is also capable of eliciting anaplastic glial tumor.[76,126,132] In some cases, both the glial and sarcomatous elements may arise concomitantly as a response to an oncogenic stimulus.[112]

Some lymphomas have, in the past, been classified as sarcomas. Perivascular sarcoma probably is a lymphoma in most instances.[21,66] Reticulum cell sarcoma of brain is discussed as a lymphoma in Chapter 87.

In most instances the cause of primary central nervous system sarcomas is unknown. Previous radiotherapy has, however, been associated with a number of meningeal fibrosarcomas.[135,149] This experience parallels the demonstrated production of sarcomas arising many years after radiotherapy to extraneural tissues.[26,152] Most patients with irradiation-induced sarcomas have undergone pituitary radiotherapy. X-ray treatment for other neoplasms has, however, also been reported to be followed by sarcoma.[90,108,135] The true incidence of sarcoma from this cause is unknown, since most patients who undergo radiotherapy to the central nervous system die of their original neoplasm before there is time for a sarcoma to develop. It is possible that some patients with presumed recurrent gliomas have unrecognized fibrosarcoma.

---

* See references 9, 12, 34, 60, 66, 129.

Incidence

The incidence of sarcomas depends on the particular subtypes of brain tumors included in their category. If neoplasms that may be of glial origin, such as "monstrocellular sarcoma," are included, up to approximately 3 per cent of brain tumors will be so identified.[157] In other series, the incidence is reported as 1 per cent.[44,107,154] These figures may be higher than would be appropriate for the narrower definition used in this chapter. A more accurate estimate of the number of sarcomas, as defined by the World Health Organization classification, is probably to be found in the reported incidence of fibrosarcomas. These neoplasms account for approximately 0.1 to 0.6 per cent of brain tumors.[20,44,107]

If the World Health Organization classification is followed, the majority of sarcomatous masses are either anaplastic meningiomas, coexistent sarcomas and gliomas, or fibrosarcomas. Anaplastic meningiomas are discussed in Chapter 90. Gliomas and sarcomas arising together are included in Chapter 86. Other types of sarcomatous tumors have been reported but are rare. These include fibromyxosarcoma, mesenchymal chondrosarcoma, and osteogenic sarcoma.*

Rhabdomyosarcoma is a rare primary central nervous system neoplasm. It is presumed to arise from multipotential mesenchymal tissues and can produce a spindle cell histological pattern as well as collections of small round or oval cells.[80,87,98] The diagnostic feature of the neoplasm is cross-striations in cells. The clinical course is one of rapid deterioration. Excision and radiotherapy may prolong survival.

Pathology

Fibrosarcoma arising from the meninges usually is firm and white. When it arises from perivascular connective tissue and occurs in the parenchyma of the brain, it may be soft and gray. Necrosis can be identified in many of the more anaplastic fibrosarcomas but is unusual in the less anaplastic ones. The interface between neoplasm

and brain is ill defined. Surrounding edema may be quite marked. The tumor may arise in any part of the brain. Approximately 20 per cent are in the posterior fossa. They may spread through the subarachnoid pathways, and operative intervention may give them access to the systemic circulation and allow systemic metastases.[2,28]

The microscopic appearance is characterized by fibroblasts with a reticulin and sometimes collagenous background (Fig. 88–5).[107] Nuclei of these cells are oval, have chromatin content similar to fibroblasts in other sites, and have little pleomorphism.[20,76] There are few mitotic figures. The cytoplasmic configuration tends to be bipolar. They usually form abundant reticulin fibers, but the amount of reticulin is not always a good criterion for establishing a diagnosis of sarcoma.[76]

On the basis of their increasing anaplasia, these tumors can be divided into three types: fibrous, spindle cell, and polymorphocellular.[34] The more anaplastic types have greater cellularity and more frequent mitoses. These factors indicate an ominous prognosis.[72,139] The more anaplastic lesions are more difficult to diagnose and are more common than the less anaplastic ones.

Clinical Presentation

Fibrosarcomas occur with equal frequency in both sexes.[20] The anaplastic forms tend to occur in younger patients; and the very anaplastic forms, in children.[34,55] Duration of symptoms is often less than six months.[18] A long history of symptoms suggests anaplasia from a previous meningioma.

There are no specific clinical manifestations that separate sarcomas from other intracranial neoplasms. Most patients have headache, and many have papilledema. Evidence of increased intracranial pressure is particularly frequent with the more anaplastic forms. Seizures occur in approximately 25 per cent.[34] Spontaneous hemorrhage may also occur.[125]

Spinal metastases are apparent in approximately 10 per cent of patients with intracranial fibrosarcomas.[34] Usually a posterior fossa sarcoma is the initial intracranial neoplasm.

Cells and protein in cerebrospinal fluid

* See references 4, 15, 57, 76, 121, 132.

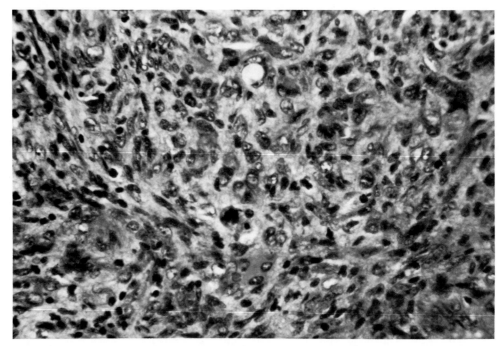

Figure 88–5 Microscopic examination of a fibrosarcoma reveals an anaplastic tumor with pleomorphism of fibroblasts. 450 ×. (Courtesy of Surl L. Nielsen, M.D., University of California, Davis.)

usually are normal. In view of the frequency of increased intracranial pressure and the danger of transtentorial or tonsillar herniation, together with the lack of diagnostic help provided by cerebrospinal fluid, lumbar puncture is not advisable. The lesion is shown on enhanced CT scans and can be identified by isotope brain scan.

Treatment and Results

The standard treatment of intracranial sarcomas has been operative. This allows tissue diagnosis and decompression of intracranial mass. Details of operative technique are covered in Chapters 31 and 86. Although gross total operative removal of the more anaplastic fibrosarcomas usually is not possible, most of the nonanaplastic ones can be totally removed.[34] Clinical impression suggests that radiotherapy is beneficial and may prolong life, but no data are available to prove the point.[12,76] Few patients with markedly anaplastic fibrosarcomas live more than six months, while few patients with nonanaplastic ones die in less than two years. Christensen and Lara found average postoperative survival in four patients with fibrous fibrosarcomas to be 74 months. Nine

patients with spindle cell fibrosarcomas survived a mean of 27 months, and nine with polymorphocellular fibrosarcomas survived a mean of only 12 months. Only 3 of their entire series of 22 patients available for postoperative follow-up survived for five years.[34]

REFERENCES

1. Abbott, K. H., and Kernohan, J. W.: Primary sarcomas of the brain: Review of the literature and report of twelve cases. Arch. Neurol. Psychiat., *50*:43–66, 1943.
2. Abbott, K. H., and Love, J. G.: Metastasizing intracranial tumors. Ann. Surg., *118*:343–352, 1943.
3. Adams, J. E.: Familial hemangioblastoma of the cerebellum: Pedigree of two families. J. Neurosurg., *10*:421–423, 1953.
4. Amine, A. R. C., and Sugar, O.: Suprasellar osteogenic sarcoma following radiation for pituitary adenoma: Case report. J. Neurosurg., *44*:88–91, 1976.
5. Averback, P.: Mixed intracranial sarcomas: Rare forms and a new association with previous radiation therapy. Ann. Neurol., *4*:229–233, 1978.
6. Bachman, K., Markwalder, R., and Seiler, R. W.: Supratentorial hemangioblastoma: Case report. Acta Neurochir. (Wien), *44*:173–177, 1978.
7. Backwinkel, K. D., and Diddams, J. A.: Hemangiopericytoma: Report of a case and compre-

hensive review of the literature. Cancer, 25:896–901, 1970.

8. Bailey, O. T., and Ford, R.: Sclerosing hemangiomas of the central nervous system: Progressive tissue changes in hemangioblastomas of the brain and in so-called angioblastic meningiomas. Amer. J. Path., 18:1–27, 1942.

9. Bailey, O. T., and Ingraham, F. D.: Intracranial fibrosarcomas of the dura mater in childhood: Pathological characteristics and surgical management. J. Neurosurg., 2:1–15, 1945.

10. Bailey, P.: Intracranial sarcomatous tumors of leptomeningeal origin. Arch. Surg. (Chicago), 18:1359–1402, 1929.

11. Bailey, P.: A propos d'une forme speciale de méningiome angioblastique. J. Neurol. Psychiat., 29:577–581, 1929.

12. Bailey, P., and Bucy, P. C.: The origin and nature of meningeal tumors. Amer. J. Cancer, 15:15–54, 1931.

13. Bailey, P., and Cushing H.: A Classification of the Tumors of the Glioma Group on a Histogenetic Basis with a Correlated Study of Prognosis. Philadelphia, J. B. Lippincott, 1926.

14. Bailey, P., Cushing, H., and Eisenhardt, L.: Angioblastic meningiomas. Arch. Path. Lab. Med., 6:953–990, 1928.

15. Baker, G. S., Dockerty, M. B., and Kennedy, R. L.: Fibromyxosarcoma of the skull and meninges: Report of case. Mayo Clin. Proc., 25:129–134, 1950.

16. Battifora, H.: Hemangiopericytoma: Ultrastructural study of five cases. Cancer, 31:1418–1432, 1973.

17. Begg, C. F., and Garret, R.: Hemangiopericytoma occurring in the meninges: Case report. Cancer, 7:602–606, 1954.

18. Bennett, W. A.: Primary intracranial neoplasms in military age group: World War II. Milit. Surg., 99:594–652, 1946.

19. Bergstrand, H.: On the classification of the hemangiomatous tumours and malformations of the central nervous system. Acta Path. Microbiol. Scand., suppl. 26:89–95, 1936.

20. Bingas, B.: On the primary sarcomas of the brain. Acta Neurochir. (Wien) suppl., 10:186–189, 1963.

21. Black, V. K., and Kernohan, J. W.: Primary diffuse tumors of the meninges (so-called meningeal meningiomatosis). Cancer, 3:805–819, 1950.

22. Bloch, S., and Danziger, J.: Hemangioblastomas presenting at the cervical medullary junction. S. Afr. Med. J., 47:2452–2456, 1973.

23. Bonebrake, R. A., and Siqueira, E. B.: Familial occurrence of solitary hemangioblastoma of the cerebellum. Neurology (Minneap.), 14:733–743, 1964.

24. Bradford, F. K.: Hemangioblastoma of the posterior fossa (Lindau's disease): Report of two cases with familial history. J. Neurosurg., 5:196–201, 1948.

25. Brown, M. H., and Kernohan, J. W.: Diffuse meningiomatosis. Arch. Path. (Chicago), 32:651–658, 1941.

26. Cahan, W. G., Woodard, H. Q., Higinbotham, N. L., Stewart, F. W., and Coley, E. L.: Sarcoma arising in irradiated bone: Report of eleven cases. Cancer, 1:3–29, 1948.

27. Cancilla, P. A., and Zimmerman, H. M.: The fine structure of a cerebellar hemangioblastoma. J. Neuropath. Exp. Neurol., 24:621–628, 1965.

28. Caner, G. C.: Case 24312, New Eng. J. Med., 219:169–173, 1938.

29. Carpenter, G., Schwartz, H., and Walker, A. E.: Neurogenic polycythemia. Ann. Intern. Med., 19:470–481, 1943.

30. Castaigne, P., David, M., Pertuiset, B., Escourolle, R., and Poirier, J.: L'Ultrastructure des hémangioblastomes du système nerveux central. Rev. Neurol. (Paris), 118:5–26, 1968.

31. Cervos-Navarro, J.: Elektronenmikroskopie der Hämangioblastome des ZNS und der angioblastichen Meningiome. Acta Neuropath. (Berlin), 19:184–207, 1971.

32. Chapman, R. C., and Diaz-Perez, R.: Pheochromocytoma associated with cerebellar hemangioblastoma: Familial occurrence. J.A.M.A., 182:1014–1017, 1962.

33. Chou, S. N., Erickson, E. L., and Ortiz-Suarez, H. J.: Surgical treatment of vascular lesions in the brain stem. J. Neurosurg., 42:23–31, 1975.

34. Christensen, E., and Lara, E.: Intracranial sarcomas. J. Neuropath. Exp. Neurol., 12:41–56, 1953.

35. Corradini, E. W., and Browder, J.: Angioblastic neoplasms of the brain. J. Neuropath. Exp. Neurol., 7:299–308, 1948.

36. Courville, C. B.: Pathology of the Central Nervous System. 2nd Ed. Mountain View, Calif., Pacific Press Pub. Ass., 1945.

37. Courville, C. B., and Abbott, K. H.: On the classification of meningiomas: A survey of 99 cases in the light of existing schemes. Bull. Los Angeles Neurol. Soc., 6:21–31, 1941.

38. Craig, W. M., and Horrax, G.: The occurrence of hemangioblastomas (two cerebellar and one spinal) in three members of a family. J. Neurosurg., 6:518–529, 1949.

39. Craig, W. M., and Keith, H. M.: Tumors of the brain occurring in childhood. Acta Psychiat. Neurol. Scand., 24:375–390, 1949.

40. Craig, W. M., and Kernohan, J. W.: Tumors of the fourth ventricle. J.A.M.A., 111:2370–2377, 1938.

41. Cramer, F., and Kimsey, W.: The cerebellar hemangioblastomas: Review of 53 cases with special reference to cerebellar cysts and the association of polycythemia. Arch. Neurol. Psychiat., 67:237–252, 1952.

42. Crompton, M. R., and Gautier-Smith, R. C.: The prediction of recurrence in meningiomas. J. Neurol. Neurosurg. Psychiat., 33:80–87, 1970.

43. Cushing, H. C.: The meningiomas (dural endotheliomas): Their source and favoured seats of origin. Brain, 45:282–316, 1922.

44. Cushing, H.: Intracranial Tumors: Notes upon a Series of Two Thousand Verified Cases with Surgical Mortality Percentages Pertaining Thereto. Springfield, Ill., Charles C Thomas, 1932.

45. Cushing, H., and Eisenhardt, L.: The Meningiomas: Their Classification, Regional Behavior, Life History, and Surgical End Results. Springfield, Ill, Charles C Thomas, 1938.

46. Davison, C., Schick, W., and Goodhart, S. P.: Cerebellar hemangioblastomas with incidental

changes of the spinal cord. Arch. Neurol. Psychiat., 25:783–802, 1931.

47. Enzinger, F. M., and Smith, B. H.: Hemangiopericytoma: An analysis of 106 cases. Hum. Path., 7:61–82, 1976.

48. Feigin, I., Allen, L. B., Lipkin, L., and Gross, S. W.: The endothelial hyperplasia of the cerebral blood vessels with brain tumors, and its sarcomatous transformation. Cancer, 11:264–277, 1958.

49. Feigin, I. H., and Gross, S. W.: Sarcoma arising in glioblastoma of the brain, Amer. J. Path., 31:633–653, 1955.

50. Fisher, E. R., Davis, J. S., and Lemmen, L. J.: Meningeal hemangiopericytoma. Arch, Neurol. Psychiat., 79:40–45, 1958.

51. Fishman, R. S., and Bartholomew, L. G.: Severe pancreatic involvement in three generations in von Hippel-Lindau disease. Mayo Clin. Proc., 54:329–331, 1979.

52. Fukui, M., Kitamura, K., Ohgami, S., Takaki, T., Kinoshita, K., Watanabe, K., and Mihara, K.: Radiosensitivity of meningioma—analysis of five cases of highly vascular meningioma treated by preoperative irradiation. Acta Neurochir. (Wien), 36:47–60, 1977.

53. Gado, M., Huete, I., and Mikhael, M.: Computerized tomography of infratentorial tumors. Seminars Roentgen., 12:109–120, 1977.

54. Garret, R.: Glioblastoma and fibrosarcoma of the brain with extracranial metastasis. Cancer, 11:888–894, 1958.

55. Globus, J. H., Levin, S., and Sheps, J. G.: Primary sarcomatous meningioma (primary sarcoma of the brain). J. Neuropath. Exp. Neurol., 3:311–343, 1944.

56. Goellner, J. R., Laws, E. R., Soule, E. H., and Okazaki, H.: Hemangiopericytoma of the meninges: Mayo Clinic experience. Amer. J. Clin. Path., 70:375–380, 1978.

57. Guccion, J. G., Font, R. L., Enzinger, F. M., and Zimmerman, L. E.: Extraskeletal mesenchymal chondrosarcoma. Arch. Path. (Chicago), 95:336–340, 1973.

58. Gullotta, F., and Wullenweber, R.: Meningiomi angioblastici ed emangiopericitomi meningei: Ricerche in situ e in vitro. Acta Neurol. (Napoli), 24:581–592, 1969.

59. Hahn, M. J., Dawson, R., Esterly, J. A., and Joseph, D. J.: Hemangiopericytoma: An ultrastructural study. Cancer, 31:255–261, 1973.

60. Hanberry, J. W., and Dugger, G. S.: Perithelial sarcoma of the brain: A clinical pathological study of 13 cases. Arch. Neurol. Psychiat., 71:732–761, 1954.

61. Harvey, S. C., and Burr, H. S.: The development of the meninges. Arch. Neurol. Psychiat., 15:545–567, 1926.

62. Harvey, S. C., Burr, H. S., and VanCampenhout, E.: Development of the meninges: Further experiments. Arch. Neurol. Psychiat., 29:683–690, 1933.

63. Hitselberger, W. E., Kernohan, J. W., and Uihlein, A.: Giant cell fibrosarcoma of the brain. Cancer, 14:811–852, 1961.

64. Hoff, J. T., and Ray, B. S.: Cerebral hemangioblastoma occurring in a patient with von Hippel-Lindau disease: Case report. J. Neurosurg., 28:365–368, 1968.

65. Horten, B. C., Urich, H., Rubinstein, L. J., and Montague, S. R.: The angioblastic meningioma: A reappraisal of a nosological problem: Light-, electron-microscopic, tissue and organ culture observations. J. Neurol. Sci., 31:387–410, 1977.

66. Hsu, Y. K.: Primary intracranial sarcomas. Arch. Neurol. Psychiat., 43:901–924, 1940.

67. Ishwar, S., Taniguchi, R. M., and Vogel, F. S.: Multiple supratentorial hemangioblastomas: Case study and ultrastructural characteristics. J. Neurosurg., 35:396–405, 1971.

68. Jamieson, K. G., Yelland, J. D. N., and Merry, G. S.: Hemangioblastomas of the hind brain: A report of 18 cases. Aust. New Zeal. J. Surg., 44:254–257, 1974.

69. Jeffreys, R.: Clinical and surgical aspects of posterior fossa hemangioblastoma. J. Neurol. Neurosurg. Psychiat., 38:105–111, 1975.

70. Jeffreys, R.: Pathological and haematological aspects of posterior fossa haemangioblastomata. J. Neurol. Neurosurg. Psychiat., 38:112–119, 1975.

71. Jellinger, K., and Denk, H.: Blood group isoantigens in angioblastic meningiomas and hemangioblastomas of the central nervous system. Virchow. Arch. [Path. Anat.], 364:137–144, 1974.

72. Jellinger, K., and Slowik, F.: Histological subtypes and prognostic problems in angiomas. J. Neurol., 208:279–298, 1975.

73. Kauffman, S. L., and Stout, A. P.: Hemangiopericytoma in children. Cancer, 13:695–710, 1960.

74. Kawamura, J., Garcia, A. H., and Kamijyo, Y.: Cerebellar hemangioblastoma: Histogenesis of stroma cells. Cancer, 31:1528–1540, 1973.

75. Kernohan, J. W., and Sayre, G. P.: Tumors of the Central Nervous System, Atlas of Tumor Pathology. Section X, Fascicle 35. Washington, D.C., Armed Forces Institute of Pathology, 1952.

76. Kernohan, J. W., and Uihlein, A.: Sarcomas of the Brain. Springfield, Ill., Charles C Thomas, 1962.

77. Krayenbühl, H., and Yasargil, G.: Das Kleinhirnhamangiom. Schweiz. Med. Wschr., 88:99–104, 1958.

78. Kruse, F.: Hemangiopericytoma of the meninges (angioblastic mengioma of Cushing and Eisenhardt): Clinical pathologic aspects and follow-up studies in eight cases. Neurology (Minneap.), 11:771–777, 1961.

79. Kuhn, C., and Rosai, J.: Tumors arising from pericytes: Ultrastructure and organ culture of a case. Arch. Path. (Chicago), 88:653–663, 1969.

80. Leedham, P. W.: Primary cerebral rhabdomyosarcoma and the problem of medullomyoblastoma. J. Neurol. Neurosurg. Psychiat., 35:551–559, 1972.

81. Levin, P. M.: Multiple hereditary hemangioblastomas of the nervous system. Arch. Neurol. Psychiat., 36:384–391, 1936.

82. Lichtenstein, B. W., and Ettleson, A.: Diffuse mesothelioma of the leptomeninges associated with cortical and ventricular glial hernias: A clinical-pathologic study and report of a case. Arch. Path. (Chicago), 24:497–507, 1937.

83. Lindau, A.: Studien über Kleinhirncysten Bau, Pathogeneses und Beziehungen zur Angiomatosis retinae. Acta Path. Microbiol. Scand. (suppl.), *1*:1–128, 1926.

84. Lindau, A.: Discussion on vascular tumors of the brain and spinal cord. Proc. Roy. Soc. Med., *24*:363–388, 1931.

85. Lindau, A.: Capillary angiomatosis of the central nervous system. Acta Genet. (Basel), 7:338–340, 1957.

86. Lindgren, E.: Percutaneous angiography of the vertebral artery. Acta Radiol. (Stockholm), *33*:389–404, 1950.

87. Lopes de Faria, J.: Rhabdomyosarcoma of cerebellum. Arch. Path. (Chicago), *63*:234–238, 1957.

88. Ludwin, S. K., Rubinstein, L. J., and Russell, D. S.: Papillary meningioma: A malignant variant of meningioma. Cancer *36*:1363–1373, 1975.

89. Lynn, J. A., Panopio, I. T., Martin, J. H., Shaw, M. L., and Race, G. J.: Ultrastructural evidence for astroglial histogenesis of the monstrocellular astrocytoma (so-called monstrocellular sarcoma of brain). Cancer, *22*:356–366, 1968.

90. Mann, I., Yates, P. C., and Ainslie, J. P.: Unusual case of double primary orbital tumor. Brit. J. Ophthal., *37*:758–762, 1953.

91. Maroon, J. C., Haines, S. J., and Phillips, J. G.: Calvarial hemangioendothelioma with intracranial hemorrhage: A case report. Neurosurgery, *4*:178–180, 1979.

92. Matakas, F., and Cervos-Navarro, J.: Die Feinstruktur sog. maligner Meningiome. Verh. Deutsch. Ges. Path., *57*:418, 1973.

93. McDonald, J. V., and Terry, R.: Hemangiopericytoma of the brain. Neurology (Minneap.), *11*:497–502, 1961.

94. McDonnell, D. E., and Pollock, P.: Cerebral cystic hemangioblastoma. Surg. Neurol., *10*:195–199, 1978.

95. McMaster, M. J., Soule, E. H., and Givins, J. D.: Hemangiopericytoma: A clinicopathologic study and long-term follow-up of sixty patients. Cancer, *36*:2232–2244, 1975.

96. Melmon, K. L., and Rosen, S. W.: Lindau's disease: Review of the literature and study of a large kindred. Amer. J. Med., *36*:595–617, 1964.

97. Merzbacher and Uyeda: Gliastudien; das reaktive Gliom und die reaktive gliose; ein Kritischer Beitrag zur Lehre vom Gliosarkom. Z. Ges. Neurol. Psychiat., *1*:285–317, 1910.

98. Min, K. W., Gorkey, F., and Halpert, B.: Primary rhabdomyosarcoma of the cerebrum. Cancer, *35*:1405–1411, 1975.

99. Mohan, J., Brownell, B., and Oppenheimer, D. R.: Malignant spread of hemangioblastoma: Report on two cases. J. Neurol. Neurosurg. Psychiat., *39*:515–525, 1976.

100. Moller, H. U.: Ophthalmic symptoms and heredity in cerebellar angioreticuloma. Acta Psychiat. Neurol. Scand., *19*:275–292, 1944.

101. Mondkar, V. P., McKissick, W., and Russell, R. W. R.: Cerebellar hemangioblastomas. Brit. J. Surg., *54*:45–49, 1967.

102. Morello, G., and Bianchi, M.: Cerebal hemangioblastomas: Review of literature and report of two personal cases. J. Neurosurg., *20*:254–264, 1963.

103. Muller, J., and Mealey, J.: The use of tissue culture in differentiation between angioblastic meningioma and hemangiopericytoma. J. Neurosurg., *34*:341–348, 1971.

104. Namba, K., Aschenbrener, C., Nikpour, M., and Van Gilder, J. C.: Primary rhabdomyosarcoma of the tentorium with peculiar angiographic findings. Surg. Neurol., *11*:39–43, 1979.

105. Neller, K., Brunngraber, C. V., and Wechsler, W.: Klinik, Pathologie und Differentialdiagnose der Groshirnangioblastome. Acta Neurochir. (Wien), *21*:227–252, 1969.

106. Nibbelink, D. W., Peters, B. H., and McCormick, W. F.: On the association of pheochromocytoma and cerebellar hemangioblastoma. Neurology (Minneap.), *19*:455–460, 1969.

107. Nichols, P., and Wagner, J. A.: Primary intracranial sarcoma: Report of nine cases with suggested classification. J. Neuropath. Exp. Neurol., *11*:215–234, 1952.

108. Noetzli, M., and Malamud, N.: Postirradiation fibroid sarcoma of the brain. Cancer, *15*:617–622, 1962.

109. Obrador, S., and Blazquez, M. G.: Benign cystic tumours of the cerebellum. Acta Neurochir. (Wien), *32*:55–68, 1975.

110. Obrador, S., and Martin-Rodriguez, J. G.: Biological factors involved in the clinical features and surgical management of cerebellar hemangioblastomas. Surg. Neurol., *7*:79–85, 1977.

111. Olivecrona, H.: The cerebellar angioreticulomas. J. Neurosurg., *9*:317–330, 1952.

112. Onofrio, B. M., Kernohan, J. W., and Uihlein, A.: Primary meningeal sarcomatosis: A review of the literature and report of twelve cases. Cancer, *15*:1179–1208, 1962.

113. Palmer, J. J.: Haemangioblastomas: A review of eighty-one cases. Acta Neurochir. (Wien), *27*:125–148, 1972.

114. Peña, C. E.: Intracranial hemangiopericytoma: Ultrastructural evidence of its leiomyoblastic differentiation. Acta Neuropath. (Berlin), *33*:279–284, 1975.

115. Penfield, W.: The encapsulated tumors of the nervous system: Meningeal fibroblastoma, perineural fibroblastoma, and neurofibromata of von Recklinghausen. Surg. Gynec. Obstet., *45*:178–188, 1927.

116. Pennybacker, J.: Recurrence in cerebellar haemangiomas. Zbl. Neurochir., *14*:63–73, 1954.

117. Perks, W. H., Cross, J. N., Sivapragasam, S., and Johnson, P.: Supratentorial haemangioblastoma with polycythaemia. J. Neurol. Neurosurg. Psychiat., *39*:218–220, 1976.

118. Pitkethly, D. T., Hardman, J. M., Kempe, L. G., and Harle, K. M.: Angioblastic meningiomas. Clinicopathologic study of eighty-one cases. J. Neurosurg., *32*:539–544, 1970.

119. Ramsey, H. J.: Fine structure of hemangiopericytoma and hemangio-endothelioma. Cancer, *19*:2005–2018, 1966.

120. Rappaport, Z. H., and Epstein, F.: Computerized axial tomography in the preoperative evaluation of posterior fossa tumors in children. Child's Brain, *4*:170–179, 1978.

121. Raskind, R., and Grant, S.: Primary mesenchy-

mal chondrosarcoma of the cerebrum: Report of a case. J. Neurosurg., *24*:676–678, 1966.

122. Rawe, S. E., van Gilder, J. C., and Rothman, S. L. G.: Radiographic diagnostic evaluation and surgical treatment of multiple cerebellar, brain stem, and spinal cord hemangioblastomas. Surg. Neurol., *9*:337–341, 1978.

123. Rivera, E., and Chason, J. L.: Cerebral hemangioblastoma: Case report. J. Neurosurg., *25*:452–454, 1966.

124. Rosse, W. F., Berry, R. J., and Waldmann, T. A.: Some molecular characteristics of erythropoietin from different sources determined by inactivation by ionizing radiation. J. Clin. Invest., *42*:124–129, 1963.

125. Rottino, A., and Poppiti, R.: Diffuse meningeal sarcoma. J. Neuropath. Exp. Neurol., *2*:190–196, 1943.

126. Rubinstein, L. J.: The development of contiguous sarcomatous and gliomatous tissue in intracranial tumours. J. Path. Bact., *71*:441–459, 1956.

127. Rubinstein, L. J.: Morphological problems of brain tumors with mixed cell population. Acta Neurochir. (Wien) suppl., *10*:141–165, 1964.

128. Rubinstein, L. J.: Microgliomatosis. Acta Neurochir. (Wien) suppl., *10*:211–217, 1964.

129. Rubinstein, L. J.: Sarcomas of the Nervous System. *In* Minckler, J., ed: Pathology of the Nervous System. New York, McGraw-Hill Book Co., 1971, pp. 2144–2164.

130. Rubinstein, L. J., and Northfield, D. W. C.: The medulloblastoma and the so-called "arachnoidal cerebellar sarcoma": A critical re-examination of a nonsological problem. Brain, *87*:379–412, 1964.

131. Russell, D. S.: Meningeal tumours: A review. J. Clin. Path., *3*:191–211, 1950.

132. Russell, D. S., and Rubinstein, L. J.: Pathology of Tumors of the Nervous System. 4th Ed. Baltimore, Williams & Wilkins Co., 1977.

133. Sargent, P., and Greenfield, J. G.: Haemangeiomatous cysts of the cerebellum. Brit. J. Surg., *17*:84–101, 1929.

134. Schmidt, M. B.: Ueber die Pacchionischen Granulationen und ihr verhältnis zu den Sarkomen und Psammomen der Dura mater. Virchow. Arch. [Path. Anat.], *170*:429–464, 1902.

135. Schrantz, J. L., and Araoz, C. A.: Radiation induced meningeal fibrosarcoma. Arch. Path. (Chicago), *93*:26–31, 1972.

136. Silver, M. L., and Hennigar, G.: Cerebellar hemangioma (haemangioblastoma): A clinicopathological review of forty cases. J. Neurosurg., *9*:484–492, 1952.

137. Simpson, D.: The recurrence of intracranial meningiomas after surgical treatment. J. Neurol. Neurosurg. Psychiat., *20*:22–39, 1957.

138. Singounas, E. G.: Haemangioblastomas of the central nervous system. Acta Neurochir. (Wien), *44*:107–113, 1978.

139. Skullerud, K., and Loken, A. C.: The prognosis in meningiomas. Acta Neuropath. (Berlin), *29*:337–344, 1974.

140. Sobin, L. H.: Personal communication, 1977.

141. Spence, A. M., and Rubinstein, L. J.: Cerebellar capillary hemangioblastoma: Its histogenesis studied by organ culture and electron microscopy. Cancer, *35*:326–341, 1975.

142. Stout, A. P.: Hemangio-endothelioma: A tumor of blood vessels featuring vascular endothelial cells. Ann. Surg., *118*:445–464, 1943.

143. Stout, A. P.: Hemangiopericytoma: A study of twenty-five new cases. Cancer, *11*:1027–1035, 1949.

144. Stout, A. P., and Murray, M. R.: Hemangiopericytoma: A vascular tumor featuring Zimmerman's pericytes. Ann. Surg., *116*:26–33, 1942.

145. Stroebe, H.: Ueber Entstehung und Bau der Gehirngliome. Beitr. Path. Anat., *18*:405–497, 1895.

146. Terry, R. D., Hyams, V. J., and Davidoff, L. M.: Combined nonmetastasizing fibrosarcoma and chromophobe tumor of the pituitary. Cancer, *12*:791–798, 1959.

147. von Hippel, E.: Über eine sehr seltene Erkrankung der Netzhaut: Klinische Beobachtungen. Graefes Arch. Ophthal., *59*:83–106, 1904.

148. Waldmann, T. A., Levin, E. H., and Baldwin, M.: The association of polycythemia with a cerebellar hemangioblastoma. Amer. J. Med., *31*:318–324, 1961.

149. Waltz, T. A., and Brownell, V.: Sarcoma: A possible late result of effective radiation therapy for pituitary adenoma: Report of two cases. J. Neurosurg., *24*:901–907, 1966.

150. Weed, L. H.: The meninges: With special reference to the cell coverings of the leptomeninges. *In* Penfield W., ed.: Cytology and Cellular Pathology of the Nervous System. Facsimile of 1932 edition. New York, Hafner Publishing Co., 1965, pp. 611–634, 1965.

151. Willis, R. A.: A diffuse leptomeningeal tumour in a child: With comments on "sarcomatosis" of the meninges. J. Path. Bact., *47*:253–256, 1938.

152. Wilson, H., and Brunschwig, A.: Irradiation sarcoma. Surgery, *2*:607–611, 1937.

153. Zeitlin, H.: Hemangioblastomas of the meninges and their relation to Lindau's disease. J. Neuropath. Exp. Neurol., *1*:14–23, 1942.

154. Zimmerman, H. M.: Introduction to tumors of the central nervous system. *In* Minckler, J., ed.: Pathology of the Nervous System. Vol. 2. New York, McGraw-Hill Book Co., 1971, pp. 1947–1951.

155. Zimmerman, H. M.: Vascular tumors of the brain. *In* Vinken, P. J., and Bruyan, G. W., eds.: Handbook of Clinical Neurology. Vol. 18. Amsterdam, North-Holland Publishing Co., 1975, pp. 269–298.

156. Zülch, K. J.: Primary sarcomas of the brain. Acta Neurochir. (Wien) suppl., *10*:185, 1964.

157. Zülch, K. J.: Brain Tumors: Their Biology and Pathology. Am Ed 2. New York, Springer-Verlag, 1965.

89

TUMORS OF PINEAL REGION

Tumors arising from the pineal gland and surrounding regions such as the posterior third ventricle and the quadrigeminal area lie in a central portion of the brain and are difficult to expose for operative removal. They often involve the deep venous system of the brain, which adds to the hazard of operation.

Although the percentage of tumors occurring in this region is relatively small, they represent a wide variety of histological types and have been a challenge to expose operatively, which has led to a comparatively voluminous literature on their treatment.*

PATHOLOGY

Although many tumors in this region are invasive and therefore not amenable to operative removal, it is well recognized that among these heterogenous lesions there is a group of encapsulated tumors and cysts.† Such lesions usually are not considered to be radiosensitive, but because of their discrete nature and lack of invasiveness, they are potentially resectable.

Approximately 10 to 25 per cent of the lesions have a well-defined margin. Ringertz and co-workers, reporting 65 cases, listed 11 encapsulated teratomas and 2 cysts.[39] The teratomas, except for two that were of a low-grade infiltrative nature, were all sharply circumscribed, without ventricular seeding or metastases. In a review of 113 cases, Haldeman reported 22 teratomas and 14 cysts.[15] Araki and Matsumoto reported 39 teratomas among 136 pineal tumors, but gave no indication as to their encapsulation.[3] Poppen and Marino found one teratoma in 20 cases, and Suzuki and Iwabuchi two in 19 cases.[35,44]

Unfortunately, a lack of uniformity regarding the histological labeling of these tumors has plagued the literature. Russell used the term "atypical teratoma" to describe the tumor that Globus labeled a pinealoma.[13,14,40] Ringertz and associates classified the tumors into: (1) seminoma-like tumors, (2) classic two-cell types, (3) tumors with fibroglial vessel-carrying stroma with small lymphocyte-like cells, (4) teratomas of low and high differentiation, and (5) miscellaneous lesions including gliomas, undifferentiated tumors, and simple cysts.[39]

The spectrum ranges from the invasive and often highly malignant atypical teratoma or dysgerminoma-like tumor to the benign dermoid. To the surgeon, a description of the discreteness and encapsulation of the lesion is most pertinent. In spite of the problem in case reporting, it is obvious that there are tumors arising in this region that are benign, encapsulated, presumably radioresistant, and potentially resectable. These neoplasms include the well-differentiated teratoma, the dermoid, the epidermoid, and other rarer tumors.

Other rare masses in the pineal region are the nonneoplastic cysts.[1,2,16,32] These cysts, whose lining cells can vary from arachnoidal to ependymal, can be the cause of aqueductal compression and secondary hydrocephalus. Being nonneoplastic, these lesions are potentially curable by operation.

---

* See references 3, 4, 11, 17–19, 21, 22, 27, 30, 32, 34, 35, 37, 41–45, 47, 49.
† See references 1, 2, 6, 15, 16, 19, 23, 25, 27, 39, 42, 45, 47.

ANATOMY

The pineal region is equidistant from most portions of the cranium. Tumors that arise in this region expand into the posterior part of the third ventricle, the pulvinar region, and the quadrigeminal portion of the midbrain. Superiorly, they are bounded by the internal cerebral veins, the vein of Galen, and the tela choroidea. Although these important vascular structures are often involved by the tumor, they usually lie on or within its dorsal surface; it is rare for them to lie within its central portion. Posteriorly, the precentral cerebellar vein borders these tumors; however, anterior portions of the cerebellum usually are not involved by them. Lateral to the tumors lie the veins of Rosenthal. Inferiorly invasive tumors may infiltrate the midbrain and the thalamus.

Pineal region tumors receive blood supply from the lateral and medial posterior choroidal arteries and from branches of the quadrigeminal, posterior cerebral, and superior cerebellar arteries. These are relatively small unimportant vessels whose interruption during tumor removal is not critical.

With the obliteration of the quadrigeminal cisterns by these tumors, adhesions, which often play a role in the production of hydrocephalus, develop about the incisura.

CLINICAL PRESENTATION

The clinical picture, although not pathognomonic, has certain features that can lead to the correct diagnosis of a pineal tumor.* Because of the strategic location of these lesions, signs of intracranial pressure appear early and are a hallmark of the syndrome. In spite of the close proximity of the tumors to the aqueduct, total obstruction of this passage, even in the presence of large tumors, is not invariable. Presumably, the absence of aqueductal obstruction in some patients is due to the slow growth and the noninvasive quality of their tumors. Nevertheless, Jennett and co-workers reported that in the majority of their cases there was aqueductal block.[24]

Cerebellar signs in the form of gait or limb ataxia frequently are present and most likely result from compression of the efferent cerebellar pathways in the superior cerebellar peduncles. Also prominent are limitation of upward gaze, convergence paresis, and inequality of pupils with impairment of reaction to light and accommodation. Components of the syndrome of Parinaud, these signs are often fragmentary, and a fully developed tectal syndrome is uncommon.[33,36,37]

Disturbances of endocrine function, previously recorded as a salient feature of pineal lesions, are more a curiosity than a significant component of the pineal tumor syndrome.[4,6,21,37,39] Precocious puberty, reported in 8 to 10 per cent of patients, when present, invariably occurs in the male.

In spite of a plethora of experimental observations, the mechanism of precocious puberty is not completely understood.[9,29,48] The syndrome has been recognized in association with a variety of intracranial disorders, including hypothalmic tumors and hydrocephalus due to causes other than pineal tumors, and therefore cannot be considered diagnostic of a pineal lesion. Gonadotrophic hormone assays are usually reported as normal. Injection of pineal extracts into animals has not led to precocious development. Reiter and Fraschini noted that recent experimental data favor inhibition of gonadal maturation by the pineal body.[38] Although little correlation has been made between the histological nature of the tumor and the presence of sexual precocity, Kitay observed a higher incidence of precocity with nonparenchymal tumors that destroyed the pineal body than with tumors arising from the pineal gland.[28] Others have suggested that precocious development is due to seeding of the hypothalmus by the tumor.[37] Because of its rarity and its varied origin, the presence of sexual precocity has rarely been a practical clue in the diagnosis of pineal tumors.

Diabetes insipidus, seen in 10 per cent of patients with pineal tumors, arises either from direct involvement of the hypothalamus by the tumor or as the secondary effect of hydrocephalus.

The following case report emphasizes the ease and value of operative resection in some lesions.

---

* See references 4, 5, 17, 20, 24, 39.

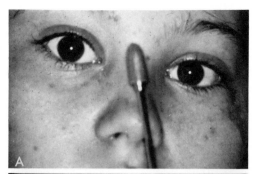

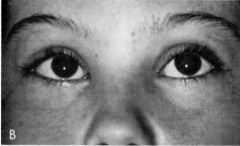

Figure 89–1 Preoperative extraocular movements. *A*. Impaired convergence and near reflex of pupils. *B*. Impaired upward gaze.

Case History

An 11-year-old girl had a nine-month history of progressively severe headache, diplopia, blurred vision, ataxia, and deterioration of scholastic ability. Admission to the hospital was prompted by trancelike states that were observed during the prior week. A cerebellar tumor was suspected. Physical examination revealed limb and truncal ataxia, marked bilateral papilledema, and a right abducens nerve palsy. In addition, convergence and upward gaze were impaired (Fig. 89–1). The pupils, which were unequal, were dilated and sluggishly reactive to light.

Skull x-rays showed evidence of chronically elevated intracranial pressure. A mercury brain scan was normal. A ventriculogram showed advanced hydrocephalus with forward displacement of the aqueduct and indentation of the posterior portion of the third ventricle (Fig. 89–2).

A posterior fossa supracerebellar exposure of the pineal region revealed a large dermoid tumor. All but a small portion of the capsule, which was adherent to the quadrigeminal region, was removed. Postoperatively the patient did well, and her extraocular difficulties gradually improved (Fig. 89–3). An eight-year follow-up shows her to be normal.

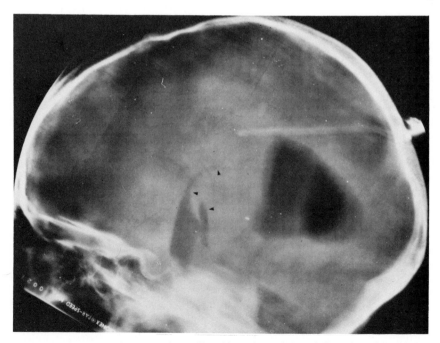

Figure 89–2 Ventriculogram demonstrating a dilated lateral ventricle and distortion of the third ventricle due to a large pineal dermoid tumor (*arrows*).

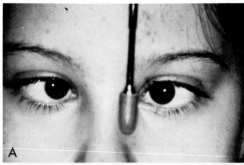

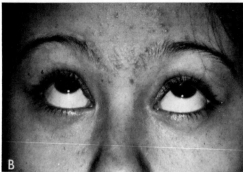

Figure 89-3 Postoperative extraocular movements. *A*. Normal convergence. *B*. Normal upward gaze.

DIAGNOSIS

X-rays of the skull that show an abnormally large or premature calcification of the pineal gland may indicate the possibility of neoplasm. An area of calcification more than 5 mm in diameter or dense calcification occurring before the age of 10 years would be considered abnormal. Radioisotope scans may identify a tumor of this region should the lesion be abnormally vascular.

Angiography may be utilized to rule out vascular anomalies of the region, such as a vein of Galen aneurysm, or to define the vascular pattern of the lesion. While angiography can reveal distortion of the deep venous system and the posterior choroidal arteries, thus suggesting a pineal tumor, it is with air ventriculography that the definitive diagnosis is made.[20,24,44] Ventriculography gives a comprehensive evaluation of the lesion by indicating its relationship to the third ventricle and aqueduct, and by giving some indication of its eccentricity. Pneumoencephalography via the lumbar route supplements ventriculography in defining the relationship of the quadrigeminal cistern, lower aqueduct, and fourth ventri-

cle to the tumor. Pneumoencephalography is, however, contraindicted as a primary procedure because of the danger of transtentorial or tonsilar herniation and the great likelihood of nonfilling of the ventricular system prior to ventricular decompression by ventriculography.

Suzuki and Hori have reported the use of positive contrast media in the diagnosis of pineal tumors and the use of residual contrast within the ventricular system as a method of gauging the effectiveness of radiotherapy.[43] The question must be raised whether dye remaining in the ventricular system may be a focus for ependymitis and thus convert marginal function into true obstruction with resultant hydrocephalus.

Of great value is the identification of these tumors by the computed tomographic (CT) scan. This modality precisely defines the limits of the tumor, its relationship to the third ventricle, midbrain, and quadrigeminal cisterns and, additionally, may indicate cysts within the tumor. At many centers, the CT scan has supplanted all other contrast studies. If, as infrequently occurs, the scan suggests a vascular lesion, angiography is used to supplement the diagnostic evaluation; otherwise it is safe to operate on the basis of the CT scan alone.

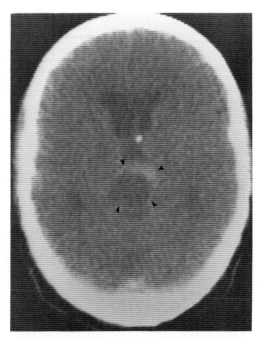

Figure 89-4 Computed tomographic scan with contrast enhancement showing a cystic atypical teratoma of the pineal (*arrows*).

Computed tomography gives the exact position and extent of the tumor, and the presence or absence of cysts and of low-density material such as a dermoid cyst (Fig. 89–4). None of these data could be obtained by the usual methods of radiographic analysis. It remains to be seen whether the diagnosis of malignancy and infiltration can be made with a high degree of accuracy by the CT scan. If this proves to be the case, it would preclude an operation done only for histological verification.

TREATMENT

Because of the deep-seated location and predominantly invasive quality of pineal tumors, endeavors to remove them have led to frequent failures and high mortality rates.[11,37,39] Cushing set a keynote for the conservative therapy of these tumors when he stated, "Personally, I have never succeeded in exposing a pineal tumor sufficiently well to justify an attempt to remove it."[8] Horrax and Daniels stated, "The radical operative extirpation of tumors situated in the region of the pineal body is a procedure of great magnitude with an extremely high mortality."[22]

The hazards of operation, with disastrous results following even a biopsy, as well as improvement in radiotherapeutic and shunting techniques, had led to the abandonment of operative intervention in favor of conservative treatment for pineal tumors.[7,22] The latter regimen usually consisted of: radiation of 4000 to 5000 rads directed to the lesion and insertion of either a Torkildsen or an extracranial cerebrospinal fluid shunt.

Certain drawbacks to nonoperative therapy are obvious. As Cushing remarked, "Treatment of these tumors is a therapeutic shot in the dark as long as the tumor's precise histological type is unknown."[8] Jennett and co-workers emphasized that the ventriculogram cannot always distinguish between encapsulated and invasive lesions, and that the clinical picture is even less accurate in determining the pathological nature of the lesion.[24,46] Katagiri describes a unique case (his patient no. 2) in which obstruction of the aqueduct, caused by a pineal mass, was relieved by a period of ventricular tapping.[26] The fact that his patient was intact, without radiotherapy, after 12 years further stresses the vagaries of these lesions. Cummins and co-workers observed, "Epidermoid and dermoid cysts present the most difficult problem. Patients with these will, under our method of treatment, be considered as having third ventricle tumors, improved by relief of obstruction yet unresponsive to irradiation."[7] They summarized by stating, "Indeed, our policy is that, if there is any doubt, the need for exploration should be emphasized despite the operative risk."

The limitations of radiotherapy and shunting procedures as the sole treatment of pineal tumors is apparent.[7,18] Cummins and associates reported a series in which the nature of pineal masses was unverified and the follow-up relatively short.[7] The results of radiotherapy in these cases, although generally satisfactory, cannot be correlated with the histological nature of the lesion. In a small series of confirmed lesions that were operated on, however, these authors reported about half the patients surviving longer than 15 years. Although survival in the majority of patients with lesions histologically confirmed by operation is limited, there are numerous case reports of benign masses occurring in the pineal region that have been excised with good results.*

If a cerebrospinal fluid diversionary procedure is required in the treatment of pineal tumors, the author prefers an extracranial shunt, ventriculoatrial or ventriculoperitoneal. The Torkildsen shunt used to be the classic method of treating hydrocephalus secondary to pineal tumors, but it has been shown, because of a compromise of the cerebrospinial fluid pathway through the incisura, to have limited value in these cases.[12,45]

In the face of a mandate for conservative therapy, not only must an operative procedure be relatively safe but a significant benefit from the procedure must be demonstrated in order to justify an operation on pineal tumors.[7,22,35,37,46]

Dandy, a master at approaching deep-seated brain tumors, was particularly interested in pineal region tumors. To gain exposure to the pineal region, he advocated an interhemispheric approach with section

---

* See references 12, 17, 18, 25, 26, 31, 35, 42, 44, 45, 47.

of the posterior portion of the corpus callosum.[10] This approach required sacrifice of a number of parietal cortical veins in order to retract the right hemisphere. In the region of the pineal tumor, difficulties were encountered in dissecting the deep venous system. Many of the fatalities appeared to result from venous thrombosis and edema of the diencephalic region.

Van Wagenen advocated an approach through a dilated right lateral ventricle.[49] Since the approach was primarily dorsal to the tumor, it also involved dissection of the deep veins. In addition, it had the disadvantages of a transcortical incision and possible hemispheric collapse when the ventricle was open.

Poppen advocated an approach under the occipital lobe.[34] The bridging veins were sacrificed, and a large portion of the hemisphere was retracted. The edge of the tentorium was divided in order to expose the deep venous plexus in a more favorable attitude in relation to the underlying tumor.

These operative approaches all have the inherent disadvantages of approaching the tumor through the crucial deep venous system; hence, there is great morbidity and a high mortality rate.

In 1926 Krause first described the infratentorial supracerebellar approach to the pineal region.[30] In one of his three cases, he was able to accomplish a significant removal of tumor. Since his report, there have been sporadic instances in which this approach was used without comment as to its merits or disadvantages.[4,11,35] Such a route to the pineal has the advantage of avoiding the deep venous system, which usually lies dorsal or lateral to the tumor. Most of the tumors are midline and are best exposed through this approach; when one is eccentric, the interhemispheric transcallosal approach to it has been chosen, since it can be reached more effectively through one or the other lateral ventricles.

Operative Technique

If the patient has severe intracranial hypertension and marked hydrocephalus, the direct approach to the pineal tumor can be preceded by a preliminary extracranial shunt in order to gradually reduce the ventricular size and compensate for the raised intracranial pressure. In most cases shunt-

ing is not necessary, and a direct approach to the tumor is performed, ventricular drainage being optional.

Unless the patient is under 2 years of age and has a severe degree of hydrocephalus, the sitting position is preferred. Strong flexion of the head is necessary to give maximal exposure of the tentorial notch with the greatest comfort to the surgeon. In addition to having the neck strongly flexed, the seated patient is tilted forward somewhat so that the surgeon actually works over the patient's back into the posterior fossa.

A long midline incision extending from C2 to high up in the occipital region is used so that the pericranium and muscle attachments can be elevated to either side without disrupting their continuity. This type of incision also greatly facilitates the closure. A wide craniectomy, which must extend above the lateral sinuses and the torcular, is performed in all instances. The opening of the dura is important, for it must be bilateral and include the region of the lateral sinuses. The dural incision should, however, not be carried too far laterally, since if it is, one is unable to retract the dural flap adequately in the region of the torcular (Fig. 89–5). A self-retaining retractor is utilized to elevate the tentorium, and the weight of cottonoids or a copper retractor is used to depress the cerebellum.

The operating microscope with a 250- or 275-mm objective is used. The use of an armrest is recommended. Because of the distance to the pineal region and the frequent extension of the tumor into the third ventricle or even to the region of the foramen of Monro, long instruments are required.

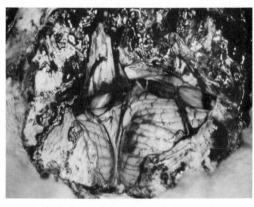

Figure 89–5 Craniectomy and dural opening for approach to pineal tumor.

All the bridging veins over the dorsal surface of the cerebellum may be sacrificed in order to open the incisural region. The arachnoid, which is almost always thickened and opaque in the presence of tumors, must be opened by microdissection in order to expose the surface of the tumor. The great vein of Galen and the internal cerebral veins are generally well above the tumor and are not encountered in these initial maneuvers (Fig. 89–6). The veins of Rosenthal lie laterally adjacent to the medial aspect of the temporal lobes. The tumor capsule is then cauterized and opened by sharp dissection. The tumor, depending on its consistency, is removed with tumor forceps, suction, and cautery.

The trajectory of the operation is toward the velum interpositum (Fig. 89–7). One must consider this point when attempting to remove portions of the tumor that lie either in the inferior portion of the third ventricle or directly over the quadrigeminal plate in relation to the anterior lobe of the cerebellum. This portion of the tumor is the most difficult to deal with, and small dental mirrors and angled instruments may be required to remove it.

Even in the case of nonresectable tumors, benefit may be derived from internal decompression of the tumor or creation of an opening through the tumor to the posterior part of the third ventricle into which a shunt between the ventricle and the cisterna magna can be placed. In cases in which significant removal of the tumor cannot be accomplished and an internal shunt

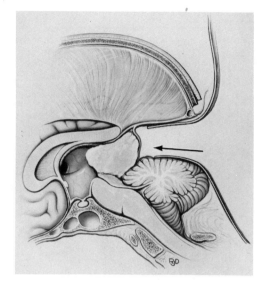

Figure 89–7 Drawing of sagittal aspect of operative exposure. With the patient's neck flexed, the trajectory of this posterior fossa approach is toward the velum interpositum (*arrow*).

cannot be placed, an extracranial shunt is used.

Usually the dura is left open, but with smaller openings into the posterior fossa and significant decompression or removal of tumor, it may be closed. Closure of the dura makes the postoperative course smoother and may limit the degree of aseptic meningitis.[42]

Personal Experience

Table 89–1 reviews the author's 21 cases. It indicates the variety of lesions that are found in the pineal region.

Direct operation, resulting in either removal of encapsulated or well-defined tumors or a confirmation of histological type in the invasive or nonresectable tumors, has led to a more enlightened approach to the treatment of patients with these tumors. Furthermore, information has been obtained regarding the response of different tumors to a variety of treatments.

As yet, there is no infallible means of diagnosing the nature of tumors in this region prior to operation. This point was underscored by two of the cases listed in Table 89–1. Both patients had large cystic tumors that were diagnosed on the CT scan. These tumors were presumed to be low-grade astrocytomas, but at the time of

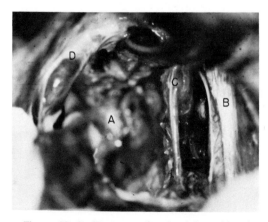

Figure 89–6 Exposure of a pineal dermoid under the operating microscope. A, Interior of the tumor; B, right edge of the tentorium; C, vein of Rosenthal; D, precentral cerebellar vein.

TABLE 89–1 OPERATIVELY TREATED PINEAL TUMORS

CASE NO.	AGE (Years)	DIAGNOSIS	PRIOR TREATMENT	RESULTS
1	8	Teratoma	—	Normal
2	24	Cystic astrocytoma	Radiotherapy	Late death
3	8 (mo.)	Arachnoid cyst	—	Normal
4	12	Dermoid	—	Normal
5	9	Teratoma	Radiotherapy	Unchanged
6	4	Teratoma	—	Improved
7	5	Atypical teratoma	—	Late death
8	25	Astrocytoma	—	Improved
9	10	Astrocytoma	Radiotherapy	Improved
10	8	Glioblastoma	—	Operative death
11	12	Atypical teratoma	—	Improved
12	37	Atypical teratoma	—	Late death
13	35	Astrocytoma	Radiotherapy	Unchanged
14	16	Atypical teratoma	—	Improved
15	43	Atypical teratoma	Radiotherapy	Improved
16	18	Atypical teratoma	—	Improved
17	22	Colloid cyst	Radiotherapy	Unchanged
18	15	Atypical teratoma	—	Unchanged
19	15	Pinealocytoma	—	Unchanged
20	26	Meningioma	Radiotherapy	Unchanged
21	28	Meningioma	—	Improved

operation they proved to be atypical teratomas. In approximately 25 per cent of the cases included in Table 89–1 the tumors were amenable to total or near-total resection and, therefore, would fall into the category of encapsulated benign tumors.

The operation is reasonably safe. There was only one operative death among the cases shown in Table 89–1. This patient had a delayed hemorrhage in a glioblastoma. It occurred one week after the primary operative procedure. There has been no significant morbidity in the remaining cases.

Since histological identification of pineal tumors has been paramount in the selection of therapy, it is advisable to expose and at least perform biopsy of all pineal tumors. With direct operation, total removal, if feasible, can be performed and, when removal is not feasible, either internal decompression or the establishment of an internal shunt from the third ventricle to the cisterna magna can be accomplished.

REFERENCES

1. Alexander, E., Jr.: Benign subtentorial supracollicular cyst as a cause of obstructive hydrocephalus. Report of a case. J. Neurosurg., *10*:317–323, 1953.
2. Alvord, E. C., Jr. and Marcuse, P. M.: Intracranial cerebellar meningoencephalocele (posterior fossa cyst) causing hydrocephalus by compression at the incisura tentorii. J. Neuropath. Exp. Neurol., *21*:50–69, 1962.
3. Araki, C., and Matsumoto, S.: Statistical re-evaluation of pinealoma and related tumors in Japan. J. Neurosurg., *30*:146–149, 1969.
4. Baggenstoss, A. H., and Love, J. G.: Pinealomas. Arch. Neurol. Psychiat. (Chicago), *41*:1187–1206, 1939.
5. Bailey, P., and Jelliffe, S. E.: Tumors of the pineal body with an account of the pineal syndrome. Arch. Intern. Med., *8*:851–880, 1911.
6. Bing, J. F., Globus, J. H., and Simon, H.: Pubertas praecox: A survey of the reported cases and verified antomical findings. With particular reference to tumors of the pineal body. J. Mount Sinai Hosp. N.Y. *4*:935–965, 1938.
7. Cummins, F. M., Taveras, J. M., and Schlesinger, E. B.: Treatment of gliomas of the third ventricle and pinealomas. With special reference to the value of radiotherapy. Neurology (Minneap.), *10*:1031–1036, 1960.
8. Cushing, H.: Intracranial tumors: Notes upon a series of two thousand verified cases with surgical mortality pertaining thereto. Springfield, Ill., Charles C Thomas, 1933, p. 64.
9. Dandy, W. E.: Extirpation of the pineal body. J. Exp. Med., *22*:237–247, 1915.
10. Dandy, W. E.: An operation for the removal of pineal tumors. Surg. Gynec. Obstet., *33*:113–119, 1921.
11. Dandy, W. E.: Operative experience in cases of pineal tumor. Arch. Surg. (Chicago), *33*:19–46, 1936.
12. Fincher, E. F., Strewler, G. J., and Swanson, H. S.: The Torkildsen procedure. A report of 19 cases. J. Neurosurg., *5*:213–229, 1948.
13. Globus, J. H.: Pinealoma. Arch. Path., *31*:533–568, 1941.
14. Globus, J. H., and Silbert, S.: Pinealomas. Arch. Neurol. Psychiat. (Chicago), *25*:937–985, 1931.
15. Haldeman, K. O.: Tumors of the pineal gland. Arch. Neurol. Psychiat., *18*:724–754, 1927.
16. Hamby, W. B., and Gardner, W. J.: An ependymal cyst in the quadrigeminal region: Report of a case. Arch. Neurol. Psychiat. *33*:391–398, 1935.

17. Harris, W., and Cairns, H.: Diagnosis and treatment of pineal tumors with report of a case. Lancet, *222*:3–9, 1932.

18. Hide, T. A. H.: Pineal region tumors. J. Neurol. Neurosurg. Psychiat., *32*:68, 1969.

19. Horrax, G.: Extirpation of a huge pinealoma from a patient with pubertas praecox. A new operative approach. Arch. Neurol. Psychiat., *37*:385–397, 1937.

20. Horrax, G.: The diagnosis and treatment of pineal tumors. Radiology, *52*:186–192, 1949.

21. Horrax, G.: Treatment of tumors of the pineal body. Experience in a series of twenty-two cases. Arch. Neurol. Psychiat., *64*:227–242, 1950.

22. Horrax, G., and Daniels, J. T.: The conservative treatment of pineal tumors. Surg. Clin. N. Amer. *22*:649–659, 1942.

23. Hosoi, K.: Teratoma and teratoid tumors of the brain. Arch. Path., *9*:1207–1219, 1930.

24. Jennett, B., Johnson, R., and Reid, R.: Positive contrast ventriculography of pineal region tumors. Acta Radiol. (Diagn.) (Stockh.), *1*:857–871, 1963.

25. Kahn, E. A.: Surgical treatment of pineal tumor. Arch. Neurol. Psychiat., *38*:833–842, 1937.

26. Katagiri, A.: Arachnoidal cyst of the cisterna ambiens. Report of two cases. Neurology (Minneap.), *10*:783–786, 1960.

27. Katsura, S., Suzuki, J., and Wada, T.: A statistical study of brain tumors in the neurosurgical clinics in Japan. J. Neurosurg., *16*:570–580, 1959.

28. Kitay, J. I.: Pineal lesions and precocious puberty: A review. J. Clin. Endocr., *14*:622–625, 1954.

29. Krabbe, K. H.: The pineal gland, especially in relation to the problem of its supposed significance in sexual development. Endocrinology, *7*:379–414, 1923.

30. Krause, F.: Operative Frielegung der Vierhügel, nebst Beobachtungen über Hirndruck und Dekompression. Zbl. Chir., *53*:2812–2819, 1926.

31. Kroening, P. M.: Pineal teratoma—before and after dentition. Amer. J. Roentgen., *88*:533–535, 1962.

32. Kunicki, A.: Operative experiences of 8 cases of pineal tumor. J. Neurosurg., *17*:815–823, 1960.

33. Parinaud, H.: Paralysie des mouvements associés des yeux. Arch. Neurol. (Paris), *5*:145–172, 1883.

34. Poppen, J. L.: The right occipital approach to a pinealoma. J. Neurosurg., *25*:706–710, 1966.

35. Poppen, J. L., and Marino, R., Jr.: Pinealomas and tumors of the posterior portion of the third ventricle. J. Neurosurg., *28*:357–364, 1968.

36. Posner, M., and Horrax, G.: Eye signs in pineal tumors. J. Neurosurg., *3*:15–24, 1946.

37. Rand, R. W., and Lemmen, L. J.: Tumors of the posterior portion of the third ventricle. J. Neurosurg., *10*:1–18, 1953.

38. Reiter, R. J., and Fraschini, F.: Endocrine aspects of the mammalian pineal gland: A review. Neuroendocrinology, *5*:219–255, 1969.

39. Ringertz, N., Nordenstam, H., and Flyger, G.: Tumors of the pineal region. J. Neuropath. Exp. Neurol., *13*:540–561, 1954.

40. Russell, D.: The pinealoma: Its relationship to teratoma. J. Path. Bact., *56*:145–150, 1944.

41. Schmidek, H. H.: Pineal Tumors. New York, Masson Publishing, U.S.A., Inc., 1977, pp. 1–137.

42. Stein, B. M.: The infratentorial supracerebellar approach to pineal lesions. J. Neurosurg., *35*:197–202, 1971.

43. Suzuki, J., and Hori, S.: Evaluation of radiotherapy of tumors in the pineal region by ventriculographic studies with iodized oil. J. Neurosurg., *30*:595–603, 1969.

44. Suzuki, J., and Iwabuchi, T.: Surgical removal of pineal tumors (pinealomas and teratomas). Experience in a series of 19 cases. J. Neurosurg., *23*:565–571, 1965.

45. Torkildsen, A.: Should extirpation be attempted in cases of neoplasm in or near the third ventricle of the brain? Experiences with a palliative method. J. Neurosurg., *5*:249–275, 1948.

46. Tytus, J. S.: Differentiation of tumors arising in area of the posterior third ventricle. Neurology (Minneap.), *10*:654–657, 1960.

47. Ward, A., and Spurling, R. G.: The conservative treatment of third ventricular tumors. J. Neurosurg., *5*:124–130, 1948.

48. Wurtman, R. J., and Axelrod, J.: The pineal gland. Sci. Amer. *213*:50–60, 1965.

49. Van Wagenen, W. P.: A surgical approach for the removal of certain pineal tumors. Report of a case. Surg. Gynec. Obstet., *53*:216–220, 1931.

90

METASTATIC
BRAIN TUMORS

The diagnosis and treatment of metastatic tumors of the nervous system is a challenge. Despite improving diagnostic methods and treatment protocols, the clinician counts palliation as a worthy effort and cure as often beyond his reach. Indeed, palliation is significant, since relief from symptoms such as paralysis, seizures, and dementia contributes substantially to the quality of life and is appreciated by both the patient and his family.

Systemic cancer can affect the intracranial contents by metastasizing to the skull, dura, leptomeninges, brain parenchyma, and related anatomical sites. In this chapter the consequences of intraparenchymal and leptomeningeal metastases only are discussed, since they occur commonly and often can benefit from neurosurgical management.

CEREBRAL METASTASES

Incidence

Table 90–1 shows the incidence of cerebral metastases in a Memorial Sloan-Kettering Cancer Center study. Patients detailed here had intraparenchymal metastases without other intracranial metastases. Thus, the incidence is slightly lower than that reported in other autopsy series that include dural and meningeal metastases, and somewhat higher than reported in several clinical series.* There are several interesting findings in these data: Carcinoma of the lung is the most frequent primary tumor producing cerebral metastases, although the percentage of cerebral metastases is higher in a less common tumor, malignant melanoma. The majority of patients with carcinoma of the lung, melanoma, and cancer of the colon had multiple cerebral metastases, whereas single metastases were more common in breast cancer, renal carcinoma, ovarian carcinoma, and osteogenic sarcoma.

Metastatic disease of the brain in children differs in several respects from that in adults. In the first place, the incidence is lower, only 6 per cent according to Vannucci and Baten in a study of 216 children dying of cancer.[99] The brain was involved with metastatic disease in 13 of those cases (the cerebral hemispheres in 12, and the cerebellar hemispheres in 1). Pulmonary involvement preceded central nervous system involvement in all cases. Neuroblastoma, rhabdomyosarcoma, and Wilms' tumor were the most common primary tumors (though more recently the incidence of osteogenic sarcoma in children appears to be on the rise).[26,76] Interestingly, while Wilms' tumor was the third most commonly diagnosed pediatric neoplasm, it metastasized to the brain two to five times as frequently as the more common neuroblastoma or rhabdomyosarcoma.[99]

Pathology

Malignant cells may reach the nervous system in several ways. The most common

---

* See references 48, 74, 79, 82, 83, 86, 89, 102, 110.

F. W. GAMACHE, JR., J. B. POSNER,
AND R. H. PATTERSON, JR.

2872

TABLE 90–1 INTRACEREBRAL METASTASES FOUND AT AUTOPSY IN SLOAN-KETTERING CANCER CENTER STUDY*

PRIMARY TUMOR	NO. OF PATIENTS	INTRACEREBRAL METASTASES No.	Per Cent[a]	SINGLE METASTASES No.	Per Cent[b]
Lung	297	61	21	25	41
Breast	324	33	9	19	58
Melanoma	125	50	40	19	38
Lymphoma	346	4	1		
Hodgkin's	119	0	0		
Non-Hodgkin's	190	4	2		
Gastrointestinal tumors	311	10	3		
Colon	130	6	5	2	33
Stomach	46	0	0		
Pancreas	44	1	2		
Genitourinary tumors	357	40	11		
Kidney	52	11	21	10	91
Prostate	49	0	0		
Testes	37	17	46		
Cervix	62	3	5		
Ovary	60	3	5	3	100
Osteosarcoma	39	4	10	3	75
Neuroblastoma	39	2	5		
Head and neck	118	7	6		

[a] Per cent of total systemic tumor.
[b] Per cent of total intracerebral metastases.

* No other intracranial lesions (i.e., dural or arachnoidal metastases) were included.

mode of spread is hematogenous; that is, the tumor is carried to the brain by the arteries and distributed according to regional blood flow and regional mass.[82,102,109] A second mode of spread is by direct extension from the skull, a situation often occurring in carcinomas of the nasopharynx or breast. A third possible mode of spread is by way of Batson's intraspinal plexus. Notwithstanding the report in 1940 by Batson in which he demonstrated in cadaver studies that tumor cells could make their way to the brain via freely communicating vertebral veins, spread by this route appears to be rather rare.[7]

The large majority of tumors reach the brain by hematogenous spread via the systemic arterial circulation. In the case of carcinoma of the lung, tumor cells invade the pulmonary veins. Tumors from other sites enter the systemic veins and then either pass through the lung capillary circulation, or bypass the lung through a patent foramen ovale, or first metastasize to and grow in the lungs. This last sequence is called the "cascade effect." Tumors (especially from the pelvis) reach the central nervous system by first metastasizing to bone and then to the lungs via Batson's plexus. From the lungs the tumor crosses the pulmonary circulation to reach the brain.[7,70,100] The implication of this theory is that several organs

(especially bone and the lungs) are involved with tumor as it spreads to the brain.

The frequency of metastases to various parts of the brain is proportional to blood flow and tissue mass.[2,74,82,102,109] Reports that the incidence of cerebellar or brain stem metastases was higher than could be accounted for by organ weight or blood flow seem to have been incorrect.[110] This issue was reviewed by Penzholz in 1968. The cerebellum is about one tenth the mass of the cerebral hemispheres, for example. Experience around the world, according to Penzholz's review, revealed a range of involvement of the cerebellum by metastatic disease of between 5 and 60 per cent.[73] The larger and more recent studies generally report the lower percentages, whereas the smaller studies and older literature tended to report a higher range of values. The relationship between metastasis frequency and blood flow and tissue mass appears to hold true for the glands associated with the brain, such as the posterior lobe of the pituitary.[19,29] Since the anterior lobe of the pituitary receives little or no direct arterial blood supply, tumor reaches it more often by direct extension. Kistler and Pribram, in their series of 11 patients with metastatic disease involving the sella, found that the most common primaries were tumors of the lung, prostate, thyroid, breast, and lympho-sarcoma.[45] Hagerstrand and Schonebeck have presented a good review of this subject.[31]

Grossly, metastatic nodules in the brain usually are well circumscribed and may be solitary or multiple. They have a propensity for the junction of the gray and white matter, and usually are solid but may be cystic, depending upon the degree of central necrosis. Metastatic tumors evoke a substantial amount of edema in the surrounding brain. The amount of edema is not necessarily a reflection of the size of the metastatic tumor, and some tumors seem to produce more edema than others. Multiple factors probably account for the degree of edema, such as the number of tumor vessels, the extent of vascular permeability, local peculiarities in metabolism, and the production of fluid by the neoplastic cells.[4,23]

Metastatic tumors appear to be well circumscribed grossly. At the microscopic level the tumor cells are relatively well demarcated from brain parenchyma in comparison with those of primary brain tumors.[76,89] Scattered clusters of metastatic tumor cells may, however, grow and develop at the microscopic fringes of the metastasis (especially in adjacent perivascular spaces) and hence invade or spread within brain (but not actually diffusely infiltrate brain the way a primary tumor would). Recent data suggest that between 26 and 84 per cent of patients with known brain metastasis have persisting disease at the local tumor site at autopsy despite operative excision or radiation treatment.[25,48,55] Perhaps as many as 50 per cent of patients believed on clinical grounds to suffer from a single metastatic brain tumor have multiple metastases that are not identified during life.[2,25,48,52,102]

Diagnosis

Cerebral metastases may make their appearance at any time during the course of the primary disease. In general, the interval between the diagnosis of the primary cancer and the cerebral metastasis is a short one for patients harboring lung, skin (melanoma), or renal primaries. It is common for patients with lung cancer to develop neurological signs before the primary tumor is

TABLE 90–2   MEDIAN INTERVAL BETWEEN DIAGNOSIS OF PRIMARY TUMOR AND CEREBRAL METASTASIS*

PRIMARY TUMOR	MEDIAN INTERVAL (MONTHS)	RANGE (MONTHS)
Lung	5.0	0–75
Melanoma	28.5	2–240
Breast	37.0	3–192
Sarcoma	26.0	9–108
Choriocarcinoma	27.5	1–45
Undetermined 1°	2.5	0–5
Kidney	6.0	0–33
Uterus	71.0	33–108
Colon	53.0	34–72
Prostate	60.0	—
Ovary	11.0	—
Neuroblastoma	23.0	—

* Data from study of 80 patients admitted to Memorial Sloan-Kettering Cancer Center.

discovered. On the other hand, patients with breast cancer, sarcoma, and gastrointestinal cancer may live for a considerable time following the discovery of the primary tumor before an intracranial tumor appears. Data from a recent review of patients with intracranial metastases at Memorial Sloan-Kettering Cancer Center illustrate the variabilities by tumor type in Table 90–2. Such variability reflects differences in host-tumor relationships, the success of therapy, and the aggressiveness of the clinician in looking for cerebral metastasis.

Signs and Symptoms

Table 90–3 lists the presenting symptoms and signs of single intracerebral metastases in 80 patients evaluated in Memorial Sloan-Kettering Cancer Center. There are several points worth emphasizing: Headache was a presenting complaint in only slightly more than half the patients. Frequently the headache was mild and not particularly dis-

TABLE 90–3   PRESENTING SYMPTOMS AND SIGNS OF INTRACRANIAL METASTASIS*

SYMPTOM	NO. OF PATIENTS
Headache	43
Mental changes	34
Seizure(s)	21
Hemiparesis	34
Increased intracranial pressure	32
Visual field abnormality	13

* Neurological findings of 80 patients admitted to Memorial Sloan-Kettering Cancer Center with a single metastasis.

abling. In most patients with headache, the symptoms strongly suggested increased intracranial pressure; i.e., the headache was present early in the morning upon awakening and before arising from bed. It often disappeared within 20 to 30 minutes after arising, whether or not the patient took analgesic agents, but returned again the following morning. As time passed the headache assumed increasing importance. Such a story is classic in brain tumor headache and therefore deserves serious consideration. Papilledema was present in only a quarter of patients, making its absence not useful diagnostically. An important point is that careful neurological examination of patients with systemic cancer often discloses unsuspected signs of central nervous system disease. For example, focal weakness and abnormal cognitive function were found more often on examination than they were reported by the patient or his family. Seizures, which were an early complaint in 26 per cent of patients, also may appear later in the evolution of the disease, even during the course of treatment. Seizures are particularly common in metastatic melanoma. They also commonly affect patients with leptomeningeal metastases without intracerebral mass lesions.

Specific symptoms and signs may result either from the local effects of the metastasis or from a remote effect due to such mechanisms as edema, hemorrhage, hydrocephalus, and ischemia. The role that edema plays in the production of neurological signs and symptoms associated with brain metastases is worth emphasizing. It not only magnifies the symptoms of relatively small metastases but probably accounts for the dramatic reduction in clinical symptoms that may follow the administration of corticosteroids.

A single small metastasis can cause signs of diffuse brain involvement if it is strategically located to obstruct cerebrospinal fluid pathways. Similarly, seizures or disorders of speech can be the consequence of tissue irritation or destruction of tissue that follows ischemia or hemorrhage from a remote metastasis. Consequently, the clinical examination has limits in precisely localizing a tumor.

Cerebral metastases at times present in unusual ways. Hayward, for example, has reported that 7 of his 20 patients with malignant melanoma presented clinically with

TABLE 90–4 CLINICAL FEATURES*

CLINICAL FEATURES	PER CENT
Gait disturbance	89
Headache	70
Dizziness	62
Vomiting	60
Gait ataxia	95
Dysdiadochokinesia	76
Nystagmus	76
Dementia	30
Papilledema	24

* Data from 37 cases treated at Memorial Sloan-Kettering Cancer Center.

subarachnoid hemorrhage.[34] Hemorrhage is even more common in the case of choriocarcinoma. Subdural hematomas or effusions have been reported as a cause of presenting symptoms in subdural metastases, particularly from carcinomas of the breast and prostate.[50] Large intracranial cysts may be produced by metastatic carcinomas of the breast or lung.

Patients with cerebellar metastases may present with subtle findings. Often they complain of headache and some difficulty with gait, but little else. The neurological signs that are usually present are often mild and easily overlooked. Table 90–4 lists the common clinical features that were observed in a series of patients with cerebellar metastases at Memorial Sloan-Kettering Cancer Center.

Laboratory Tests

The diagnostic work-up of a patient suspected of harboring a cerebral metastasis should begin with computed tomography performed without and then with the injection of iodinated contrast material. The reason for performing both procedures is that some metastatic lesions are isodense with brain and will not be apparent on the CT scan unless they shift the ventricular system. Such lesions are often enhanced after the injection of contrast and become more dense than the surrounding normal brain (Fig. 90–1). Some lesions demonstrate increased density on the CT scan prior to the administration of contrast agent; in this situation the addition of contrast agent may aid in differentiating calcium from hemorrhage. Rarely, other lesions are radiolucent without contrast but are enhanced just enough by the injection of contrast to become isodense with the contrast-enhanced brain and thus appear

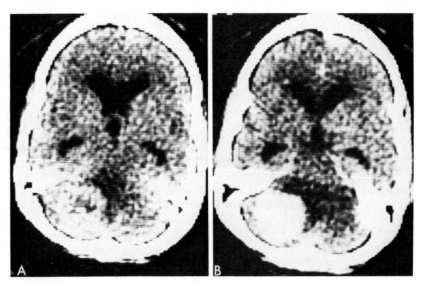

Figure 90–1 CT brain scan of a patient with biopsy-proved metastatic disease of the brain. *A*. The noncontrast scan appears relatively normal. *B*. Following the injection of contrast agent, gross abnormalities are clearly apparent. (Courtesy of Dr. Gerald F. Abbott.)

normal in the contrast scan. Enhancement of the tumor by iodinated contrast is the result of neovascularity, abnormalities in the blood-brain barrier locally (secondary to abnormal tight junctions), or frank tissue destruction with associated changes in local metabolism.[44,51,101,108] These factors are believed to account for alterations in radioisotope density in radionuclide scanning as well.

The smallest nodules that can be detected by computed tomography are probably 6 to 9 mm in diameter.[66,72] Melanoma and choriocarcinoma, because of their high blood content and propensity to hemorrhage, and adenocarcinoma of the stomach and colon (for unclear reasons) are likely to appear radiodense before contrast. Epidermoid carcinomas of the breast and lung are often of low density on the unenhanced scan. Almost all metastatic tumors are enhanced with contrast agent.

The exact percentage of symptomatic metastases that will be missed on the CT scan without and with contrast is in dispute. Reported figures vary from 3 to 40 per cent for lesions greater than 1 cm, but data from an in-progress national cooperative study suggest that about 7 per cent of lesions greater than 1 cm may be missed.[24,62] Lesions in the posterior fossa, near the base of the skull, and high on the convexity are most likely to be missed and require special attention on the part of the radiolo-

gist (Fig. 90–2). If a lesion in that area is suspected but not identified on the routine scan, then a repeat scan with overlapping cuts or sections taken at various angles relative to the orbitomeatal baseline or coronal plane may yield further information. False positive findings are less common than false negative findings and likely result from misinterpretation or overinterpretation of the CT scan.[24]

The CT scan can identify a lesion, but it does not indicate its histological type. Lesions that mimic metastatic tumors include meningiomas (usually dense before contrast and close to the surface rather than in the white matter), cerebral abscesses (particularly in patients with lymphomas and Hodgkin's disease), and even multiple sclerosis.[81] The radionuclide brain scan or the CT scan may be positive even in the absence of symptoms of cerebral disease when patients with known cancer are screened for metastases. Hayes and coworkers found brain scans to be positive for 8 per cent of patients with carcinoma of the lung who were neurologically asymptomatic.[33] Jacobs and associates, even after excluding asymptomatic patients with positive radionuclide brain scans, have reported a 6 per cent incidence of positive CT scans for asymptomatic patients with carcinoma of the lung. All these patients had what appeared to be normal radionuclide brain scans.[42]

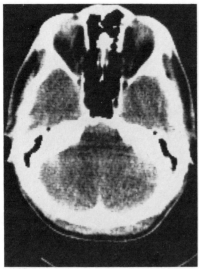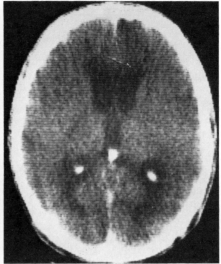

Figure 90–2 CT brain scan that failed to demonstrate obvious lesions in a patient in whom cerebellar metastases from choriocarcinoma of the testis were suspected clinically. Operative exploration with biopsy revealed glial reaction. Autopsy revealed bilateral, deep hemispheric masses in both the cerebrum and cerebellum. (Courtesy of Dr. Michael D. F. Deck.)

If the physician suspects a metastatic cerebral lesion and the CT scan is negative or not available, a radionuclide brain scan should be performed. Although less accurate than computed tomography (false negative results occur about 20 per cent of the time), nuclide scans will occasionally be positive when the CT scan is unrevealing.[9,15,24,44,72] A nuclide scan, however, is unable to differentiate between a lesion of the skull and a lesion of the underlying cortex when it is a superficial one. A variety of radionuclide substances have been used for brain scanning; [67]gallium may be superior to [99m]technetium in the detection of tumors in the brain.[104] If both studies are negative, rather than pursue further tests, the physician should follow the patient for two to three weeks and repeat the CT scan.

Even in evaluation of bony skull metastases, computed tomography is probably the best diagnostic technique. If the radiologist adjusts the window properly to look for bony lesions, abnormalities that are not apparent on plain skull x-rays may be detected both at the base of the skull and over the convexity, particularly if overlapping cuts are taken (Fig. 90–3).

Other diagnostic tests may occasionally be useful in the evaluation of metastatic disease. Arteriography is less effective in defining cerebral lesions than computed tomography.[64,66,110] It assumes importance as a preoperative procedure, however, for two reasons: it assists the surgeon in planning his approach to the metastatic tumor by displaying vascular landmarks, and it indicates the presence of a mass lesion through a shift in the blood vessels. On several occasions the authors have encountered lesions that appeared to be tumors on the CT scan but that failed to produce any mass effect. Although this can happen with metastatic tumors, the surgeon should be cautious that he is not dealing with some other disease process, for example, multiple sclerosis.

Sometimes skull roentgenograms are useful in identifying skull metastases in cases of cranial nerve palsy or facial pain. Young and co-workers found, however, that they were rarely helpful in evaluating intracranial metastases.[111]

In the past, air encephalography was most useful for the demonstration of extra-axial basal tumors, extraventricular tumors, and masses in the posterior fossa, brain stem, corpus callosum, and diencephalon.[92,107] Computed tomography has, however, supplanted pneumographic techniques in most of these cases.

The electroencephalogram is sometimes helpful in differentiating metabolic from structural brain disease. In the case of tumors, various degrees of delta activity (persistent focal, intermittent focal, persistent lateralizing) often are seen when a

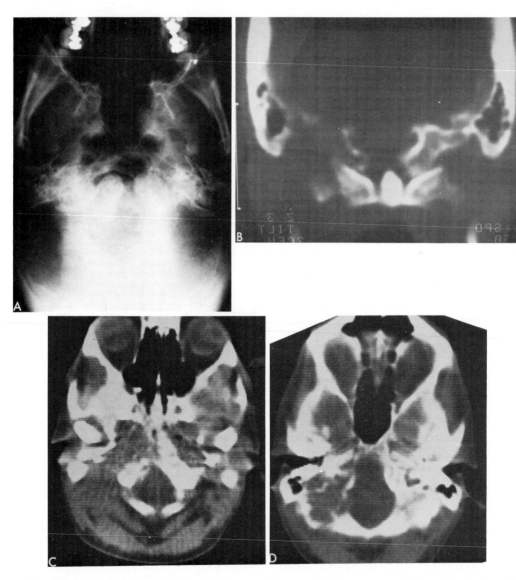

Figure 90–3   *A*. Skull film of a patient with suspected metastatic disease was entirely normal. *B*, *C*, and *D*. With overlapping and coronal cuts the CT scan revealed evidence of metastatic disease in the left occipital bone, jugular foramen, and clivus with soft-tissue extension into the foramen magnum. (Courtesy of Dr. Michael D. F. Deck.)

lesion of 2 cm or larger is present.[88] Posterior fossa lesions are occasionally missed entirely, and electroencephalographic changes are quite nonspecific in the presence of deep-seated metastatic tumors.[87]

Most recently kilovolt peak CT scans (i.e., CT scans performed at two different kilovoltage settings in order to evaluate changes in CT numbers associated with the lesion) have been recommended to evaluate single radiodense lesions that might thus be distinguished as being calcium, iodine, or blood by the differences in atomic number.[59] By means of this technique, six cases of metastatic brain tumor that presented as intraparenchymal hemorrhage were correctly identified. While encouraging, the experience with this technique is too limited to be fully evaluated at this time.

Evaluation of Extent of Disease

If a cerebral metastasis is identified in a patient known to have or have had cancer, the extent of the disease should be evaluated before definitive therapy of the cerebral lesion is decided upon. The work-up includes: (1) hematological and chemical evaluation of the blood for electrolytes, liver chemistry, urea, and biochemical markers of neoplasia (carcinoembryonic antigen [CEA], alpha-fetoprotein, and the like) and high-quality chest roentgenograms; (2) a radionuclide or CT scan of the liver; and (3) a radionuclide bone scan, followed by roentgenographic study of areas positive on the bone scan.

Liver metastases should be suspected if the liver is enlarged, if more than two liver function tests are abnormal, or if focal abnormalities are present on the liver scan. The bone scan is more useful than standard routine bone survey films for metastases, since it is positive 30 per cent more often.[44]

In some instances, a cerebral metastasis is suspected either from the clinical story or from laboratory findings, even when no known primary neoplasm has been identified. For example, a middle-aged heavy smoker may develop the subacute onset of headache and focal neurological signs, and a contrast-enhanced CT scan may reveal one or more lesions surrounded by edema.

In such cases the primary tumor most often lies in the lung or gastrointestinal tract. Vieth and Odom demonstrated in such cases, as have others, that months or years may pass between the time when cerebral metastases are diagnosed and when the primary is finally identified.[25,77,79,102]

For the patient with a suspected intracranial metastasis but no known primary tumor, the work-up should include a *complete* physical examination (including rectal, bimanual vaginal, scrotal, and total skin surface examinations). In addition to the tests outlined earlier, CT scan of the abdomen, without and with contrast, if available, may be used in place of the traditional liver scan, intravenous pyelograms, barium enema, and upper gastrointestinal series.

The foregoing routine will need to be varied to suit the circumstances. For example, in a patient with a single intracranial metastasis without a demonstrable primary, the studies of the intestinal tract might be omitted and a craniotomy performed in hopes of providing both a tissue diagnosis and treatment. Should the biopsy be consistent with a gastrointestinal primary, the intestinal x-rays may be done postoperatively.

For a few patients, even after an unrewarding search for a primary tumor, the excision of the cerebral lesion provides tissue that narrows the probable location of the primary down to several possibilities. These patients must be followed closely until the primary tumor finally declares itself.

Differential Diagnosis

Several conditions can mimic metastatic tumors, both clinically and by laboratory test. Such conditions include meningioma, which occurs with greater frequency in patients with carcinoma of the breast than in the general population; cerebral abscesses, which are more common among patients with Hodgkin's disease and other patients whose immune responses are suppressed or who have subdural hematomas; primary brain tumors; intraparenchymal hematomas; or even cerebral aneurysms.[6,80,90] In a patient known to have systemic cancer, a typical clinical history combined with a lesion enhanced by contrast on CT scan is sufficient for a presumptive diagnosis of cerebral metastasis. The likelihood of metastases increases if multiple lesions are demonstrated on the CT scan. One should always consider the possibility that the identified lesion may have another cause, however, and if the clinical history or the computed tomographic findings are unusual, then further diagnostic evaluation including cerebral angiography, radionuclide scanning, and even pneumoencephalography may be indicated. In rare instances, a question still may remain after these diagnostic tests have been performed, and biopsy is necessary to establish the diagnosis of cerebral metastasis.

In a patient not known to have a systemic neoplasm, the situation is even more difficult. If extensive diagnostic work-up does not reveal a primary neoplasm, then biopsy to establish a diagnosis is indicated. An exception to this is the case in which multiple lesions on the CT scan, all enhanced by contrast and surrounded by edema, strongly suggest cerebral metastases, a situation in which operation might be dangerous.

Treatment of Brain Metastases

The authors' approach to treatment of patients with cerebral metastases is outlined in Table 90–5. Patients are divided into three groups: (1) patients who are acutely deteriorating (cerebral herniation), (2) patients in stable condition who have multiple metastases or systemic disease, and (3) patients in stable condition who have a single metastasis and no systemic disease.

TABLE 90–5 TREATMENT OF CEREBRAL METASTASES

Acutely decompensating patients
  Mannitol 1.5 to 2.0 gm per kilogram intravenously immediately, followed by 25 gm as required
  Dexamethasone 100 mg intravenously immediately, then 25 mg four times a day
  Lower Pa_{CO_2} to 25 to 30 mm of mercury if patient is comatose
Stable patients with multiple cerebral metastases or systemic disease
  Dexamethasone 4 mg every 6 hours orally (or more if needed to control symptoms)
  Radiation therapy
    500 rads every day for 3 days
    4 days rest
    300 rads every day for 8 days
    Total—3900 rads in 2 weeks
  Taper steroids as tolerated after radiation therapy is completed
Stable patients with single cerebral metastasis and no systemic disease
  Dexamethasone 4 mg every 6 hours orally (or more if needed)
  Operative removal, radiation therapy, or both
  After treatment, taper steroids as tolerated

For the first group of patients, the initial treatment is directed toward decreasing cerebral edema and shrinking both the brain and its vascular space in order to reverse the cerebral herniation. With this treatment, the condition of about two thirds of patients can be expected to stabilize, and then they can be treated with either radiation therapy or operation. Approximately one third of the patients will die of cerebral herniation despite the treatment program outlined in Table 90–5. The results of emergency operative treatment in the face of herniation usually are disappointing.[25]

For the stable patient with multiple metastatic disease, radiation therapy has been generally accepted as the treatment of choice.[10,75,108] For the stable patient with a single cerebral metastasis, some have advocated operative removal and others, radiation therapy.* There is no controlled study that compares these two treatment modalities, but relevant data from the authors' series and those in the literature are presented in Tables 90–6, 90–7, and 90–8.

Corticosteroids

Despite the fact that corticosteroids have been used to treat patients with cerebral metastasis for almost 20 years, their mechanism of action remains to be defined. Weinstein and co-workers observed that clinical improvement in eight patients with metastatic tumors was related to a fall in lumbar cerebrospinal fluid pressure.[105] Kulberg and West, on the other hand, were less impressed with the effect of steroids on the basic level of pressure but thought that episodes of high pressure (plateau waves) were ameliorated.[46]

The authors' experience and that of others is that 60 to 75 per cent of patients with intracerebral metastases experience significant amelioration of their symptoms when treated with adrenocorticosteroids.† Usually the more severe and striking the symptoms, the greater the relief. Headache and alterations in consciousness are particularly likely to respond, but all symptoms, including hemiparesis and dementia, may improve. It is generally believed that adrenocorticosteroids exert their effect by decreasing the edema around metastatic

---

* See references 10, 18, 21, 61, 77, 83, 109.
† See references 12, 23, 37, 60, 67, 79, 85, 108–110.

TABLE 90-6 OPERATIVE TREATMENT OF CEREBRAL METASTASIS

SERIES	YEAR PUBLISHED	NO. OF CASES	MORTALITY RATE (PER CENT)	SURVIVAL				PER CENT NEUROLOGICALLY IMPROVED
				Median (Months)	1 Year (Per Cent)	Long-Term		
						No. of Patients	Years	
Stortebecker*	1954	125	25 (20 days)	3.6	21	3	>4	32[b]
Richards and McKissock†[a]	1963	108	32	5.0	17	8	>2	—
Lang and Slater‡	1964	208	22	4.0	20	27	>2	40[c]
Vieth and Odom§	1965	155	15 (2 weeks)	6.0	13.5	12	>2	52[c]
Raskind et al.‖	1971	51	12 (2 weeks)	6.0	30	4	>3	79
Haar and Patterson¶	1972	167	11	6.0	22	7	>5	—
Ransohoff**	1975	100	10	6+	28	12	>1	—
Magilligan et al.††[d]	1976	22		9.5	45	2	>3	77 (3 months)

[a] Total excision only.
[b] Back to work.
[c] Alive and well at six months following operation.
[d] Patients were disease-free except for solitary cerebral metastasis; 16 of the 22 patients received whole brain radiation therapy, some more than once.

* Metastatic tumors of the brain from a neurosurgical point of view: a follow-up study of 158 cases. J. Neurosurg., 11:84-111.
† Intracranial metastases. Brit. Med. J., 1:15-18.
‡ Metastatic brain tumors. Results of surgical and non-surgical treatment. Surg. Clin. N. Amer., 44:865-872.
§ Intracranial metastases and their neurosurgical treatment. J. Neurosurg., 23:375-383.
‖ Survival after surgical excision of single metastatic brain tumors. Amer. J. Roentgen. 111:323-328.
¶ Surgery for metastatic intracranial neoplasm. Cancer, 30:1241-1245.
** Surgical management of metastatic tumors. Seminars Oncol., 2:21-27.
†† Pulmonary neoplasm with solitary cerebral metastasis. J. Thorac. Cardiovasc. Surg., 72:690-698.

TABLE 90–7　RADIATION THERAPY OF CEREBRAL METASTASIS

SERIES	YEAR PUBLISHED	NO. OF CASES	30-DAY MORTALITY RATE (PER CENT)	SURVIVAL Median (Months)	SURVIVAL 1-Year (Per Cent)	LONG-TERM Per Cent	LONG-TERM Years	PER CENT NEUROLOGICALLY IMPROVED
Order et al.*	1968	108	—	<6.0[c]	16	—	—	60
Deeley and Edwards†[a]	1968	61	—	9 (mean)	14	6	>3	—
Brady et al.‡	1974	138	—	4.5	—	—	—	64[e]
Berry et al.§	1974	102	—	~4 months	9	—	—	63
Young et al.||	1974	162	25	3.0	3	—	—	~60
Deutsch et al.¶	1974	88	36[b]	<6.0[c]	9	—	—	"Majority"
Glanzmann et al.**	1976	118	—	6.0[d] (mean)	12.9	4.2	≥2	58

[a] Lung only.
[b] Includes patients unable to complete therapy because of death or rapid clinical deterioration.
[c] At 3 months, 60 per cent alive; at 6 months, 30–32 per cent alive.
[d] Survival at 6 months, 27 per cent.
[e] Excludes patients unable to complete therapy because of death or rapid clinical deterioration.

* Improvement in quality of survival following whole-brain irradiation for brain metastasis. Radiology, 91:149–153.
† Radiotherapy in the management of cerebral secondaries from bronchial carcinoma. Lancet, 1:1209–1213.
‡ Radiation therapy for intracranial metastatic neoplasia. Radiol. Clin. (Basel), 43:40–47.
§ Irradiation of brain metastases. Acta. Radiol. Ther. (Stockholm), 13:535–544.
|| Rapid-course radiation therapy of cerebral metastases: results and complications. Cancer, 34:1069–1076.
¶ Radiotherapy for intracranial metastases. Cancer, 34:1607–1611.
** Radiotherapy results in brain metastases (118 cases). Strahlentherapie, 152:352–357.

TABLE 90–8 COMPARISON OF RESULTS FROM BEST RADIATION THERAPY WITH BEST OPERATION PLUS RADIATION THERAPY*

SERIES	YEAR PUBLISHED	NO. OF CASES	30-DAY MORTALITY RATE (PER CENT)	SURVIVAL		PER CENT IMPROVED
				Median (Months)	1 Year (Per Cent)	
Glanzmann et al.†	1976	118	—	3 < x < 6	12.9	58
Ransohoff‡	1975	100	10	6+	38	majority
MSKCC	1977	80	11	6	33	79

* "Best" refers to what are currently the best results as published in the literature. Various primary tumors were contained in each study.
† Radiotherapy results in brain metastases (118 cases). Strahlentherapie, 152:352–357.
‡ Surgical management of metastatic tumors. Seminars Oncol., 2:21–27.

tumors rather than by producing a direct effect on the tumor itself.[12] The particular glucocorticoid used does not seem to make a major difference. Dexamethasone and methylprednisolone appear to be the favorites of neurologists and neurosurgeons. The dosage of adrenocorticosteroids for the best relief of symptoms is unknown, and possibly varies from patient to patient. In general, most clinicians use approximately 16 mg of dexamethasone (Decadron) per day in divided doses. Dosages up to 96 mg per day have been advocated, however, and some have employed as much as 1000 mg per day of prednisone.[85] Corticosteroids in these high dosages may be epileptogenic.[13]

Anticonvulsants

The metabolism of glucocorticoids and anticonvulsants interact in such a way that patients receiving large doses of steroids often require larger than usual doses of hydantoin in order to achieve therapeutic levels of anticonvulsants. The metabolism of glucocorticoids appears increased by diphenylhydantoin, according to the studies by Werk and associates reviewed by Buchanan and Sholitan.[13] Whether or not the reverse is true has not been proved, though it has been suspected clinically. Diphenylhydantoin intoxication becomes a distinct possibility when steroid doses are tapered after treatment of the brain tumor. For this reason, careful monitoring of the blood levels of anticonvulsant drugs is necessary in patients with brain tumors who are receiving corticosteroids.

Operative Treatment

Treatment for cerebral metastases depends primarily on the use of cortico-steroids, radiation therapy, and operation, and it is decisions about the advisability of an operation that are the most difficult (Table 90–9). Certainly, an operation is indicated when tissue biopsy is necessary to establish the diagnosis. This circumstance arises in patients in whom the primary is yet undiscovered and also in patients in whom a primary tumor has been identified, treated, and apparently cured in the past. In the first instance, removing a solitary mass in the head from a patient with no other disease, even if the mass is compatible with a cerebral metastasis, establishes the diagnosis. In the instance in which the patient has a past history of cancer but no evident disease at the time the cerebral tumor is discovered, removing the tumor not only establishes the diagnosis but also may provide long-term palliation or even cure.

Sometimes patients with extracranial metastasis will develop a nonmetastatic cerebral mass such as brain abscess, gliosis as the result of radiation or chemotherapy, or a new primary brain tumor. In such patients, operative excision or biopsy may be appropriate.

Occasionally a single cerebral metastasis will develop in a patient with a slowly growing tumor that may be radioresistant but would in any case be compatible with a rel-

TABLE 90–9 INDICATIONS FOR OPERATION ON METASTATIC BRAIN TUMORS

Uncertain diagnosis
Failure of conservative therapy to control symptoms
Recurrence or persistence of severe neurological disability following radiation or chemotherapy
Certain indolent but radioresistant tumors (e.g., alveolar soft-part sarcomas)
?Accessible, single cerebral metastasis
  No other disease
  Large cerebral metastases with small extracranial tumor burden

TABLE 90–10   CONDITION AT TIME OF CRANIOTOMY AND SURVIVAL

SITE	ELECTIVE CRANIOTOMIES			EMERGENCY CRANIOTOMIES*		
	No. of Patients	Median Survival (Months)	30-Day Mortality Rate	No. of Patients	Median Survival (Months)	30-Day Mortality Rate
Supratentorial	58	11	3/58	7	2	2/7
Posterior fossa	6	2	2/6	9	4	2/9
Total	64	7.7		16	3	
		Overall median			Overall median	

* Patients in stupor or coma; clinical herniation.

atively long life span if cerebral metastases were not present. Such a patient may receive maximum palliation through operative excision as documented later.

Operation should be avoided under a number of circumstances, particularly in patients with multiple cerebral metastases, extensive or disseminated extracerebral disease, or those who are in stupor or coma. (Table 90–10).

Operative Technique

If an operation is to be performed, accurate anatomical preoperative localization of the metastasis is imperative. Localization on the basis of the ordinary CT scan may be difficult because of differences in the planes of laminographic sections. Accurate localization can, however, be achieved by a combination of ordinary roentgenograms and computer tomography.[16] Seeing the tumor from another perspective, perhaps by obtaining coronal sections on the CT scan or by a radionuclide brain scan, also aids in localization. Angiography is particularly helpful with small tumors that may be deep underneath the cortex. By comparing distribution of superficial veins and arteries in the angiogram and on the cerebral cortex at operation, precise localization is usually possible. Occasionally the surgeon may feel obliged to place air in the ventricles and use an image intensifier during the operation in order to identify the position of the tumor deep in the hemisphere near the ventricle.

To decrease intracranial pressure at operation, the authors' practice is to pretreat patients with corticosteroids and to place a spinal needle or catheter in the lumbar subarachnoid space, anticipating the need to withdraw spinal fluid. The patient often is given small doses of an osmotic diuretic (12.5 to 50 gm of mannitol) at the induction of anesthesia to increase the possibility that the brain will be slack when the dura is exposed. If the brain is still tight at this juncture, the withdrawal of 15 to 30 ml of spinal fluid usually will relax the dura so that the brain can be exposed without herniation. In the case of subcortical tumors, the area of the brain overlying the tumor is identified by comparing the pattern of arteries and veins on the surface with an angiogram. The authors prefer to excise a core of brain perhaps 3 to 4 cm in diameter down to the tumor site. This avoids retraction of the brain that may lead to postoperative edema. In addition, the view through the tract created by removing the core is substantially better than that which is achieved through a simple cortical incision. If possible, all the tumor should be removed, since the postoperative course is smoother and the mortality rate lower if this is accomplished.[30,79,86] At the end of the operation the dura is closed in order to eliminate extracranial sources from which blood can leak into the site of the tumor. In general, the bone plate is replaced except in the posterior fossa.

Results of Operative Treatment

The benefits of operative therapy are outlined in Table 90–11. The postoperative outcome depends on a number of factors. If the tumor can be only biopsied or partially removed, the operative morbidity and mortality rates are likely to be high owing to the effects of the residual tumor.[30,79,86] The preoperative neurological deficit is also related to postoperative outcome. Patients with severe neurological dysfunction such as dementia, coma, or hemiplegia are less likely to achieve a satisfactory level of function

TABLE 90–11 BENEFITS OF OPERATIVE THERAPY

Diagnosis is secured when primary is uncertain or unknown

Benign lesions may be properly identified and treated

Treatment may be offered for recurrent or radioresistant tumors

Perhaps longer median and 1-year survivals may be obtained

Occasional long-term survivors may be obtained

Perhaps a larger percentage of patients is improved

than those with only mildly to moderately incapacitating neurological deficits. Among the authors' patients who underwent emergency craniotomy because of cerebral herniation median survival was three months as compared with those who underwent elective craniotomy and in whom median survival was almost eight months.[25]

The extent of the extracranial metastases has a lesser relationship to survival than might be anticipated. The median survival for patients in good general condition who are tolerating their disease well approximates the survival of those who are thought to be free of extracranial diseases at the time of craniotomy. Survival also depends on the tumor type, being shorter in patients with melanoma and lung cancer and longer in those with breast cancer and various sarcomas (Table 90–12). Cure, though rare, is possible. One patient has been reported who has survived more than 10 years since removal of a carcinoma of the lung and bilateral cerebral metastases.[30] Occasional long-term survivors have been reported by others as well.*

---

* See references 14, 35, 48, 63, 65, 82, 83.

TABLE 90–12 MEDIAN AND ONE-YEAR SURVIVAL FROM TIME OF CRANIOTOMY BY TUMOR TYPE*

PRIMARY TUMOR	SURVIVAL	
	Median (Months)	One Year (Per Cent)
Lung	5.5	32
Melanoma	3.5	31
Sarcoma	11.0	45
Breast	13.0	63
Choriocarcinoma	8.0	33
Undetermined	9.0	50
Kidney	4.0	0
Uterus	8.0	33
Colon	5.5	0

* Data from 80 patients treated at Memorial Sloan-Kettering Cancer Center.

Operative treatment of metastatic brain tumor is not without complications. Sometimes the tumor is difficult to find, and often removal is incomplete even though all gross tumor appeared to have been removed. Determining whether residual tumor is present may be difficult. Figure 90–4 shows pre- and postoperative CT scans of a patient with a metastatic brain lesion. The scans demonstrate contrast enhancement postoperatively; residual tumor was documented at necropsy at the site of previous operation despite the fact that all tumor had been removed grossly. In contrast, Figure 90–5 shows pre- and postoperative contrast enhancement on the CT scan of a patient who at necropsy had no residual tumor. Apparently the contrast enhancement resulted from disruption of the blood-brain barrier and alterations in local vascularity and metabolism.[4,23,51] Currently there is no simple way to determine the true nature of the area of contrast enhancement found on CT scanning immediately following a tumor operation.

Thirty-day mortality rates reported from series in which metastatic brain tumors were treated with operation range from 5 to 32 per cent, with most studies reporting 10 to 15 per cent.† At Memorial Sloan-Kettering Cancer Center, for example, the 30-day operative mortality rate is approximately 11 per cent; but if patients dying from pulmonary emboli two to four weeks after operation are excluded, and if patients treated following development of herniation and coma are excluded, the so-called operative mortality rate drops to approximately 1 to 3 per cent.

The usual complications following extirpation of cerebral metastases include intracranial hematoma, brain swelling, loculation of cerebrospinal fluid, and infection. Haar and Patterson reported a postoperative complication rate of 24 per cent and an 8 per cent reoperation rate.[30] Of 77 patients recently reviewed following operative removal of a tumor at Memorial Sloan-Kettering Cancer Center, 17.5 per cent underwent re-exploration. Subdural hematomas, though in all cases less than 50 cc in volume, were present in 7 of 17 explorations, and were associated with brain swelling. Cerebrospinal fluid loculation was found in

---

† See references 25, 30, 48, 57, 79, 83, 86, 97, 102.

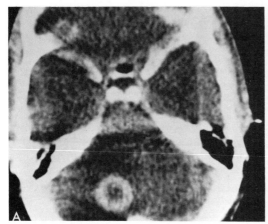

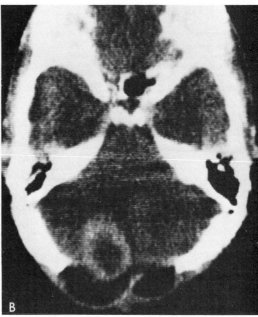

Figure 90–4 *A*. Preoperative CT brain scan. *B*. Postoperative scan demonstrating ring enhancement of a posterior fossa lesion. Residual tumor was suspected clinically and confirmed at autopsy. (Courtesy of Dr. Michael D. F. Deck.)

two patients, intraparenchymal hematoma in two others, and one had a brain abscess.[25]

Whole brain radiation following operation appears appropriate in most cases, both to treat the bed of the tumor and also to treat any other unrecognized metastases. In necropsy series of patients treated for metastatic brain tumors, occasionally as many as 71 to 84 per cent have been found to have tumor still present in the brain despite treatment (operation or radiation). In 21 to 29 per cent of patients who were operated on, residual tumor was present at the operative site, and in those patients who were harboring intracerebral metastasis at necropsy, 15 to 50 per cent of lesions were multiple.[25,47,48,75,77]

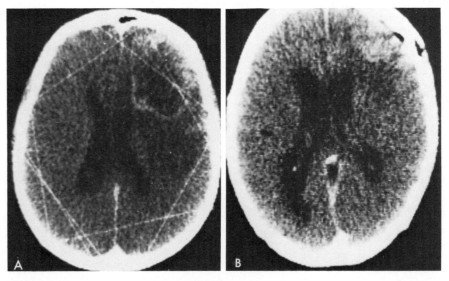

Figure 90–5 *A*. Preoperative CT brain scan. *B*. Postoperative scan demonstrating ring enhancement of a supratentorial lesion. Operative exploration confirmed the presence of metastatic tumor. All tumor was believed to have been excised. Autopsy revealed no residual tumor despite the postoperative contrast enhancement. (Courtesy of Dr. Michael D. F. Deck.)

Radiation Therapy

Radiation therapy is indicated for the patient with multiple metastases to brain and for those with single metastases that are particularly radiosensitive, such as lymphoma, seminoma, testicular carcinoma, and childhood embryonal cell carcinoma. Under these circumstances, patients who improve most are those with headache, seizures, vertigo, and evidence of increased intracranial pressure. Those patients who improve least demonstrate cranial nerve palsies, cerebellar dysfunction, or motor weakness prior to therapy.

While single-dose radiation therapy has been advocated by some, it generally has not been found as useful as fractionated radiation therapy and has been associated with a higher incidence of complications, most notably brain swelling, herniation, and hemorrhage.[43,96,111] The dose recommended has been 1000 R. Most patients receiving radiation therapy receive instead between 2000 and 4000 R fractionated by various methods (dose or time) over various port sizes.[36,37,71] The schedule outlined in Table 90–13 is the one used by the authors. Response to therapy is often reported in terms of a "palliative index" (ratio of the duration of improvement to the duration of survival for a given time, x), which was introduced by Hindo and Order and their co-workers.[40,71]

Hendrickson recently reported the results of a study evaluating the possible complementary role of steroids and chemotherapy in patients receiving radiation therapy.[37] He found steroids increased the promptness of improvement but did not change the proportion of patients who actually improved, nor did steroids alter the duration of improvement from radiation therapy. Chemotherapy did not appear to modify the course of the response to radiation therapy favorably.

The results of radiation therapy series abound in the literature, and an overview of recent reports is included in Table 90–7. Complications of radiation therapy at usual dosages are rare but include hemorrhage, necrosis, brain swelling with herniation, and abscess formation.[67,77,80,111] Radiation therapy appears to injure brain by inducing vascular thrombosis and inflammation with an associated change in the permeability of blood vessels, and also by damaging myelin sheaths, which may lead eventually to an autoimmune response.[69,113]

Like operative therapy, radiation therapy usually offers palliation for cerebral metastases, although occasionally it sterilizes the cerebral tumor.[74,75] Figure 90–6 shows the pre- and postradiation CT scans from one such patient. In some of these patients no residual tumor has been found at necropsy.

One argument frequently put forward for operative removal of the single metastasis is that biopsy at least guarantees that the pretreatment diagnosis was in fact correct. Because histological verification of the cerebral metastasis treated with radiation is not obtainable except at autopsy, if one is performed, occasional long-term survivors in the radiation therapy series may represent errors in diagnosis. Raskind and co-workers have emphasized such errors in their report of 12 patients believed to have a cerebral metastasis who at operation were found to have other lesions.[83] On the other hand, with careful pretreatment neurological evaluation, errors in diagnosis are rare.[74]

Chemotherapy

The role of chemotherapy in the treatment of intraparenchymal metastasis to the brain remains unclear. In general, the results of treating metastatic brain tumors with chemotherapeutic agents have been disappointing.[38,39,77,110]

Immunotherapy

Immunotherapy to treat cancer has little role in the treatment of cerebral metastases at present. For extracranial tumors, the most effective therapy appears to be the direct injection of an immunological agent into a lesion. Substances that potentiate im-

TABLE 90–13 CURRENT RADIATION THERAPY PROTOCOL

Glucocorticoids (dexamethasone 16 mg every day, then therapy
Radiation
   500 Rads every day, days 1, 2, 3
   No radiation therapy, days 4 to 7
   300 Rads every day, days 8 to 12
   No radiation therapy, days 13, 14
   300 Rads every day, days 15 to 17
   Total dose: 3900 rads in 21 days
   Equivalent to 5200 rads in 5 weeks (200 × 26)
Taper glucocorticoids to tolerance

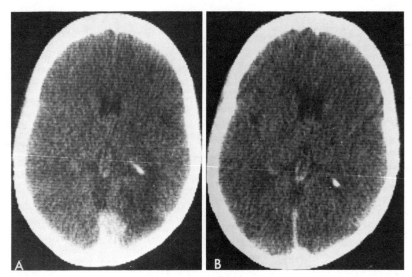

Figure 90–6 *A*. CT brain scan before a course of whole brain radiation therapy. *B*. Tumor that is obvious on the pretreatment scan has disappeared following therapy. (Courtesy of Dr. Michael D. F. Deck.)

mune mechanisms such as BCG, PPD, Freund's adjuvent, or C-parvum may also be effective.[58] Unfortunately, little evidence exists that metastatic brain tumors respond to this form of therapy.

Results

For untreated patients, the median survival of patients with a cerebral metastasis from time of diagnosis is approximately one to two months.[56,63,77] While the majority of patients receiving corticosteroids improve temporarily, the median survival with steroids alone is about two to three months.[52,54,63,77] The combination of corticosteroids plus radiation therapy provides a median survival of three to five months, and the combination of cortocosteroids plus operation usually provides a median survival of approximately four to six months (see Tables 90–6 and 90–7). Finally, the median survival following corticosteroids plus operation plus radiation appears to be about six months (see Table 90–8). More data—and in particular, controlled prospective studies—are necessary to establish the relative merits of different forms of therapy, but at present, the combination of corticosteroids, operation, and radiation is probably the most effective therapy for a single metastasis to the brain if the patient meets the prerequisites for operation.

LEPTOMENINGEAL METASTASES

"Leptomeningeal metastases" ("meningeal carcinomatosis," "meningeal sarcomatosis," "meningeal leukemia") refers to diffuse or widespread multifocal seeding of the leptomeninges by systemic cancer.[68] Leptomeningeal metastases may occur in the absence of other metastatic intracranial disease or may coexist with mass lesions of the brain or the subdural or epidural spaces.[11] In some instances, the metastases reach a size that is apparent on gross inspection at postmortem examination or can be identified by pneumoencephalographic or myelographic examination. More often, the tumor is apparent only microscopically, although hydrocephalus produced by the tumor's blocking of subarachnoid pathways may suggest its existence on gross inspection at autopsy. The presence of leptomeningeal tumor may excite an inflammatory response of white cells, usually lymphocytes, within the meninges that exfoliate into the cerebral spinal fluid. This inflammatory response has led some to use the term "carcinomatous meningitis" to designate this metastatic complication of cancer.

The first case of leptomeningeal metastases was probably that of Eberth, reported in 1870; more recently, several reviews have documented the clinical findings and treatment of this condition, which may be a complication of any systemic cancer.[20,53,68,95]

Incidence

For the century after the original description, leptomeningeal metastases were thought to be a rare metastatic curiosity, the diagnosis of which could only be made at postmortem examination. Such lesions were the subject of case reports and small case series. The same was true of leptomeningeal leukemia, as this entity was rare until effective parenteral chemotherapy began to prolong the lives of children with acute lymphoblastic leukemia. Ultimately, this disorder affected approximately 50 per cent of all children with acute lymphoblastic leukemia. Protocols calling for prophylactic treatment of the neuraxis either by radiation therapy or chemotherapy or both have since been developed that once again have made meningeal leukemia an uncommon disorder.

Leptomeningeal metastases from solid tumors are not a rare problem. Current evidence indicates that this metastatic complication of systemic cancer is increasing in frequency. In one series, leptomeningeal metastases were present in 8 per cent of patients with systemic cancer who came to autopsy, and in 3 per cent of them leptomeningeal metastases represented the only central nervous system involvement.[76] The incidence of leptomeningeal metastases counted at autopsy has doubled in the years between 1970 and 1976, and the clinical incidence at Memorial Sloan-Kettering Cancer Center has risen as well.[28,76] The increasing incidence of leptomeningeal metastases has been noted by other observers.[26] In children, the most common primary neoplasms producing tumor infiltration of the leptomeninges are leukemia and medulloblastoma; in adults, carcinoma of the breast, lymphoma, carcinoma of the lung, and melanoma are the most frequent systemic tumors seeding the leptomeninges, in that order.[41,76]

Pathophysiology

Tumor cells may reach the leptomeninges in one of several ways. One mode of entrance into the leptomeninges is via hematogenous metastasis to the choroid plexus, from which cells reach the ventricular system and float with the flow of spinal fluid until they lodge in one of the interstices of the arachnoid membrane at the base of the brain or in the spinal canal. Another potential mode of spread to the leptomeninges is by direct extension from a mass lesion either in the brain or in the subdural space. In the first instance, the intraparenchymal brain tumor must reach the surface of the cortex, rupture through the pia mater, and then seed the meninges via the cerebrospinal fluid. An alternate method is for the brain tumor to breach the pia at the Virchow-Robin spaces and grow along blood vessels to the surface of the cortex. It is surprising how rarely mass lesions in the brain lead to leptomeningeal seeding, probably because the pia is an effective barrier against the growing tumor mass. Subdural tumors probably represent the most frequent origin of spread. Subdural tumors do not frequently produce diffuse leptomeningeal spread, however, perhaps because the arachnoid membrane keeps them localized to the subdural space. A third potential route of entrance to the nervous system is by growth of paravertebral tumors along nerve roots into the spinal canal. This is probably a common mode of entrance to the leptomeninges for Hodgkin's disease and other lymphomas. Finally, tumor cells can spread hematogenously to the arachnoid vessels and insinuate themselves through arachnoid membranes into the subarachnoid space. This mode of entrance of leukemia into the nervous system has been demonstrated by Price and Johnson, and perhaps occurs with solid tumors as well.[78]

Once tumor has gained entrance to the subarachnoid space, it disseminates widely, showing a predilection for sticking and growing in specific areas. Thus, in many instances the tumor growth is thickest at the base of the brain, in the sylvian fissure, and down the posterior aspects of the spinal canal. Less growth is apparent around anterior roots and over the surface of the hemispheres. Although ventricular metastases are observed from time to time, they are rare compared with the number in the subarachnoid space. Tumor grows in sheetlike fashion, eliciting a variable inflammatory response in the pia and arachnoid. Rarely, small amounts of tumor incite a great deal of pial and arachnoidal fibrosis and inflammation, and at other times large amounts of tumor fail to stimulate much pial or arachnoidal reaction. The tumor may invade the parenchyma of the brain or spinal cord, reaching the brain by growth down the Virchow-Robin spaces to produce perivascular infiltrates of tumor within the substance of the cerebral cortex, and reaching the spinal cord often by growth along the posterior root into the substance of the cord. Hydrocephalus from obstruction either of the foramina of Luschka or of the basal cisterns is a common pathological accompaniment of meningeal carcinomatosis. When melanoma seeds the meninges, the local vascular endothelium develops abnormal fenestrations, and thus the tumor may be hemorrhagic, at times leading to a false diagnosis of subarachnoid hemorrhage; except for choriocarcinoma, or even more rarely lymphoma, other tumors generally do not produce a similar change.[55,103]

Leptomeningeal metastases produce their signs and symptoms in one of several ways: (1) *Hydrocephalus* develops as a consequence of blocking of the subarachnoid pathways, leading to typical, nonspecific signs and symptoms. (2) *Direct invasion* of cranial nerves, spinal roots and parenchyma of the brain and spinal cord by tumor from the subarachnoid space first demyelinates and then completely destroys the cranial and spinal roots by infiltrating into their substance. Similarly, the invasion of tumor from the subarachnoid space into the brain or spinal cord can produce focal neurological signs. Because the cortex is invaded first, seizures are a common accompaniment of meningeal carcinomatosis. At times, leptomeningeal metastases grow to such size that they cause cranial nerve or spinal root dysfunction from compression rather than direct invasion. (3) *Ischemia* caused by involvement of Virchow-Robin spaces with tumor growing from the subarachnoid space into the cortex of the brain, although not clearly established as a cause of symptoms, has the potential of interfering with microcirculation to the area of cortex. Pathological changes in humans and in experimental animals have been found that are suggestive of ischemia in areas where the Virchow-Robin spaces were invaded by tumor, and it is postulated that this mechanism sometimes produces symptoms in humans.[98] (4) *Metabolic dysfunction* is a more speculative possibility, i.e., that the tumor and the neurons lying near the tumor compete for the same metabolic substances, neurological symptoms being produced by neurons losing out to the more voracious tumor cells. Hypoglycorrhachia occurs in a significant percentage of patients with leptomeningeal metastases, and whether parts of the brain itself are glucose-deprived has not been established. An intriguing clinical finding that suggests the possibility that this may be the case is the so-called hypothalamic obesity reported in some children with meningeal leukemia.[5] In these children, inexplicable weight gain is associated with a voracious appetite but without other signs or symptoms of central nervous dysfunction. In some children who have died, the hypothalmus has been invaded by leukemia cells. One of the authors' patients (an 18-year-old girl in systemic remission from leukemia) had a 20-kg weight gain, which led to a lumbar puncture that revealed malignant cells and a glucose concentration of 7 mg per 100 ml. After treatment with intrathecal methotrexate, the glucose returned to normal, the cells disappeared, and the patient lost 20 kg, which restored her to her ideal weight.

Diagnosis

Signs and Symptoms

Because the entire neuraxis can be seeded by leptomeningeal metastases, signs and symptoms can involve almost any part of the central nervous system. Two clues lead to the diagnosis in patients suffering from systemic cancer and with neurological symptoms: (1) Neurological symptoms are more widespread than can be explained on the basis of a single lesion. For example, the patient may complain of diplopia resulting from a third or sixth nerve palsy and simultaneously complain of numbness or weakness in a root distribution in one upper or lower extremity. (2) Although patients may have unifocal complaints, careful neurological examination often reveals neurological signs unexplainable by a lesion at the site of the major complaint. For example, a patient with headache and papilledema suggesting increased intracranial pressure may, on careful examination, have absence of the left ankle jerk and weakness of plantar flexion of that foot also, suggesting in addition to the cerebral problem a coexisting root problem. Specific signs and symptoms produced by leptomeningeal metastases can be arbitrarily attributed to three areas of origin: cerebral, cranial nerve, and spinal root. In the first group, common signs and symptoms are headache, focal seizures, lethargy, and cognitive changes, probably resulting from hydrocephalus. In the second group, optic and oculomotor difficulties and patchy involvement of multiple cranial nerves (especially the seventh) are observed. In the third group, weakness and sensory changes (in the distribution of the spinal roots) typically involve both lower extremities in a patchy fashion and produce early autonomic dysfunction. In some patients, because of meningeal inflammation, neck and back pain and nuchal rigidity are early signs. Specific signs and symptoms and their frequency have been reviewed elsewhere.[11,22,53,68]

Because the disease responds better to therapy when treated in its early stages, early diagnosis is important and can often be made by examination of the spinal fluid even in the absence of clear neurological evidence of multifocal dysfunction.

Laboratory Examination

The most important laboratory test for the diagnosis of meningeal carcinomatosis is the lumbar puncture. Because mass lesions within cerebral substance may coexist with leptomeningeal tumor, making the lumbar puncture hazardous, other diagnostic procedures such as computed tomography should precede lumbar puncture in any patient with symptoms or signs suggesting increased intracranial pressure. The findings on spinal fluid examination are often characteristic. Often the pressure is elevated, white cells are increased in number (representing the inflammation that the tumor engenders), protein concentration is increased, and the glucose concentration is reduced. Malignant cells may be found on cytological examination of the cerebrospinal fluid, but they may be absent even in the presence of striking symptoms of meningeal invasion. Repeated spinal taps may be necessary to identify malignant cells, and large quantities of spinal fluid often have to be examined. The presence of malignant cells in the fluid is strong evidence

that the leptomeninges have been invaded by the tumor, since isolated intracerebral or intraspinal metastases do not usually seed malignant cells into the cerebrospinal fluid. At the present time there are no clear biochemical markers to identify leptomeningeal seeding in the absence of malignant cells, although Schuttleworth and Allen have reported that beta-glucuronidase levels are often elevated in the spinal fluid of patients with leptomeningeal metastases.[91] Evaluation of serum and cerebrospinal fluid chorionic gonadotropin (HCG) ratios or cerebrospinal fluid carcinoembryonic antigen (CEA) levels may also aid in monitoring disease metastatic to the central nervous system.[3,112]

Other laboratory tests may be helpful as well. The CT scan frequently reveals hydrocephalus in the absence of mass lesions, suggesting that the subarachnoid pathways are blocked. In addition, in some patients contrast enhancement is present in the cisterns surrounding the brain stem, providing strong evidence for neoplastic invasion. Parenthetically, the presence of contrast enhancement probably indicates that the blood-arachnoid barrier in that area is no longer normal (Fig. 90-7). The myelogram also may be a useful diagnostic test, since careful inspection of the films often will reveal small tumor nodules studding nerve roots. These myelographic findings in association with the contrast enhancement of the subarachnoid space on CT scan are adequate evidence of meningeal seeding by tumor even in the absence of identification of malignant cells in the spinal fluid.

Treatment of Leptomeningeal Metastases

Despite the fact that diffuse leptomeningeal metastases are not amenable to direct operative therapy, the neurosurgeon has an important role to play in the treatment of this metastatic complication of systemic cancer. Two procedures that are important in the therapy of this disorder are the placement of a ventricular cannula attached to a subcutaneous reservoir for the injection of chemotherapeutic agents into the ventricular system and, less often, the shunting of the ventricles to alleviate the symptoms of hydrocephalus. Technical considerations in the performance of these procedures in pa-

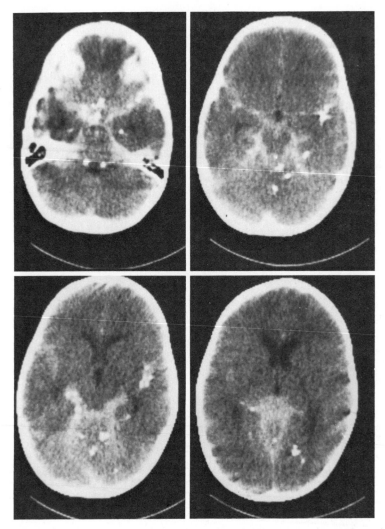

Figure 90–7 CT brain scan after intravenous administration of contrast agent in a patient with documented meningeal carcinomatosis. Contrast enhancement of the subarachnoid cisterns and hydrocephalus are apparent. (Courtesy of Dr. Michael D. F. Deck.)

tients with cancer are considered later. Treatment of leptomeningeal metastases must be directed toward the entire neuraxis, since the seeding is so widespread. Thus, operative extirpation of a single lesion is not useful. It is likely that the most effective treatment would be high-dosage radiation therapy delivered to the entire neuraxis, but since this would produce severe bone marrow depression, and since many patients require chemotherapy for control of their systemic tumor, the authors have elected to deliver radiation therapy only to the site of major neurological symptoms and treat the remainder of the neuraxis with intrathecal drugs. The use of intrathecal drugs was chosen because of

prior experience that systemic chemotherapy failed to treat meningeal leukemia effectively. Even though there is both clinical and experimental evidence of blood-brain barrier breakdown when the leptomeninges are seeded by tumor, experience with systemic chemotherapy in this circumstance has been disappointing. The drug commonly used is methotrexate in the dosage and by the schedule detailed in Table 90–14. The route of administration is into the lateral ventricle through a ventricular cannula attached to a subcutaneous reservoir under the scalp (Ommaya device). Use of an Ommaya device is preferable to repeated lumbar puncture for three reasons: (1) the drug distribution throughout the neuraxis is

TABLE 90–14 TECHNIQUE FOR INTRAVENTRICULAR INSTILLATION OF DRUGS VIA OMMAYA RESERVOIR

1. Check hematocrit, white blood count (WBC), platelet count, and blood urea nitrogen (BUN)
   Do not give methotrexate (MTX) if
   BUN > 20 mg per 100 ml, or
   WBC < 2500 or falling, or
   Platelets < 100,000 or falling
   Do not give methotrexate if there are mouth ulcers
2. Preparation of drugs
   Usual dose
   Methotrexate, 7.0 mg per square meter
   Arabinosylcytosine (ara-C) 30 mg per square meter
   Dilute arabinosylcytosine with nonbacteriostatic sterile water (100-mg vial with 5 ml water). Discard that which will not be used, leaving the appropriate dose in the vial
   For methotrexate treatment, use the 5-mg vial. Remove appropriate volume for dose into a 20-ml syringe.
   Add arabinosylcytosine to methotrexate syringe if combined drugs are to be used
3. Have available
   Sterile towel for under head
   Iodine
   4 4- by 4-inch sponges
   1 22-gauge or pediatric lumbar puncture needle (a 23-gauge butterfly needle may be used but is more likely to drag fragments of skin into the Ommaya reservoir and hence invite infection)
   1 5-ml syringe
   1 5- to 10-ml syringe for samples
   Syringe with methotrexate plus arabinosylcytosine
   Alcohol wipes
4. Shave area over reservoir
5. Clean Ommaya reservoir with iodine, wiping off excess
6. With 5-ml syringe attached, insert lumbar puncture needle (or butterfly) and slowly remove 2.5 to 3.0 ml cerebrospinal fluid. Keep sterile for later "tube flush" (see step 9)
7. Change syringes and slowly remove appropriate volume for desired samples (5- to 10-ml syringe)
8. Attach 20-ml syringe containing drugs to needle. Withdraw sufficient cerebrospinal fluid into drug mixture to make up a total volume of 15 to 20 ml; do this slowly, as some patients have transient headache; then slowly instill entire volume
9. Replace syringe with initial syringe and inject back into Ommaya reservoir the first 3 ml of cerebrospinal fluid
10. Remove needle. Stop any bleeding (do not apply pressure to reservoir). Wipe off iodine with alcohol

better when the drug is injected into the ventricles than into the lumbar sac; (2) the intraventricular cannula assures that the drug is being injected into the subarachnoid space, whereas injection by lumbar puncture fails 5 to 10 per cent of the time, the drug reaching the subdural or epidural space rather than the subarachnoid space; and (3) the drug can be easily administered via the Ommaya device through a small-bore pediatric spinal needle and syringe (or if necessary a No. 23 scalp vein needle)

without the necessity for repeated lumbar punctures (Fig. 90–8).[49,94]

The results of treatment by this method are detailed elsewhere.[28,84,95] In general, patients with lymphomas respond quite well, those with carcinoma of the breast relatively well, and those with other solid tumors less well. If the patient has severe neurological signs before treatment is undertaken, the response to therapy is less good than if neurological signs are mild. Thus, as with other central nervous system metastatic complications of cancer, early treatment yields much better results. The condition of many patients can be stabilized without increasing neurological symptoms until they succumb to their systemic disease.

The treatment is not without its complications. The complications fall into two groups: those related to the toxicity of the drugs and those of the Ommaya device. Drug complications include aseptic meningitis and encephalopathy, an acute idiosyncratic reaction of the patient to the drug or its impurities.[106] This acute response generally clears in two or three days and may not recur if the patient is treated again. A second, more serious, complication, partic-

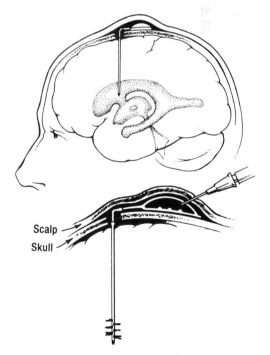

Figure 90–8 Ommaya reservoir connected to a ventricular catheter in the frontal horn of the right lateral ventricle. (Courtesy of Dr. William R. Shapiro.)

Scalp

Skull

ularly with the injection of methotrexate, is leukoencephalopathy.[93] This complication occurs more commonly when the patient has received prior brain irradiation. It is heralded by vague abnormalities of cognitive function and often mild tremulousness. At this stage, if the drug is discontinued, the condition is usually reversible. If treatment is continued, the patients often go on to develop severe neurological signs, including hemiplegia or quadriplegia and stupor or coma. Because methotrexate leukoencephalopathy is more common in patients with ventricular obstruction, the drug should not be given into the ventricles unless it is known that spinal fluid pathways between the ventricular system and the subarachnoid space are open. This is usually assured by doing a preoperative pneumoencephalogram. The third complication of the drug is focal leukoencephalopathy produced by backtracking of the methotrexate along the pathway of the ventricular cannula. This results in an area of focal low density on the CT scan that may or may not be associated with signs of neurological dysfunction. This complication appears to occur in patients with high intracranial pressure and has led the authors to lower intracranial pressure by removal of spinal fluid before injection of the drugs if the patient's pressure is elevated, and to inject the drugs while the patient is in the head-upright position if he has had a preexisting elevated spinal fluid pressure. Other aspects of the technique of injection of drugs into the ventricular system are included in Table 90–14.

Complications of the Ommaya device, which include infections, incorrect placement, and occasionally development of new neurological signs, are quite rare when strict attention is paid to the technical aspects of its installation. Since the ventricles are not enlarged, placing the catheter blindly in the frontal horn sometimes can be difficult. Placement is simplified if the ventricles are filled with air prior to the procedure, either by performing a pneumoencephalogram or by sitting the patient on the edge of the operating table and instilling perhaps 20 cc of air into the ventricles via lumbar injection. The patient is then positioned supine, and an image intensifier is used to identify the ventricles. A flanged ventricular catheter then is placed in the frontal horn through a burr hole anterior to

the coronal suture. The image intensifier helps again in gauging the proper length of the catheter, as shown in Figure 90–8. Admittedly the use of air and an image intensifier may not be required in some cases, but their routine use reduces complications to an absolute minimum. Since the authors have been using this frontal placement, they have had few instances of malfunctioning reservoir systems after placement.[32] Intracranial infection, usually mild and often asymptomatic, is surprisingly uncommon even in patients whose immune responses are suppressed. The infecting organism invariably has been *Staphylococcus epidermidis*. When the Ommaya device becomes infected, the patient is given systemic antibiotics, and an antibiotic (methicillin 50 to 100 mg a day) is injected directly into the ventricular system via the reservoir. In three of the five most recent infections encountered by the authors, the antibiotic treatment was successful and removal of the reservoir was not required. Because the infected prostheses are often asymptomatic, spinal fluid should be cultured with each sampling.

SUMMARY

Tumor metastatic to the brain is a common and devastating complication of cancer. The brain parenchyma or any of its various coverings may be involved by tumor, which most commonly is carried to the central nervous system by cerebral arteries. Edema, hemorrhage, obstruction of cerebrospinal fluid pathways, and mass effect may each participate in producing the headache, motor weakness, or mental changes that most often prompt the patient with metastatic involvement of the brain to consult a physician. Age, tumor type, and general toleration of disease all interact to produce variations from patient to patient in the "disease-free interval" between primary tumor discovery and the development of secondary involvement of the brain. When signs and symptoms of nervous system involvement occur, the differential diagnosis includes hemorrhage, abscess, infarction, and primary or secondary brain tumor. The CT scan with contrast agent is usually the single most useful test in evaluating such a problem. For the patient with a single brain metastasis who is tolerating his disease well (or is disease-free), for the patient with no known primary tumor, or the one who is a radiation failure, corticosteroids followed by operation followed by radiation therapy (if not already received) represents probably the best available treatment. Otherwise corticosteroids followed by radiation therapy is best, particularly when the lesion is radiosensitive or when the patient has multiple metastases. In the instance of meningeal carcinomatosis, following the documentation of positive cytological findings in the cerebrospinal fluid and evaluation of subarachnoid pathways, installation of an Ommaya reservoir for intrathecal delivery of chemotherapeutic agents followed by supplemental radiation therapy in appropriate cases provides the best currently available therapy. In all cases, the therapy is essentially palliative. Considering the devastating nature of tumor involvement of the central nervous system, however, even palliation is worthwhile for the patient and gratifying for the physician.

REFERENCES

1. Alderson, P. O., Gadd, M. H., and Siegel, B. A.: Computerized cranial tomography and radionuclide imaging in the Seminars Nucl. Med., 7:161–173, 1977.
2. Arseni, C., and Constantinescu, A. I.: Considerations on the metastatic tumours of the brain with reference to a statistics of 1217 cases. Schweiz. Arch. Neurol. Neurochir. Psychiat.117:179–195, 1975.
3. Bagshawe, K. D., and Harland, S.: Detection of intracranial tumours with special reference to immunodiagnosis. Proc. Roy. Soc. Med., 69:51–53, 1976.
4. Bakay, L.: Changes in barrier effect in pathological states. Progr. Brain Res., 29:315–341, 1968.
5. Barak, Y., and Liban, E.: Hypothalamic hyperphagia, obesity, and disturbed behavior in acute leukemia. Acta Paediat. Scand., 57:153–156, 1968.
6. Barnett, A.: Clinical differentiation between primary and secondary brain tumor. Lancet, 2:1344–1346, 1966.
7. Batson, O. V.: The function of the vertebral veins and their role in the spread of metastases. Ann. Surg., 112:138–149, 1940.
8. Berry, H. C., Parker, R. G., and Gerdes, A. J.: Irradiation of brain metastases. Acta Radiol. Ther. (Stockholm), 13:535–544, 1974.
9. Boller, F., Patten, D. H., and Howes, D.: Correlation of brain-scan results with neuropathological findings. Lancet, 1(813):1143–1146, 1973.
10. Brady, L. W., Mancall, E. L., Lee, D. K., Neff, L. B., Shockman, A. T., Faust, D. S., Antoniades, J., Prasavinichai, S., Torpie, R. J., and

Glassburn, J. R.: Radiation therapy for intracranial metastatic neoplasia. Radiol. Clin. (Basel), 43(1):40–47, 1974.
11. Bramlet, D., Giliberti, J., and Bender, J.: Meningeal carcinomatosis. Case report and review of the literature. Neurology (Minneap.), 26:287–290, 1976.
12. Brennen, M. J.: Corticosteroids in the treatment of solid tumors. Med. Clin. N. Amer., 57:1225–1230, 1973.
13. Buchanan, R. A., and Sholiton, J. J.: Diphenylhydantoin. In Woodbury, D. M., Penry, J. K., and Schmidt, R. P., eds.: Antianaleptic Drugs. New York, Raven Press, 1972, pp. 181–191.
14. Dandy, W. E.: Surgery of the Brain. Hagerstown, Md., W. F. Prior Co., Inc., 1945, pp. 671–688.
15. Deck, M. D. F., Messina, A. V., and Sackett, J. F.: Computed tomography in metastatic disease of the brain. Radiology, 119:115, 1976.
16. Deck, M. D. F.: Computed tomography for localization of brain metastases. In Gilbert H., Weiss, L., and Posner, J., eds.: Brain metastases. Boston, G. K. Hall, 1980, pp. 276–286.
17. Deeley, T. J., and Edwards, J. M.: Radiotherapy in the management of cerebral secondaries from bronchial carcinoma. Lancet, 1:1209–1213, 1968.
18. Deutsch, M., Parsons, J. A., and Mercado, R., Jr.: Radiotherapy for intracranial metastases. Cancer, 34:1607–1611, 1974.
19. Duchen, L. W.: Metastatic carcinoma involving the pituitary. J. Path. Bact., 91:347–355, 1966.
20. Eberth, C. J.: Zür Entwicklung des Epithelioms (Cholesteatoms) der Pia und der Lunge. Virchow. Arch., 49:51–63, 1870.
21. Fager, C. A.: Indications for neurosurgical intervention in metastatic lesions of the central nervous system. Med. Clin. N. Amer., 59:487–494, 1975.
22. Fischer-Williams, M. B., Sanquet, F. D., and Daniel, P. M.: Carcinomatosis of the meninges: A report of three cases. Brain, 78:42, 1958.
23. Fletcher, J. W., George, E. A., Henry, R. E., and Donati, R. M.: Brain scans, dexamethasone therapy, and brain tumors. J.A.M.A., 232:1261–1263, 1975.
24. Fordham, E. W.: The complementary role of C.A.T.T. and radionuclide imaging of brain scan. Seminars Nucl. Med., 7(2):137–159, 1977.
25. Gamache, F. W., Jr., Posner, J. B., and Galicich, J. H.: Treatment of brain metastases by surgical extirpation. In Gilbert, H., Weiss, L., and Posner, J., eds.: Brain Metastases. Boston, G. K. Hall, 1980, pp. 390–414.
26. Gercovich, F. G., Luna, M. A., and Gottlieb, J. A.: Increased survival in sarcoma patients. Cancer, 36:1843–1851, 1975.
27. Glanzmann, C., Jutz, P., and Horst, W.: Radiotherapy results in brain metastases (118 cases). Strahlentherapie, 152:352–357, 1976.
28. Glass, J. P., Shapiro, W. R., and Posner, J. B.: Treatment of leptomeningeal metastases (Meeting abstract). Neurology (Minneap.), 28:350–351, 1978.
29. Goldman, H., and Sapirstein, L. A.: Nature of the hypophysical blood supply in the rat. Endocrinology, 71:845–858, 1962.

30. Haar, F., and Patterson, R. H., Jr.: Surgery for metastatic intracranial neoplasm. Cancer, *30*:1241–1245, 1972.

31. Hagerstrand, I., and Schonebeck, J.: Metastases to the pituitary gland. Acta. Path. Microbiol. Scand., *75*:64–70, 1969.

32. Haghbin, M., and Galicich, J. H.: Use of the Ommaya reservoir in the prevention and treatment of CNS leukemia. Amer. J. Pediat. Hematology. Oncology, *1*:111–117, 1979.

33. Hayes, T. P., Davis, L. W., and Raventos, A.: Brain and liver scans in the evaluation of lung cancer patients. Cancer, *27*:362–363, 1971.

34. Hayward, R. D.: Secondary malignant melanoma of the brain. Clin. Oncol., *2*:227–232, 1976.

35. Hendricks, G. L., Barnes, W. T., and Hood, H. L.: Lung J.A.M.A., *220*:127, 1972.

36. Hendrickson, F. R.: Radiation therapy of metastatic tumors. Seminars Oncol., *2*:43–46, 1975.

37. Hendrickson, F. R.: The optimum schedule for palliative radiotherapy for metastatic brain cancer. Int. J. Radiat. Oncol. Biol. Phys., *2*:165–168, 1977.

38. Hildebrand, J., Brihaye, J., Wagenknecht, L., Michel, J., and Kenis, Y.: Combination chemotherapy with 1-(2-chloroethyl-3-cyclohexyl-1-nitrosourea) (CCNU), vincristine and methotrexate in primary and metastatic brain tumors—a preliminary report. Europ. J. Cancer, *9*:627–634, 1973.

39. Hildebrand, J., Brihaye, J., Wagenknecht, L., Michel, J., and Kenis, Y.: Combination chemotherapy with CCNU, vincristine and methotrexate in primary and metastatic brain tumors. Europ. J. Cancer, *11*:585–587, 1975.

40. Hindo, W. A., Detrana, F. A., Lee, M. S., and Hendrickson, F. R.: Large dose increment irradiation in treatment of cerebral metastases. Cancer, *26*:138–141, 1970.

41. Horenstein, S.: Miscellaneous forms of meningitis. Advances Neurol., *6*:205–221, 1974.

42. Jacobs, L., Kinkel, W. R., and Vincent, R. G.: Silent brain metastasis from lung carcinoma determined by computed tomography. Arch. Neurol. (Chicago), *34*:690–693, 1977.

43. Jazy, F., and Aron, B. S.: Single dose irradiation in treatment of cerebral metastases from bronchial carcinoma. Cancer, *34*:254–256, 1974.

44. Kagan, A. R., and Gilbert, H. A.: Detection of occult metastases with imaging studies. Int. J. Radiat. Oncol. Biol. Phys., *1*(5-6):529–533, 1976.

45. Kistler, M., and Pribram, H. W.: Metastatic disease of the sella turcica. Amer. J. Roentgen., *123*(1):13–21, 1975.

46. Kullberg, G., and West, K. A.: Influence of corticosteroids in the ventricular fluid pressure. Part II. Acta Neurol. Scand., *41*:suppl. 13:445–452, 1965.

47. Lang, E. F., Jr.: Neurosurgical management of intracranial metastatic malignancy. Surg. Clin. N. Amer., *47*:737–742, 1967.

48. Lang, E. F., and Slater, J.: Metastatic brain tumors. Results of surgical and non-surgical treatment. Surg. Clin. N. Amer., *44*:865–872, 1964.

49. Larson, S. M., Schall, G. L., and DiChiro, G.: The influence of previous lumbar puncture and pneumoencephalography on the incidence of unsuccessful radioisotope cisternography. J. Nucl. Med., *12*:555–557, 1971.

50. Leech, R. W., Welch, F. T., and Ojemann, G. A.: Subdural hematoma secondary to metastatic dural carcinomatosis. Case report, J. Neurosurg., *41*:610–613, 1974.

51. Leppik, I. E., Thompson, C. J., Ethier, R., and Sherwin, A. L.: Diatrizoate in computed cranial tomography: A quantitative study. Invest. Radiol., *12*:21–26, 1977.

52. Lesse, S., and Netsky, M. G.: Metastasis of neoplasms to the central nervous system and the meninges. Arch. Neurol. Psychiat., *72*:133–153, 1954.

53. Little, J. R., Dale, A. J., and Okazaki, H.: Meningeal carcinomatosis. Clinical manifestations. Arch. Neurol. (Chicago), *30*:138–143, 1974.

54. Lokich, J. J.: Management of cerebral metastases. J.A.M.A., *234*:748–751, 1975.

55. Lovings, E. T.: Endothelial fenestrations and other vascular alterations in primary melanoma of the nervous system. Cancer, *34*:1982–1991, 1974.

56. MacGee, E. E.: Surgical treatment of cerebral metastasis from lung cancer. J. Neurosurg., *35*:416–420, 1971.

57. Magilligan, D. J., Jr., Rogers, J. S., Knighton, R. S., and Davila, J. C.: Pulmonary neoplasm with solitary cerebral metastasis. J. Thorac. Cardvasc. Surg., *72*:690–698, 1976.

58. Mahaley, M. S.: Immunotherapy of brain tumors. Seminars Oncol., *2*:75–78, 1975.

59. Marshall, W. H., Jr., Easter, W., and Batz, L. M.: Analysis of the dense lesion at computed tomography with dual kVp scans. Radiology, *124*:109–112, 1977.

60. Marty, R., and Cain, M.: Effects of corticosteroid administration on the brain scan. Radiology, *107*:117–121, 1973.

61. Mayer, E. G., Boone, M. L., and Aristizabal, S. A.: Role of radiation therapy in the management of neoplasms of the central nervous system. Advances Neurol., *15*:201–220, 1976.

62. Messian, A. V.: Cranial computerized tomography: A radiologic-pathologic correlation. Arch. Neurol. (Chicago), *34*:602–607, 1977.

63. Modesti, L. M., and Feldman, R. A.: Solitary cerebral metastasis from pulmonary cancer. Prolonged survival after surgery. J.A.M.A., *231*:1064, 1975.

64. Moore, J. S., Kieffer, S. A., Goldberg, M. E., and Loken, M. K.: Intracranial tumors: Correlation of angiography with dynamic radionuclide studies. Radiology, *115*:393–398, 1975.

65. Mosberg, W. H., Jr.: 12 year cure of lung cancer metastatic to brain. J.A.M.A., *235*:2745–2746, 1976.

66. New, P. F., Scott, W. R., Schnur, J. A., Davis, K. R., Taveras, J. M., and Hochberg, F. H.: Computed tomography with the EMI scanner in the diagnosis of primary and metastatic intracranial neoplasms. Radiology, *114*:75–87, 1975.

67. Nisce, I. Z., Hilaris, B. S., and Chu, F. C. H.: A review of experience with irradiation of brain metastasis. Amer. J. Roentgen., *111*:329–333, 1971.

68. Olson, M. E., Chernik, N. L., and Posner, J. B.: Infiltration of the leptomeninges by systemic

cancer. A clinical and pathologic study. Arch. Neurol. (Chicago), *30*:122–137, 1974.

69. Olsson, Y., Klatzo, I., and Carsten, A.: The effect of acute radiation injury on the permeability and ultrastructure of intracerebral capillaries. Neuropath. Appl. Neurobiol., *1*:59–68, 1975.

70. Onuigbo, W. I.: Batson's theory of vertebral venous metastasis: A review. Oncology, *32*:145–150, 1975.

71. Order, S. E., Hellman, S., Von Essen, C. F., and Kligerman, M. M.: Improvement in quality of survival following whole-brain irradiation for brain metastasis. Radiology, *91*:149–153, 1968.

72. Pendergrass, H. P., McKusick, K. A., New, P. F., and Potsaid, M. S.: Relative efficacy of radionuclide imaging and computed tomography of the brain. Radiology, *116*:363–366, 1975.

73. Penzholz, H.: Die metastatischen Erkrankungen des Zentralnervensystems bei bösartigen Tumoren. Acta Neurochir. (Wien), suppl. *16*:1–205, 1968.

74. Posner, J. B.: Diagnosis and treatment of metastases to the brain. Clin. Bull., *4*:47–57, 1974.

75. Posner, J. B.: Management of central nervous system metastases. Seminars Oncol., *4*:81–91, 1977.

76. Posner, J. B., and Chernik, N. L.: Intracranial metastases from systemic cancer. Advances Neurol., *19*:575–587, 1978.

77. Posner, J. B., and Shapiro, W. R.: The management of intracranial metastases. *In* Morley, T. P., ed.: Current Controversies in Neurosurgery. Philadelphia, W. B. Saunders Co., 1976, pp. 356–366.

78. Price, R. A., and Johnson, W. W.: The central nervous system in childhood leukemia. I. The arachnoid. Cancer, *27*:247–256, 1971.

79. Ransohoff, J.: Surgical management of metastatic tumors. Seminars Oncol., *2*:21–27, 1975.

80. Raskind, R.: Central nervous system damage after radiation therapy. Int. Surg., *48*:430–441, 1967.

81. Raskind, W., and Weiss, S. R.: Conditions simulating metastatic lesions of the brain. Report of eight cases. Int. Surg., *43*:40–43, 1970.

82. Raskind, R., Weiss, S. R., and Wermuth, R. E.: Single metastatic brain tumors: Treatment and follow-up in 41 cases. Amer. Surg., *35*:510–515, 1969.

83. Raskind, R., Weiss, S. R., Manning, J. J., and Wermuth, R. E.: Survival after surgical excision of single metastatic brain tumors. Amer. J. Roentgen. *111*:323–328, 1971.

84. Ratcheson, R. A., and Ommaya, A. K.: Experience with a subcutaneous CSF reservoir: A preliminary report of 60 cases New Eng. J. Med., *279*:1025–1034, 1968.

85. Renaudin, J., Fewer, D., Wilson, C. B., Boldrey, E. A., Calogero, J., and Enot, K. J.: Dose dependency of Decadron in patients with partially excised brain tumors. J. Neurosurg., *39*:302–305, 1973.

86. Richards, P., and McKissock, W.: Intracranial metastases. Brit. Med. J., *1*:15–18, 1963.

87. Roman, I., Cristian, C., and Terzi, A.: EEG data in intracranial metastases. Electroencephalogr. Clin. Neurophysiol., *27*:635, 1969.

88. Rowan, A. J., Rudolk, N. De. M., and Scott, D.

F.: EEG prediction of brain metastases. A controlled study with neuropathological confirmation. J. Neurol. Neurosurg. Psychiat. *37*:888–893, 1974.

89. Russell, D. S., and Rubinstein, L. J.: Secondary neoplasms of the nervous system. In Pathology of Tumors of the Nervous System. Baltimore, Williams & Wilkins, Co., 1977, pp. 355–356.

90. Schoenberg, B. S., Christine, B. W., and Whisnant, J. P.: Nervous system neoplasms and primary malignancies of other sites. Neurology (Minneap.), *25*:705–712, 1975.

91. Schuttleworth, E. C., and Allen, N.: Early differentiation of chronic meningitis by enzymatic assay. Neurology (Minneap.), *18*:534–542, 1968.

92. Sellwood, R. B.: The radiological approach to metastatic cancer of the brain and spine. Brit. J. Radiol., *45*:647–651, 1972.

93. Shapiro, W. R., Chernik, N. L., and Posner, J. B.: Necrotizing encephalopathy following intraventricular methotrexate. Arch. Neurol. (Chicago), *28*:96–102, 1973.

94. Shapiro, W. R., Young, D. F., and Mehta, B. M.: Methotrexate: Distribution in cerebrospinal fluid after intravenous, ventricular and lumbar injections. New Eng. J. Med., *293*:161–166, 1975.

95. Shapiro, W. R., Posner, J. B., Ushio, Y., Chernik, N. L., and Young, D. F.: Treatment of meningeal neoplasms. Cancer Treat. Rep., *61*:733–743, 1977.

96. Shehata, W. M., Hendrickson, F. R., and Hindo, W. A.: Rapid fractionation technique and retreatment of cerebral metastases by irradiation. Cancer, *34*:257–261, 1974.

97. Stortebecker, T. P.: Metastatic tumors of the brain from a neurosurgical point of view: a follow-up study of 158 cases. J. Neurosurg., *11*:84–111, 1954.

98. Ushio, Y., Chernik, N. L., Posner, J. B., and Shapiro, W. R.: Meningeal carcinomatosis: Development of an experimental model. J. Neuropath Exp. Neurol., *36*:228–244, 1977.

99. Vannucci, R. C., and Baten, M.: Cerebral metastatic disease in childhood. Neurology (Minneap.), *24*:981–986, 1974.

100. Varrarakis, M. J., Winterberger, A. R., Gaeta, J., Moore, R. A., and Murphy, G. R.: Lung metastases in prostatic cancer. Urology, *3*:447–452, 1974.

101. Vick, N. A., Khandekar, J. D., and Bigner, D. D.: Chemotherapy of brain tumors. Arch. Neurol. (Chicago), *34*:523–566, 1977.

102. Vieth, R. G., and Odom, G. L.: Intracranial metastases and their neurosurgical treatment. J. Neurosurg., *23*:375–383, 1965.

103. Ward, J. D., Hatfield, M. G., Becker, D. P. and Lovings, E. T.: Endothelial fenestrations and other vascular alterations in primary melanoma of the nervous system. Cancer, *34*:1982–1991, 1974.

104. Waxman, A. D., Siemsen, J. K., Lee, G. C., Wolfstein, R. S., and Moser, L.: Reliability of gallium brain sacnning in the detection and differentiation of central nervous system lesions. Radiology, *116*:675–678, 1975.

105. Weinstein, J. D., Toy, F. J., Jaffe, M. E., and Goldberg, H. I.: The effect of dexamethasone

on brain edema in patients with metastatic brain tumors. Neurology (Minneap.), *23*:121–129, 1973.

106. Weiss, H. D., Walker, M. D., and Wiernik, P. H.: Neurotoxicity of commonly used antineoplastic agents. New Eng. J. Med., *291*:75–81, 127–133, 1974.

107. Wilson, C. B.: Diagnostic procedures. Seminars Oncol., *2*:9–10, 1975.

108. Wilson, C. B.: Bran metastases: Basis for surgical selection. Int. J. Radiat. Oncol. Biol. Phys., *2*:169–172, 1977.

109. Wilson, C. B., and Fewer, D.: Role of neurosurgery in the management of patients with carcinoma of the breast. Cancer, *28*:1681–1685, 1971.

110. Wilson, C. B., Yorke, C. H., Jr., and Levin, Y. A.: Intractranial malignant growth, primary and metastatic. Curr. Probl. Cancer, *1*:1–46, 1977.

111. Young, D. F., Posner, F. B., Chu, E., and Nisce, L.: Rapid-course radiation therapy of cerebral metastases: Results and complications. Cancer, *34*:1069–1076, 1974.

112. Zubrod, C. G.: Cerebral metastases and carcinoembryonic antigen in CSF. New Eng. J. Med., *293*–:1101, 1975.

113. Zulch, K. J.: Roentgen sensitivity of cerebral tumours and so-called late irradiation necrosis of the brain. Acta Radio. Ther., *8*:92–110, 1969.

91

BRAIN TUMORS OF DISORDERED EMBRYOGENESIS IN ADULTS

The tumors that arise as a result of abnormal nervous system development are a heterogeneous group of masses. Some have so little anaplasia that their growth potential approaches that of hamartomas. The World Health Organization classification of this group is given in Table 91–1.[216]

Many of these tumors that arise from malformation, among them Rathke's cleft cyst and choristoma, which are pituitary masses, intraspinal enterogenous cysts, arachnoid cysts, and nasal glial heterotopias, are discussed in other chapters (e.g., 84, 85, 89, and 98). In this chapter, epidermoid cysts, dermoid cysts, teratomas, craniopharyngiomas, colloid cysts, and lipomas are discussed. As a group they have been described by Kernohan as congenital tumors of the central nervous system.[114] Epidermoid cysts, dermoid cysts, and teratomas are considered under the heading of Inclusion Tumors.

CRANIOPHARYNGIOMA

At the beginning of the twentieth century, cystic suprasellar tumors of embryonic origin were recognized as a discrete entity separate from gliomas and pituitary adenomas.[6,64,159] The name "craniopharyngioma" was popularized by Cushing, by McKenzie and Sosman, and by McLean.[54,152,155] Many authors have criticized it because it suggests an origin from primitive pharynx. Even if one assumes

that the neoplasm arises from Rathke's pouch, the inferior portion of Rathke's pouch is related to the buccal cavity, not to the primitive pharynx.[102,198] The widespread use and understanding of this name, however, argues for its preservation, and in spite of embryological criticism, it remains generally accepted.

These tumors have been presumed to arise from Rathke's pouch, which develops from a superior diverticulum of the stomodeum, which in turn will form the buccal cavity.[188] As this diverticulum matures, the neck narrows and eventually is obliterated. The remnant, Rathke's pouch, matures into the anterior pituitary and the pars intermedia (Fig. 91–1).[50,61,167]

There is histological similarity between craniopharyngioma and adamantinoma (a neoplasm of the primitive buccal cavity). Since the embryonic formation of Rathke's pouch brings primitive buccal tissue to the sella, and since craniopharyngioma occurs in an age group prone to maldevelopmental tumors, it has been assumed to arise from Rathke's pouch.[64,159] This assumption is reinforced by the finding of rudimentary teeth in craniopharyngiomas.[208] These tumors have also been found along the course of invagination taken by Rathke's pouch—in the sphenoid bone and in the nasopharynx.[48,185]

Some craniopharyngiomas arise later in life. Remnants of Rathke's pouch might be represented by epithelial cells, which have been identified in one third to one fourth of

C. A. COBB AND J. R. YOUMANS

**TABLE 91–1   WORLD HEALTH
ORGANIZATION CLASSIFICATION OF
MALFORMATIVE BRAIN TUMORS**

Craniopharyngioma
Rathke's cleft cyst
Epidermoid cyst
Dermoid cyst
Colloid cyst of the third ventricle
Enterogenous cyst
Other cysts
  Arachnoid cysts
  Ependymal lined cysts
  Neuroglial lined cysts
Lipoma
Choristoma (granular cell myoblastoma, pituicytoma)
Hypothalamic neuronal hamartoma
Nasal glial heterotopia (nasal glioma)

adults.[38,65,144] These cells are found in only 3 per cent of newborns, however, suggesting that they are acquired.[78] Perhaps they are immature in neonates and were not recognized, or more likely, they represent metaplasia of anterior pituitary cells.[65,100,196]

It is possible that this tumor is a variant of the epidermoid or dermoid inclusion cyst.[198] An intrasellar and suprasellar tumor resembling both an inclusion tumor and a craniopharyngioma has been reported, and the suggestion has been made that it demonstrates a link between them. There is insufficient pathological detail in the original report, however, to be certain of the correct classification of this tumor.[245]

If the tumor does arise from Rathke's pouch, it is surprising that its epithelium is so different from that of Rathke's cleft cyst, which is also presumed to arise from the pouch.[50,96,192] Perhaps these cysts are not derived from Rathke's pouch even though their epithelium is nearly identical.[211] Alternative suggestions are that the absence of either the adjacent notocord or posterior pituitary allows Rathke's pouch epithelium to become squamous (as in craniopharyngioma) or that Rathke's cleft cyst is a nonneoplastic condition and that anaplasia of this type of tissue can give rise to craniopharyngioma.

Incidence

Craniopharyngiomas make up approximately 2.5 per cent of brain tumors, although they account for a greater percentage in centers attracting a large number of patients with pituitary tumors.[4,54,173] They may be slightly more frequent in Japan.[202] They make up approximately 20 per cent of sellar-chiasmal tumors of adults.[152,221] In children, they make up about 7 per cent of brain tumors, are the most common nonglial tumor, and constitute approximately half of sellar-chiasmal tumors.[102,120,150]

Although in general they tend to occur in children, they may develop in patients of all ages. Approximately 50 per cent occur in persons less than 20 years of age, but they are not uncommon in old age, and a large calcified one has been reported in a newborn.[223] Both sexes are affected with equal frequency.*

---

* See references 4, 13, 75, 95, 110, 132, 157, 167, 173, 174, 182, 194, 198, 210, 220, 221, 258.

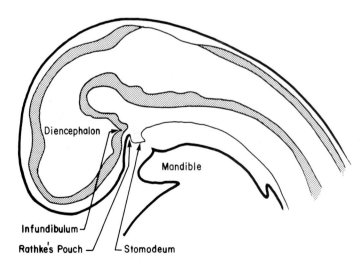

Figure 91–1 Rathke's pouch arises as a diverticulum of the stomodeum, the forerunner of the buccal cavity. It joins with the infundibulum to form the pituitary gland.

Pathology

Macroscopic Changes

Craniopharyngiomas are suprasellar tumors and usually contain both solid and cystic portions (Fig. 91–2). The solid tissue is smooth, firm, and gray or pink. The cystic portion is softer. Its consistency and color are determined by the thickness of the wall, which may be thin and translucent or may resemble the solid portion. Calcium deposition may make the tumor hard. The mass may be lobulated and may be extensive.

In approximately 15 per cent of them, degenerative changes produce large cysts.[173] Even the portions that are called solid usually contain small cysts. The inner wall of the cyst may be smooth or may contain multiple papillae.[221] The cysts are filled with brownish, muddy fluid containing suspended cholesterol crystals.

Most craniopharyngiomas occur in the suprasellar subarachnoid space or intrasellar areas or the third ventricle. A few occur in the sphenoid bone, the sinus, or intranasally. The usual size is 2 to 10 cm in diameter.[221] In most cases they remain localized to the suprasellar region. They extend under the frontal or temporal lobe in approximately 2 per cent and into the posterior fossa in 1 per cent of cases. In the posterior fossa they may present as clivus tumors. They can also pass through the foramen magnum.[4,173,190] The cyst of a craniopharyngioma has been accidentally entered when a ventriculogram was being performed through an occipital burr hole.[150]

When found incidentally at autopsy, they usually are located at the tuber cinereum, the site where symptomatic ones are most adherent to adjacent tissue.[95,198] Although Matson and Crigler denied that craniopharyngiomas invade brain, other authors have noted that projections of tumor interdigitate with gliotic nonfunctioning hypothalamus.[150,182,237] This penetration can extend 5 to 6 mm.[17,195]

A few craniopharyngiomas have been reported in the third ventricle.[29,41,237] Usually they only appear to arise in the third ventricle, however; in fact, they arise beneath the hypothalamus and displace a film of hypothalamus up into the third ventricle.[237]

Most of these tumors are located in the subarachnoid space just above the sella. The infundibulum of the pituitary gland usually lies posterior to them.[182] They are posterior to the chiasm in approximately one third of cases, the rest lying either beneath or anterior to the chiasm.[75,183,220] When prechiasmatic, they displace the chiasm posteriorly, whereas if retrochiasmatic, they lift up the floor of the third ventricle. Despite the intimate relation between tumor and chiasm, visual pathways are not infiltrated by tumor.[182]

The presence of congenitally short optic

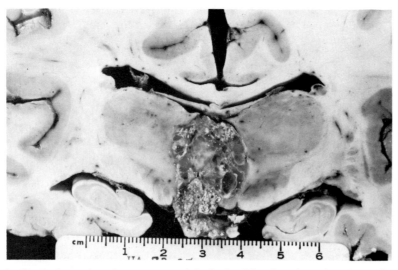

Figure 91–2 Craniopharyngioma is a tumor containing both solid and cystic portions. It usually arises beneath the third ventricle but may extend superiorly, lifting a film of hypothalamus into the third ventricle. (Courtesy of Surl L. Nielson, M.D., University of California, Davis.)

nerves displaces the chiasm anteriorly, creating the condition referred to as a prefixed chiasm. This occurs in approximately 5 to 10 per cent of the general population.[173] A prefixed chiasm is, however, found in one third of patients with craniopharyngiomas, suggesting that the chiasm may be displaced forward by the tumor rather than as the result of a congenital variation in optic nerve length.[173,220]

Approximately 15 to 20 per cent of craniopharyngiomas are intrasellar.[173,220] An intrasellar lesion may be associated with a suprasellar component or may be isolated from the subarachnoid space. The tumor may produce a very large sella containing a typical cystic or a solid lesion.

The arterial supply commonly is from many small vessels.[173] Small internal carotid artery branches in the sella, probably the dorsal capsular arteries, supply any sellar portion of the tumor. The suprasellar portion is supplied by arterial branches from the posterior communicating artery and the anterior cerebral artery. The posterior portion usually is without independent arterial supply.[182]

Rapidly growing craniopharyngiomas tend to have an invasive margin and extensive gliosis. The more indolent ones are separate from the hypothalamus and are not adherent. The slowly growing ones also tend to contain denser and more extensive calcium.[17]

Microscopic Changes

The solid portions consist of epithelial tissue with a columnar or cuboidal basal layer, an intermediate layer of rounded or polygonal cells, and a central mass of epithelial cells (Fig. 91–3).[50] The supporting stroma is connective tissue. Cystic areas have a wall of variable thickness that is histologically like the solid portion. A collagenous basement membrane forms a boundary between the tumor and surrounding meninges or brain.[198]

An attempt has been made to separate craniopharyngiomas into histological types. The usual type has the columnar basal layer and other features already noted and can be seen in either adults or children. An epithelial type has also been identified. Its squamous epithelium mimics that of the buccal cavity, and it does not have palisading of the basal layer. This latter type occurs only in adults and does not calcify.[110] The validity of this subclassification has not been confirmed by other authors.

The distinction between craniopharyngiomas and epidermoid cysts has been disputed by Russell and Rubinstein.[198] They argue that the cyst contents and epithelium are too variable to allow a discrete separation. This variability does not seem sufficient to outweigh the long-standing opinion that the epithelium of these two lesions differs, that the neoplasm with an epithelium characteristic of craniopharyngioma occurs only in the sellar region (whereas epidermoid cyst is found in many locations), that large solid portions of craniopharyngioma never contain dermal skin elements, that they have different cyst contents, or that they have a vastly different prognosis.

Degenerative changes may lead to cell death, formation of foreign body giant cells, or lymphocytic infiltration.[110,198] As these degenerative changes progress, cysts form and may coalesce. Degeneration may also produce confluent keratin masses that calcify. Calcium is shown histologically in approximately 80 per cent of all craniopharyngiomas, and in all craniopharyngiomas in children.[132,182]

There is no convincing evidence that craniopharyngiomas are subject to anaplasia. Tumor invading areas of gliosis sometimes suggests carcinomatous invasion, but this interpretation probably is incorrect.[198]

The external fibrous surface of a craniopharyngioma may produce either no significant response in subjacent glia or an intense glial reaction with Rosenthal fibers.[50,150] Some authors have stated that glial cells are present in craniopharyngiomas remote from brain involvement, but astrocytic protein analysis has not yet been used to document or disprove this suggestion.[129,150]

Tissue culture usually shows cells with little mitotic activity and a tendency to form cysts.[47] Approximately one fourth of the tumors have an atypical pattern with irregular cell growth, increased mitotic rate, and other histological signs of anaplasia.[138] Tumors with this anaplastic behavior in tissue culture also have more aggressive clinical behavior.

Signs and Symptoms

The duration of symptoms prior to diagnosis of craniopharyngioma is quite variable. The mean is about one year; however,

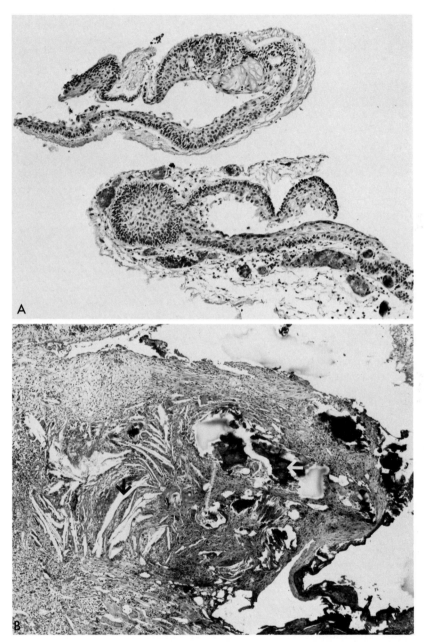

Figure 91–3 Microscopic pathological changes of craniopharyngioma. *A*. There is stratified squamous epithelium in cystic areas. *B*. Solid portions contain cholesterol clefts (*black arrow*) and calcium deposits (*white arrow*). 80 ×.

symptoms may be present for as long as 30 years and are not uncommonly present for as little as one month.[4,13,221] They are apparent for nearly the same length of time in adults and children.[210] There is usually no known inciting event, and symptoms develop insidiously and are progressive. Head injury triggers their onset in approximately 4 per cent of cases.[4] The rate of growth of the tumor can be estimated by the duration of symptoms. If the outcome for patients with symptoms for more than two years is compared with that for those having symptoms for less than two years, the longer durations of symptoms correlates with longer survival after treatment.[17]

The suprasellar region is surrounded by potentially symptomatic central nervous system structures. The visual system is anterior and to each side, the pituitary gland beneath, the mesencephalon and pons behind, and the hypothalamus and third ventricle (with the foramina of Monro) above. These structures allow symptoms to be classified into several general categories: visual symptoms, endocrine disturbances, increased intracranial pressure, and psychiatric symptoms. Extensive growth of the tumor can involve the frontal or temporal lobes, producing anosmia or seizures, or can involve posterior fossa structures, causing abnormality in the function of the fourth, fifth, and sixth cranial nerves, the pyramidal tract, and the cerebellum. Rarely, craniopharyngiomas can present with bizarre neurological deficits such as eighth cranial nerve dysfunction.[13] There is a general tendency for children and adolescents to present with increased intracranial pressure, while older patients more commonly have visual or endocrine complaints.[20]

The most common initial symptom in all patients is headache; it is the first symptom in approximately half of them. Abnormal vision is also a common first symptom. By the time diagnosis is made, 75 to 90 per cent of patients have headache, 30 to 38 per cent have vomiting, and approximately 67 per cent have visual disturbances.[4,221] Other symptoms such as growth arrest, diabetes insipidus, psychiatric disturbances, and seizures are present in 10 to 20 per cent.

If adults and children are considered separately, adults are found to present with visual symptoms in up to 93 per cent of cases.[13] Adults also may complain of head-

aches, gonadal dysfunction, and mental abnormalities.[75,194] About 40 per cent of children have initial symptoms in the visual system.[240] This may not reflect normal vision in the remainder but only the failure of children to complain of visual dysfunction.

By the time of diagnosis, 80 per cent of children have headache, and most of them also have vomiting.[127,150,157] Visual deficit is present in approximately 60 per cent of patients. Eighty to ninety per cent of adults have visual abnormalities. Vomiting is present in 40 to 60 per cent. Mental abnormalities are also common in adults.[13,75]

Neurological signs are most commonly in the visual system, and only 6 per cent of patients with craniopharyngiomas have normal visual function by testing.[167] Sixty per cent have abnormalities in neurological function outside the visual system.[80] These include cranial nerve palsies, which are seen in one fourth of children and one third of adults, and nystagmus and pyramidal and cerebellar signs.[94,210,221] The presence of paresis of cranial nerves (other than the first and second), of pyramidal tract signs, or of cerebellar signs suggests a tumor in a retrochiasmatic location.

Papilledema is present in 30 to 50 per cent of children, but in only 10 to 15 per cent of adults.[4,94,110] Although usually bilateral, it is unilateral in approximately 10 per cent of patients.[221] The presence of papilledema confirms hydrocephalus and obstruction of the cerebrospinal fluid spaces.

Patients without papilledema usually have optic atrophy. In only 8 per cent is funduscopic examination normal bilaterally.[4,127] Optic atrophy is particularly common in children, being present in about 55 per cent.[94] Approximately 40 per cent of adults have optic atrophy.[13,75]

Visual field defects are present in 60 to 80 per cent of children and between 90 and 95 per cent of adults.[94,95,194] Visual acuity is reduced in 75 per cent.[4] This reduction may be transitory, simulating retrobulbar neuritis.[194] The most common visual field deficit is bitemporal hemianopia, which accounts for two thirds of all field defects.[4,20,95] Paracentral scotomas are seen occasionally, and homonymous hemianopias are present in about 15 per cent of patients.[13,75,221] The suggestion that optic nerve involvement is common has not been borne out by other investigators, although unilateral blindness is occasionally present.[4,167,221]

Approximately 80 per cent of children with craniopharyngiomas have headache, which is their most common initial symptom.[15,102] Absence of headache does not rule out ventricular enlargement, since about 20 per cent of children whose ventricles are expanded by this tumor have neither headache nor vomiting.[15] The headache is diffuse and generalized, which is characteristic of increased intracranial pressure. Adults may present without headache or evidence of increased intracranial pressure. When headache is present, it may be either diffuse or localized in the forehead or above or behind the eyes, suggesting local dural involvement around the sella.[20]

The incidence of endocrine dysfunction that is reported varies with the sophistication of the evaluation techniques. In most series some 70 per cent of all patients have endocrine abnormalities, and the incidence is higher in children.[15,102,221] If elaborate endocrine studies are performed, it can be found that all patients have a deficiency of gonadotropins, 65 per cent have decreased growth hormone, 45 per cent have decreased adrenocorticotropic hormone, and 15 per cent have decreased thyroid function.[121] These findings correlate well with the 60 per cent frequency of menstrual irregularity in women of child-bearing age who have this tumor.[13] Intrasellar lesions produce severe panhypopituitarism, often without significant visual dysfunction.[173] Growth is impaired in approximately one fourth of children.[95,102,150] Obesity is also relatively frequent, occurring in about 20 per cent of patients.[13,80,221] Diabetes insipidus is a well-known postoperative problem, but occurs before operation in only 15 per cent.

Most patients with psychiatric abnormalities have tumors located behind the chiasm and have enlarged ventricles.[13,102,195] A variety of symptoms may occur, the most common being hypersomnia, apathy, and spatial disorientation.[4] Incontinence, memory disturbances, depression, and other psychiatric changes may also occur. According to Kahn and associates, Korsakoff's syndrome is seen in as many as 25 per cent of adults.[110] The presence of mental symptoms suggests an ominous prognosis.[17]

Chemical meningitis may result from release of toxic cyst contents.[50] This produces headache, neck stiffness, and photophobia.[4] Recurrent attacks are especially suggestive of craniopharyngioma.[194]

Investigation

Craniopharyngioma is one of the few intracranial tumors in which a tissue diagnosis can be made with reasonable certainty on the basis of plain skull x-rays. Sixty-six per cent of adults and ninety-five per cent of children with them have abnormal skull x-rays.[13,110,157] Radiographic changes are most prominent in the sella turcica and often include calcification of the tumor. Other changes include enlargement of the optic canals, seen in approximately 5 per cent of patients; widening of intracranial sutures; and digital markings in the skull.[4,150]

Changes in the sella turcica are seen in approximately half the patients.[94,110,157] These changes distinguish intrasellar from suprasellar craniopharyngiomas. Suprasellar tumor and its associated hydrocephalus press downward on the dorsum sellae and anterior clinoids and may enlarge the sella.[137,182,228] Sellar enlargement occurs in approximately 50 per cent of children.[110,150] Even in children with known hydrocephalus, the x-ray changes of increased intracranial pressure are not always present.[15]

If all ages are considered, about 60 per cent of patients with craniopharyngioma have radiographically visible calcium.[4,127,137] Even when not seen by x-ray, calcium is present in more than half the craniopharyngiomas examined under the microscope.[132] Its frequency is much greater in children, approximately 80 to 85 per cent of whom have radiographically identifiable calcification.[15,95,150,157] Only 40 per cent of adults have radiographically demonstrable tumor calcification.[75,194] Many of these adults have a history of symptoms since childhood.[110]

The calcification is in the suprasellar region in 75 per cent of patients and in the intrasellar space in 33 per cent. Occasionally, it can be identified in the temporal lobe.[4] It consists of aggregates of small flecks of calcium in 80 per cent of cases and is curvilinear, outlining a portion of the cyst wall, in 15 per cent of cases.[15,16] Unfortunately, even when curvilinear, it may not outline the periphery of the tumor.[110,137,150]

Intrasellar craniopharyngiomas produce

a "ballooned sella."[137,173] In this condition, the dorsum is bowed posteriorly and is thinned. A double floor is usually present.[182] The sella is usually huge, and flecks of calcium are present.[173]

Matson and Crigler have reommmended that plain x-rays be obtained for every child with small stature, retarded sexual development, persistent headache, or unexplained visual disturbance.[150] If a calcified suprasellar mass is identified in a child, it is very likely to be a craniopharyngioma.[102]

Some authors have thought radioisotope scans to be unhelpful, but in two reports 95 per cent of patients had abnormal scans, and the only patient in whom there was no isotope uptake had a tumor that was entirely cystic.[106,157,182] Scans delayed three hours after isotope injection may be more helpful than immediate scans.

The CT scan is abnormal in almost all patients with craniopharyngiomas.[164] A calcified suprasellar mass is identified in 75 per cent, and only a suprasellar soft-tissue density is seen in 25 per cent of them (Fig. 91–4). Contrast enhancement occurs in three fourths of children and in one third of adults.[69] The tumors that cannot be enhanced are cystic and without a detectable solid component.

When calcified, a craniopharyngioma appears as a round or smoothly lobulated mass with diffuse or focal calcium deposits. The cyst fluid is usually of a density in the range between cerebrospinal fluid and brain, but it can be very dense or of low density as a result of containing cholesterol.[69,164] In the adult with a suggestion of a cystic mass without enhancement, computed tomography after the injection of water-soluble iodinated contrast material in the cerebrospinal fluid should outline the "isodense" cyst. Coronal scanning may assist in defining the intrasellar extent of the tumor. Meningiomas and pituitary adenomas can be differentiated by their denser enhancement and by the cystic areas usually seen in craniopharyngiomas.

The electroencephalogram is abnormal in most patients with craniopharyngioma.[4,182] The abnormalities are more pronounced in children than in adults. Most frequently the abnormality is diffuse, although low voltage and slowing are also seen. Ventricular drainage does not alter the changes, suggesting that they may be not a direct effect of hydrocephalus but due to hypothalamic dysfunction.[182]

B-scan echoencephalography can identify a craniopharyngioma cyst.[150] The value of this diagnostic option has been reduced by the ready availability of computed tomography.

The investigation must define the relation

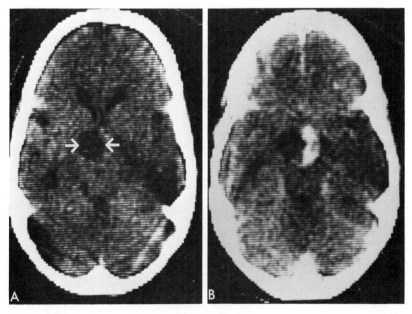

Figure 91–4 *A*. Computed tomographic scan of craniopharyngioma reveals a cystic mass. *B*. An adjacent solid component is enhanced with intravenous contrast material.

of the cyst and the chiasm, the ventricular size, and the relation between tumor and sellar contents. It may also be helpful to determine the arterial supply, although this is relatively constant. Vascular displacement includes superior and lateral stretching of the supraclinoid carotid artery with upward and forward displacement of the anterior choroidal arteries and the basilar vein of Rosenthal.[182] Angiography also demonstrates ventricular enlargement. In approximately 25 per cent of patients, the tumor is so small that angiograms are normal.[4]

In the past, the standard technique for investigation of patients with craniopharyngioma was the study of cerebrospinal fluid spaces. Air ventriculography was the procedure of choice until the 1960's. Matson and Crigler have recommended lumbar air encephalograms, even when papilledema is present, so that the basal cisterns can be studied. (Fig. 91–5).[149] If pneumoencephalographic study is chosen despite evidence of increased intracranial pressure, it probably is safest to establish external ventricular drainage before the encephalogram. Ventriculography is still considered safer by some authors.[182] If an oil is used, more manipulation may be required to outline the anterior part of the third ventricle. This manipulation can be avoided by using water-soluble positive contrast media. Pertuiset recommends twist drill holes, measurement of intracranial pressure, and placement of external drainage if intracranial pressure is

elevated.[182] Contrast materials should be placed, and if the two sides do not communicate, bilateral external drains should be used.

The most sensitive change in radiographs of the ventricular system is deformation of the anterior recesses of the third ventricle. This is seen in 95 per cent.[4,15,150] Hydrocephalus is seen in about 66 per cent, although a complete block of the foramen of Monro is seen in only 10 per cent.[16,110,221] Hydrocephalus can result from narrowing or obstruction of the foramen of Monro or from compression of the third ventricle (Fig. 91–6). The differential diagnosis of masses simulating craniopharyngioma includes pituitary adenoma, meningioma, epidermoid or dermoid cyst, saccular aneurysm, optic nerve or hypothalamic glioma, germinoma, glioma, and metastasis.

Because of the risk of herniation of the cerebellar tonsils, lumbar puncture rarely is justified in these patients. If analyzed, cerebrospinal fluid contains increased protein in three fourths of adults.[194] If the tumor's cyst leaks, it produces chemical meningitis that can sometimes be distinguished from other types of meningitis by finding lipid droplets and increased cholesterol concentration in the cerebrospinal fluid.[177]

Although not important in the diagnosis of craniopharyngioma, endocrine assessment to aid in management usually includes tests of hormonal reserve. Radiographic

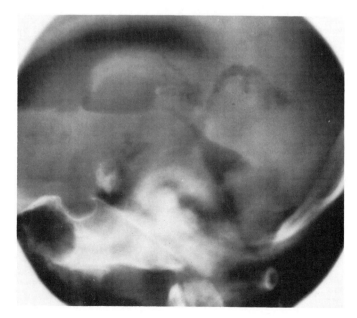

Figure 91–5 Pneumoencephalography demonstrates a calcified mass in the subarachnoid space above and behind the sella turcica. The dorsum sellae has been eroded. (Courtesy of Thomas H. Newton, M.D., University of California, San Francisco.)

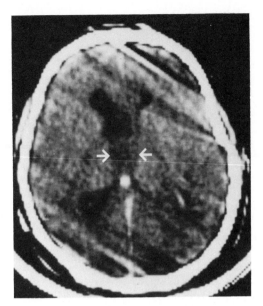

Figure 91–6 Cystic craniopharyngioma (*arrows*) can obstruct the third ventricle and produce unilateral (as in this case) or bilateral hydrocephalus.

evaluation of bone age may be important in children, and assessment of height, weight, and sexual maturity is necessary.[102,150]

Treatment and Results

Analysis of the various recommendations for treatment of craniopharyngioma is made difficult by several factors. The natural history varies greatly from patient to patient. Different investigators, applying similar treatment regimens to similar series of patients, can obtain very different results. There are a few clinicians who have gained considerable experience in treating this type of tumor and are able to achieve results that cannot be obtained by clinicians with less experience. Treatment techniques are improving rapidly, so reports of results obtained 15 to 20 years ago may no longer be applicable, and series that include patients treated earlier than that may not be representative of current expectations.

The variability in the natural history of craniopharyngiomas is shown by the report of Weber and co-workers of a patient with an eight-year history of nonprogressive bitemporal hemianopia who died of an unrelated gastrointestinal infection.[245] Other authors have reported clinical observation for 20 years or more without treatment or clinical change.[17,194] Although these indolent

craniopharyngiomas probably are uncommon, they illustrate the variability of prognosis and warn against attaching too great a significance to small series with unusual results.

Age influences the outcome with craniopharyngioma. In children they are more rapidly progressive than in adults.[94,110,189] Some authors have attributed this phenomenon to a histological difference.[110] A long history of symptoms before treatment probably suggests a more slowly growing tumor. Bartlett reported seven patients with long histories, followed without treatment. One patient died after six years, and the other six were alive and well an average of 20.5 years later. Among patients undergoing all types of treatment, those who live to complete treatment survive almost three times as long if the pretreatment history of symptoms was long, and a much greater proportion of patients with long histories are alive at late follow-up.[17]

The type of symptoms also correlates with prognosis. Patients with prominent mental symptoms do not survive as long as those without mental symptoms.[17] The comparative effects of this factor are illustrated in Table 91–2. The presence of motor signs is also ominous.[210]

The standard treatment for a craniopharyngioma has been operative. In earlier decades excision was successful occasionally, but it did not become a practical treatment until glucocorticoid protection against the postoperative loss of adrenocorticotropic hormone became available.[103] The tumor can be approached through a subfrontal, subtemporal, transsphenoidal, or transventricular route. Most authors agree

TABLE 91–2 CHANCE OF SURVIVAL AFTER TREATMENT FOR CRANIOPHARYNGIOMA*

	BRIEF DURATION OF SYMPTOMS		LONG DURATION OF SYMPTOMS	
	Per Cent alive	*Average Follow-up (Years)*	*Per Cent alive*	*Average Follow-up (Years)*
Mental changes	9	3	14	$3\frac{1}{2}$
No mental changes	50	7	63	$10\frac{1}{2}$

* After Bartlett, J.R.: Craniopharyngiomas: An analysis of some aspects of symptomatology, radiology and histology. Brain, *94*:725–732, 1971.

that exposure should be from the nondominant side of the brain.[80,173,221] The exception to this is the large unilateral frontal tumor, which should be approached from the side of the tumor.[182]

Dissection of the tumor capsule may be difficult, but with care, optic nerves and most of the adjacent brain can be freed from tumor. It may be possible to recognize and preserve the pituitary stalk.[182] It is likely that at least at the tumor attachment to the tuber cinereum, some brain will be injured. Traction on the tumor capsule must be gentle, since the tumor may be adherent to large arteries and forceful removal may tear them. One of the most important advances in the treatment of craniopharyngiomas has been the widespread use of the operating microscope, which allows much more precise and meticulous dissection of the tumor–nervous system interface.

Most craniopharyngiomas are best approached through a low frontal bone flap on the nondominant side. Spinal or ventricular drainage may be helpful. The approach can be extradural in the anterior frontal fossa, allowing the dura to protect the frontal lobe. An L-shaped dural opening is made 1 cm anterior to the sphenoid wing and 1 cm lateral to the olfactory tract. The olfactory tract and optic nerves are then exposed. If the chiasm is prefixed, removal of tumor from between the optic nerves may be difficult. In this circumstance, the approach is between the optic nerve and the carotid artery, since these structures usually are separated by the tumor. When it is visualized, it should be drained of cyst fluid through a needle, and then the capsule can be dissected free from surrounding structures. A free portion of the capsule should be held during the entire dissection so that the tumor does not retract out of the surgeon's reach.

Craniopharyngiomas may develop posterior to the chiasm in a location that cannot easily be seen from the subfrontal approach. These lesions may be approached through the lamina terminalis if no other avenue of visualization is possible.[220] Little tumor can be visualized through an incision in the lamina terminalis, but the mass can be displaced downward and removed from between the optic nerves.[148] A subtemporal approach may give access to the posterior portion of a craniopharyngioma, but dissec-

tion from optic nerves may be difficult. Section of the tentorium sometimes improves visualization of posterior fossa contents.[182] Although the best view of intrasellar craniopharyngiomas can probably be obtained transsphenoidally, this approach may not be safe if the tumor extends above the diaphragma sellae.

There is considerable controversy regarding the advisability of transventricular approach to craniopharyngiomas. Objections to it are that it may be difficult to distinguish the rare craniopharyngioma that is entirely within the third ventricle from the much more common one that arises beneath the ventricle and indents its floor. If a craniopharyngioma arising below the third ventricle is excised via a transventricular approach, hypothalamic injury is sure to result.[182,237] Even for those restricted to the third ventricle, intraventricular approaches are hazardous.[110,140,150]

Symptoms of craniopharyngioma may be due to the tumor cyst or to the solid tumor. Although the cyst is relatively easy to decompress, it may re-expand rapidly. Solid tumor grows very slowly, but may be more difficult to decompress. The safest and easiest operative procedures are either burr hole or craniotomy and cyst aspiration. These procedures can be used to diagnose craniopharyngiomas or to decompress the ventricles and visual system before or after other types of treatment.[154] Transventricular approach to a cyst and marsupialization of the cyst into the frontal horn may be relatively safe and provide long symptomatic relief.[203] A large cyst opening (up to 2 cm in diameter) is preferable, and the cyst should be evacuated before marsupialization.

In most patients, operative exposure can be aided by ventricular drainage.[150,182] This may also be helpful in alleviating the symptoms of hydrocephalus before operation and may be necessary for postoperative control of intracranial pressure. Ventricular shunting is probably preferable in some patients, since the brain can be decompressed several days before the tumor is approached. Communication between the lateral ventricles must be assessed before drainage of the ventricular system, since bilateral shunts or drains may be required.

Some surgeons have advised total excision as the best treatment.[95,150,182] In experienced hands, excision can be accomplished in three fourths of all patients.[80] It is possible in more than 90 per cent of previously untreated patients, but in only approximately 50 per cent of those who have had previous incomplete excisions.[150] Even though it may at first appear that total resection is impossible, persistence may be successful because as more tumor is removed, visualization continually improves.

The reluctance of some surgeons to attempt total excision results from consideration of the delicate structures in the suprasellar region and anticipation of tumor adherence to the hypothalamus.[132,157,173,182] Clinical experience has not always been as favorable as the results of those who advocate aggressive operation. This difference may be in part due to the age of the patients treated, since in children, adhesions between tumor and hypothalamus are not as extensive and operations are not as difficult or as dangerous. Operative excision is also much safer and easier in patients who have not undergone previous operations or radiotherapy, since these manipulations produce adhesions between tumor and optic nerves, carotid arteries, and hypothalamus.

The proportion of the tumor that is cystic also influences its resectability. Total excision of approximately 90 per cent of cystic lesions is possible, but only 50 per cent of those with a large solid portion can be entirely removed.[210] Few tumors more than 3 cm in diameter can be excised totally. Similarly, excision of craniopharyngiomas that are intrasellar or prechiasmatic is much more likely to be complete than excision of those with a subchiasmatic or retrochiasmatic component.[75]

There is little doubt that if total excision can be performed safely, it is the treatment of choice. Young patients, particularly those who have cystic tumors less than 3 cm in diamater and who have not had prior treatment, probably should have an excision by a surgeon who is experienced with the operating microscope and has a good knowledge of the removal of these tumors. In other patients, choice of treatment may be more difficult.

Cyst evacuation alone has been recognized as inadequate for long-term management of most patients.[53] Partial tumor removal does not prevent ultimate recurrence of symptoms, although approximately one third of patients whose tumors are partially removed survive several years.[102,150] If most of the tumor can be removed, most patients survive for many years even without radiotherapy (87 per cent of one series of children were alive at follow-up an average of 6.4 years after operation).[95] Subtotal excision is even more successful in adults.[110]

Patients who survive the operation still may die from recurrent tumor, which can be fatal more than 20 years after initial treatment.[210,221] If symptoms recur, total excision at a second operation may allow cure and protect against further recurrence.[94,182] Recurrent tumor may be solid even though the original lesion was cystic.

In earlier series, in which operative techniques may have been less sophisticated than currently, symptomatic recurrence followed one third of radical excisions.[80] More recently, rates of 0 to 20 per cent have been reported.* Matson and Crigler encountered recurrent tumor in only 1 of 44 patients with total excision, and Hoffman and co-authors have not had recurrence in any of 17 patients in whom total removal was accomplished and who have been followed for an average of five years.[95,150]

Death due to tumor many years after operative treatment much more commonly follows less extensive resection than it does more radical excision.[17,75,221] Between 50 and 80 per cent of patients who have cyst aspiration or partial removal fail to survive for long.[150] Early postoperative symptomatic recurrence is more of a hazard in the presence of a large solid component and is more likely in children than in adults.[94,210] Olivecrona has suggested that the much better outcome with total excision may be in part because patients with the difficult large tumors that cannot be totally removed are included in the partial-excision group, while those with the smaller more manageable tumors are in the group with total excision.[173] The ability of some surgeons to excise craniopharyngiomas completely in almost all childhood cases and achieve good results partially refutes this criticism.

Vision is improved in approximately half the patients who undergo operative treatment—in 67 per cent undergoing total excision, in 40 per cent undergoing subtotal excision, but in only 17 per cent in whom aspiration is used.[95] Return of vision is

---

* See references 4, 75, 95, 150, 210, 221.

more likely if the tumor is prechiasmatic than if it is retrochiasmatic.[182] Vision is occasionally worse after operation than before.[4,94] Long-standing visual loss and severe optic atrophy suggest that improvement is unlikely.

The risk of death after radical excision varies widely, but is approximately 5 to 10 per cent in most series.[157,210] Some authors have reported mortality rates as low as zero in 40 consecutive patients not previously treated, 1 in 63 consecutive operations, and none in eight consecutive micro-operative removals.[94,150] The number of deaths in some series is fairly high, even with partial excision, and may reach 25 per cent.[221] Mortality rates may be significant even among patients undergoing aspiration and biopsy. Early series produced few useful survivals.[50,80,167] Retrochiasmatic and subchiasmatic craniopharyngiomas are more difficult to excise and pose greater operative risk.[75]

Operative deaths are usually due to hypothalamic injury, although the surgeon must not neglect the possibility of hematoma, infection, or metabolic derangement in a patient who deteriorates after operation.[40,221] Intrasellar craniopharyngiomas are much less dangerous than suprasellar craniopharyngiomas, and very low mortality rates should be expected.[173] The initial operation is safer than reoperations, but if subtotal resection is accepted, some surgeons can operate on recurrent tumors without any deaths.[94,150] Endocrine testing is also a cause of postoperative death.[95]

Radical excision of craniopharyngioma is almost always followed by diabetes insipidus.[75,95,150] This may rarely have its onset in the operating room and is only temporary in 10 to 20 per cent of patients.[75,150,182] It also follows subtotal excision in many cases.[95] Diabetes insipidus after operation probably is best managed with fluid replacement for the first postoperative days. If Pitressin is given very early after operation, there may be a risk of renal failure, although not all authors agree that this hazard is possible.[150,182] If diabetes insipidus recovers spontaneously, urinary output will decrease rapidly, and overhydration, promoting brain swelling, is a risk.[150] Daily measurement of body weight and comparison with preoperative weight is helpful in the assessment of hydration, as are frequent evaluations of serum and urine electrolytes and osmolalities. The fluid used for intravenous replacement should match the urine in electrolytes.

Hypothalamic injury can interfere with electrolyte balance, and hypernatremia may result.[150] This may be permanent and should be treated by increasing fluid intake. Impaired temperature regulation, abnormal sleep patterns, and episodic emotional behavior may also follow hypothalamic injury subsequent to craniopharyngioma removal.[117]

As might be expected, excision of a craniopharyngioma usually results in at least some endocrine deterioration.[4,125,150] For this reason, all patients whose tumors have been excised should be treated as if they have had total hypophysectomy until they have recovered from the immediate effects of operation, at which time they can be tested. In some cases glucocorticoid replacement can be discontinued several months after operation.[75,95,150] Replacement of thyroid hormone and gonadotropins usually is needed following total excision and is required in more than half the cases after subtotal excision.[95]

Retardation of growth may follow operation, but most children grow at a normal rate as long as postoperative endocrine substitution is appropriate.[150,182] Accelerated growth may occur even in the absence of detectable growth hormone.[68,109,193] This continued growth may be a response to changes in insulin levels, production of an altered growth hormone that is not detected by immunological assay systems, continued production of very low levels of growth hormone (too low to be assayed), or production of somatomedin. Other endocrine deficits are more common, and sexual maturation and fertility are rare after radical excision of the tumor.[150,182] Perhaps with improved endocrine support, these deficits can be avoided. Mental symptoms may not improve postoperatively.[110,182] The role of treatment of hydrocephalus in the management of mental changes has not been determined.

Despite the serious complications that can occur postoperatively, Matson and Crigler reported that more than 85 per cent of patients who survived operation were functioning well and only three were invalids.[150] Half of Nakagawa and Tsuru's patients had no or minimal residual symptoms.[165] In another series, one fourth of the patients were doing well at follow-up after biopsy and aspiration.[157]

Combination of radiotherapy and operative treatment prolongs survival and delays recurrence of tumor.* Unfortunately, subtotal resection even when combined with radiotherapy only delays and does not prevent eventual recurrence of symptoms due to tumor alone. This delay may be in part related to relatively small radiation doses in many of the series in which it was used with operation. The frequency of recurrent symptoms increases as patients are followed for longer periods of time, and eventually the majority of those who have had both operative treatment and radiotherapy develop recurrent symptoms (Fig. 91–7).[94] Of 32 patients treated with excision and radiotherapy, only 12 had good-quality survival at follow-up and one third had died in one series.[174] Some authors state that there is no microscopic change in tumor that has been irradiated, although one group believes fibrosis occurs.[132,150,174] Backlund demonstrated tumor necrosis after intensive interstitial radiation.[8]

The possibility of successful radiotherapy was popularized by Kramer and coworkers. They reported six children who received 5500 rads in six weeks and four adults who received 7000 rads in seven weeks.[123] The six children were alive at follow-up, 13.5 to 15 years later. The four

adults did less well. One died of causes unrelated to tumor six months after treatment; a second died 10 years, and a third died 14 years, after operation.[124] Three of ten other adults with craniopharyngiomas treated by irradiation died, one from radionecrosis, one during an operation for recurrent symptoms, and one of causes not related to tumor. The survivors in this last group had been followed for six months to 8.6 years, and some had symptomatic recurrences during follow-up. In a later series of six children, there were two deaths from recurrent tumor during a follow-up of two to five and one third years.[122] Although these results suggest that radiotherapy may be beneficial for craniopharyngiomas, they do not support the conclusion that radiotherapy after biopsy and cyst aspiration is "curative in most of these patients."[124]

Cyst evacuation followed by radiotherapy has also been advocated.[25,111,206] Radiotherapy may be beneficial in decreasing the production of cyst fluid.[40,95,132] Recent 5- and 10-year survivals with modern radiotherapy techniques were 85 and 72 per cent in a series of approximately 100 patients, of whom half were children and half were adults. If radiotherapy data for patients requiring more aggressive operations are included, 5- and 10-year survival rates are 76 and 61 per cent.[24] Radiotherapy with the linear accelerator may produce better results.[25]

Radiotherapy can damage brain, meninges, and optic nerves and can be fatal.[124]

---

* See references 94, 95, 132, 174, 182, 210.

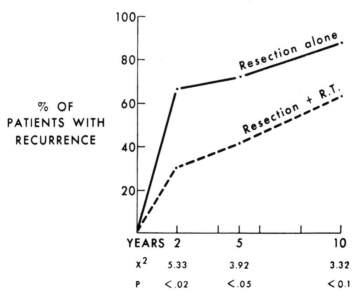

Figure 91–7 Risk of symptomatic recurrence of craniopharyngioma treated by resection alone or in combination with radiotherapy (R.T.). (From Hoff, J. T., and Patterson, R. H.: Craniopharyngiomas in children and adults. J. Neurosurg., *36*:299–302, 1972. Reprinted by permission.)

Meningioma in the region of the sella has developed long after radiotherapy for craniopharyngioma.[42,243]

Not all series demonstrate the degree of radiotherapy effectiveness seen in the patients just reported. The tumor recurred in approximately 50 per cent of those who had cyst aspiration and radiotherapy in a mean of 4.4 years in the series of Shapiro and associates.[210] Other authors have reported a clinical impression that radiotherapy is not curative.[4,80,95] Perhaps some craniopharyngiomas are sensitive to irradiation while others are not.[132] Certainly the long survivals after cyst decompression and radiotherapy are not necessarily due to the radiotherapy, since long-term survivals occur after cyst decompression and biopsy without it.[157,160]

It is frequently a large cystic portion, rather than the solid portion, that produces symptoms. An innovative technique for cyst treatment was described by Leksell and Lidén.[10,134,135] A stereotaxic frame directs a small needle for the cyst puncture. Cyst volume is determined by isotope dilution, and a measured dose of a beta-emitting isotope with a short half-life is injected. The distribution of isotope in the head and the concentration in the liver are followed for several times the half-life of the isotope, and the cyst is then aspirated.[8,10] Insertion of an Ommaya reservoir in the cyst may make aspiration easier and may allow detection of a leak from the cyst before placement of the therapeutic isotope.[166] An Ommaya reservoir requires a larger hole in the cyst wall than a needle and may be more likely to leak.

The isotope recommended by Backlund and co-workers is ^{90}yttrium.[10] It has a short half-life, is almost entirely without gamma emission, and has greater penetration than ^{32}phosphorus. ^{198}Gold has also been recommended, but emits gamma as well as beta rays.[166] If gamma emission is present, the radiation effect will extend beyond the cyst wall, which is an advantage for treating solid tumor, but exposes the surrounding neural structures to significant dosages and does not have much advantage over external focused radiotherapy. Other agents have also been recommended.[234]

The advantages of intracyst isotope radiotherapy are that the dosimetry allows very large doses of radiation to the entire cyst capsule and, theoretically, little exposure to functioning brain.[10,134] Initially doses of approximately 100,000 rads were recommended, although a more recent report recommends doses of only 20,000 to 40,000 rads.

Kramer and associates have argued that intracyst isotope radiotherapy may lead to cyst distention and deterioration in vision, but these have not been problems.[123] Slightly increased temperature may result from intracyst isotope injection and was seen in 2 of 15 cases in one series. "Mild diabetes insipidus" was also seen in 2 of the 15 patients.[8] Multiloculated cysts are a potential problem, since each loculus must be separately treated and each will require a separate dose calculation.

Radioisotope therapy of craniopharyngioma cysts can improve vision and decreases the size of the cyst in 85 per cent of cases in which moderate therapeutic doses are given and in all patients who are given more than 100,000 rads.[8,134,135] A major problem with intracyst isotope treatment is treatment of the remaining solid tumor. There is no information regarding the effect of radiotherapy on the boundary between cyst and hypothalamus. This area may become adherent as it does after external irradiation. Intensive external radiotherapy delivered to a very small volume of tissue may be the treatment of choice for the rest of the tumor.[10,134]

Some authors have recommended only aspiration of a childhood craniopharyngioma cyst until puberty, with definitive treatment after growth is completed.[75,110] Repeated aspiration can be accomplished through the transphenoidal route, through a balloon-tipped catheter with the balloon inflated in the cyst, or with a stereotaxic approach.[234,254] Cyst visualization may be aided by placing a barium suspension in the cyst. Occasionally an abscess arises spontaneously in a craniopharyngioma, a very ominous event associated with a high mortality rate.[168,169] The management of this problem has not yet been defined.

Purely intrasellar craniopharyngioma is an exception to many of the principles just outlined. This tumor can usually be completely excised, particularly if the operating microscope and transphenoidal approach are used.[89,90]

The treatment of patients with craniopharyngioma must be individualized, and a combination of the various modalities may be needed. All types of therapy have risk, and those that are most effective have the greatest immediate risk. Some older patients may be able to live a normal life span without treatment, but in childhood the risks of aggressive resection may be justified in view of the fatal outcome with other forms of treatment. In children the operative excision as currently performed is the most effective treatment, and supplemental irradiation usually is not justified. An attempt to remove all of the tumor should be made in these cases.

INCLUSION TUMORS

Teratomas are listed as germ cell tumors in the World Health Organization classification. The other members of the germ cell group (germinoma, embryonal carcinoma, and choriocarcinoma) are primarily tumors of the pineal region and are discussed in Chapter 89; teratomas are discussed with malformative tumors. There is general agreement that there is a continuum of histological complexity from the stratified squamous epithelium of an epidermoid cyst to the embryologically diverse tissues of a teratoma or even an embryoma.[114,198,222]

The least complex of these tumors, the epidermoid cyst, is a soft mass that insinuates itself through the subarachnoid space, gently distorting and compressing neural elements. The external appearance usually consists of a glistening, shining surface, for which Cruveilhier named them tumeurs perlées.[51] These masses have also been termed cholesteatomas. This is a poor name because it refers to a chemical byproduct not only of the cyst but also other types of tumors.[52,163,187] A variety of different tumor types have been included in the category of cholesteatoma.[49] The terms "epidermoid" and "dermoid" were suggested by Bostroem in 1897 and are the preferred names.[31,49,163]

The cholesteatoma found in the middle ear resembles the intracranial epidermoid cyst, and the two may have a common origin, although most otologists believe middle ear cholesteatoma usually arises as a result of chronic otitis media.[79,231] In order to avoid confusing these possibly different entities, common usage has termed the ear mass cholesteatoma and the central nervous system mass epidermoid cyst.

These cysts consist of only epidermal elements. It can be argued either that epidermoid cysts are neoplasms or that they are simply included dysplastic tissues or hamartomas. In neoplastic potential they range from a mass enlarging by desquamation of normally formed epidermal cells to epidermoid carcinoma.[114,231]

If hair and dermal glands are included, the cyst is called a dermoid.[49,222] Some investigators have devised a classification of "teratoids" to apply to masses that contain histological elements not found in the dermis or epidermis but do not contain derivatives of all three germ layers.[222] Most authors broaden the term "teratoma" to include a tumor deriving from more than one germ cell layer. Teratoma has been defined by Willis as a neoplasm "composed of multiple tissues of kinds foreign to the part in which it arises."[248] Anaplastic germ cell tumors, such as germinomas or embryonal carcinomas, may arise in teratomas, further confusing the discrete classification of these masses.

Patten has described a tumor he refers to as embryoma. It includes organs and all three germ layers. This tumor begins as an identical twin that develops poorly and is included by the thriving twin. Other teratomas, such as those of the gonads, may arise from totipotential germinal tissue, while sacral teratomas (and presumably intracranial teratomas) might arise from "unorganized growth of totipotential cells from the primitive streak region of the embryo."[178]

A variety of tumors could be classified as teratomas according to the description used in this chapter. Ependymomas and other gliomas containing cartilage, as well as medulloblastoma containing smooth muscle cells, are all technically teratomas, although their structure is predominantly that of a typical tumor type and they have the clinical behavior characteristic of that tumor type. Russell believes that pineal germinomas are "atypical teratomas," and the association of dermoids or typical teratomas with 20 of 144 atypical teratomas supports this idea.[60,197] Medulloepithelioma may also be associated with teratoma.[233]

The relationship between lipomas and teratomas is emphasized by the finding of cartilage and muscle fibers in lipomas.[204,227] Lipomas may coexist with teratomas or with other cerebral malformations.[36] Particularly common is the coexistence of lipoma and agenesis of the corpus callosum.[255]

Epidermoid cysts were among the first neoplasms identified and classified, perhaps because their macroscopic appearance is so distinctive. Critchley and Ferguson credit a 1745 report by Verattus with being the first description of a dermoid tumor.[49] A description of epidermoid in 1807 has been attributed to Pinson, and these tumors were reportedly noted to resemble mother-of-pearl by LePrestre in 1828 and by Cruveilhier in 1829.[49,147] Muller is credited with describing the microscopic structure of epidermoid cysts in 1838, and in 1854 VonRemak is reported to have suggested they might arise from misplaced epithelial cells.[11] Bostroem coined the terms "pial dermoid" and "pial epidermoid" and suggested an origin from embryonic inclusion of epithelial tissue at an early (dermoid) or a late (epidermoid) stage of development.[31]

Pathogenesis

The obvious relationship between epidermoid cyst, dermoid cyst, and normal skin suggested to nineteenth century pathologists that these cysts arose from epithelial fragments included in the brain. This could represent either embryonic malformation or the result of trauma. The favored theory in the late nineteenth century was that trauma was the cause of inclusion tumors, and experimental evidence still suggests this may at times be possible. Epidermis implanted in the central nervous system will form masses resembling epidermoid and dermoid cysts. Indeed, lumbar puncture can implant skin into the spinal canal and cause an epidermoid cyst.[44,217,238]

Many findings, however, demonstrate that most inclusion tumors are congenital malformations rather than of traumatic origin. A dermal sinus in association with a dermoid cyst demonstrates a congenital origin, as does the occurrence of apocrine glands in an intracranial dermoid (glands not normally present in the scalp).[142,226,235] The indistinct boundary between dermoid and teratoma also suggests that dermoid cysts are of maldevelopmental origin.

Several embryological theories have been advanced to explain the difference between epidermoid and dermoid cysts. The more primitive epithelium may be capable of a more diverse differentiation. This factor would allow the epithelium included in the nervous system during neural tube closure to differentiate into dermal as well as epidermal elements. Epithelium included at a later time would have fewer potential lines of differentiation and would be more likely to form an epidermoid cyst.[31,49]

The depth of included epithelium could also explain the presence or absence of dermal structures. If only epidermal tissue were included, an epidermoid cyst would result, but if dermal tissue were also included, a dermoid cyst would result.[49,97,231]

Inclusion tumors also may arise after closure of the neural tube during formation of the flexures of the brain.[49] Thus the pontine flexure might include epithelial cells in the region of the cerebellopontine angle. An alternative explanation for epidermoid cysts in the cerebellopontine angle, however, is that these cysts are derived from the ectodermal precursors of the labyrinth, which are separated from the developing embryonic brain by only the eighth cranial nerve.[158,231]

The origin of teratomas is difficult to explain. The selective involvement of the pineal region suggested to Sweet that the great variety of cellular types found in the developing pineal region might account for subsequent teratomas.[222] Extragonadal midline teratomas may also represent an included twin pregnancy that has been overgrown by the host.[5]

Incidence

Epidermoid cysts make up 0.5 to 1.5 per cent of brain tumors in most series, although the incidence in Japan may be greater, and in one series they constituted 2.2 per cent of the intracranial tumors that came to autopsy. Dermoid cysts are less common than epidermoid cysts and make up about 0.3 per cent of brain neoplasms.*

Teratomas are nearly twice as common as dermoid cysts and account for approximately 0.5 per cent of brain tumors.[222,258] They make up around 2.0 per cent of brain tumors of children.[101] Japanese series show a higher incidence of all teratomas, perhaps because of the greater frequency of the sub-

---

* See references 70, 81, 85, 105, 114, 146, 170, 184, 198, 236, 258.

group of germinomas.[105] In a recent series in Japan in which germinomas were excluded from the teratoma group, 1.2 per cent of brain tumors were teratomas, suggesting that these nongerminoma teratomas are more frequent in Japan just as are the germinomas.[230]

Epidermoid cysts can occur at any age, although approximately 50 per cent of patients are between 20 and 40 years old.[147,170,236] Dermoid cysts tend to be symptomatic and diagnosed at a younger age than epidermoid cysts, and approximately half of the patients in whom dermoid cysts have been identified are in the pediatric age group.[70,85,146]

Teratomas are particularly likely to occur in children, as many as one fourth of intracranial tumors detected or symptomatic in the first year of life being of this type.[101,108,230] A teratoma replacing most of the cerebral hemispheres has been reported in an infant delivered two weeks prematurely.[242] The average age of patients with this tumor is approximately 12 years.[230]

Epidermoid cysts occur with equal frequency in both sexes.[81,147,170] Dermoid cysts also probably occur with equal frequency in the two sexes.[85,146] Teratomas are probably more common in males, even if germinomas are excluded from the teratoma group, although teratomas in neonates and suprasellar teratomas may be more common in females.[82,222,230]

Pathology

Macroscopic changes

An epidermoid cyst contains concentric layers of desquamated epithelium surrounded by a capsule of stratified squamous epithelium. The surface is smooth, often nodular, and resembles mother-of-pearl (Fig. 91–8).[11,49,51] Dermoid cysts include dermal elements, such as hair and sebaceous glands, in part or all of their capsule. If dermal elements occur in only a small area of capsule, the dermoid may closely resemble an epidermoid cyst. If sebaceous glands are included in the capsule, their secretion will mix with the desquamated epithelium, producing greasier contents.

In contrast with epidermoid and dermoid cysts, which have a predictable appearance, teratomas are variable. They may consist of a large cyst, may be multicystic, or may be solid. Cysts may contain desquamated epithelium or fluid that is yellow or brown as a result of hemorrhage or serous transudation. Solid portions also vary in appearance and consistency, depending on the tissues present, and may contain all elements of primitive tissue, including teeth.[26]

Epidermoid cysts occur in a variety of locations in the nervous system. Only approximately half are intradural and intracranial, the remainder being in the diploë of the skull or in the spine.[146] One fourth to one half of epidermoid cysts arise in the cerebellopontine angle and the posterior fossa basal cisterns.[146,147,170] The suprasellar region is nearly as commonly involved.[70,170,172] Approximately 20 per cent of epidermoid cysts are in the sylvian fissure and 10 to 20 per cent are in either the lateral or fourth ventricle. The precise location of a subarachnoid epidermoid cyst is often difficult to define, since the cyst is likely to involve adjacent subarachnoid cisterns extensively.

Dermoid cysts tend to occur in the midline. Approximately one third are in or adjacent to the fourth ventricle.[85,146,222] An equal number lie in the subarachnoid space at the base of the brain.[258] The remainder occur over the convexities and in other locations.

Although dermoids are infrequent in the pineal region, approximately half of all teratomas are located there.[161,222,230] Other common sites are the pituitary area and the floor of the third ventricle.[66,161,230]

Part of the difficulty in characterizing the location of epidermoid cysts lies in the extent and the pervasive nature of the mass. They are situated in the subarachnoid space and are very soft. This characteristic allows them to insinuate themselves gently through the subarachnoid cisterns, flowing around vessels and cranial nerves and filling all available space.[170,172,236] Extensions of tumor may fill depressions in the brain parenchyma. Some epidermoids, initially developing in the subarachnoid space, may burrow into cerebral tissue and appear to be in the cerebral hemispheres.[2,184,235]

The brain surrounding an epidermoid cyst may be compressed, the result being gliosis and loss of ganglion cells.[142] Small groups of epithelial cells may be found adjacent to epidermoid cysts.[115] The cyst capsule may be adherent to vessels that course

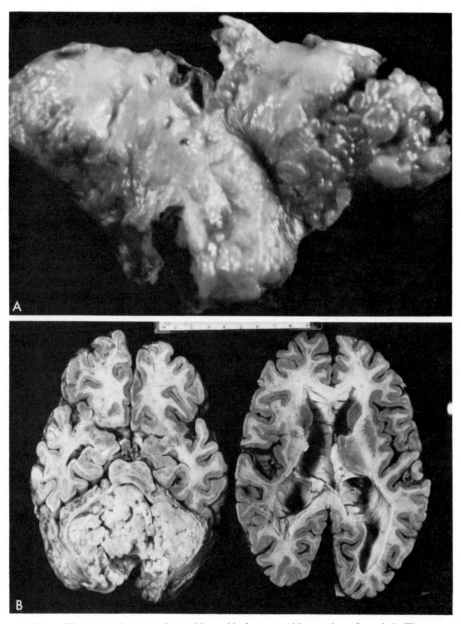

Figure 91–8   *A*. The external aspect of an epidermoid often resembles mother-of-pearl. *B*. The tumor may fill the fourth ventricle and distort the brain stem. (Courtesy of Surl L. Nielsen, M.D., University of California, Davis.)

on its surface or to brain or cranial nerves.[235,236] Widespread involvement of the basal cisterns and arachnoidal scarring, which may follow epidermoid or dermoid cyst rupture into the subarachnoid space, account for the frequency of hydrocephalus in patients with these tumors.[236]

The effects of dermoid cysts on surrounding structures are similar to those of epidermoid cysts. Fifty per cent of dermoid cysts are also associated with embryonic midline fusion defects such as vertebral failure of segmentation, cleft lip, spina bifida, and sacral dermal sinus.[146] A connection between the cyst and the skin through a dermal sinus is found in approximately one fourth of dermoid cysts of the posterior fossa but does not occur in epidermoid cysts or teratomas.[222]

Anaplastic change in an epidermoid cyst has been reported and can give rise to meningeal carcinomatosis.[119,250]

Microscopic Changes

The major portion of an epidermoid cyst consists of dead cellular debris. This is surrounded by a thin epithelial envelope. Bailey separated the histological layers of epidermoid cysts into four strata.[11] The most external of these layers consists of a fibrous membrane with few cells and is called the stratum durum. This fibrous membrane serves as the supporting framework for the essential portion of the tumor, the stratified squamous epithelium called the stratum granulosum. As the epithelial cells lose their nuclei and desquamate, they make up the bulk of the tumor. This central portion was originally divided into two layers, the stratum fibrosum and the stratum cellulosum. Critchley and Ferguson considered these inner layers as one under the name "area cornea."[49] Other authors have agreed with the three-layer concept of epidermoid cysts. (Fig. 91–9).[35,184]

The most external layer of an epidermoid is composed of collagen and reticulin with few cells.[11,35,187] The leptomeningeal connective tissue becomes thickened and may be infiltrated with foreign-body giant cells, histiocytes, and lymphocytes.[236] These leptomeningeal changes are particularly prominent in patients with long-standing clinical symptoms. Calcium may develop in the cyst wall.[141,184]

The epithelial cells of an epidermoid cyst

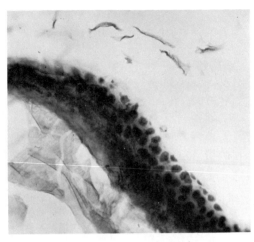

Figure 91–9 Microscopic examination of an epidermoid cyst wall demonstrates an external fibrous membrane (the stratum durum) supporting a stratified squamous epithelium (stratum granulosum). As epithelial cells desquamate, they collect in the area cornea. Some of these cells have been artifactually displaced outside the stratum durum. 980 ×.

can become anaplastic, and in this case, mitoses are seen, the basal layer is disorganized, and nuclear pleomorphism occurs.[231] This anaplastic change justifies a diagnosis of squamous cell carcinoma.

Dermoid cysts differ from epidermoid cysts only by the inclusion of dermal structures and can be thought of as a variant of an epidermoid cyst (Fig. 91–10).[114] There is also a gradual transition from dermoid cyst to teratoma, beginning with a cyst that is typically dermoid except for the inclusion of a single nondermal structure. Technically, this would be classified as a teratoma, although its macroscopic structure would resemble a dermoid more than one of the very complex teratomas, which may include muscle, respiratory epithelium, gastrointestinal epithelium, cartilage, bone, fat, and even neuroepithelial plaques (Fig. 91–11).[249]

Clinical Presentation

Symptoms in patients with epidermoid cysts and other inclusion tumors may result from involvement of important structures by the tumor or from obstruction of the cerebrospinal fluid circulation.[142] The symptoms usually have been present for many years before diagnosis. Their duration for more than 10 years is not unusual,

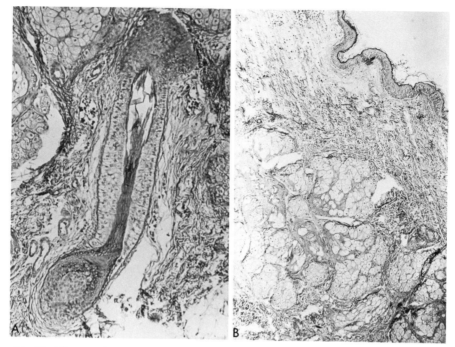

Figure 91–10   Microscopic pathological changes of dermoid cyst. *A*. Hair follicles are revealed. 50 ×. *B*. Sebaceous glands and stratified squamous epithelium are also present. 20 ×.

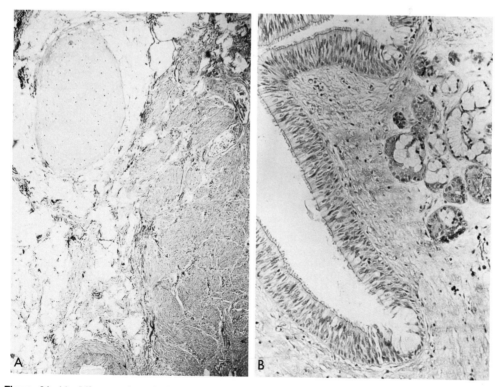

Figure 91–11   Microscopic pathological changes of a mature teratoma. *A*. Cartilage and muscle are demonstrated. 30 ×. *B*. Respiratory epithelium is also present. 100 ×.

and a duration of 53 years has been reported.[146,170,236]

Alvord has noted that while solid tumors have an exponential growth rate, epidermoid cysts grow at a linear rate. This is because the daughter cells produced by the granular layer of an epidermoid are destined for desquamation and death, and are incapable of progressively increasing the number of dividing cells as occurs in other tumor types.[3]

Dermoid cysts are likely to cause more rapid progression of symptoms, the average duration being approximately eight years prior to diagnosis.[85,142] Inclusion tumors may have short clinical histories, however, if the ability to regulate intracranial pressure is lost, if the tumor becomes anaplastic, or if a cyst ruptures and chemical meningitis develops.[222]

Although intradiploic epidermoid cysts can compress brain, they usually present as asymptomatic masses.[35,52] The epidermoid cysts that arise in the petrous bone may result in slowly progressive seventh nerve dysfunction and can erode through dura or follow the fifth cranial nerve into the orbit.[19,107,180]

Intracranial epidermoid cysts cannot be identified on the basis of clinical presentation alone in most cases.[2] Although there is a wide variety of symptoms and signs, patients often present with a many-year history of abnormal cranial nerve activity, particularly trigeminal neuralgia, hemifacial spasm, or cranial nerve deficits.[170,236] The more delicate cranial nerves, such as the optic nerve, are more likely to be affected. This may be because the soft, slowly growing tumor can displace or encompass more heavily myelinated cranial nerves without causing neurological deficit. Mental symptoms, probably due to hydrocephalus, also are common.[184] In spite of their diversity, the clinical symptoms and signs usually do not reflect the full extent of the mass.[236] They depend on the location of the tumor. In the fourth ventricle it produces hydrocephalus, and in the cerebellopontine angle it produces cranial nerve symptoms and signs. Most epidermoid cysts arise in the basal cisterns. They have been divided into four categories: suprasellar-chiasmatic, parasellar–sylvian fissure, retrosellar–cerebellopontine angle, and basilar–posterior fossa. The suprasellar cysts produce visual impairment with optic atrophy and often bitemporal hemianopia. The parasellar ones induce seizures and may result in hemiparesis and trigeminal nerve deficits. Those in the retrosellar cerebellopontine angle interfere with function of the fifth, seventh, and eighth cranial nerves, while those in the basilar area interfere with function of lower cranial nerves and cause cerebellar deficits and pyramidal tract abnormalities.[170]

Optic atrophy usually is seen when epidermoid cysts occur in the sellar region. Approximately 50 per cent of all patients with intracranial epidermoid cysts have seizures. The percentage is much higher when the mass is in the region of the temporal lobe. Seizures are uncommon in patients with dermoid cysts, probably because these usually are not adjacent to epileptogenic cortex.[85,146,171]

Approximately 18 per cent of patients with epidermoid cysts develop trigeminal neuralgia, and if only cerebellopontine angle cysts are considered, the incidence is as high as 40 per cent. The tic may be present for years prior to diagnosis of the cyst.[85,146,170,172] A cyst should be suspected in a young patient who develops trigeminal neuralgia or hemifacial spasm.

Leakage of epidermoid cyst contents probably occurs frequently without clinical sequelae, but if large amounts of cyst contents are spilled, chemical meningitis may develop. The patient may have repeated attacks of meningitis, probably owing to the cholesterin or fatty acids that are spilled. As many as one third of the patients who have aseptic meningitis after operation for epidermoid cyst will develop communicating hydrocephalus. Hydrocephalus following spontaneous rupture of epidermoid cysts probably accounts for the dementia that has been estimated to occur in three fifths of cases.*

If bacterial meningitis develops in the presence of a midline tumor in the posterior fossa, dermoid cyst with a congenital sinus tract must be suspected. Approximately 50 per cent of patients with fourth ventricular and cerebellar dermoid cysts have a congenital dermal sinus.[85,151,222]

The clinical presentation of patients with teratomas is even more diverse than that of epidermoids and dermoids. The history

---

* See references 21, 85, 131, 147, 207, 236, 239.

may be long, as illustrated by the case of a 27-year-old patient with hydrocephalus who had been retarded since infancy because of a teratoma in the fourth ventricle.[99] Germinomas and anaplastic teratomas may progress rapidly with clinical findings as outlined in Chapter 89 if the pineal region is involved and with diabetes insipidus, hypopituitarism, optic atrophy, and visual field deficits if the suprasellar region is involved.[230]

Investigation

Routine radiographs of the skull are diagnostic of intradiploic epidermoid cysts.[35,52] With intradural epidermoid cysts, they may reveal bony erosion and occasionally enlargement of the optic foramina.[172] Tumor calcification is only rarely seen in patients with intracranial epidermoids, although approximately 20 per cent of dermoid cysts and 50 per cent of mature teratomas (teratomas without evidence of anaplasia) contain areas of calcification.[39,85,184] Calcification is uncommon in teratomas that lack mature areas. Radiographs may reveal a linear groove in the occipital bone, marking the site of a dermal sinus in patients with fourth ventricular dermoid cysts.[235]

Computed tomography of an extradural epidermoid cyst reveals a densely enhanced rim of contrast around a low-density lesion.[224] Intradural epidermoid cysts contain a low-density central area surrounded by a capsule that may contain calcium but cannot be enhanced (Fig. 91–12).

Scanning with radioisotopes may reveal an epidermoid or dermoid cyst and usually demonstrates teratomas.[28,205,230]

Pneumoencephalography often not only discloses the tumor mass but also, since air may gain access to the tumor center through tears in the capsule, may show it as streaks or as a reticulated lacework in the tumor (Fig. 91–13).[62,126,141] Iodinated contrast agents may reveal a similar pattern.

Cerebrospinal fluid usually is normal with epidermoid and dermoid cysts, although in approximately 15 per cent of patients the protein level is elevated.[116,170,235] In unusual cases, it may be elevated to approximately 100 mg per 100 ml, glucose may be reduced to 30 to 40 mg per 100 ml, and as many as 2500 cells per cubic millimeter may be present, with polymorphonu-

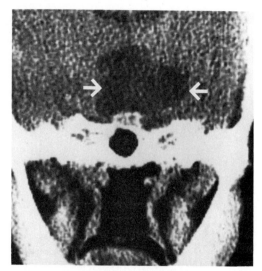

Figure 91–12 Computed tomographic scan of an epidermoid demonstrates a low-density mass just above the sella turcica. (Courtesy of Thomas H. Newton, M.D., University of California, San Francisco.)

clear leucocytes predominating.[207] If histological anaplasia occurs, cerebrospinal fluid may contain malignant cells.[119]

Treatment and Results

Treatment of epidermoid cysts, dermoid cysts, and mature teratomas is operative. Epidermoid and dermoid cysts of the skull can usually be totally excised without difficulty. Extradural epidermoid cysts at the petrous apex may be difficult to excise, but can be marsupialized into a labyrinthectomy defect.[74] Operative difficulty with intradural epidermoid cysts is variable. Some can be removed easily, particularly those in the fourth ventricle.[11] Dandy has commented that epidermoid cysts in the cerebellopontine angle are "not large, are very slow growing, are bloodless and easily removed"; however, other authors have noted that they may be adherent to arteries and important neural structures, which prevents total excision.[118,172,235] MacCarty and his coauthors reported total excision of 3 of 5 cerebellopontine angle epidermoid cysts and 11 of 19 (58 per cent) epidermoid cysts of all locations.[146] Even large ones in the pineal region can be successfully excised.[201] It is less likely that dermoid cysts can be totally excised, but they can be subtotally removed.

Teratomas are even more difficult to treat

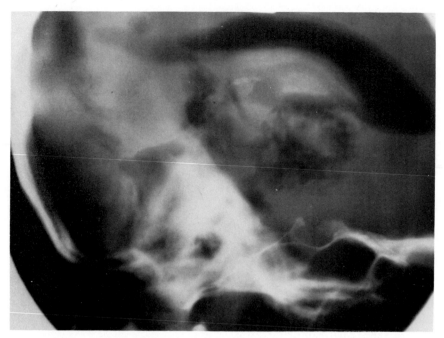

Figure 91–13 Pneumoencephalography of a suprasellar epidermoid cyst demonstrates displacement of the brain stem and third ventricle by a mass in which the injected gas has produced a reticulated pattern. (Courtesy of Thomas H. Newton, M.D., University of California, San Francisco.)

than epidermoids and dermoids. In newborn children they may be fatal at delivery owing to very large size (up to 2100 gm).[82,242] If they present later, excision may be possible. When teratomas contain anaplastic elements such as choriocarcinoma or germinoma, radiotherapy may be helpful.

Although some authors have recommended radiotherapy without biopsy for presumed teratomas, this course of action makes it possible to overlook a neoplasm more appropriately treated by excision.[219] It is reasonable to place an Ommaya reservoir with a catheter through the foramen of Monro into the third ventricle (unless the anterior part of the ventricle is obstructed by tumor) and to sample ventricular fluid for cytological analysis. If this examination is nondiagnostic, stereotaxic biopsy or biopsy through a craniotomy can establish a tissue diagnosis. If a mature teratoma is identified, it should be excised in most cases. If radiotherapy is utilized, the response of the tumor to it can be followed by CT scan (see Chapter 95).

Operative mortality rates have been dramatically reduced over the years. Prior to 1936 the rate was 67 per cent for operations on intracranial epidermoid cysts.[147] By the 1950's, it was approximately 20 per cent for intracranial epidermoid and dermoid cysts.[146,235] Guidetti and Gagliardi reported an operative death rate of only 10 per cent for epidermoid cysts and no deaths in nine cases of dermoid cysts operated on since 1952.[85]

Chemical meningitis occurs after operation in approximately 40 per cent of patients. It is more common if the tumor is near the ventricle and if the excision is incomplete.[85,226,235] Intraventricular spillage of cyst contents is not, however, always followed by chemical meningitis.[91,131] Meningeal reaction may lead to arachnoiditis that encases and compresses cranial nerves. If progressive neurological deficit results from arachnoidal compression, removal of constricting adhesions may be beneficial.[19]

Although some authors have said that total excision of tumors is required to prevent clinical recurrence of symptoms, others have found such recurrence to be rare.[2,19,172] In one series, only two of eight patients who had operative treatment of epidermoid cysts developed clinical symptoms again over a mean follow-up of 7.3

years, and one patient who had subtotal excision of a cerebellopontine angle epidermoid was asymptomatic when seen 22 years later.[146] There was no clinical recurrence after complete removal in another series, and of eight incompletely removed epidermoid cysts, recurrent symptoms developed in three patients at 7, 8, and 13 years, with no demonstrated recurrence in the other five patients at a mean follow-up of 8 years.[235] A third series revealed no identifiable recurrence of any of 11 incompletely removed epidermoid cysts. The duration of follow-up was not stated.[81]

Few authors have commented on the neurological function of patients undergoing operative treatment for epidermoid and dermoid cysts. Alpers noted that six of eight patients with operative treatment of epidermoid cysts made "good recoveries."[2] In another series, 29 intracranial epidermoid and dermoid cysts were treated operatively. Twenty-one patients (72 per cent) were able to return to work or school, two (7 per cent) were able to work but developed seizures, four (14 per cent) were unable to work because of neurological deficits, and only two (7 per cent) died of recurrence of the tumor.[85]

Undoubtedly there are occasional patients in whom no treatment is needed because of the minor degree of tumor symptoms and the age of the patient. There is no evidence that radiotherapy is beneficial for either epidermoid or dermoid cysts or for mature teratomas. Likewise, chemotherapy has not been of demonstrated benefit for these lesions.

COLLOID CYST

A colloid cyst is a unilocular cystic tumor lined with epithelium on its inner surface and usually arising from the roof of the third ventricle. The first patient in whom a colloid cyst was described was a 50-year-old man who presented with a staggering gait and involuntary micturition and defecation.[244] Although many necropsy cases had been reported, a premorbid diagnosis could not be made prior to the advent of ventriculography. In 1921, this technique was used to diagnose ventricular obstruction in a 24-year-old woman with headache, papille-

dema, and a right sixth nerve palsy. A colloid cyst was successfully removed.[55] In his monograph in 1933, Dandy reported treating five colloid cysts operatively, with four of the patients surviving removal of the tumor.[56]

Incidence

Colloid cysts constitute about 2 per cent of all gliomas.[198] Although they have been reported in persons as young as three weeks and as old as 72 years, patients usually are between 20 and 50 years of age.[34,130,252] There is no sex preponderance.[252]

Pathology

The tumor consists of a spherical unilocular mass. The wall encapsulates a thick gelatinous colloidlike material. Symptomatic cysts vary from 6 mm to 9 cm in diameter, but usually range from 1 to 3 cm. They usually take origin from the roof of the third ventricle just posterior to the foramen of Monro; on rare occasions, however, they also occur between the leaves of the septum pellucidum or in the fourth ventricle.[45,46,175,176,181]

The cyst lining is somewhat variable, consisting of either simple or stratified epithelium with columnar, cuboidal, or squamous cells (Fig. 91–14). These cells may be ciliated and may contain blepharoplasts. Mucus-secreting cells, goblet cells, granular cells, foamy cells, and vacuolated cells have all been described.[212]

Pathogenesis

In 1910 Sjovall suggested that colloid cysts might arise from the paraphysis.[214] This was suspected because the paraphysis arises at the site favored by colloid cysts. This structure is an evagination of the roof of the third ventricle that occurs during embryogenesis at the site that will come to lie just posterior to the foramen of Monro. In amphibians this organ is secretory and empties into the anterior part of the third ventricle.[112] In humans it is rudimentary,

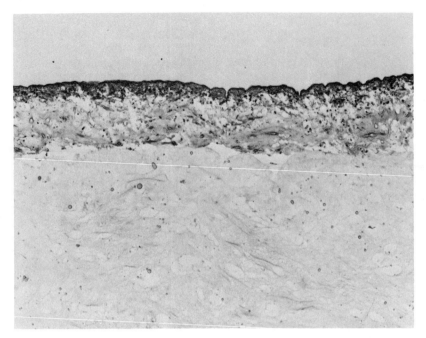

Figure 91–14 Microscopic pathological changes of colloid cyst. A uniform, thin cyst wall with cilia on its surface is shown. 233 ×.

being present from the 17- to the 100-mm stage. The paraphysis usually degenerates by the 100-mm stage, although vestiges may persist as the paraphyseal vesicle.

A second evagination from the neuroepithelial roof of the third ventricle, occurring just caudal to the paraphysis, is named the diencephalic recess of the postvelar arch, and this structure is believed by some to be the source of typical colloid cysts.[112] Cysts in other locations would then arise from other diverticula of the neuroepithelial roof. Electron microscopy has suggested an entodermal origin.[77,92]

The suggestion that colloid cyst may not arise from the paraphysis is encouraged by morphological differences in the epithelium of colloid cysts and of the paraphysis. Although colloid cyst epithelium may contain cilia, as may the epithelium of the diencephalic recess, the paraphysis does not contain cilia. Also, the occasional occurrence of colloid cyst in the middle and posterior parts of the third ventricle and the rare occurrence between the leaves of the septum pellucidum would be difficult to explain on the basis of origin from the paraphysis. Perhaps the term "neuroepithelial cysts" suggested by Fulton and Bailey is more appropriate, since it does not specify the exact embryological anlage for colloid cysts.[73]

Clinical Presentation

Although there are characteristic symptoms and signs of colloid cysts, there are no reliable means of clinical diagnosis. Headache is the presenting complaint in 85 per cent of patients and is present in up to 96 per cent. It may occur in a variety of locations, being initially or primarily frontal in 50 per cent, occipital in 15 per cent, and generalized in 25 per cent.[252] The headache often is severe and usually occurs during the day. In 16 of 29 patients with this lesion who were reviewed by Kelly, it lasted only seconds or minutes, whereas a history of headaches of brief duration was found in only 9 of 361 patients with other types of tumors. In Kelly's series of colloid cyst cases, the headaches were improved by lying down or changing position in 8 of the 29 patients. Although other signs were often present, nearly 25 per cent presented with headache and papilledema without any other signs or symptoms.[113] In the majority of cases with these symptoms, no tumor can be identified and benign intracranial hypertension will be diagnosed.[247]

In approximately 15 per cent of patients in one series the initial attack was acute and fatal; 63 per cent had repeated attacks with short intermissions, and the remaining 22 per cent had repeated attacks with long intermissions.[252] This history of repeated episodes of headache or neurological deficit, which usually consists of paroxysms of headache with vomiting and sometimes amblyopia, has been considered to be classic for colloid cysts.[84] The attacks may be followed by loss of consciousness and prolonged coma or profound mental changes that last for hours or days and then completely subside. These paroxysms of disability are thought to be related to intermittent ventricular obstruction by a pendulous cyst, although episodes of increased intracranial pressure without cyst movement may also be responsible.

Sudden attacks of leg weakness occurred in 6 of the 29 patients reported by Kelly, and each of these patients had massive hydrocephalus.[113] Episodes of leg weakness may also be related to intermittent ventricular obstruction with sudden ventricular enlargement or episodes of increased intracranial pressure. In a series of 361 tumors, similar attacks of leg weakness occurred in only three patients who did not have colloid cyst.[113]

Fluctuating or progressive dementia may also occur with colloid cyst.[113] This can accompany hydrocephalus and increased pressure or hydrocephalus without increased pressure. The occurrence of dementia with ventricular enlargement due to anterior third ventricular tumors, in the absence of increased pressure, was first described by Riddoch and again emphasized by Adams and co-workers and given the designation "normal pressure hydrocephalus."[1,191] Each of these authors reported a patient with a colloid cyst as well as other patients with dementia and hydrocephalus but apparently normal intracranial pressure. Fourteen of the thirty-eight patients described by Little and MacCarty had "disturbed mentation," and eight of these patients presented with chief complaints of progressive dementia and gait disturbance. Some of them had elevated intracranial pressure.[139]

Other signs and symptoms are less common. Approximately 20 per cent of patients have epilepsy, the seizures usually being generalized.[252] Temperature regulation may be abnormal, and there have been reports of fever to 102° F and hypothermia to 94° F.[84,253]

Investigation

Two questions must be answered in the evaluation of a patient suspected of having a colloid cyst. The presence of a mass in the anterior portion of the third ventricle must be determined, and masses arising within the ventricle must be distinguished from those arising from the diencephalon and projecting into the ventricle.

Plain skull x-rays are normal in 60 per cent of patients with colloid cyst and reveal stigmata of hydrocephalus with erosion of the dorsum sellae in 40 per cent.[200] Posterior-inferior displacement of the pineal gland occurs in 13 per cent of the patients.[139] Although electroencephalography is abnormal in approximately 70 per cent of patients, the abnormalities are of a nonfocal character and reflect a deep-seated lesion or increased intracranial pressure.[139] Cerebrospinal fluid usually has normal protein and cells. Its pressure is elevated in 80 per cent.[252] In the presence of ventricular obstruction, lumbar puncture is dangerous. Little and MacCarty have reported two deaths that may have been contributed to by lumbar puncture and pneumoencephalography.[139] Radioisotope brain scan occasionally reveals an area of uptake at the site of the tumor.[179]

Angiography, aside from demonstrating hydrocephalus, may also be suggestive if the cyst displaces the anterior portion of the internal cerebral vein, causing a hump in this vein at the level of the foramen of Monro. Downward displacement of the posterior portion of the internal cerebral vein and flattening of its normally upward convex curve suggests lateral ventricular enlargement without third ventricular enlargement and thus suggests anterior third ventricular obstruction.[18]

In the past, the definitive diagnostic procedure has been ventriculography.[37] This reveals hydrocephalus, which may be symmetrical or asymmetrical, as well as a filling defect in the anterior part of the third ventricle and obstruction of communication between one lateral ventricle and the other or between the lateral and the third ventricles. The third ventricle may also be wider than normal. To outline the tumor, it is helpful to hyperextend the neck, making the vertex of the head most dependent so that air selectively fills the anterior part of the frontal horns and the region of the foramen of Monro.

The advent of computed tomography has simplified the diagnosis of colloid cyst. This study reveals hydrocephalus that is either symmetrical or asymmetrical and may reveal the presence of a mass in the anterior portion of the third ventricle.[86,199] If a cyst is suspected but is not seen on routine CT scans, the cerebrospinal fluid density may be enhanced by intraventricular injection of an iodinated contrast agent. This enhancement has made it relatively simple to demonstrate anterior third ventricular tumors (Fig. 91–15).[213]

Therapy

Nonoperative treatment is not useful. Although ventricular shunting without tumor removal has been advocated, the favorable results in most patients who are operated on argue in favor of removal of the tumor.[232] Most colloid cysts occur just pos-

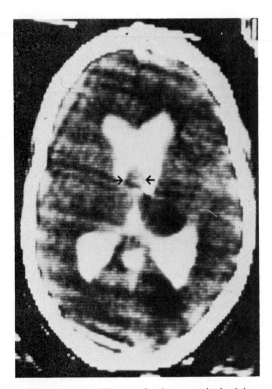

Figure 91–15 CT scan after intraventricular injection of contrast material demonstrates a filling defect in the anterior part of the third ventricle. (From Sivalingam, S., Dublin, A. B., and Youmans, J. R.: Computer assisted ventriculography. J. Comput. Assist. Tomogr., 2:162–164, 1978. Reprinted by permission.)

terior to the foramen of Monro. In the unusual patient who has a colloid cyst in some other location, the operative approach to the tumor will be dictated by the location of the tumor.

The most commonly used approach to the anterior aspect of the third ventricle is a modification of the one devised by Dandy.[56] A unilateral right frontal craniotomy is performed, exposing the cortex just anterior to the coronal suture. A 2-cm cortical incision is made in the middle frontal gyrus and carried down to the ventricle. Subependymal veins are followed to the foramen of Monro. The tumor is usually seen as a domed grayish or bluish structure presenting in the foramen. Occasionally the surgeon is fortunate enough to encounter a small tumor and an enlarged foramen of Monro. If this occurs and the stalk of the tumor can be identified, clipped, and divided, the cyst may not need to be opened prior to removal. In the majority of cases, it will not be possible to deliver the cyst safely without evacuation of its contents. In this circumstance, the tumor is gently freed from the margins of the foramen of Monro and is opened with sharp dissection. The cyst contents are evacuated with suction. These contents will be found to be thick and tenacious. The tumor wall is then delivered through the foramen of Monro in the collapsed state. The remnant of tumor usually is attached to either the roof of the third ventricle or the choroid plexus. This attachment may be either sessile or pedunculated. If a long neck is present, it may be rather easy to deliver the cyst wall in its entirety through the foramen of Monro and clip and divide the attachment to the choroid plexus or the roof of the ventricle. If the cyst wall is sessile, a remnant of cyst wall may be left in the third ventricle with only a 10 per cent risk of cyst recurrence.[153] If greater access to the anterior part of the third ventricle is required, the column of the fornix can be divided unilaterally where it makes up the anterior and superior margins of the foramen of Monro. If the right fornix is divided and the left fornix is injured during tumor removal, however, the patient will develop serious affective and memory disturbances that may be permanent.

The structures at greatest risk during tumor dissection and removal are the fornix, the thalamostriate vein, the internal cerebral vein, and the choroid plexus. Bleeding from vascular structures may be difficult to control if it comes from an inaccessible portion of the third ventricle. For this reason great care must be taken to protect these structures during tumor removal. If venous bleeding occurs and the thalamostriate vein must be obliterated, hemorrhagic infarction in the basal ganglia may result.[153] Should tumor removal be difficult and postoperative obstruction of the foramen of Monro by intraventricular clot seem possible, fenestration of the septum pellucidum may be helpful.[186]

Following tumor removal, the ventricles should be irrigated with warm saline to remove blood and tumor contents that have spilled. If these contaminants are not carefully removed, postoperative confusion, fever, and chemical meningitis may occur. If the ventricles are very large, the postoperative course may be complicated by ventricular collapse. Risk of this complication can be lessened by sealing the cortical incision with Gelfoam.[34]

The authors have had good results with the conventional approach as described by Dandy and also with the transcallosal approach as recommended by Greenwood.[83] The latter requires a craniotomy at the level of the coronal suture. The medial surface of the frontal lobe is retracted laterally, exposing the corpus callosum. The exact midline is sought so that the pericallosal arteries are spared. The corpus callosum is divided in the midline to allow the operating surgeon access to the frontal horn of the right lateral ventricle. The cyst is then removed through the foramen of Monro in a fashion similar to that used for the transcortical approach. The advantages of the transcallosal approach are that it does not require ventricular enlargement for good vision and that little cortical injury is produced, thus avoiding the seizure focus that ensues after transcortical approaches.[186]

The most frequent other location of colloid cyst is in the middle or posterior part of the third ventricle. Little and MacCarty have reported a cyst missed at transfrontal operation in a patient who later died. At autopsy a colloid cyst was found in an unusually posterior location in the third ventricle. If a colloid cyst is far enough posterior to prevent removal through the foramen of Monro, an operation through the roof of the third ventricle may be required.[56] The approach to the midportion of the ventricle requires a bone flap centered at the coronal suture and crossing the midline. This is removed, and the dura is opened and hinged on the sagittal sinus. The brain is retracted from the falx, care being taken to preserve bridging veins in the region of the central sulcus. The corpus callosum is divided exactly in the midline, sparing both anterior cerebral arteries. If the exposure is not directly in the midline, the operating surgeon will find himself in one lateral ventricle after opening the corpus callosum. At this point it is not difficult to trace subependymal veins to the foramen of Monro. The midline is then again sought, and staying directly between the leaves of the septum pellucidum, dissection is carried down through the roof of the third ventricle between the two internal cerebral veins. Great care must be taken to preserve these veins. The colloid cyst can then be directly visualized and incised, and its contents evacuated. Its attachment to the roof of the third ventricle can then be clipped and divided. The operating surgeon must realize that this approach can be difficult and hazardous.

Aspiration of cyst contents by stereotaxic placement of a needle in the cyst has been successful and carries little risk. A needle with an inner diameter of at least 1.5 mm is required. If the cyst refills, repeat aspiration can be accomplished. No evidence of recurrent cyst has been noted in four patients treated by this method and followed up to seven years.[30] Aspiration can be followed by placement of a shunt from the cyst to the peritoneum. This technique has been used successfully to treat five anterior third ventricle cysts. No evidence of recurrence has been identified, although the average follow up time is only 33 months.[87]

Results

Removal of colloid cysts can result in several postoperative complications. These include stupor or coma vigil, confusion, hyperthermia, Korsakoff's syndrome, seizures, and rare cases of diabetes insipidus. In spite of these potential complications, Dandy was able to operate on the first five patients with colloid cysts with only one death.[56] Among the 25 patients in whom preoperative diagnosis was correct and who underwent operations prior to 1938, there were only three deaths.[84] With the use of modern operative methods, including micro-operative techniques, patients have "generally witnessed rapid and uncomplicated recovery."[179]

INTRACRANIAL LIPOMA

Intracranial lipomas are rare masses of mature fat, usually discovered as incidental autopsy or CT scan findings. They are of relatively little clinical importance, being so slowly growing that they are more nearly malformations or hamartomas than neoplasms.[36,63,215]

There is general consensus that lipomas are the result of abnormal formation of the central nervous system.[198,204,255] This origin is suggested by the midline site of most lipomas, the very indolent, nonneoplastic clinical behavior, and the commonly associated central nervous system malformations (particularly agenesis of the corpus callosum).[241]

Although in an early series four lipomas were identified in 5000 autopsies, the frequency is probably greater; nine lipomas were identified in a selected series of 1956 autopsies.[36,241] They constitute 0.1 per cent of brain tumors in pathological series and occur in patients of all ages.[248,256] The average age of patients with diagnosed lipomas is early in the fifth decade.[36] The incidence is nearly equal in the two sexes, although women may be affected slightly more frequently.[255]

Intracranial lipomas are usually identified in the region of the corpus callosum, the tuber cinereum, or the corpora quadrigemina. The lipoma is always connected to the leptomeninges, but there are also connections to the adjacent brain. The leptomeninges and surrounding brain may become calcified.[36,225,258] The tumor may contain cartilage or osseous tissue.[12,204,241]

Lipomas consist of mature adipose tissue with variable amounts of collagen. Ganglion cells and areas of neuroglia may be included in them.[198]

Symptoms due to intracranial lipomas are uncommon. Most of these masses are incidental autopsy findings. Patients with corpus callosum lipomas have seizures in approximately 65 per cent of cases and may also have other neurological deficits, but

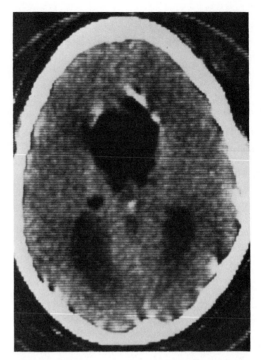

Figure 91–16   Computed tomography of a lipoma of the corpus callosum demonstrates a central area of low density with a calcific rim. (Courtesy of Arthur B. Dublin, M.D., University of California, Davis.)

these symptoms may be due to associated brain malformations rather than to the lipoma.[215,255] Rarely lipomas are sufficiently large to compress cerebrospinal fluid pathways and produce hydrocephalus.[114,198,225,241]

Corpus callosum lipomas produce a striking plain skull x-ray appearance in which a central lucent space is bounded on each side by a calcific shell that consists of the summation of small areas of calcification. Computed tomography demonstrates a central area of low density with a calcific rim (Fig. 91–16).[225]

Since an intracranial lipoma rarely produces mass effect, operative treatment is usually not necessary. Excision of the lipoma is difficult owing to vessels incorporated in the fatty mass, and if hydrocephalus develops, it is probably sufficient to place shunts in the lateral ventricles without directly treating the lipoma.[63,225]

REFERENCES

1. Adams, R. D., Fisher, C. M., Hakim, S., Ojemann, R. G., and Sweet, W. H.: Symptomatic occult hydrocephalus with "normal" cerebro-

spinal fluid pressure: A treatable syndrome. New Eng. J. Med., *273*:117–126, 1965.

2. Alpers, B. J.: The cerebral epidermoids (cholesteatomas). Amer. J. Surg., *43*:55–65, 1939.

3. Alvord, E. C.: Growth rates of epidermoid tumors. Ann. Neurol., *2*:367–370, 1977.

4. Arseni, C., and Maretsis, M.: Craniopharyngioma. Neurochirurgia (Stuttgart), *1*:25–32, 1972.

5. Ashley, D. J. B.: Origin of teratomas. Cancer, *32*:390–394, 1973.

6. Babinski, M. J.: Tumeur du corps pituitare sans acromégalie et avec arrèt. de développement des organes génitaux. Rev. Neurol. (Paris), *8*:531–533, 1900.

7. Backlund, E.-O.: Studies on craniopharyngiomas. I. Treatment: Past and present. Acta Chir. Scand., *138*:743–747, 1972.

8. Backlund, E.-O.: Studies on craniopharyngiomas. III. Stereotaxic treatment with intracystic yttrium-90. Acta Chir. Scand. *139*:237–247, 1973.

9. Backlund, E.-O.: Studies on craniopharyngiomas. IV. Stereotaxic treatment with radiosurgery. Acta Chir. Scand., *139*:344–351, 1973.

10. Backlund, E.-O., Johansson, L., and Sarby, B.: Studies on craniopharyngiomas. II. Treatment by stereotaxis and radiosurgery. Acta Chir. Scand., *138*:749–759, 1972.

11. Bailey P: Cruveilhier's "tumeurs perlées." Surg. Gynec. Obstet., *31*:390–401, 1920.

12. Bailey, P., and Bucy, P. C.: The origin and nature of meningeal tumors. Amer. J. Cancer, *15*:15–54, 1931.

13. Banna, M.: Craniopharyngioma in adults. Surg. Neurol., *1*:202–204, 1973.

14. Banna, M.: Intracranial cholesteatoma. Clin. Radiol., *28*:161–164, 1977.

15. Banna, M., Hoare, R. D., Stanley, P., and Till, K.: Craniopharyngioma in children. J. Pediat., *83*:781–785, 1973.

16. Barnett, D. J.: Radiologic aspects of craniopharyngiomas. Radiology, *72*:14–18, 1959.

17. Bartlett, J. R.: Craniopharyngiomas: An analysis of some aspects of symptomatology, radiology and histology. Brain, *94*:725–732, 1971.

18. Batnitzky, S., Sarwar, M., Leeds, N. E., Schechter, M. M., and Behroz, A.-K.: Colloid cysts of the third ventricle. Radiology, *112*:327–341, 1974.

19. Baumann, C. H. H., and Bucy, P. C.: Paratrigeminal epidermoid tumors. J. Neurosurg., *13*:455–468, 1956.

20. Beckmann, J. W., and Kubie, L. S.: A clinical study of twenty-one cases of tumour of the hypophyseal stalk. Brain, *52*:127–170, 1929.

21. Bender, L.: Experimental production of gliosis: Effects on the nervous system of the rabbit of intravenous and intraspinal injections of cholesterol emulsion. Amer. J. Path., *1*:657–665, 1925.

22. Berry, R. G., and Schlezinger, N. S.: Rathke-cleft cysts. Arch. Neurol. (Chicago), *1*:48–58, 1959.

23. Block, M. A., Goree, J. A., and Jiminez, J. P.: Craniopharyngioma with optic canal enlargement simulating a glioma of the optic chiasm: Case report. J. Neurosurg., *39*:523–527, 1973.

24. Bloom, H. J. G.: Combined modality therapy for intracranial tumors. Cancer, *35*:111–120, 1975.

25. Bloom, H. J. G., and Harmer, C. L.: Craniopharyngiomas. Brit. Med. J., *2*:288–289, 1972.

26. Bochner, S. J., and Scarff, J. E.: Teratoma of the pineal body: Classification of the embryonal tumors of the pineal body; report of a case of teratoma of the pineal body presenting formed teeth. Arch. Surg. (Chicago), *36*:303–329, 1938.

27. Bock, E.: Beitrag zur Pathologie der Hypophyse. Virchow. Arch. Path. Anat., *252*:89–112, 1924.

28. Bogdanowicz, W. M., and Wilson, D. H.: Dermoid cyst of the fourth ventricle demonstrated on brain scan: Case Report. J. Neurosurg., *36*:228–230,1972.

29. Bollati, A., Giunta, F., Lenzi, A., and Marini, G.: Third ventricle intrinsic craniopharyngioma. J. Neurosurg. Sci., *17*:316–317, 1973.

30. Bosch, D. A., Rähn, T., and Backlund, E. O.: Treatment of colloid cysts of the third ventricle by stereotactic aspiration. Surg. Neurol., *9*:15–18, 1978.

31. Bostroem, E.: Ueber die pialen Epidermoide, Dermoide und Lipome und duralen Dermoide. Centralbl. Allg. Path. Path. Anat., *8*:1–98, 1897.

32. Boyd, J. D.: Observations on the human pharyngeal hypophysis. J. Endocr., *14*:66–77, 1956.

33. Brock, S., and Klenke, D. A.: A case of dermoid overlying the cerebellar vermis. Bull. Neurol. Inst. N.Y., *1*:328–342, 1931.

34. Buchsbaum, H. W., and Colton, R. P.: Anterior third ventricular cysts in infancy: Case report. J. Neurosurg., *26*:264–266, 1967.

35. Bucy, P. C.: Intradiploic epidermoid (cholesteatoma) of the skull. Arch. Surg. (Chicago), *31*:190–199, 1935.

36. Budka, H.: Intracranial lipomatous harmartomas (intracranial "lipomas"). Acta Neuropath. (Berlin), *28*:205–222, 1974.

37. Bull, J. W. D., and Sutton, D.: The diagnosis of paraphysial cysts. Brain, *72*:487–516, 1949.

38. Carmichael, H. T.: Squamous epithelial rests in the hypophysis cerebri. Arch. Neurol. Psychiat., *26*:966–975, 1931.

39. Carney, J. A., Thompson, D. P., Johnson, C. L., and Lynn, H. B.: Teratomas in children: Clinical and pathologic aspects. J. Pediat. Surg., *7*:271–282, 1972.

40. Carpenter, R. C., Chamberlin, G. W., and Frazier, C. H.: The treatment of hypophyseal stalk tumors by evacuation and irradiation. Amer. J. Roentgen., *38*:162–177, 1937.

41. Cashion, E. L., and Young, J. M.: Intraventricular craniopharyngioma: Report of two cases. J. Neurosurg., *34*:84–87, 1971.

42. Chadduck, W. M., and Roberts, M.: Long term survival with craniopharyngioma: Report of patient in 29th year after treatment, seen for a second intracranial tumor. J. Neurosurg., *25*:312–314, 1966.

43. Childe, A. E., and Young, A. W.: Pneumographic diagnosis of intraventricular epidermoid. Radiology, *48*:56–60, 1947.

44. Choremis, C., Economos, D., Papadatos, C., and Gargoulas, A.: Intraspinal epidermoid tumours (cholesteatomas) in patients treated for

tuberculous meningitis. Lancet, *271*:437–439, 1956.

45. Ciric, I.: Neuroepithelial cysts. J. Neurosurg., *44*:134, 1976.

46. Ciric, I., and Zivin, I.: Neuroepithelial (colloid) cysts of the septum pellucidum. J. Neurosurg., *43*:69–73, 1975.

47. Cobb, J. P., and Wright, J. C.: Studies on a craniopharyngioma in tissue culture. I. Growth characteristics and alterations produced following exposure to two radiomimetic agents. J. Neuropath. Exp. Neurol., *18*:563–568, 1959.

48. Cooper, P. R., and Ransohoff, J.: Craniopharyngioma originating in the sphenoid bone: Case report. J. Neurosurg., *36*:102–106, 1972.

49. Critchley, M., and Ferguson, F. R.: The cerebrospinal epidermoids (cholesteatomata). Brain, *51*:334–384, 1928.

50. Critchley, M., and Ironside, R. N.: The pituitary adamantinomata. Brain, *49*:437–481, 1926.

51. Cruveilhier, J.: Anatomie Pathologique du Corps Humain: Ou, Descriptions, avec Figures Lithographiees et Coloriées, des Diverses Alterations Morbides dont le Corps Humain est Susceptible. Paris, J.-B. Bailliere, 1835–1842, Vol. 2, p. 341.

52. Cushing, H.: A large epidermal cholesteatoma of the parietotemporal region deforming the left hemisphere without cerebral symptoms. Surg. Gynec. Obstet., *34*:557–566, 1922.

53. Cushing, H.: Studies in Intracranial Physiology and Surgery. London, Oxford University Press, 1926.

54. Cushing, H.: Intracranial Tumors. Notes upon a Series of Two Thousand Verified Cases with Surgical-Mortality Percentages Pertaining Thereto. Springfield, Ill., Charles C Thomas, 1932.

55. Dandy, W. E.: Diagnosis, localization and removal of tumors of the third ventricle. Bull. Johns Hopkins Hosp., *33*:188–189, 1922.

56. Dandy, W. E.: Benign Tumors in the Third Ventricle of the Brain: Diagnosis and Treatment. Springfield, Ill., Charles C Thomas, 1933.

57. Dandy, W. E.: Operative experience in cases of pineal tumor. Arch. Surg. (Chicago), *33*:19–46, 1936.

58. Davidson, S. I., and Small, J. M.: Malignant change in an intracranial epidermoid. J. Neurol. Neurosurg. Psychiat., *23*:176–178, 1960.

59. Davis, K. R., Roberson, G. H., Taveras, J. M., New, P. F. J., and Trevor, R.: Diagnosis of epidermoid tumor by computed tomography: Analysis and evaluation of findings. Radiology, *119*:347–353, 1976.

60. Dayan, A. D., Marshall, A. H. E., Miller, A. A., Pick, F. J., and Rankin, N. E.: Atypical teratomas of the pineal and hypothalamus. J. Path. Bact., *92*:1–29, 1966.

61. Duffy, W. C.: Hypophyseal duct tumors. Ann. Surg., *72*:537–555, 725–757, 1920.

62. Dyke, C. G., and Davidoff, L. M.: Encephalographic appearance of intraventricular epidermoid. Bull. Neurol. Inst. N.Y., *6*:489–493, 1937.

63. Ehni, G. J., and Adson, A. W.: Lipoma of the brain: Report of cases. Arch. Neurol. Psychiat., *53*:299–304, 1945.

64. Erdheim, J.: Zur normalen und pathologischen Histologie der Glandula thyreoidea, parathyreoidea und Hypophysis. Beitr. Path. Anat., *33*:158–236, 1903.

65. Erdheim, J.: Über Hypophysenganggeschwülste und Hirncholesteatome. S. B. Acad. Wiss. Wien, 113, Abt 3, p. 537, 1904.

66. Ernst, P.: Häufung dysontogenetischer Bildungen am Zentralnervensystem. Verh. Deutsch. Ges. Path., *15*:226–234, 1912.

67. Evans, R. A., Schwartz, J. F., and Chutorian, A. M.: Radiologic diagnosis in pediatric ophthalmology. Radiol. Clin. N. Amer., *1*:459–495, 1963.

68. Finkelstein, J. W., Kream, J., Ludan, A., and Hellman, L.: Sulfation factor (somatomedin): An explanation for continued growth in the absence of immunoassayable growth hormone in patients with hypothalamic tumors. J. Clin. Endocr., *35*:13–17, 1972.

69. Fitz, C. R., Wortzman, G., Harwood-Nash, D. C., Holgate, R. C., Barry, J. F., and Boldt, D. W.: Computed tomography in craniopharyngiomas. Radiology, *127*:687–691, 1978.

70. Fleming, J. F. R., and Botterell, E. H.: Cranial dermoid and epidermoid tumors. Surg. Gynec. Obstet., *109*:403–411, 1959.

71. Frazier, C. H., and Alpers, B. J.: Tumors of Rathke's cleft (hitherto called tumors of Rathke's pouch). Arch. Neurol. Psychiat., *32*:973–984, 1934.

72. Frölich, A.: Fall von Tumor der Hypophyse ohne Akromegalie. Wien Klin. Wschr., *15*:27, 1902.

73. Fulton, J. F., and Bailey, P.: Contribution to the study of tumors in the region of the third ventricle: Their diagnosis and relation to pathological sleep. J. Nerv. Ment. Dis., *69*:1–25, 145–164, 261–277, 1929.

74. Gacek, R. R.: Diagnosis and management of primary tumors of the petrous apex. Ann. Otol., suppl. 18:1–20, 1975.

75. Garcia-Uria, J.: Surgical experience with craniopharyngioma in adults. Surg. Neurol., *9*:11–14, 1978.

76. Ghatak, N. R., Hirano, A., and Zimmerman, H. M.: Ultrastructure of a craniopharyngioma. Cancer, *27*:1465–1475, 1971.

77. Ghatak, N. R., Kasoff, I., and Alexander, E.: Further observation on the fine structure of a colloid cyst of the third ventricle. Acta. Neuropath. (Berlin), *39*:101–107, 1977.

78. Goldberg, G. M., and Eshbaugh, D. E.: Squamous cell nests of the pituitary gland as related to the origin of craniopharyngiomas: A study of their presence in the newborn and infants up to age four. Arch. Path. (Chicago), *70*:293–299, 1960.

79. Goodhill, V.: Ear Disease, Deafness, and Dizziness. Hagerstown, Md., Harper & Row, 1979, pp. 333–334.

80. Gordy, P. D., Peet, M. M., and Kahn, E. A.: The surgery of the craniopharyngiomas. J. Neurosurg., *6*:503–517, 1949.

81. Grant, F. C., and Austin, G. M.: Epidermoids: Clinical evaluation and surgical results. J. Neurosurg., *7*:190–198, 1950.

82. Greenhouse, A. H., and Neuburger, K. T.: Intracranial teratomata of the newborn. Arch. Neurol. (Chicago), *3*:718–724, 1960.

83. Greenwood, J.: Paraphysial cysts of the third ventricle: With report of eight cases. J. Neurosurg., 6:153–159, 1946.

84. Grossiord, A.: Le kyste colloide du trosième ventricule. Thèse de Paris, 1941.

85. Guidetti, B., and Gagliardi, F. M.: Epidermoid and dermoid cysts: Clinical evaluation and late surgical results. J. Neurosurg., 47:12–18, 1977.

86. Guner, M., Shaw, M. D. M., Turner, J. W., and Steven, J. L.: Computed tomography in the diagnosis of colloid cyst. Surg. Neurol., 6:345–348, 1976.

87. Gutierrez-Lara, F., Patiño, R., and Hakim, S.: Treatment of tumors of the third ventricle: A new and simple technique. Surg. Neurol., 3:323–325, 1975.

88. Haig, P. V.: Primary epidermoids of the skull: Including a case with malignant change. Amer. J. Roentgen., 76:1076–1080, 1956.

89. Hamberger, C. A., Hammer, G., Norlén, G., and Sjögren, B.: Surgical treatment of craniopharyngioma: Radical removal by the transantrosphenoidal approach. Acta Otolaryng. (Stockholm), 52:285–292, 1960.

90. Hardy, J., and Wigser, S. M.: Trans-sphenoidal surgery of pituitary fossa tumors with televised radiofluoroscopic control. J. Neurosurg., 23:612–619, 1965.

91. Hash, C. J., and Ritchie, D. J.: Ruptured intraventricular dermoid cyst without clinical inflammation. Arch. Neurol. (Chicago), 34:61, 1978.

92. Hirano, A., and Ghatak, N. R.: The fine structure of colloid cysts of the third ventricle. J. Neuropath. Exp. Neurol., 33:333–341, 1974.

93. Hirano, A., Ghatak, N. R., and Zimmerman, H. M.: Fenestrated blood vessels in craniopharyngioma. Acta Neuropath. (Berlin), 26:171–177, 1973.

94. Hoff, J. T., and Patterson, R. H.: Craniopharyngiomas in children and adults. J. Neurosurg., 36:299–302, 1972.

95. Hoffman, H. J., Hendrick, E. B., Humphreys, R. P., Buncic, J. R., Armstrong, D. L., and Jenkin, D. T.: Management of craniopharyngioma in children. J. Neurosurg., 47:218–227, 1977.

96. Holbach, K.-H., and Gullotta, F.: Zur Formalgenese intrasellärer und intraventrikulärer Zysten. Neurochirurgia (Stuttgart), 20:186–188, 1977.

97. Horrax, G.: A consideration of the dermal versus the epidermal cholesteatomas having their attachment in the cerebral envelopes. Arch. Neurol. Psychiat., 8:265–285, 1922.

98. Horrax, G.: Benign (favorable) types of brain tumor: The end results (up to twenty years), with statistics of mortality and useful survival. New Eng. J. Med., 250:981–984, 1954.

99. Hosoi, K.: Teratoma and teratoid tumors of the brain. Arch. Path. (Chicago), 9:1207–1219, 1930.

100. Hunter, I. J.: Squamous metaplasia of cells of the anterior pituitary gland. J. Path. Bact., 69:141–145, 1955.

101. Ingraham, F. D., and Bailey, O. T.: Cystic teratomas and teratoid tumors of the central nervous system in infancy and childhood. J. Neurosurg., 3:511–532, 1946.

102. Ingraham, F. D., and Scott, H. W.: Craniopharyngiomas in children. J. Pediat., 29:95–116, 1946.

103. Ingraham, F. D., Matson, D. D., McLaurin, R. L.: Cortisone and ACTH as an adjunct to the surgery of craniopharyngiomas. New Eng. J. Med., 246:568–571, 1952.

104. Innes, J. R. M., and Saunders, L. Z.: Comparative Neuropathology. New York, Academic Press, 1962.

105. Ito, T.: Pathology of brain tumors. Acta Path. Jap., 8:415–416, 1958.

106. James, A. E., Jr., DeLand, F. H., Hodges, F. J., 3rd, and Wagner, H. N.: Radionuclide imaging in the detection and differential diagnosis of craniopharyngiomas. Amer. J. Roentgen. 109:692–700, 1970.

107. Jefferson, G., and Smalley, A. A.: Progressive facial palsy produced by intratemporal epidermoids. J. Laryng., 53:417–443, 1938.

108. Jellinger, K., and Sunder-Plassmann, M.: Connatal intracranial tumours. Neuropaediatrie, 4:46–63, 1973.

109. Job, J. C., Lambertz, J., Sizonenko, P. C., and Rossier, A.: La croissance des enfants atteints de craniopharyngiome. Arch. Franc. Pediat., 27:341–353, 1970.

110. Kahn, E. A., Gosch, H. H., Seeger, J. F., and Hicks, S. P.: Forty-five years experience with the craniopharyngiomas. Surg. Neurol., 1:5–12, 1973.

111. Kaplan, I. I.: Clinical Radiation Therapy. 2nd Ed. New York, Paul B. Hoeber, Inc., 1949.

112. Kappers, J. A.: The development of the paraphysis cerebri in man with comments on its relationship to the intercolumnar tubercle and its significance for the origin of cystic tumors in the third ventricle. J. Comp. Neurol., 102:425–510, 1955.

113. Kelly, R.: Colloid cysts of the third ventricle: Analysis of twenty-nine cases. Brain, 74:23–65, 1951.

114. Kernohan, J. W.: Tumors of congenital origin. In Minckler, J., ed.: Pathology of the Nervous System. New York, McGraw Hill Book Co., 1971, pp. 1927–1937.

115. Kernohan, J. W., and Sayre, J. P.: Tumors of the Central Nervous System: Atlas of Tumor Pathology. Fascicle 35. Washington Armed Forces Institute of Pathology, 1952.

116. Keville, F. J., and Wise, B. L.: Intracranial epidermoid and dermoid tumors. J. Neurosurg., 16:564–569, 1959.

117. Killeffer, F. A. and Stern, W. E.: Chronic effects of hypothalamic injury: Report of a case of near total hypothalamic destruction resulting from removal of a craniopharyngioma. Arch. Neurol. (Chicago), 22:419–429, 1970.

118. King, J. E. J.: Extradural diploic and intradural epidermoid tumors (cholesteatoma). Ann. Surg., 109:649–688, 1939.

119. Kömpf, D., and Menges, H.-W.: Maligne Entartung eines parapontinen Epidermoids. Acta Neurochir. (Wien), 39:81–90, 1977.

120. Koos, W. T., and Miller, M. H.: Intracranial Tumors of Infants and Children. Stuttgart, Georg Thieme, 1971.

121. Korsgaard, O., Lindholm, J., and Rasmussen, P.: Endocrine function in patients with supra-

sellar and hypothalamic tumours. Acta Endocr. (Kobenhavn), *83*:1–8, 1976.

122. Kramer, S.: The value of radiation therapy for pituitary and parapituitary tumours. Canad. Med. Ass. J., *99*:1120–1127, 1968.

123. Kramer, S., McKissock, W., and Concannon, J. P.: Craniopharyngiomas: Treatment by combined surgery and radiation therapy. J. Neurosurg., *18*:217–226, 1961.

124. Kramer, S., Southard, M., and Mansfield, C. M.: Radiotherapy in the management of craniopharyngiomas: Further experiences and late results. Amer. J. Roentgen., *103*:44–52, 1968.

125. Krayenbühl, H., and Prader, A.: Traitement endocrinien des troubles de la croissance chez des malades opérés d'un craniopharyngiome. Neurochirurgie, *8*:223–233, 1962.

126. Krieg, W.: Aseptische Meningitis nach Operation von Cholesteatomen des Gehirns. Zbl. Neurochir., *1*:79–86, 1936.

127. Kunicki, A., Lechowski, S., Madroszkiewicz, E., and Szwagrzyk, E.: Rathke's pouch tumors of childhood in the material of the Department of Neurosurgery, Medical Academy in Cracow. Pol. Med. J., *11*:985–990, 1972.

128. Landers, J. W., and Danielski, J. J.: Malignant intracranial epidermoid cysts. Arch. Path. (Chicago), *70*:419–423, 1960.

129. Landolt, A. M.: Die Ultrastruktur des Kraniopharyngeoms. Schweiz. Arch. Neurol. Neurochir. Psychiat., *111*:313–329, 1972.

130. Larson, C. P.: Colloid (paraphysial) cyst of third ventricle with rupture into caudate nucleus and internal capsule. J. Nerv. Ment. Dis., *91*:557–565, 1940.

131. Laster, D. W., Moody, D. M., and Ball, M. R.: Computerized cranial tomography of free intracranial fat in congenital tumors. Comput. Tomogr., *2*:257–265, 1978.

132. Leddy, E. T., and Marshall, T. M.: Roentgen therapy of pituitary adamantinomas (craniopharyngiomas). Radiology, *56*:384–393, 1951.

133. Leksell, L.: Stereotaxis and Radiosurgery: An Operative System. Springfield, Ill., Charles C Thomas, 1971.

134. Leksell, L., and Lidén, K.: A therapeutic trial with radioactive isotopes in cystic brain tumour. *In* Radioisotope Techniques. Oxford, H. M. Stationery Office, 1951, pp. 76–78.

135. Leksell, L., Backlund, E. O., and Johansson, L.: Treatment of craniopharyngiomas. Acta Chir. Scand., *133*:345–350, 1967.

136. Lewis, D. D.: A contribution to the subject of tumors of the hypophysis: I. Tumors developing from cranio-pharyngeal duct inclusions. JAMA, *55*:1002–1008, 1910.

137. Lindgren, E., and Di Chiro, G.: Suprasellar tumours with calcification. Acta Radiol., *36*:173–195, 1951.

138. Liszczak, T., Richardson, E. P., Phillips, J. P., Jacobson, S., and Kornblith, P. L.: Morphological, biochemical, ultrastructural, tissue culture and clinical observations of typical and aggressive craniopharyngiomas. Acta Neuropath. (Berlin, *43*:191–203, 1978.

139. Little, J. R., and MacCarty, C. S.: Colloid cysts of the third ventricle. J. Neurosurg., *39*:230–235, 1974.

140. Long, D. M., and Chou, S. N.: Transcallosal removal of craniopharyngiomas within the third ventricle. J. Neurosurg., *39*:563–567, 1973.

141. Long, J. M., Kier, E. L., and Schechter, M. M.: The radiology of epidermoid tumors of the cerebellopontine angle. Neuroradiology, *6*:188–192, 1973.

142. Love, J. G., and Kernohan J. W.: Dermoid and epidermoid tumors (cholesteatomas) of central nervous system. JAMA, *107*:1876–1883, 1936.

143. Love, J. G., and Marshall, T. M.: Craniopharyngiomas (pituitary adamantinomas). Surg. Gynec. Obstet., *90*:591–601, 1950.

144. Luse, S. A., and Kernohan, J. W.: Squamous-cell nests of the pituitary gland. Cancer, *8*:623–628, 1955.

145. Lushka, H.: Der Hirnanhang und Die Steissdrüse des Menschen. Berlin, Georg Reimer, 1860.

146. MacCarty, C. S., Levens, M. E., Love, J. G., and Kernohan, J. W.: Dermoid and epidermoid tumors in the central nervous system of adults. Surg. Gynec. Obstet., *108*:191–198, 1959.

147. Mahoney, W.: Die Epidermoide des Zentralnervensystems. Z. Ges. Neurol. Psychiat., *155*:416–471, 1936.

148. Matson, D. D.: Craniopharyngioma. *In* Matson, D. D., ed.: Neurosurgery in Infancy and Childhood. 2nd Ed. Springfield, Ill., Charles C Thomas, 1969, pp. 544–574.

149. Matson, D. D., and Crigler, J. F.: Radical treatment of craniopharyngioma. Ann. Surg., *152*:699–704, 1960.

150. Matson, D. D., and Crigler, J. F.: Management of craniopharyngioma in childhood. J. Neurosurg., *30*:377–390, 1969.

151. Matson, D. D., and Ingraham, F. D.: Intracranial complications of congenital dermal sinuses. Pediatrics, *8*:463–474, 1951.

152. McKenzie, K. G., and Sosman, M. C.: The roentgenological diagnosis of craniopharyngeal pouch tumors. Amer. J. Roentgen., *11*:171–176, 1924.

153. McKissock, W.: The surgical treatment of colloid cysts of the third ventricle: A report based upon twenty-one personal cases. Brain, *74*:1–9, 1951.

154. McKissock, W., and Ford, R. K.: Results of treatment of the craniopharyngiomas. J. Neurol. Neurosurg. Psychiat., *29*:475, 1966.

155. McLean, A. J.: Die Craniopharyngealtaschentumoren (Embryologie, Histologie, Diagnose und Therapie). Zbl. Ges. Neurol. Psychiat., *38*:468–471, 1930.

156. McLean, A. J.: Pineal teratomas: With report of a case of operative removal. Surg. Gynec. Obstet., *61*:523–533, 1935.

157. Michelsen, W. J., Mount, L. A., and Renaudin, J.: Craniopharyngioma: A thirty-nine year survey. Acta Neurol. Lat. Amer., *18*:100–106, 1972.

158. Montgomery, G. L., and Finlayson, D. I. C.: Cholesteatoma of the middle and posterior cranial fossae. Brain, *57*:177–183, 1934.

159. Mott, F. W., and Barratt, J. O. W.: Three cases of tumour of the third ventricle. Arch. Neurol. Psychiat., *1*:417–440, 1899.

160. Muller, P. J., Russell, N. A., and Morley, T. P.: Craniopharyngioma: Results of surgical treat-

ment without radiotherapy. *In* Morley, T. P., ed.: Current Controversies in Neurosurgery. Philadelphia, W. B. Saunders, Co., 1976, pp. 344–350.

161. Müller, R., and Wohlfart, G.: Intracranial teratomas and teratoid tumors. Acta Psychiat. Neurol. Scand., *22*:69–95, 1947.

162. Müller, R., and Wohlfart, G.: Craniopharyngiomas. Acta Med. Scand., *138*:121–138, 1950.

163. Munro, D., and Wegner, W.: Primary cranial and intracranial epidermoids and dermoids. New Eng. J. Med., *216*:273–279, 1937.

164. Naidich, T. P., Pinto, R. S., Kushner, M. J., Lin, J. P., Kricheff, I. I., Leeds, N. E., and Chase, N. E.: Evaluation of sellar and parasellar masses by computed tomography. Radiology, *120*:91–99, 1976.

165. Nakagawa, Y., and Tsuru, M.: Studies on postoperative course of craniopharyngioma. No To Shinkei, *23*:993–1002, 1971.

166. Nakayama, T., Kodama, T., and Matsukado, Y.: Treatment of inoperable craniopharyngioma with radioactive gold. No To Shinkei, *23*:509–513, 1971.

167. Northfield, D. W. C.: Rathke-pouch tumours. Brain, *80*:293–311, 1957.

168. Obenchain, T. G., and Becker, D. P.: Head bobbing associated with a cyst of the third ventricle: Case report. J. Neurosurg., *37*:457–459, 1972.

169. Obrador, S., and Blazquez, M. G.: Pituitary abscess in craniopharyngioma: Case report. J. Neurosurg., *36*:785–789, 1972.

170. Obrador, S., and Lopez-Zafra, J. J.: Clinical features of the epidermoids of the basal cisterns of the brain. J. Neurol. Neurosurg. Psychiat., *32*:450–454, 1969.

171. Olivecrona, H.: On suprasellar cholesteatomas. Brain, *55*:122–134, 1932.

172. Olivecrona, H.: Cholesteatomas of the cerebellopontine angle. Acta Psychiat. Neurol. Scand., *24*:639–643, 1949.

173. Olivecrona, H.: The surgical treatment of intracranial tumors. *In* Olivecrona, H., and Tönnis, W., eds.: Handbuch der Neurochirurgie. Volume IV. Heidelberg–New York, Springer-Verlag, 1967, pp. 1–301.

174. Onoyama, Y., Ono, K., Yabumoto, E., and Takeuchi, J.: Radiation therapy of craniopharyngioma. Radiology, *125*:799–803, 1977.

175. Palacios, E., Azar-Kia, B., Shannon, M., and Messina, A. V.: Neuroepithelial (colloid) cysts: Pathogenesis and unusual features. Amer. J. Roentgen., *126*:56–62, 1976.

176. Parkinson, D., and Childe, A. E.: Colloid cyst of the fourth ventricle: Report of a case of two colloid cysts of the fourth ventricle. J. Neurosurg., *9*:404–409, 1952.

177. Patrick, B. S., Smith, R. R., and Bailey, T. O.: Aseptic meningitis due to spontaneous rupture of craniopharyngioma cyst: Case report. J. Neurosurg., *41*:387–390, 1974.

178. Patten, B. M.: Patten's Human Embryology. New York, McGraw-Hill Book Co., 1976.

179. Pecker, J., Guy, G., and Scarabin, J.-M.: Third ventricle tumours: Including tumours of the septum pellucidum, colloid cysts and subependymal glomerate astrocytoma. *In* Vincken, P.

J., and Bruyn, G. W., eds.: Handbook of Clinical Neurology. Vol. 17. Amsterdam, North-Holland Publishing Co., 1974, pp. 440–489.

180. Pennybacker, J.: Cholesteatoma of the petrous bone. Brit. J. Surg., *32*:75–78, 1944.

181. Pennybacker, J., and Russell, D.: Necrosis of the brain due to radiation therapy: Clinical and pathological observations. J. Neurol. Neurosurg. psychiat., *11*:183–198, 1948.

182. Pertuiset, B.: Craniopharyngiomas. *In* Vinken, P. J., and Bruyn, G. W. eds.: Handbook of Clinical Neurology, Part III, Tumours of the Brain and Skull. Amsterdam, North-Holland Publishing Co., 1975.

183. Pertuiset, B., Metzger, J., Houtteville, J. P., Caruel, N., and Ernest, C.: Indications et résultats de la ventriculographie cérébrale au sel méthylglucamine du dimer iotalamique. Rev. Neurol. (Paris), *126*:299–304, 1972.

184. Peyton, W. T., and Baker, A. B.: Epidermoid, dermoid and teratomatous tumors of the central nervous system. Arch. Neurol. Psychiat., *47*:890–917, 1942.

185. Podoshin, L., Rolan, L., Altman, M. M., and Peyser, E.: "Pharyngeal" craniopharyngioma. J. Laryng., *84*:93–99, 1970.

186. Poppen, J. L., Reyes, V., and Horrax, G.: Colloid cysts of the third ventricle: Report of seven cases. J. Neurosurg., *10*:242–263, 1953.

187. Rand, C. W., and Reeves, D. L.: Dermoid and epidermoid tumors (cholesteatomas) of the central nervous system: Report of twenty-three cases. Arch. Surg. (Chicago), *46*:350–376, 1943.

188. Rathke, H.: Ueber die Entstehung der Glandula pituitaria. Arch. Anat. Physiol. Wissensch., M:482, 1838.

189. Ray, B. S.: Surgery of recurrent intracranial tumors. Clin. Neurosurg., *10*:1–30, 1964.

190. Riccio, A.: Su di un caso di craniofaringioma del clivus. Minerva Neurochir., *13*:13–15, 1969.

191. Riddoch, G.: Progressive dementia, without headache or changes in the optic discs, due to tumours of the third ventricle. Brain, *59*:225–233, 1936.

192. Ringel, S. P., and Bailey, O. T.: Rathke's cleft cyst. J. Neurol. Neurosurg. Psychiat., *35*:693–697, 1972.

193. Rosenberg, D., David, L., Bertrand, J., Ruitton-Ugliego, A., Lapras, C., Picot, C., and Monnet, P.: Craniopharyngiome. Reprise de croissance après l'intervention malgré déficit en hormone somatotrope. Arch. Franc. Pediat., *27*:355–369, 1970.

194. Ross-Russell, R. W., and Pennybacker, J. B.: Craniopharyngioma in the elderly. J. Neurol. Neurosurg. Psychiat., *24*:1–13, 1961.

195. Rougerie, J., and Fardeau, M.: Les Craniopharyngiomes. Paris, Masson & Cie, 1962.

196. Roussy, G., and Mosinger, M.: Les ilots paramalpighiens de l'hypophyse humaine. Leur histogénèse et leur intérêt. Rev. Neurol. (Paris), *63*:731–738, 1935.

197. Russell, D. S.: The pinealoma: Its relationship to teratoma. J. Path. Bac., *56*:145–150, 1944.

198. Russell, D. S., and Rubinstein, L. J.: Pathology of Tumours of the Nervous System. 4th Ed. Baltimore, Williams & Wilkins Co., 1977.

199. Sackett, J. F., Messina, A. V., and Petito, C. K.: Computed tomography and magnification vertebral angiotomography in the diagnosis of colloid cysts of the third ventricle. Radiology, *116*:95–100, 1975.

200. Sage, M. R., McAllister, V. L., Kendall, B. E., Bull, J. W. D., and Moseley, I. F.: Radiology in the diagnosis of colloid cysts of the third ventricle. Brit. J. Radiol., *48*:708–723, 1975.

201. Sambasivan, M., and Nayar, A.: Epidermoid cyst of pineal region. J. Neurol. Neurosurg. Psychiat., *37*:1333–1335, 1974.

202. Sano, S.: Intracranial Tumors. Tokyo, Igaku Shoin, 1972, pp. 101–103.

203. Scarff, J. E.: A new method for treatment of cystic craniopharyngioma by intraventricular drainage. Arch. Neurol. Psychiat., *46*:843–867, 1941.

204. Schmid, A. H.: A lipoma of the cerebellum. Acta Neuropath. (Berlin), *26*:75–80, 1973.

205. Schulhof, L. A., and Heimburger, R. F.: Frontal lobe epidermoid tumor with a positive brain scan. Surg. Neurol., *1*:265–266, 1973.

206. Schwartz, C. W.: Tumors of the hypophysis cerebri from a roentgenologic viewpoint. Amer. J. Roentgen., *40*:548–570, 1938.

207. Schwartz, J. F., and Balentine, J. D.: Recurrent meningitis due to an intracranial epidermoid. Neurology (Minneap.), *28*:124–129, 1978.

208. Seemayer, T. A., Blundell, J. S., and Wiglesworth, F. W.: Pituitary craniopharyngioma with tooth formation. Cancer, *29*:423–430, 1972.

209. Shanklin, W. H.: On the presence of cysts in the human pituitary. Anat. Rec., *104*:379–399, 1949.

210. Shapiro, K., Till, K., and Grant, D. N.: Craniopharyngiomas in childhood: A rational approach to treatment. J. Neurosurg., *50*:617–623, 1979.

211. Shuangshoti, S., Netsky, M. G., and Nashold, B. S.: Epithelial cysts related to sella turcica: Proposed origin from neuroepithelium. Arch. Path. (Chicago), *90*:444–450, 1970.

212. Shuangshoti, S., Roberts, M. P., and Netsky, M. G.: Neuroepithelial (colloid) cysts. Arch. Path. (Chicago), *80*:214–224, 1965.

213. Sivalingam, S., Dublin, A. B., and Youmans, J. R.: Computer assisted ventriculography. J. Comput. Assist. Tomogr., *2*:162–164, 1978.

214. Sjovall, E.: Über eine Ependymcyste embryonalen Charakters (Paraphyse?) im dritten Hirnventrikel mit tödlichem Ausgang. Beitr. Path. Anat., *47*:248–269, 1910.

215. Slooff, A. C. J., and Slooff, J. L.: Supratentorial tumours in children. *In* Vinken, P. J., and Bruyn, G. W. eds.: Handbook of Clinical Neurology. Vol. 18. Amsterdam, North-Holland Publishing Co., 1975, pp. 305–386.

216. Sobin, L. H.: Personal communication, 1977.

217. Spencer, A. T., and Smith, W. T.: Behaviour of intracerebral autografts of mouse tail skin pretreated with a single application of 20-methylcholanthrene. Nature, *207*:649–650, 1965.

218. Spencer, F. R.: Primary cholesteatoma of the sinuses and orbit: Report of a case of many years duration followed by carcinoma and death. Trans. Amer. Laryng. Rhin. Otol. Soc., *36*:543–549, 1930.

219. Spiegel, A. M., Di Chiro, G., Gorden, P., Ommaya, A. K., Kolins, J., and Pomeroy, T. C.: Diagnosis of radiosensitive hypothalamic tumors without craniotomy: Endocrine and neuroradiologic studies of intracranial atypical teratomas. Ann. Intern. Med., *85*:290–293, 1976.

220. Svien, H. J.: Surgical experiences with craniopharyngiomas. J. Neurosurg., *23*:148–155, 1965.

221. Svolos, D. G.: Craniopharyngiomas: A study based on 108 verified cases. Acta Chir. Scand., suppl. *403*:1–44, 1969.

222. Sweet, W. H.: A review of dermoid, teratoid and teratomatous intracranial tumors. Dis. Nerv. Syst., *1*:228–238, 1940.

223. Tabaddor, K., Shulman, K., and Dal Canto, M. C.: Neonatal craniopharyngioma. Amer. J. Dis. Child., *128*:381–383, 1974.

224. Tadmor, R., Davis, K. R., Roberson, G. H., New, P. F. J., and Taveras, J. M.: Computed tomography in extra-dural epidermoid and xanthoma. Surg. Neurol., *7*:371–375, 1977.

225. Tahmouresie, A., Kroll, G., and Shucart, W.: Lipoma of the corpus callosum. Surg. Neurol., *11*:31–34, 1979.

226. Tan, T. I.: Epidermoids and dermoids of the central nervous system. Acta Neurochir. (Wien), *26*:13–24, 1972.

227. Taniguchi, T., and Mufson, J. A.: Intradural lipoma of the spinal cord. J. Neurosurg., *7*:584–586, 1950.

228. Taveras, J. M., and Wood, E. H.: Diagnostic Neuroradiology. Baltimore, Williams & Wilkins Co., 1964.

229. Taylor, J. C.: Craniopharyngioma: A radiological technique for outlining the anatomy of large cysts. J. Neurol. Neurosurg. Psychiat., *34*:105, 1971.

230. Tekeuchi, J., Mori, K., Moritake, K., Tani, F., Waga, S., and Handa, H.: Teratomas in the suprasellar region: Report of five cases. Surg. Neurol., *3*:247–255, 1975.

231. Toglia, J. U., Netsky, M. G., and Alexander, E.: Epithelial (epidermoid) tumors of the cranium: Their common nature and pathogenesis. J. Neurosurg., *23*:384–393, 1965.

232. Torkildsen, A.: Should extirpation be attempted in cases of neoplasm in or near the third ventricle of the brain? Experiences with a palliative method. J. Neurosurg., *5*:249–275, 1948.

233. Treip, C. S.: A congenital medulloepithelioma of the midbrain. J. Path. Bact., *74*:357–363, 1957.

234. Trippi, A. C., Garner, J. T., Kassabian, J. T., and Shelden, C. H.: A new approach to inoperable craniopharyngiomas. Amer. J. Surg., *118*:307–310, 1969.

235. Tytus, J. S., and Pennybacker, J.: Pearly tumours in relation to the central nervous system. J. Neurol. Neurosurg. Psychiat., *9*:241–259, 1956.

236. Ulrich, J.: Intracranial epidermoids: A study on their distribution and spread. J. Neurosurg., *21*:1051–1058, 1964.

237. Van Den Bergh, R., and Brucher, J. M.: L'abord transventriculaire dans les crâniopharyngiomes du troisième ventricule: Aspects neurochirurgicaux et neuro-pathologiques. Neurochirurgie, *16*:51–65, 1970.

238. Van Gilder, J. C., and Schwartz, H. G.: Growth of dermoids from skin implants to the nervous system and surrounding spaces of the newborn rat. J. Neurosurg., 26:14–20, 1967.

239. Verbiest, H.: Die Epidermoide des Rückenmarkes, Analyse eines Falles, Zugleich Beitrag zur Frage der Entstehung der aseptischen Meningitis nach Epidermoidoperationen. Zbl. Neurochir., 4:129–141, 1939.

240. Vladykova, J.: Kraniofaryngeom z hlediska oftalmologa. Cesk. Oftal., 29:109–116, 1973.

241. Vonderahe, A. R., and Niemer, W. T.: Intracranial lipoma: A report of four cases. J. Neuropath. Exp. Neurol., 3:344–354, 1944.

242. Vraa-Jensen, J.: Massive congenital intracranial teratoma. Acta Neuropath. (Berlin), 30:271–276, 1974.

243. Waga, S., and Handa, H.: Radiation-induced meningioma: With review of literature. Surg. Neurol., 5:215–219, 1976.

244. Wallman, H.: Eine Colloidcyste im dritten Hirnventrikel und ein Lipom im Plexus choroides. Virchow. Arch. [Path. Anat.], 11:385–388, 1858.

245. Weber, F. P., Worster-Drought, C., Dickson, W. E. C.: Cholesterol tumour (craniopharyngioma) of the pituitary body. J. Neurol. Psychopath., 15:39–45, 1934.

246. Weil, A., and Blumklotz, B.: Experimental intracranial epithelial cysts. J. Neuropath. Exp. Neurol., 2:34–44, 1943.

247. Weisberg, L., and Nice, C. N.: Computed tomographic evaluation of increased intracranial pressure without localizing signs. Radiology, 122:133–136, 1977.

248. Willis, R. A.: Pathology of Tumours. 4th Ed. London, Butterworths Inc., 1967.

249. Willis, R. A.: Nervous tissue in teratomas. In Minckler, J., ed.: Pathology of the Nervous System. New York, McGraw-Hill Book Co., 1971, pp. 1937–1943.

250. Wong, S. W., Ducker, T. B., and Powers, J. M.: Fulminating parapontine epidermoid carcinoma in a four-year-old-boy. Cancer, 37:1525–1531, 1976.

251. Wycis, H. T., Robbins, R., Spiegel-Adolf, M., Meszaros, J., and Spiegel, E. A.: Studies in stereoencephalotomy. III. Treatment of a cystic craniopharyngioma by injection of radioactive P³². Confin. Neurol., 14:193–202, 1954.

252. Yenermen, M. H., Bowerman, C. I., and Haymaker, W.: Colloid cyst of the third ventricle: A clinical study of 54 cases in the light of previous publications. Acta Neuroveg., 17:211–277, 1958.

253. Zeitlin, H., and Lichtenstein, B. W.: Cystic tumor of the third ventricle containing colloid material. Arch. Neurol. Psychiat., 38:268–287, 1937.

254. Zervas, N. T.: Stereotaxic radiofrequency surgery of the normal and the abnormal pituitary gland. New Eng. J. Med., 280:429–437, 1969.

255. Zettner, A., and Netsky, M. G.: Lipoma of the corpus callosum. J. Neuropath. Exp. Neurol., 19:305–319, 1960.

256. Zimmerman, H. M.: Brain tumors: Their incidence and classification in man and their experimental production. Ann. N.Y. Acad. Sci., 159:337–359, 1969.

257. Zimmerman, H. M.: Introduction to tumors of the central nervous system. In Minckler, J., ed.: Pathology of the Nervous System. Vol. 2. New York, McGraw-Hill Book Co., 1971, pp. 1947–1951.

258. Zülch, K. J.: Brain Tumors: Their Biology and Pathology. 2nd Amer. Ed. New York, Springer-Verlag, 1965.

92

MENINGEAL TUMORS OF THE BRAIN

The meningioma, more than any other intracranial tumor, has been involved in the development of neurological surgery. Approximately 100 years after Louis first described this tumor, Francesco Durante, Professor of Clinical Surgery at the University of Rome, performed the first successful operation for intracranial tumor when he removed a meningioma of the olfactory groove in June 1885. This operation was done only six months after Bennett and Godlee's removal of an intracranial glioma had resulted in a fatality, probably secondary to a wound infection.[15]

The introduction of ''electrosurgery'' by Cushing and Bovie was a major advance in modern surgery as well as in neurosurgery. Its application to removal of meningiomas of the olfactory groove was described by Cushing in his 1927 Macewen Memorial Lecture.[16] Since then, the development of modern neuroanesthesia, steroids, the operating microscope, selective cerebral angiography, and computed tomography have further enhanced the treatment of meningiomas. Their successful operative management, however, continues to challenge even the most skilled and experienced surgeon.

INCIDENCE

Cushing and Eisenhardt found that meningiomas constituted 13.4 per cent of all intracranial tumors in their series.[15] Castellano and Ruggiero reported an incidence rate of 19.2 per cent.[10] In an effort to evaluate the true incidence of neoplasms of the central nervous system, Percy and co-workers studied their occurrence in a community population during the years of 1935 through 1968. A total of 297 cases of intracranial and intraspinal neoplasms were identified; approximately 59 per cent of the intracranial neoplasms were primary and 41 per cent were metastatic. Thirty-eight per cent of the primary intracranial neoplasms were meningiomas. The ratio of all meningiomas to all gliomas was 1.2 to 1, which is significantly different from the ratio in most neurosurgical and hospital series, in which gliomas usually outnumber meningiomas 2 to 1 or 3 to 1.[33] The age-specific rates demonstrated that the incidence of meningiomas increases with increasing age (Table 92–1). The ratio of females to males is 2 to 1.

The possibility that head trauma predisposes to meningioma formation has been a subject of controversy for many years. Cushing, probably in part as a result of his struggle with the meningioma of General Leonard Wood, was convinced that the coincidence of head trauma and subsequent brain tumor occurs too often to be ignored. Both Bailey and Wilson, on the contrary, denied any significant association between head injury and brain tumor.[3,42] This question was recently studied in a prospective analysis of a community population by Annegers and associates. They found no difference between the observed and the expected numbers of all brain tumors, and the

C. S. MacCARTY, D. G. PIEPGRAS,

AND M. J. EBERSOLD

TABLE 92–1 AGE-SPECIFIC INCIDENCE RATES FOR MENINGIOMAS*

AGE (YEARS)	NO. OF TUMORS	RATE
0–24	1	0.2
25–44	5	1.6
45–64	19	9.2
≥65	36	39.4

* Rate is per 100,000 population, Rochester, Minnesota, 1935–1968. (Modified from Percy, A. K., Elveback, L. R., Okazaki, H., et al: Neoplasms of the central nervous system: Epidemiologic considerations. Neurology (Minneap.), 22: 40–48, 1972.)

occurrence of subsequent brain tumors was not associated with the severity or location of head injury. No etiological relationship between head trauma and meningioma was found.[1]

LOCATION

Intracranial meningiomas are most frequently located in the parasagittal region; however, the regions of the sphenoidal ridge, the convexity, and the posterior fossa are also common sites of origin (Table 92–2). Middle fossa, gasserian ganglion, foramen magnum, intraorbital, optic sheath, ventricular, tentorial, and multiple tumors occur more rarely. Of 214 parasagittal meningiomas seen at the Mayo Clinic from 1960 through 1975, 99 arose anteriorly, 26 arose in the posterior portion of

the falx or sinus, and 84 arose from the midportion. For five patients, the location was not recorded. During this same period, 143 sphenoidal ridge meningiomas were seen, of which 50 were medial, 23 middle, 53 lateral, 1 bilateral, 3 middle and medial, and 13 unclassified.[29]

PATHOLOGICAL FEATURES

Meningiomas have been recognized as dural tumors for more than 200 years, but their cell of origin and therefore their classification and the terminology applicable to them have been subjects of controversy. Several pathologists, the first being Bright in 1831, recognized the similarity between the histological appearance of cells of the arachnoid villus and those of these tumors, and proposed that the cell of origin derived from the arachnoid layer. These opinions did not gain general acceptance until Harvey Cushing again advanced the concept in his 1922 Cavendish Lecture and introduced the name "meningioma" to encompass several tumor types that had previously been separated on a histological basis.[14]

Bailey and Bucy's subsequent classification of meningiomas described nine types: mesenchymal, angioblastic, meningotheliomatous, psammomatous, osteoblastic, fibroblastic, melanoblastic, sarcomatous, and lipomatous.[4] Cushing and Eisenhardt's

TABLE 92–2 INTRACRANIAL MENINGIOMAS, MAYO CLINIC, 1914 THROUGH 1975*

LOCATION	OPERATION		AUTOPSY		TOTAL	
	Number	Per Cent	Number	Per Cent	Number	Per Cent
Parasagittal	582	30.3	42	18.8	624	29.1
Sphenoidal ridge	357	18.6	20	8.9	377	17.6
Convexity	247	12.8	41	18.3	288	13.4
Posterior fossa	190	9.9	21	9.4	211	9.8
Tuberculum sellae	180	9.4	17	7.6	197	9.2
Olfactory groove	105	5.5	9	4.0	114	5.3
Middle or temporal fossa	69	3.6	12	5.4	81	3.8
Foramen magnum	48	2.5	1	0.4	49	2.3
Multiple tumors	28	1.4	16	7.1	44	2.0
Intraorbital	39	2.0	4	1.8	43	2.0
Gasserian ganglion	24	1.2	2	0.9	26	1.2
Tentorial	20	1.0	0	. . .	20	0.9
Ventricle	16	0.8	0	. . .	16	0.7
Mixed tumors	6	0.3	7	3.1	13	0.6
Optic sheath	7	0.4	0	. . .	7	0.3
Unspecified	5	0.3	32	14.3	37	1.7
Total	1923	100	224	100	2147	100

* Identified at operation and postmortem examination. (From MacCarty, C. S., and Taylor, W. F.: Intracranial meningiomas: Experiences at the Mayo Clinic. Neurol. Med. Chir. (Tokyo), 19:569–574, 1979. Reprinted by permission.)

classification was considerably more elaborate, whereas Courville and subsequently
Russell and Rubinstein simplified the classification to five main categories: syncytial,
transitional, fibrous, angioblastic, and sarcomatous.[13,15,34]

The authors have followed an even more
simplified classification based on that of
neuropathologists Kernohan and Sayre.[24]
Basically, meningiomas have been divided into meningotheliomatous, fibroma-
tous, and malignant types. Psammomatous
tumors are considered a subtype of the
meningotheliomatous group, and most "angioblastic" tumors have been considered to
be hemangiopericytomas because, histologically, they appear identical to similar
tumors in the soft tissues and they are aggressive.[19]

The meningotheliomatous meningiomas
have a microscopic appearance characterized by sheets or islands of cells with varying amounts of stroma (Fig. 92–1A). Cell
nuclei are large and usually oval, and cytoplasmic boundaries are indistinct. There
may be frequent small, dark pyknotic nuclei, but mitotic figures are usually absent.
The stroma is typically very vascular. In
the psammomatous subtype, the cells tend

to assume a whorl arrangement, the center
of the whorl becoming hyalinized. Mineral
salts frequently are deposited in these areas
in a concentric fashion, forming the psammoma, or "sandlike," bodies (Fig. 92–1B).

Fibroblastic meningiomas are characterized by streams and less definite whorls of
long narrow cells and a heavy stroma containing reticulin and collagen fibers (Fig.
92–2). The latter give the tumor a "toughness" that is noticeable when it is palpated
or cut at operation. Intraventricular tumors
are commonly of this type.

As stated earlier, the authors and their
neuropathologist colleagues have held the
opinion first advanced by Begg and Garrett
in 1954 that the entity of angioblastic meningioma described by Bailey and by Cushing and Eisenhardt was in fact the now-rec-
ognized tumor hemangiopericytoma.[3,6,15,19]
The controversies over this categorization
have been well summarized by Russell and
Rubinstein in their text and need not be
elaborated.[34] These tumors, arising from a
cell of origin normally present in the external mural layer of capillaries (the so-called
pericyte), are typically very vascular radiographically, grossly at operation, and microscopically. Like meningiomas, heman-

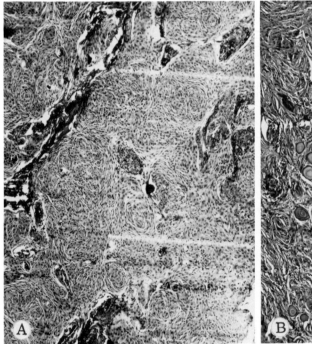
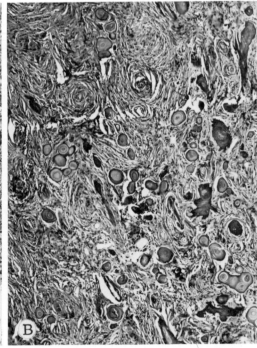

Figure 92–1 *A.* Meningotheliomatous meningioma. (Hematoxylin and eosin, 64 ×.) *B.* Psammomatous meningioma. Hematoxylin and eosin, 64 ×.

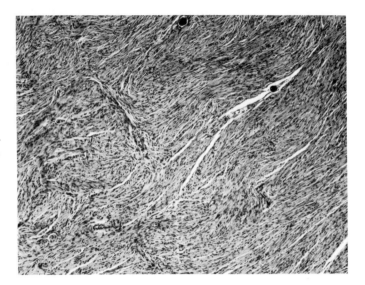

Figure 92–2 Fibroblastic meningioma. Hematoxylin and eosin, 64 ×.

giopericytomas when they occur in the central nervous system are solid tumors and are generally attached to the meninges, more commonly in the parasagittal region but also along the tentorium or petrous and sphenoidal ridges. They tend to compress rather than invade the brain. The symptoms likewise are similar to those of meningiomas, but most of these lesions occur in men rather than in women and at a somewhat younger age, most frequently in the fourth decade.[19]

The diagnosis is made on the basis of histological features, characterized microscopically by masses of closely packed cells with round, ovoid, or elongated nuclei that form swirls and frondlike projections in the intervascular spaces (Fig. 92–3). There are multitudinous thin-walled, irregular vascular channels forming a spongy network within the tumor. Reticulin stain shows a typical pattern of fine reticulin fibers around either a single cell or small groups of tumor cells, and mitotic figures are frequent. "Total" operative removal is the treatment of choice for these tumors, yet the recurrence rate is high and distant metastasis is not uncommon. In a series of patients treated at the Mayo Clinic, Goellner and associates found the rate of recurrence to be 80 per cent and the rate of metastasis to be 23 per cent, the mean length of survival being 84 months.[19] Although postoperative radiation therapy has been commonly used, its value is questionable.

The hemangiopericytoma aside, malignant meningioma, although rare, is a well-documented entity that should be recognized by the pathologist and neurosurgeon for its prognostic importance. Jellinger's review of more than 1200 meningiomas showed that 1.2 per cent were malignant, a rate similar to Cushing and Eisenhardt's 1.9 per cent, but Zülch and Mennel found that 9 per cent of 1400 meningiomas were "histologically not benign."[15,20,44] Indications of malignancy include cellular pleomorphism and increased numbers of mitotic figures as well as local invasion of the adjacent brain tissue. Much rarer is the occurrence of distant metastasis of meningioma in the cerebrospinal fluid pathways and extracranially. The lungs and abdominal viscera tend to be the sites most frequently affected by the latter.[21] Most lesions have occurred in patients who have previously undergone operation for the tumor, although metastasis has been found in patients who have not had operations as well as in patients who have died on the day of operation.

CLINICAL PRESENTATION

Like other extra-axial intracranial tumors, meningiomas cause symptoms and signs primarily due to compression of adjacent brain tissue and cranial nerves, and in this sense there is no specificity to the presenting clinical pattern that indicates the tumor type with certainty. Because the le-

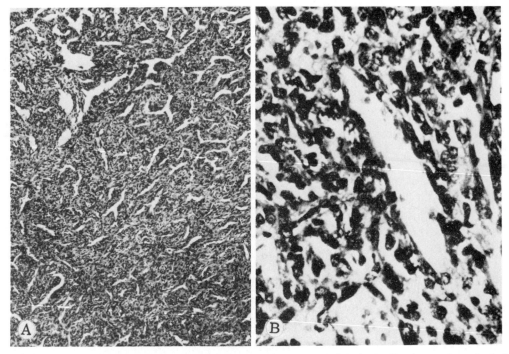

Figure 92–3   *A.* Typical histological features of hemangiopericytoma of the brain. There are a sheet of spindle cells and numerous irregular vascular spaces. (Hematoxylin and eosin, 100 ×.) *B.* Higher magnification of hemangiopericytoma of brain shows endothelial lining of vessels and proliferation of surrounding pericytes. Hematoxylin and eosin, 640 ×.

sions tend to arise in certain locations, however, and grow slowly, sometimes inciting hyperostosis in adjacent bone, several syndromes have been identified that are characteristic for meningiomas at those sites.

Sphenoidal Ridge

Especially when located along the sphenoid wing, meningiomas may produce a clinical pattern that, when full-blown, is pathognomonic. In this instance, however, it is related as much to the tumor's tendency to cause hyperostosis of the adjacent bone as to the neoplasm itself. More common in middle-aged women, the thickening of the sphenoid wing, reduction of the orbital volume, and vascular compression at the orbital fissure produce a nonpulsating, painless unilateral exophthalmos. Particularly along the lateral sphenoid wing, the meningioma tends to grow as a flat, spreading tumor that induces considerable hyperostosis, the so-called en plaque meningi-

oma. Externally, fullness in the temporal fossa as well as proptosis is associated with such tumors.

Effects of the tumor on the nervous system relate to its location along the sphenoid wing, which Cushing divided into three segments: inner or clinoidal, middle or alar, and outer or pterional (Fig. 92–4). Tumors that arise at the clinoid process typically cause unilateral loss of vision and primary optic atrophy owing to optic nerve compression. If the optic tract or chiasm is also involved, there may be an incongruous homonymous-type field defect typically, but loss of vision is more pronounced in the ipsilateral eye.[22] Cranial nerve involvement in the superior orbital fissure may produce ophthalmoplegia, with the abducens nerve being affected most frequently. Hypesthesia in the distribution of the first division of the trigeminal nerve also may occur.[2]

Meningiomas of the middle and lateral thirds of the sphenoid wing generally reach a larger size before making their presence known, either with the secondary external changes already mentioned or with brain ef-

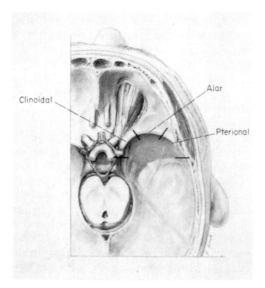

Figure 92–4 Topography of the sphenoidal ridge showing the three portions (clinoidal, alar, and pterional) described by Cushing. (From MacCarty, C. S.: Meningiomas of the sphenoidal ridge. J. Neurosurg., *36*:114–120, 1972. Reprinted by permission.)

fects such as seizures or symptoms of increased intracranial pressure.

Parasagittal and Falcial Meningiomas

Parasagittal and falcial meningiomas present most classically when they arise in the central area near the sensorimotor cortex. In this location, the tumors commonly make themselves known by causing epilepsy, which is frequently of focal onset, typically initiated in the lower extremity, before spreading to the upper extremity or becoming generalized. Likewise, hemiparesis may develop in a progressive fashion, frequently affecting the lower extremity to a greater degree than the upper. Large bilateral parasagittal tumors in the central region may cause severe spastic paraplegia, which may be incorrectly diagnosed as a possible spinal cord lesion if other symptoms and signs pointing to a cerebral cause are absent or not recognized. Anteriorly- and posteriorly-arising tumors are associated with a higher incidence of headache and mental symptoms because of the size they may reach before becoming manifest. Hemianopia, caused by

compression of the occipital lobe by posterior tumors, is commonly not recognized by the patient.[18]

Cerebral Convexity

These slowly growing tumors may present with nonlocalizing symptoms and signs of altered mentation, increased intracranial pressure, or epilepsy, depending on their location, which Cushing and Eisenhardt subclassified as precoronal, coronal, postcoronal, paracentral, parietal, occipital, and temporal.[15]

The diagnosis may not be apparent from the clinical findings alone but often is clarified by radiographic changes on plain roentgenograms of the head. In Cushing and Eisenhardt's series, 70 per cent of the tumors of the convexity lay anterior to the rolandic fissure.[15]

Intraventricular Meningioma

Intraventricular meningiomas most commonly lie in the trigone of the lateral ventricle and, unlike those previously mentioned, do not produce a clearly diagnostic complex of symptoms and signs. The patient's symptoms are often vague, reflecting the mass of the tumor or obstruction of cerebrospinal fluid flow. In a series of patients reviewed at the authors' institution, headaches, mental change, and visual symptoms were frequent, and the most specific finding on examination was homonymous hemianopia, which was noted in most of the patients.[26] Spontaneous hemorrhage of an intraventricular meningioma has been reported by several authors.[36]

Olfactory Groove

The syndrome related to meningioma of the olfactory groove is best known under the eponym of Foster Kennedy, who in 1911 described its occurrence with various frontal lesions, including endothelioma (meningioma), abscess, and glioma.[23] As widely recognized today, Kennedy's symptom complex includes central scotoma and primary optic atrophy on the side of the lesion and papilledema in the opposite eye. Ipsilateral loss of smell and mental and motor system changes ascribable to involvement of the frontal lobe also were described. Cushing emphasized the syndrome's occurrence with meningiomas of the olfactory groove and the importance of its recognition for operative treatment.[16]

Tuberculum Sellae

Like that of the olfactory groove meningioma, the syndrome related to the meningioma arising from the tuberculum sellae was recognized early by Cushing:

> . . . a lesion, scarcely known even to pathologists except as an accidental postmortem finding, which elicits a clean-cut and hardly mistakable syndrome, whose ophthalmological features usually lead to the mistaken diagnosis of "retrobulbar neuritis."[16]

The features of this syndrome as exemplified in Cushing's discussion can be summarized: a middle-aged patient with progressive loss of vision and findings on examination of either papilledema or optic atrophy, bitemporal hemianopia, and normal sella turcica on roentgenogram.

The necessity for recognition of the syndrome and its operative treatment to preserve vision cannot be stressed enough because there continue to be too many patients whose condition is diagnosed only after advanced, irreversible loss of vision has occurred. It should be remembered that meningiomas may swell in pregnancy and produce a visual loss that may improve after termination of the pregnancy.[40]

Other Basilar Sites

Infratemporal meningiomas may arise anywhere along the floor of the middle fossa, though much less commonly than from the sphenoidal ridge. Because of the relatively silent area of their growth, these tumors may attain considerable size before making their presence known with symptoms of increased intracranial pressure. In contrast to this, very small or en plaque tumors impinging on the gasserian ganglion or trigeminal root in Meckel's cave may present with typical trigeminal neuralgia or atypical face pain.[30]

Meningiomas arising from the tentorium may grow primarily supratentorially, into the posterior fossa, or at the falcial-tentorial junction. Those with primarily supratentorial extension tend to present as lateralized cerebral lesions. Infratentorial tumors may produce obstructive hydrocephalus when growing in the midline, lateralized cranial nerve deficits typically with trigeminal nerve involvement when the impingement is into the cerebellopontine angle, or less specific findings of gait difficulty and cerebellar signs with more posterior or posterolateral growth.[5]

Clivus meningiomas may present clinically like other posterior fossa tumors and may mimic intrinsic brain stem neoplasms. Symptoms and signs of cranial nerve involvement, cerebellar and cortical spinal tract compression, and increased intracranial pressure are typical.[11]

Cerebellar Convexity and Cerebellopontine Angle

Meningiomas arising from the tentorium, the lateral sinus, or simply the posterior fossa dura may compress the cerebellar hemisphere and typically, after attaining a large size, present with symptoms of increased intracranial pressure or progressive cerebellar deficit.

Arising from the dura of the petrous bone near the porus acusticus, meningiomas may grow into the cerebellopontine angle to mimic an acoustic neuroma. Hearing loss is a less constant feature with meningioma, however, and the petrous bone rarely shows radiographic evidence of erosion.

Foramen Magnum

The most common benign extramedullary tumor of the foramen magnum region is the meningioma, and its recognition is paramount to proper treatment—which is its removal. Unfortunately, the clinical presentation of foramen magnum tumors is protean, and misdiagnosis is commonplace, the progressive condition not infrequently being erroneously diagnosed as carpal tunnel syndrome, syringomyelia, cervical spondylosis, myelopathy, or multiple sclerosis. Among a series of patients treated for foramen magnum tumors, the most frequent initial symptoms were pain in the suboccipital region or neck and dysesthesias of the upper extremities, the next most frequent being clumsiness, stereoanesthesia of the hands, and gait disturbance.[43] Neurological findings may be absent early in the course, but severe deficits occur later. Spastic paresis of one or both upper extremities or hemiparesis progressing to tetraparesis is typical. Atrophy of the hand muscles is common, but its mechanism is poorly understood. Sensory loss also tends to involve the upper more than the lower extremities, and of particular importance is the finding of involvement of the upper cervical dermatomes. Findings more commonly seen with intramedullary lesions, "cape distribution" sensory loss and Horner's syndrome, also may be seen with foramen magnum tumors.

A high index of suspicion for this lesion must be followed by adequate radiographic study, the most important method being complete myelography with the patient in the prone and supine positions, with the contrast agent (preferably Pantopaque) being carried through the foramen magnum. Meningiomas of this region typically are attached ventrolaterally at the rim of the foramen magnum with an intimate relationship to the vertebral artery.[37]

Hyperostosis is the most frequent direct radiographic sign of meningioma, the inner table being most often involved; the diploë and outer table may, however, be affected as well. The hyperostosis may be a focal enostotic process at the site of the tumor's attachment or, as is seen most frequently with en plaque meningioma, a more diffuse homogeneous sclerosis. The latter may be difficult to distinguish from fibrous dysplasia (Fig. 92–5).

Increased vascular markings associated with meningioma may be localized to the area of tumor origin or involve the meningeal vascular channels in their course through the foramen spinosum and across the cranial vault. To be considered significant, vascular prominence should be unilateral, although certain parasagittal and falcial meningiomas may produce the changes bilaterally. Diploic veins also may be enlarged owing to meningioma, but normal variations in their radiographic appearance make this a less reliable sign.

Calcification of meningiomas that is apparent radiographically appears in less than 10 per cent of cases but, when present, may dramatically demonstrate the whole tumor. Other less specific calcific deposits may be seen, however, but may represent only a small area within the tumor and in them-

DIAGNOSTIC TESTS

Plain Films of Skull

In approximately 75 per cent of the patients with intracranial meningiomas, plain films of the skull are suggestive of the presence of an intracranial tumor, and the specific diagnosis of meningioma can reportedly be made in 30 to 60 per cent of cases.[38] Indirect radiographic signs of the tumor (not specifically of meningioma) include those associated with increased intracranial pressure, such as sellar pressure changes, displacement of the calcified pineal gland or choroid plexus, and less frequently, widening of the sutures or atrophy of the cranial vault.

Direct evidence for intracranial meningioma on the skull films includes hyperostosis, increased vascularity, tumor calcification, and rarely bone destruction.

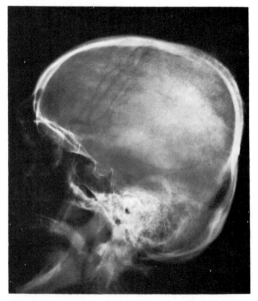

Figure 92–5 Characteristic roentgenographic skull changes due to meningioma, including hyperostosis, exostosis, and large vascular channels.

selves may not be diagnostic of meningioma.[32]

Computed Tomography

In the few years since the first edition of
this text was published, computed tomography (CT) has essentially replaced radioisotope scanning, echoencephalography,
pneumoencephalography, and ventriculography in the diagnosis of intracranial
tumors of all types. It has proved to be particularly sensitive in the demonstration of
meningiomas. Not only does the CT scan
allow detection of tumors approaching 1 cm
in size but it often permits a specific diagnosis of meningioma to be made.[12] Tumors
smaller than 1 cm in size may escape detection, the orbits and parasellar and parasagittal areas being particularly difficult in
this regard.

The characteristic features of meningioma on computed tomography include the
tumor's enhancement with contrast medium and an appearance of a homogeneous
high-density mass with distinct, round borders. Computed tomography will also identify associated cranial hyperostosis, bone
destruction, and tumor calcification and
clearly demonstrates areas of surrounding
brain edema, which is common with meningiomas. Also, and of particular importance
to the neurosurgeon, computed tomography identifies ventricular dilatation that
may be secondary to the tumor's obstruction of cerebrospinal fluid pathways (Fig.
92–6).

Angiography

Although the CT scan has assumed a
major role in the diagnosis and demonstration of intracranial meningiomas, cerebral
angiography remains the definitive test for
complete evaluation of the tumor and planning of the operation. Because meningiomas tend to be vascular and derive this
vascular supply at least in part from meningeal vessels, angiography characteristically
can indicate the specific diagnosis of meningioma, the tumor's site of origin, and its
vascular supply and relationship to the normal intracranial arteries, which may be
markedly displaced by the tumor. All of
this information, supplied only by the an-

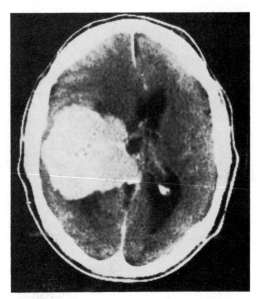

Figure 92–6   CT scan of giant intraventricular meningioma.

giogram, is essential to the planning of
tumor removal.

In addition to the meningioma's tendency
to derive its blood supply from meningeal
vessels, other typical angiographic signs include the "sunburst appearance," or radial
spread of tumor vessels from a central
hilus, and a homogeneous tumor blush or
stain, which may appear in the arterial
phase but is usually more prominent in the
venous phase.[41] The uniform opacification
of a well-defined, rounded mass is indicative of a benign neoplasm and typical of meningioma.

Selective angiography of the external and
internal carotid and vertebral arteries by
the Seldinger method and magnification and
subtraction techniques has not only enabled radiologists to obtain more specific
information regarding the vascular supply
of meningiomas but has also improved
demonstration of small tumors that may not
be visualized on the CT scan.

OPERATIVE TECHNIQUES

Preparation of Patient

Prior to proceeding with craniotomy for
removal of the intracranial meningioma,
certain preoperative measures for preparation of the patient may be indicated. If com-

puted tomography has demonstrated profound edema around a large tumor with much mass effect, or if a tumor is arising in the parasellar region, corticosteroid administration preoperatively may be of benefit. If the patient has had epileptic seizures related to the tumor, the anticonvulsants should be maintained at therapeutic levels during the perioperative period. Even though clinical seizures have never occurred, in such patients as those with cerebral convexity and parasagittal tumors near the sensorimotor cortex, it is reasonable to administer prophylactic anticonvulsant medication, usually diphenylhydantoin, to minimize the likelihood of seizure activity during the postoperative period.

If excessive brain retraction is expected for exposure of the tumor (e.g., tumor in the region of the tuberculum sellae or tentorial notch), cerebrospinal fluid drainage or the use of an osmotic diuretic such as mannitol or urea may be indicated, necessitating prior placement of a lumbar needle or bladder catheter. Placement of the lumbar needle for drainage of cerebrospinal fluid is contraindicated in any patient with a very large tumor and increased intracranial pressure. The routine use of an antistaphylococcal antibiotic during the immediate perioperative period is recommended, the first dose preferably being given intravenously before the skin incision is made. Because of the often extreme vascularity of meningiomas and their frequent attachment to major dural sinuses, hemorrhage during tumor removal can constitute a major risk, and provisions must be made to have adequate whole blood available for transfusion. If the operation is going to be done with the patient in the sitting position or if the tumor approaches a venous sinus, the possibility of air embolism from an opening in that sinus should be considered and appropriate precautions taken, including intraoperative Doppler monitoring and placement of a right atrial catheter for detection and removal of intracardiac air.

Skin Incisions and Bone Flaps

Because of the meningioma's vascularity and its common relationship to the major dural sinus, the planning of the skin incision and the location of the bone flap is of utmost importance. Whenever possible, the tumor should be approached so as to allow early control of the vascular channels—to quote Cushing and Eisenhardt, to "get windward of the lesion."[15] Skin flaps must be designed to give adequate circulation for healing, generous exposure of the skull at the desired location, and when at all possible, an acceptable cosmetic result. There are many different scalp incisions available for unilateral and bilateral craniotomies and suboccipital craniectomy (Figs. 92–7 through 92–10). Free bone flaps rather than osteoplastic flaps are advocated in order to minimize intraoperative bleeding and reduce the risk of postoperative hemorrhage.[27]

Parasagittal and Falcial Meningiomas

In the exposure of parasagittal meningiomas, the scalp flap that crosses the midline should be elevated so that bone can be removed from both sides of the sagittal sinus if necessary. In most patients, only a unilateral bone flap will be necessary, but in patients with sagittal sinus or bilateral falcial involvement, the need for bilateral exposure and control of the sagittal sinus is to be expected. In addition to a standard horseshoe incision, an S-shaped incision can be used to expose a parasagittal meningioma (Fig. 92–11). Frequently, it is helpful to make multiple burr holes that can be joined by using a rongeur or Gigli saw, this technique being especially useful when there is a large associated osteoma. Bleeding from the bone edges is controlled with the generous use of bone wax, and the dura is opened unilaterally or bilaterally, reflected toward the midline and ultimately excised completely in order to expose the tumor. The tumor is then removed either piecemeal or in toto. If the sagittal sinus is thrombosed by the tumor, it can be ligated on either side and excised with the neoplasm (Figs. 92–12 and 92–13). If the sinus is patent, however, it can be safely sacrificed only as far posteriorly as the rolandic veins. Sacrifice of the patent sinus posterior to this point carries a very high risk of cerebral damage owing to venous infarction and cerebral edema. If the tumor invades the sinus in its posterior two thirds, it is safer to leave the sinus intact by amputating the tumor just lateral to the sinus and coagulat-

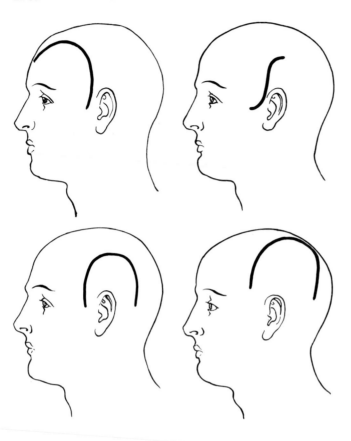

Figure 92–7   Scalp incisions used for the frontal, temporal, and parieto-occipital craniotomies. (From Mac-Carty, C. S.: The Surgical Treatment of Intracranial Meningiomas. Springfield, Ill., Charles C Thomas, 1961. Reprinted by permission.)

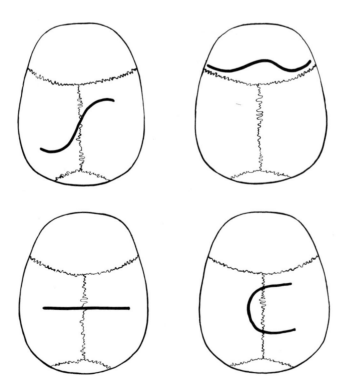

Figure 92–8   Scalp incisions for bilateral exposure. (From MacCarty, C. S.: The Surgical Treatment of Intracranial Meningiomas. Springfield, Ill., Charles C Thomas, 1961. Reprinted by permission.)

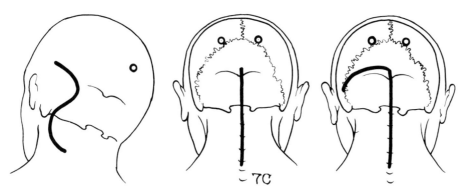

Figure 92–9   Scalp incisions for approaching the posterior fossa tumor. (From MacCarty, C. S.: The Surgical Treatment of Intracranial Meningiomas. Springfield, Ill., Charles C Thomas, 1961. Reprinted by permission.)

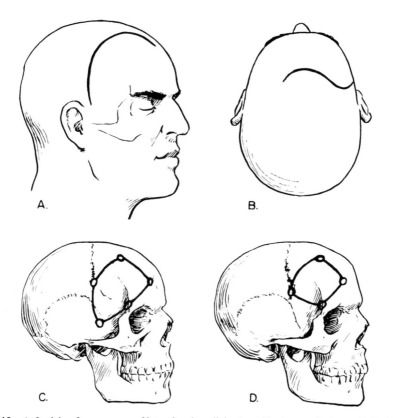

Figure 92–10   *A*. Incision for exposure of lateral and medial sphenoid wing meningioma. *B*. Incision for clinoidal meningioma. *C*. Craniotomy for exposure of lateral and medial sphenoid wing meningioma. *D*. Craniotomy for exposure of clinoidal meningioma by subfrontal approach. (From MacCarty, C. S.: Meningiomas of the sphenoidal ridge. J. Neurosurg., *36*:114–120, 1972. Reprinted by permission.)

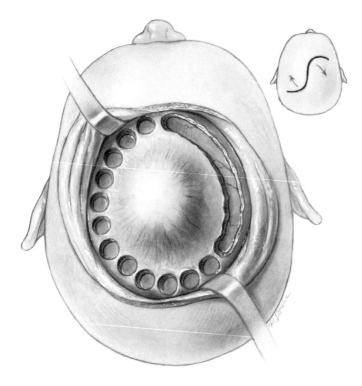

Figure 92–11 Removal of an osteoma by using an S-shaped incision and multiple burr holes, and connecting the burr holes by using a rongeur. (From MacCarty, C. S.: The Surgical Treatment of Intracranial Meningiomas. Springfield, Ill., Charles C Thomas, 1961. Reprinted by permission.)

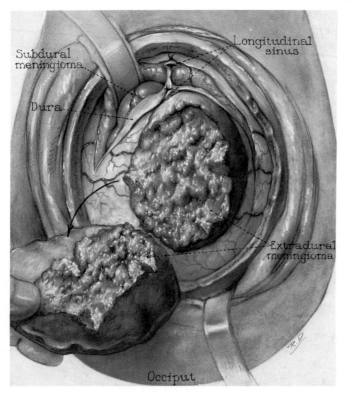

Figure 92–12 Removal of a parasagittal osteoma prior to removal of the neoplasm. (From MacCarty, C. S.: The Surgical Treatment of Intracranial Meningiomas. Springfield, Ill., Charles C Thomas, 1961. Reprinted by permission.)

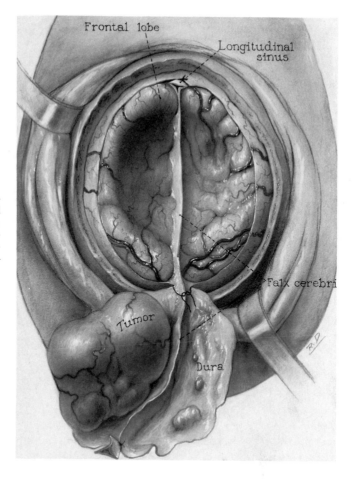

Figure 92-13 Removal of a parasagittal meningioma and the involved dura, longitudinal sinus, and falx. (From Adson, A. W.: The surgical considerations of brain tumor. Northwestern Univ. Bull. Med. School, *35*:16:1–42, 1934. Reprinted by permission.)

ing the sites of attachment. Subsequent tumor recurrence that will have to be treated with reoperation is accepted in such an instance rather than risking serious morbidity or death related to sacrifice of the sinus. In some patients, a portion of the sinus wall can be removed or opened to achieve total tumor removal, and the incision in the sinus can be sutured or a venous patch graft or dural flap can be used to restore its integrity.[8]

Falcial tumors unattached to the sagittal sinus usually can be removed through a unilateral dural opening, although in this instance as well, access across the midline should be planned because it may become necessary. The tumor is approached from the side of the major mass, and the involved dura is excised to achieve bilateral tumor removal. The close proximity of the pericallosal arteries must be considered while the deepest portion of the tumor is being excised.

Convexity Meningioma

Convexity meningiomas are common and generally are amenable to complete removal and cure. Usually, the dura around the site of tumor attachment is opened, encircling the tumor, thereby interrupting most if not all of the vascular supply to the tumor as well as exposing the tumor's whole periphery. Removal of a small meningioma of the convexity is usually not difficult and is achieved by slowly elevating the tumor out of its bed with gentle dissection and by coagulating and dividing the feeding and draining vessels as the dissection progresses (Fig. 92–14). Care must be exercised to minimize injury to adjacent cerebral tissue, which might result in postoperative neurological deficit or seizures. For larger meningiomas of the convexity, the center of the tumor should be cored out, as was originally described by Cushing and Eisenhardt.[15] With this accomplished, the

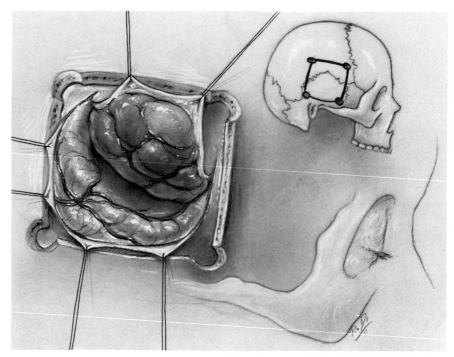

Figure 92–14   Removal of a convexity meningioma. (From MacCarty, C. S.: The Surgical Treatment of Intracranial Meningiomas. Springfield, Ill., Charles C Thomas, 1961. Reprinted by permission.)

edges of the tumor can be folded inward and it can be easily removed.

Sphenoid Wing

As in the clinical presentation, meningiomas of the sphenoid wing must be considered according to their site of origin along that structure and also on the basis of their growth characteristics, which may be either globular or en plaque. Generally, operations for the globular tumor are primarily directed at the removal of the tumor, whereas the goals for the en plaque tumor are often removal of the involved dura and osteoma and decompression of the orbit. If the tumor has been associated with severe proptosis of the eye, a preliminary temporary blepharorrhaphy may be performed to protect the eye during postoperative orbital swelling.

A meningioma at the lateral aspect of the sphenoid wing is often relatively easily removed, but removal of a meningioma at the medial aspect may be among the most challenging of operations to the neurosurgeon and the riskiest for the patient. These tumors must be approached along the base

of the skull through a low frontotemporal craniotomy, often requiring removal of the pterion itself (Figs. 92–15 and 92–16). Brain relaxation with intravenously administered mannitol or urea is often desirable, and the tumor is then exposed transdurally. The soft portion of the tumor is reduced in piecemeal fashion, with care being taken to protect the middle cerebral artery, which can then be followed to the internal carotid bifurcation and optic mechanism. In tumors of the inner sphenoid wing or clinoidal region, injury to the carotid artery and optic nerve, chiasm, and tract poses the greatest risk and must be guarded against by identification of these structures early in the operation (Fig. 92–17). For most neurosurgeons, the operating microscope greatly facilitates this difficult dissection for removal of the tumor and protection of the neurovascular structures. Small perforating branches of the carotid and middle cerebral arteries must be identified and preserved as well. Once the soft tumor has been eradicated, the dural and bony attachments of the lesion and any portion of it invading the orbit must be removed. This means that the involved portion of the dura and bony tissue of the middle fossa and along the

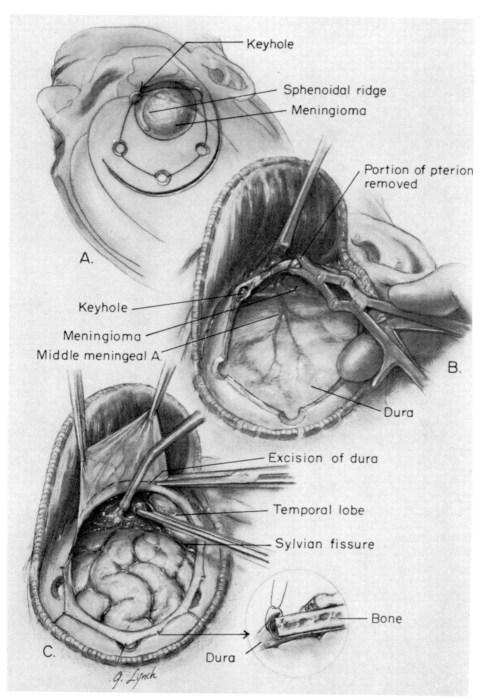

Figure 92–15   *A*. Exposure of a lateral and medial sphenoidal meningioma with emphasis on a properly placed "keyhole" to allow ready access to the lateral sphenoid wing and orbit. *B*. Removal of an osteoma of the lateral wing of the sphenoid. *C*. Method of securing hemostasis of the dura. Initial steps in removal of the tumor. (From MacCarty, C. S.: Meningiomas of the sphenoidal ridge. J. Neurosurg., *36*:114–120, 1972. Reprinted by permission.)

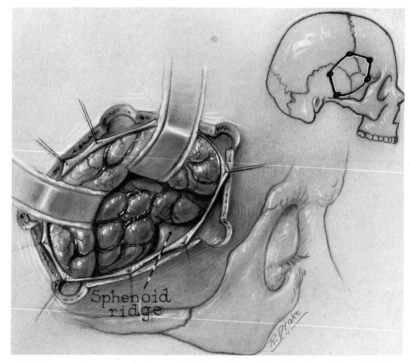

Figure 92–16 Exposure for removal of a meningioma of the sphenoidal ridge. (From MacCarty, C. S.: The Surgical Treatment of Intracranial Meningiomas. Springfield, Ill., Charles C Thomas, 1961. Reprinted by permission.)

greater and lesser wings of the sphenoid bone and orbital roof must be removed (Fig. 92–18).[28] In medial tumors extending through the optic foramen, the dura over the roof of the foramen can be incised and the bony canal roof removed with a small rongeur or angled punch. Tumor infiltrating the cavernous sinus usually must be left, as should also any tumor so completely encasing the optic nerves and carotid and middle cerebral arteries that these structures cannot be identified or freed from it without very great risk. In several cases of the latter, when there has been severe stenosis of the internal carotid artery related to tumor compression, the authors have employed a superficial temporal–middle cerebral artery bypass to treat the hemodynamic cerebral ischemia rather than attempting total removal of the tumor that encircled the artery.

Olfactory Groove

Meningiomas of the olfactory groove may present primarily as unilateral or midline masses, and the operative approach should be planned accordingly. In either case, administration of an osmotic diuretic may facilitate the necessary retraction of the frontal lobe for tumor exposure and may minimize trauma due to traction or the necessity of frontal lobe resection, as has been advocated by some.[31]

Smaller unilateral tumors can be adequately exposed and removed by unilateral frontal craniotomy, but larger midline tumors are best exposed through a bifrontal craniotomy that is placed as low as possible on the brow (Fig. 92–19). The bifrontal approach usually necessitates entering the frontal sinuses, which is managed simply by reflecting the sinus mucosa to the orifice, packing the sinus with Gelfoam or muscle, and then closing the sinus with overlapping reflected pericranial and dural flaps. In these cases, the advantages of low exposure far outweigh the disadvantages related to opening the sinuses. The longitudinal sinus is ligated anteriorly, and the sinus and falx are then divided to expose the tumor. The mass of the tumor is reduced to permit the surgeon to roll the posterior portion of the tumor forward to expose the anterior cerebral arteries and their

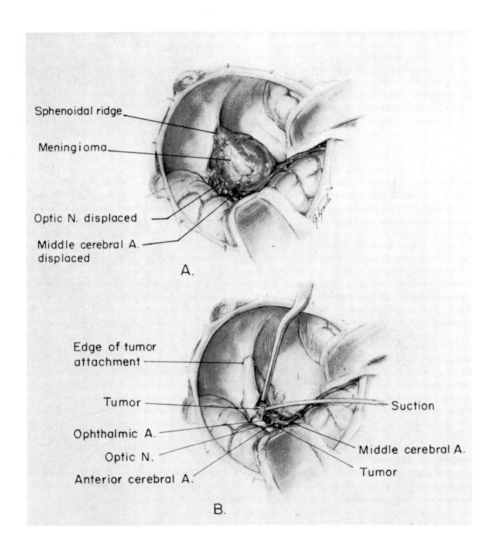

Figure 92–17 Removal of a clinoidal meningioma. Its proximity to the optic nerve, optic tract, and carotid and middle cerebral arteries is shown. (From MacCarty, C. S.: Meningiomas of the sphenoidal ridge. J. Neurosurg., *36*:114–120, 1972. Reprinted by permission.)

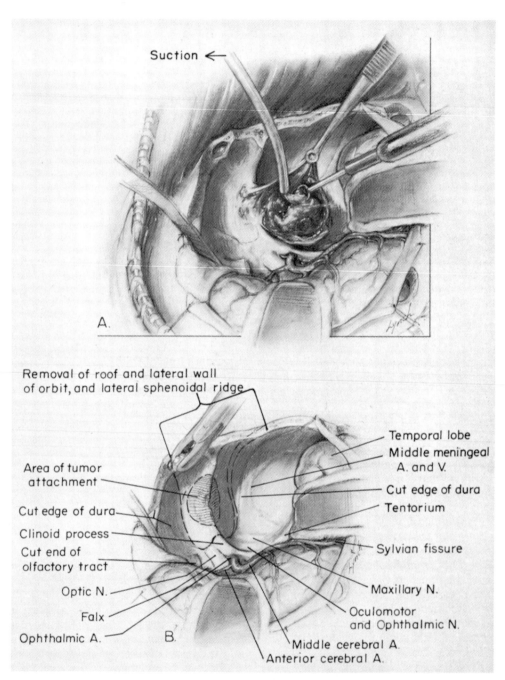

Suction ←

A.

Removal of roof and lateral wall
of orbit, and lateral sphenoidal ridge

Temporal lobe
Middle meningeal
A. and V.

Area of tumor
attachment

Cut edge of dura
Tentorium

Cut edge of dura

Clinoid process

Cut end of
olfactory tract

Sylvian fissure

Optic N.

Maxillary N.

Falx

Oculomotor
and Ophthalmic N.

B.

Ophthalmic A.

Middle cerebral A.
Anterior cerebral A.

Figure 92–18   Removal of the intracranial extension of the meningioma, the involved dura, and an osteoma of the sphenoid wing and roof and lateral wall of the orbit to insure eradication of dural and bony attachments of the lesion. (From MacCarty, C. S.: Meningiomas of the sphenoidal ridge. J. Neurosurg., *36*:114–120, 1972. Reprinted by permission.)

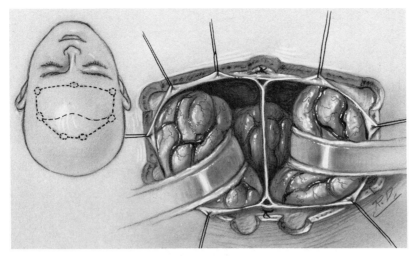

Figure 92–19 Exposure for removal of an olfactory groove meningioma. (From MacCarty, C. S.: The Surgical Treatment of Intracranial Meningiomas. Springfield, Ill., Charles C Thomas, 1961. Reprinted by permission.)

branches, which are then protected. After further reduction and mobilization of the tumor, the optic nerves are noted and the chiasm is identified beneath its deepest aspect, after which the remaining tumor can be amputated from its site of attachment. The olfactory nerves cannot be spared in the excision of bilateral tumors of this type. The dural attachment is removed if possible but otherwise is cauterized. Unless the tumor has actually broken through the cribriform plate into the ethmoidal sinuses, vigorous removal of bone should be avoided to minimize the risk of postoperative cerebrospinal fluid rhinorrhea.

Tuberculum Sellae

Usually presenting with progressive loss of vision, meningiomas of the tuberculum sellae must be treated aggressively with operative removal, before the condition progresses to complete loss of vision. Likewise, the diagnostic evaluation of such patients must be thorough, and if a compressive lesion is suspected, even though unconfirmed by contrast studies or computed tomography, craniotomy or exploration of the optic chiasm and nerve must be performed.

Most meningiomas arising from the tuberculum sellae can be removed via a unilateral craniotomy on the side of the greater mass (Fig. 92–20). If there is advanced visual loss on one side, the authors prefer an

approach from this side so that the tumor is dissected across the most involved nerve, and if sacrifice of the nerve is necessary for complete tumor removal, it is done on the side of the greatest visual deficit. Again, exposure is facilitated by low frontotemporal craniotomy, with removal of the pterion and with cerebral relaxation achieved through osmotic diuresis or removal of cerebrospinal fluid via a lumbar needle (or both). If the tumor is very large and extends bilaterally beyond the optic nerve or carotid arteries, a bilateral craniotomy may be advisable. Preferably under the operating microscope, the tumor is removed piecemeal until its bulk is sufficiently reduced to allow it to be rolled forward away from the optic nerves and anterior cerebral arteries. The site of attachment is then progressively coagulated and divided, and the remaining portions of the tumor are carefully dissected away to permit its total removal. Additional discussion of parasellar tumors and meningioma is given in Chapter 98.

Lateral Ventricle

Usually originating in the posterior portion of the ventricle, meningiomas of the lateral ventricle can be removed with acceptable morbidity and a low mortality rate (Fig. 92–21).[26] This requires an approach that minimizes the adverse effects of the necessary cortical incision and yet allows

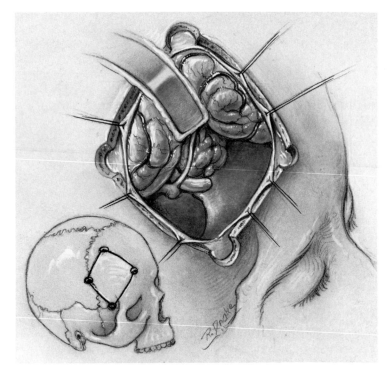

Figure 92–20 A method for exposure of a tuberculum sellae meningioma. (From MacCarty, C. S.: The Surgical Treatment of Intracranial Meningiomas. Springfield, Ill., Charles C Thomas, 1961. Reprinted by permission.)

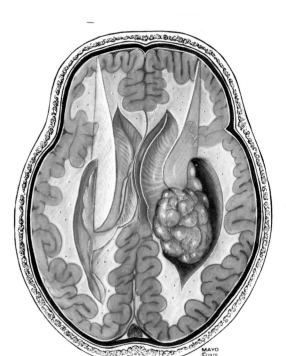

Figure 92–21 Diagrammatic representation of an intraventricular meningioma.

access to the vascular supply, which should be demonstrated by preoperative angiography. In most patients, this supply is from the choroidal arteries.[7]

The cortical incision is made either directly over the tumor or over the cortices of either the posterior parietal or the posterior temporal lobes. Dominant supramarginal and angular gyri and motor cortex should be avoided to prevent aphasia or other untoward effects. De La Torre and co-workers preferred an incision at the most posterior portion of the middle temporal gyrus.[17] The authors prefer the posterior parietal approach just above the lambdoidal suture (Fig. 92–22). This approach allows access to the temporal horn as well as to the anterior and posterior horns of the ventricle. In this manner, both the arterial supply from the temporal horn and the medial vascular supply can be visualized.

Tentorial Meningiomas

Management of meningiomas attached to the tentorium must be individualized, the operative approach being determined by the location of the main mass of the tumor.

There are essentially three approaches to such a tumor: supratentorially, infratentorially, and by a combination of these. For the tumor situated primarily in the middle fossa, a temporo-occipital craniotomy should be done, the tumor then being attacked from above. The patient should be reclining with the head turned laterally with some lateral flexion away from the side of the lesion. The operative field should include the suboccipital areas so that infratentorial access through a suboccipital craniectomy can be gained if necessary (Fig. 92–23). Again, exposure may be facilitated by the use of an osmotic diuretic. After piecemeal reduction of the tumor and dissection away from the brain stem, cranial nerves, and vessels, the involved tentorium should be excised if possible. Bleeding is best controlled by initially incising the tentorium around the tumor.

Subtentorial tumors attached to the tentorium are predominantly unilateral and are best approached from a unilateral suboccipital craniectomy, though again the field should be prepared for a supratentorial approach if indicated. The authors prefer to achieve this with the patient in the sitting position. Precautions as previously de-

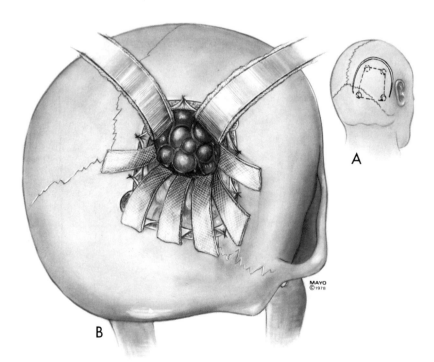

Figure 92–22   *A*. Supralambdoidal posterior parietal incision and craniotomy. *B*. Approach to an intraventricular meningioma.

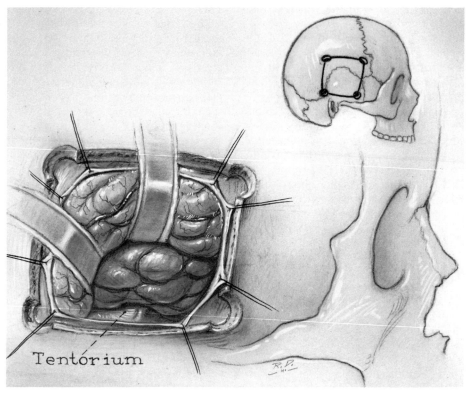

Figure 92–23 Exposure of a tentorial (primarily supratentorial) meningioma. (From MacCarty, C. S.: The Surgical Treatment of Intracranial Meningiomas. Springfield, Ill., Charles C Thomas, 1961. Reprinted by permission.)

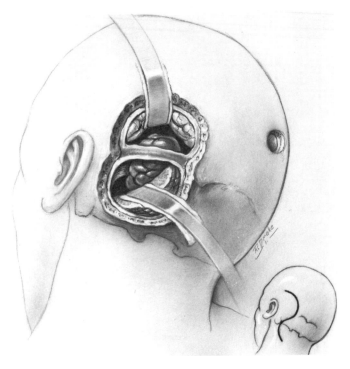

Figure 92–24 Exposure of a tentorial meningioma that has large supratentorial and infratentorial components. Resection of a portion of the cerebellar hemisphere may be desirable to facilitate exposure. (From MacCarty, C. S.: The Surgical Treatment of Intracranial Meningiomas. Springfield, Ill., Charles C Thomas, 1961. Reprinted by permission.)

scribed should be taken for detection and treatment of air embolism should it occur. An S-shaped incision, extending from above the ear and curving behind the mastoid and then medially toward the foramen magnum, is used. The suboccipital craniectomy is carried to the transverse and lateral sinuses, and the dura is opened and reflected toward the sinus. Retraction of the cerebellar hemisphere may be greatly facilitated by osmotic diuresis to expose the tumor. Once again the basic objectives are extensive decompression of the tumor and its careful dissection away from the adjacent brain, cranial nerves, and vessels. If complete removal requires the supratentorial approach, the craniectomy is extended upward and the dura is opened without interfering with the sinus. The occipital lobe can then be retracted upward to expose the superior aspects of the tumor and allow its resection along with the involved tentorium (Fig. 92–24).

Cerebellar Convexity

Meningiomas of the cerebellar convexity may be attached to the transverse sinus or

torcular Herophili. Sinus involvement or obstruction, as well as the pattern of venous drainage through the sinuses, should be determined by preoperative angiography if possible, as management of the site of tumor attachment to the sinus may be a difficult problem. If it is on the nondominant side or is occluded by a tumor, the sinus usually can be resected if necessary. If the tumor incompletely involves the dominant sinus or torcular, it is best to leave these channels intact, allowing residual tumor to remain. Again, the authors' preference is to do the suboccipital craniectomy with the patient in the seated position (Fig. 92–25).

Cerebellopontine Angle

As previously mentioned, the site of attachment of the meningioma in the cerebellopontine angle is most frequently along the posterior aspect of the petrous bone, although the tentorium also may be involved. These tumors are approached in a fashion similar to that for acoustic neuroma, although the tendency for the meningioma to attach itself intimately to adjacent neurovascular structures often makes its com-

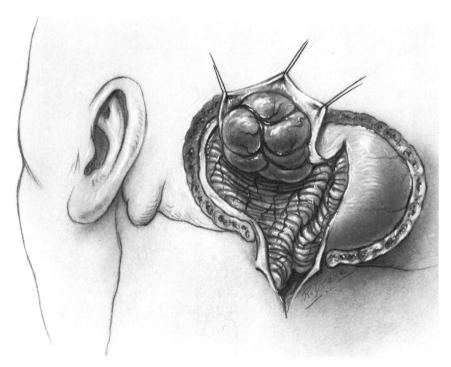

Figure 92–25 Exposure of a cerebellar convexity meningioma. (From MacCarty, C. S.: The Surgical Treatment of Intracranial Meningiomas. Springfield, Ill., Charles C Thomas, 1961. Reprinted by permission.)

plete removal more difficult and hazardous. Occasionally, meningiomas presenting in the cerebellopontine angle may arise from the clivus, in which case it may not be possible to do more than partially remove them. Clivus tumor also may be approached transtentorially via the middle fossa.

Foramen Magnum

Meningiomas arising at the foramen magnum are approached through a midline incision, and a suboccipital craniectomy and upper cervical laminectomy are done with the patient in the sitting position (Fig. 92–26). It is advantageous to have the patient's head somewhat flexed, but this position may be hazardous to the patient with advanced brain and spinal cord compression, and the patient's tolerance to sustained neck flexion should be tested before the induction of anesthesia. As has been already noted, most of these tumors are attached anterolaterally with respect to the spinal cord and medulla, and often there is an intimate relationship to the vertebral artery. For their removal, it is necessary to divide the dentate ligaments and occasionally the

upper cervical nerve rootlets to mobilize the upper part of the spinal cord for access to the tumor. Intracranially, the tumor may lie anterior to the ninth, tenth, and eleventh cranial nerves, sacrifice of which should be avoided if at all possible. If the dural attachment is directly anterior to the medulla, a more lateral approach should be used, as in removing a cerebellopontine angle tumor.

Intraorbital Meningioma

Intraorbital meningiomas are discussed in Chapter 95. The transcranial exposure of the intraorbital meningioma is accomplished by utilizing a small frontotemporal scalp flap and entering the orbit through the lateral aspect of the roof (Fig. 92–27). Although this procedure is best accomplished by an extradural approach, it becomes necessary to open the dura to inspect the proximal optic nerve.

TUMOR RECURRENCE

It is axiomatic in neurological surgery that tumor removal should be as radical as is safe for the patient. With intracranial me-

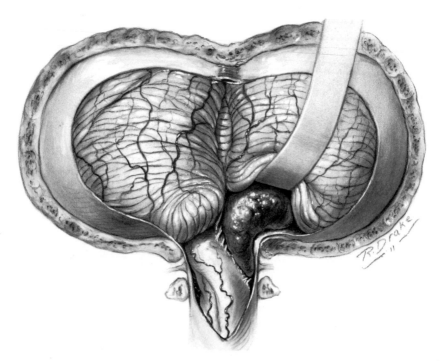

Figure 92–26 Exposure of a foramen magnum meningioma via a suboccipital craniectomy and cervical laminectomy. (From MacCarty, C. S.: The Surgical Treatment of Intracranial Meningiomas. Springfield, Ill., Charles C Thomas, 1961. Reprinted by permission.)

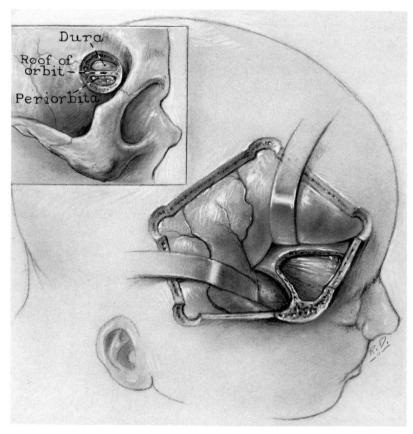

Figure 92–27 Transcranial approach to the orbit. (From MacCarty, C. S.: The Surgical Treatment of Intracranial Meningiomas. Springfield, Ill., Charles C Thomas, 1961. Reprinted by permission.)

ningiomas, occasionally it is both possible and safe to achieve complete removal of the tumor with its site of dural attachment, but probably more commonly it is necessary that the site of attachment be left in situ after the involved dura is cauterized. In rare situations, decompression of the tumor is all that can be safely accomplished. It should not be unexpected, therefore, that there are tumor recurrences.

A thorough study of the frequency of meningioma recurrence was made by Simpson. For patients with "total removal" of the tumor, including the site of attachment, the recurrence rate was 9 per cent. For patients with total removal of the tumor except for the site of dural attachment, which was cauterized, the recurrence rate was 19 per cent. Interestingly, recurrences were usually manifested, on an average, 5 years after operation, and recurrences 10 to 15 years after operation were unusual. Tumor recurrences in patients who had gross total removal of the intradural tumor mass but

no resection or coagulation of the dural attachment site or involved bone, as is often done with en plaque tumors, were noted in 29 per cent. Only partial removal of the intradural tumor resulted in a significant recurrence rate of 40 per cent for patients so treated. Simpson attributed recurrences to unnoticed tumor invasion of the dural venous sinus (found to be present in 40 per cent of all patients with parasagittal tumors), spread occurring across a dural septum (present in 10 per cent), and detached tumor nodules, subdural tumor fringe, and bone infiltration.[35]

Particularly in patients with neurofibromatosis, the possibility of multiple meningiomas or associated central nervous system tumors of other cell types must be kept in mind when there are symptoms and signs of meningioma recurrence. In the authors' experience, young women presenting with a meningioma frequently will ultimately develop multiple meningiomas.

The treatment for clinically significant

meningioma recurrence usually is operative, the timing of the reoperation being dictated by a number of considerations, including the patient's condition, the site and nature of the tumor, and the operative risks.

The role of radiation therapy in the treatment of subtotally removed or recurrent meningioma has yet to be clarified. Although meningiomas generally are considered to be radioresistant tumors, radiation therapy has been advocated for patients with incompletely excised tumors that have malignant characteristics and, rarely, for patients with incompletely removed typical meningioma.[9,25] A wider role for radiation therapy has been advocated by Wara and associates, who found a recurrence rate of 74 per cent for patients with subtotally removed meningiomas that were not irradiated compared with a rate of 29 per cent for patients who had subtotal removal followed by radiation therapy.[39] They advocated a tumor dose of at least 5000 rads for incomplete meningioma resection and certain previously nonirradiated recurrent tumors and also preoperatively in an attempt to improve resectability of certain highly vascular meningiomas.

PROGNOSIS

The prognosis for patients with intracranial meningiomas depends on many factors, including the age of the patient, the site of the tumor, the completeness of its removal, and the presence or absence of malignancy. MacCarty and Taylor studied some of these factors in their review of patients treated at the Mayo Clinic for intracranial meningioma between 1960 and 1975. In that series, 739 patients underwent 790 craniotomies, and of these, 682 patients were operated on for the first time. Despite many of these patients being more than 60 years of age, the one-month postoperative mortality rate was 5.1 per cent for the group that had their first operation. For patients operated on during the span from 1960 through 1964, the mortality rate was 8.9 per cent, but from 1965 through 1969, only 3.1 per cent (Fig. 92–28). From 1970 to 1975, the one-month postoperative mortality rate was 2.9 per cent.[29]

Significantly higher first-month mortality rates were noted for patients who were more than 70 years of age (11.9 per cent) and for patients with meningiomas in the tentorial (25 per cent) or posterior fossa

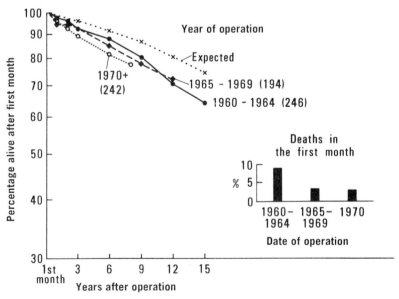

Figure 92–28 Survival curves from one month postoperatively for patients undergoing operation in the periods 1960 through 1964, 1965 through 1969, and 1970 through 1975. The expected survival curve based on regional actuarial tables is also shown. Percentages of patients who died in the first month postoperatively are shown in inset at right. (Modified from MacCarty, C. S., and Taylor, W. F.: Intracranial meningiomas: Experiences at the Mayo Clinic. Neurol. Med. Chir. (Tokyo), *19*:569–574, 1979.)

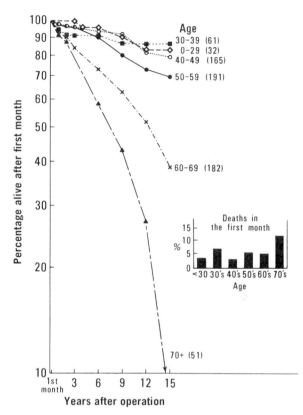

Figure 92–29 Survival curves from one month postoperatively for patients at various ages. Percentages of patients who died in the first month postoperatively are shown in inset at right. (Modified from MacCarty, C. S., and Taylor, W. F.: Intracranial meningiomas: Experiences at the Mayo Clinic. Neurol. Med. Chir. (Tokyo), *19*:569–574, 1979.)

sites (13.2 per cent) (Figs. 92–29 and 92–30). Understandably, operative and postoperative deaths are somewhat more frequent among patients who have undergone previous operations for their tumors. The comparison of hospital mortality rates among Mayo Clinic patients operated on for the first time and those undergoing reoperation for intracranial meningiomas between 1960 and 1975 is summarized in Table 92–3.

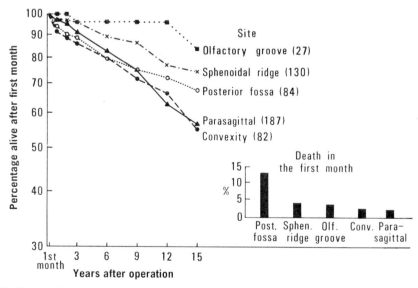

Figure 92–30 Survival curves from one month postoperatively for patients whose tumor site was the olfactory groove, sphenoidal ridge, posterior fossa, parasagittal area, or convexity. Percentages of patients who died in the first month postoperatively are shown in inset at right. (Modified from MacCarty, C. S., and Taylor, W. F.: Intracranial meningiomas: Experiences at the Mayo Clinic. Neurol. Med. Chir. (Tokyo), *19*:569–574, 1979.)

TABLE 92–3 HOSPITAL MORTALITY
RATES IN INTRACRANIAL
MENINGIOMAS, MAYO CLINIC,
1960–1975*

	NUMBER OF OPERATIONS	DEATH	
		Number	Per Cent
At first operation	682[a]	27	4.0
For all operations	790[a]	34	4.3

[a] Number of patients having first operation during specified period (1960 through 1975).

* From MacCarty, C. S., and Taylor, W. F.: Intracranial meningiomas: Experiences at the Mayo Clinic. Neurol. Med. Chir. (Tokyo), 19:569–574, 1979. Reprinted by permission.

Of those 682 patients operated on for the first time between 1960 and 1975 and surviving for at least one month thereafter, 96 per cent survived the first year and 63 per cent survived 15 years (see Fig. 92–28).

MacCarty and Taylor also found that age had a profound effect on the long-term prognosis (see Fig. 92–29). For patients living longer than one month after operation, the observed 15-year survival of patients who were in their 70's was 9 per cent, whereas the expected 15-year survival of a similar age population without meningiomas is 27 per cent.[29]

It was found that women had a significantly better prognosis than did men (Fig. 92–31).

Likewise, the relationship between tumor site and prognosis was significant. For patients with convexity, tentorial, or parasagittal tumors, the 15-year survival rate was 53 to 57 per cent, whereas for patients with sphenoidal ridge, olfactory groove, and foramen magnum tumors, the rate was 74 to 86 per cent (see Fig. 92–30). Interestingly, the authors found no significant alteration in survival rates for patients with parasagittal tumors when the tumors were subclassified according to their location in anterior, middle, and posterior regions, or for those with sphenoidal ridge tumors when the tumors were located in its lateral, middle, and medial thirds.

In MacCarty and Taylor's series of the 682 meningiomas operated on initially, 76 were considered to be "cellularly active with mitosis present" (the histological criteria for meningioma malignancy), whereas 606 tumors did not demonstrate such malignant changes. The one-month mortality rates were 7.9 per cent for patients with malignant lesions and 4.8 per cent for those with benign lesions. This difference was statistically significant. The 15-year survival rate was only 34 per cent for patients

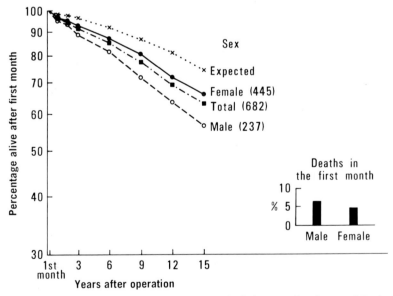

Figure 92–31 Survival curves from one month postoperatively by sex of patients and for both sexes combined. Expected survival curve is also shown. Percentages of patients who died in the first month postoperatively are shown in inset at right. (Modified from MacCarty, C. S., and Taylor, W. F.: Intracranial meningiomas: Experiences at the Mayo Clinic. Neurol. Med. Chir. (Tokyo), 19:569–574, 1979.)

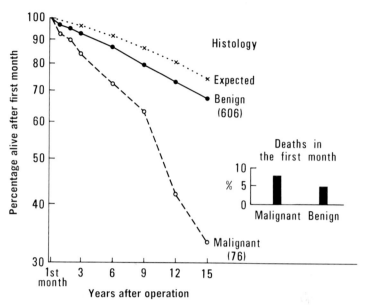

Figure 92-32 Survival curves from one month postoperatively for patients with benign or malignant tumors. Expected survival curve is also shown. Percentages of patients who died in the first month postoperatively are shown in inset at right. (Modified from MacCarty, C. S., and Taylor, W. F.: Intracranial meningiomas: Experiences at the Mayo Clinic. Neurol. Med. Chir. (Tokyo), *19*:569–574, 1979.)

with malignant tumors, in contrast to 68 per cent for those with benign tumors (Fig. 92–32).[29]

REFERENCES

1. Annegers, J. F., Laws, E. R., Jr., Kurland, L. T., et al.: Head trauma and subsequent brain tumors. Neurosurgery, *4*:203–205, 1979.
2. Ausman, J. I., French, L. A., and Baker, A. B.: Intracranial neoplasms. *In* Baker, A. B., and Baker, L. H., Eds.: Clinical Neurology. Vol 1. Hagerstown, Md., Harper & Row, 1974, pp. 1–103.
3. Bailey, P.: Intracranial Tumors. Springfield, Ill., Charles C Thomas, 1933.
4. Bailey, P., and Bucy, P. C.: The origin and nature of meningeal tumors. Amer. J. Cancer, *15*:15–54, 1931.
5. Barrows, H. S., and Harter, D. H.: Tentorial meningiomas. J. Neurol. Neurosurg. Psychiat., *25*:40–44, 1962.
6. Begg, C. F., and Garrett, R.: Hemangiopericytoma occurring in the meninges: Case report. Cancer, *7*:602–606, 1954.
7. Bernasconi, V., and Cabrini, G. P.: Radiological features of tumours of the lateral ventricles. Acta Neurochir. (Wien), *17*:290–310, 1967.
8. Bonnal, J., and Brotchi, J.: Surgery of the superior sagittal sinus in parasagittal meningiomas. J. Neurosurg., *48*:935–945, 1978.
9. Bouchard, J.: Central nervous system. *In* Fletcher, G. H., ed.: Textbook of radiotherapy. 2nd Ed. Philadelphia, Lea & Febiger, 1973, pp. 366–418.
10. Castellano, F., and Ruggiero, G.: Meningiomas of the posterior fossa. Acta Radiol. [Suppl.] (Stockholm), *104*:1–177, 1953.
11. Cherington, M., and Schneck, S. A.: Clivus meningiomas. Neurology (Minneap.), *16*:86–92, 1966.
12. Claveria, L. E., Sutton, D., and Tress, B. M.: The radiologic diagnosis of meningiomas, the impact of EMI scanning. Brit. J. Radiol., *50*:15–22, 1977.
13. Courville, C. B.: Pathology of the Central Nervous System. 3rd ed. Mountain View, Calif., Pacific Press Publishing Association, 1950.
14. Cushing, H.: The meningiomas (dural endotheliomas): Their source, and favoured seats of origin. Brain, *45*:282–316, 1922.
15. Cushing, H., and Eisenhardt, L.: Meningiomas: Their Classification, Regional Behavior, Life History, and Surgical End Results. Springfield, Ill., Charles C Thomas, 1938.
16. Cushing, H. W.: The meningiomas arising from the olfactory groove and their removal by the aid of electrosurgery. *In* Matson, D. D., and German, W. J., eds.: Harvey Cushing: Selected Papers on Neurosurgery. New Haven, Conn., Yale University Press, 1969, pp. 246–273.
17. De La Torre, E., Alexander, E., Jr., Davis, C. H., Jr., et al.: Tumors of the lateral ventricles of the brain: Report of eight cases, with suggestions for clinical management. J. Neurosurg., *20*:461–470, 1963.
18. Gautier-Smith, P. C.: Parasagittal and Falx Meningiomas. New York, Appleton-Century-Crofts, 1970.
19. Goellner, J. R., Laws, E. R., Jr., Soule, E. H., et al.: Hemangiopericytoma of the meninges: Mayo Clinic experience. Amer. J. Clin. Path., *70*:375–380, 1978.
20. Jellinger, K.: Histological subtypes and prognostic problems in meningiomas. J. Neurol., *208*:279–298, 1975.
21. Karasick, J. L., and Mullan, S. F.: A survey of metastatic meningiomas. J. Neurosurg., *40*:206–212, 1974.
22. Kearns, T. P., and Wagener, H. P.: Ophthalmologic diagnosis of meningiomas of the sphenoid ridge. Amer. J. Med. Sci., *226*:221–228, 1953.
23. Kennedy, F.: Retrobulbar neuritis as an exact diagnostic sign of certain tumors and abscesses

in the frontal lobes. Amer. J. Med. Sci., *142*:355–368, 1911.

24. Kernohan, J. W., and Sayre, G. P.: Tumors of the central nervous system. *In* Atlas of Tumor Pathology. Fascicles 35 and 37. Washington, D.C., Armed Forces Institute of Pathology, 1952.

25. King, D. L., Chang, C. H., and Pool, J. L.: Radiotherapy in the management of meningiomas. Acta Radiol. [Ther.] (Stockholm), *5*:26–33, 1966.

26. Kobayashi, S., Okazaki, H., and MacCarty, C. S.: Intraventricular meningiomas. Mayo Clin. Proc., *46*:735–741, 1971.

27. MacCarty, C. S.: The Surgical Treatment of Intracranial Meningiomas. Springfield, Ill., Charles C Thomas, 1961.

28. MacCarty, C. S.: Meningiomas of the sphenoidal ridge. J. Neurosurg., *36*:114–120, 1972.

29. MacCarty, C. S., and Taylor, W. F.: Intracranial meningiomas: Experiences at the Mayo Clinic. Neurol. Med. Chir. (Tokyo), *19*:569–574, 1979.

30. Nijensohn, D. E., Araujo, J. C., and MacCarty, C. S.: Meningiomas of Meckel's cave. J. Neurosurg., *43*:197–202, 1975.

31. Northfield, D. W. C.: The Surgery of the Central Nervous System: A Textbook for Postgraduate Students. Oxford, Blackwell Scientific Publications, 1973.

32. Ozonoff, M. B., and Burrows, E. H.: Intracranial calcification. *In* Newton, T. H., and Potts, D. G., eds.: Radiology of the Skull and Brain. St. Louis, C. V. Mosby Co., 1971, vol 1, bk 2, pp. 823–873.

33. Percy, A. K., Elveback, L. R., Okazaki, H., et al.: Neoplasms of the central nervous system: Epidemiologic considerations. Neurology (Minneap.), *22*:40–48, 1972.

34. Russell, D. S., and Rubinstein, L. J.: Pathology of Tumours of the Nervous System. 4th Ed. Baltimore, Williams & Wilkins Co., 1977.

35. Simpson, D.: The recurrence of intracranial meningiomas after surgical treatment. J. Neurol. Neurosurg. Psychiat., *20*:22–39, 1957.

36. Smith, V. R., Stein, P. S., and MacCarty, C. S.: Subarachnoid hemorrhage due to lateral ventricular meningiomas. Surg. Neurol., *4*:241–243, 1975.

37. Stein, B. M., Leeds, N. E., Taveras, J. M., et al.: Meningiomas of the foramen magnum. J. Neurosurg., *20*:740–751, 1963.

38. Taveras, J. M., and Wood, E. M.: Diagnostic Neuroradiology. 2nd Ed. Baltimore, Williams & Wilkins Co., 1976.

39. Wara, W. M., Sheline, G. E., Newman, H., et al.: Radiation therapy of meningiomas. Amer. J. Roentgen. *123*:453–458, 1975.

40. Weyand, R. D., MacCarty, C. S., and Wilson, R. B.: The effect of pregnancy on intracranial meningiomas occurring about the optic chiasm. Surg. Clin. N. Amer., August, 1951, pp. 1225–1233.

41. Wickbom, I.: Tumor circulation. *In* Newton, T. H., and Potts, D. G., eds.: Radiology of the Skull and Brain. St. Louis, C. V. Mosby Co., 1971, vol 2, bk 4, pp. 2257–2285.

42. Wilson, S. A. K.: Neurology. Edited by A. N. Bruce. Baltimore, Williams & Wilkins Co., 1940.

43. Yasuoka, S., Okazaki, H., Daube, J. R., et al.: Foramen magnum tumors: Analysis of 57 cases of benign extramedullary tumors. J. Neurosurg., *49*:828–838, 1978.

44. Zülch, K. J., and Mennel, H. D.: The question of malignancy in meningiomas. Acta Neurochir. (Wien), *31*:275–276, 1975.

93

ACOUSTIC NEUROMAS

HISTORICAL BACKGROUND

Cushing made a historical review of early reports of acoustic tumors.[9] He believed that Sandifort's (presumptive) case reported in 1777 was the earliest descriptive account. Sandifort stated:

. . . as I examined the base of the brain, with the origins of the nerves, I discovered a small body clinging to the right auditory nerve, of such toughness that it was supposed surely to be cartilage. It was not so firmly attached to the inferior part of the said nerve, but it clung tightly to the proximal portion of the medulla oblongata, at that point where this nerve (VIII), together with the VIIth, makes its exit, *likewise insinuating into the foramen* as one obstruction in the interior of the petrous portion of the temporal bone, which said nerve enters. *Its surface was exceedingly* uneven—especially that part which was in relation with the base of the skull and various larger and smaller nodules arose from its surface. It was not possible to separate the nerve from the lesion and neither was it possible to free it entirely from the foramen which the nerve enters, but it was more easily separated from the part of the medulla to which, as stated before, it adhered.

Having cut into the body, it presented a tough cortex or exterior part: the interior, however, was somewhat softer, although in this also there were hard particles interspersed.

The situation and firm lodging of this little body demonstrate without doubt that *it compressed the auditory nerve.* The depression seen at the point noted in the medulla and neighboring soft parts proves it, and the extension of the nodules into the foramen of the nerve still further confirms it. This lessened the nerve greatly in its capacity, as seen by a comparison of the right auditory nerve with the left.

And so this little body, hiding in the recess of the brain, is to be considered as the cause of deafness in this case. To it there was neither medical nor manual access, the case being therefore entirely incurable. . . .[53]

Most surgeons agreed with Cushing that Sandifort's patient undoubtedly had an acoustic neurinoma that somewhat compressed the medulla oblongata and compromised function of the right auditory nerve.

In 1810 Leveque-Lasource reported the case of a 38-year-old woman whose primary symptoms were vertigo, headache, loss of vision, tinnitus followed by deafness in the left ear, instability, numbness of the extremities, dysarthria, and deviation of the tongue.[37]

At autopsy, a fibrous tumor was found apparently arising from the auditory meatus. It was further attached to the petrous bone. The acoustic nerve was pressed and pushed aside but not destroyed, which raised the question whether this was a meningioma and not a true acoustic neuroma or perhaps a rare tumor of the facial nerve.

Cushing pointed out that if hearing returned after such a tumor was removed it tended to signify that the tumor in the cerebellopontine angle was usually a meningioma and not an acoustic neuroma. Preservation of hearing in these early operations for tumors was practically unheard of; currently in acoustic tumor surgery, the facial nerve can usually be saved and hearing occasionally preserved.

The first accredited clinical report of an acoustic tumor was given in 1830 by Charles Bell.[5] The following account was submitted in a letter from John Whiting; Cushing described it as "a good illustration of the clinical acumen and descriptive powers of this physician of a century ago. . . ."

R. W. RAND, D. D. DIRKS, D. E. MORGAN, AND J. R. BENTSON

Mrs. F. . . . The burning sensation commenced on the left side of her tongue, and has gradually increased for the twelve months, until now it extends over half of the tongue, and mouth, and face, and head . . . she has lost the sense of taste in the affected side of her tongue. . . . Since the age of twenty-one a violent headache had frequently distressed her . . . accompanied with sickness and vomiting of bile; this headache has continued to return at intervals since the commencement of her present ailment.

A year later in September 1828,

Her speech had become indistinct, her face was drawn to the right side, the masseter and temporal muscles of the left side had ceased to act, the tongue was protruded toward the left side, the hearing in the left ear had ceased . . . she was emaciated and bed-ridden and complained of great and constant pain at the back part of her head . . . she seemed to die at length from difficult respiration, and want of the power of swallowing.

Post mortem appearance . . . a tumor containing fluid of the color of urine about the size of pigeon's egg, was discovered . . . on the left side, bounded by the petrous portion of the temporal bone, the pons varolii, and the left lobe of the cerebellum . . . and had by its pressure produced considerable indentation of the left side of pons . . . the fifth cranial nerve was flattened and then as if from pressure . . . but the seventh, both portio dura (facial nerve) and mollis (acoustic nerve), was completely involved and lost in the tumor from a quarter of an inch from the origin to the meatus internus: and into the foramen . . . could be seen to enter. . . the membranous portion of the tumor . . .[5]

This was clearly a cystic type of acoustic nerve tumor.

Cruveilhier gave another complete description of these lesions in 1842.[8]

In 1894 Ballance operated upon what may have been an acoustic neuroma, although he called it a fibrosarcoma of the meninges.[4] His description of the operation, which was done in two stages, is graphic.

To prove that operation for cerebellar tumor in the adult may be completely successful, I may mention that in 1894 I removed an encapsulated fibro-sarcoma from the right cerebellar fossa of a woman aged forty-nine years, and that she is alive and now well (12 years later). The following is an account of the operations.
Operation: November 19, 1894.
Scalp flap thrown down in right occipital re-

gion and bone removed. Toward the external occipital protuberance an exostosis presented toward the dura as well as externally. The inward projection had occluded the lateral sinus. When, therefore, the exostosis was removed the sinus filled up causing a considerable alteration in the venous circulation. The result was the patient collapsed, and respiration ceased. Patient was revived with much difficulty.
Operation: November 26, 1894.
Flap thrown down, and then dural flap thrown down. Solid tumour found attached to dura over inner part of posterior surface of petrous. Somewhat firmly fixed, and the finger had to be inserted between pons and tumour to get it away.

Patient, after a somewhat protracted convalescence, recovered. The fifth and seventh nerves were injured at the operation, and the right eye ulcerated and had to be removed. The optic neuritis in the left eye cleared up with recovery of good eyesight. Some trophic ulceration occurred at the angle of the mouth and at the right ala nasi, this ultimately healed.[4]

Development of Operations for Acoustic Tumors

Cushing first encountered an acoustic tumor in 1906. The experience was a memorable one, and 11 years later he described the difficulties of this operation in the following words:

. . . The operation was abandoned in the hope of completing it at a second session for the situation as now recalled brings up a picture of the patient's head insecurely held by an assistant, the anesthetic awkwardly administered to a subject having respiratory embarrassment, and an inexperienced operator attempting to expose the cerebellum in a wobbly and bloody field.[9]

After this experience it is no wonder that Dr. Cushing called exploration of the cerebellopontine angle "the gloomy corner of neurologic surgery." In 1954, however, McKenzie and Alexander, quoting List, stated that in his series of 176 acoustic neuromas Cushing had 13 cases in which complete removal was accomplished with a mortality rate of 7.7 per cent.[39,42]

Cushing analyzed the more direct operative approach to the acoustic neuroma by operations upon the labyrinth, as had been performed by otologists. Panse in 1904 suggested an operation by an approach directly through the petrous bone.[46] This approach involved destruction of the middle ear and led to homolateral facial paralysis. He mentioned as obvious drawbacks the depth of the wound and the narrow field of action, circumscribed as it is externally by such important vascular structures as the sigmoid and superior petrosal sinuses, and deeper by the carotid artery. He believed that only a small acoustic tumor confined to the internal auditory canal could be removed successfully.

Two other serious disadvantages of the translabyrinthine approach were mentioned. It does not serve as a palliative measure if removal of the lesion is incomplete, while the suboccipital approach, although less direct, provides room for decompressive measures. The resultant cerebrospinal fluid leak through the wound or ear increases the probability of the development of meningitis.

In 1910 Kummel of Heidelberg reported a case operated upon by the translabyrinthine approach with recovery and temporary improvement.[34] In 1911 Quix in Utrecht removed a small tumor the size of a pea.[47] Six months later intracranial symptoms appeared. At autopsy a tumor was seen projecting into the porus. In 1915 Zange reported partial removal of "a neuroblastoma of the acusticus," and in 1915 Schmiegelow added two more cases in which fragmentary intradural tissue was extirpated that in each instance proved to be a glioma.[56,63]

Cushing finally concluded:

It is . . . within the realm of possibility that in case of a very early and minute tumor limited to the internal canal, the translabyrinthine operation may in time be the operation of choice, but this will necessitate far more precocious and more exact diagnosis than we as yet are capable of.[9]

The translabyrinthine operation of Panse was perfected by House and his associates, and the results were published as monographs in 1964 and 1968.[24,25] These authors learned that total removal was not uniformly attainable by this translabyrinthine approach when the tumors were of medium or large size. The limited field of action and the lack of operative exposure of the mesial aspect of the tumor and its blood supply has been responsible for the failure of otological surgeons to perform routinely the total resection of many acoustic tumors by this approach. Other disadvantages included: production of total hearing loss prior to direct tumor identification; inability to observe directly and dissect the tumor capsule from the brain stem vessels, especially the anterior inferior cerebellar artery, compromising the opportunity for safe total tumor removal; and the impossibility of or difficulty in reconstructing the facial nerve if it was involved by the acoustic tumor.

It was Cushing's belief that total extirpation of these tumors was impossible because of the high attending mortality rate.[9] Consequently, he resorted to an intracapsular procedure to remove as much of the contents as possible. He was aware that in every instance the tumor would recur and might require a second operation later. Forty per cent of his patients died within five years of their original operation because of continued growth of the residual tumor. This led Cushing to develop his so-called "bilateral exposure of the cerebellar hemispheres through a crossbow incision," a method that was almost universally followed until Dandy reverted to the unilateral approach for the total removal of these tumors.[10]

To Cushing goes the full credit for being the first to reduce the mortality rate drastically—by meticulous technique and great care in controlling bleeding. He gave the following figures. After the first 10 cases the death rate was lowered to 40 per cent; after 15 cases it had dropped to 33.3 per cent; after 20 cases to 30 per cent; after 25 cases to 24 per cent; and after 30 cases to 20 per cent. These early statistics represent his operative experience. McKenzie stated before the Congress of Neurological Surgeons in 1955: "It is not generally known that Cushing in his series of 176 acoustic neuromas (as reported by List in 1932) had 13 cases of complete removal with a mortality of 7.7 per cent."[42] His former assistant, Dandy, reduced the figure even more. During the last five years of his life, Dandy did a complete tumor removal in 41 cases with a mortality rate of only 2.4 per cent—a figure that has never been equaled.[10]

Total versus Partial Tumor Resection

In 1917 Cushing published his important monograph *Tumors of the Nervus Acusticus*. In it he stated, "I doubt very much, unless some more perfected method is devised, whether one of these tumors can safely be enucleated."[9] However, in that same year, 1917, Dandy presented a patient from whom he had successfully totally removed an acoustic neuroma.[10] It was a great step forward, for it stimulated other neurosurgeons to attempt these complete removals. Between 1917 and 1941 Dandy published a series of papers outlining the technique he employed with an ever increasing number of total successes.

Dandy's description of his first successful total extirpation is rather dramatic.

. . . our first experiences with intracapsular enucleation were unfortunate in being less satisfactory than had been anticipated. Following an uneventful and quick recovery from the effects of the operation the first patient seven days later became listless and drowsy, and during the succeeding three days all symptoms became progressively worse and finally alarming. The late appearance of these symptoms seemed to exclude the postoperative complications which might have been expected, such as hemorrhage or infection, and suggested that in some way the reaction about the stump of tumor which remained was responsible for the condition. The wound was reopened and the shell of tumor extirpated with the index finger. There was surprisingly little hemorrhage which was readily controlled. The patient's condition then steadily improved. Diminished drowsiness was at once apparent, the vomiting at once ceased, and five days later she was able to swallow. From the result of this case it seemed logical to infer that if the shell of the tumor could in some way be removed at the first operation, this dangerous course following subtotal removal might be avoided.[10]

In succeeding cases in which the entire tumor was removed at one operation the results amply supported this inference.

Valiant attempts at total removal of these tumors followed, mostly with devastating results prior to 1920. The results of operations for acoustic nerve tumors were summarized in the article "Fifty Years of Neurosurgery, 1905–1955" by Scarff (Table 93–1).[55] Gradually it became apparent that incomplete removal of acoustic neuromas almost invariably led to their recurrence and the death of the patient.

In 1905 Krause described his unilateral osteoplastic operation that was performed in two stages and primarily for the purpose of exposing and dividing the auditory nerve for persistent tinnitus.[32] Borchardt, in 1906, reported 18 cases of acoustic tumor with 13 fatalities, 72.2 per cent.[6] At the Seventeenth International Congress in 1913, A. Von Eiselberg reported 16 cases with 12 immediate fatalities, 75 per cent, and at the same meeting Krause reported 26 deaths among his 31 cases, 83.8 per cent.

Olivecrona reported 304 unilateral acoustic tumors, or 9.5 per cent of a total of 3265 brain tumors verified to December 31, 1946.[19,44] This covered the entire material on acoustic tumors from December 1922 until the end of 1946. He regretted that up to 1946 recognition of these tumors in their early stage had not improved much, a condition that, thanks to present-day otological tests and special contrast neurolradiological procedures, has been greatly improved. At operation most of the patients had large tumors and choked discs, and many showed blindness or vision much reduced. There was only one instance of a very early tumor—in a patient who was believed to have Ménière's disease. In four instances the tumor was not disclosed; suboccipital decompression only was performed in three cases, and in the fourth the tumor was considered too vascular to be attacked. The re-

TABLE 93–1 RESULTS OF OPERATIONS FOR ACOUSTIC NERVE TUMORS AS REPORTED IN THE LITERATURE–1917*

SURGEON	NUMBER OF CASES	OPERATIVE MORTALITY (PER CENT)
Henschen (collected cases, 1910)	43	80
Leischner (1911)	10	70
Krause (personal cases, 1912, reported by Fumarola)	30	86.6
Eiselsberg (1912)	12	66.6
Horsley et al. (1912, reported by Tooth)	24	70
Henschen (collected cases, 1910–1915)	70	68.7
Cushing (personal cases)		
Baltimore series (1902–1912)	11	35
Boston series (1912–1917)	18	11

* From Scarff, J. E.: Fifty years of neurosurgery. Surg. Gynec. Obstet., *101*:417–513, 1955. Reprinted by permission.

maining 300 were subjected to partial or total removal of the tumor. The unilateral Dandy approach was always used.

In 83 cases the tumor was incompletely removed. In the remaining 217 cases all visible tumor tissue was extirpated. In 69 cases, or about 30 per cent, the anatomical continuity of the facial nerve was preserved. The mortality rate associated with the incompletely removed tumors was 29 per cent; that with the completely removed tumors, 23.5 per cent. In two thirds of the cases, when the facial nerve was saved, good or satisfactory regeneration occurred.

Among the survivors of the operations in which removal was incomplete, recurrence of the tumor was observed in 50 per cent and led to death or to a second operation three to four years after the first operation. The mortality rate with and without a second operation was 40 per cent of those surviving the first operation. When the tumors were completely removed no recurrences were observed.

CLINICAL DIAGNOSIS OF ACOUSTIC TUMORS

History and Neurological Findings

As learned from the aforementioned historical review, hearing loss of gradual onset, often associated with tinnitus, is one of the earliest symptoms of an acoustic tumor. The loss of hearing is unilateral and may be partial or complete. Episodes of true vertigo that may be difficult to distinguish from that of Ménière's disease may occur. In addition, periods of unsteadiness experienced by patients in the early stages can have been forgotten. Word discrimination ability is decreased, a characteristic finding. This difficulty in understanding the meaning of words is often noticeable to the patient before hearing loss and is most evident when using the telephone. These early symptoms occur as the neoplasm involves the cochlear and vestibular divisions of the eighth nerve when the tumor is confined to the internal auditory canal and is beginning to grow out of the porus acusticus.

Compression of the facial nerve within the internal auditory canal occurs early, but a motor deficit is rarely obvious clinically. An electromyogram of the facial muscles may show electrical abnormalities of facial

nerve function before clinical findings such as reduction in time of blink response are apparent. Change in taste perception can be determined by a special taste unit using electrical stimulation or by more standard clinical techniques.

Decrease or loss of the corneal response on the ipsilateral side of an acoustic tumor is generally not observed by the patient. Such a finding suggests a moderate- to large-sized tumor with upward and medial growth against the pontine trigeminal nuclei and the entering nerve fibers. Occasionally the patient will notice paresthesias and numbness of the face (the tumor is quite large by this time). Motor dysfunction of the trigeminal nerve is rarely found even in the presence of massive tumors.

Vestibular Tests

Nystagmus is a frequent neurological finding of acoustic tumors. The Hallpike caloric test or a modification of it using both warm and cool water is an essential part of the neurological work-up.[38,43] Loss of or decrease in the response on the ipsilateral side is usually found with acoustic tumors. If decrease of response is observed on the side opposite the suspected tumor, it may indicate involvement of the contralateral vestibular nuclei and their pathways from brain stem compression and distortion or a second tumor on the unsuspected side. The electrical activity of the eye as it moves in various directions is recorded by electronystagmography. This technique can detect subclinical nystagmus and record the response to caloric stimulation of the vestibular nerves more accurately.

This technique, which has become more widespread as its value and commercial availability have become more appreciated, should be a routine procedure in patients who are suspected of harboring an acoustic neuroma. It has the advantage of making a permanent record of the nystagmus patterns that can be compared with future results if the test is repeated. Therefore subtle changes in the function of the vestibular nerves and brain stem systems may be discerned.

Cerebellar dysfunction is a rather late syndrome of an acoustic tumor. The patient usually complains of a progressively staggering gait and ipsilateral incoordination of the hand. For example, one patient noticed an inability to strike the piano keys accurately and to control the force of the touch when she did strike them. The neurological examination will bring out such problems by objective signs of dysmetria, ataxia, tremor, and change of muscle tone.

Auditory Tests of Eighth Nerve Impairment

Assessment of the magnitude of the hearing loss can be accomplished by pure tone air- and bone-conduction audiometry. The results of conventional pure tone audiometry, however, offer no definitive diagnostic information regarding the anatomical site of the lesion beyond a gross differentiation between a conductive and a sensorineural hearing loss. For this reason, so-called "special auditory tests" have been developed.

The primary purpose of the "special auditory tests" is a precise differential diagnosis of the locus of the pathological change within the sensorineural system. Results of such tests do not indicate whether the person has Ménière's disease or an eighth nerve tumor, but rather they indicate whether the lesion is located in the cochlea or the eighth nerve. From this and other diagnostic and case history information the physician may conclude that the hearing loss, as well as the other physical symptoms, is the result of an eighth nerve tumor or of disease involving other structures of the auditory system.

Prior to 1970, the auditory diagnostic test battery was principally composed of behavioral measures such as Békésy audiometry, the threshold tone decay test, the short increment sensitivity index (SISI), the alternate binaural loudness balance test and speech audiometry, especially the performance-intensity function for words or sentences. During the past decade other more objective measures of auditory function have been applied to the diagnosis of eighth nerve disorders. These procedures, including impedance measures and brain stem auditory evoked response (BSER) measures have proved to be especially sensitive to changes in the retrocochlear auditory system. As a result, early identification of subtle retrocochlear disorders has become possible.

Impedance Studies

In the auditory system, changes in acoustic impedance are obtained by the insertion of an air-tight probe into the external auditory canal. A "probe-tone" is introduced into the ear canal. From the same probe tip, a microphone measures the sound pressure level in the ear canal. Any change in impedance at the plane of the tympanic membrane will be observed as a change in sound pressure level of the "probe tone." Two types of acoustic impedance measures are commonly employed: tympanometry and stapedius muscle contraction. Tympanometry is a measure of relative impedance changes that occur as air pressure (via a manometer) is systematically varied in the ear canal. The tympanogram provides an objective measure of the mechanical integrity of the middle ear mechanism and is most useful in ruling out the possibility of a middle ear disorder. When the tympanogram is normal, the stapedius muscle reflex is measured by monitoring acoustic impedance over time while periodically inducing a contraction of the stapedius muscle. When the muscle contracts, a concomitant change in acoustic impedance is measured. The contraction of the stapedius muscle may be induced by tactile or acoustic stimulation, although the latter is by far the most commonly used activating signal.[14a] The "acoustic reflex" threshold is determined by increasing the intensity of an acoustic signal until a change in impedance coincidental with the onset of the activating stimulus is observed.

In patients with cochlear disorders the reflex threshold may be observed at normal or slightly elevated activating levels.[46b] In contrast, among patients with eighth nerve disorders, the reflex is often absent or dramatically increased. Impedance studies provide objective measures of the integrity of the middle ear mechanism (tympanometry) and the acoustic reflex arc, including eighth (acoustic) nerve function and seventh (stapedius innervation) nerve function. The impedance studies are noninvasive and can be accomplished in less than 20 minutes in a cooperative or sedated patient.

Auditory Evoked Response Measures

"Auditory brain stem response" (ABR) is a term used to describe five to seven electrical events that occur in rapid succession (less than 10 msec) following presentation of an acoustic signal to the ear.[30a] The events are time-locked to the beginning of the signal. Although the amplitudes of the auditory evoked potentials are minute, an array of three (or more) surface electrodes featuring an active electrode at the vortex (or on the forehead) can detect them. The procedure requires repetitive signal presentations, amplification, filtering and signal averaging (by computer) to separate the time-locked electrical activity from "background noise." The averaged response can be characterized in terms of the amplitude and latency of each potential and the overall shape of the waveforms. Although the issue of generator sites for the five to seven potentials is not completely resolved, there is general consensus that wave I reflects the eighth nerve action potential; wave II, the cochlear nucleus; wave III, the superior olivary complex; waves IV and V, the areas of the lateral lemniscus and inferior colliculus; and waves VI and VII, thalamic sites.[46a,56a-56c]

Space-occupying lesions that affect the eighth nerve or the brain stem disrupt the latency and overall shape of the evoked response.[56a] When first-order neurons of the eighth nerve are affected by the lesion, wave I and all subsequent waves may be altered. When the lesion involves the auditory pathways in the brain stem, later waves (especially III to V) may be the only ones affected. The alterations in the evoked response typically include absence of identifiable waves, increases in the latency of specific waves, and increases in interwave latency times ("conduction time"). In contrast, patients with cochlear disorders usually evidence near-normal wave latencies and interwave latencies at suprathreshold levels.

Threshold Tone Decay Test

In 1961 Jerger demonstrated that predictions of the site of a lesion may be enhanced if other auditory tests are utilized. One such technique is the threshold tone decay test, which measures the rate of adaptation of the auditory system.[7] This procedure may be accomplished with a conventional pure tone audiometer. The tone may be presented initially at a level 5 db greater than the threshold of the patient. The pa-

tient is instructed to signal as long as he can hear the stimulus. Individuals with normal hearing or conductive hearing impairments can maintain the signal at near threshold levels for at least 60 seconds. Persons with sensorineural loss due to cochlear impairment may require a 15- to 20-db increase in the intensity of the stimulus in order to hear the signal for 60 seconds. The patient with an eighth nerve impairment, however, may be expected to demonstrate abnormal tone decay or the inability to hear the tone for 60 seconds until the intensity level of the signal is 30 to 35 db or more above the threshold level.[44a]

Alternate Binaural Loudness Balance Test

Another useful diagnostic measurement is the alternate binaural loudness balance (ABLB) test of recruitment, originally reported by Fowler in 1936.[15] The phenomenon of loudness recruitment is fundamentally an abnormally rapid increase in the sensation of loudness. It is characteristically found among patients with cochlear disorders. The test involves the stimulation of the two ears alternately with a pulsing stimulus of identical frequency. The intensity is fixed at a predetermined level above threshold in one ear. The patient is instructed to adjust the intensity on the opposite ear until the tones in the two ears are equally loud. The diagnostic value of the ABLB test lies in the fact that if the disorder is in the cochlea, either partial or complete recruitment is observed. In contrast, lesions that occur only in the middle ear or the eighth nerve ordinarily do not show recruitment.

Application of Test Results

Figure 93–1 summarizes the auditory test results for a patient with a 0.8-cm operatively confirmed cerebellopontine angle tumor on the left side. Routine auditory tests revealed near-normal auditory findings bilaterally. The differential diagnostic tests revealed no abnormal tone decay but an elevated acoustic reflex threshold when the acoustic signal was presented to the left ear. The brain stem evoked response waveform and wave latencies are within normal limits for the right ear. The left ear, how-

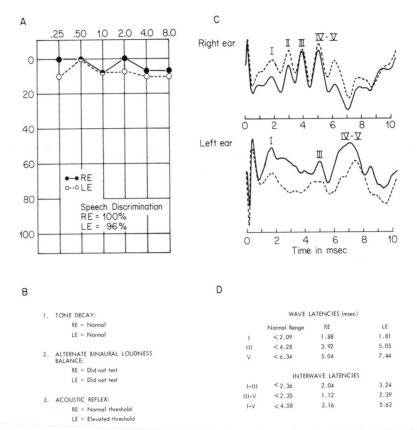

Figure 93–1 Preoperative auditory test results for a patient with an operatively confirmed cerebellopontine angle tumor on the left side. *A*. Pure tone air conduction and speech audiometry results were nearly normal. *B*. Differential diagnostic test results show normal tone decay and an elevated acoustic reflex threshold on the left. *C*. Brain stem evoked response recordings for an 0.1-msec click are within normal limits (- test; - · - replication run). *D*. Absolute and interwave latencies from brain stem evoked response measures.

ever, is characterized by a grossly abnormal waveform and abnormally increased wave latencies.

The elevated acoustic reflex threshold and abnormal brain stem response for the left ear together suggest the probability of a lesion of retrocochlear origin. It is important that the standard battery of auditory tests did not reveal abnormalities strongly suggestive of a retrocochlear lesion in this case. The results from this patient are consistent with the principle that any single auditory test result, when viewed in isolation, may lead to ambiguous conclusions regarding the possible site of the lesion. The accuracy with which the site of an auditory lesion can be predicted is significantly improved when the examiner has access to the results of a battery of auditory tests.

Cushing's assessment of the clinical stages of acoustic tumors remains valid today, and it is therefore worth reading Chapters III and VI of *Tumors of the*

Nervus Acusticus, which give the case reports of verified acoustic tumors and the chronology of symptoms in these cases. Needless to say, early diagnosis and operation with total removal of the acoustic tumor is or should be the goal.

Radiological Diagnosis of Acoustic Tumors

The prinipal neuroradiological studies used at present for evaluating the cerebellopontine angles include plain films, laminagraphy, positive contrast (Pantopaque) encephalography, cisternography, vertebral angiography, fractional pneumoencephalography and computed tomographic (CT) brain scanning. The CT technique has greatly reduced the number of the other positive contrast neuroradiological procedures that are needed. It is noninvasive, and it has a high degree of diagnostic accuracy for medium- and large-sized acoustic tumors, especially when combined with intravenous iodine contrast solutions such as those used for intravenous pyelograms. Even some small acoustic neuromas can be identified.

This variety of studies makes the question of test selection a legitimate concern. An attempt is made here to give the relative advantages and disadvantages of each. The acoustic neurinoma, by far the most common tumor mass found in this region, is dealt with first, and some examples of other angle masses follow.

Anatomy

The cerebellopontine angle is the junctional area between the pons, medulla oblongata, and cerebellum. The pontocerebellar cistern, which occupies this space, is continuous medially with the prepontine cistern. Its boundaries are the posterior surface of the petrous pyramid anteriorly and laterally, the tentorium anteriorly and superiorly, and the cerebellar hemisphere above and posteriorly. The medial border is formed by the pons, brachium pontis, and the ventral lateral surface of the upper medulla oblongata. The laterally directed apex of this triangular cistern extends a variable distance beyond the porus acusticus, or opening of the internal auditory canal. The flocculus of the cerebellum indents the posteromedial portion of the pontocerebellar cistern from above. Posterior to the flocculus, the ninth and tenth cranial nerves pass laterally into the posterior part of the cistern. The seventh and eighth cranial nerves exit from the sulcus between the medulla and pons anterior to the flocculus and pass forward and laterally to the porus acusticus of the internal auditory canal. A projection of the cistern enters the canal itself. The fifth cranial nerve arises from the lateral pons and passes anteriorly through the anteromedial portion of the cistern. The anterior inferior cerebellar artery is related closely to the seventh and eighth nerves. The petrosal vein arises near the origin of the fifth nerve and passes laterally through the anterolateral portion of the cistern.[1]

Plain Roentgenograms

Though earlier reports stated that up to 80 per cent of acoustic neuromas could be diagnosed from plain films, the present tendencies of patients toward earlier presentation and of their physicians toward earlier radiological evaluation have lowered this percentage.[12] Valvassori reported in 1969 that he was able to make the correct plain film diagnosis of acoustic neuroma in only 50 per cent of his cases.[62] The most helpful conventional projections are the anteroposterior view with the petrous bones projected through the orbits, the half-axial or Towne view, the basal view, and Stenver's view. Stenver's view is helpful in evaluating the porus but gives a foreshortened view of the internal auditory canal (Fig. 93–2). The canal is demonstrated in its full length by the other views listed but is unfortunately often obscured by superimposed structures. The main reason to continue to obtain plain films is to rule out abnormalities outside the petrous pyramids, which could be missed on the closely coned laminagrams.

Laminagraphy

Laminagraphy of the petrous pyramids remains the most useful screening test for the suspected acoustic neuroma because it can now also be done by the CT scanner using a 320 matrix as well as by the more conventional radiological tomography. Valvassori reported he had made the correct diagnosis of acoustic neuroma by laminagraphy in 78 per cent of operatively proved cases prior to positive contrast studies.[61] Laminagraphy should be done in two projections. The frontal projection shows the canal in its entire length and is the most helpful. The second projection may be a lateral or a basal view, either of which will give additional information about the porus. The superior and inferior walls of the internal auditory canals are approximately parallel on the frontal projection. Graf, in his 1952 monograph, reported that the ventricular diameter of the canal was usually about 1 mm larger than that of the porus acusticus, and that the porus was never larger than the canal in this dimension.[20] On the basal projection most internal auditory canals are funnel-shaped with the medial end being wider, while a minority have parallel walls.

The range of normal dimensions of the canals is so great that absolute measurements are of little use, but the two canals of

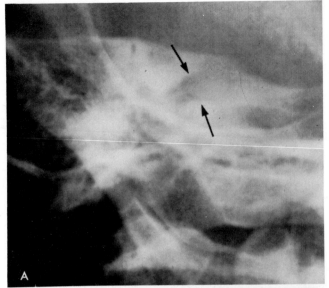

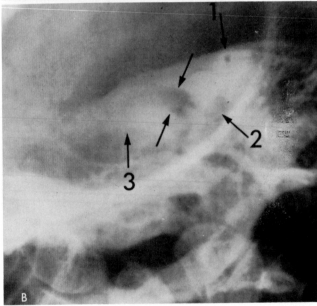

Figure 93-2 *A.* Stenver's projection showing enlargement of porus acusticus (*arrows*). *B.* The normal porus acusticus (*unmarked arrows*) of the opposite side. The internal auditory canal may be identified with certainty by first noting the superior semicircular canal (1), then the vestibule (2), which is just lateral to the canal. The superior wall of the carotid canal (3) is sometimes mistaken for a wall of the internal auditory canal.

any one patient are fortunately nearly always symmetrical and of similar dimensions. The first laminagraphic sign of acoustic neuroma is usually erosion of the lips of the porus acusticus, while widening of the porus occurs later (Fig. 93–3). Valvassori states that the internal auditory canal is considered abnormal whenever we find: (1) erosion of the cortical or capsular lines surrounding the lumen of the canal, (2) widening of 2 mm or more of any portion of the internal auditory canal under investigation in comparison to the corresponding segment of the opposite canal, (3) shortening

of the posterior wall by at least 3 mm in comparison to the opposite side, (4) the crista falciformis running closer to the inferior than to the superior wall of the internal auditory canal, as the crista should normally be located at or above the midpoint of the vertical diameter of the canal.[60]

The tomographic study is considered suggestive but not conclusive whenever we find: (1) demineralization of the cortical outline of the canal, (2) widening of 1 to 2 mm of any portion of the canal in comparison to the corresponding segment of the opposite side, (3) shortening of 2 to 3 mm of

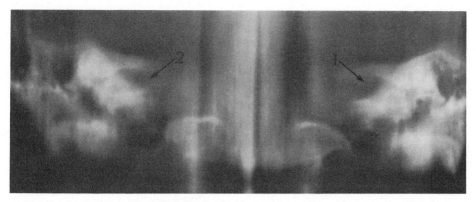

Figure 93–3 Laminagram in frontal plane demonstrates widening of left porus acusticus (1) and erosion of its superior lip compared with the normal right porus (2).

the posterior wall, and (4) the position of the crista falciformis on the side of investigation differing by at least 1 mm from the normal side.

Computed Tomographic Brain Scan

The 160-matrix scan of the brain, including the posterior fossa, can best be achieved by a body scanner because this instrument allows scanning through the foramen magnum into the cervical vertebrae. It gives an excellent overall view of the brain and its ventricular and cisternal anatomy. Enhancement of tumor images usually is accomplished with the intravenous injection of an iodine contrast material of the type used for intravenous pyelograms.

If one uses an instrument capable of scanning in less than 20 seconds to avoid movement artifact, with a 320 matrix, a magnified view of the petrous bone can be achieved and the abnormalities in the size and shape of the porus acusticus and the internal auditory canal can be distinguished. Once these areas are defined on a particular level of the CT san, the contrast material is given to enhance a soft-tissue mass such as an acoustic tumor. By using this technique, even small acoustic tumors can be identified as they start growing out of the porus acusticus into the cistern of the cerebellopontine angle.

Most medium-sized and large acoustic tumors can be readily identified on a CT scan of the posterior fossa (Fig. 93–4). The differential diagnosis between other tumors and aneurysms is best investigated by additional neuroradiological studies, especially

the vertebral and carotid angiograms on the ipsilateral side, using subtraction film technique.

The noninvasive nature of a CT brain scan and its very slight exposure of the brain to radiation because of fine collimation of the x-ray beam allow repeated studies. Thus in a patient with a quite small tumor who has lost hearing ipsilaterally, an early operation to preserve hearing would not be an issue. The biological growth pattern can be determined by serial scans sev-

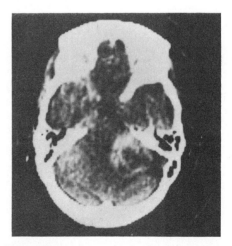

Figure 93–4 Computed tomographic (CT) brain scan with contrast demonstrating an extremely large acoustic neuroma on the right side in the cerebellopontine angle. The white area within the tumor represents the solid portion, while the dark areas are cystic degeneration within the neoplasm. Trapped cerebrospinal fluid is present in the right cerebellopontine angle cistern. The tumor was completely excised, with preservation of the facial nerve.

eral months apart, and if the tumor is shown to be enlarging in a young or middle-aged patient, then an operation can clearly be recommended.

Because the operative mortality rate and morbidity are less with small and medium-sized tumors, every patient with a proved unilateral sensorineural loss should have a 320-matrix contrast enhancement scan of the petrous bone to rule out an early tumor or discover the presence of an unsuspected mass. Air should be used for contrast in the cerebellopontine angle if necessary.

Positive Contrast Cisternography

Though many minor modifications have been described, there are two basic techniques of posterior fossa cisternography with iophendylate (Pantopaque). In the first, as described by Baker, Gass, Scanlon, and others, the Pantopaque is passed into the pontocerebellar angle cistern under fluoroscopic control.[2,18,54] The exact amount injected is not critical, and volumes ranging from 3 to 15 ml have been recommended. Moderate amounts, such as 4 to 6 ml, completely fill the cistern, but the chance of spillage into the middle fossa is less than with larger amounts. The fluoroscopy table is tilted to a head-downward position, and the contrast material collects in the cervi-

cal canal. The table is returned to a more nearly horizontal position, and passage of the medium into the posterior fossa is accomplished by using short head-downward tilts. This may be done with the head in extension, in which case the Pantopaque first flows into the clivus and then into the dependent angle cistern when the head is rotated. Another method consists of pooling the contrast medium in the cervical canal, rotating the extended head to the side, and then tilting the table to run the contrast medium into the dependent angle. Spot films will show the contrast material in the angle cistern as a triangular collection with its medially placed base being the vertebral and basilar arteries (Fig. 93–5). The fingerlike collection of Pantopaque in the internal auditory canal may be obscured by that in the cistern above it (Fig. 93–5B). The special view described by Reese and Bull, in which a cross-table lateral x-ray beam is used and the patient's head is turned 45 degrees to the side, will show the contrast-filled canal as a diverticulum projecting downward into the petrous bone (Fig. 93–6).[51] If there is some question regarding the degree of filling of the canal, horizontal beam tomography is helpful to achieve better definition (Fig. 93–7B). When filming of the first angle is completed, the contrast material is returned to the cer-

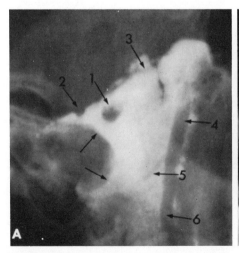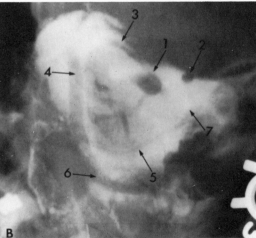

Figure 93–5 Pantopaque cisternogram of same patient as Figure 93–3. *A*. Spot film of left angle cistern shows Pantopaque outlining acoustic neuroma (*unnumbered arrows*). *B*. The normal right angle cistern. Overlying Pantopaque obscures the filling of the right internal auditory canal, expected at site indicated by arrow (7). Other arrows indicate trigeminal nerves (1), petrosal veins (2), superior cerebellar arteries (3), basilar arteries (4), anterior inferior cerebellar arteries (5), and vertebral arteries (6).

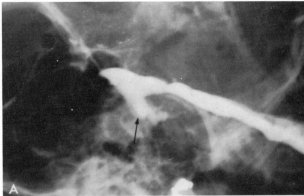

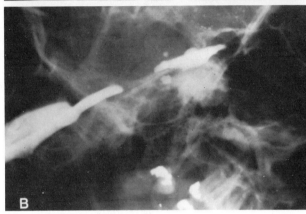

Figure 93–6 Pantopaque cisternogram, cross-table lateral oblique view. *A.* The arrow indicates filling of the internal auditory canal. *B.* Lack of filling of the opposite canal is due to an acoustic tumor.

vical canal and the opposite side is filled in the same manner. The head should be kept extended throughout the procedure to prevent spillage of contrast medium into the middle fossa, from which it cannot be retrieved.

The second technique of Pantopaque cisternography, the Polytome-Pantopaque study, was described by Hitselberger and House.[23] Only 1 ml of Pantopaque is injected into the lumbar canal, and the patient is then placed on his side. The table is tilted head downward approximately 35 degrees, allowing the Pantopaque to collect in the dependent angle cistern. The table is returned to horizontal position, and the patient's head is turned about 45 degrees to the side. A series of Polytome films are taken through the internal auditory canal. The authors do not recommend the study for tumors believed to be of moderate or large size.

Pantopaque cisternography has become very popular and, until the advent of the CT scan, was considered by some to be the contrast procedure of choice for the evaluation of angle masses.[18,23,61] Good detail is readily obtained with relatively simple radiographic equipment. It is the only contrast study at present that will demonstrate small intracanalicular masses. Though Olivecrona reported no intracanalicular masses in his series of 415 acoustic tumors, some are mentioned in more recent reports.[44,60] Of interest here is the finding by Hardy and Crowe of four histologically verified acoustic tumors in 250 temporal bones from consecutive autopsies.[22] On the other hand, Baker and Reese reported in 1968 to the Radiological Society of North America on 10 patients in whom the internal auditory canals did not fill but who did not have acoustic tumors, showing that a canal that does not completely fill is not necessarily pathological.[3]

Though Pantopaque is generally considered a reasonably safe contrast medium, there are numerous reports describing arachnoiditis following its use.[14,40,41,52,59] This possibility may be of somewhat

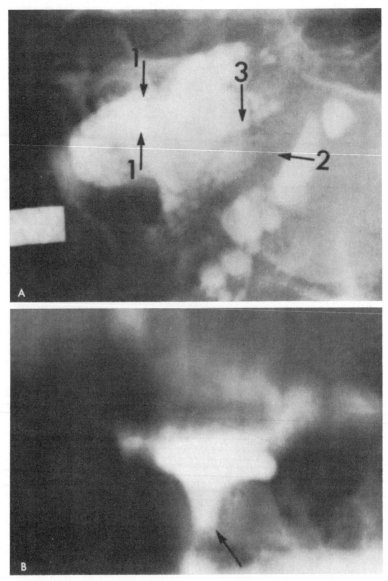

Figure 93–7   Pantopaque cisternogram, using a smaller amount of contrast medium than in Figure 93–4. *A*. Left cerebellopontine cistern. Fingerlike projection of Pantopaque into the internal auditory canal (1) was barely visible on original film. Basilar (2) and anterior inferior cerebellar (3) arteries are shown. *B*. Horizontal tomogram demonstrates good filling of the left internal auditory canal (*arrow*).

Illustration continued on opposite page

greater concern in cisternography than in routine myelography, considering that spillage of Pantopaque above the posterior fossa in cisternography is not rare. Pantopaque gives less information than air contrast does whether the tumor mass is large or small. The best results are obtained by combining air with computed tomography and taking overlapping views.

Vertebral Angiography

Numerous angiographic changes have been described related to pontocerebellar

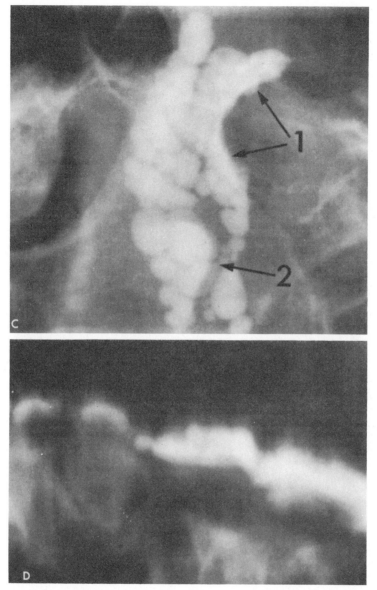

Figure 93–7 (*continued*)   *C*. Right cerebellopontine cistern. Pantopaque outlines medial border of small acoustic neuroma (1). Tortuous artery (2) is right vertebral. *D*. Lateral laminagram of the right cistern (not really needed) again showing lack of canal filling.

angle tumors. In his first report of vertebral angiography by catheterization in 1947, Radner showed an illustration that demonstrated the superior displacement of arterial branches by an acoustic tumor.[48] Most accounts have emphasized the displacement of the superior cerebellar artery. Olsson described the catheter vertebral angiograms of 14 proved acoustic neuromas, 13 of which showed superior displacement of the superior cerebellar artery and 9 of which showed small vessels encompassing the tumor.[45] Leman and co-workers distinguished two types of displacement of the superior cerebellar artery.[36] In the first, the initial segment of the artery is straightened and elevated. In the second, a longer and more distal segment of the vessel passing around the brain stem is displaced toward the midline (Fig. 93–8). Khilnani and Silverstein emphasized that superior displacement of the first portion of the superior cerebellar artery is highly suggestive of an extra-axial mass.[31]

Large neoplasms may result in posterior and contralateral displacement of the cephalic loops of the posterior inferior cerebellar arteries and the inferior portions of their vermian branches (Fig. 93–8). These displacements may occasionally be more prominent than those of the superior cerebellar artery.

The significance of displacement of the anterior inferior cerebellar artery was emphasized by Takahashi and co-workers.[58] This vessel is best evaluated on subtraction

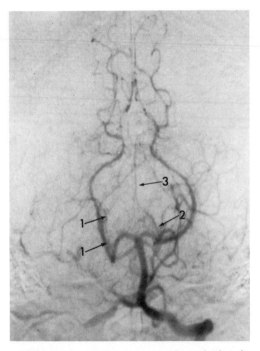

Figure 93–8 Subtraction print of vertebral angiogram, half-axial projection. A large right acoustic neuroma has displaced the right superior cerebellar artery (1) and low-lying right posterior cerebral artery medially. The cephalic loop and inferior vermian branch (2) of the left posterior inferior cerebellar artery are displaced to the left, but the superior continuation of the vermian artery returns to the midline (3).

prints of straight anteroposterior films, rather than the routine half-axial projection (Figs. 93–9 and 93–10). These paired arteries originate from the basilar artery at the junction of its middle and lowest thirds and pass laterally and slightly downward within the pontocerebellar angle cistern. The trunk vessel divides into the lateral branch, which loops around the flocculus and passes laterally to give branches to the middle cerebellar peduncle and cerebellar hemisphere, and the medial branch, which passes downward on the medial and anterior border of the cerebellar hemisphere. Takahashi found displacements of the cisternal segment of the anterior inferior cerebellar artery in 9 of 14 angle tumors of various types. The majority of displacements were superior, though inferior displacements and simple straightening were also seen. Cerebellar and pontine masses may produce similar displacements of this vessel, though much less frequently.

Atkinson's study of patients who died following removal of acoustic neuromas points out another value of evaluating the anterior inferior cerebellar artery preoperatively.[1] He found that occlusion of this vessel resulting in lateral pontine infarction was an important cause of postoperative death, particularly when the artery was larger than usual. There tends to be an inverse relationship between the sizes of the anterior inferior cerebellar and the ipsilateral posterior inferior cerebellar arteries. Vertebral angiography is the best means of demonstrating these congenital variations and the position of the displaced anterior inferior cerebellar artery, facts of importance to the neurosurgeon.

Changes in the course and degree of opacification of the petrosal vein and its tributaries are usually the earliest detectable signs of angle tumors on vertebral angiograms (Figs. 93–11 and 93–12B). The petrosal vein is a short trunk that originates just posterior and cephalad to the root of the fifth nerve, then runs anterolaterally through the angle cistern to enter the superior petrosal sinus, usually just above and lateral to the porus of the internal auditory canal. It receives tributaries from all directions. Some of the major tributaries are the transverse pontine vein medially, the branchial vein and anastomotic mesencephalic vein superomedially, and the cerebellar

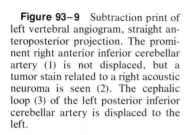

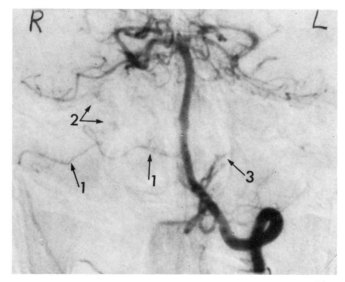

Figure 93–9 Subtraction print of left vertebral angiogram, straight anteroposterior projection. The prominent right anterior inferior cerebellar artery (1) is not displaced, but a tumor stain related to a right acoustic neuroma is seen (2). The cephalic loop (3) of the left posterior inferior cerebellar artery is displaced to the left.

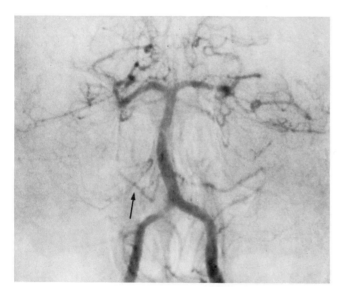

Figure 93–10 Subtraction print of vertebral angiogram, straight anteroposterior projection. The right anterior inferior cerebellar artery (*arrow*) is displaced superiorly and medially.

Figure 93–11 Venous phase of vertebral angiogram, half-axial projection. The left petrosal vein (1), just above and lateral to the internal auditory canal, is well seen. No filling of the right petrosal vein is visible. Patient had a large right acoustic neuroma. The circummesencephalic veins (2) outline the cerebral peduncles.

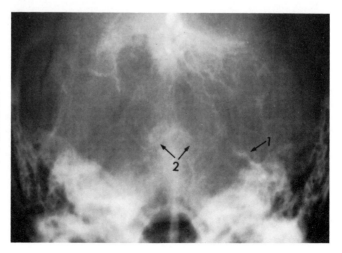

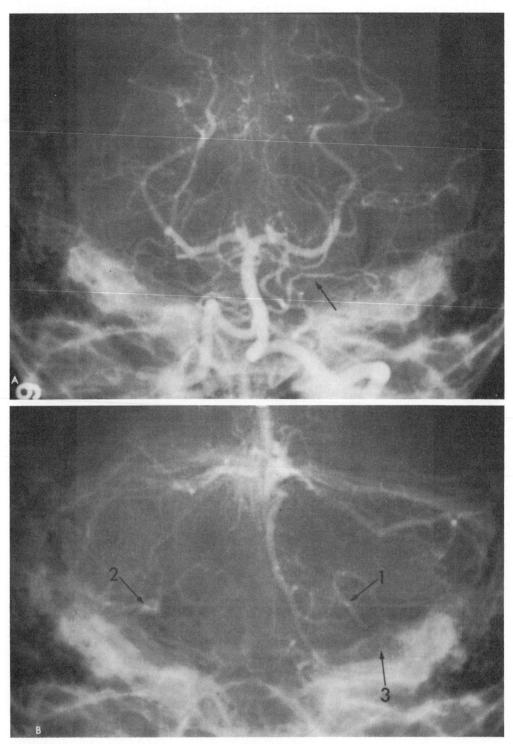

Figure 93–12   Left acoustic neuroma. *A*. Left vertebral arteriogram, modified half-axial projection. The only abnormality is the superior displacement (*arrow*) of the left anterior inferior cerebellar artery. *B*. Same projection as *A*, venous phase. The left petrosal vein (1) is stretched and elevated relative to the normal right petrosal vein (2). Note the close relationship of the left petrosal vein to the internal auditory canal (3).

Illustration continued on opposite page

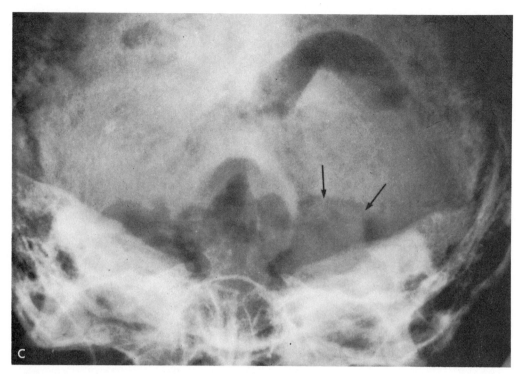

Figure 93-12 (*continued*) *C.* Pneumoencephalogram, same patient, similar projection. Air caps the tumor (*arrows*).

hemisphere veins laterally.[57] Takahashi and associates observed that of 11 patients with angle masses, 6 showed displacement or compression of the petrosal vein and 5 showed poor or no filling of that vessel on the side of the mass. These changes too are not specific for angle masses, but occur less frequently from tumors elsewhere in the posterior fossa. Reflux into the contralateral vertebral artery with resultant filling of both posterior inferior cerebellar arteries commonly occurs in selective catheter studies and is necessary if the degree of filling of the petrosal veins is to be evaluated.

The values of vertebral angiography in providing information regarding the location of the tumor in the presence of anatomical variations have been described. A third reason for doing this study is to rule out vascular lesions presenting as masses.

Pneumoencephalography

Filtered air (or oxygen) is generally regarded to be the least noxious contrast medium used intracranially. Dissatisfaction with the pneumoencephalogram in the diagnosis of angle masses in the past has been related to the relatively slight contrast obtained with air and the consequent difficulty in appreciating cerebellopontine angle cistern anatomy. The use of anteroposterior tomography of the posterior fossa during pneumoencephalography has largely corrected this defect of visualization, making this technique the most valuable study for most cerebellopontine angle tumors. The main defect of the air study is that tumors confined within the internal auditory canal cannot be detected.

Filling of the pontocerebellar angle cisterns by air can usually be accomplished with the head well flexed and by adding small increments of air and withdrawing enough cerebrospinal fluid to lower the fluid level below the clivus. If this is unsuccessful, air may be injected with the head extended, after which the head is again flexed and serial tomograms are obtained. If one angle cistern still does not fill, air is injected with the head inclined so that the side in question is high. If tomography continues to show failure of filling of that pontocerebellar cistern, a lesion can generally be assumed to be present.

The pneumoencephalographic findings

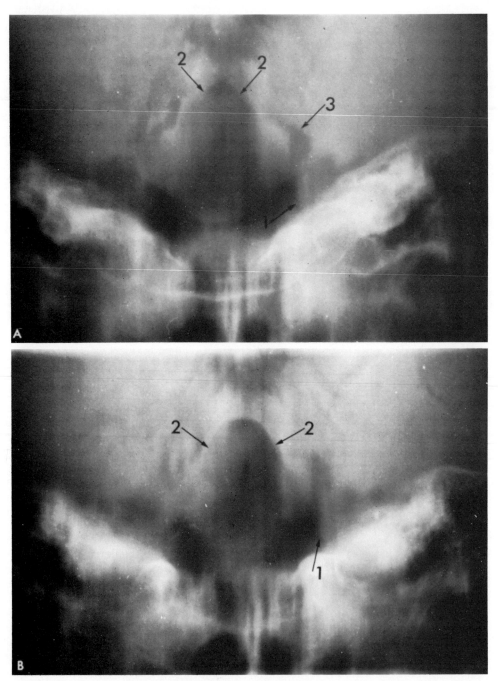

Figure 93–13 *A.* Anteroposterior laminagram through level of internal auditory canals. Air caps the medial margin (1) of the left acoustic neuroma. Note the good filling by air of the right angle cistern. The walls of the superior fourth ventricle (2) appear undisplaced. The left ambient cistern (3) is slightly widened by the tumor in comparison with the opposite side. *B.* This laminagram, at a plane 1 cm caudad to the former, shows no displacement of the fourth ventricle (2) by the small tumor (1).

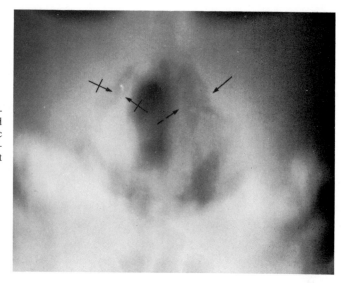

Figure 93–14 Anteroposterior laminagram at level of junction of pons and mesencephalon. This larger left acoustic neuroma markedly widens the left ambient cistern (*plain arrows*) relative to that of the opposite side.

are dependent upon the size of the angle mass. A small tumor about the porus acusticus may be completely capped with air. Larger neoplasms are occasionally completely capped (Fig. 93–12C), but more commonly only the medial surface of the tumor is seen (Fig. 93–13). As the mass size increases, the ventral-lateral surface of the pons is flattened and the angle and medullary cisterns adjacent to the mass are enlarged. The ambient cistern on the side of the mass may be dilated and the opposite may be compressed (Fig. 93–14). Contralateral displacement and rotation of the fourth ventricle so that its base faces the mass eventually occurs (Fig. 93–15). Pos-

terior displacement of the fourth ventricle that is recognizable on lateral films occurs only with quite large tumors. Marked aqueductal displacement and elevation of the posterior third ventricle indicate extension of the mass upward through the tentorial notch. The superior surface of the mass may sometimes be visible on lateral tomograms.

Other Angle Masses

Other types of cerebellopontine angle masses may be impossible to differentiate from acoustic tumors. Suspicion of their presence is usually aroused by an unusual

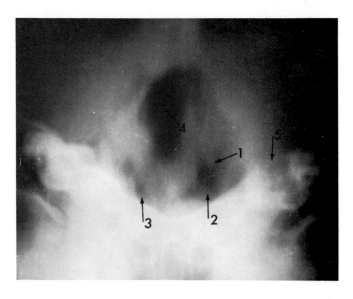

Figure 93–15 Anteroposterior laminagram through level fourth ventricle. This large left acoustic neuroma (1) has displaced the brain stem to the right, widening the left pontomedullary cistern (2) and narrowing the right (3). The fourth ventricle (4) is displaced to the right and rotated. The left internal auditory canal (5) is destroyed.

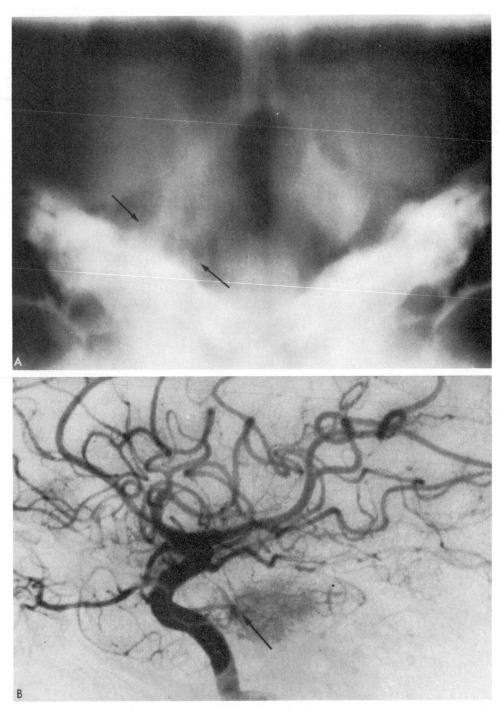

Figure 93–16   Meningioma involving upper right angle cistern. *A*. Anteroposterior laminagram just cephalad to plane of internal auditory canals shows mass (*arrows*) in right angle cistern. Midline structures were not displaced. *B*. Subtraction print of selective right internal carotid arteriogram, later view. An enlarged tentorial branch arising from the cavernous portion of the carotid artery supplied the tumor stain of the meningioma.

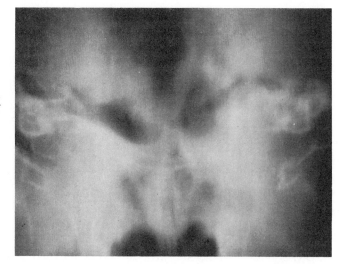

Figure 93–17 Chordoma. Antero-posterior laminagram through level of pons shows marked destruction of the left petrous bone by a mass that is growing upward into the left cerebellopontine angle cistern and elevating the left ventrolateral pons.

clinical presentation and may be substantiated radiologically by angiography or pneumoencephalography.

The most important differentiation is between a vascular abnormality and a tumor. Jannetta and his co-workers, describing two patients who had posterior fossa aneurysms, listed several findings that aroused suspicion of vascular lesions.[26] These included sharp delineation of the lesion, obliteration of the lateral recess of the fourth ventricle, little shift of the fourth ventricle and vallecula, normal filling of the ventricular system, and lack of cerebellar tonsilar herniation. The similarity of these findings to those of other extra-axial posterior fossa masses points out the advisability of performing vertebral angiography in diagnosis of extra-axial masses of all types.

Meningiomas of the cerebellopontine angle may be suspected when there is erosion of the petrous bone away from the porus and particularly when there is local hyperostosis. Calcification of the mass also suggests meningioma. Carotid angiography may demonstrate an enlarged tentorial branch, confirming the diagnosis (Fig. 93–16).

Metastatic tumors to the angle may show any of the signs already listed. There often are bone erosions away from the porus acusticus, which may suggest meningioma, but no characteristic stain is seen on the angiogram. The correct diagnosis frequently is made only at the time of operation.

The marked destruction of the petrous bone shown in Figure 93–17 may suggest a malignant tumor, but the four-year history would not be consistent with that diagnosis. A chordoma was found at operation. The lateral laminagram of another patient demonstrates the mottled air pattern characteristic of cholesteatoma (Fig. 93–18).

The patient in Figure 93–19 had multiple unilateral cranial nerve deficits suggesting an angle mass. Pantopaque studies showed thinning of the contrast collection in the right angle, but the canal filled. The laminagram obtained at the time of pneumoencephalography showed a pontine tumor bulging into the angle.

Selection of Studies

In summary, plain films and laminagrams of the petrous bone should be obtained whenever a pontocerebellar angle mass is suspected. The choice of further tests depends upon the clinical presentation.

The computed tomographic scan of the posterior fossa, with enhancing contrast of an appropriate intravenous iodine compound, using a 320 matrix and rapid scanning times, and centered at the internal auditory canal would be the next radiological procedure of choice. It should probably include a general 160-matrix scan of the supratentorial regions to try to find other related or unrelated and separate pathological entities as well as acoustic tumors.

If a small acoustic tumor is suggested but not adequately detailed by a CT scan, an air contrast CT scan is the next procedure of choice. If clinical findings suggest exten-

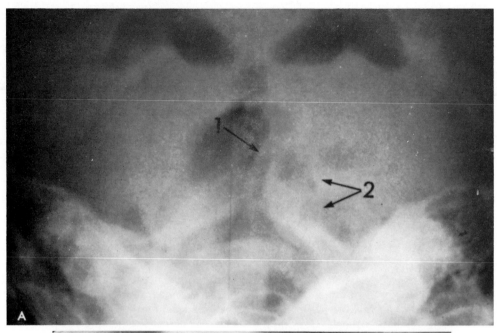

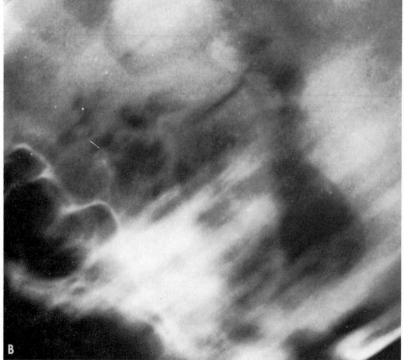

Figure 93–18   Epidermoid tumor. *A*. Fourth ventricle (1) is displaced by large angle mass, in which accumulations of air (2) are seen. *B*. Lateral laminagram clearly shows characteristic "bubbly" appearance.

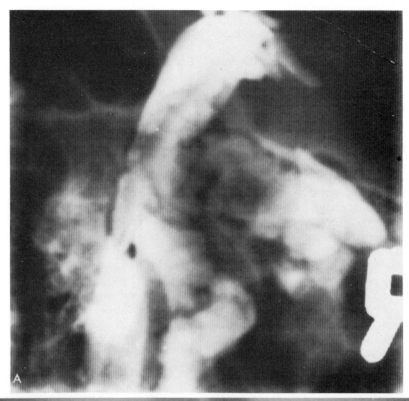

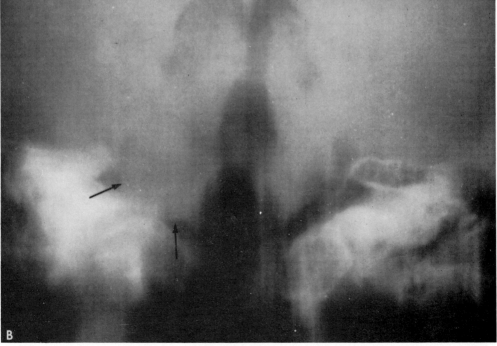

Figure 93–19   Pontine glioma invading angle cistern. *A.* The layer of Pantopaque in the midportion of the right angle cistern is thinned. *B.* Anteroposterior laminagram through level of internal auditory canals shows mass invading right angle cistern. The mass (*arrows*) seems broader superiorly, consistent with its pontine origin.

sion of the mass beyond the canal, air enhanced computed tomography is more informative. Vertebral angiography is possibly advisable before operative treatment of all but the very small cerebellopontine angle tumors, especially to rule out aneurysms and study the potential collateral circulation of the brain stem between the posterior and anterior inferior cerebellar arteries.

POSTERIOR FOSSA TRANSMEATAL OPERATION

Whether a person found to be harboring an acoustic tumor should, therefore, have an immediate operation, or perhaps should never have operative treatment is a question taken up in the discussion at the end of this chapter. At the moment the authors would like to review briefly the background and operative technique of the procedure that is believed to be most suitable to patients suffering from this benign and yet deadly neoplasm.

The suboccipital transmeatal operation is Dandy's original acoustic tumor operation as modified by Rand and Kurze. It allows not only total removal of all acoustic tumors regardless of size but also the possibility of preserving function of uninvolved cochlear, vestibular, and facial nerves (Figs. 93–20 and 93–21).[49,50] This is accomplished by a microsurgical dissection of the internal auditory canal after the posterior wall has been removed by diamond drill re-section under the binocular operating microscope.

This suboccipital transmeatal technique has a number of advantages over the middle fossa and translabyrinthine approaches used by otologists. These include a wide field of operative action; direct visualization of the anterior inferior cerebellar artery and other brain stem arteries; identification of the acoustic tumor prior to risk of damage of the facial nerve, the labyrinth, and the cochlear systems; dissection of all surfaces of the acoustic tumor always under direct vision; and finally direct facial nerve anastomosis and reconstruction of the facial nerve with a nerve graft if or when necessary.

A review of the surgical principles and major steps of the suboccipital transmeatal operation is worthwhile. The supine and semilateral positions of the patient can be used and may indeed be indicated in a particular situation. Rand has consistently used a semisitting posture and pin fixation of the head to immobilize the patient rigidly. The major advantage of this position for a unilateral suboccipital approach is that the cerebrospinal fluid and blood drain away from the site of dissection, thus allowing continually good visualization of the tumor and its relationship to the brain stem arteries. The disadvantages include the risk of air embolism and hypotension. He has used both the American Sterilizer table and the Gardner chair, preferring the latter because it allows the surgeon to come closer

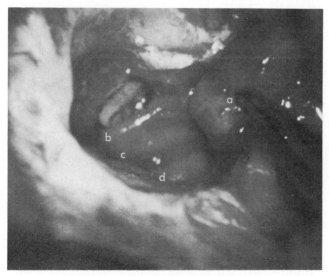

Figure 93–20 Left internal auditory canal unroofed, exposing the acoustic tumor (a) being lifted out of the canal and away from the facial nerve (c), cochlear nerve (d), and uninvolved vestibular nerve (b). Function of the facial and vestibular nerves was retained postoperatively.

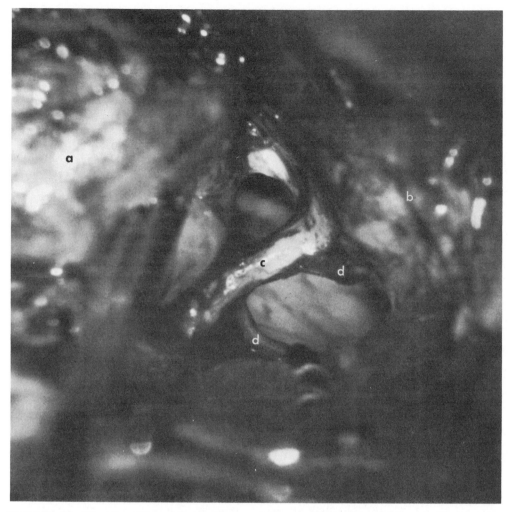

Figure 93-21 Dissection of large left acoustic tumor (a) from brain stem (b) under the operating microscope. Note preserved facial nerve (c) and anterior inferior cerebellar artery (d).

to the operative field with the patient in a sitting posture.[17]

The usual diuretic agents, including either intravenous urea or mannitol, and intravenous dexamethasone are given at the beginning of the operation. Blood is administered as required to replace loss in order to maintain a systolic pressure above 100 mm of mercury. The maintenance of normal blood pressure is essential to prevent infarction of the brain stem and can be assisted by using Gardner's modified G-suit or wrapping the legs with Ace bandages or both. The preoperative positioning of a venous catheter in the right side of the heart is now done in all cases to allow removal of any air embolus. Expired alveolar carbon dioxide is continually monitored as an early indicator of embolization into the venous system. In addition, ultrasonic monitoring of the cardiac sounds is used as another sensitive technique to detect quite small air emboli.

In the past hypothermia was used, but has been abandoned by this author because of its potential for causing cardiac irregularities and because with the patient in this particular sitting posture, cardiac resuscitation is difficult. The results of French and colleagues, however, using bretylium to prevent cardiac irregularity with cooling of the body core to 26° to 28° C, would encourage one to resume the use of hypothermia in certain selected cases, particularly when large tumors make brain stem compression and possible ischemia more likely to occur.[16]

For suboccipital craniectomy a unilateral

inverted J-shaped incision is made and the bone is removed between the mastoid and the foramen magnum until the floor of the posterior fossa is horizontal. It is then elevated superiorly to expose the lateral sinus. It may be necessary in certain patients with herniation of the cerebellar tonsil to resect the lateral wall of the foramen magnum and the arch of the atlas.

The dura is incised either in a cruciate or curvilinear manner to expose the cerebellar lobe, which generally is loose in the posterior fossa as a result of the diuretic agents. A self-retaining retractor over cottonoid sponges or regular and mini-sized Rand neuropledgets* elevates the lobe superiorly, exposing the tumor in the cerebellopontine angle. The superior cerebellar veins should be carefully preserved in order to reduce cerebellar lobe swelling in the immediate postoperative period. Resection of the lateral portion of the cerebellar lobe is not necessary for small and medium-sized tumors but may be indicated for large tumors.

As the cerebellar lobe is being elevated at the beginning of the exposure of the cerebellopontine angle, in the subarachnoid space the lower cranial nerves are freed from the acoustic tumor and covered with a mini-sized neuropledget or a strip of thin rubber sheeting and then a cottonoid sponge (Fig. 93–22). This dissection is generally done under the binocular operating microscope. Attention is then directed to the porus acusticus. The dura is coagulated along the posterior wall of the petrous bone and then resected; the jugular sinus must be avoided. The diamond and cutting drill dissection is done by an air turbine or electric drill, starting at the edge of the porus acusticus and working laterally (Fig. 93–23). The further lateralward the bone resection is done, the deeper the bone channel because of the anatomical position of the internal auditory canal in the petrous bone. The canal must be opened widely, leaving no overlapping edges either superiorly or inferiorly, and extending laterally to the transverse bar. Care must be exercised not to open the labyrinth system. If air cells in the petrous bone are opened by the drill dissection they must be sealed with bone wax

* Surgeon's International Inc., Los Angeles, California.

or muscle before wound closure to avoid cerebrospinal otorrhea.

Once the canal is opened, the acoustic tumor resection is commenced at the lateral extreme. These neoplasms originate either from the superior or inferior vestibular nerve. Characteristically the facial nerve is located anteriorly and superiorly in the canal and has a white glistening appearance. The anesthesiologist must watch the patient's facial muscles during this portion of the tumor section and inform the surgeon of any changes so that he may avoid excessive traction on the facial nerve. Bipolar stimulation for identification of the facial nerve is an important adjunct during operation. As Greenwood pointed out, extreme care must be taken not to stimulate the spinal accessory nerve with unipolar current, as it may cause violent shoulder movements that will change the patient's position on the operating table.[21]

It is important to free the acoustic tumor capsule completely from the facial nerve in the subarachnoid space at and beyond the porus acusticus toward the brain stem. This is best done by sharp microdissection. In large tumors this may be a bit tedious because the capsule often becomes attached to the dura along the lateral wall of the posterior fossa. If this dissection is not done immediately after the internal auditory canal is cleared of the tumor, however, the surgeon will find it more difficult to preserve the facial nerve at the completion of the dissection of the capsule from the brain stem.

The uninvolved vestibular and cochlear nerves may also be preserved during the resection of small tumors within the internal auditory canal, also staying within the subarachnoid space (see Fig. 93–20). It is essential to preserve the internal auditory artery if cochlear function is to be maintained. Rand has preserved the uninvolved vestibular nerve in two patients and the cochlear nerve in two patients. Kurze has described the preservation of the cochlear nerve in a third case in which the suboccipital transmeatal operative approach was used.[35,49]

Internal decompression of small acoustic tumors is generally unnecessary (Fig. 93–24). In tumors of larger size, internal decompression is required in order to provide adequate operative exposure of the junc-

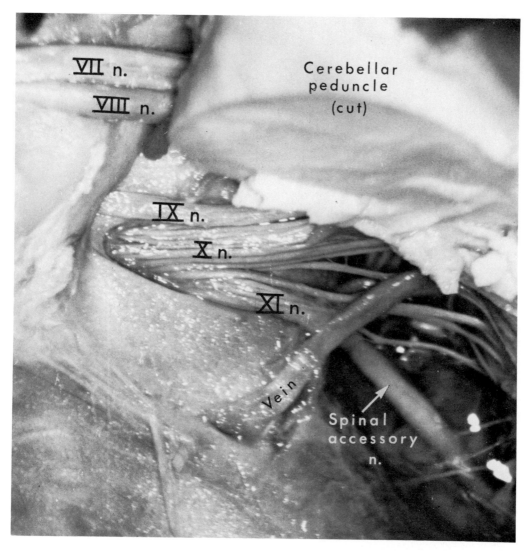

Figure 93–22 Anatomical dissection of cerebellopontine angle as seen under the binocular operating microscope. Note the relation of cranial nerve VII to cranial nerve VIII as seen from the posterior fossa approach.

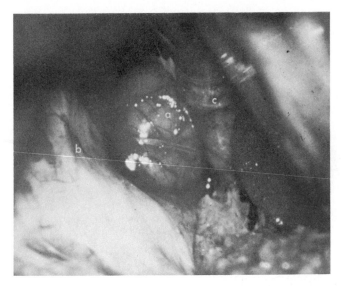

Figure 93–23   Small acoustic tumor (a) in left cerebellopontine angle protruding from porus acusticus (b) and beginning to compress cerebellum (c).

tion between the mesial aspect of the neoplasm and the brain stem. This part of the operation can be accomplished by suction and curettage, an Urban rotodissector, or, with quite firm tumors, the use of an electrosurgical loop.

The dissection of the acoustic tumor from the brain stem is the most hazardous and delicate phase of the suboccipital transmeatal operation. Attention is first directed to the angle between the lower pole of the tumor and the medulla oblongata. The lower cranial nerves that were previously dissected free from the tumor capsule and

covered with thin layers of rubber dam and cottonoid sponge mini neuropledgets are left undisturbed. A small spatula type of dissector is used to elevate the tumor laterally from the brain stem and arachnoid, which are then gently teased off the mesial surface of the tumor. Those arteries that pass directly into the tumor capsule are coagulated with low bipolar current, using a straight or bayonettype Gerald fine-tipped forceps. Rather than tear the coagulated artery from the capsule, it is preferable to cut it with microscissors.

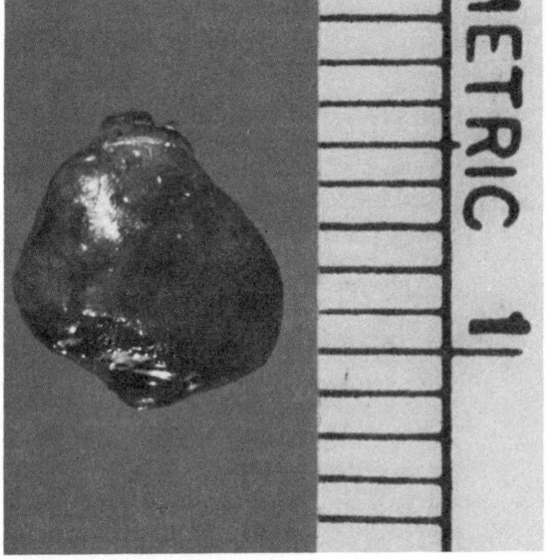

This dissection procedure is repeated until the tumor is freed from the brain stem. The author has found it dangerous to leave cottonoid sponges along the brain stem because they may be quite difficult to remove from this position at the time of closure even when copious amounts of irrigation fluid are used. If cottonoid sponges are to be left in place for any length of time they should be covered with thin rubber sheets or mini neuropledgets. Suction during this dissection must be done with great care. The hole in the suction-irrigation tip should not be covered lest it damage a small brain stem arteriole. The irrigation is useful because it prevents small blood clots from forming and obscuring the plane of dissection as seen under the operating microscope.

The anterior inferior cerebellar artery and its branches constitute one of the most critical sources of blood to the lateral aspect of the brain stem. Damage to this and

Figure 93–24   Small acoustic tumor excision completed as demonstrated in Figure 93–23.

related arteries invariably causes brain stem infarction and usually death of the patient. The anterior inferior cerebellar artery gives several branches to the tumor, however, which can be safely coagulated and cut without harm to the brain stem by using a bipolar coagulation system and microscissors (see Fig. 93–21).

The cochlear and the uninvolved vestibular nerves can be identified and preserved by microdissection in small and even in some medium-sized tumors. They may never function, however, because of impairment of their blood supply. Nevertheless, they should be sought and an effort made to dissect them from the tumor. In medium-sized and large tumors the components of the auditory nerve are totally involved by tumor.

The facial nerve may lie either superiorly or inferiorly to the anterior inferior cerebellar artery. Either structure is a guide to the other, but generally the operator comes on the anterior inferior cerebellar artery before the facial nerve. The tumor capsule is gently lifted away from the seventh nerve with a suction tip on a cottonoid pledget. A Rosen knife curet will then allow sharp dissection to the point where the nerve was previously freed from the tumor capsule during the transmeatal portion of the resection. The nerve is carefully covered with a thin rubber sheet (Figs. 93–25, 93–26, 93–27, and 93–28). Attention is then directed to the region of the trigeminal nerve.

In large acoustic tumors that have passed superiorly through the incisura it may be necessary to open the tentorium to free this portion of the tumor. Generally, with adequate internal decompression this step is not needed. The petrosal vein may be troublesome during this part of the cerebellopontine angle dissection of large tumors; usually it can be dissected from the capsule without requiring coagulation. Its preservation is important to reduce cerebellar swelling following operation.

When total removal of the acoustic tumor is not possible because of the anatomical relationship of the residual tumor fragments to the brain stem, its blood supply, or regional cranial nerves, a cryosurgical technique may be used to freeze repeatedly and thus destroy these small fragments of tumor tissue. It is necessary to take the temperature to below $-60°$ C in order to achieve this result. Often it is necessary to use temperatures in the range of -80 to $-90°$ C and to make multiple overlapping lesions.

The margin between the ice and normal tissue is very precise and can be seen clearly under the operating microscope. In this way the fragment of tumor attached to the brain stem and its associated vessels can be destroyed and left in place to be phagocytized. A carbon dioxide laser can also vaporize small fragments.

In small and medium-sized tumors the dura of the posterior fossa is closed carefully after a thorough search of the wound for neuropledgets and bleeding points. Hemostasis should be assured with the blood pressure at normotensive levels. Either the dura is left open or a dural graft is used to allow for the inevitable swelling of the cerebellar lobe with large tumors and prolonged cerebellar retraction. The head is then extended and the wound closed in anatomical layers.

POSTOPERATIVE CARE

Postoperative care following removal of an acoustic neuroma is virtually identical to that for patients who have undergone a posterior fossa operation for resection of another type of tumor. The prevention of massive cerebellar swelling and brain stem infarction in acoustic tumor resection depends primarily upon gentle intraoperative manipulation and the preservation of these vital structures. Mild edema is controlled by head elevation, a 7- to 10-day course of dexamethasone in large doses, and limited intravenous hydration.

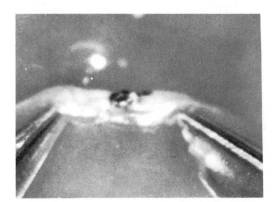

Figure 93–25 End-to-end anastomosis of the facial nerve after resection of a segment of nerve found to be involved by large acoustic tumor.

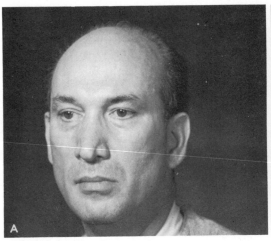
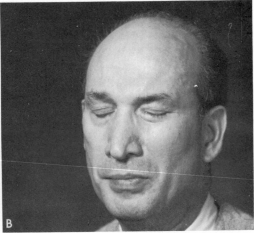

Figure 93–26 *A* and *B*. Left facial movements restored to near normal after direct intracranial anastomosis of facial nerve involved by acoustic tumor.

The resection of an acoustic neuroma puts the fifth, seventh, and tenth cranial nerves at risk. Transient dysfunction of the vagus nerve will cause dysphagia and potential aspiration of fluid and food. In such patients, pharyngeal function must be evaluated carefully before oral fluids are instituted. If severe or permanent disability occurs, which would be rare indeed, esophagostomy and tracheostomy may be necessary.

The ipsilateral anesthetic cornea, unprotected by lid closure owing to facial palsy,

may develop keratitis; therefore mediolateral tarsorrhaphy is indicated. The facial nerve, although anatomically intact, may take as long as 18 months to regain sufficient function to close the lid. Additional care will include daily facial massage and electrical stimulation. If corneal sensation remains intact and facial paresis appears transient, then simpler measures may be used to protect the involved eye.

Direct intracranial reconstruction can be performed when the facial nerve has been transected because of severe stretching or

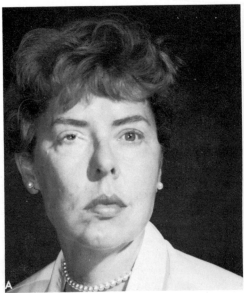
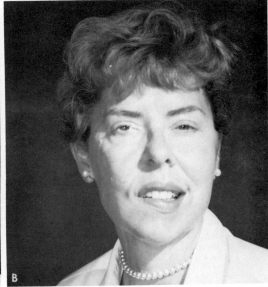

Figure 93–27 *A* and *B*. Right facial movements partially returned 13 months after direct intracranial anastomosis of facial nerve fragmented by massive acoustic tumor.

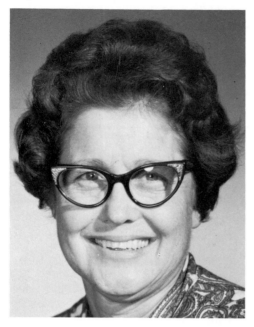

Figure 93–28 Patient's normal facial expression and movements immediately after transmeatal microdissection and removal of moderate-size left acoustic neuroma with preservation of the facial nerve.

tumor invasion. This has been accomplished in several of the authors' patients. Facial movement returned by 16 months after operation in the first case, and the patient achieved almost normal use within four years. In the second case, motor activity became evident within seven months and was normal two and a half years later. In the event that intracranial reconstruction is precluded by a significant loss of the seventh nerve, more classic repair may be accomplished by the hypoglossal anastomosis or by cable grafting. In the latter method, a segment of transected sural nerve is anastomosed to the proximal stump of the previously severed facial nerve. The remainder of the graft is brought out through the craniotomy and stored in a subcutaneous tunnel overlying the mastoid region. After a sufficient period has elapsed to allow adequate regeneration, the distal end of the graft is removed from the tunnel and united with a distal portion of the facial nerve as it exits from the stylomastoid foramen, by passing the petrous portion of the facial nerve.

Postoperative problems may also include a cerebrospinal fluid fistula. The condition should be treated immediately by elevating the head, daily lumbar punctures, and the giving of prophylactic antibiotics to avoid meningitis. If this type of therapy proves unsuccessful, operative closure of the middle ear with small pieces of muscle, especially of the opening of the eustachian tube, will be necessary because the leak is usually through this tube.

Increased intracranial pressure in the early postoperative period will be heralded by a change in the level of consciousness or the vital signs, or both. The cause may be a hematoma, which would require immediate reopening of the wound, or it may involve obstructive hydrocephalus, which would require a decompressive shunt. These conditions can be well visualized on a CT brain scan.

RESULTS OF OPERATION

The techniques described were employed by the authors to treat 140 patients between 1964 and 1980.

Although a significant number of these (90 per cent) had radiologically and intraoperatively verified medium- or large-sized acoustic neuromas, the outcome was superior to that obtained with other operative techniques.

Smaller tumors (less than 2 cm) were totally removed and there was complete physiological preservation of the facial nerve in 100 per cent of cases. Half of this group of patients evidenced some residual function in both superior and inferior vestibular nerves postoperatively.

Although 95 per cent of those patients with medium-sized lesions (2 to 4 cm) underwent complete eradication of the tumors, 80 per cent showed no subsequent facial weakness. Included in this category was one patient whose seventh nerve had to be sacrificed because of direct involvement by a 4 cm acoustic neuroma. Intracranial anastomosis was performed, and normal function returned within 30 months. A small number of patients (10 per cent), although the facial nerve appeared intraoperatively to be anatomically intact, eventually suffered a partial loss of voluntary facial motor activity; in an equal number (10 per cent) the loss was complete.

In those individuals with large neuromas (greater than 4 cm), complete tumor extirpation was performed in 93 per cent of cases. Postoperatively the physiological function was normal in 32 per cent and slightly paretic in 50 per cent of patients. Fewer than 18 per cent did experience complete and irreversible facial paralysis. Four of these patients showed some evidence of motor activity, but they died of complications in the early postoperative course. The remaining few patients, who survived, had had massive tumors that had invaded and virtually obliterated the involved seventh nerve.

Thus 94 per cent of the 140 patients had complete resection of their acoustic neuromas. Following the operation, facial motor activity was normal in 60 per cent, and there were slight partial deficiencies in an additional 30 per cent of patients. In the 6 per cent of patients in whom complete resection was not possible, residual tumor tissue was destroyed by using cryosurgical techniques and leaving the small necrotic fragment in situ against the brain stem or other structure from which it could not be separated by micro-operative dissection. The overall mortality rate was 40 per cent, but all deaths occurred among those acous-

tic tumor patients who had neoplasms that were larger than 4 cm in size.

DISCUSSION

The binocular operating microscope has caused a re-evaluation of operation on brain tumors in the cerebellopontine angle, especially acoustic neuromas. Cushing noted that a translabyrinthine operation might one day become an accepted operative approach to small acoustic tumors more or less limited to the internal auditory canal (Fig. 93–29). This has been possible because of the development and use of the operating microscope. The Panse translabyrinthine approach, introduced in 1904, has been refined and used by House and his colleagues in the total removal of quite small acoustic tumors with preservation of the anatomical and functional integrity of the facial nerve in most cases.

This translabyrinthine operation is also employed by House and co-workers for moderate-sized acoustic tumors.[24,25] They have pointed out, however, that the separa-

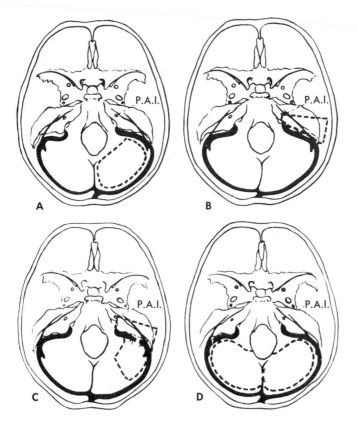

Figure 93–29 Operation for the exposure of the porus acusticus internus in acoustic tumors. *A*. Unilateral suboccipital approach. *B*. Translabyrinthine approach. *C*. Combined petrosal-occipital operation. *D*. Bilateral suboccipital operation. (From Cushing, H.: Tumors of the Nervus Acusticus and the Syndrome of the Cerebellopontine Angle. Philadelphia, W. B. Saunders Co., 1917.)

tion of the tumor from the brain stem still remains the most dangerous aspect of any of these (translabyrinthine) operations. In addition, it should be re-emphasized that this translabyrinthine approach does not allow preservation of hearing and creates the definite risk of cerebrospinal otorrhea with possible meningitis. The Rand-Kurze suboccipital transmeatal operation, in experienced hands, overcomes these disadvantages of the translabyrinthine operation.

The subtemporal extradural approach to the internal auditory canal is accomplished by a tedious diamond drill dissection between the semicircular canals and the cochlear system within the petrous bone. The removal of rather tiny intracanalicular tumors can be accomplished by this operation with preservation of the uninvolved facial and vestibular nerves, including at times the integrity of the cochlear nerve. However, a major question is raised: Should the tiny intracanalicular acoustic tumors be treated by operation at all? The surgeon must ask the basic question: Do the benefits of the operation, such as possibly preserving the residual hearing on the affected side, outweigh the potential hazards, including meningitis, brain hemorrhage, general anesthesia, sensitivity to drugs, and the like? It must be remembered that the growth, or lack of it, of these tiny intracanalicular tumors can be followed by repeated posterior fossa myelography and cisternography. Planographic x-rays of the internal auditory canal with only small amounts of Pantopaque are required to do this follow-up study. The risk of myelographic petrous laminagraphy is certainly less than that of any operation on the internal auditory canal, whether it be via the subtemporal, translabyrinthine, or posterior fossa approach. This is particularly true in middle-aged and older patients. An exception might be a youngster or young adult with rather good cochlear nerve function on the affected side. The Leksell gamma cobalt knife has now been used successfully to arrest or destroy small acoustic neuromas, and improved cochlear and vestibular nerve function has been achieved in about 30 to 50 per cent of a series of 32 cases.[35a]

On the other hand, neither a neurosurgeon nor an otological surgeon would like to have a tiny intracanalicular tumor become a massive acoustic neoplasm that caused brain stem failure, papilledema, and blindness. This can be avoided with proper follow-up neurological and roentgenographic studies in patients harboring these tiny tumors, provided they are educated to this point of view.

Once an acoustic tumor has broken out of the confines of the internal auditory canal and penetrated into the cerebellopontine angle, operation should be recommended for young and middle-aged patients because the benefit at this time would be worth the operative risk. Whether it should be done in patients over 60 years old depends on the general health of the patient and the rate of growth of the particular tumor. This can be determined by repeated pneumoencephalograms or, better, by CT enhanced scans with air contrast.

House and Hitselberger speak of a "system of operations" for acoustic tumors and have outlined their principles and criteria for gauging the effectiveness of a particular operative technique to be used in the management of acoustic tumors. These principles include: (1) avoidance of further cranial nerve damage, (2) adequate decompression of the posterior fossa, (3) avoidance of injury to the brain stem or cerebellum, (4) satisfactory access for the removal of the tumor, and (5) management of any postoperative complications.[23]

Although they recommend the translabyrinthine operations, they point out that the separation of the tumor from the brain stem still remains the most dangerous aspect of any of these operations. The authors of this chapter submit that the House-Hitselberger third surgical principle is difficult to accomplish by the translabyrinthine operation.

House and Hitselberger also point out that the middle fossa subtemporal approach gives very limited access to any area beyond the porus acusticus. Therefore, they conclude, "If operative or postoperative hemorrhage were to occur in the cerebellopontine angle, the limited access imposed by this procedure would be quite serious." In other words, this would be a violation of their surgical principles 2 and 4.

In order to fulfill their criteria and surgical principles, especially in large tumors, the combined suboccipital-petrosal operation was reintroduced by House and his associates. This is generally done in two stages with ligation of the sigmoid venous sinus and is a potential hazard to the venous drainage of the brain.

After 18 years' experience, the authors are convinced that the Rand-Kurze suboccipital transmeatal microsurgical operation satisfies all the surgical criteria and principles for successful removal of small, medium-sized, and large to massive acoustic tumors.

REFERENCES

1. Atkinson, W. J.: The anterior inferior cerebellar artery, J. Neurol. Neurosurg. Psychiat., *12*:137–151, 1949.
2. Baker, H. L., Jr.: Myelographic examination of the posterior fossa with positive contrast medium, Radiology, *81*:791–801, 1963.
3. Baker, H., and Reese, D. F.: Non-tumors of the C-P angle demonstrated by Pantopaque myelography. Presented to the 54th Annual Meeting of the Radiological Society of North America, December, 1968.
4. Ballance, C.: Some Points in the Surgery of the Brain and Its Membranes. London, Macmillan & Co., 1907. p 276.
5. Bell, C.: The Nervous System of the Human Body. London, 1830. Appendix of cases, pp. 112–114.
6. Borchardt, M.: Über Operationen in der hinteren Schädelgrube inkl. der operation von Tumoren des Kleinhirnbrückenwinkels. Arch. Klin Chir., *81*:386–432, 1906.
7. Carhart, R.: Clinical determination abnormal auditory adaptation. A.M.A. Arch. Otolaryng., *65*:32–39, 1957.
8. Cruveilhier, J.: Anatomie Pathologique du Corps Humain. Paris, 1835–1842, 2 part 26, pp. 1–8.
9. Cushing, H.: Tumors of the Nervus Acusticus and the Syndrome of the Cerebellopontine Angle. Philadelphia, W. B. Saunders Co., 1917.
10. Dandy, W. E.: Results of removal of acoustic tumors by the unilateral approach. A.M.A. Arch. Surg., *42*:1026–1033, 1941.
11. Davies, F. L.: Effect of unabsorbed radiographic contrast media in the central nervous system. Lancet, *2*:747–748, 1956.
12. Ebenius, B.: The result of examination of the petrous bone in auditory nerve tumors, Acta Radiol., *15*:284, 1934.
13. Eiselsberg, A.: Über die chirurgische Behandlung der Hirntumoren. Trans. Int. Cong. Med. Lond., 1913, Sec. VII, pp. 203–207.
14. Erickson, T. C., and van Baaren, H. J.: Late meningeal reaction to Pantopaque used in myelography (report of a case which terminated fatally). Trans. Amer. Neurol. Ass., *77*:134–135, 1952; J.A.M.A., *135*:636–639, 1953.
14a. Feldman, A., and Wilber, L.: Acoustic Impedance and Admittance. Baltimore, Williams & Wilkins Co., 1976.
15. Fowler, E. P.: Method for early detection of otosclerosis; study of sounds well above threshold. Arch. Otolaryng., *24*:731–741, 1936.
16. French, L. A., Chou, S. N., and Buckley, J. J.: Control of hypothermic cardiac irritability with bretylium. Presented at Amer. Assoc. Neurol. Surgeons, April 15, 1969, Cleveland.
17. Gardner, W. J.: A neurosurgical chair. J. Neurosurg., *12*:81–86, 1955.
18. Gass, H.: Pantopaque anterior basal cisternography of the posterior fossa. Amer. J. Roentgen., *90*:1197–1204, 1963.
19. Givre, H., and Olivecrona, H.: Surgical experiences with acoustic tumors. J. Neurosurg., 6:396–407, 1949.
20. Graf, K.: Geschwülste des Ohres und des Kleinhirnbrückenwinkels. Stuttgart, Georg Thieme Verlag, 1952.
21. Greenwood, J.: Personal communication, 1970.
22. Hardy, M., and Crowe, S. J.: Early asymptomatic acoustic tumor. Report of six cases. Arch. Surg., *32*:292–301, 1936.
23. Hitselberger, W. E., and House, W. F.: Polytome-Pantopaque: A technique for the diagnosis of small acoustic tumors. J. Neurosurg., *29*:214–217, 1968.
24. House, W. F.: Monograph I: Transtemporal bone microsurgical removal of acoustic neuromas. Arch. Otolaryng., *80*:597–756, 1964.
25. House, W. F.: Monograph II: Acoustic neuroma. Arch. Otolaryng., *88*:576–715, 1968.
26. Jannetta, P. J., Hanafee, W., Weidner, W., and Rosen, L.: Pneumoencephalographic findings suggesting aneurysm of the vertebral-basilar junction. J. Neurosurg., *24*:530–535, 1966.
27. Jerger, J. F.: Békésy audiometry in analysis of auditory disorders. J. Speech Hearing Res., *3*:275–287, 1960.
28. Jerger, J. F.: Recruitment and allied phenomena in differential diagnosis. J. Auditory Res., *2*:145, 1961.
29. Jerger, J. F.: Hearing tests in otologic diagnosis. ASHA *4*:5, 1962.
30. Jerger, J. F., Shedd, J., and Harford, E.: On the detection of extremely small changes in sound intensity. A.M.A. Arch. Otolaryng., *69*:200, 1959.
30a. Jewett, D. L., and Williston, J. S.: Auditory-evoked far fields averaged from the scalp of humans. Brain, *94*:681–696, 1971.
31. Khilnani, M., and Silverstein, A.: Displacement of the superior cerebellar artery. Arch. Neurol., *8*:502–505, 1963.
32. Krause, F.: Zur Freilegung der hinteren Felsenbeinfläche und des Kleinhirns. Beitr. Klin. Chir., *37*:728–764, 1905.
33. Krause, F.: Discussion of Eiselberg's paper. Trans. Int. Cong. Med. Lond., 1913, Sec. VIII, p. 214.
34. Kummel, W.: Otologische Gesichtspunkte bei der Diagnose und Therapie von Erkrankungen der hinteren Schädelgrube. Deutsch. A. Nervenheilk., *36*:132–142, 1909.
35. Kurze, T.: Personal communication, 1969.
35a. Leksell, L.: Personal communication, 1977.
36. Leman, P., Cohadon, F., and Leifer, C.: Valeur de l'artériographie vertébrale dans les tumeurs de l'angle ponto-cérébelleux. Ann. Radiol., *10*:791–802, 1967.

37. Leveque-Lasource, A.: Observation sur un amaurosis et un cophosis, avec perte ou diminution de la voix, des mouvements, etc, par suite de lésion organique apparente de plusieurs parties du cerveaux. J. Gen. Med. Chir. Pharm., *37*:368–373, 1810.

38. Linthicum, F. H., and Churchill, D.: Vestibular test results in acoustic neuroma cases. Arch. Otolaryng., *88*:604, 1968.

39. List, C. F.: Die operative Behandling der Acusticusneurinom. Arch. Klin. Chir., *171*:282–325, 1932.

40. Luce, J. C., Leith, W., and Burrage, W. S.: Pantopaque meningitis due to hypersensitivity. Radiology, *57*:878–881, 1951.

41. Mason, M. S., and Raaf, J.: Complications of Pantopaque myelography; case report and review. J. Neurosurg., *19*:302–311, 1962.

42. McKenzie, K. G., and Alexander, E., Jr.: Acoustic neuroma. Clin. Neurosurg., *2*:21–36, 1955.

43. Nelson, J. R.: The minimal ice water caloric test. Neurology, *19*:577–585, 1969.

44. Olivecrona, H.: Acoustic tumors. J. Neurosurg., *16*:6–13, 1967.

44a. Olsen, W., and Noffsinger, D.: Comparison of one new and three old tests of auditory adaptation. Arch. Otolaryng. (Chicago), *99*:94–99, 1974.

45. Olsson, O.: On technique of the lumbar pneumomyelography. Acta Radiol., *29*:107–111, 1948.

46. Panse, R.: Ein Gliom des Akustikus. Arch Ohrenheilk., *61*:251–255, 1904.

46a. Picton, T. W., Hillyard, S. A., Krausz, H. I., and Galambos, R.: Human auditory evoked potentials: I. Evaluation of components. Electroenceph. Clin. Neurophysiol., *36*:179–190, 1974.

46b. Popelka, G., Margolis, R., and Wiley, T.: Effect of activating signal bandwidth on acoustic-reflex thresholds. J. Acoust. Soc. Amer., *59*:153–159, 1976.

47. Quix, F. H.: Ein Acusticustumor. *In* III. Niederlandische Gesellschaft für Hals, Nasen und Ohrenheilkunde. Arch. Ohr. Nas. Kehlkopfheilk., *84*:252–253, 1911.

48. Radner, S.: Intracranial angiography via the vertebral artery. Acta Radiol., *28*:838–842, 1947.

49. Rand, R. W.: Microneurosurgery for acoustic tumors. *In* Microneurosurgery. St. Louis, C. V. Mosby Co., 1969, pp. 126–155.

50. Rand, R. W., and Kurze, T.: Facial nerve preservation by posterior fossa transmeatal microdissection in total removal of acoustic tumors. J. Neurol. Neurosurg. Psychiat., *28*:311–316, 1965.

51. Reese, D. F., and Bull, J. W. D.: Positive contrast demonstration of normal internal acoustic me-

atus, Meckel's cave, and jugular foramen. Amer. J. Roentgen. *100*:650–655, 1967.

52. Reinhardt, K.: Aktuelle Problems in der Kontrastmitteluntersuchung des Wirbelkanals. Fortschr. Röntgenstr., *83*:809–819, 1955.

53. Sandifort, E.: Observations anatomicopathologicae. Lugduni Batvarorum, 1777, Chap. IX, pp. 116–120.

54. Scanlon, R. C.: Positive contrast medium (iophendylate) in diagnosis of acoustic neuroma. Arch. Otolaryn., *80*:698–706, 1964.

55. Scarff, J. E.: Fifty years of neurosurgery, 1905–1955. Surg. Gynec. Obstet. *101*:417–513, 1955.

56. Schmiegelow, E.: Beitrag zur translabyrintharen Entfernung der Akustikustumoren. Z. Ohrenheilk., *73*:1–21, 1915.

56a. Selters, W. A., and Brackmann, D.: Acoustic tumor detection with brainstem electric response and audiometry. Arch. Otolaryng. (Chicago), *103*:181–187, 1977.

56b. Sohmer, H., Feinmesser, M., and Szabo, G.: Sources of electrocochleographic responses as studied in patients with brain damage. Electroenceph. Clin. Neurophysiol., *37*:663–669, 1974.

56c. Starr, A., and Hamilton, A. E.: Correlation between confirmed sites of neurological lesions and abnormalities of far field auditory brainstem response. Electroenceph. Clin. Neurophysiol., *41*:595–608, 1976.

56d. Stockard, J. J., and Rossiter, V. S.: Clinical and pathological correlates of brainstem auditory response abnormalities. Neurology (Minneap.) *27*:316–325, 1977.

57. Takahashi, M., Wilson, G., and Hanafee, W.: The significance of the petrosal vein in the diagnosis of cerebellopontine angle tumors. Radiology, *89*:834–840, 1967.

58. Takahashi, M., Wilson, G., and Hanafee, W.: The anterior inferior cerebellar artery: Its radiographic anatomy and significance in the diagnosis of extra-axial tumors of the posterior fossa. Radiology, *90*:281–287, 1968.

59. Tarlov, I. M.: Pantopaque meningitis disclosed at operation. J.A.M.A., *129*:1014–1016, 1945.

60. Valvassori, G. E.: The radiological diagnosis of acoustic neuromas. Arch. Otolaryng., *83*:582–587, 1966.

61. Valvassori, G. E.: The abnormal internal auditory canal: The diagnosis of acoustic neuroma. Radiology, *92*:449–459, 1969.

62. Valvassori, G. E.: The diagnosis of acoustic neuromas. Seminars Roentgen., *4*:171, 1969.

63. Zange, J.: Translabrinthare Operationen von acusticus und Kleinhirnbrückenwinkeltumoren. Klin. Wschr., *52*:1334, 1915.

94

LESIONS OF
THE CAVERNOUS
PLEXUS REGION

HISTORICAL BACKGROUND

Winslow is credited with naming this space "cavernous sinus" because he thought it resembled in structure the corpus cavernosum of the penis. He should have known better, as the two structures serve no similar purpose and nature does nothing in vain.[5,72]

The first report of a mass lesion in this area, a giant aneurysm, was made by Holmes in 1860.[21] In 1920 Foix described the syndrome of a mass in this location and frequently is credited with having been the first to do so.[13] Bartholow, however, had given a detailed account of the signs and symptoms of a mass in this region in 1872. He also described a giant aneurysm that presented with trigeminal neuralgia, exophthalmos, anosmia, and extraocular palsies.[4] Inasmuch as anosmia has not been noted by any subsequent author, it seems possible that this was coincidental deficit in Bartholow's patient. In 1875 Hutchinson proposed ligation of the carotid for these lesions, and Krogius, in 1896, first operated on a mass, presumably a neuroma, at this site.[23,32]

Jefferson's classic descriptions of the various presentations have remained as the standard to date.[24–26]

INCIDENCE

The incidence of masses in this space that may be treated by operation remains putative, based on reports that of necessity reflect the variations in pattern of practice, interest, and referral base of the authors. For instance, most cases of nasal pharyngeal carcinoma will never be seen by neurosurgeons. This in part explains the variations ranging from 20 to 75 per cent in the reported incidence of malignant primary tumors.[17,20]

The two largest brain tumor series reported to date indicate that from 0.1 to 0.2 per cent of all intracranial tumors involve the space known as the "cavernous sinus."[2,59] Again it is difficult to interpret involvement of this space. For instance, sphenoid ridge meningiomas and tentorial notch meningiomas may well involve the third, fourth, fifth, and sixth cranial nerves at the extremes of their extension and yet are clearly not tumors of the space. The two large series indicate equal male to female and right to left ratios.

The most common and in fact the only mass originating within this space is a giant saccular aneurysm. The only other tissues normally present there are fat, the sixth cranial nerve, and fine blood vessels. Interestingly enough, there are no reports of lipomas, neuromas, or hemangiomas arising here.

The neuromas of the fifth cranial nerve arise within Meckel's cave or its extension along the three divisions of the nerve and thus actually arise within the lateral wall of this lateral sellar space. The meningiomas seen by the authors have appeared to extend into the sinus from a lateral origin. Pituitary tumors extend in from a medial origin. Of 294 of Cushing's meningiomas reported by Gordy, only 5 involved this

---

space, and again, it is not known whether the word "involve" here means presented as a mass primarily in this space or as a mass obviously originating elsewhere and extending into it.[18] The incidence of craniopharyngiomas and epidermoids involving the space must be virtually nil. Metastases and the direct extensions of malignant nasopharyngeal tumors are probably the most common neoplasms affecting this region.[16] The neurofibromas of the fifth nerve are usually benign, there being only three in the world literature that have been reported as malignant.[10]

Chordomas are the only other neoplasms entering the cavernous plexus with significant frequency, and operatively they may be considered as malignant tumors.

It is probable that from 50 to 75 per cent of all tumors involving the cavernous plexus are malignant nasopharyngeal extensions, distant metastases, or chordomas. Of the primary tumors affecting the area, saccular aneurysms probably account for 80 per cent. Neurofibromas and meningiomas would account for approximately 10 per cent each, with pituitary tumors constituting less than 1 per cent if one excludes the pituitary tumor that is clinically evident as such and has merely bulged into the space. It should be noted, however, that in some series pituitary tumors outnumber meningiomas 3 to 1.[5,18,25-29,68] Again the discrepancies would be in the reporting author's determination of what constitutes "involvement" of this space. It must be remembered that all these figures are percentages of a total that constitutes no more than 0.2 per cent of all intracranial tumors.

In the authors' series they have excluded any tumor that, after suitable investigation, declared itself as arising elsewhere, i.e., pituitary, sphenoid ridge, or tentorial notch meningioma, even though the presenting sign or symptom might have been involvement of a structure traversing the cavernous plexus. The series includes a total of 19 aneurysms in this space out of a total of 435 saccular aneurysms coming to operation over the same period of time. Fourteen tumors were diagnosed preoperatively as arising within the cavernous sinus or within its wall out of a total of seventeen hundred intracranial tumors operated on over the same time span. Even after thoroughly screening to exclude malignant neoplasms, at operation 5 of the 14 proved to be malig-

nant. One was a fibrosarcoma, one a lymphoma, one a distant pulmonary metastasis, and two were nasopharyngeal carcinomas.

There were two meningiomas evidently arising within the lateral wall of this space and three neurofibromas of the fifth nerve, one of which was a dumbbell tumor extending into the posterior fossa. During the same period there were 37 acoustic neuromas, making the authors' ratio of trigeminal to acoustic neuromas much greater than the quoted 1 to 100.[42]

There were two pituitary tumors that presented in such a way as to masquerade as tumors originating here even after suitable investigation. One of the patients had undergone operation for an acoustic neuroma two years earlier. Eleven other pituitary tumors involved this space, but the pituitary origin of all of them became clinically evident after suitable investigation.

Thus in the authors' series, a total of 31 masses have been operated on in the cavernous sinus, of which saccular aneurysms constitute 60 per cent. If the wrongly operated on malignant tumors and chordomas were subtracted, the aneurysms would constitute about 80 per cent of the benign masses presenting in this space.

The age distribution is similar to that of all other central nervous system tumors.

ANATOMY

The anatomy of the small, compact, rigid space commonly called the cavernous sinus varies minimally in size and shape, although rarely do two patients have identical curvatures of the parasellar segment of the internal carotid artery, which this space accommodates. The artery tends to form an S in the sagittal plane and another more tightly coiled S in the coronal plane, starting at the point where it comes up through the foramen lacerum and ending where it runs through the dura above the anterior clinoid process. The entering segment of the carotid is firmly anchored, and its point of dural exit is also firmly anchored, but it lies unsupported in the intervening space known as the "cavernous sinus."[45,46] For its diameter it is relatively thin-walled throughout its course, and atheroma is relatively uncommon in this segment (cf. Fig. 94–12). The rich collateral circulation that

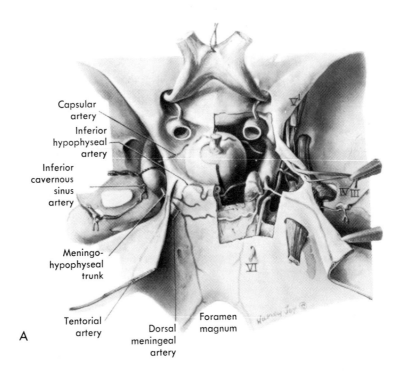

Capsular
artery

Inferior
hypophyseal
artery

Inferior
cavernous
sinus
artery

Meningo-
hypophyseal
trunk

Tentorial
artery

A

Dorsal
meningeal
artery

Foramen
magnum

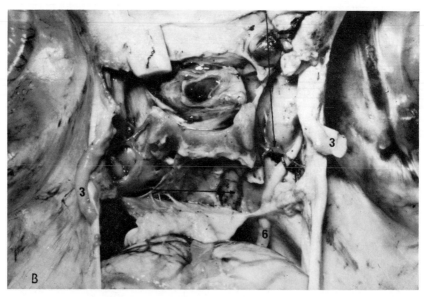

B

Figure 94–1   *A.* The relationships between the arterial anastomoses, the cranial nerve, and the dural coverings
in the lateral sellar space. *B.* Cadaver dissection in similar perspective. The third cranial nerves, 3, on each side are
hanging over the free margin of the tentorium. The sixth cranial nerve, 6, is visible coming from the brain stem up
through Dorello's canal, then turning around the carotid artery on the right beneath the branches of the meningohypophyseal trunk, which is indicated by the descending thin vertical arrow. The right tentorial artery leaves from
this point and goes to the right across the sixth nerve, giving a small branch down to the sixth nerve, and then
branches again just before entering the tentorium. The left meningohypophyseal trunk is less completely exposed,
but the inferior hypophyseal artery and dorsal meningeal artery are visible in their proximal portions. The right
dorsal meningeal artery indicated by the horizontal arrow is visible throughout a considerable length, descending
along the clivus, which is exposed beneath the dura, which has been cut and folded backward and downward.
(From Parkinson, D.: Collateral circulation of cavernous carotid artery: Anatomy. Canad. J. Surg., 7:251, 1964.
Reprinted by permission.)

exists between the two parasellar segments of the internal carotid arteries has been previously described and is well pictured in Figure 94–1A.[45]

The venous anatomy has been classically described as a trabeculated venous cavern connected anteriorly with the orbital veins and the sphenoid sinus and posteriorly with the petrosal veins and the sinus running down the dorsum and the clivus (Fig. 94–2). Although anatomy texts describe superior and inferior orbital veins, the superior orbital vein is dominant and has often been the only one seen in the authors' specimens. There are small venous connections across the midline in front of, behind, and beneath the pituitary. Taptas states that the veins in this region form a plexus.[62] Solassol and associates, working with 4-month-old fetuses, always found a plexus of veins in this space.[60] Hamby expressed the belief that the veins here were in the form of a plexus rather than a single sinus, and the authors' work indicates that the venous channels in the parasellar region are multiple branching and rejoining channels that pass without change of character into the plexus of veins along the floor of the middle fossa.[19] Significantly, the internal

carotid is never completely sheathed with venous channels; there are always bare areas (Figs. 94–3 through 94–6.[50,51] Some of these bare areas are occupied by fat.

The cranial nerves in the parasellar region converge to the superior orbital fissure consistently, leaving a triangular space between the third and fourth nerves above and the sixth and the first division of the fifth below (cf. Figs. 94–1 and 94–7 through 94–12). The third and fourth nerves carry small sleeves of arachnoid into small dural tunnels in the roof of this space. Their point of entrance is at the base of a shallow groove formed by the lateral extension of the dura of the tentorium going forward to the anterior clinoid and the medial extension of the tentorium joining the posterior clinoid. The third and fourth nerve maintain the relative relationship adjacent to each other throughout their course in the parasellar region, with a very thin medial dural cover and a thick upper and lateral dural cover. The sixth nerve enters down low through Dorello's canal and courses upward and laterally around the carotid and is the only nerve lying within this space aside from the sympathetics (Figs. 94–10 and 94–11).

Text continued on page 3014

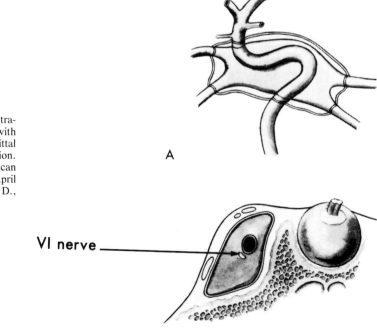

Figure 94–2 Schema of trabeculated cavern concept with trabeculae removed. *A.* Sagittal section. *B.* Coronal section. (From Poster Session, American Association of Anatomists. April 1978, Vancouver. Parkinson, D., Hunt, B., and Zeal, A.)

A

VI nerve

B

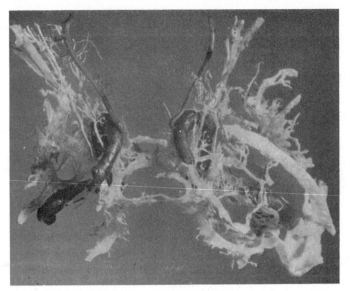

Figure 94–3 Corrosion specimen with carotid siphon (*dark*) and the venous channels (*light*). The two ophthalmic arteries are visible running upward and forward, and on the lateral aspect of each is the superior orbital vein and its branches. Running down off to the right is a clearly defined superior sphenoid sinus. The pituitary fossa is outlined with the connecting venous channels. Note that the venous channels around the carotid and the lateral sellar region are in no way different from the venous channels along the floor of the middle fossa or out in the orbit. They do not completely surround the carotid nor do they form a discrete single "sinus" or even a trabeculated "sinus."

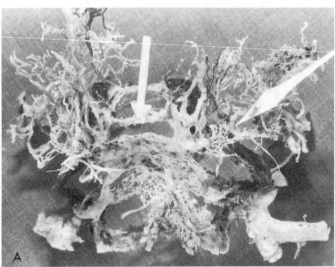

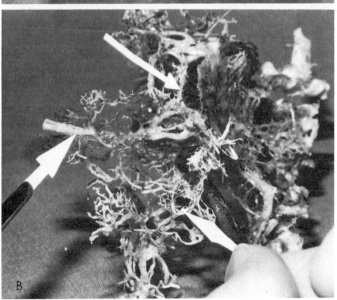

Figure 94–4 *A*. Corrosion specimen viewed from above with a vertical arrow resting in the space of the pituitary fossa. Just behind it the oblong vacant space would have been occupied by the dorsum sellae. The oblique arrow on the right is in the foramen ovale. On the left the ophthalmic artery and the superior orbital vein have been preserved. Again note that the veins in the lateral sellar region form a plexus, particularly on the left, and that these venous channels are in no way distinguishable from their continuation along the floor of the middle fossa. Note in the right lower corner, by way of contrast, the distal portion of the sigmoid with the single distinct smooth-walled channel characteristic of this and all the other intracranial sinuses. *B*. Same specimen viewed from the left and above. The uppermost white arrow points to the connecting venous channels behind the pituitary. The lower right white arrow points to the left foramen ovale, and the left white arrow points to the left superior orbital vein, beneath which is seen the left ophthalmic artery. (From Parkinson, D.: *In* Smith, J. L., Ed.: Neuro-ophthalmology. St. Louis, C. V. Mosby Co., 1972. Reprinted by permission.)

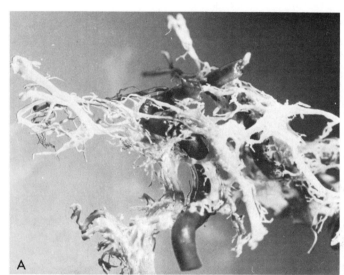

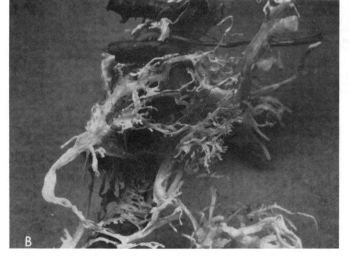

Figure 94–5 *A*. Corrosion specimen showing extreme example of the carotid being bare of coverage by venous channels. The superior petrosal veins are the largest channels visible in this specimen. The left superior orbital vein and ophthalmic artery are in clear focus in the upper left corner, and the right superior orbital vein and ophthalmic artery are slightly out of focus in the upper central field. *B*. Same specimen viewed from the right. Note the thin plexus of veins on the proximal portion of the carotid siphon giving way to a much less complete coverage of the carotid in the lateral sellar space.

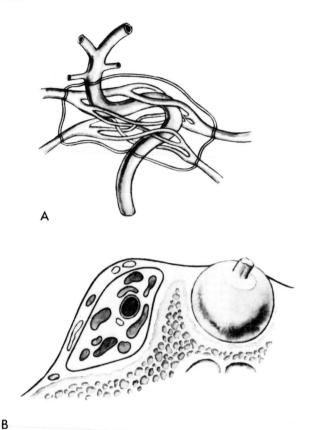

A

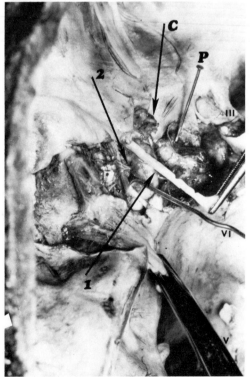

B

Figure 94-6 *A.* Sagittal section schema of parasellar venous anatomy indicated from the authors' study. *B.* Coronal section of parasellar venous anatomy. (From Poster Session, American Association of Anatomists. April 1978, Vancouver. Parkinson, D., Hunt, B., and Zeal, A.)

Figure 94-7 Dissection of the left lateral sellar region. The dura has been removed over the left lateral sellar space as well as over Meckel's cave and down along the floor of the middle fossa beyond the foramen ovale and foramen rotundum. The pin, P, is in the pituitary. C, the cut end of the carotid above the clinoid; *arrow 1,* the meningohypophyseal trunk; *arrow 2,* the artery to the inferior cavernous sinus running over the sixth nerve, which is held upward by the bent wire hook. The jaws of the large forcep, V, hold the posterior root of the fifth cranial nerve as it goes into Meckel's cave. The first division of the fifth cranial nerve has been removed to expose the underlying sixth nerve, which it would normally parallel and cover. The uppermost forceps hold the third nerve in its normal position, and the triangular space is outlined between the third nerve above and the sixth below. (From Parkinson, D.; Collateral circulation of cavernous carotid artery: Anatomy. Canad. J. Surg., 7:251, 1964. Reprinted by permission.)

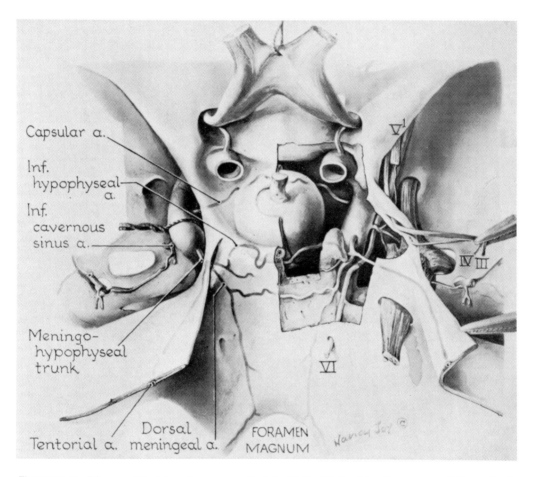

Figure 94–8   Diagram of the triangular space on the left with the third and fourth nerves paralleling each other above. (From Parkinson, D.: A surgical approach to the cavernous portion of the carotid artery. Anatomical studies and case report. J. Neurosurg., *23*:474–483, 1965. Reprinted by permission.)

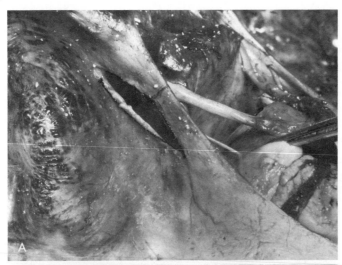

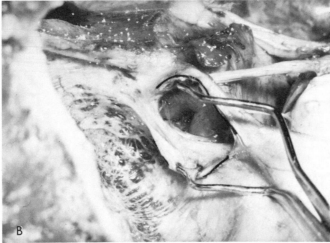

Figure 94–9 *A*. Incision outlined in the triangular space. The third and fourth nerves are visible departing from the brain stem, which is held back from the dorsum by the forceps. *B*. Incision opened with the retractors, showing that the third nerve and the fourth (just visible beneath the upper jaw of the retractor) remain protected in the thick dura of the upper part of the incision. The first division of the fifth is visible through the dura propria at the bottom of the incision. The sixth can be seen just beyond, wrapping around the carotid siphon. (From Parkinson, D.: A surgical approach to the cavernous portion of the carotid artery. Anatomical studies and case report. J. Neurosurg., *23*:474–483, 1965. Reprinted by permission.)

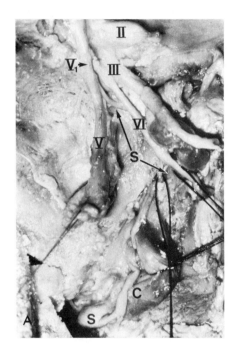

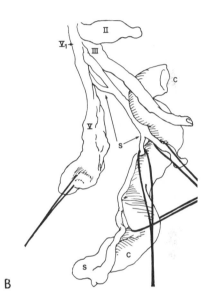

Figure 94–10 *A*. Extensive dissection of left parasellar space. II, cut end of left optic nerve above clinoid; III, third cranial nerve converging with sixth cranial nerve, VI, and first division of the fifth, V_1, at the superior orbital fissure. The gasserian ganglion, V, has been turned down and out and held with a suture. The carotid, C, has a suture drawing it to the right just as it comes through the carotid foramen, and its cut end is visible just above the third cranial nerve where it comes up beneath the clinoid, which structure has been largely removed in this specimen. S, the superior sympathetic ganglion at the bottom drawn up through the carotid foramen. From this ganglion can be traced up the sympathetic nerve to the right and left arrows from the uppermost, S. These arrows point to the sympathetic nerve joining the sixth and then leaving to join the first division of the fifth. Just beneath this left arrow tip is the second division of the fifth going through the foramen rotundum. *B*. Diagram of structures shown in *A*. (From Parkinson, D., Johnston, J. A., and Chaudhuri, A.: Sympathetic connections to the fifth and sixth cranial nerves. Anat. Rec., *191*:221–226. 1978. Reprinted by permission.)

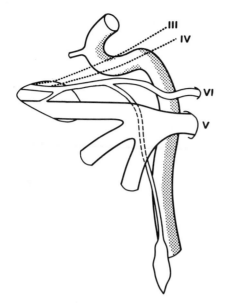

Figure 94–11 Schema of large sympathetic nerve connection to the sixth nerve and then to the first division of the fifth. The courses of the third and fourth cranial nerves are indicated by dotted lines. The sixth nerve is portrayed as being considerably above the posterior root and first division of the fifth, although in actuality it is slightly medial and roughly parallel to this structure.

The fifth cranial nerve enters from the posterior fossa through the large opening, which resembles a pocket that might be formed by invaginating a three-fingered hand through the dura and arachnoid. The invaginated portion is known as Meckel's cave and contains the ganglion and the first portions of the three divisions of the fifth cranial nerve (Fig. 94–12). The dura between the fifth nerve and the space is exceedingly thin, as shown in Figure 94–10. The relationship of the gasserian ganglion and its three branches to the dura differs in no way from that of the third and fourth cranial nerves except that it is in a larger pouch or tunnel (see Figs. 94–1A, 94–7, 94–8, and 94–12).

In addition to the cranial nerves, the sympathetic fibers come up into this area. The largest residual sympathetic nerve arising from the superior sympathetic ganglion joins the sixth nerve and runs with it for a short distance, then leaves it and joins the first division of the fifth. This sympathetic nerve is so large in many cadavers that it led some early observers to believe the sympathetics originated as a branch of the sixth nerve (Figs. 94–11 and 94–12).[30,52]

Except for the three main arteries and their multiple branches that depart from this segment of the internal carotid, the sympathetic fibers, the extremely thin-walled venous channels, and some fat, there are no other structures in this region. Quite probably the "septi" or "trabeculi" described as transversing this space are in actuality the small vessels and sympathetic fibers.[30,49–52]

In cross section, this space forms a blunted triangle. Anteriorly it twists and tapers down to a narrow horizontal triangle constituting the superior orbital fissure. Posteriorly it narrows to a twisting, curving slit as the lateral and medial surfaces curve and join to become the superior and inferior surface of the tentorium. (Figs. 94–1 and 94–13A and B). Whether the medial wall is formed by a division of the dura from the floor of the middle fossa or whether it is formed as a separate fibrous layer is not known (cf. Fig. 94–12). The medial fibrous layer, which is extremely thin, covers the roof of the bones of the sphenoid sinus and the lateral portions of the body of the sphenoid and the pituitary gland. The dural continuation on the lateral aspect of this space is thick and becomes even thicker superiorly as a continuation of the free margin of the tentorium, as shown in Figures 94–1, 94–9, and 94–12.

DIAGNOSIS

Signs and Symptoms

A lesion in the lateral sellar region can be suspected when any one of the cranial nerves from the second to the sixth inclusive is involved. This suspicion becomes a certainty when any two or more are involved.[56,63] The combinations of involvement are not of great diagnostic value beyond allowing one to guess at the direction of progression and the extent. For example, if the second is involved, the lesion must extend at least that far forward, and if the third division of the fifth is involved, it extends at least that far posteriorly and inferiorly, whereas if the seventh or eighth is involved, it is obviously into the posterior fossa.[2,28] The sixth nerve is the only nerve free in this space, yet it is rarely the first involved, although several authors have noted that it is the most likely to be affected along with the fifth.[37,39,40,57,71]

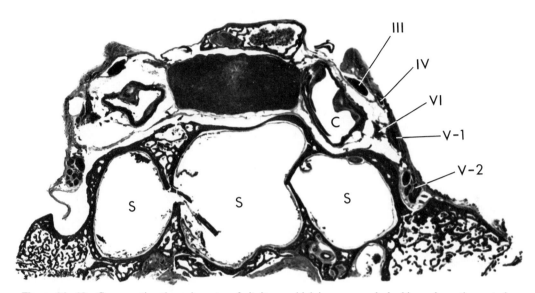

Figure 94–12   Cross section through center of pituitary, which is seen as a dark oblong above the central one of the three sphenoid sinus cavities, S. Both internal carotid arteries, C, show marked atherosis, rather uncommon in this location. On the right, cranial nerves III and IV and the first division of V, V-1, are marked lying in the lateral wall with a very thin layer separating them from this space. Cranial nerve VI is irregular in cross section, lying just medial to V-1. The second division of the fifth, V-2, is seen on its way toward the foramen rotundum. The third division of the fifth has already departed through the foramen ovale posterior to the plane of this section. Between the sixth nerve and the wall of the carotid artery on the right can be seen three distinct venous channels in cross section and another venous channel in longitudinal section beneath them and above the bone. On the left is a large venous channel in the lateral wall just lateral to the first division of the fifth nerve and the sixth cranial nerve. On both sides adipose tissue is visible just below and medial to the third and fourth cranial nerves.

When sympathetic nerve function has been disturbed, some investigators have implicated a plexus of nerves on the internal carotid or sympathetic fibers from the carotid directly to the first division of the fifth or to the third cranial nerve.* The authors' findings indicate that there are no sympathetic pathways going to the third nerve and that the involved pathways probably are not a plexus on the wall of the internal carotid but a nerve several millimeters away that joins the sixth for a short distance and leaves it to join the first division of the fifth, as shown in Figures 94–11 and 94–12.[30,52] There is, however, no nerve structure in this space more than a few millimeters away from another nerve at any given point, making very discrete clinical localization most tempting (cf. Figs. 94–1 and 94–7).[46,47]

The severity of disability has more to do with the suddenness of onset than with the extent of neurological deficit. A very minimal diplopia of sudden onset is quite disabling, as opposed to a much more extensive diplopia of gradual onset.[63]

A sudden onset is not diagnostic of neoplasm nor of aneurysm. Remission and response to steroids do not exclude tumors or aneurysms, nor do they prove an inflammatory process.[22,63,64,66]

A high sedimentation rate strongly suggests malignancy or an inflammatory process. Short intervals between remissions favor neoplasms. The presence of enlarged cervical nodes confirms a malignant naso-

_____
* See references 7, 25, 26, 29, 39, 54.

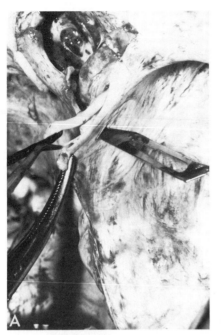

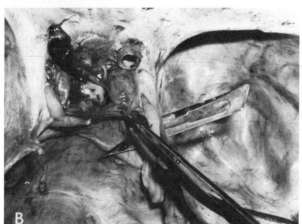

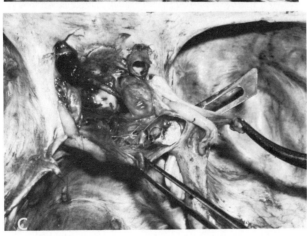

Figure 94–13 *A*. Cadaver specimen viewed from above and right. Curved forceps holding cut edge of tentorium. Angled forceps holding fourth nerve. Third nerve draped over the blunt hook. Knife blade entering triangular space too far posteriorly. *B*. Same specimen viewed from directly above dorsum. The cut edge of the tentorium is pulled laterally with the curved forceps. The third nerve is held in its normal position with the straight forceps. The knife has been pushed on in demonstrating the proximity of the posterior fossa to the lateral wall of the parasellar space. Note that the medial wall of this space posteriorly is formed by the dura sweeping in a curved fashion laterally and posteriorly from the dorsum. This in turn fuses with the middle fossa dura as it sweeps back from the lateral wall of this space. The knife blade is coming through the entrance to Meckel's cave from the posterior fossa. The cut root of the fifth nerve is visible behind it. *C*. Same specimen showing the course of the knife blade with the two walls pulled apart. The cut edge of the tentorium and the third nerve are pulled laterally with the curved forceps, and the dura from the dorsum is pulled down off the dorsum. The cut end of the carotid artery on the right is empty; that on the left has a clot extruding. Note the multiple stretched-out venous channels just above the knife blade.

pharyngeal neoplasm in the presence of a lateral sellar syndrome unless it can be proved otherwise.[17] Statistically, one would have to suspect malignant growth at the top of the list in any case. Trotter's triad, deafness, face pain, and palatal paresis, is virtually diagnostic of malignant nasopharyngeal tumor.[65]

There is considerable variation noted in the method of presentation with involvement of the fifth nerve. Some authors emphasize that numbness is the most common, while others have found that pain is the most common.[*] The pain has been tic-like in the experience of some.[†] A few authors argue that pain indicates involvement of the ganglion, whereas numbness indicates involvement of the root.[10,31,59] Jefferson disagreed with both of these arguments.[29]

The sequence of the appearance of each additional deficit suggests the site of origin and direction of growth in the anteroposterior plane and also in the coronal plane.[26-29,33]

One author has made the statement that the diagnosis is a simple task when the extraocular muscles and fifth nerve are involved.[61] Nevertheless, Jefferson's admonition is well worth remembering:

Anyone with the presumption that fifth nerve neuromas will be easy to diagnose because pain and numbness will be demonstrated is set for disillusionment.[29]

Radiography

The x-ray changes associated with a mass in the lateral sellar region have been progressively well documented, starting with Cohen, who first reported erosion of the superior orbital fissure in 1933.[8] His description was followed closely by those of McKinney and co-workers and Jefferson in 1936, and it was soon accepted by most that destruction of the sphenoid wing favored a tumor, whereas erosion of the lower and outer wall of the optic foramen with loss of the strut favored an aneurysm.[‡] Erosion of the posterior clinoid or petrous tip, or both, indicates posteriorly located masses.[43] Iso-

lated erosion of the foramen ovale is more suggestive of upward extension of nasopharygneal carcinoma than it is of isolated third division neuroma.[34] Tomography has been considered worthwhile by some, while others were not impressed.[44,55,58] The value of angiography is firmly established, however.[§] The direction of displacement of the carotid as well as evidence of compression of the wall of the carotid is of value. A tumor blush provides an absolute diagnosis.[6,44]

The venous pattern is diagnostically helpful if a poor flow into the lateral sellar veins is demonstrated or if the basilar vein of Rosenthal is elevated.[9,35,67] Oxygen encephalography on occasion is useful.[44] When present, curvilinear calcification, so diagnostic of aneurysm, may give a better indication of the size of the aneurysm than angiography, as large portions of the lumen are often occupied by laminar clot.[36,39,40,55] As time goes on, computed tomography will no doubt play an increasing role in diagnosis of masses in this region.

TREATMENT

Indications

An operative approach to this space is indicated when it is anticipated that the lesion can be removed. A preoperative diagnosis of either an aneurysm, a meningioma, or a neurofibroma would justify this belief. With rare exceptions, pituitary tumors extending into this space are best decompressed by removal of the tumor mass from within the sella and not through the space known as the cavernous sinus. The authors have had two cases that presented with a mass in this region, and at operation the neoplasms were discovered to be of pituitary origin.

Malignant tumors arising from the nasopharynx, metastases, and chordomas should not be approached in this space, since the entire lesion cannot be removed. If a mistake in diagnosis has led the surgeon into this space, he should stop once he finds the mass is malignant or is a chordoma extending from beyond his reach. Continuing the operation can only do more harm and will not cure the patient.

---

* See references, 16, 18, 28, 31, 39, 54, 66, 70.
† See references 2, 4, 8, 11, 14, 37, 59.
‡ See references 1, 7, 20, 24, 39, 41, 44, 55, 69.

§ See references 6, 12, 16, 18, 33, 69, 70.

Operative Approach

The patient is placed in the lateral position. A lumbar puncture needle is inserted, and the stylet is removed as brain retraction is initiated. The sagittal suture should be parallel with the horizon, and the long axis of the head tilted down slightly. Gravity then assists the surgeon, as the temporal lobe falls away from the floor of the middle fossa. Mannitol or urea is routinely used. The approach is along the floor of the middle fossa. Some patients have a very shallow middle fossa, and very minimal retraction is necessary. Other patients have a very deep middle fossa with a very prominent overhanging lesser wing of the sphenoid. If after adequate lumbar puncture drainage and the full effect of the dehydrating agent firm retraction is still necessary, it is best to amputate the tip of the temporal lobe. At all costs one wishes to avoid the postoperative complication of a bruised, swelling temporal lobe.

The first landmark is the free margin of the tentorium, and the next is the third nerve appearing over the horizon of the free margin of the tentorium (Fig. 94–14). The fourth nerve may not readily be visualized but is always parallel to and approximately 1 mm beneath the third nerve throughout

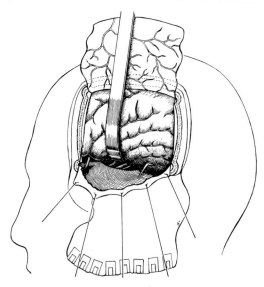

Figure 94–14 Operative approach. Temporal lobe is elevated. The carotid artery and the third and fourth nerves are appearing at the end of the retractor, the bridging vein from the temporal lobe to the tentorium is visible posteriorly, and the sylvian veins are represented anteriorly, running to the sphenoid ridge.

its course prior to and after entering the dura. The triangular space should be identified by these landmarks and the incision planned at least 4 mm beneath the projected course of the third nerve, centering at the point where the third nerve appears over the horizon of the free margin of the tentorium (see Figs. 94–8, 94–9, and 94–13). An incision so placed may be extended 1 cm forward and backward without fear of running into the converging nerves anteriorly or running through into the posterior fossa posteriorly. Beyond this length it should be extended anteriorly by simply advancing a blunt hook ahead. This maneuver "ploughs" apart the third and fourth nerve above, converging with the sixth and the first division of the fifth below as they approach the superior orbital fissure. Posteriorly the risk is not of cutting the nerves, as they are getting farther apart, but rather that the incision will extend through the medial wall forming the two leaves of the tentorium, as shown in Figures 94–1, 94–9, and 94–13.

Whenever in doubt, a surgeon should always go lower than he might have measured and never higher. It is far better to split a few fibers of the first division of the fifth nerve than it is to cut into the third or fourth. If the surgeon rubs up and down with the handle of the knife he can often feel the ridge of the first division of the fifth nerve and sometimes can actually see the fibers through the outer layer of dura. If the dura is relatively avascular, as over a neurofibroma or aneurysm, it is quite possible to visualize the fibers of the first division of the fifth nerve through a very shallow incision through the outer layer of the dura. If these fibers do appear at the bottom of the incision, they can then be brushed downward with the knife handle so that the continuing incision through the next layer goes above them.

If the desired exposure extends to the anterior portion of the space or if there is a very deep middle fossa with a large overhanging lesser wing of the sphenoid, it is well worthwhile to rongeur away the lesser wing extradurally, as shown in Figure 94–15. The few minutes of extra time required are well rewarded with the dramatic extra exposure and extra illumination that become available. It is also possible to elevate the brain a few millimeters further with safety, as the point of tethering of the sylvian vein folds upward once the bony ridge is removed. Most surgeons are justifiably wary of entering this space for two reasons: first, the fear of cutting the cranial nerves, and second, the fear of torrential venous bleeding. If there is a mass within the space, both these risks are minimized (Fig. 94–16). The mass will have obliterated the venous channels and in addition will have widened out the triangular space between the nerves. Thus the surgeon's adversary becomes his ally in these two respects. He should, however, never become overconfident, and no one should approach this space without verifying the landmarks several times on autopsy cadavers.

If a mass has originated laterally and is growing into the space, of course, all the relationships are distorted and one must be extremely careful as one approaches the surface wherein these cranial nerves would normally lie. It should again be emphasized that they will remain within their dural tunnels with the exception of the sixth nerve. It is unlikely that there is any indication for pursuing a tumor of known malignancy on into this space. Hence one is considering only a meningioma or neurofibroma for all practical purposes. The venous bleeding will be no more severe than it would from dura elsewhere, and one should have no more fear of venous bleeding with a meningioma in this region than he would of a meningioma along the petrous pyramid, and certainly not as much as with one along the sagittal sinus. The surgeon should take the same fastidious care and progressively cautious approach as he gets to the bottom of the tumor as he does, for example, with a cerebellopontine angle meningioma.

Results of Treatment

The evolution of a rational treatment for these lesions has been gradual, starting with Hutchinson's first proposal of carotid ligation for an aneurysm in 1875 and the first direct approach for a tumor by Krogius in 1896.[23,32] Carotid ligation continues to be promoted as a treatment of choice for an aneurysm, even though hemiplegia and death have been common accompaniments.[7,39,40,55,71] McKinney and co-workers report three common carotid ligations with survival and two internal carotid ligations, in both of which the patient became hemiplegic.[39] This emphasizes the fact that a common carotid ligation does not take away the blood supply as does ligation of the internal carotid.

Radiation emerges to date as the treatment of choice for malignant nasopharyngeal tumors. The mortality and morbidity rates remain very high, with a 17 per cent 10-year survival rate in nasopharyngeal carcinoma when the parasellar space is clinically involved.[17]

The operative approach to a tumor in this region will depend on the extent. If it is entirely limited to the middle fossa, then the middle fossa approach is the only one, and

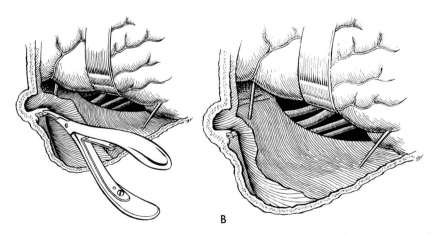

A   B

Figure 94–15 *A*. Diagram of the extradural approach to rongeuring away the sphenoid ridge. *B*. The additional exposure available with the sphenoid ridge removed. The optic nerve is indicated as the first structure now visible with the carotid artery behind it and the third and fourth cranial nerves next. The point of tethering of the sylvian veins has moved slightly upward and forward as the dural fold flattens out.

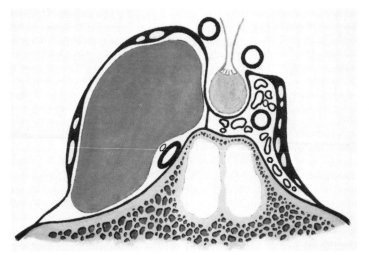

Figure 94–16 Schema indicating how a mass, be it saccular aneurysm or neoplasm, will have obliterated the venous channels and widened the triangular space. The sixth nerve will have been moved inward against the compressed carotid in the case of any tumor originating laterally. It will be displaced laterally with an aneurysm originating from the lateral sellar segment of the carotid. With a tumor starting medially, both the carotid and the sixth nerve will be displaced laterally. It is difficult to conceive that either the fifth or sixth could become medial to the artery.

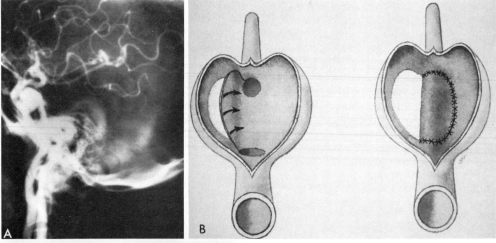

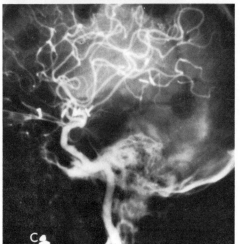

Figure 94–17 *A.* Angiogram of saccular aneurysm in the lateral sellar space. *B.* Schema of method of repair. Aneurysm sac is entered through the triangular space. Sufficient clot is removed to expose enough of the wall to turn a flap down over the entering and leaving ostia of the carotid. *C.* Postoperative angiograms showing site of repair. The remaining wall of the aneurysm has been left in situ to avoid risk of cranial nerve damage.

this may be either extradural or intradural of both.* During the posterior fossa approach for trigeminal neuralgia, Dandy encountered 18 unsuspected tumors involving the fifth nerve.[11] Cohen also reports such tumors as an incidental finding during operations for trigeminal neuralgia.[7] As Jefferson has so well pointed out, the posterior fossa extent of a neurofibroma originating from the fifth nerve can be reached from the middle fossa by sectioning the tentorium and quite safely delivered, whereas it is extremely difficult, if starting in the posterior fossa, to get any tumor from the middle fossa.[28,29] Thus the middle fossa approach evolves as the best for a tumor in this space, commonly called the cavernous sinus, and as the approach of choice to any mass that arises here and has extended posteriorly.[16,18,31,43]

Data concerning results from any form of treatment are virtually unobtainable, as no reports of any significant number of any type of lesion treated by any given method have been published. Significant mortality and morbidity rates have been noted over the years from carotid ligation and trapping for the saccular aneurysms.[7,36,39,71]

On three occasions the authors have been able to enter a saccular aneurysm and reconstruct the carotid artery after removing enough of the laminated clot to provide room. They used profound hypothermia with temporary circulatory arrest. One of the patients died, but the other two are entirely well and have recovered from their preoperative cranial nerve palsies (Fig. 94–17). Possibly such a repair could be done by temporarily trapping the carotid in an individual with an adequate anterior communicating or posterior communicating artery, or possibly it could be done over a bypass tube. Wire-induced thrombosis must be a consideration. Whether this would cure the ocular palsies is not known.

A morbidity rate of 25 to 33 per cent has been noted for the benign tumors, with a sixth nerve palsy the most common deficit.[2,17,18,27,28] In the authors' series there have been no deaths and no increase in any pre-existing neurological deficit from removal of benign tumors from this space. With five malignant tumors that were not evident as such preoperatively, the operation was stopped before producing any increase in preoperative morbidity.

Two patients with pituitary tumors presented with findings primarily in this region. One patient died, and the survivor has not improved from his preoperative state.

REFERENCES

1. Alajouanine, T., Thurel, R. Nehlil, J., and Baldacci, Y.: L'anéurysme du siphon carotidien et son retentissement osseux (réunion du trou optique et de la fente sphénoidale). Rev. Neurol. (Paris), 92:249–253, 1955.
2. Arseni, C., Dumitrescu, L., and Constantinescu, A.: Neurinomas of the trigeminal nerve. Surg. Neurol., 4:497–503, 1975.
3. Barr, H. W. K., Blackwood, W., and Meadows, S. P.: Intracavernous carotid aneurysms—a clinical pathological report. Brain, 94:607–622, 1971.
4. Bartholow, R.: Aneurysms of the arteries at the base of the brain: Their symptomatology, diagnosis, and treatment. Amer. J. Med. Sci., 64:374–386, 1872.
5. Bedford, M. A.: Cavernous sinus. Brit. J. Ophthal., 52:41–46, 1966.
6. Chase, N. E., and Taveras, J. M.: Carotid angiography in the diagnosis of extradural parasellar tumors. Acta Radiol. (Diagn.) (Stockholm), 1:214–224, 1963.
7. Cogan, D. G., and Mount, H. T. J.: Intracranial aneurysms causing ophthalmoplegia. Arch. Ophthal. (Chicago), 70:757–771, 1963.
8. Cohen, I.: Tumors involving the Gasserian ganglion. J. Nerv. Ment. Dis., 78:492–499, 1933.
9. Cophignon, J., Doyon, D., Djindjian, R., and Vignaud, J.: Les tumeurs du sinus caverneux et de la région: Opacification artérielle et veineuse. Neurochirurgie, 19:7–27, 1973.
10. Cuneo, H. M., and Rand, C. W.: Tumors of the Gasserian ganglion. Tumor of the left Gasserian ganglion associated with enlargement of the mandibular nerve. A review of the literature and case report. J. Neurosurg., 9:423–431, 1952.
11. Dandy, W. E.: The treatment of trigeminal neuralgia by the cerebellar route. Ann. Surg., 96:787–795, 1932.
12. Dilenge, D., Metzger, J., Ramee, A., and Simon, J.: L'angiographie des tumeurs de la région du sinus caverneux. J. Radiol. Electr., 47:615–628, 1966.
13. Foix, M.: Syndrome de la paroi externe du sinus caverneux. Ophtalmoplégie unilatérale à marche rapidement progressive. Bull. Mém. Soc. Méd. Hôp. Paris, 36:1355–1361, 1920.
14. Frazier, C. H.: An operable tumor involving the Gasserian ganglion. Amer. J. Med. Sci., 156:483–490, 1918.
15. Glasauer, F. E., and Tandan, P. N.: Trigeminal neurinoma in adolescents. J. Neurol. Neurosurg. Psychiat., 32:562–568, 1969.
16. Glaser, M. A.: Tumors arising from the sensory root of the trigeminal nerve in the posterior fossa. Perineurial fibroblastoma. Ann. Surg., 101:146–155, 1935.

---

* See references, 14, 16, 27–29, 31, 51, 53, 59.

17. Godtfredsen, E., and Lederman, M.: Studies on the cavernous sinus syndrome. 2. Diagnostic and prognostic roles of ophthalmoneurological signs and symptoms in malignant nasopharyngeal tumors. Acta Neurol. Scand., *41*:53–51, 1965.

18. Gordy, P. D.: Neurinoma of the Gasserian ganglion. Report of a case and review of the literature. J. Neurosurg., *22*:90–94, 1965.

19. Hamby, W. B.: Carotid cavernous fistulae. Springfield, Ill., Charles C Thomas, 1966.

20. Hedeman, L. S., Lewinsky, B. S., Lochridge, G. K., and Trevor, R.: Primary malignant schwannoma of the Gasserian ganglion. J. Neurosurg., *48*:279–283, 1978.

21. Holmes, T.: Aneurysms of the internal carotid artery in the cavernous sinus. Trans. Path. Soc., London, *12*:61, 1860–61.

22. Hunt, W. E., Meagher, J. S., Le Fever, H. E., and Zeman, W.: Painful ophthalmoplegia. Its relation to indolent inflammation of the cavernous sinus. Neurology (Minneap.), *11*:56–62, 1961.

23. Hutchinson: Quoted by Meadows, S. P.; see ref. 40.

24. Jefferson, G.: Discussion on the value of radiology in neurosurgery. Proc. Roy. Soc. Med., *29*:1169–1172, 1936.

25. Jefferson, G.: Compression of the chiasma, optic nerves, and optic tracts by intracranial aneurysms. Brain, *60*:444–497, 1937.

26. Jefferson, G.: On the saccular aneurysms of the internal carotid artery in the cavernous sinus. Brit. J. Surg., *26*:267–302, 1938.

27. Jefferson, G.: Extrasellar extensions of pituitary adenomas. Proc. Roy. Soc. Med., *38*:433–458, 1940.

28. Jefferson, G.: Concerning injuries, aneurysms, and tumors involving the cavernous sinus. Trans. Ophth. Soc. U.K., *73*:117–152, 1953.

29. Jefferson, G.: Trigeminal neurinomas with some remarks on the malignant invasion of the Gasserian ganglion. Clin. Neurosurg., *1*:11–54, 1955.

30. Johnston, J. A., and Parkinson, D.: Intracranial sympathetic pathways associated with the sixth cranial nerve. J. Neurosurg., *39*:236–242, 1974.

31. Krayenbühl, H.: Primary tumors of the root of the fifth cranial nerve: Their distinction from tumors of the Gasserian ganglion. Brain, *59*:337–352, 1936.

32. Krogius: Quoted by Peet, M. M.; see ref. 53.

33. Legré, J., Dufour, M., Debaene, A., et al.: Signes angiographiques des tumeurs de la région du sinus caverneux. Neurochirurgie, *19*:29–48, 1973.

34. Lin, S. R., Lin, Z. S., and Tatoian, J. A.: Trigeminal neurinoma with extracranial extension. Neuroradiology, *8*:183–185, 1974.

35. Lloyd, G. A. S.: The localization of lesions in the orbital apex and cavernous sinus by frontal venography. Brit. J. Radiol., *45*:405–414, 1972.

36. Lombardi, G., Passerini, A., and Migliavacca, F.: Intracavernous aneurysms of the internal carotid artery. Amer. J. Roentgen., *89*:361–371, 1963.

37. Love, J. G., and Woltman, H. W.: Trigeminal neuralgia and tumors of the Gasserian ganglion. Proc. Staff Meet. Mayo Clin., *17*:490–496, 1942.

38. Malis, L. I.: Tumors of the parasellar region. Advances Neurol., *15*:281–299, 1975.

39. McKinney, J., Acree, T., and Soltz, S. E.: Syndrome of unruptured aneurysm of intracranial portion of internal carotid artery. Bull. Neurol. Inst. N.Y., *5*:247–277, 1936.

40. Meadows, S. P.: Intracavernous aneurysms of the carotid artery, Arch. Ophthal., *62*:566–574, 1959.

41. Mello, L. R., and Tänzer, A.: Some aspects of trigeminal neurinomas. Neuroradiology, *4*:215–221, 1972.

42. Northfield, D. W. C.: Surgery of the Central Nervous System. Oxford, Blackwell Scientific Publications, 1973.

43. Olive, I., and Svien, H. G.: Neurofibromas of the fifth cranial nerve. J. Neurosurg., *14*:484–505, 1957.

44. Palacios, E., and MacGee, E. E.: The radiographic diagnosis of trigeminal neurinomas. J. Neurosurg., *36*:153–156, 1972.

45. Parkinson, D.: Collateral circulation of cavernous carotid artery: Anatomy. Can. J. Surg., *7*:251–268, 1964.

46. Parkinson, D.: A surgical approach to the cavernous portion of the carotid artery. Anatomical studies and case report. J. Neurosurg., *23*:474–483, 1965.

47. Parkinson, D.: Transcavernous repair of carotid cavernous fistula. J. Neurosurg., *26*:420–424, 1967.

48. Parkinson, D.: Carotid cavernous fistula. *In* Vinken, P. J., and Bruyn, G. W., eds.: Handbook of Clinical Neurology, Vol. 12. Amsterdam, North-Holland Publishing Co., 1972.

49. Parkinson, D.: Carotid cavernous fistula: Direct repair with preservation of the carotid artery. J. Neurosurg., *38*:99–106, 1973.

50. Parkinson, D.: Carotid cavernous fistula: Direct repair with preservation of carotid artery. Surgery, *76*:882–889, 1974.

51. Parkinson, D.: Carotid cavernous fistula, direct approach with repair of fistula and preservation of the artery. *In* Morley, T. P., ed.: Current Controversies in Neurosurgery. Philadelphia, W. B. Saunders Co., 1976, pp. 237–249.

52. Parkinson, D., Johnston, J. A., and Chaudhuri, A.: Sympathetic connections to the fifth and sixth cranial nerves. Anat. Rec., *191*:221–226, 1978.

53. Peet, M. M.: Tumors of the Gasserian ganglion. With the report of two cases of extracranial carcinoma infiltrating the ganglion by direct extension through the maxillary division. Surg. Gynec. Obstet., *44*:202–207, 1927.

54. Raeder, J. G.: Paratrigeminal paralysis of oculopupillary sympathetic. Brain, *47*:149–158, 1924.

55. Rischbieth, R. H. C., and Bull, J. W. D.: The significance of enlargement of the superior orbital (sphenoidal) fissure. Brit. J. Radiol., *31*:125–135, 1958.

56. Rucker, C. W.: The causes of paralysis of the third, fourth, and sixth cranial nerves. Amer. J. Ophthal., *61*:1293–1298, 1966.

57. Sakalas, R., Harbison, J. W., Vines, F. S., and Becker, D. P.: Chronic sixth nerve palsy. An initial sign of basisphenoid tumors. Arch. Ophthal. (Chicago), *93*:186–190, 1975.

58. Schatz, N. J., Savino, P. J., and Corbett, J. J.: Primary aberrant oculomotor regeneration. A sign of intracavernous meningioma. Arch. Neurol. (Chicago), *34*:29–32, 1977.

59. Schisano, G., and Olivecrona, H.: Neurinomas of the Gasserian ganglion and trigeminal root. J. Neurosurg., *17*:306–322, 1960.

60. Solassol, A., Zidane, C., Slimane-Taleb, S., et al.: The veins of the cavernous sinus in the four month old human fetus. C. R. Ass. Anat., *149*:1009–1015, 1970.

61. Stopford, J. S. B.: The arteries of the pons and medulla oblongata: Part III. J. Anat., *12*:250–277, 1917.

62. Taptas, J. N.: Étiologie et pathogénie des exophtalmies d'origine vasculaire dites exophthalmies pulsatiles. Arch. Ophtal. (Paris), *10*:22–50, 1950.

63. Thomas, J. E., and Yoss, R. E.: The parasellar syndrome. Problems in determining etiology. Mayo Clin. Proc., *45*:617–623, 1970.

64. Talosa, E.: Periarteritic lesion of the carotid syphon with the clinical features of a carotid intraclinoid aneurysm. J. Neurol. Neurosurg. Psychiat., *17*:300–302, 1954.

65. Trotter, W.: Symptoms of malignant tumors of the nasopharynx. Lancet, *1*:1277, 1911.

66. Verbruggen, A.: Subarachnoid hemorrhage. Mississippi Valley Med. J., *77*:95–101, 1955.

67. Waga, S., Kikuchi, H., Handa, J., and Handa, H.: Cavernous sinus venography. Amer. J. Roentgen., *109*:130–137, 1970.

68. Weinberger, L. M., Adler, F. H., and Grant, F. C.: Primary pituitary adenoma and the syndrome of the cavernous sinus. A clinical and anatomic study. Arch. Ophthal. (Chicago), *24*:1197–1236, 1940.

69. Westberg, G.: Angiographic changes in neurinoma of the trigeminal nerve. Acta Radiol. (Diagn.) (Stockholm), *1*:513–520, 1963.

70. White, J. C., and Ballantine, H. T.: Intrasellar aneurysms simulating hypophyseal tumors. J. Neurosurg., *18*:34–50, 1961.

71. Wilson, C. B., and Myers, F. K.: Bilateral saccular aneurysms of the internal carotid artery in the cavernous sinus. J. Neurol. Neurosurg. Psychiat., *26*:174–177, 1963.

72. Winslow, J. B.: Exposition Anatomique de la Structure du Corps Human. Vol. 2, p. 31. London, Prevost, 1732.

95

TUMORS OF THE ORBIT

The orbit claims the interest of at least three surgical disciplines: opthalmology, otorhinolaryngology, and neurological surgery. A number of tumors overlap the borders of these specialties. A clear understanding of orbital anatomy will assist the neurological surgeon in selecting those cases with unilateral exophthalmos that can be treated best by a transcranial approach and those cases that require the cooperation of more than one surgical discipline.

SURGICAL ANATOMY*

Viewed from above, the orbit is a pear-shaped cavity with its apical portion directed medially: The optic canal, representing the stem of the pear, is 5 to 10 mm long and enters the intracranial cavity medial to the anterior clinoid process. Of principal interest to neurosurgeons is the apical portion of the orbit, which is crowded with structures that cannot be safely approached by anterior or lateral routes. A precise knowledge of the orderly relations of the retro-ocular nerves, arteries, and muscles is essential to provide safe access both to tumors within the muscle cone and to disease lying between the muscles and the periosteum of the orbit (the periorbita) (Fig. 95–1). Of special importance is the confluence of the periorbita with the dura at the superior orbital fissure and at the optic canal. Once these structures are involved by tumor, it is difficult if not impossible to obtain total tumor resection without injury to the structures traversing them.

---

* See references 6, 13, 38, 48.

Bony Confines of the Orbit

The quadrangular orbital rim is formed by the frontal, maxillary, and zygomatic bones. The supraorbital margin is continuous medially with the crest of the lacrimal bone. The roof of the orbit is formed by the orbital plate of the frontal bone, which also forms the major portion of the floor of the intracranial anterior fossa. The floor of the orbit is formed primarily by the orbital plate of the maxillary bone. There is a small contribution to the floor by the palatine bone at the orbital apex and anterolaterally by the zygomatic bone.

The 5- to 10-mm long optic canal is situated at the apex of the orbital cavity. It is formed by the two roots of the lesser wing of the sphenoid and it passes medially to the intracranial cavity. The lateral orbital margin is formed by the greater wing of the sphenoid and the frontosphenoidal process of the zygomatic bone. There is a horizontal obliquity to the canal at its cranial end, after which it becomes round and, at the orbital end, forms a vertical oval.

The superior and inferior orbital fissures bound the medial margin of the greater wing of the sphenoid. The superior orbital fissure, lying near the apex of the orbit, provides the passage for the oculomotor, trochlear, and abducens nerves and the ophthalmic division of the trigeminal nerve from the cranial cavity to the orbit. Sympathetic branches from the cavernous plexus nerves also accompany the ophthalmic artery. Small orbital branches of the middle meningeal artery enter, and a recurrent branch of the lacrimal artery and the ophthalmic vein leave the orbit through this space. The recurrent meningeal arteries supply the dura covering the posterior as-

---

E. M. HOUSEPIAN, S. L. TROKEL, F. O. JAKOBIEC, AND S. K. HILAL

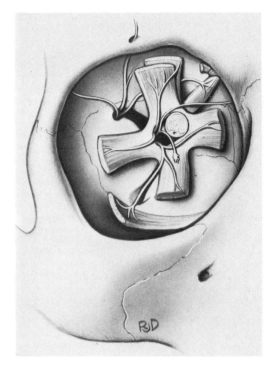

Figure 95–1   Diagram of the structures at the apex of the orbit showing: optic nerve and ophthalmic artery entering at the optic foramen; origins of all the extraocular muscles at the annulus of Zinn (with the exception of the inferior oblique); and the lacrimal, frontalis, and trochlear nerves entering the superior orbital fissure in that order. Superior ramus of the third nerve, nasociliary nerve, sixth nerve, and inferior ramus of the third nerve enter between the two roots of origin of the lateral rectus muscle.

pect of the greater wing of the sphenoid. The inferior orbital fissure separates the floor and lateral wall of the orbit and transmits the maxillary nerve, the infraorbital vessels, and ascending branches from the sphenopalatine ganglion. The medial wall of the orbit is formed by a number of fragile bones, including the lacrimal bone and the lamina papyracea of the ethmoid bone.

Optic Nerve

In conformity with the shape and size of the optic canal, the optic nerve has a flattened horizontal oval shape in its cranial course and measures approximately 4 by 6 mm (Fig. 95–2). After entering the cranial end of the optic canal it is 5 mm and circular, and continues to the globe as a 6- by 4-mm vertically oval structure. A vascularized pial membrane accompanies the nerve

from the chiasm to the sclera. The intracranial arachnoid is also a discrete structure investing the optic nerve throughout its course, fusing with the pia at the globe. Loose trabeculations are found in this subarachnoid space. At the apical orbital portion of the nerve, however, the pia and arachnoid are fused dorsomedially and ventrally with the dura and the fibrous annulus of Zinn, tethering the optic nerve and partially obliterating the subarachnoid space.

The Periorbita

The periosteum of the orbit known as the periorbita is loosely connected to and easily separated from the bony margins. It is continuous with the intracranial dura at the superior orbital fissure and the dura of the optic nerve at the orbital end of the optic canal. It is this confluence of the periorbita with the intracranial dura that often makes total resection of tumors invading the periorbita impossible without injury to the important nerves passing through the superior orbital fissure. Anteriorly, the periorbita is continuous with the periosteum at the orbital margin; structural modifications in the periorbita enclose the lacrimal gland and fix the pulley of the superior oblique tendon.

The lacrimal gland lies in a fossa just inside the roof of the orbital process of the frontal bone. A portion of the tear fluid is secreted via the canaliculi in the upper fornix. Many other conjunctival glands contribute to the formation of the tears. Tears drain via the upper and lower puncta at the medial end of the lids, via two canaliculi, into the nasolacrimal sac and duct. They are carried into the nasal cavity under the inferior turbinate.

Extraocular Muscles

As the optic nerve with its pial, arachnoid, and dural sheath exits from the optic canal, it is invested with a fibrous band called the anulus tendineus (annulus of Zinn), which, encircles the dural sheath of the optic nerve, the upper and lower divisions of the third, the abducens nerve, and the nasociliary nerve. The fourth nerve enters superior to this structure and to the origins of the levator and superior rectus

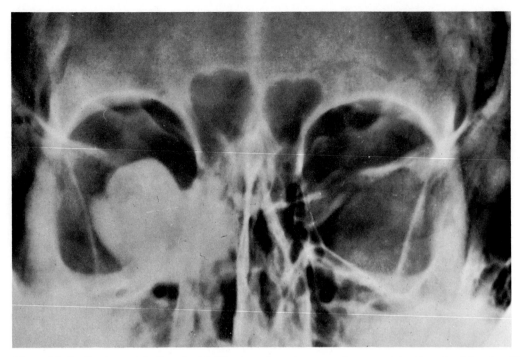

Figure 95–2 Osteoma, plain film of orbit: The dense bone tumor can be seen arising from the right ethmoid sinus.

muscles. The levator muscle arises from the upper medial margin of the annulus, the superior rectus muscle beneath the levator and on the upper surface. The anulus tendineus also forms the origin of the superior oblique and medial rectus muscles on its medial side, and the lateral rectus muscle on its lateral side; the inferior rectus muscle arises on its inferior border. The inferior oblique is the only ocular muscle that does not have this fibrous sheath as its origin. The lateral rectus muscle arises by two narrow heads between which pass the two divisions of the oculomotor nerve, the nasociliary nerve, the abducens nerve, and the ophthalmic vein.

Arteries of the Orbit

The ophthalmic artery usually arises from the supracavernous portion of the internal carotid at its emergence from the cavernous sinus. The point of origin of the ophthalmic artery may be entirely within the cavernous sinus, but it is most frequently found just below the level of the anterior clinoid where the internal carotid artery becomes intradural. It passes on the

medial side of the anterior clinoid process and enters the orbit through the optic canal. It then curves over the lateral margin of the optic nerve as it enters the orbit and crosses to the medial wall and forward to its two terminal branches along the lower border of the superior oblique muscle. While beneath the optic nerve, it gives off two long posterior ciliary arteries, one to either side of the globe. These run between the sclera and choroid to anastomose with the anterior ciliary arteries derived from muscular branches. The central artery of the retina, one of the smallest and earliest branches of the ophthalmic artery, runs within the dural sheath of the optic nerve for a short distance but then pierces the nerve obliquely, approximately 1 cm behind the globe, and courses within the center of the nerve to the retina. There are six or eight short posterior ciliary arteries, most of which supply the choroid, which in turn nourishes a portion of the retina. Besides the ocular branches, the ophthalmic artery gives rise to six orbital branches: supratrochlear and supraorbital to the forehead; a dorsal nasal branch to the face; a lacrimal branch to the lacrimal gland, eyelid, and cheek, and to the temporal region through its zygomatic branches; and finally, anterior and posterior ethmoidal branches to the nasal cavity.

There are also two small muscular branches arising from the ophthalmic artery that supply the ocular muscles near their insertion at the annulus. All these vessels anastomose freely with branches of the external carotid artery. The lacrimal artery frequently anastomoses with the middle meningeal artery by a recurrent branch passing through the lacrimal foramen or superior orbital fissure.

It is clear from this description that there is a rich arterial anastomosis supplying the structures of the orbit. Although obstruction of the central retinal artery results in severe loss of visual acuity, obstruction or occlusion of the ophthalmic artery may not lead to any visual impairment because of these abundant external anastomoses with the ophthalmic artery; these anastomotic channels can be sufficient to preserve the ocular blood supply.

Veins of the Orbit

The superior and inferior ophthalmic veins are the primary valveless channels that drain the orbital cavity. The superior ophthalmic vein communicates anteriorly with the nasofrontal and thence the angular vein, and drains along a course similar to that of the ophthalmic artery, receiving tributaries corresponding to branches of the ophthalmic artery. It passes between the two heads of the lateral rectus muscle and the medial portion of the superior orbital fissure, ending in the cavernous sinus. There are many anastomoses with the inferior ophthalmic vein, which is formed of a network of veins in the floor and medial wall of the orbit. In its course it receives venous channels from the eyelids, inferior muscles, and lacrimal sac. It then divides, one branch passing through the inferior orbital fissure to join the pterygoid plexus, the other joining the superior ophthalmic vein as it traverses the superior orbital fissure.

Communications between the angular and deep facial veins and pterygoid plexus allow for minor alterations in venous drainage. Apical disease, resulting in occlusion of the superior ophthalmic vein, may lead to orbital venous congestion. Rupture of an intracavernous aneurysm or the development of an arteriovenous shunt introducing blood under arterial pressure into this system can lead to the development of chemosis, exophthalmos, and ocular bruit.

Orbital Nerves

The passage of the third, fourth, fifth, and sixth cranial nerves to the orbit follows an orderly route that allows the surgeon, familiar with the anatomy, to approach a variety of lesions in the orbit safely. The small size of and the difficulty in visualizing these structures in the presence of expanding disease make it imperative that the normal course of the nerve supply to the muscles and ocular structures be well in mind. Fortunately there is a paucity of fatty tissue in the apex of the orbit in the presence of expanding disease, and most of the structures are displaced, not destroyed, by enlarging tumors. Careful manipulation and a planned surgical approach to a tumor in the apex can be safely accomplished by the transcranial route.

The third, fourth, fifth, and sixth cranial nerves, in that order, from above downward, traverse the cavernous sinus (see Fig. 95–1). They are reoriented as they pass through the dura and enter the superior orbital fissure, entering the orbital cavity in almost the inverse order: From above downward and lateromedially are the lacrimal and frontalis branches of the ophthalmic division of the fifth nerve, the fourth nerve, the superior ramus of the third nerve, the nasociliary nerve, the sixth nerve, and the inferior ramus of the third nerve.

Upon unroofing of the orbit, the frontalis branch of the sensory ophthalmic division of the trigeminal nerve is often visible through the thin periorbita. Just before entering the orbit through the superior orbital fissure, the ophthalmic nerve divides into the frontalis, nasociliary, and lacrimal nerves.

The lacrimal nerve, the smallest branch of the ophthalmic, enters the orbit through the narrowest lateral part of the superior orbital fissure in a separate dural sheath. It follows the lacrimal artery at the upper border of the rectus lateralis muscle, innervates the lacrimal gland, and supplies filaments to the upper lid.

The frontalis nerve runs above the levator palpebrae muscle, dividing into the supratrochlear and supraorbital branches. The smaller supratrochlear nerve passes above the pulley of the superior oblique and exits from the orbit after giving off a branch to join the infratrochlear branch of the nasociliary nerve. It supplies the skin of the lower part of the forehead close to the midline. The supraorbital nerve exits through the supraorbital foramen, giving filaments to the upper lid, and then ascends to the scalp of the forehead.

The nasociliary nerve enters the orbit between the two heads of the lateral rectus muscle between the superior and inferior rami of the oculomotor nerve, passes across the optic nerve obliquely beneath the superior rectus and superior oblique muscles to the medial wall of the orbital cavity. From there it re-enters the cranial cavity through the anterior ethmoidal foramen and descends through a slit at the side of the crista galli into the nasal cavity. The infratrochlear branch arises just before the nasociliary nerve enters the anterior ethmoid foramen and supplies the skin of the eyelids and side of the nose, the conjunctiva, and the lacrimal sac. In its passage, this sensory nerve gives off a long root to the ciliary ganglion and a long ciliary nerve that accompanies short ciliary nerves from the ganglion forward to the iris and cornea through the posterior part of the sclera. Injury to this branch will result in corneal anesthesia.

The ciliary ganglion is a structure less than 1 mm in size, situated behind and lateral to the globe in loose areolar tissue between the optic nerve and the lateral rectus muscle. This is a parasympathetic ganglion containing preganglionic fibers derived from the visceral nuclei of the oculomotor complex in the midbrain. In the ciliary ganglion, these fibers synapse with neurons whose postganglionic fibers pass to the ciliary muscle and sphincter of the pupil. Six to ten short ciliary nerves arise from the ganglion in two bundles and run forward in a curving manner with the ciliary arteries above and below the optic nerve. They are accompanied by the long ciliary branches of the nasociliary nerve. They pierce the sclera and are distributed to the ciliary muscle, iris, and cornea. Injury to the ciliary ganglion results in dilatation of the pupil. The ganglion also is traversed by a few

sympathetic fibers passing from the superior cervical ganglion to the dilator muscles of the eye.

The trochlear nerve pierces the dura mater in the free border of the tentorium just behind and lateral to the posterior clinoid. It passes through the cavernous sinus between the opthalmic and oculomotor nerves. As it enters the orbit through the superior orbital fissure it crosses the oculomotor nerve, becoming superior to it, and then courses medial to the frontalis nerve, from whence it passes medially above the origin of the levator palpebrae muscle to enter the orbital surface of the superior oblique muscle. Because of its small size and its relation to the origin of the levator palpebrae muscle, it is frequently torn by lateral retraction of the levator and superior oblique muscles.

If the levator insertion is torn or deliberately sectioned during resection of an optic nerve tumor through the annulus, the trochlear nerve is sacrificed but the functional deficit is not cosmetically deforming.

The oculomotor nerve is the principal somatic motor nerve supplying the ocular muscles with the exception of the superior oblique and the lateral rectus. It also contributes to the ciliary ganglion and supplies preganglionic parasympathetic motor fibers to the pupillary sphincter and ciliary muscles. Within the cavernous sinus, the oculomotor nerve lies above all the other cranial nerves, and here receives several filaments from the sympathetic plexus and a communicating sensory branch from the ophthalmic division of the trigeminal nerve.

As it enters the orbit through the superior orbital fissure, between the two insertions of the lateral rectus muscle, the oculomotor nerve passes inferior to the trochlear nerve and the frontal and lacrimal branches of the ophthalmic nerve. The nasociliary nerve passes between its superior and inferior rami.

It is of significance to the surgeon that the smaller superior ramus supplying the superior rectus and levator palpebrae muscles passes above the optic nerve, while the branches of the inferior ramus supplying the medial and inferior recti and the inferior oblique muscles pass beneath the optic nerve. It is clear that direct access to the optic nerve through the medial compartment of the orbit may be gained by lateral retraction of the levator and superior rectus muscles without injury to their nerve supply.

The small, long abducent nerve penetrates the dura mater near the dorsum sellae. It runs through a small notch below the posterior clinoid and passes through the cavernous sinus on the lateral side of the internal carotid artery. It enters the orbital fissure above the ophthalmic vein, from which it is separated by a lamina of dura mater. Passing between the two heads of the lateral rectus, it enters the ocular surface of that muscle.

In summary: The lacrimal and frontal branches of the ophthalmic nerve and the trochlear nerve enter in this order from the lateral to the medial side of the superior orbital fissure and, upon entering the orbital cavity, lie above the levator and superior rectus muscles. The remaining nerves enter the orbit between the two heads of the lateral rectus in the following order: the superior division of the oculomotor, the nasociliary branch of the ophthalmic nerve, the abducent nerve, and the inferior division of the oculomotor. Once in the orbit, the trochlear, frontal, and lacrimal nerves lie directly beneath the thin periosteum. The superior division of the oculomotor nerve lies immediately beneath the superior rectus muscle while the nasociliary nerve crosses the optic nerve to reach the medial wall of the orbit. Beneath this is the optic

nerve with the ciliary ganglion on its lateral side. Between it and the lateral rectus muscle is the abducent nerve and the inferior division of the oculomotor nerve.

INCIDENCE OF ORBITAL TUMORS

The incidence of orbital disease found by a neurosurgeon is compared in Table 95–1 with a series of consecutive cases reported by an ophthalmological surgeon at the same institution. As in most series, an unavoidable bias reflecting the interests and viewpoints of the differing disciplines is evident. Only 12 per cent of the cases in the ophthalmological series were of particular interest to the neurosurgeon, while half the cases referred to the neurosurgeon were found to have orbital disorders best treated by nonneurosurgical methods. Mucocele is probably one of the most common causes of unilateral proptosis seen in otolaryngological practice.

Approximately one third of the patients in a random series of consecutive cases of unilateral proptosis seen at the Columbia–Presbyterian Medical Center proved to have hemangioma; another third had pseudotumor, thyrotoxic myositis, granuloma, or other mass lesions that are not primarily neurosurgical problems; and the remaining

TABLE 95–1 UNILATERAL EXOPHTHALMOS—CONSECUTIVE CASES

	CONSECUTIVE NEUROSURGICAL CASES*	CONSECUTIVE OPHTHALMOLOGICAL CASES†
Optic glioma	51	8
Meningioma	40	11
Cylindroma	12	17
Neurofibroma, metastatic malignant tumors	20	15
Sarcoma	9	6
Osteoma, mucocoele	14	8
Fibrous dysplasia, carotid cavernous fistula	12	1
Granuloma, pseudotumor, ossifying fibroma, unverified cause	20	41
Hemangioma, trauma, arteriovenous malformation, thyroid ophthalmopathy	16	65
Encephalocoele, hemangiopericytoma, melanoma, lymphangioma, histiocytoma	15	13
Myopathy, internal carotid aneurysm, cavernous sinus thrombosis, osteogenic sarcoma, foreign body	10	5
Lymphoma, dachryoadenitis, hemangioma of bone, neuresthesio-epithelioma, dermatomyositis, aneurysmal bone cyst, dermoid, lymphosarcoma, chondrosarcoma, odontoma, calcified optic nerve (tumors?)	11	30
Angiosarcoma, sarcoid, myxoma, tuberculosis, posterior scleritis	0	10
TOTAL	230	230

* Consecutive patients with unilateral proptosis examined by the senior author.
† Data from Reese, A. B.: Tumors of the Eye. 2nd Ed. New York, Hoeber Medical Division, Harper & Row, 1963, p. 553.

third of these patients who presented with unilateral exophthalmos proved to have optic glioma, neurofibroma, meningioma, osteoma, encephalocele or carotid-cavernous fistula.[51,62]

DIAGNOSIS OF ORBITAL TUMORS

In the past decade, improvement in diagnostic radiology and the development of newer diagnostic methods have made it possible to obtain more critical pretreatment evaluation.

The results of the preoperative history, physical examination, radiographic evaluations (including contrast studies and pleuridirectional tomography), computed tomography (CT), radioactive scanning, and ultrasonography help to limit the differential diagnosis and lead to the selection of proper therapy. The recent introduction of high-resolution computed tomography of the orbit has greatly increased the accuracy of detection of retrobulbar masses and the definition of their exact relationships to the optic nerve, extraocular muscles, and orbital wall.

Symptoms and Signs

Exophthalmos

The cardinal sign of an orbital tumor is exophthalmos. It may develop over a period of time ranging from days to years. Seldom is it accompanied by pain unless there is invasion of the orbital wall by a lesion such as a carcinoma arising in a sinus or the nasopharynx. Pain may be a late symptom, especially if there is corneal exposure and irritation.

Deep palpation of the ocular fornices will often allow a mass to be felt. The patient is instructed to look toward the fornix that is being palpated. This rotation of the globe toward the examining finger will relax the orbital septum and allow surprisingly deep palpation. Tumors of the lacrimal gland, mucoceles, and tumors along the orbital floor may be felt in this manner. Lymphomas and pseudotumors often extend sufficiently anteriorly so that they too may be palpable. The superior oblique tendon

and its trochlea may mimic a mass in the upper nasal quadrant of the orbit.

Prominence of the lateral orbital wall strongly suggests the presence of a sphenoid wing meningioma when there is hyperostosis of the sphenoid wing and invasion of the orbit.

Any lesion near the orbital apex can affect the nerves in this region, with a resultant defect in motility of the eye causing diplopia; even large tumors, however, particularly those anterior to the narrow apical part of the orbit, may not affect motility. Invasive tumors at the apex, such as carcinoma or meningioma invading the superior orbital fissure, may produce the syndrome of the superior orbital fissure: total external ophthalmoplegia with variable pupillary involvement. Ocular motility can also be limited by tumors arising within the muscle cone at the apex or by invasive tumors or inflammatory processes involving the extraocular muscles. Thus, idiopathic myositis or myositis due to thyroid disease or minimal exophthalmos can limit eye movements, whereas large extraperiorbital tumors, such as osteomas, will not hinder movement even when proptosis is severe.

A clue to the location and nature of an orbital tumor is given by the direction of the exophthalmos. Tumors in the muscle cone, optic nerve, or orbital apex will push the globe forward along the axis of the orbit. Even small lesions here can cause a considerable degree of exophthalmos. Tumors in the anterior part of the orbit tend to displace the globe away from the mass. For example, a mucocele of the frontal sinus will displace the globe down and laterally, while a tumor of the lacrimal gland will displace the globe down and medially.

Chemosis

Chemosis indicates severely increased pressure in the veins of the orbit. This sign may be caused by venous obstruction due to inflammation or an orbital tumor, or by an arteriovenous communication in or behind the orbit. Carotid-cavernous fistulae, usually the result of rupture of an intracavernous aneurysm is the more common form of arteriovenous communication and produces chemosis by increasing intraorbital venous pressure. These shunts are most frequently due to trauma, but arteriovenous malformations in this area, often arising from branches of the external carotid artery, may produce the same clinical syndrome.

An early sign of orbital arteriovenous communication is the appearance of dilated episcleral vessels that extend up to the corneal limbus. On close (biomicroscopic) inspection these vessels appear quite tortuous. This type of vascular injection should not be confused with chronic conjunctivitis, in which the vascular engorgement stops before the vessel reaches the limbus. The patient with an orbital arteriovenous malformation or carotid-cavernous fistula may complain of bruit, which can be auscultated by the examiner.

Ophthalmoscopy

Ophthalmoscopy is important. The observance of retro-ocular striae is evidence that the globe is being deformed extrinsically. Striae of the posterior pole indicate a mass in the muscle cone of the orbit. Unilateral papilledema may be present as a result of venous engorgement, or rarely there may be actual invasion of the nerve head by a glioma of the optic nerve that can be seen with the ophthalmoscope. Optic atrophy may be found in some patients with optic nerve and chiasmal glioma with vision loss even in the absence of proptosis. Optociliary shunting is a characteristic funduscopic finding in patients with primary nerve sheath meningioma.[19]

Orbital tumors show considerable variation in visual symptoms. Surprisingly, large tumors may not alter the visual acuity or field of vision in the affected eye, especially if anteriorly located. Tumors in the orbital apex and those that involve the optic canal are usually accompanied by disturbances of vision early in their development. Intracanalicular lesions may disturb vision and cause no exophthalmos. Large gliomas of the optic nerve may affect only the visual acuity and spare the peripheral field. The presence of a peripheral field defect with optic glioma suggests chiasmal involvement.

Related Syndromes

A number of systemic disease states may be present and readily suggest the cause of the exophthalmos. One of the most common conditions causing exophthalmos is hyperthyroidism. A careful search should be made for possible signs of thyroid dysfunction. This includes observation of lid lag, stare, or restriction of extraocular motility. Intensive clinical laboratory testing should include the Werner test (T_3 suppression) to evaluate thyroid function fully. Clinical examination supplemented by computed tomography usually allows this diagnosis to be made.

Von Recklinghausen's syndrome should be looked for in children with exophthalmos. The presence of café-au-lait spots suggests the diagnosis. Optic nerve glioma, orbital neurofibroma, orbital dehiscence, malignant schwannoma, meningioma, and congenital glaucoma are frequent causes of a prominent globe associated with this condition. Orbital hemangioma in infancy may be accompanied by cutaneous angiomas of a typical appearance.

In children, the possibility of a metastatic neuroblastoma must be borne in mind, as these tumors frequently metastasize to one or both orbits. Metastatic disease to the orbit in adults is a less common cause of exophthalmos. Tumors of the lung, breast, and pancreas, and melanomas can metastatize to the orbit. A general examination is indicated to consider the possible existence of an unsuspected primary tumor.

Diagnostic Tests

When studying the patient with unilateral proptosis, the following questions must be answered by clinical examination and special studies:

1. Is a tumor mass present displacing the globe anteriorly?

2. Is the tumor mass restricted to the orbit?

3. Does the tumor mass involve an adjacent cranial fossa?

4. Does the tumor mass involve a neighboring sinus?

5. Is the tumor part of a generalized disease process?

The symptoms and signs as outlined here will help define the problem; in most cases of exophthalmos, however, further diagnostic studies are necessary to answer these questions. The differential diagnosis can only be clearly discussed in terms of the physical findings supplemented by special studies. In the past, operative exploration *primarily* for diagnosis has been required for diagnosis in a small number of patients. This has become less true with the advent of computed tomography.

Plain X-Ray Films

Plain x-ray films constitute an important diagnostic study of the skull and orbits. To visualize the orbits optimally, it is essential to modify the usual Caldwell view so the petrous pyramids are at or slightly below the orbital floors. Optic canal views should be taken routinely in the evaluation of patients with exophthalmos. The optic canal view also demonstrates the orbital apex, the planum sphenoidale, the medial wall of the orbit, and the fossa of the lacrimal gland.

The x-rays may be normal or may show increased soft-tissue density, increase in orbital volume, changes involving the orbit and adjacent cranial fossae, changes involving the orbit and an adjacent sinus, or miscellaneous changes in the contour and density of the orbital walls.

There are a number of lesions that will cause specific changes in the plain x-rays.[15,49] One of the most common is mucocele involving the orbit and arising from an adjacent sinus. Dermoids and lacrimal gland tumors can cause the formation of a characteristic indentation (fossa formation) in the orbital wall. A hemangioma will, occasionally, show phleboliths, which are considered specific for this tumor. The characteristic dense bone of an orbital osteoma is readily appreciated on the x-ray (see Fig. 95–2). Osteitis may be associated with sinus disease, as may carcinoma that has a sinus origin.

Meningiomas and fibrous dysplasia may show bony changes of the skull that differ only by history, age, and distribution (Fig. 95–3). Arteriography may be required to make the diagnosis in some cases.

Neurofibromatosis may present with dehiscence of the greater wing of the sphenoid, or may be associated with an orbital neurofibroma. Orbital neurofibroma is usually part of the generalized syndrome but may also occur as a solitary tumor.

A unilateral enlargement of the optic foramen strongly suggests the presence of an optic glioma (Fig. 95–4). Rounding of the contour of the canal or an asymmetrical enlargement greater than 1 mm is considered abnormal.

Encephaloceles are readily recognized in children. They may, at times, be difficult to distinguish from mucoceles when these are coexisting anomalies involving the paranasal sinuses.

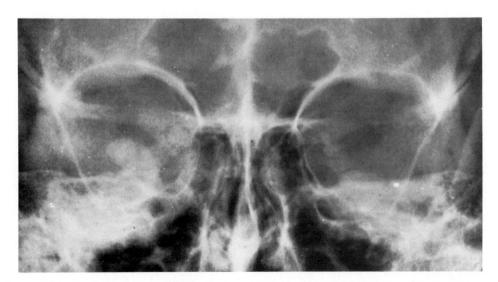

Figure 95–3 Hyperostosing en plaque meningioma involving the lesser wing of the right sphenoid and the greater wing adjacent to the superior obital fissure. This tumor caused vision loss and exophthalmos by direct extension into the orbit.

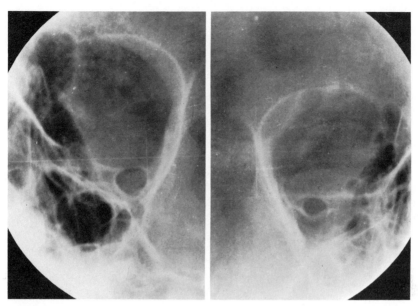

Figure 95–4 Optic glioma, optic foramen views. The enlarged, rounded canal in the left orbit strongly suggests the presence of an optic nerve glioma.

Special Studies

Tomography

The findings in plain radiographs may be elaborated and extended by tomographic examination.[50] Pleuridirectional tomographic examination may show the clouded ethmoid sinus to be surrounded by bone destruction (Figs. 95–5 and 95–6). At times tomograms provide the only evidence of bone destruction associated with mucocele, carcinoma, or granuloma arising in a sinus. Thickening of the orbital plate found in lacrimal gland tumor can be delineated in this way.

Pleuridirectional tomography is most helpful in evaluating the optic canal. Widening of the cranial end of the canal indicates extension of an optic nerve neoplasm into the intracranial cavity, or it may represent the only evidence of a glioma involving the intracranial segment of the optic nerve. High-resolution computed tomography is less sensitive for the detection of intracranial tumors of the optic nerve than those involving the nerve in its intraorbital course. Polytomography may therefore be crucial in evaluating the intracranial optic nerve by demonstrating widening of the cranial end of the optic canal.

Computed Tomography

Computed tomography permits the pictorial differentiation between vitreous, aqueous lens, sclera, optic nerve, extraocular muscles, and orbital fat as well as visualization of the surrounding bones. Small amounts of calcium not visible on the plain x-rays are readily detected by this method. As in studies of brain tumors, intravenous iodinated contrast material will enhance areas of pathological change in the orbit, primarily because of the alteration of the blood-brain barrier by the pathological process. Usually an intravenous injection of 100 ml of a 75 per cent solution of a mixture of meglumine and sodium salts of diatrizoate is administered in a bolus.

High-resolution computed tomography scanning of the orbit can be achieved by decreasing the thickness of the slices from the standard 1 cm to 3.5 mm. It is only with thin sections that details of the orbital apex can be resolved with sufficient accuracy to be useful. Figure 95–7 shows a high-resolution computed tomogram of a normal midorbit. Because orbital fat is naturally radiolucent, a high-contrast image is produced, which is responsible for the extraordinary sensitivity of the method in the diagnosis of orbital tumors.

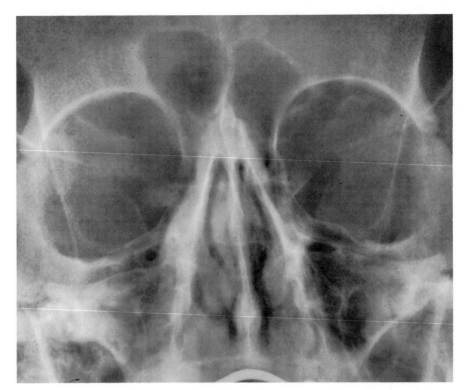

Figure 95–5 This patient with left exophthalmos and severe orbital pain was shown to have a carcinoma of the left anterior ethmoid. The minimal findings of increased ethmoid density may well be overlooked in this plain film view of the orbits.

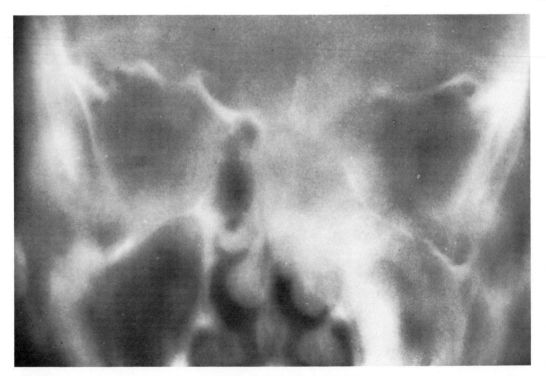

Figure 95–6 Polytomogram of the same patient shown in Figure 95–5. The extensive bone destruction involving the structures of the medial wall of the orbit is clearly seen.

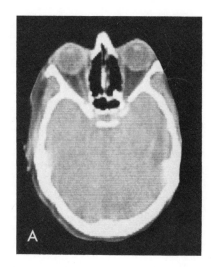

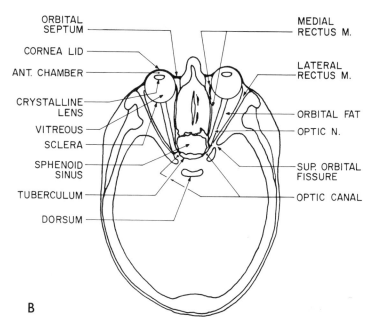

ORBITAL SEPTUM

MEDIAL RECTUS M.

CORNEA LID

ANT. CHAMBER

LATERAL RECTUS M.

CRYSTALLINE LENS

VITREOUS

ORBITAL FAT

SCLERA

OPTIC N.

SPHENOID SINUS

SUP. ORBITAL FISSURE

TUBERCULUM

OPTIC CANAL

DORSUM

B

Figure 95–7   *A*. Normal high-resolution computed tomographic scan through the midorbit. *B*. A labeled diagram of the same section. The globe, vitreous, lens, optic nerve, retrobulbar fat, and extraocular muscles can all be detected and differentiated, even near the apex of the orbit.

As noted elsewhere, unilateral exophthalmos is frequently associated with thyroid dysfunction. Figure 95–8 shows the midorbital scan of an 85-year-old woman with Graves' disease. Clinically, metastatic breast cancer was the suspected cause of her exophthalmos and vision loss. The swollen medial and lateral rectus muscles are clearly visualized in this study. The optic nerve sheath is enlarged owing to compression by the swollen extraocular muscles. It is important to distinguish edematous extraocular muscles, especially the superior and inferior rectus muscles seen in this projection, from orbital masses.

Only one of the authors' series of 131 tumors of the orbit studied with high-resolution computed tomography failed to be visible on the scan. That patient proved to have a lymphangioma. Usually it is possible to determine whether an orbital tumor surrounds or infiltrates the normal orbital structures. Also it is possible to determine whether a tumor is limited to the orbital

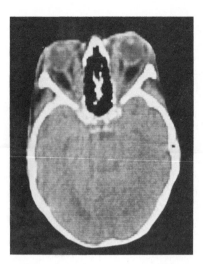

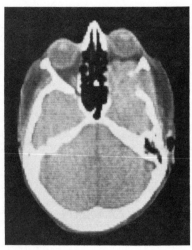

Figure 95-8 Graves' disease. A midorbit high-resolution scan of a patient with Graves' disease shows the characteristic swelling of the extraocular muscles as well as the proptosis. The swollen muscles may enlarge sufficiently to compress the optic nerve and reduce vision. A swollen inferior rectus when obliquely sectioned, particularly if the sections are thick, may mimic an orbital tumor. Great caution must be exercised when an apical tumor is detected on a thick CT section obtained in the lower part of the orbit.

Figure 95-9 Orbital metastasis from a primary tumor in the breast. This patient presented with exophthalmos and vision loss one year following mastectomy for cancer. The orbital mass has caused destruction of the lateral orbital wall and extended intracranially. Bone destruction is a common occurrence in metastatic disease.

cavity or is extending intracranially to the extracranial temporal fossa or to an adjacent paranasal sinus. Further, it is usually possible to establish whether a lesion lies outside the muscle cone or within it; and as a rule, it is possible to determine whether an intraconal mass is arising from the optic nerve or just displacing it.

The patient whose CT scan appears in Figure 95-9 is a 59-year-old woman with a history of mastectomy eight months before. She had an eight-week history of progressive vision loss. The plain film views of the orbit showed slight destruction of the orbital floor at the apex. The CT scan shows a large soft-tissue mass invading the orbit and the middle cranial fossa, destroying the greater wing of the sphenoid. The true extent of the tumor was unsuspected on clinical evidence alone. This example is a good illustration of the importance of computed tomography in the study of lesions of the orbit, particularly those invading adjacent compartments. Figure 95-10 shows a meningioma arising from the left greater wing of the sphenoid bone, displacing the lateral rectus muscle and the optic nerve. The anterior clinoid is also involved by this tumor. Computed tomog-

raphy in this case has established the extent and nature of this extraconal meningioma.

Tumors of the intraorbital portion of the optic nerve have, heretofore, been difficult to diagnose. No bone changes are produced by these tumors if they do not reach the optic canal, and vascular displacements are

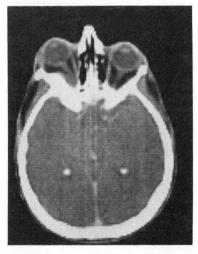

Figure 95-10 Meningioma of the lateral orbital wall. There is hyperostosis and thickening of the greater wing of the sphenoid of the left orbit. The lateral rectus muscle and the optic nerve are both displaced medially. The proptosis is well demonstrated. The meningioma also involves the anterior clinoid process and the region of the optic foramen.

unreliable. Computed tomography has contributed greatly to the diagnosis of optic nerve tumors. Specifically, one can establish whether any given tumor meets the following diagnostic criteria.

1. Enlargement of the intraorbital segment of the optic nerve can be readily detected. The optic nerve normally measures 2 mm on the Polaroid print in the standard computed tomography head unit. A nerve that is 4 mm in diameter or is irregular in outline is abnormal.

2. It is possible on a CT scan to detect the intracranial extension of a tumor, particularly after the administration of intravenous contrast medium. The sensitivity of computed tomography in detecting small intracranial extensions, however, is not as good as its sensitivity in the orbit. Accurate evaluation of the intracranial component can only be achieved by the intravenous administration of contrast medium, and even with such contrast, a few gliomas are not enhanced sufficiently to be differentiated from the surrounding brain tissue.

3. The involvement of the optic chiasm is easier to detect with computed tomography than the involvement of the intracranial part of the optic nerve. The optic chiasm is surrounded by the basal cisterns, which can be detected readily on the scan, and a tumor in the optic chiasm region is usually appreciated, particularly after contrast enhancement.

Multicentric tumors arising from both

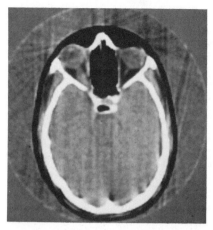

Figure 95–12 Left optic nerve glioma. The left optic nerve is thickened and nodular and is involved from the globe to the orbital apex.

optic nerves are readily detected by CT scanning. Computed tomography appears, therefore, to be the investigative procedure of choice for the evaluation of tumors of the optic nerve. This technique may be supplemented by pneumoencephalography with tomography to appreciate small extensions of a tumor in the intracranial portion of the optic nerve and chiasm that cannot be enhanced.

Figure 95–11 shows a scan of a 42-year-old woman with progressive vision loss. The fusiform swelling of the optic nerve is suggestive of a nerve sheath meningioma, which was confirmed at operation in this case. The scan in Figure 95–12 is that of a young patient with neurofibromatosis, exophthalmos, and vision loss, who proved to have an optic nerve glioma.

Since the clinical introduction of computed tomography, it has become the single most important test for the evaluation of patients with exophthalmos. The technique is noninvasive, is highly reliable in the retrobulbar space, and can differentiate between masses arising from the various anatomical structures in the orbit. Its development has led to a decrease in the use of arteriography, almost complete replacement of phlebography, and limitation of the use of pneumoencephalography to a very few cases.

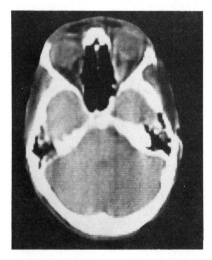

Figure 95–11 Meningioma of the optic nerve. The intraorbital segment of the optic nerve is enlarged by a fusiform mass that proved to be an optic nerve sheath meningioma.

Pneumoencephalography

Pneumoencephalography is helpful in studying exophthalmos.[12] Air in the supra-

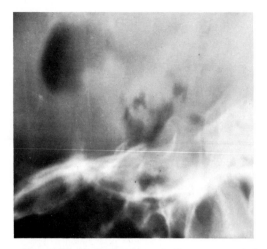

Figure 95–13 Optic chiasmal glioma surrounded by air with obliteration of infundibular and optic recesses.

sellar cisterns and anterior third ventricle can outline the optic nerve and chiasm; obliteration of the chiasmatic recess is characteristic of tumor invading the optic chiasm (Fig. 95–13). This is the most critical indication of small chiasmal tumors; thus far more sensitive than computed tomographic scanning.

The intracranial extent of orbital tumors invading the cranial cavity can be delineated by air study. Visualization of the anterior tips of the temporal horns provides an indication of significant extension of tumor into the middle cranial fossa.

Angiography*

Because the ophthalmic artery has a variable course through the orbit, arteriography is not a sensitive indicator for mass displacement. Vascular tumors in the orbit show neovascularization and a stain, and some large orbital tumors will cause visible displacement of the ophthalmic artery.

Arteriography may still prove useful in the study of tumors that involve the orbital apex as well as an adjacent cranial fossa. The common tumor of this region, meningioma, usually will have a well-developed vascular supply and stain.

Selective internal and external carotid angiograms are helpful in assessing the rela-

tive contributions of the two circulations. Selective study is especially useful in analyzing arteriovenous malformations. The demonstration of a significant external carotid supply can influence the selection of a therapeutic approach.

Venography frequently yields positive findings in tumors restricted to the orbit because the venous pattern is frequently displaced by these tumors. Venous disease can be assessed by means of venography: Varices are readily visible, venous inflammatory disease can be studied, and the cavernous sinus can be visualized. Nevertheless these contrast studies have become less necessary since high-resolution CT scans have become available.

Isotope Scanning

Many cases of unilateral exophthalmos are associated with inflammatory disease and thyroid dysfunction. Isotope scanning of the orbits has proved to be an effective way to separate these patients from those harboring tumors. There is an impressive difference in isotope concentration between patients with tumors and those with thyroid disease.

Scanning of the orbits has proved useful not only in detecting cellular tumors, but also in following these patients after treatment. The single exception is neurofibroma of the orbit, which is not detectable by radioisotope study. These tumors do, however, usually show enhancement on computed tomography.

Ultrasonography

Ultrasonography is a diagnostic modality for detecting orbital tumors. The acoustic image of an orbital tumor pressing on the posterior aspect of the globe is seen in Figure 95–14. This technique is, in its current state of development, most useful in detecting tumors in or close to the globe. It is least sensitive for tumors in the orbital apex. Clearly the computed tomography scanner has superseded the ultrasonogram in the routine examination of the patient with exophthalmos. The ultrasonogram does present characteristic patterns in inflammatory disease that are helpful in the evaluation of the patient with pseudotumor.[8]

* See references 22, 42, 61.

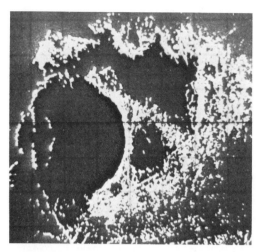

Figure 95–14   Ultrasonogram: B-scan at 10 MHz. The homogeneous acoustic density behind the globe is caused by a muscle cone tumor.

TREATMENT OF ORBITAL TUMORS

Ophthalmologists, otolaryngologists, internists, and neurosurgeons have shared an interest in the diagnosis and treatment of patients with unilateral exophthalmos, but their differing experience has led to controversy as to the best therapy or the proper operative approach. Some ophthalmologists have advocated orbital exploration as the primary diagnostic method, and some neurosurgeons believe a primary transcranial procedure is indicated when an orbital tumor is suspected.[10,11]

The neurosurgeon must recognize that many types of exophthalmos can be treated by systemic medical therapy, chemotherapy, or radiotherapy. The preferred treatment for others, particularly tumors in the anterior and lateral sections of the orbit, may require an orbital or nasal approach for diagnosis and simple or radical excision. Tumors involving the orbital apex and optic canal, including optic glioma, meningioma, neurofibroma, encephalocele, and carotid-cavernous fistula are of particular importance to the neurosurgeon and should be recognized clinically because primary transcranial operation is indicated.

Orbital Approaches

Orbital operation may be performed primarily to confirm or to make a diagnosis.[3,39,45] Excisional biopsy by this approach is, of course, achieved whenever possible. If no discrete orbital mass is found, biopsy of the lacrimal gland and extraocular muscles should be performed. Infiltration of inflammatory cells in the muscles and the lacrimal gland in the absence of other findings indicates myositis or dacryoadenitis as a cause for the exophthalmos. The absence of inflammation raises the suspicion that a tumor mass has been missed.

The orbital approach should be considered when the tumor is located anterior to the equator of the eye. In this position tumors can usually be palpated and are readily approachable by one of the standard transconjunctival or skin incisions at the suitable orbital margin.

Tumors behind the equator of the globe require more extensive procedures. A lateral orbitotomy or a modified Krönlein resection of the lateral orbital wall will provide excellent exposure of the retrobulbar contents. In Berke's modification of the Krönlein operation, a lateral canthotomy is extended beyond the edge of the zygomatic bone, the lateral canthal ligaments are divided, and the periosteum is incised at the upper and lower borders of the lateral wall. The lateral wall is cut with a Stryker saw, broken free, and retracted laterally to expose the orbital contents. Tumors of the orbital apex can be exposed by this approach, and safe excision of tumors in the lateral quadrants of the orbit may be achieved. With the use of micro-operative techniques, even tumors that crowd the lateral apex can be excised without injury to the extraocular muscles or their nerve supply by lateral orbitotomy. Diagnostic exploration by this route should be considered in those few cases of exophthalmos in which the suspicion of a tumor persists when results of diagnostic work-up have been inconclusive. Tumors of the optic nerve or medial to the optic nerve and near the apex can more safely be approached by the transcranial route.

Transcranial Approach

The primary advantages offered by the transcranial route to the orbital apex and optic canal are access to both the orbital and cranial cavities, and superior exposure of the superior medial and lateral quadrants of the orbit with an expectation of preservation of function and a good cosmetic result.[24,24a,43,46]

It is obvious that when treating a malignant neoplasm, eradication of the disease may be the primary aim, and preservation of function and cosmetic considerations become secondary. It naturally follows that preoperative investigations that can narrow the differential diagnosis are essential in deciding which case should be explored primarily by the transcranial route and which should not.

If invasive orbital malignant disease is confined to structures within the periorbita, it should be treated by radical exenteration. Hesitancy in applying this principle frequently results in local recurrence of tumor with extension through the superior or inferior orbital fissure to the cranial cavity or base of the skull. A primary transcranial approach is unwise, as the orbital unroofing can expose the intracranial space to a malignant neoplasm.

Only half of 100 neurosurgical cases of unilateral exophthalmos were found to be suitable for primary exploration (Table 95–2). It is perhaps of greater significance that after thoughtful preoperative work-up no patient with pseudotumor, myopathy, inflammatory disease, or malignant disease of the orbit underwent primary exploration by the transcranial route.

Transorbital exploration for diagnosis is sometimes indicated in cases of solitary orbital neurofibroma, because of the relative difficulty in making this diagnosis clinically. A primary transcranial exploration is preferred when optic glioma, meningioma, osteoma, or encephalocele can be recognized. In addition to superior exposure and preservation of cranial nerve function, there are a number of other advantages offered by this approach. The coronal incision and frontal craniotomy are cosmetically acceptable. The extradural approach affords little risk of injury to the cerebral cortex. The use of osmotic diuretics or drainage of cerebrospinal fluid from the chiasmatic cistern permits the safe development of an adequate operative field for orbital unroofing. This in turn provides access to the apex and the medial and superior lateral compartments of the orbit (Fig. 95–15).

Following transcranial orbital exploration for tumor, it is recommended that the periorbita be closed with fine silk or synthetic suture and that tantalum or stainless steel screen be used to bridge the defect in the orbital roof to avoid transmission of cerebral pulsation to the globe.

A tarsorrhaphy performed at the time of operation will protect the eye, and a pressure dressing over the orbit helps to reduce orbital swelling in the immediate postoperative period. Systemic steroid therapy is also useful in reducing postoperative swelling.

Radical Operative Procedures

When ocular or adenexal malignant tumors have recurred following transorbital or transnasal operations, more extensive and radical procedures may be considered.

TABLE 95–2 TREATMENT OFFERED IN 100 CASES REFERRED TO NEUROSURGEON FOR PRIMARY MANAGEMENT

	THERAPY AND NUMBER OF CASES						
TYPE OF TUMOR	Primary Intracranial Operation	Primary Transorbital or Transnasal Operation	Radiotherapy Only	Carotid Infusion and Radiotherapy	Shunt and Radiotherapy	Other Therapy	Total
Optic glioma	22		10		2		34
Meningioma	18	3	5	1		1	28
Neurofibroma	6	2					8
Osteoma	2	2					4
Carcinoma		2	1	3			6
Mucocele		2					2
Pseudotumor		3					3
Granuloma	2	3					5
Melanoma		2					2
Carotid-cavernous fistula	3					2	5
Hemangioma		3					3
Total	53	22	16	4	2	3	100

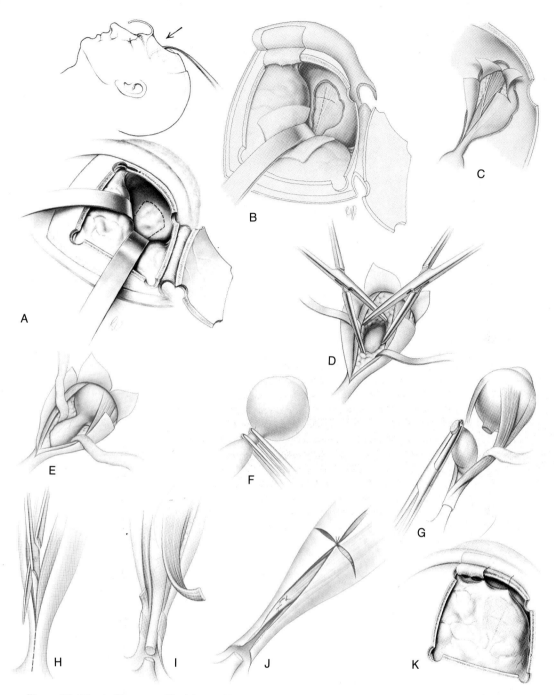

Figure 95–15 *A.* The coronal incision and low frontal osteoplastic craniotomy flap are used to expose the floor of the anterior fossa. *B.* A flap of pericranium is pulled over the bone margin and sutured to the dura to seal the frontal sinus. An epidural approach to the anterior fossa insures preservation of the olfactory nerve and minimizes retraction injury to the frontal lobe. *C.* The periorbita is incised medial to the levator and superior rectus muscles as identified by the location of the frontalis nerve. *D.* A direct trajectory is made toward the optic nerve and tumor capsule without dissection of intraorbital fat. *E.* Moist cottonoids are used to separate the orbital fat at a plane directly on the tumor capsule. *F.* The nerve is sectioned between forceps. *G.* The nerve can be lifted from its bed. *H.* The levator muscle must be sectioned at its origin to avoid tearing. *I.* The entire intracanalicular portion of the nerve is removed. *J.* The levator origin is reattached to the annulus of Zinn with atraumatic 6-0 figure-of-eight suture. *K.* Upon completion of tumor removal the periorbita is closed with fine atraumatic sutures; Gelfoam is placed over the periorbita; a wire mesh bridge is formed and placed at the orbital roof defect to avoid postoperative pulsation of the globe. Dural tenting sutures are then placed. (*A* and *K* from Housepian, E. M.: Intraorbital tumors. *In* Schmidek, H. H., and Sweet, W. H., eds.: Current Techniques in Operative Neurosurgery. New York, Grune & Stratton, 1977. *B* through *J* from Housepian. E. M.: The surgical treatment of optic nerve sheath meningiomas. Modern Technics in Surgery, Vol. 21, Neurosurgery. Mt. Kisco, N.Y., Futura Publishing Co., 1981. Reprinted by permission.)

For example, the fortunately infrequent choroidal malignant melanoma is usually treated by simple enucleation. For those cases in which it recurs locally, wide en bloc resection must be used. In this instance, following subperiosteal excision of the orbital structures (radical exenteration), the bony margins of the orbit must be meticulously excised. When there is preoperative evidence of invasion of bone at the roof, intracranial dura should also be resected. Extension of the operative procedure through all structures bordering on, not harboring, pathological process must be achieved. The residual deformity is then covered by mobilization of tissue from the forehead.

It is equally apparent that when there is evidence of extension of tumor beyond a safe operative field, radical excision cannot be successful and should not be undertaken.

OPTIC GLIOMA

Optic nerve gliomas represent between 0.1 and 1 per cent of conditions responsible for the production of unilateral exophthalmos in the general population. The incidence is higher, approximately 3 to 6 per cent, in children. They occur most frequently in the first decade and are often associated with neurofibromatosis.

It may be highly significant that although there is an overall 20 per cent incidence of neurofibromatosis in patients with optic glioma, the association is only 5 per cent in chiasmal glioma but over 50 per cent in single optic nerve glioma without chiasmal involvement. This observation correlates well with the occurrence of two morphologically different types of astrocytomas. One type, found in over half the patients with neurofibromatosis and single optic nerve glioma, is characterized by preservation of the gross appearance of the nerve, which is invaded by tumor and surrounded by hyperplastic fibrous stroma and tumor. A second type, found in the absence of neurofibromatosis, is characterized by a diffuse replacement of optic nerve elements by astrocytic tumor. These observations may provide a clue to the etiology of tumors found in association with von Recklinghausen's disease. In addition, should a difference be found in the natural history of

these two types, it may alter current concepts on management.

Although it is well known that the growth characteristics of optic glioma are quite variable, it is surprising that any controversy exists as to the neoplastic nature of this condition.[25,27,56] Throughout the literature on this topic, the low-grade pilocytic astrocyte has been described as the predominant cell type.[14,40,44,63] These tumors are composed of elongated astrocytic cells that are compactly arranged in some areas and loosely arranged in myxomatous foci containing mucosubstances in other areas (Figs. 95–16 and 95–17). The demonstration of Rosenthal fibers is useful in distinguishing these tumors from schwannomas, which also may exhibit compact and looser foci. The concept of "benign arachnoidal hyperplasia" occurring in association with optic glioma and extending beyond the tumor is controversial. Enlargement of an optic canal by such a process has not been proved. "Fibromatosis" of the optic nerve sheath has been seen in association with glioma of the optic nerve but not alone. This finding may be responsible for some confusion regarding the clinical behavior of these tumors.

Several cases of glioblastoma have been found in both infants and adults.[26,65] Oligodendroglia-like cells have been described in a few isolated reports but none were found in 57 histologically studied optic gliomas at the Columbia–Presbyterian Medical Center.

A glioma of the optic nerve may be confined to its orbital, intracanalicular, or intracranial portion, or it may arise in or extend to the chiasm. While glioma of the optic nerve is usually unilateral, chiasmatic tumors may spread to both nerves. In the authors' most recent study of 114 cases of optic glioma, 25 per cent were found to involve a single optic nerve alone, whereas the majority (83 cases) involved the chiasm alone or the chiasm and one or both optic nerves. The optic tracts were involved in three cases. Two patients were found to have gliomas of multicentric origin with involvement of both optic nerves and sparing of the chiasm. One case was proved by operative exploration and the other by CT scanning. The gliomas that appear to be confined to the orbit are usually found by histological examination to extend into or through the optic canal. Frequently when

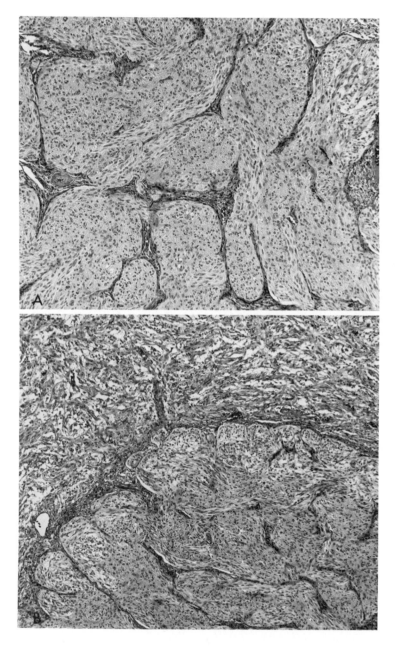

Figure 95–16 Optic nerve gliomas in children are pilocytic astrocytomas, juvenile type, sharing many morphological and behavioral features with similar tumors of the periventricular and cerebellar regions. *A*. The tumor has separated the septa of the optic nerve and, *B*, has grown in the subarachnoid space.

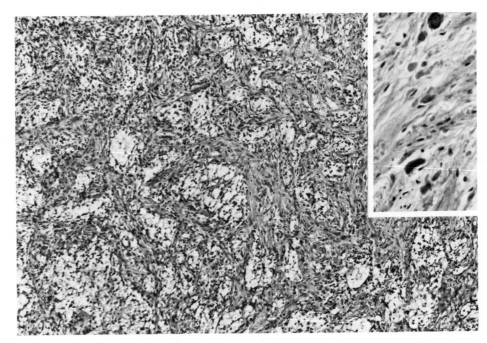

Figure 95–17 Optic nerve gliomas display compactly arranged pilocytic astrocytes and stellate astrocytes in a myxoid background. The demonstration of Rosenthal fibers (*inset*) helps to distinguish the tumor from a schwannoma.

gross tumor is limited to one optic nerve on the intracranial aspect of the optic foramen, astrocytes are found as far as the optic chiasm. Technically, a tumor can be resected if it is limited to a single optic nerve and does not appear to involve the chiasm. Tumors that obviously involve the chiasm are rarely removed because of the severe visual impairment associated with partial chiasm resection. In addition, resection of the optic chiasm offers no assurance that total tumor removal has been achieved. Because this neoplasm is often radiosensitive, radiotherapy is the treatment of choice in chiasmal or multicentric lesions.

The diagnosis of optic glioma can be made preoperatively in almost every case. Chiasmal involvement can be determined without operative exploration. The diagnosis is made by the characteristic x-ray appearance of an enlarged and rounded optic canal. The normal optic canal is elliptical with the long axis vertical at the orbital end and horizontal at the cranial end. Tomography can show which end of the canal is largest and indicate where the major part of the tumor will be found. A chiasmal tumor will deform the anterior third ventricle as seen by pneumoencephalography. The computed tomographic scan may show

a large chiasmal tumor but is not as sensitive for small chiasmal lesions that do not show enhancement. At times the hyperplastic type of tumor associated with von Recklinghausen's disease can be visualized by computed tomography. An enlarged intracranial optic nerve sometimes can be outlined by air in the suprasellar cistern. Visual field testing is difficult in children, helpful in older patients. Surprisingly, a large chiasmal tumor may not produce a chiasmal syndrome, and only the vision of one eye may be affected.

Table 95–2 shows that of a group of 34 cases of optic glioma, 22 were explored transcranially, 10 others were irradiated primarily because of clinical evidence of chiasmal tumor, and 2 required shunting procedures prior to radiotherapy because of the presence of obstructive hydrocephalus. Of the 22 patients operated on by the transcranial route, 3 of the earlier ones were found to have extension of tumor to the chiasm; biopsies were obtained, and the patients received radiotherapy. Today these three patients would not have been subjected to exploration, as they all showed blunting of the chiasmatic recess on pneumoencephalography. In 19 cases, the glioma was confined to a single optic nerve and was resected in its entirety; in none of these cases has there been recurrence of tumor.

There is general agreement that operative excision is indicated in those cases of unilateral optic nerve glioma associated with proptosis and visual impairment. To fulfill the criteria, there must be no evidence of chiasmal involvement on pneumoencephalography and no tumor (multicentric) on the other optic nerve by computed tomography. Under these conditions, operative excision should extend from the globe to the chiasm.

A detailed discussion of the operative approach in the treatment of optic glioma will clarify the accessibility of the orbital apex by the transcranial route.[24] The coronal incision is favored for cosmetic reasons. Following the unilateral frontal craniotomy, the chiasm is inspected intradurally. If there is chiasmal involvement, orbital exploration is usually not indicated. If the tumor is confined to a single optic nerve, the nerve should be sectioned as close to the chiasm as possible. There is no virtue in saving a stump of optic nerve in front of the chiasm. The farther from the tumor that the nerve is sectioned, the less the chance that straggling glial tumor cells will appear at the resection margin. If tumor has not been identified intracranially, it is wise to wait until the orbit is explored and the presence of a tumor verified before sectioning the prechiasmal nerve.

In either case, the dura is then replaced and an extradural approach made toward the anterior clinoid, uncovering the floor of the anterior fossa. The orbital unroofing is started with a drill or small chisel and completed with small rongeurs and must be extended through the optic canal so that the dural sheath can be uncovered. The periorbita, particularly in young children, is very thin but can be carefully opened in a cruciate fashion. An operating microscope often is helpful because the orbital structures are difficult to identify in young patients, particularly when they are thinned and attenuated by compression. The frontalis branch of the ophthalmic division of the fifth nerve can be seen lying over the levator and the superior rectus muscles, and these structures must be identified. The trochlear nerve is found with difficulty because of its small size and cannot always be spared when optic nerve resection is indi-

cated. The deficiency of superior oblique muscle function, however, is hardly recognized and, of course, of no functional consequence in a blind eye.

In older children, when the structures are of sufficient size and exposure is wide enough to allow manipulation, it is possible to identify the levator origin and place a suture through it. Although the superior rectus muscle arises directly from the midportion of the annulus, the levator curves laterally over the superior rectus muscle and the optic nerve from its origin on the superior medial side of the annulus of Zinn (Fig. 95–18). To open the annulus, the levator origin should be sectioned and the muscle with its nerve supply retracted laterally. The annulus may then be opened without disturbing the superior rectus origin to allow removal of the tumor-bearing intraorbital optic nerve (Fig. 95–19). If there is bleeding from the ophthalmic artery or one of its small posterior ciliary branches, it can easily be controlled by bipolar electrocoagulation. It must be remembered that the third nerve enters the orbit lateral to the optic nerve and then branches to the inferior and medial rectus muscles by passing under the optic nerve. Following section

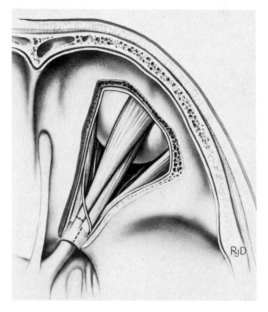

Figure 95–18 Diagram of operative exposure of the right orbit following unroofing. The filamentous trochlear nerve is seen coursing over the bodies of the levator and superior rectus muscles. Perforated lines represent the plane of sectioning of the levator muscle origin and the annulus of Zinn.

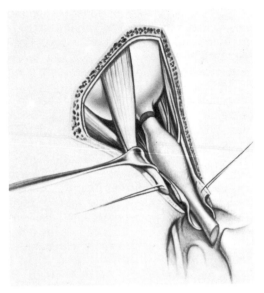

Figure 95–19 Diagram of operative exposure of the right optic nerve. The limits of resection at the globe and chiasm are illustrated. Sectioning of the levator insertion and opening of the annulus of Zinn with lateral retraction of the levator and superior rectus muscles and their nerve supply are shown.

and resuturing of the levator origin, there is prompt recovery of the levator and superior rectus function, usually beginning in one to three weeks with full recovery in three to six months (Fig. 95–20).

In children under 3 or 4 years of age, the structures and spaces are too small for ade-

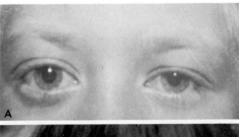
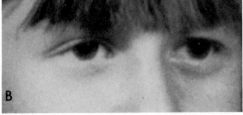

Figure 95–20 Nine year-old girl with glioma of the right optic nerve. She is shown preoperatively, *A*, and three years after resection of the optic nerve, *B*. The excellent preservation of extraocular muscle function following levator section and resuturing is seen.

quate operative exposure, and the optic nerve should be removed in two pieces—from the globe to the annulus and from the annulus to the chiasm.

Although radiotherapy has been shown to be highly effective in the treatment of some gliomas of the optic nerve, long-term follow-up study indicates that late recurrences have occurred.[7,28,60] For this reason, when the tumor is confined to a single optic nerve, operative resection is believed to be the treatment of choice. Resection of the globe is not necessary. It is important to perform histological examination on the proximal margin of the resected optic nerve, since straggling astrocytes may be found extending as far as the chiasm. In these cases, it is deemed wise to supplement the resection with radiotherapy of 4500–5000 rads tumor dose to the optic chiasm over a five-week period.

Postoperative isotope scans provide a useful index of clinical activity and revert to normal following tumor resection or radiotherapy. The mercury scan can thus indicate recurrence of tumor growth. The CT scan has shown a reduction of the size of the mass following radiotherapy in some cases.

ORBITAL MENINGIOMA

Meningioma accounts for from 5 to 17 per cent of orbital disease producing exophthalmos.[52] This tumor most frequently occurs in the fourth and fifth decades, but primarily orbital meningioma has been found in the first and second decades. There is a greater preponderance in females, on the order of 2:1. In the older age group, meningiomas of the sphenoid wing are most often responsible for the development of proptosis and exophthalmos. Between 20 and 30 per cent of meningiomas that produce exophthalmos arise in the orbit and are confined to the optic nerve sheath. Meningioma of the orbit in children is frequently associated with neurofibromatosis, and the occurrence of meningioma and neurofibroma of the orbit or meningioma and cerebellopontine angle neurofibroma has been reported in children with von Recklinghausen's disease. Childhood meningiomas are more aggressive than those in adults. They grow more rapidly in an invasive manner and may be difficult to eradicate when involving the periorbita. Virtually all primary intraorbital meningiomas begin initially under the dura of the optic nerve anywhere from the optic foramen to the globe.[9,57] Sheath meningiomas occur within the intraorbital portions of the optic nerve more commonly than within the canal, but microscopic extension of tumor through the optic canal may occur without accompanying hyperostosis or enlargement of the canal.[58] Many apparently primary sheath meningiomas may indeed have their true origin at the cranial end of the optic canal between the optic nerve and carotid artery, a region normally rich in arachnoid rests and possibly a "spawning ground" for meningioma. Intracranial exploration of this region is therefore mandatory when dealing with optic nerve sheath meningioma.[59] Axial proptosis is an early sign of lesions near the globe but may appear late in apical lesions. Opticociliary veins may develop on the optic nerve head as blood is shunted away from the obstructed central retinal vein into the choroidal veins (Fig. 95–21).[19]

Meningiomas involving the periorbita usually occur in the upper lateral quadrant and arise from arachnoid rests in the superior orbital fissure.

In some instances, they have been found to erode through the lateral sphenoid wing in continuity with en plaque dural tumor at the pteryon. In these cases it may be difficult to define the origin and direction of extension of the tumor. Whether a meningioma may begin in the orbit initially unattached to the optic nerve or at the superior orbital tissue is a controversial subject. In the review by Karp and associates, not a single instance of an ectopic meningioma originating in the soft tissue of the orbit was encountered.[35] If this type of lesion does rarely occur, it is presumed to originate from ectopic arachnoid cells within the perineurium of an orbital peripheral nerve.

Histopathologically, intrasheath meningiomas are of the syncytial or transitional varieties, featuring polygonal cells with indistinct cytoplasm and vesicular nuclei (Fig. 95–22). Angioblastic and fibroblastic variants of meningioma are not seen among primary intraorbital meningiomas. Psammoma bodies are frequently present in these tumors.

The characteristic radiographic finding of hyperostosis strongly suggests the presence of a meningioma. Cloudlike calcification may be demonstrated on x-ray studies. A particularly difficult type of optic nerve meningioma to diagnose is the intracanalicular meningioma, which may present as progressive optic neuritis over months or years.[36,54] Pleuridirectional tomography is the best way of diagnosing intracanalicular meningiomas. Computed tomography with enhancement often delineates the location and extent of the tumor, and angiography demonstrates its blood supply and vascularity, confirming this diagnosis.

The preferred treatment for sphenoid ridge meningioma is craniotomy and total or partial removal of the tumor.[9] If partial excision with enucleation or exenteration has already been done by the transorbital route, craniotomy may not be indicated for eradication of residual tumor at the apex. In an exenterated orbit, this can be achieved with a dissecting microscope, and a clean optic sheath left at the optic canal. Split-thickness skin grafting must follow such radical exenteration. Radioactive isotope scanning is not only helpful in the preoperative diagnosis and localization of meningioma of the orbit, but is extremely useful as an index of recurrent growth following operative removal. Although not usually considered, radiotherapy has been successful in retarding the regrowth of residual meningioma in some cases in which the tumor cannot be totally extirpated. Radiotherapy should be considered for palliation in patients who are very elderly or in poor-risk

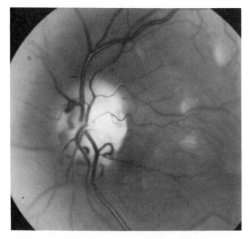

Figure 95–21 Optic atrophy, opticociliary shunt vessels on the nervehead, and retinal striae developed in a patient with an intrasheath meningioma.

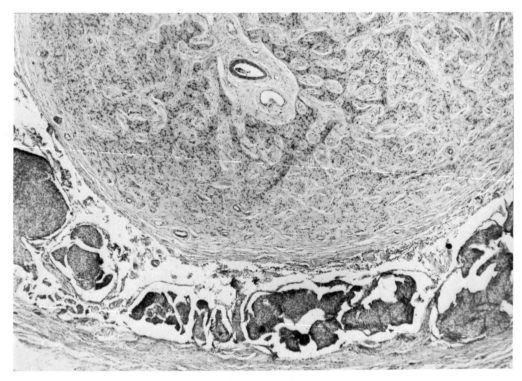

Figure 95–22   Sheets and nests of meningothelial cells are present beneath the dura in this intrasheath meningioma. Note the atrophy of the optic nerve.

patients with extensive sphenoid ridge meningioma.

Meningioma involving the periorbita can rarely be locally extirpated. In young children particularly, this tumor appears to grow more rapidly than meningiomas found elsewhere. All too frequently it spreads radially, infiltrating the apical periorbita. It invades structures at the base of the skull once it reaches the confluence of the orbital dura and the inferior orbital fissure, or extends to the intracranial dura through the superior orbital fissure. Local gross total removal of periorbital meningioma in children too frequently leads to "recurrence." When at the time of transcranial exploration, meningioma in a child is found to extend beyond the structures at the apex of the orbit and to involve the periorbita, it is reasonable to recommend that the optic sheath and nerve be sectioned at the orbital entrance to the optic canal and that the apical periosteum be separated from the orbital bone and excised as cleanly as possible. For these reasons, when orbital meningioma is suspected and a primary transcranial operation is planned, the possible necessity for optic nerve section and later radical exenteration must be discussed preoperatively. The surgeon must be aware that transection of the periorbita at the superior orbital fissure not only destroys the nerve supply to the extraocular muscles but almost always results in severe orbital swelling because of interruption of the major orbital venous drainage, the superior ophthalmic vein. In preparation for a second-stage orbital exenteration, a Silastic and wire mesh barrier can be placed over the orbital roof defect to exclude the possibility of meningioma seeding to the intracranial dura. When biopsy of a meningioma has been performed through a Krönlein approach, "seeding" of tumor within the temporalis muscle has occasionally occurred.

Primary optic nerve sheath origin was found in 9 of 28 cases of proptosis produced by meningioma. The typical patient is a woman in the second or third decade who presents with gradual, painless proptosis and with or without visual impairment (Fig. 95–23). Plain films and orbital tomograms are negative. There is frequently a positive radioisotope scan and an optic nerve tumor

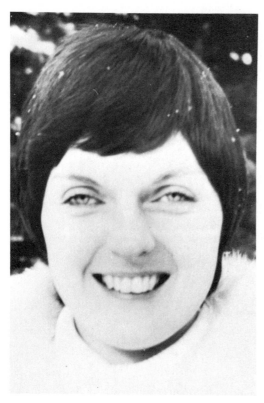

Figure 95–23 Twenty-three-year-old woman six months after a transcranial orbital exploration and gross total removal of a primary optic nerve sheath meningioma.

that can be enhanced with contrast on computed tomography. Angiographic evidence of a mass with a tumor stain is frequently confirmatory.

Lateral orbitotomy, though at times successful in dealing with nerve sheath meningioma located far distal to the apex, is not the preferred treatment for meningioma. The medial approach to the tumor is safer near the apex. Intracranial microinspection may reveal tumor at the cranial end of the canal. Although continuity of the optic nerve can at times be preserved by piecemeal tumor removal, nevertheless vision is usually lost because of interruption of the collateral blood supply that is shared by the retina and the tumor. When vision is impaired before operation, tumor removal is facilitated by resection of the optic nerve together with the tumor from the globe to the orbital apex, or to the chiasm if intracranial tumor is seen at the optic canal. Once this is achieved, inspection of the origins of the muscles at the annulus of Zinn

and oculomotor foramen with high magnification (the operating microscope) will determine whether gross total tumor removal has been achieved. In this location, the meningioma usually grows slowly and the pathologic changes may be confined to within the muscle cone remote from the periorbita. In these cases, it is reasonable to avoid a radical resection of all the apical structures, as may be necessary to effect an operative cure. This manner of management of the problem also avoids the functional and cosmetic deficit that accompanies the radical resection. In such cases, serial radioisotope and computed tomography scanning supplementing clinical evaluation may be permissible in following the course of a possible recurrence.

PERIPHERAL NERVE TUMORS

The orbit is richly endowed with nerves that are destined for the extraocular muscles as well as with sympathetic, parasympathetic, and trigeminal sensory fibers. Any of these nerve supplies can conceivably give rise to peripheral nerve tumors, although the absence of significant motor deficits after removal of these tumors and their frequently lateral location suggest that they may most commonly arise from the ciliary branches of the nasociliary nerve. Peripheral nerve tumors are essentially those of Schwann cells with variable participation of axons. These lesions in aggregate constitute approximately between 5 and 15 per cent of all orbital tumors.

Simple Neurofibroma

Simple neurofibromas are usually isolated orbital lesions unassociated with neurofibromatosis. They occur from the second to the fifth decades, are unencapsulated but usually circumscribed growths with a pseudocapsule, and are commonly located in the superior lateral orbital quadrant. The tumors are composed of axons and enveloping fascicles of Schwann cells separated by endoneurial fibroblasts (Fig. 95–24). These lesions are readily removed in toto through a direct lateral orbital approach or a transcranial approach.

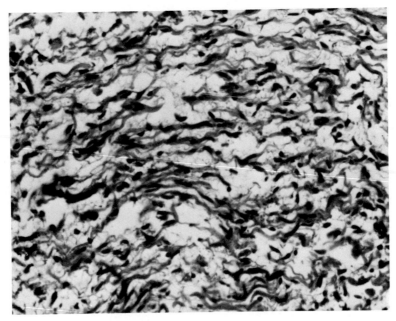

Figure 95–24 Simple neurofibroma. Wavy, slender fascicles of Schwann cells surround axons and are separated from each other by a myxoid interstitium.

Diffuse Neurofibroma

In contrast to simple neurofibromas, diffuse neurofibromas permeate and dissect throughout the orbital tissues. They therefore are more extensive and less delimited lesions than simple neurofibromas and are more difficult to eradicate. They may be seen as part of neurofibromatosis or as isolated lesions.

Plexiform Neurofibroma

This lesion is pathognomonic of von Recklinghausen's neurofibromatosis. The lesion is composed of bundles of diffusely enlarged and neoplastic nerves, each neuromatous unit being delimited by a perineurial sheath (Fig. 95–25). These lesions commonly produce "elephantiasis neuromatosa" or diffuse hyperplasia of the soft tissues of the lid and orbit and can be palpated as wormy growths. A defect of the sphenoid bone is commonly associated with the plexiform neurofibroma of the orbit and results in pulsating exophthalmos and more rarely in enophthalmos.[4] Congenital glaucoma with an enlarged globe can occur. There is usually diffuse hyperplasia of the schwannian and melanocytic elements of the choroid, and the glaucoma has been ascribed to an associated anterior chamber angle anomaly. Because of their extensive growth, these tumors are impossible to eradicate. Subtotal removal through an orbital approach is performed when the tumor mass becomes deforming. Optic nerve glioma or meningioma may on occasion be associated with plexiform orbital neurofibromas. Sarcomatous degeneration of these tumors in the orbit is extremely rare.

Schwannoma (Neurilemoma)

In contrast to the preceding tumors, which are composed of an intermixture of axons, Schwann cells, and endoneurial cells, the schwannoma is exclusively composed of Schwann cells. Enormous degrees of proptosis can be accommodated by the lids, since the tumors grow slowly. A solid, encapsulated orbital tumor seen on ultrasonography or computed tomography is most likely a schwannoma. The tumors are encapsulated by the perineurium of the nerve of origin and consequently can be easily removed in the course of the operation. Gross examination may show them to be cystic and yellow owing to the presence

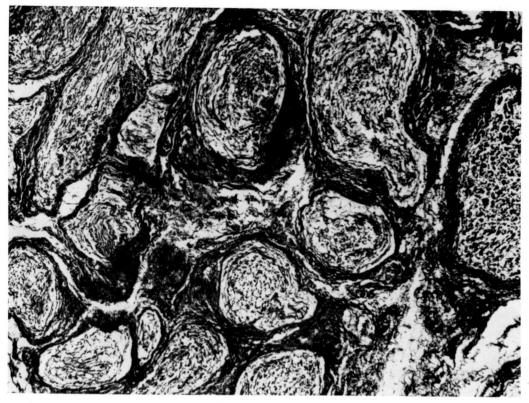

Figure 95–25 Plexiform neurofibroma. Each of the proliferating neuromatous units is ensheathed by a perineurium.

of xanthoma cells. They are composed of Schwann cells in compact Antoni A and loose Antoni B patterns (Fig. 95–26). There may be striking palisading (Verocay bodies) (Fig. 95–27). These tumors are believed to be even less likely to undergo malignant degeneration than neurofibromas.

Malignant Schwann Cell Tumors (Neurofibrosarcoma)

Malignant tumors of Schwann cells that are primary in the orbit are exceedingly rare. It is usually taught that malignant degeneration of peripheral nerve tumors will occur more often in neurofibromas associated with von Recklinghausen's disease than in isolated lesions. In the orbit, malignant degeneration of a plexiform neurofibroma into a malignant schwannoma is a curiosity. As isolated lesions, malignant schwannomas sometimes originate along the supraorbital nerve.[21] Such tumors in the superior nasal quadrant can easily gain access to the anterior cranial fossa if they are

not adequately excised en bloc. Histologically, these tumors are composed of spindle cells with oval, vesicular nuclei (Fig. 95–28). Differentiation from a mesenchymal tumor depends upon the demonstration of an attachment to a nerve or of a pre-existent neurofibroma.

Management of Peripheral Nerve Tumors

Since the advent of the computed tomographic scan, the diagnosis of a solitary neurofibroma or schwannoma may be suspected before operation. These lesions characteristically present with painless proptosis with preservation of exocular movement and vision. Plain films and pleuridirectional tomograms of the skull, orbit, and optic canals are normal. There is no radioisotope uptake. The lateral location and contrast enhancement under these circumstances should lead one to suspect the diagnosis.

These tumors can be approached safely

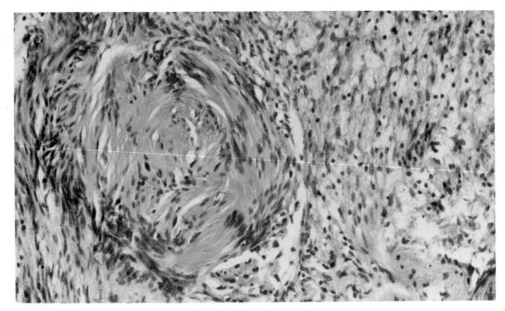

Figure 95–26 Schwannoma. The cells on the left are arranged into a compact whorl with palisading (Antoni A pattern) while those on the right are more loosely arranged (Antoni B pattern).

through the upper lateral quadrant of the orbit, either transcranially or by lateral canthotomy.[3,45] If care is taken in the medial retraction of the superior rectus muscle and its nerve supply by the cranial route, and in lateral retraction of the lateral rectus muscle and its nerve supply by the Berke modification of the Krönlein operation,

little cosmetic deformity may result. Injury to the parasympathetic innervation may produce postoperative pupillary dilatation following tumor resection by either route.

Radiotherapy plays no part in the treatment of neurofibromatosis. The prognosis following excision of a solitary neurofibroma of the orbit is excellent.

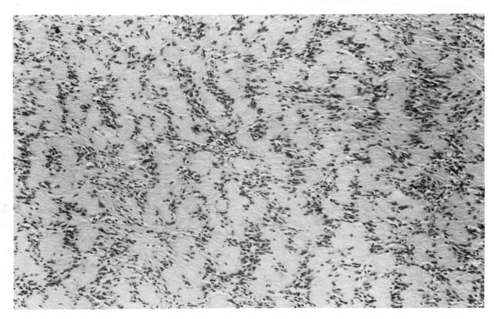

Figure 95–27 Schwannoma. High degree of nuclear palisading creates a field of Verocay bodies.

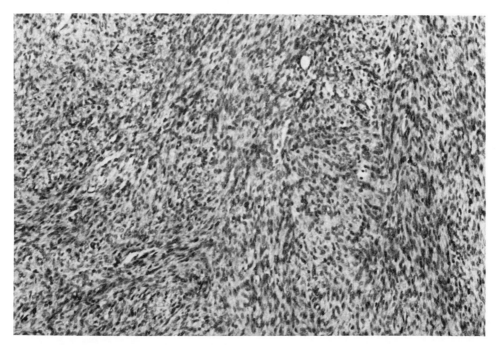

Figure 95–28 Malignant schwannoma. A diffuse myxoid neurofibroma recurred many times over a 25-year period and finally transformed into this malignant spindle cell schwannian tumor that invaded the anterior cranial fossa.

Although the authors have preferred the transcranial route in treating the solitary orbital neurofibroma and have attained excellent results in preserving vision and cosmetic appearance by sparing extraocular muscle function, as shown in Figure 95–29, a carefully performed micro-operative lateral orbitotomy approach can also provide excellent access to this laterally occurring tumor. There may, however, be a greater risk of injury to the abducens nerve by this approach. The lateral skin incision used in orbitotomy may be cosmetically acceptable, but it should be stressed that there should be little other difference in the morbidity associated with a transcranial epidural approach to the orbit and the Krönlein approach to the lateral orbit.

ENCEPHALOCELE AND MENINGOCELE

Congenital malformations are a rare cause of unilateral exophthalmos. More frequently, orbital encephalocele is associated with a post-traumatic defect in the orbital roof. Together they account for 0.5 to 3 per cent of cases presenting with unilateral exophthalmos. The congenital defects appear in early infancy or childhood and become apparent because of slowly progressive, frequently pulsating, proptosis. A characteristic defect usually is visible radiographically at the junction of an orbital bone with a cranial fossa. Pneumoencephalography will confirm the diagnosis.

Obviously the primary treatment for

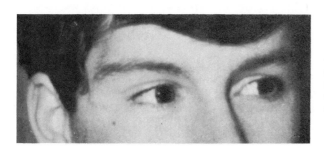

Figure 95–29 Eleven-year-old patient with solitary neurofibroma of the right orbit shown three years following transcranial orbital operation. Excellent functional and cosmetic result following transcranial apical exploration is illustrated.

these orbital lesions is transcranial operation for dural repair and reconstruction of the orbital roof to prevent proptosis and pulsation of the globe.

VASCULAR TUMORS

All varieties of vascular tumors constitute from 12 to 15 per cent of orbital tumors.[52] The principal vascular tumors that may involve the orbital soft tissues are the capillary hemangioma of infancy, the cavernous hemangioma of adults, lymphangioma, hemangiopericytoma, and arteriovenous malformations. Malignant hemangioendotheliomas virtually never involve the orbit.

Capillary Hemangioma (Benign Hemangioendothelioma)

This orbital tumor usually presents within the first six months after birth. The tumor may be located deep within the orbit or more anteriorly, where it can be palpated as a compressible, soft, poorly delimited lesion in the upper quadrants, usually superonasally. There may be inconstantly associated cutaneous lesions characterized as strawberry nevi because of their bright red hue and their upraised, dimpled surface. Although histologically benign, these tumors may grow in an infiltrative fashion and quite rapidly. If there are no telltale lid or facial lesions, a rhabdomyosarcoma of the orbit can be closely simulated. There is a natural tendency for these lesions to undergo spontaneous involution over three to five years following their appearance. Nonetheless, they are capable of creating cosmetic disfigurement and amblyopia if closure of the lids develops. Histopathologically, these tumors are composed of plump endothelial cells forming compressed lumina, a feature that is best brought out with the reticulum stain.

It is almost impossible to extirpate all of the tumor surgically because it is unencapsulated and dissects throughout much of the orbital tissues. Most biopsies are accomplished through the lid in order to rule out rhabdomyosarcoma. The cutaneous lesions can be managed by ligation of the feeding arteries, and lately large doses of corticosteroids have been recommended for their pharmacological effect on these orbital tumors.[23,64] Low-dosage orthovoltage radiotherapy (500 rads) can retard tumor growth and encourage involution.

Cavernous Hemangioma

While the capillary hemangioma presents in the newborn period or first six months of life, cavernous hemangioma is primarily a tumor of young and middle-aged adults and is one of the most common lesions producing proptosis in this age group (10 to 30 per cent). This encapsulated growth is often situated behind the globe and within the muscle cone, so that it may compress the optic nerve and indent the globe, thereby producing visual loss and retinal striae respectively. Lying in the loose areolar tissue of the anterolateral orbit, the cavernous hemangiomas occur as endothelium-lined spaces with no recognizable afferent vessel; thus, there is little bleeding following operative removal. These lesions are easily excised by lateral canthotomy or orbitotomy and do not recur. Ultrasonographic evaluation discloses a rounded, well-encapsulated "cystic" lesion, owing to the presence of the large blood-filled spaces within the tumor.

Lymphangioma

The orbit does not possess a lymphatic drainage system. Nevertheless lymphangiomas do occur in this area. Children and young adults are most commonly affected.[34] The tumor grows slowly, diffusely infiltrating the orbital tissues. It is composed of flattened endothelial cells creating ectatic, bloodless spaces separated by a delicate stroma containing lymphoid follicles. Spontaneous hemorrhage into the substance of the tumor creates abrupt and worrisome proptosis and the formation of "chocolate cysts." Upper respiratory viral infections may lead to an increase in proptosis owing to hypertrophy of the lymphoid tissue. Diagnostic biopsy and judicious subtotal excisions are best handled via an orbital approach.

Hemangiopericytoma

This tumor occurs primarily in young and middle-aged adults.[33] It arises from the pericyte of the microvasculature. In the orbit the tumors are usually slowly progressive and encapsulated. The capsule is less well developed than in cavernous hemangioma and can be broken during operative delivery. Ultrasonography discloses an encapsulated, partially cystic tumor closely mimicking the acoustic pattern of a cavernous hemangioma. Histologically, the tumor is composed of oval cells packed solidly around prominent capillaries. The tumor cells are embedded in a meshwork of reticulin fibers. They differ from those of cavernous hemangioma, however, since they can metastasize, although this happens very rarely in orbital cases. If not completely excised, usually by a direct orbital approach, hemangiopericytoma will recur even many years later and require exenteration. These tumors have also been found to invade the orbital roof and the cranial cavity, in which case a transcranial approach is necessary to achieve total excision.

Arteriovenous Malformations

These tumors are, by definition, composed of arterial elements that directly communicate with venous channels without an intervening capillary bed. They are quite rare in the orbit and are most dramatically described in the Wyburn-Mason syndrome.[66,67] Pulsating exophthalmos and subarachnoid hemorrhage may be encountered in these cases. Typically there are corkscrew episcleral vessels extending on the globe up to the limbus. Arteriovenous malformations should be distinguished from carotid-cavernous sinus fistulae, which may occur spontaneously or after trauma from rupture of a small aneurysm in the cavernous sinus. True orbital malformations should also be distinguished from simple fistulae between the orbital arteries and veins. Arteriography is required to distinguish precisely among these various kinds of lesions.

Varices may be primary in the orbit or may be secondary to the presence of an intracerebral arteriovenous malformation, in which case blood is shunted from within the anterior or middle cranial fossa and through the superior orbital fissure into the low-resistance valveless orbital veins, which subsequently dilate.[41]

Dilatation of epibulbar veins may result from an arteriovenous lesion in the orbit and also from a distant intracranial lesion.[18]

Primary or secondary orbital varices, as well as primary orbital venous angiomas, cause a diagnostic type of exophthalmos that is affected by position. When the patient bends forward or performs a Valsalva maneuver the proptosis is increased. True positional proptosis should be distinguished from "intermittent proptosis" due, for example, to a ruptured dermoid or a hemorrhage into a lymphangioma. Intermittent proptosis disappears slowly as the hemorrhagic or inflammatory complication subsides.

FIBRO-OSSEOUS TUMORS

Osteoma of the Orbit

Osteoma of the orbit may arise from embryonic rests, most frequently found in the anterior ethmoid cells. This slowly growing extraperiosteal lesion of cancellous bone may invade the orbit, producing proptosis, and eventually visual loss, often with little interference with ocular motility. The base of the lesion is frequently narrow and the mass is pedunculated. Many of these lesions may be removed by an orbital route. Because of their origin from anterior ethmoid cells, they may grow posteriorly or, at times, arise from posterior ethmoid or sphenoid cells. They may also arise from frontal and maxillary sinuses. When the tumor has invaded the intracranial cavity at the base of the skull or when it lies in a posterior position near the orbital apex, orbital unroofing by the transcranial route is indicated. In extreme cases, a two-staged transcranial and transorbital procedure may be necessary to achieve total removal.

Fibrous Dysplasia

When it has an orbital presentation, fibrous dysplasia involves the sphenoid bone or the orbital plate of the frontal bone. In such cases the tumor usually is a monostotic lesion, unassociated with Albright's syndrome or multifocal polyostotic disease.[47]

Pathologically the lesion is composed of a fibrous stroma displaying focal areas of osteoid. Because of the absence of osteoblasts surrounding the bony trabeculae the osteoid is arrested at the stage of woven bone and does not mature into lamellar bone.[20] This lesion has been likened to a hamartomatous disturbance in the maturation of bone.

Children and young adults are most commonly affected. There is one report of a case of cranial fibrous dysplasia occurring in neurofibromatosis.[53] There may be headache, facial asymmetry, and painless swelling of the cheek or orbital regions. Proptosis usually develops slowly and is rarely severe enough to warrant orbital unroofing. Optic atrophy and visual dysfunction will result if a sphenoid lesion encroaches on the optic canal. When this occurs a transcranial epidural approach to unroof the optic canal may be helpful. While the radiographic appearance of hyperostosis may mimic that of meningioma of the sphenoid, it is uncommon for sphenoidal meningiomas to occur in the pediatric age group. Radiotherapy has no role in the treatment of this disease, and in fact, in rare instances, it may transform the lesion into an osteogenic sarcoma.

Ossifying Fibroma

This tumor has created considerable confusion and controversy. It appears to be a distinctive lesion restricted to the facial and skull bones.[20] Females are more frequently affected than males; the average age of presentation is around 15 years. When the maxillary sinus or bone, ethmoid sinus, and frontal or sphenoid bones are affected, there is a painless facial swelling, exophthalmos, and displacement of the eye. Radiographically, the lesion tends to be somewhat more circumscribed than fibrous dysplasia. It has a rather cellular but benign fibroblastic stroma in which osteoid is found. A significant pathological difference from fibrous dysplasia is the presence of osteoblasts (denticulocytes) that rim the osteoid material and bring about the maturation of woven bone to lamellar bone. There

is also a significant clinical difference between ossifying fibroma and fibrous dysplasia. An ossifying fibroma tends to be progressive. It may recur if it is incompletely excised. In rare instances it may grow into the middle cranial fossa and cause death. Complete operative removal of the lesion by a transcranial epidural approach is the treatment of choice.

Aneurysmal Bone Cyst

This lytic lesion may affect the frontal bone of the orbit in children from 5 to 15 years of age.[16] Proptosis usually develops rather rapidly. The cyst is composed of large cavernous spaces filled with blood, between which are found areas containing hemosiderin-laden macrophages and new bone formation. The biopsy material should be closely scrutinized for evidence of osteogenic sarcoma, a true hemangioma of bone, and giant cell tumor of bone, all of which may undergo cystic changes.[39] Operative removal of the lesion done by the epidural transcranial approach will adequately treat the tumor.

Osteogenic Sarcoma

It is rare for osteogenic sarcoma to present around the orbit. Osteogenic sarcoma does, however, sometimes develop in patients with the bilateral, inherited form of retinoblastoma who have received radiotherapy.[1] These patients are prone to develop other malignant neoplasms away from the orbit and they are especially likely to develop osteogenic sarcoma in the orbital bones after radiotherapy. Osteogenic sarcoma may also rarely develop spontaneously in the orbital bones in younger individuals in the second decade and after radiotherapy in patients with fibrous dysplasia or giant cell tumors.[20] Furthermore, Paget's disease of the skull may rarely degenerate into an osteogenic sarcoma.[5] Radical operative procedures combined with chemotherapy and radiotherapy have been effective in controlling the disease. Needless to say, radical operation should not be performed unless a careful clinical evaluation shows that a wide excision beyond the tumor can be performed safely. Bone and dura can be excised by a direct approach at the time of radical exenteration; whereas involvement of the cavernous sinus or the carotid artery by tumor, or evidence of metastases would constitute a contraindication of this type of procedure.

MESENCHYMAL TUMORS

Rhabdomyosarcoma

Rhabdomyosarcoma is the most common primary orbital malignant tumor of childhood. It constituted 7 per cent of one series of orbital biopsies.[52] Although it may present congenitally, it is usually a tumor of childhood and adolescence. The average age of presentation is 7 years. The male to female ratio is 5 : 3. The typical history is that of a rapidly progressive proptosis over several weeks, which in some cases, may reach hideous proportions. An immediate biopsy is essential because radiotherapy and adjuvant chemotherapy may be curative in 70 per cent of cases.[37] Diagnostic tissue is obtained either through a lid approach for anterior tumors or by lateral orbitotomy for retrobulbar tumors. The transcranial approach is contraindicated because of the potential for seeding the intracranial compartments. Pleuridirectional tomograms of the orbit, computed tomography, and ultrasonography can help to define the extent of the tumor spread beyond the orbit. The latter situation does not necessarily imply a poor prognosis if radiotherapy is tailored to encompass the extraorbital tumor. Histopathologically most of the tumors in children are of the embryonal type composed of nondescript hyperchromatic spindle cells. Trichrome stain discloses cytoplasmic acidophilia due to the presence of myofilaments in the cytoplasm. Cross-striations are difficult to find in the more poorly differentiated tumors. Occasionally a more differentiated or pleomorphic rhabdosarcoma may be seen in older individuals and may have a somewhat better prognosis.

Fibrous Histiocytoma

Fibrous histiocytoma is the most common mesenchymal orbital tumor of adults. Usually it is an unencapsulated infiltrative growth, but occasionally it may be circumscribed.[32] It develops insidiously over months or years. These lesions have often been misdiagnosed in the past as neurogenic tumors or other mesenchymal tumors. The orbit is the site of predilection for this particular soft-tissue tumor. Although locally infiltrating, most fibrous histocytomas of the orbit are benign. Rare instances of malignant tumors with nuclear anaplasia and a high mitotic rate with metastatic potential have been reported. Microscopically the tumor is composed of spindle cells with an admixture of lipidized histiocytic elements. The spindle cells adopt an unusual cartwheel or spiral nebular configuration.

An orbital or lid approach is the preferred way of obtaining diagnostic tissue. The tumor should be completely and widely excised. If incompletely excised, it will recur, possibly requiring exenteration at a later time.

Other mesenchymal orbital tumors, such as fibroma and fibrosarcoma, leiomyoma and leiomyosarcoma, lipoma and liposarcoma, are very rare.

LYMPHOMA

Lymphomas affecting the orbits of adults account for up to 10 per cent of biopsies of orbital tumors.[30] Previous reports of lymphoma of the orbit in children most likely were in error and were misinterpreted instances of deposits of leukemia or granulocytic sarcoma. Orbital lymphomas have a tendency to present in the anterior orbit and may be palpable in the majority of cases. Also they are likely to be seen in the fornices, especially in the inferior fornix. When present under the conjunctiva, these tumors present as salmon pink or flesh-colored lesions. Biopsy is easy and confirmatory of the diagnosis. Retrobulbar lesions, however, pose a dilemma. By ultrasonography or computed tomography they may show a diffusely infiltrative pattern or a localized mass with irregular contours, simulating an inflammatory pseudotumor or a metastatic carcinoma. Biopsy of these lesions should be obtained by an orbital approach. Most cytologically malignant orbital lymphomas are part of the systemic disease, although in some cases it may take years for the other sites of involvement to declare themselves. For this reason, patients who have evidence of cytologically proved malignant lymphoma in the orbit should be subjected to a rigorous systemic work-up, including lymphangiography, bone marrow biopsy, biopsy of suspicious lymph nodes, and serum immunoelectrophoresis.

LEUKEMIA AND GRANULOCYTIC SARCOMA

Orbital leukemia deposits in patients with known leukemia may be bilateral and generally occur in children with acute lymphoblastic leukemia. Granulocytic leukemia more rarely involves the orbital tissues. There is, however, a rare form of leukemic involvement of the orbital soft tissues, bones, and periosteum referred to as granulocytic sarcoma ("chloroma").[68] In this disease there is initially a soft-tissue deposit composed of immature myeloid leukemia cells without overt evidence of leukemia or bone marrow involvement. The latter generally occur within a matter of months after the orbital mass develops. It is important to bear this tumor in mind, since it may initially suggest a rhabdomyosarcoma to the clinician or a lymphoma to the histopathologist. Since lymphoma rarely affects the orbits of children, a report of this diagnosis by the pathologist should raise the question of the possibility that granulocytic sarcoma is the true diagnosis. The Leder stain for peroxidase in the cytoplasm will confirm the diagnosis. The disease is uniformly fatal unless chemotherapy can be introduced before the leukemic stage with bone marrow involvement develops.

MUCOCELES OF THE PARANASAL SINUSES

Mucoceles that arise from a paranasal sinus and produce unilateral proptosis are a common cause of exophthalmos. They may occur with or without pain. Usually they are not associated with extraocular muscle palsy. The condition may be suspected when there is a history of recurrent sinus infection; however, it can occur without this problem preceding it. Usually there is radiographic demonstration of opacification of a sinus with a characteristic deformity of the orbital bone. Tomography can confirm destructive changes at the orbital border even when plain films are normal. A characteristic resilient mass may be palpated at the site of the mucocele. The globe is usually displaced away from the sinus that is diseased.

Mucoceles can be excised. They rarely recur when drainage into the nasal cavity is established. Transfrontal cranial exploration must be considered when there are symptoms and findings consistent with intracranial extension of the disease process.

DERMOID TUMORS

Orbital dermoids are most commonly found in the anterior portion of the frontal bone. They have, however, been reported in all positions in the orbit. They produce a characteristic radiolucent defect, and usually they are diagnosed radiogaphically. An orbital operative approach usually gives adequate exposure and permits complete eradication of the mass. If there is evidence of intracranial extension, a primary cranial approach should be made.

LACRIMAL GLAND TUMORS

Most clinically obvious swellings of the lacrimal gland are inflammatory and noninfectious. The globe is displaced downward and medially more than forward. The lateral portion of the upper lid may be full. Idiopathic inflammatory pseudotumor, the benign lymphoepithelial lesion (formerly called Mikulicz's disease), and Sjogren's syndrome are inflammatory nonneoplastic causes of lacrimal gland enlargement. Epithelial tumors of the lacrimal gland are responsible for only 5 per cent of orbital tumors. The encapsulated benign mixed tumor is the most common. If this tumor is incompletely removed or seeded into the orbital bone during operation, it can continue to grow over many years and may eventually gain entrance to the cranial fossae. The next most common epithelial tumor of the lacrimal gland is the adenocystic carcinoma (cylindroma). This malignant tumor is unusual among orbital neoplasms in that it often causes pain. Pain is rare in orbital tumors except for those that are metastatic from elsewhere. Preferential growth of the adenocystic carcinoma along nerves accounts for the pain and the dismal long-term results of treatment. The authors' longest "cure" of 15 years of a patient with a lacrimal gland tumor was ended when a computed tomogram performed for recurrent pain disclosed tumor in the temporal fossa. Primary radical en bloc resection and exenteration should be considered to be the most effective treatment for this tumor when studies exclude widespread local invasion. Those patients who survive two years do well, even with later recurrence.

CARCINOMA

Undifferentiated carcinoma arising in a paranasal sinus accounts for from 4 to 9 per cent of cases in which the presenting symptom is unilateral exophthalmos. Although carcinoma of the maxillary antrum is most frequent, tumors that arise in the ethmoid sinuses are most often responsible for the proptosis.

The diagnosis of invasive carcinoma should be suspected in the presence of multiple cranial nerve signs accompanying proptosis and by the radiographic demonstration of destructive changes at the medial margins of the orbit. This tumor is frequently accompanied by severe pain. Chronic inflammatory changes are often seen by x-ray but are not always an accompaniment of carcinoma of the sinus. Tomography is very helpful in establishing the diagnosis of sinus carcinoma by showing dissolution of the orbital bony margins of the ethmoid, sphenoid, frontal, or maxillary sinuses. Computed tomography may help delineate the extent of the disease process. The diagnosis may be confirmed by transnasal sinus biopsy. Often multiple biopsies are necessary to obtain a representative sample of the tumor.

When a diagnosis of carcinoma of the sinus invading the orbit has been made, the treatment of choice is radiotherapy and regional chemotherapy. The excellent results that have followed this combined therapy make radical operative procedures for undifferentiated carcinoma in the sinus seem unwarranted.

Metastatic orbital disease has been described but is relatively rare. Carcinomas of the breast and bronchi have most frequently been reported metastasizing to the choroid. Because of their rarity and because they often present with visual impairment before producing proptosis, they seldom are encountered by the neurosurgeon.

Metastatic tumors develop in the globe 8 to 10 times as frequently as in the orbit. In adults the most common primary tumors are in the breast in women and in the lung in men.[17] Metastatic breast tumors may appear many years after the primary breast carcinoma has been removed. Thus, it is important to inquire about past operations. In men, bronchogenic carcinoma may spread early.

Proptosis may be the first sign of a silent primary tumor. Spread of gastrointestinal and female genitourinary tumors to the orbit is uncommon. Proptosis, pain, and extraocular motility disturbances with ptosis occur more rapidly in metastatic disease to the orbit than in primary orbital tumors. Patients who present with any of these signs early in the course of their orbital disease should be suspected of harboring a metastatic tumor whether or not x-rays show bone destruction.

Neuroblastoma and Ewing's sarcoma are the primary sources for the two most common orbital metastases in children.[2] Rosettes usually are not seen in the orbital metastases of neuroblastomas. The presence of glycogen in Ewing's sarcoma cells is helpful in making the diagnosis. The metastasis of retroperitoneal neuroblastoma to the orbit usually is a late event in the disease. Most of the patients with this problem will present with a palpable abdominal mass and osseous metastases. The proptosis in both tumors develops rapidly and often is due to hemorrhage. Proptosis is bilateral in 50 per cent of cases of orbital neuroblastoma, whereas it is always unilateral in Ewing's orbital tumors. The primary tumor in Ewing's sarcoma usually is located in a long bone, but primaries in the ribs and metatarsals have been found to metastasize to the orbit.

INFLAMMATION

Graves' Disease

Graves' disease is one of the commonest causes of proptosis in adults.[31] Females are more commonly affected than males. An early sign is lid retraction. Patients may be hyperthyroid, euthyroid, or even hypothyroid. The proptosis and lid retraction may be the first signs of impending or actual thyrotoxicosis, or may appear after the disease has been brought under control by treatment. Other subtle clues to be looked for are edema and injection over the insertions of the rectus muscles behind the limbus. Ultrasonography can be useful in showing that there is thickening of the extraocular muscles without a discrete orbital mass. Indeed, if one orbit is more affected than the other, ultrasonography of the less involved orbit may still show diagnostic signs of extraocular muscle thickness. This disease should always be considered in patients, especially women, who present with proptosis, and particularly when ultrasonography or computed tomography fails to disclose a discrete orbital mass. The triiodothyronine (Werner) test, which establishes the metabolic autonomy of the thyroid gland, is positive in 75 per cent of cases; however, a negative test does not rule out the disease. It should be performed on all patients suspected of Graves' disease. Late fibrosis of the extraocular muscles can occur. It especially affects the inferior muscles and may result in an inability to look up in a manner that simulates a neurogenic or double superior rectus palsy. The traction test, however, in which forceps are placed on the globe and resistance is encountered to passive movement, will confirm that the motility disturbance is mechanical or restrictive (inflammatory) rather than neurogenic in origin.

Fortunately, the clinical diagnosis can be made readily if suspected, and appropriate medical treatment can be instituted. Frequently the proptosis is self-limited and rarely progressive after two years. Should severe proptosis threaten the globe, large doses of steroids in combination with low-dosage radiotherapy often is effective in controlling the symptoms. Operative decompression by a transcranial route, unroofing the orbit, or a transantral one for downward decompression has been used effectively at times when medical treatment has failed to control proptosis or for cosmetic reasons after the disease process has been stabilized.

Idiopathic Inflammatory Pseudotumor

In the opththalmological literature the terms "pseudotumor" and "chronic granu-loma" frequently appear interchangeably. Orbital pseudotumor is a strictly localized inflammatory disease without identifiable local or systemic cause and is a challenging mimicker of true neoplasms.[31] It is the reason for up to 20 per cent of orbital biopsies. The term "pseudotumor" actually means pseudoneoplasm, since the clinician's impression of a neoplasm is invalidated when biopsy of the orbital condition reveals only a nonspecific chronic inflammation. As defined at present, this entity is probably a spectrum of different diseases with different causes (e.g., viral or autoimmune) but sharing similar location, symptom complexes, and histopathologic changes.

Patients characteristically present with a fairly rapid proptosis, early pain, and extraocular motility disturbances. Usually they have epibulbar inflammation or injection, notably engorgement of the vessels overlying the rectus muscle insertion. Patients of all ages may be affected, but usually the disease presents in the third to the sixth decades. Males may be somewhat more affected than females. Children in the first and second decades have been affected, and the disease should not be overlooked in this age group.

Pseudotumor can affect any of the orbital tissues. The process more commonly involves the superior orbit, and the mass, if anteriorly located, can be palpated through the lids, thereby helping to distinguish the disease from Graves' disease, in which no mass is palpable. The untreated disease may take several courses. It may be self-limiting with a variable degree of permanent ocular motility disturbance or visual loss after the acute inflammation subsides. Another course is that of inexorable progression involving all the extraocular structures, resulting in a frozen globe and intractable pain necessitating exenteration for palliation. Yet another course, especially in children, is one of multiple recurrences with spread to the other orbit. While pseudotumor typically is a unilateral process, it may be bilateral in a minority of cases. Bilateral proptosis should bring to mind the possibility of a systemic disease, such as Graves' disease, vasculitis, or a collagen disease. Compared with pseudotumor, Graves' disease usually displays less pain, less paresis, and fewer visual difficulties early in its course.

X-ray studies usually are normal. Occasionally lesions located near the periosteum may cause reactive changes and erosion. These parosteal lesions are also apt to be quite painful because they impinge on the periosteal nerves. The diagnosis of pseudotumor has been greatly facilitated with the advent of ultrasonography and computed tomography. Each of these diagnostic techniques may disclose multiple sites of orbital inflammation, e.g., around Tenon's capsule (the loose fascial membrane enveloping the globe), thickening of the extraocular muscles, ragged perioptic shadows signifying inflammation in this zone, and enlargement of the lacrimal gland. In a minority of cases, pseudotumor may produce a rather localized orbital mass without evidence of multifocal involvement. These localized lesions are virtually impossible to distinguish from a true neoplasm without exploration and biopsy. As a general rule both the ophthalmic surgeon and the neurosurgeon should try to avoid operation in cases of orbital pseudotumor. Particularly with respect to posterior orbital lesions located within the muscle cone, perioptically, and at the orbital apex; operative intervention will most likely bring about an exacerbation of the inflammatory process and compromise the ultimate outcome for ocular motility and visual function. If an operation is performed on deep orbital lesions, the patient should receive large doses of steroids immediately postoperatively.

The histological picture of idiopathic orbital inflammation usually consists of nonspecific chronic inflammation featuring fibroplasia, endothelial capillary proliferation, lymphocytes, plasma cells, and occasionally eosinophils and polymorphonuclear leukocytes (the latter two especially in younger individuals). The lymphocytic component may display scattered follicle formation. Granulomas created by epithelioid cells are a rare feature of this disease. The designation of this process as "orbital granuloma," as was done in the past, is a misnomer in the majority of cases. These lesions resolve through progressive fibrosis culminating in dense hyalinized scars.

Another type of idiopathic inflammation is referred to as reactive lymphocytic hyperplasia. In this type of pseudotumor, sheets of mature lymphocytes, often displaying follicle formation and an intermixture of plasma cells, might easily be interpreted as a lymphoma. The follow-up data on these lesions, the predominance of the lymphocytes, and the presence of plasma cells indicate that they are reactive rather than neoplastic lesions.

One topographic variant of pseudotumor is the Tolosa-Hunt syndrome, comprising painful external ophthalmoplegia, congestion of the upper lid, and variable visual loss. In this group of patients the chronic nonspecific inflammation, sometimes exhibiting granulomatous features, is located in the vicinity of the superior orbital fissure and involves the cranial nerves and draining veins that traverse this structure. The inflammation may extend into the cavernous sinus and along the cranial surface of the sphenoid bone. The Tolosa-Hunt complex of symptoms is quite sensitive to corticosteroids. The disease must be distinguished from neoplastic causes of progressive cranial nerve palsies, which generally lack the explosive onset of the inflammatory disease and the exquisite sensitivity to steroid treatment.

The preferred treatment for all varieties of orbital pseudotumor is with 60 to 80 mg of prednisone per day. Regression of the proptosis and improvement in visual acuity and extraocular motility are monitored and the dosage is adjusted appropriately. Treatment in the more serious cases may have to be maintained for several months at 30 to 40 mg per day with slowly tapering doses. Since there may be rebound phenomena, the drug should not be discontinued abruptly. Lesions of reactive lymphocytic hyperplasia can be treated with 1000 to 2000 rads of ionizing radiation. These patients should be routinely studied for any other signs of lymphoproliferative disorders.

In addition to neoplasm, the differential diagnosis includes other inflammatory diseases of the orbit, such as Graves' disease, vasculitis, and sarcoidosis. Sarcoidosis usually affects the conjuctiva and lacrimal gland and not the connective tissues and muscles of the orbit. Histologically, it is virtually impossible to distinguish Graves' disease from pseudotumor. The diagnosis must be based on clinical and laboratory findings.

GRANULOMA

Of specific interest to the neurosurgeon is a second group of chronic granulomas that may present with unilateral exophthalmos. They can be considered true granulomas and differentiated from other types by the presence of pain, radiographic destructive changes of the bony orbit, and an elevated sedimentation rate.

Wegener's granulomatosis is a vasculitic disease that can involve the orbit and produce bone destruction. Sinus lesions, pulmonary cavitation, and glomerulonephritis are cardinal features of this disease. "Limited" Wegener's granulomatosis can, however, also involve the orbit and exhibit respiratory system lesions without renal disease. Histologically the only characteristic differentiating this from nonspecific chronic inflammatory disease (pseudotumor) is the abundance of destructive changes in the tissues involved. The clinical diagnosis may be suspected when extensive necrosis is noted. Enucleation may be necessary because of infarction of the ocular blood supply, but resection does not arrest the process. The most effective treatment appears to be long-term administration of corticosteroids.

Aspergillus infection may arise in the sphenoid sinus and extended intracranially, surrounding one or both optic nerves and carotid arteries. Operative drainage of this indolent process is indicated despite the fact that its location makes the procedure a complicated one. The use of a combination of parenteral flucytosine and systemic amphotericin-B for four to six weeks has been recommended.

CONCLUSIONS

Only a portion of the lesions occurring in the orbit and responsible for the production of unilateral exophthalmos may be of interest to the neurosurgeon. Preselection of cases will increase the incidence of optic nerve glioma, meningioma, neurofibroma, and encephalocele seen in a neurosurgical practice. Currently available clinical studies, including computed tomographic and radioactive scanning, tomography, and angiography are important supplements to the clinical diagnosis of conditions producing proptosis. With these improvements in methods for preoperative diagnosis of orbital lesions, transcranial procedures can be selected as the primary treatment only when warranted.

It is important to recognize that a large number of conditions producing exophthalmos can be eradicated by transorbital or transnasal exploration, radiotherapy, or medical management. Malignant tumors confined to structures within the periorbita should not be approached transcranially because of the danger of seeding the cranial cavity.

The primary advantage of the transcranial frontal approach to the orbit is the excellent exposure of the superior lateral and medial compartments of the orbit, providing safe access to tumors near the apex. Familiarity with the anatomy of this region allows the neurosurgeon to operate with excellent functional and cosmetic results.

REFERENCES

1. Abramson, D., Ellsworth, R., and Zimmerman, L.: Non-ocular cancer in retinoblastoma survivors. Trans. Amer. Acad. Ophthal. Otolaryng., *81*:459, 1976.
2. Albert, D., Rubinstein, R., and Scheie, H.: Tumor metastases to the eye. A clinicopathologic study in infants and children; Amer. J. Ophthal., *63*:727, 1967.
3. Berke, R. N.: A modified Kronlein operation. Trans. Amer. Ophthal. Soc., *51*:193–231, 1953.
4. Binet, E., Kieffer, S., Martin, S., and Peterson, H.: Orbital dysplasia in neurofibromatosis. Radiology, *93*:829, 1969.
5. Blodi, F.: Unusual orbital tumors and their treatment. *In* New Orleans Academy of Ophthalmology: Symposium on Surgery of the Orbit and Adnexa. St. Louis, C. V. Mosby Co., 1974, pp. 53–73.
6. Brash, J. P., ed.: Cunningham's Manual of Practical Anatomy. London, Oxford University Press, 1948.
7. Chutorian, A. M., Schwartz, J. F., Evans, R. A., and Carter, S.: Optic gliomas in children. Neurology (Minneap.), *14*:83–95, 1967.
8. Coleman, D. J., Konig, W. F., and Kata, L.: A hand-operated ultrasound scan system for ophthalmic evaluation. Amer. J. Ophthal., *68*:256–263, 1969.
9. Cushing, H., and Eisenhardt, L.: Meningiomas. Springfield, Ill., Charles C Thomas, 1938.
10. Dandy, W. E.: Results following transcranial attack on orbital tumors. Arch. Ophthal., *25*:191–216, 1941.
11. Davis, F. A.: Primary tumors of the optic nerves. Arch. Ophthal. (Chicago), *23*:735–821, 957–1022, 1940.
12. Di Chiro, G.: An Atlas of Pathologic Pneumoencephalographic Anatomy. Springfield, Ill., Charles C Thomas, 1967.
13. Duke-Elder, S., and Wybar, K. C.: The anatomy of the visual system. *In* System of Ophthalmology. Vol. 2. St. Louis, C. V. Mosby Co., 1961.

14. Eggers, H., Jakobiec, F. A., and Jones, I. S.: Tumors of the optic nerve. Docum. Ophthal., *41*:43–128, 1976.
15. Evans, R. A., Schwartz, J. F., and Chutorian, A. M.: Radiologic diagnosis in pediatric ophthalmology. Radiol. Clin. N. Amer., *1*:459–495, 1963.
16. Fite, J., Schwartz, J., and Calhoun, F.: Aneurysmal bone cysts of the orbit. Trans. Amer. Acad. Ophthal. Otolaryng., *73*:614, 1968.
17. Font, R., and Ferry, A.: Carcinoma metastatic to the eye and orbit. A clinicopathologic study of 28 cases metastatic to the orbit. Cancer, *38*:1326–1335, 1976.
18. Forman, A. R., Luessenhop, A. J., and Limaye, S. R.: Ocular findings in patients with arteriovenous malformations of the head and neck. Amer. J. Ophthal., *79*:626–633, 1975.
19. Frisen, L., Hoyt, W., and Tengroth, B.: Opticociliary veins, disc pallor and visual loss: A triad of signs indicating spheno-orbital meningioma. Acta Ophthal., *51*:241, 1973.
20. Fu, Y., and Perzin, K.: Non-epithelial tumors of the nasal cavity, paranasal sinuses and nasopharynx. Osseous and fibroosseous lesions. cancer, *33*:1289, 1974.
21. Grinberg, M., and Levy, N.: Malignant neurilemoma of the supraorbital nerve. Amer. J. Ophthal., *78*:489, 1974.
22. Hanafee, W. N., Shiu, P. S., and Dayton, G. O.: Orbital venography. Amer. J. Roentgen., *104*:29, 1968.
23. Hiles, D., and Pilchard, W.: Corticosteroid control of neonatal hemangiomas of the orbit and ocular adnexa. Amer. J. Ophthal., *71*:1003, 1971.
24. Housepian, E. M.: Surgical treatment of unilateral optic nerve gliomas. J. Neurosurg., *31*:604–607, 1969.
24a. Housepian, E. M.: Intraorbital tumors. *In* Schmidek, H. H., and Sweet, W. H., eds.: Current Techniques in Operative Neurosurgery. New York, Grune & Stratton, Inc., 1977.
25. Hoyt, W. F., and Bagdassarian, S. A.: Optic glioma of childhood. Brit. J. Ophthal., *53*:793, 1969.
26. Hoyt, W. F., Amshel, L. G., Lessell, S., Schatz, N. J., and Suckling, R. D.: Malignant optic glioma of adulthood. Brain, *96*:121–132, 1973.
27. Hudson, A. C.: Primary tumors of the optic nerve. Roy. Ophthal. Hosp. Rep., *18*:317–439, 1912.
28. Ingalls, R. G.: Orbital tumors. Amer. J. Ophthal., *32*:1595, 1949.
29. Jackson, H.: Orbital tumors. Proc. Roy. Soc. Med., *38*:587–594, 1945.
30. Jakobiec, F. A., and Jones, I. S.: Lymphomatous, plasmocytic, histiocytic and hematopoietic tumors of the orbit. *In* Duane, T., ed.: Clinical Ophthalmology. Hagerstown, Md., Harper & Row, 1976.
31. Jakobiec, F. A., and Jones, I. S.: Orbital inflammations. *In* Duane, T., ed.: Clinical Ophthalmology; Hagerstown, Md., Harper & Row, 1976, Chapter 35.
32. Jakobiec, F. A., Howard, G., Jones, I. S., and Tannenbaum, M.: Fibrous histiocytomas of the orbit. Amer. J. Ophthal., *77*:333, 1974.
33. Jakobiec, F. A., Howard, G., Jones, I., and Wolff, M.: Hemangiopericytoma of the orbit. Amer. J. Ophthal., *78*:816, 1974.
34. Jones, I. S.: Lymphangioma of the ocular adnexa; an analysis of 62 cases. Trans. Amer. Ophthal. Soc., *57*:602, 1959.
35. Karp, L., Zimmerman, L., Borit, A., and Spencer, W.: Primary intraorbital meningiomas. Arch. Ophthal., *91*:24, 1974.
36. Kennerdell, J. S., and Maroon, J. C.: Intracanalicular meningioma with chronic optic disc edema. Ann. Ophthal., *7*:507–512, 1975.
37. Knowles, D., Jakobiec, F., Potter, G., and Jones, I. S.: Ophthalmic striated muscle neoplasms. A clinicopathologic review. Survey Ophthal., *21*:219–261, 1976.
38. Last, R. J.: Wolff's Anatomy of the Eye and Orbit. 6th Ed. Philadelphia, W. B. Saunders Co., 1968.
39. Levy, W., Miller, A., Bonakdarpour, A., and Aegerter, E.: Aneurysmal bone cyst secondary to other osseous lesions. Amer. J. Clin. Path., *63*:1, 1975.
40. Lloyd, G.: Gliomas of the optic nerve and chiasm in childhood. Trans. Amer. Ophthal. Soc., *71*:488–535, 1973.
41. Lloyd, G., Wright, J., and Morgan, G.: Venous malformation of the orbit. Brit. J. Ophthal., *55*:505, 1971.
42. Lombardi, G.: Radiology in Neuroophthalmology. Baltimore, Williams & Wilkins Co., 1967.
43. Love, J. G., and Benedict, W. L.: Transcranial removal of intraorbital tumors. J.A.M.A., *121*:777–784, 1945.
44. Luce, S. A.: An electron microscopic study of normal optic nerve and an optic nerve glioma. J. Neurosurg., *18*:466–478, 1961.
45. Maroon, J. C., and Kennerdell, J. S.: Lateral microsurgical approach to intraorbital tumors. J. Neurosurg., *44*:556–561, 1976.
46. Matson, D. D.: Unilateral exophthalmos in childhood. Clin. Neurosurg., *5*:116–126, 1958.
47. Moore, R.: Fibrous dysplasia of the orbit. Survey Ophthal., *13*:321, 1969.
48. Pernkopf, E.: Atlas of Topographical and Applied Human Anatomy. Vol. 1. Philadelphia, W. B. Saunders Co., 1963.
49. Pfeiffer, R. L.: Roentgenography of exophthalmos, with notes on the roentgen ray in ophthalmology. Trans. Amer. Ophthal. Soc., *39*:492–560, 1941.
50. Potter, G. D., and Trokel, S.: Tomography of the optic canal. Amer. J. Roentgen., *106*:530–535, 1969.
51. Reese, A. B.: Tumors of the Eye. New York, Hoeber Medical Division, Harper & Row, 1963.
52. Reese, A. B.: Expanding lesions of the orbit. Trans. Ophthal. Soc. U.K., *91*:85–104, 1971.
53. Rosenberg, P., Sarsin, J., Zimmerman, E., and Carter, S.: The interrelationship of neurofibromatosis and fibrous dysplasia. Arch. Neurol., *18*:363, 1968.
54. Sanders, M. D., and Falconer, M. A.: Optic nerve compression by an intracanalicular meningioma. Brit. J. Ophthal., *48*:13–18, 1964.
55. Schlesinger, E. B., Trokel, S. L., and Baily, S.: Radioactive scanning in the analysis of unilateral exophthalmos. Trans. Amer. Acad. Ophthal. Otolaryng., *73*:1005–1011, 1969.
56. Spencer, W. H.: Primary neoplasms of the optic nerve and its sheaths: Clinical features and current concepted pathogenetic mechanisms. J. Amer. Ophthal. Soc., *70*:490–528, 1972.

57. Stern, W. E.: Meningiomas of the cranio-orbital junction. J. Neurosurg., *38*:428–437, 1973.
58. Susac, J. O., Martins, A. N., and Whaley, R. A.: Intracanalicular meningioma with normal tomography. J. Neurosurg., *45*:659–662, 1977.
59. Susac, J. O., Smith, L. J., and Walsh, F. B.: The impossible meningioma. Arch. Neurol., *34*:36–38, 1977.
60. Taveras, J. M., Mount, L. A., and Wood, E. H.: The value of radiation therapy in the management of glioma of the optic nerves and chiasm. Radiology, *66*:518–528, 1956.
61. Tenner, M. S., and Trokel, S. L.: Radiologic methods in neuroophthalmologic problems. Amer. J. Ophthal., *68*:883–895, 1969.
62. Van Buren, J. M., Poppen, J. L., and Horrax, G.: Unilateral exophthalmos: A consideration of symptom pathogenesis. Brain, *80*:139–175, 1957.
63. Verhoeff, F. H.: Primary intracranial tumors (gliomas) of the optic nerve. Arch. Ophthal. (N.Y.), *51*:120–140, 239–254, 1922.
64. Walsh, T.: Giant strawberry nevi of the orbital arteries; treatment by ligation. Surgery, *65*:659, 1969.
65. Wilson, W. B., Feinsod, M., Hoyt, W. F., et al.: Malignant evolution of childhood chiasmal pilocytic astrocytomas. Neurology (Minneap.), *26*:322–325, 1976.
66. Wolter, J.: Arteriovenous fistulas involving the eye region. J. Pediat. Ophthal., *12*:22, 1975.
67. Wyburn-Mason, R.: Arteriovenous aneurysm of midbrain and retina, facial nevi and mental changes. Brain, *66*:163, 1943.
68. Zimmerman, L., and Font, R.: Ophthalmologic manifestations of granulocytic sarcoma (myeloid sarcoma or chloroma). Amer. J. Ophthal., *80*:975–990, 1975.

96

CHEMOTHERAPY OF
BRAIN TUMORS

Many past presentations of clinical chemotherapy for brain tumors began with an apology. Predictably the author would state the magnitude of the problem; recite the success of chemotherapy in modifying the course of childhood leukemia and selected solid tumors, e.g., choriocarcinoma, Burkitt's lymphoma, and Wilms' tumor; point out the limited value of operation and irradiation; and with a note of optimism, describe the theoretical potential of chemotherapy. Until quite recently scattered reports and anecdotal accounts failed to justify chemotherapy except as an investigational pursuit. Clearly, in the routine management of patients with malignant brain tumors, chemotherapy had no established role, and even the value of radiotherapy for anaplastic astrocytomas was questioned by many neurosurgeons.

Admittedly, advances in brain tumor chemotherapy have been modest, but evidence in hand supports the following statements: (1) the availability of a wide range of animal models and a clearer concept of their use in developing strategies for clinical application have influenced the designing of drug schedules, multiple-drug protocols, and multimodality approaches; (2) current knowledge of glioma cell population kinetics and the pharmacokinetics of active drugs provides a basis for bringing promising drugs into clinical trials; (3) although not a specific marker for neural tumors, polyamines are produced by brain tumors, and their appearance in cerebrospinal fluid reflects the presence of proliferating tumor cells; (4) several agents effective against recurrent tumors have been identified and either have undergone or will undergo controlled clinical trials; and (5)

for treating malignant astrocytomas, postoperative adjuvant radiotherapy added to BCNU has a statistically significant advantage over radiotherapy alone, BCNU alone, or no postoperative therapy.

The tumor of greatest concern is the malignant astrocytoma (astrocytoma grades III and IV, glioblastoma, anaplastic astrocytoma, and their variants), and except where other tumor types are mentioned specifically, this chapter is concerned primarily with supratentorial malignant astrocytomas. One would expect histologically identical tumors in the brain stem and the rarer tumors in the cerebellum and spinal cord to respond in a similar manner, but the authors' experience with tumors in these locations has been disappointing.

The following sections provide a scientific basis for a chemotherapeutic approach and a description of the currently used and available drugs (Table 96–1). In particular, differences in treating recently diagnosed as opposed to recurrent tumors are emphasized.

ANIMAL MODELS

In 1962, an experiment using an unlikely model, mouse L1210 leukemia, established a critical first principle in selecting drugs for use against tumors residing within the central nervous system.[13] When cyclophosphamide was administered to mice bearing subcutaneous implants, the drug exhibited significant oncolytic activity, yet it was ineffective against intracerebral implants, presumably because the drug failed to reach the brain in adequate concentration. Subsequently, numerous models of primary

C. B. WILSON, V. LEVIN, AND T. HOSHINO

TABLE 96-1   ABBREVIATIONS FOR CURRENTLY AVAILABLE CHEMOTHERAPEUTIC AGENTS

ABBREVIATION	NAME OF DRUG
HU	Hydroxyurea
5-FU	5-Fluorouracil
PCV	PCB, CCNU, and VCR
PCNU	NSC-95466; CAS reg. No. 13909-02-9; urea, 1(2-chloro-ethyl)-3(2,6-dioxo-3-piperidyl)-
BCNU	Carmustine; NSC-409962; CAS reg. No. 154-93-8; urea, 1,3-*bis*(2-chloroethyl)-1-nitroso-
CCNU	Lomustine; NSC-79037; CAS reg. No. 13010-47-4; urea, 1-(2-chloroethyl)-3-cyclohexyl-1-nitroso-
Methyl-CCNU	Semustine; NSC-95441; CAS reg. No. 33073-59-5; urea, 1-(2-chloroethyl)-3-(4-methylcyclohexyl)-1-nitroso-
PCB	Procarbazine; NSC-77213; CAS reg. No. 491-88-3; p-tolu-amide, N-isopropyl-α-(2-methylhydrazine)-, monohydro-chloride
VCR	Vincristine
MTX	Methotrexate
DAG	Dianhydrogalactitol

neural tumors have been developed in both small and large animals, and today investigators can select the intracerebral tumor model best suited to a specific problem.

A discussion of details concerning available models is beyond the scope of the present chapter. In a recent review of the subject, however, Crafts and Wilson described the principal models.[15] Tables 96-2 and 96-3 have been taken from that review and show the range of models suitable for particular investigative purposes. Rubinstein has examined the neuropathological characteristics of animal brain tumors and their relationship to human tumors. His work should be consulted for this important correlation.[111]

The model defined in greatest detail is a rat bearing a transplantable gliosarcoma originally induced with methyl nitrosourea (N-nitrosomethylurea, MNU).[3] Because this tumor line grows equally well in vitro and in vivo, it is well suited to quantitative studies of in vivo cell kill. In subsequent sections data generated with this model are mentioned because of their direct bearing on the designing of clinical trials.

ANATOMICAL CONSIDERATIONS

The infiltrating nature of malignant gliomas precludes accurate estimates of their total mass. Even if this estimate were possible, the mass would contain unpredictable proportions of viable tumor cells, nonviable tumor cells, necrotic debris, non-

TABLE 96-2   CLASSIFICATION OF MODELS*

TUMOR	MODEL Chemical	Viral
Autochthonous	Polycyclic hydrocarbons Methylcholanthrene and others	ASV, MSV, simian SV 40 Human JC Papova virus Human adenovirus 12
	MNU given intravenously to adult rats, rabbits ENU given transplacentally to rats	
Transplanted	Methylcholanthrene-induced ependymoblastoma, glioma 26, glioma 261 Rat MNU-induced tumor lines, e.g., 9L	ASV-induced gliosarcoma in beagles

Key: MNU = methyl nitrosourea
      ENU = ethyl nitrosourea
      ASV = avian sarcoma virus
      MSV = murine sarcoma virus

* From Crafts, D. C., and Wilson, C. B.: Animal models of brain tumors. *In* Modern Concepts in Brain Tumor Therapy. National Cancer Institute Monograph 46, 1977. pp. 11-17.

cent to tumor.[66] This
rounding the grossl
tumor contains the
mass in the form
cells. This peripher
brain constitutes the
and within it is a po
with a large growth f
vorable capillary to
Because brain adjac
this population of
most probably in a
rate of cell death,
disproportionate to i
cause of its signific
tumor's growth but
ability of capillarie
govern the entry of
tered drugs. Levin
the brain adjacent t
ing rats, found that
for hydrophilic mol
of that for compar
brain. This unexpec
illary exchange cou
differences in capil
limited capillary pe
cent to tumor is par
entry of water-solu
earlier, the edema
adjacent to tumor r
diffusion of plasma
extracellular comp
tumor mass.

Having gained ac
tracellular space,
enter the tumor c
water-soluble drug
and molecular exch
cellular space and t
almost unrestricte
tracellular space in
to normal brain,
tumor occupies an

The preceding
translated into ge
the selection and
based upon their
teristics, and this i
cell kill capabilitie
nonspecific) should
vestigating promisi

With the assum
agent will have m
entry into much o
the critical differe
cross and those th

per
per
reti
plai
figu
tum
witl
tum
sho
cen
soli
and
cycl
cell
the
divi

Tl
was
gliot
cally
ual t
10⁸
fract
lariz
close
obta

In
man,
have
cells
(100
nenti
nonp
mal
other
gliobl
per c
such
cell
tarde
expla
the n
rate c
tion (
tumo
duced
sumin
tumor
sional
cell cy
prove
therap
signifi
netic
tion. F
of irra
reoxyg

TABLE 96-3 APPLICATIONS OF MODELS*

METHOD	ADVANTAGES	DISADVANTAGES	MAJOR USE AT PRESENT
Methyl cholanthrene implant	Economical Type of tumor can be some-what controlled by site of chemical implant	40%–60% incidence of tumors Latency long and variable Variety of tumors	
Methyl nitrosourea (MNU) to adult rats	No trauma to brain Histology and cell kinetics similar to human tumors	Laborious induction Multiple tumors and tumor types Only fair standardization of temporal course of disease	Biochemistry Peritumoral edema Immunology
Ethyl nitrosourea (ENU) trans-placentally	No trauma to brain Histology and cell kinetics similar to human tumors Less work than MNU	Multiplicity of tumors and tumor types Only fair standardization of temporal course of disease	Chemical carcinogenesis Biochemistry Immunology
Mouse ependymoblastoma lines (transplanted)	Economical Reproducible Standard tumor predictable Statistically amenable time course	Trauma to brain Tumor has questionable relation to human tumors, histologically and by cellular kinetics	Chemotherapy screen
Transplanted MNU-induced tumor	Moderate expense Reproducible Tissue culture available	Trauma to brain Uncertainty as to neuroglial nature of tumor	Chemotherapy Radiotherapy Evaluation for cell kill
Virus-induced tumors	Less trauma to brain Autochthonous tumor with natural blood supply Fairly long but predictable course Cell kinetics similar to human	Multiplicity of tumors and tumor types Expense and care of working with viruses	Immunology Chemotherapy Viral tumorigenesis
Transplantable virus-induced tumor (Only one in use is beagle)	Large brain for blood-brain-barrier pharmacokinetic studies Consistent tumor type	Trauma to brain Expense for studies requiring large number of animals Question whether blood-brain barrier of dog similar to that of human	Pharmacokinetics Chemotherapy

* From Crafts, D. C., and Wilson, C. B.: Animal models of brain tumors. In Modern Concepts in Brain Tumor Therapy. National Cancer Institute Monograph 46, 1977. pp. 11–17.

neoplastic reactive cellular constituents, blood vessels, and extravasated blood, quite apart from the variable accumulation of extracellular fluid. Histologically healthy tumor cells can be found within the brain at great distances from the grossly evident tumor mass. In recognition of this knowledge, radiotherapists have treated increasingly larger brain volumes to the point, at present, of whole brain irradiation.

Unlike the highly selective and restrictive capillaries in normal brain, the abnormal vessels within a tumor allow entry of large, water-soluble, and ionized molecules as well as plasma proteins into the extravascular extracellular compartment. Although the ineffective blood-tumor barrier permits the extravascular passage of diagnostic radionuclides and is advantageous in this respect, the detrimental consequence of abnormal permeability is the leakage of plasma constituents into the tumor and from its extracellular compartment into the adjacent brain, where it constitutes peritumoral edema. The net result is inflation of the tumor and an additional mass effect caused by the accumulation of fluid, primarily extracellular, in the surrounding brain.

Necrosis, a hallmark of glioblastomas, implies a failure of the vascular system to supply essential nutrients, the most critical deficiency being oxygen. For practical purposes, necrosis represents hypoxic cell death. Less evident is sublethal hypoxia affecting apparently healthy cells less distant from a capillary. Whether the vascular network fails to proliferate in parallel with the tumor cell population or whether occlusion of neoplastic vessels or shunting of blood within the tumor interrupts the blood supply to its field of distribution, the consequence is a group of hypoxic tumor cells surviving on a marginal supply of oxygen.

ing radio
the durati
lation of
proach,
weeks, S
gated one
cycle tin
growth fr
cellent a£
data.

The se
tomated
Nuclei
acriflavin
eter. A l
data ind
DNA coι
glioblastι
suspensiι
shino is
isolation
lem. The
files of hι
means o
tion on ε

PHARM.
PHARM.

In the
teristics
and relaι
basis of
cycling
cell cyι
specific
(unfortu
colytic
small pι
the requ
effectivι
Given a
cal testi
tential fι
system
its phaι
charactι
cologicε
behaviο
oncolyt
tial effeι
tem are

The
cussed
extracε
brain. S

---

tent or continuous infusion, or carotid-jugular perfusion. Intra-arterial administration should achieve a high drug concentration within a tumor that is confined to the carotid territorial distribution. The ideal drugs for intra-arterial administration are lipid soluble or small nonionized molecules with relatively rapid rates of chemical transformation to an active oncolytic species. These drugs would have the maximum entry into brain and brain adjacent to tumor and would achieve the highest tumor drug levels. In addition, with cross-compression of a contralateral vertebral or carotid artery, even greater tissue entry could be obtained. This approach would permit administration of smaller doses and hence lessen systemic toxicity.

Limitations

Intra-arterial administration has two major limitations: neurotoxicity, i.e., direct damage to brain within the infused area; and anatomical limitations of the field of infusion. Quite apart from the pH and osmolarity of the substance infused, a drug may be directly neurotoxic. Probably the major limitation of intra-arterial infusion is the bilaterality of a substantial number of gliomas and their frequent location within areas supplied by two or more major cerebral arteries, e.g., middle cerebral artery and posterior cerebral artery.

Technique

Infusion

For intra-arterial infusion, correct localization is imperative. In the vertebral artery, correct placement is determined either by open operation or by injection of radiopaque medium. In the carotid system, whether the technique is percutaneous cannulation or open arteriotomy, flow into the internal carotid artery must be verified by injection of either an opaque medium or a substance that can be visualized in the ophthalmic artery distribution. The authors have used fluorescein, but dyes visible under ambient light are equally satisfactory.[21,115,143]

A drug can be administered intermittently over days or weeks, or by continuous infusion over minutes to days. Percutaneous placement of either needle or catheter

---

is suitable for administration over a matter of several minutes to an hour. For longer administration (i.e., infusion), placement of a catheter is essential to prevent damage to the intima by the inflexible needle and to prevent displacement of the needle from the artery. The Seldinger technique of catheterization is suitable for cervical placement of an internal carotid catheter, and the authors have used a large-bore needle without the more refined Seldinger technique.[19,143] Transfemoral catheterization of the internal carotid artery has not been used for long-term infusion, perhaps because of the increased danger of infection in the genital-rectal area and the risk of deep venous thrombosis in the catheterized extremity. Many authors advocate the direct placement of a catheter, introducing it through either the common carotid artery or the superior thyroid artery. Nelson and co-workers gave an excellent description of catheter fixation.[82]

Injection by hand is suitable for short-term administration. For injections over a period of time and for long-term infusions, several techniques are available, ranging from gravity methods to a variety of pumps.* An excellent and easily managed infusion apparatus is the Fenwal bag, which employs an inflated cuff surrounding a plastic bag containing the solution to be infused.[143] This method is easily managed by the nursing staff and, when the bag is properly filled, avoids the potential complication of air embolism.

Certain agents, because of decomposition, cannot be mixed and administered over long periods of time. Unfortunately, many of the effective cell cycle–nonspecific agents currently in use are not stable in solution for extended periods.

Perfusion

Woodhall and Mahaley, with their collaborators at Duke, were pioneers in the isolated perfusion technique for the chemotherapy of brain tumors.[74,153,154] Discouraged by their initial results, they later switched to arterial infusion. Unfortunately, the isolation-perfusion technique using one or both internal carotid arteries and jugular veins does not approach a

---

* See references 22, 75, 128, 135, 136, 143.

closed system because of spillover of the infused solution to pericranial tissues and the return of venous blood to the systemic circulation by way of the perivertebral venous plexus. Further, isolation of both carotid arteries involves risks and poses technical difficulties.[95] Feind and co-workers, using bilateral common carotid and internal jugular vein cannulation, improved vascular isolation of the head and neck by applying a tourniquet to the base of the neck while occluding the internal vertebral venous plexus with an epidural balloon.[23] Because of the technical difficulties attending this procedure, it has not been pursued. Moss accomplished total perfusion of the brain in the calf by infusing one common carotid artery at a pressure 20 mm of mercury greater than systemic pressure, and angiograms demonstrated reverse flow in the distribution of the contralateral carotid artery and both vertebral arteries.[81] This method has not been applied to man. There seems to be little advantage in using intra-arterial perfusion instead of infusion when risks are weighed against potential benefits.

Complications

The intra-arterial administration of chemotherapeutic agents has been attended by many complications, the great majority being associated with long-term infusions through indwelling catheters. Neurological deficits, both transient and permanent, can be attributed in some cases to arterial spasm either from the drug or from the effect of the indwelling catheter.[127] With all long-term infusions, an additional problem has been infection at the cutaneous exit of the catheter, whether in the cervical or in the thoracic regions.

The major complication of arterial catheterization has been thrombosis of the internal carotid artery. In the majority of instances, carotid thrombosis has been an unexpected finding by angiography or at postmortem examination.[143] The frequency of thrombosis is related to the type of catheter and the duration of its presence in the artery. Benson and co-workers have advised the use of catheters of the smallest possible size, since a small catheter becomes excluded from the blood stream by a circumferential sheath of fibrin thrombus that fixes it to the vessel wall.[5] Occlusion of the catheter tip by blood products is avoidable by using a mechanism providing constant efflux from the catheter tip and by adding heparin to the solution. Meticulous attention to detail can significantly reduce the occurrence of air embolism and thrombosis.

Another common and potentially serious complication is displacement of the catheter tip from the vessel lumen with consequent bleeding and leakage of the drug into the perivascular soft tissues. Leakage may cause swelling and the risk of venous and airway obstruction.

Increased intracranial pressure subsequent to treatment is not unique to intra-arterial therapy, but it is possible the drug concentrations achieved by intra-arterial administration pose a particular problem in this regard.[30,35] Increased intracranial pressure can occur as a consequence of tumor necrosis, with or without additional cerebral edema caused by neurotoxicity of the infused agent. The current availability of effective means to combat cerebral edema lessens this threat.

Transitory and permanent ophthalmoplegia have occurred in patients receiving intracarotid infusions of nitrogen mustard and the vinca alkaloids.[94,143] Vasculitis has been reported recently in dogs given a large intra-arterial dose of BCNU, which may dampen enthusiasm for intracarotid therapy with BCNU in man, although Crafts and co-workers did not observe this complication in monkeys.[16,20]

Agents Administered by Intra-Arterial Methods

A number of agents have been administered by various intra-arterial techniques, none with outstanding success. Among the agents used have been methotrexate, vinblastine sulfate, vincristine sulfate, nitrogen mustard, phenylalanine mustard, triethylenethiophosphoramide, and 5-bromo-2'-deoxyuridine (BUdR).* BUdR has been used only in conjunction with radiation therapy, whereas several of the other agents listed have been used both singly and with radiation therapy. In pharmacokinetic studies of radiolabeled BCNU

---

* See references: methotrexate, 35; vinblastine, 80, 143; vincristine, 92–94; nitrogen mustard, 30, 95; phenylalanine mustard, 1; triethylenethiophosphoramide, 18, 76; BUdR, 114.

in squirrel monkeys, Levin and associates demonstrated potential benefit of intra–carotid artery BCNU therapy. They found that BCNU administered via the carotid artery achieved nucleic acid–bound drug levels in the treated brain four to five times as high as that achieved following conventional intravenous administration. These same benefits did not follow intra-carotid CCNU administration.[68] In studies in rhesus monkeys, BCNU showed no central nervous system, vascular, or ophthalmic toxicity following intracarotid administration.[16]

Intraventricular and Intrathecal Routes

Rationale

Since the ependyma and arachnoid appear to present little restriction to the movement of molecules between cerebrospinal fluid and brain extracellular space, intrathecal and intraventricular routes of administration of chemotherapeutic agents have been advocated for molecules too large to pass the blood-brain barrier as well as for drugs producing excessive systemic intoxication or drugs that are rapidly inactivated in blood.[46,52] The obvious advantage of achieving and maintaining a high level of drug in the cerebrospinal fluid is, in most cases, lessened by the tumor's location deep within the brain, at a distance 2 to 4 cm from the cerebrospinal fluid.

Simple lumbar injection of methotrexate has been highly successful in the treatment of meningeal leukemia. Meningeal leukemia is, however, almost invariably accompanied by communicating hydrocephalus with its abnormal flow pattern and reflux into the cerebral ventricles; and access of the drug to cells that are either free-floating or enmeshed in leptomeninges presents a problem entirely different from drug delivery to a solid tumor. Although methotrexate controls meningeal leukemia, as determined by cytological studies of the cerebrospinal fluid, recurrences (unexplainable by hematogenous metastasis) indicate survival of at least a few leukemic cells either because the drug failed to reach all leukemic cells at effective concentrations or because treatment was stopped before elimination of the last cell.

The authors have conducted a study of continuous (36-hour) high-dosage methotrexate infusion via either the spinal subarachnoid space or a ventricular reservoir, followed by systemic leucovorin (citrovorum factor) rescue. They have abandoned this approach, although it may be applicable to selected cases of central nervous system leukemia and meningeal carcinomatosis.[26]

Intrathecal therapy offers little advantage unless the tumor is in the path of subarachnoid cerebrospinal fluid because the normal fluid dynamics are such that intrathecally administered drugs do not enter the ventricular system to a significant extent.[11] Although this can be circumvented with a reservoir or by ventricular-lumbar perfusion, the effectiveness of the drug entering from cerebrospinal fluid into brain and tumor will still be limited and dependent on: (1) the diffusion coefficient of the drug, (2) capillary permeability, (3) drug stability in cerebrospinal fluid, (4) the location of the tumor relative to the ventricular surface, and (5) the drug's neurotoxicity.

Limitations

Intrathecally administered polar molecules move by bulk flow from the lumbar subarachnoid space to the basal cisterns and then to the cerebral convexities. Absorption then occurs through the arachnoid villi into the venous blood of the sagittal sinus. This pattern can be modified unpredictably by intracranial tumors, and proper distribution requires special techniques to insure movement of the drug to its intended site of action.

In addition to arachnoid villus absorption, capillary permeability in tumor and even in normal brain can lead to significant systemic absorption of drug from brain and tumor extracellular space, with resultant systemic intoxication. For a drug with the molecular size of fluorouracil, at least 13 per cent of intraventricular drug could leak across normal capillaries, and possibly 10 per cent could leak across tumor capillaries.[2]

One goal of ventricular perfusion is to achieve significant tumoricidal drug levels in brain adjacent to the tumor. To do this with a drug such as methotrexate, with the tumor at a depth of 2 cm from the ventricle, a piece of brain 4 cm in ventricular-subarachnoid breadth would have to be perfused on both the ventricular and subarachnoid surfaces for 48 hours to achieve, at a depth of 2 cm, 8 per cent of the concentration in the cerebrospinal fluid.[63]

Neurotoxicity constitutes a significant factor in selecting drugs for intrathecal administration. For instance, vinblastine sulfate, while well tolerated following vascular injection, is markedly neurotoxic when administered intracisternally in the dog.[44] It is well established that intrathecal and intraventricular methotrexate can, particularly with cerebrospinal fluid stasis, be seriously and life-threateningly neurotoxic.[109,122,133]

Drugs that readily cross the blood-brain barrier (i.e., lipid-soluble and small-molecule nonionized drugs) lose much of their advantage following intraventricular administration because of their rapid exit across the capillaries in normal brain.

Technique

Drugs can be injected intermittently by lumbar puncture, by cisternal puncture, through a previously placed burr hole, or through a reservoir. All these routes are available for infusion over a longer period of time. Perfusion, using separate sites for inflow and outflow, can be performed by using combinations of sites related to the target area.

Infusion

Newton and co-workers, treating childhood tumors with methotrexate, used lumbar puncture and previously placed burr holes for injection into the ventricular system.[85] Ommaya described a subcutaneous reservoir and pump for sterile access to ventricular cerebrospinal fluid, and this has become a popular apparatus for intraventricular administration, intermittent injection, and continuous infusion.[90] Although the reservoir was designed for the treatment of cryptococcal meningitis, oncolytic agents are ideally suited for percutaneous injection.[7] To assure adequate mixing and distribution of methotrexate, Norrell and

Wilson used the Pudenz shunting system with unidirectional flow.[87] A unidirectional shunting system creates a current that can be directed to the desired area over a broad surface.

The authors have infused methotrexate into the lumbar subarachnoid space via an indwelling catheter and into the lateral ventricle through an Ommaya reservoir with a Harvard infusion pump. When the patient is protected by anticonvulsant medication, they have observed no ill effects from massive doses of methotrexate followed in 24 to 36 hours by systemic leucovorin rescue. In this and other systems, one can obtain an approximation of the bulk flow of the administered molecules by observing the distribution of concomitantly injected or infused radioiodinated serum albumin on serial scintiscans.

Perfusion

Cerebrospinal perfusion provides a novel approach for the delivery of substances normally excluded by the blood-brain barrier. The complexity of the method detracts from its general applicability, but in certain special situations it may provide an effective method of adjuvant chemotherapy.

Ommaya and associates first reported the perfusion of oncolytic agents by means of techniques long practiced by physiologists. Depending upon the tumor's site, they established a perfusion system from ventricle to lumbar subarachnoid space, from lateral ventricle to lateral ventricle, from temporal horn to the body of the lateral ventricle, and from the tumor cavity to the lateral ventricle.[91]

Subsequently, Rubin and co-workers reported further experience with cerebrospinal fluid perfusions. A cannula was placed either in the frontal horn or in the tumor bed (in cases in which a fistula had been created between the tumor bed and the adjacent ventricle), and a second cannula was placed elsewhere in the cerebrospinal fluid space to provide an outflow route. They reported their experience with using methotrexate and 8-azaguanine perfused through combinations of Ommaya reservoirs and spinal cannulas. In the case of lipid-insoluble and highly ionized substances, e.g., methotrexate, egress of the molecule from cerebrospinal fluid occurs largely by bulk flow, and the rate of bulk flow is determined by the effective hydrostatic pressure, i.e., the difference between intraventricular and superior sagittal sinus venous pressures. They minimized systemic leakage of drug by perfusing with the outflow cannula set at the level of the right side of the heart (0 cm of water).[108,110]

Although perfusion techniques were envisioned as a means of exploiting relative pharmacological barriers to retain rather than exclude active compounds, in practice, and from our current understanding of brain tumor physiology and pharmacology, we can find little to recommend use of ventricular perfusion.

Complications

With long-term infusions and perfusions, the danger of infection is evident. Demyelination and seizures have occurred.[122] The chemical nature of the drug as well as the effect of the diluent may be responsible for side effects with individual agents, such as meningeal irritation and paraplegia occurring with methotrexate.[4,114] In a recent paper Bleyer gives an excellent review of the complications of intrathecal methotrexate with emphasis on necrotizing leukoencephalopathy.[7]

Another complication that could occur is injury to neural tissue secondary to manipulation of the cerebrospinal fluid. Bunge and Settlage produced lasting neurological deficits and histological lesions in cats by forcibly injecting cerebrospinal fluid into the cisterna magna.[12] More recently, forceful injection of fluid withdrawn from the lumbar subarachnoid space has been reported as a means of relieving pain.[22] In light of these reports, intrathecal injection should be made slowly.

Intra-Tumoral Route

Rationale

Effective local (topical) chemotherapy presumes that an agent will move freely throughout the tumor from its point of application and at the same time produce no adverse effects on uninvolved intradural structures. If experience with topical chemotherapy of extracranial tumors serves as any guide, this method has little potential for the treatment of intracranial tumors.

Limitations

Theoretically, a water-soluble drug, unless it binds tightly to brain tumor cell membranes or enters cells and rapidly biotransforms to its active species, would leak across tumor capillaries into the systemic circulation and into the cerebrospinal fluid sink, lowering its concentration within the tumor. This might be of little practical importance if the dose were large enough to exert an antitumor effect, but a lipid-soluble drug would move especially rapidly from intratumoral sites to the systemic circulation.

Technique

Selverstone described a stereotaxic technique for the local injection of 8-azaguanine.[6] Ringkjob treated gliomas and metastatic carcinomas by the local application of triethylenethiophosphoramide and 5-fluorouracil.[102]

Raskind and Weiss injected methotrexate into tumor cavities through an Ommaya reservoir placed at the time of operation.[139] Although the heterogeneity of their patient population precluded an evaluation of the drug's effectiveness, one of the authors examined their postmortem specimens and was impressed with the striking necrosis present in the shell of tumor surrounding the operatively created cavity. More recently, Garfield and Dayan have given up to 1250 mg of methotrexate daily for 4 to 10 days by postoperative intracavitary catheter and have reported modest chemotherapeutic responses in nine patients.[31]

Methotrexate may be an ideal drug in this respect, since it moves well through the extracellular space of both tumor and surrounding brain, and one can achieve extremely high local concentrations within the limits of systemic toxicity. Its disadvantage as a primary mode of therapy lies in its cell-cycle specificity in tumors with a small growth fraction. As an immediate adjunct to operative removal, the local application of oncolytic drugs probably deserves some further experimental study.

CLINICAL TRIALS AND THEIR RELATIONSHIP TO INITIAL AND RECURRENT TUMORS

Clinical evaluation of a drug is preceded by extensive laboratory investigation, and only after the drug's oncolytic activity and toxicity have been established in animal screens is the drug introduced into clinical trials. Given a promising drug on the basis of preclinical testing, clinical evaluation proceeds through three phases (Table 96–5). To facilitate the description of clinical studies involving specific chemotherapeutic agents, these phases are described.

Phase I studies establish tolerable doses and dosage schedules and in the process define a drug's spectrum of toxicity, e.g., bone marrow depression. Although the drug's activity may become evident, this is not the purpose of a phase I trial. With dosage and toxicity established, the *phase II* trial is designed to determine a drug's activity, if any, against specific tumors. Patients harboring measurable (evaluable) tumors are treated and observed for evidence of tumor regression. If the patient receives an adequate dosage over an adequate period of treatment, response to treatment is determined by objective criteria, usually by direct measurement of tumor mass.

A *phase III* trial compares an active new drug with the best known treatment for the tumor under study. Entry requirements are established (pathology, extent of disease, prior treatment, general condition, allowable concurrent therapy, e.g., steroids), and acceptable patients are assigned randomly to two (or more) arms of the protocol, one arm being the best known treatment and the other arm or arms being the new drug (or drugs) under study.[131] Comparability of the patients in each arm should be achieved by random assignment, and to improve the intergroup similarity many studies stratify patients according to recognized prognostic factors prior to randomization. Patients are followed to an end point: either progression (or recurrence) or death. Retrospectively, the comparability of patients in the different treatment arms should be analyzed to be certain that one arm was not weighted with "unfavorable" patients. For example, Gehan and Walker analyzed the characteristics of patients who entered a clinical trial conducted by the Brain Tumor Study Group and defined those factors most related to survival: age (young, favorable), biopsy (biopsy only unfavorable when compared with subtotal removal), seizures (favorable), and parietal location of tumor (unfavorable).[32]

Most studies involving brain tumor chemotherapy have been uncontrolled phase II trials seeking to determine the activity, if any, of a single agent. The majority of patients qualifying for entry into these phase II trials have harbored large recurrent tumors. This is an unfavorable group of patients because of their advanced disease. In view of the kinetic characteristics of large tumors, one would anticipate an observable response to effective cell cycle–nonspecific agents while conceding that response to an active cell cycle–specific agent, even though a significant cell kill (e.g., 1 log, or 90 per cent) was achieved, might be missed. The record supports this line of reasoning.

Phase III trials are more complex and necessarily involve large numbers of patients accrued and followed over longer periods of time. Because phase III trials determine the *relative* value of a particular form of therapy, the results of these trials establish the best available treatment and therefore set the standard of practice for the disease. For this reason the reader must distinguish between the results of phase II

TABLE 96–5 PHASES IN CLINICAL EVALUATION OF A NEW DRUG

PHASE	SUBJECTS	PURPOSE
I Clinical pharmacology	Patients with advanced cancer	To establish maximal tolerated dose and spectrum of toxicity
II Determination of activity	Patients with objectively measurable tumors, usually advanced	To establish activity against specific tumor types
III Definition of therapeutic value	Patients with established tumors entered into study soon after diagnosis	To compare the new drug with the best known treatment for the tumor under study

and phase III trials, because while the former may indicate the beneficial effects of a form of therapy, only the latter determine optimal therapy.

Response to Treatment and Recurrence (Regrowth) After Treatment

The authors justified a detailed consideration of these subjects for several reasons.

1. As the chemotherapy of brain tumors becomes practiced on a wider scale, neurosurgeons should become familiar with the criteria for evaluating newly introduced forms of therapy.

2. When undertaking the treatment of a patient harboring a recurrent tumor (in a phase II setting) the neurosurgeon must be able to determine the tumor's response in order to continue effective therapy and to change ineffective therapy.

3. When following the patient whose course is stable or improving (in both phase II and phase III settings), the time of regrowth should be established at the earliest time possible in order to consider therapeutic alternatives, e.g., reoperation or crossover to another drug, before the patient suffers irreversible neurological deterioration.

4. For the neurosurgeon engaged in (or who may become engaged in) clinical investigation, a clear concept of response and recurrence is essential.

Phase II and phase III trials are referred to because these terms communicate purpose and circumstances, i.e., patients with recurrent (and on occasion histologically unverified) tumors belong in a phase II setting, and patients with newly verified tumors (preferably immediately after operation) will receive adjuvant chemotherapy and radiotherapy in a phase III setting.

The terms "response" and "recurrence" (used interchangeably with "regrowth") refer to recognizable changes in the bulk of an intracranial mass composed of proliferating and nonproliferating tumor cells, nonviable tumor cells and debris, extracellular fluid, hematoma, and supporting non-neoplastic stroma.

The ideal indicator of a tumor's behavior would be a quantitative measurement of its clonogenic* cell population, but at present this approach is restricted to laboratory models. Methods for clinical use in determining either a decrease or an increase in tumor mass are relatively crude; first, they are insensitive to changes smaller than 20 to 30 per cent of the tumor mass; and second, present techniques are seldom of value in defining a mass containing fewer than 10^{10} (10 gm) cells. Translated into practice this means that present methods can be applied only to tumors with a bulk of 10 gm or more, and that they will not detect changes of less than 25 per cent.

Certain small tumors (for example, in the brain stem) produce devastating deficits, yet their local infiltrations may escape detection by radionuclide and computer-assisted tomographic (CT) scans—the two procedures currently used to follow the course of an intracranial tumor. In this situation, "response" or "recurrence" can be determined best by meticulous serial neurological examinations.

Finally, if neural structures, including gray and white matter, have been irreversibly damaged, a therapeutically-induced reduction in tumor mass may not be accompanied by improved neurological function. Although the authors have observed very few instances of this sort, reliance *solely* on the neurological examination may lead the physician to misinterpret the tumor's behavior.

Viewed simply, response and recurrence represent extreme poles of the actual situation: response is the outcome of a therapeutic reduction in tumor mass, while recurrence is a manifestation of a tumor's progression with or without concurrent treatment. At present the tools by which we make these judgments are the same for both: clinical neurological examination, radionuclide brain scanning, computed tomographic scanning, special neuroradiological procedures (angiography, pneumography, and myelography), and examination of the cerebrospinal fluid. Response is less difficult to define than recurrence, and of lesser importance. In the following sections the authors define response and recurrence on

---

* *Clonogenic*—in experimental systems, a single cell capable of producing a colony (clone) in vitro or in vivo; in the present context, a single cell capable of infinite proliferation.

the basis of their experience with 500 patients observed from the beginning of treatment to the time of death.

Criteria of Response (Phase II Trials)

Table 96–6 lists the requirements for entry into the phase II trials. The majority of entering patients have recurrent tumors. Also eligible for phase II trials are patients who, on the basis of clinical evidence short of operative confirmation, harbor either primary or metastatic brain tumors. In the latter circumstance neuroradiological procedures must provide *unequivocal* evidence of a mass, the history and neurological examination must confirm the presence of a tumor, and all available evidence must support no alternative diagnosis. The majority of primary tumors in the histologically unverified category have been located in the brain stem, the deep midline (basal ganglia and corpus callosum), and speech areas in the dominant hemisphere. In our series of patients treated without histological diagnosis, subsequent postmortem examination has not failed to verify the presence of a tumor.

Care in evaluation can usually exclude metastatic brain involvement on the basis of the presence of one or more intracranial tumors in a patient with a known primary source outside the central nervous system. Leptomeningeal carcinomatosis presents a special problem, and because the condition is both uncommon and often unaccompanied by measurable tumor mass it is excluded from further discussion.

Deterioration beginning more than two months after operation constitutes presumptive evidence of tumor regrowth if complications, e.g., hydrocephalus, are excluded. Reasons for the lapse of three months after completion of radiotherapy are considered later. Because response to a chemotherapeutic agent may be delayed, the interval of six weeks following administration of a drug should be observed (see Table 96–6). When a nitrosourea is being tested, six to eight weeks should elapse before therapy with a new agent is initiated because of the delayed response and myelotoxic effects observed in patients receiving either BCNU or CCNU.

Evaluable patients are those who fulfill all requirements for entry, complete at least one full course of therapy, and live for at least two months after initiation of treatment.

In Table 96–7 the procedures that constitute the basis for entry into a phase II trial and also provide a baseline for later comparison in evaluating response to treatment are indicated. The procedures that are repeated at the time of each re-evaluation and retreatment are identified by an asterisk. Certain of these, e.g., myelography and cytological evaluation of cerebrospinal fluid, are applied selectively under special circumstances. Although the work is still in an investigative stage, analysis of cerebrospinal fluid for polyamines has provided data that indicate that these substances are reliable though nonspecific indicators of replicating cell mass and tumor cell kill.[40,77,78] The authors have not used assay of cerebrospinal fluid sterols as a biochemical test for following the course of patients undergoing treatment, and the recent paper of Ransohoff and Weiss should be con-

TABLE 96–6 PHASE II ENTRY REQUIREMENTS

1. Unequivocal neurological deterioration secondary to tumor growth and a tumor that is demonstrable by neurodiagnostic procedures
2. Either a pathological diagnosis or a clinical picture supporting no alternative diagnosis
3. At least two months after preceding operation (if performed)
4. At least three months after preceding radiotherapy (if administered)
5. At least six weeks (eight weeks for nitrosoureas) after preceding chemotherapy (if administered)
6. Life expectancy of two months or longer

TABLE 96–7 PROCEDURES USED FOR DETERMINING ENTRY AND RESPONSE*

1. Neurological examination
2. Radionuclide scanning
3. Computed tomography
4. Neuroradiological procedures[a]: angiography and pneumography
5. Examination of cerebrospinal fluid[b]: cytology, polyamines
6. Myelography[c]

---

   a. Rarely repeated.
   b. Used selectively.
   c. Seldom used except in medulloblastoma with suspected or known spinal implants.

---

* Procedures repeated at the time of each re-evaluation and retreatment.

sulted for an account of their experience.[99] Early experience with serial cerebral angiography revealed its limited value as an indicator of tumor regression, and because of morbidity and expense its use has been discontinued.

In determining the oncolytic effectiveness of an agent, i.e., response, first importance is assigned to the neurological examination. The correlation between clinical improvement and improved radionuclide and CT scans (and the converse) is good but imperfect.[14,54,70,86]

The authors use radionuclide and CT scans in conjunction with the neurological examination as indicators of drug effect for the following reasons: (1) an improved scan may precede neurological improvement, and *vice versa;* (2) with tumors in neurologically "silent" areas, e.g., the frontal pole, neurological examination may provide little clinical indication of a change in tumor mass; (3) certain neurological deficits, e.g., hemianopsia, represent irreversible damage, and unequivocal tumor regression may be accompanied, although rarely, by no improvement in neurological function; and (4) experience has established the reliability of sequential scans in determining response to treatment.[70]

Evaluable patients are assigned to one of three categories of response on the basis of a review of two or more recorded sequential neurological examinations and corresponding brain scans.

Response

Unequivocal clinical neurological improvement *and* brain scans demonstrating reduction in tumor mass or, in the case of multiple metastatic tumors, unequivocal shrinkage of one tumor and stability of other tumors are acceptable. In addition, these changes must be observed while the patient is receiving nonescalating doses of steroid.

Probable Response or Stable Disease

Either one of two responses qualifies patients for this cateogry: (1) improvement in clinical status and unchanged scans, or an improved scan and a stable clinical course; (2) arrest of a deteriorating course, with neither progression nor improvement in

TABLE 96–8   CRITERIA OF RESPONSE (PHASE II)

RESPONSE	CRITERIA
Unequivocal	1. Unequivocal improvement in neurological function and 2. Unequivocal improvement in radionuclide and/or CT scans and 3. Nonescalating maintenance dose of glucocorticoid
Stable disease	1. Improvement in either neurological function or scans without deterioration in the other or Stability of neurological function and scans for three months and 2. Nonescalating maintenance dose of glucocorticoid

neurological condition and scans, with stability for a period of three months or longer in a patient harboring a malignant tumor (glioblastoma, malignant astrocytoma, medulloblastoma and cerebral metastasis).

No Response

Worsened clinical condition and scans.

The criteria for determining response and probable response are summarized in Table 96–8.

Criteria of Regrowth (Phase III Trials)

The *time* of recurrence (regrowth) indicates that point when regrowth of a previously treated tumor is established by techniques available at present. Unequivocal evidence of recurrence is used in two ways: first, recurrence is one requirement for entry into a phase II trial, and in this situation recurrence is established by a history of deteriorating neurological function and the demonstration of a mass with the characteristics of a recurrent tumor; and second, the time of first recurrence is a highly desirable end point for phase III trials in which serial examinations should provide an ideal basis for making this determination.

The diagnosis of recurrence is made difficult because of the anatomical distortions produced by earlier treatment and residual neurological deficits.[137] Customary diagnostic tests are less reliable because abnormality must be judged relative to previous abnormal studies. Loss of brain substance, scarring, and in some cases residual but not actively regrowing tumor may obscure the manifestations of tumor regrowth.

In establishing tumor recurrence in the patient under continuing observation, serial examinations provide the basis for defining two points: "recurrence suspected" and "recurrence confirmed." In most cases recurrence will be suspected two to three weeks before it becomes obvious, but the interval is variable. In at least one third of patients in whom recurrence is suspected, subsequent events indicate that the suspicion was a false alarm. This has been true whether the suspicion was based upon subtle neurological symptoms and signs or upon minor changes in radionuclide and CT scans. The reasons for the misleading indications of early recurrence relate to well-known variability in the functional capacity of patients with central nervous system disease, and in the case of misleading scans, the explanation is either observer error, technical error in the timing of the study, or differences in equipment and positioning of the patient. Consequently, "recurrence suspected" is not a reliable end point, although it serves to alert the investigator.

"Recurrence confirmed" indicates unequivocal evidence of regrowth; because it can, and should, provide a clear end point in phase III studies, the criteria must be strict. Proposed criteria for recurrence are indicated in Table 96–9.

Distal implants are uncommon with tumors other than medulloblastomas and anaplastic ependymomas, but their appearance at any time after initial radiotherapy indicates treatment failure. Many symptoms such as headache and lethargy are nonspecific and unreliable as indicators of recurrence. Evidence of increased intracranial pressure without accompanying deteri-

TABLE 96–9   CRITERIA FOR CONFIRMED RECURRENCE

1. Deterioration in neurological function and worsening of either radionuclide or CT scan or worsening of both the radionuclide and CT scan.*

or

2. Unequivocal evidence of distal tumor implantation, intracranial or intraspinal

---

* If both scans have remained normal or are uninterpretable because of artifact, angiography and pneumography should be performed but with the disadvantage of lacking a preceding study for comparison.

oration in another sphere is also an unreliable indication of regrowth. The same is true of cytological examination of the cerebrospinal fluid and the electroencephalogram. Additional experience may modify the author's present position in defining recurrence, but the proposed criteria will avoid mistaken diagnosis.

Differential Diagnosis of Regrowth

In the *immediate postoperative period,* deterioration raises the surgical problem of cerebral edema or hematoma versus continued growth of inadequately decompressed tumor. Cerebral edema reaches its peak in the first two to four days after operation, and hematomas usually become evident within the first few days. As a rule, improvement following the administration of steroids supports the initial diagnosis of edema, although steroids also benefit the patient with a postoperative hematoma. Postoperative impairment of cerebrospinal fluid flow or the tumor itself can cause hydrocephalus, which may appear several weeks after operation or even much later. Drowsiness and decreased mentation may develop in the absence of any new abnormality seen on the brain scan. For all the preceding diagnostic possibilities, the CT scan provides a noninvasive means of identifying the problem.

Postoperative radiotherapy can create diagnostic confusion in four ways:

1. During the course of radiation, there may be *reactive edema* with nausea, drowsiness, and worsening of deficit, especially when a tumor has been inadequately decompressed. Ordinarily this is not a serious diagnostic problem, and the edema resolves with a temporary increase in steroid dosage and a lapse of several days without radiotherapy.

2. A more difficult diagnostic problem is the *transient encephalopathy* that may appear 1 to 15 weeks (usually 6 to 10) after the end of x-ray therapy.[97] It can develop after exposure to as little as 2400 rads in children who are receiving central nervous system prophylaxis for leukemia.[29] The syndrome is usually manifested by drowsiness, nausea, and malaise, but can include ataxia, dysphasia, and exaggeration or reappearance of previous neurological deficits. It does not require a pre-existing brain le-

sion and probably reflects demyelination produced by either a direct effect on oligodendroglia or an autoimmune reaction.[57,101] The tissue is edematous, friable, and vascular, and operation is not helpful.[8] The only way to differentiate this condition from tumor recurrence is to suspect it because of the time of appearance in relation to radiotherapy and to temporize by providing symptomatic treatment with steroids, often requiring large doses. The patient with radiation encephalopathy will improve without any other specific treatment, usually within four to six weeks. The encephalopathy is ordinarily self-limited and reversible (although one patient of Lampert and coworkers died with patchy areas of demyelination disseminated in the irradiated area of brain).[57] The patient may then do well without steroids for many months or years before actual tumor regrowth.

3. Better known is the condition of *radiation necrosis,* although it is less frequent now owing to the standardization of doses and improving dosimetry. This condition may develop as early as four months or as late as nine years after radiotherapy.[53] The symptoms may mimic tumor regrowth.[130] Usually late studies will show atrophy, but coagulative necrosis can create a mass that, even on gross tissue examination, resembles a tumor.[88,111,152] Scan and angiogram may show a mass, but not neovascularity. The diagnosis may be suspected from the history of radiotherapy, but sometimes operation is required both for definitive diagnosis and to remove the mass. Steroids may help transiently, but the damage is irreversible and the result, whether disability or death, is unfavorable.

4. Necrosis of tumor after x-ray can leave a *pseudocyst* that itself can cause symptoms by mass effect.[53]

The late onset of *seizures,* or the aggravation of pre-existing seizures, may or may not be the consequence of tumor regrowth. While seizures, viewed as a symptom, can first appear or increase in severity and frequency as a manifestation of tumor recurrence, with equal probability the underlying cause is an epileptogenic focus independent of recurrent tumor. Seizures can produce neurological symptoms suggestive of recurrence, especially in the postictal state. Ordinarily, postconvulsive deficits disappear

within a few hours, but they may persist for several days. Uncommonly, deficits may be caused by an ongoing seizure unaccompanied by overt signs of seizure (subclinical status epilepticus). Electroencephalography establishes the diagnosis, and neurological improvement will follow seizure control. The possibility that an unexpected seizure heralds tumor regrowth requires appropriate investigation and treatment.

Another cause of seizures is an inadequate anticonvulsant level. This can result from chemical complexing of diphenylhydantoin with antacids in the stomach and small intestine, which thereby reduces absorption. Some of the chemotherapeutic agents may induce liver microsomal metabolism of diphenylhydantoin, although this has not been well studied in man.

Metabolic and other generalized systemic problems can cause neurological disorders, including focal deficits, if there is underlying brain damage. Hypoglycemia, acidosis, hypotension, uremia, hepatic failure, anemia, electrolyte imbalance, respiratory insufficiency, fever, and infection can increase focal deficit with or without alteration in consciousness. It is surprising how much worse a patient with severe deficit can appear even a week after a urinary tract infection. These conditions can be ruled out during the course of a thorough evaluation.

Depressant drugs, for example, phenobarbital and primidone, can have similar effects, and other drugs such as diphenylhydantoin may have neurological side effects. In this respect, information about serum drug levels may be invaluable.

SPECIFIC DRUGS

Many drugs have been examined in phase II trials. Some have exhibited no activity, and others have not received an adequate trial. The authors describe those agents they have evaluated and, beyond this, indicate those that either have undergone adequate trial or show promising activity.

Nitrosoureas

In 1970 two reports introduced BCNU as an effective agent in the treatment of primary and metastatic brain tumors.[140,148] Either as a tribute to their activity or as an example of ineptness in discovering other active drugs, the nitrosoureas, particularly BCNU, remain the most effective agents.[64]

The major antitumor action of the three available nitrosoureas (BCNU, CCNU, and MeCCNU) is not entirely clear, although alkylation correlates well with activity and carbamoylation may be an important factor in effective drug combinations.[62] Whatever the mode of action, they function as cell cycle–nonspecific agents. All are lipid-soluble and readily cross normal brain capillaries. Levin and Kabra, in comparing the effectiveness of six nitrosoureas against the 9L rat gliosarcoma as a function of their lipid solubility, concluded that the optimum log P (1-octanol/water partition coefficient), a measure of lipid solubility, was 0.37.[62] (PCNU, an agent not yet introduced into clinical trials, possessed a log P of 0.37.) They found that antitumor activity actually decreased with increasing lipid solubility in the following order: BCNU, CCNU, and MeCCNU. Clinical experience appears to substantiate their laboratory observations, BCNU being most active, MeCCNU least active, and CCNU occupying a position of intermediate activity.

The nitrosoureas, like most alkylating agents, depress the bone marrow, peripheral platelet counts decreasing in three weeks and white blood cells, principally granulocytes, decreasing a few days thereafter. The peripheral counts recover six to eight weeks after drug administration, at which time treatment can be repeated but with dose modification as indicated by platelet and white cell nadirs during the preceding course. Long-term administration of BCNU frequently leads to chronic erythropoietic depression, although it rarely requires transfusions. Aside from transient nausea and vomiting on the day of administration, other toxic manifestations (i.e., pulmonary, hepatic, and renal), although observed in laboratory animals, are exceedingly rare.

In an ongoing phase III trial, MeCCNU has shown little activity, and, in fact, it may interfere with the known effectiveness of radiotherapy.[131] Because of MeCCNU's inferiority, the following discussion of the nitrosoureas is restricted to BCNU and CCNU.

BCNU

The authors' phase II experience with BCNU in 57 patients who could be evaluated has shown a 47 per cent response rate (includes responses and probable responses) for a median duration of nine months.[151] Against malignant gliomas the response rate has been 50 per cent (22 of 43 patients) for a median duration of nine months.[64] The drug has been administered at a dosage of 80 mg per square meter of body surface on three consecutive days with succeeding courses at intervals of six to eight weeks.

The Brain Tumor Study Group has evaluated BCNU in two phase III trials. Both trials admitted patients who had undergone subtotal removal of a malignant glioma and who did not require maintenance steroids. In the first study those patients receiving no postoperative therapy had a median survival of 17 weeks. Median survivals for the three treatment arms were 25 weeks (BCNU), 37.5 weeks (radiotherapy), and 40.5 weeks (BCNU plus radiotherapy). Although the median survival with combined therapy was only slightly longer than with radiotherapy alone, at the end of 18 months one fifth of patients receiving both BCNU and radiotherapy survived, in contrast to virtually none of those receiving a single mode of therapy.

The second phase III study has been closed, but final analysis has not been completed. Preliminary results are indicated in Table 96–10. The improved survival of patients receiving BCNU plus radiotherapy in this study is thought to reflect more diligent and effective management of complications as a consequence of favorable experience in the preceding study. If final analysis sub-

TABLE 96–10   PHASE III STUDY (PROJECTED ANALYSIS)*

THERAPY	MEDIAN SURVIVAL (WEEKS)
MeCCNU	31
MeCCNU[a] + radiotherapy[b]	31
Radiotherapy[b]	36
BCNU[c] + radiotherapy[b]	51

a. 220 mg per square meter every six to eight weeks
b. Radiotherapy: 6000 rads, whole brain
c. 80 mg per square meter every six to eight weeks

* From the Brain Tumor Study Group.

stantiates these results, BCNU plus radiotherapy will be established as the best available treatment for malignant gliomas. Additional support for the value of BCNU combined with radiotherapy has been reported by Shapiro and Young.[121]

Four recently completed laboratory studies of BCNU are relevant to future clinical trials.[150]

BCNU Dose Schedule

The dose schedule most widely in use is 80 mg per square meter of body surface on three successive days with an interval of six to eight weeks between courses. A recently concluded series of in vivo–in vitro experiments concerned with quantitative tumor cell kill and post-treatment clonogenic cell kinetics indicates the superiority of a single dose of BCNU over the customary schedules of divided doses.[103,104,106] The most significant experiments are summarized as follows:

1. A small dose (0.25 LD_{10}) of BCNU achieves a 0.85 $\log_{10}$ cell kill (86 per cent of clonogenic cells), but the 9L rat brain tumor is repopulated to its original size in three days with a doubling time of 15 hours for surviving clonogenic cells and no significant increase in life span over untreated controls. In contrast, a large dose (1.0 LD_{10}) achieves a 3.441 $\log_{10}$ cell kill (99.96 per cent of the clonogenic cell population), and repopulation requires 23 days at a tumor cell doubling time of 38 hours for a 97 per cent increase in life span.

2. When a 0.5 LD_{10} dose is administered on four successive days, the first dose achieves a 1.65 $\log_{10}$ cell kill, the second dose an additional log, and the third and successive doses have no additional cytotoxic effect. A single LD_{10} dose was more effective (determined by cell kill, post-treatment kinetics, and animal survival) than any tolerated divided (multiple) dose schedule.

Although the clinical effectiveness of three successive doses is unquestioned, the preceding experiments strongly suggest that a single equitoxic dose (180 to 200 mg per square meter) may give superior results.[60a]

Schedule Dependency of BCNU in Drug Combinations

In an effort to duplicate the superiority of drug combinations in the treatment of other solid tumors, clinical pilot studies combining BCNU with 5-FU and BCNU with procarbazine were conducted. Because the results were disappointingly inferior to the success of BCNU alone, an explanation was sought in the laboratory, with the following findings:

1. A two-day course of 5-FU (45 to 100 mg per kilogram total dose) achieved a 0.58 $\log_{10}$ (74 per cent) cell kill, but this was not reflected in a significant increase in animal life span. Although a single LD_{10} dose of BCNU doubled life span, it produced no long-term survivors and no cures.

2. When 5-FU was administered 3 to 15 days after a single LD_{10} dose of BCNU, long-term survivors and occasional cures (survival > 360 days) were observed in animals receiving 5-FU at various times between 3 and 12 days following BCNU.[60]

3. A matrix design with the day of BCNU administration remaining constant was used, and procarbazine was administered at various times at two dose levels. The combination was markedly more effective in terms of long-term survivors than either drug alone, but only when the dose of BCNU was relatively large (30 mg per kilogram), the dose of procarbazine was relatively small (10 or 20 mg per kilogram times five days), and the procarbazine was administered four to eight days following BCNU. In the model, simultaneous administration of both agents was highly toxic, duplicating clinical experience. Similar results were found with a CCNU-procarbazine combination.

In the light of these experimental results, revised protocols have been introduced in the hope that principles developed in the laboratory can be applied successfully to patients.

BCNU and Irradiation

Two phase III trials have indicated that combined treatment with BCNU and irradiation is superior to either irradiation or BCNU alone when treatment is started soon after operative verification of a malignant glioma. BCNU in a three-day course was administered immediately before and after completion of irradiation, and at six to eight week intervals thereafter.

Two experiments indicate a striking schedule dependency of BCNU as an adjuvant to irradiation.

1. Because 9L rat brain tumor cells do not repair BCNU-induced sublethal and potentially lethal damage, Wheeler and co-workers tested small doses of BCNU for possible interaction

with radiation.[141,142] When small doses of BCNU were administered to cultured cells at various times before, during, and after irradiation, a reduction in the shoulder region of the dose-response curve was observed only for treatments given 6 and 16 hours before irradiation. The therapeutic gain obtained at these times ranged from 1.2 to 1.6, depending on the amount of BCNU administered. Comparable doses of BCNU could be given to patients on alternate days and perhaps even every day during a course of radiotherapy with added cell kill and no significant toxic effects.

2. In preliminary experiments conducted in collaboration with Dr. Don Baker, 1.995 rads delivered to the whole head of 9L tumor-bearing rats produced an 11 per cent increase in life span, whereas BCNU alone produced an 84 per cent increase. BCNU administered six hours following irradiation, during irradiation, or six hours before irradiation produced respective increases in life span of 29 per cent, 66 per cent, and 154 per cent, indicating a marked schedule dependency consistent with that observed for cultured cells.[2a]

BCNU and Operation

There is an even more striking schedule dependency when BCNU is administered before, during, and after subtotal operative removal of tumor in the rat glioma model, life span being increased 55 per cent, 112 per cent, and 200 per cent over that with operation alone, BCNU alone, and BCNU given one hour before or one to two hours after operation, respectively.

CCNU

Two phase II trials have demonstrated the effectiveness of CCNU, a nitrosourea that, like MeCCNU, has the advantage of being administered orally in a single dose of 120 to 130 mg per square meter at intervals of six to eight weeks.[27,105] In the authors' accumulated experience with CCNU as a single agent, the overall response rate was 44 per cent (16 of 36 patients) for a median duration of six months.[151] Patients unresponsive to BCNU did not respond to CCNU. Although inferior to BCNU in both frequency and median duration of response, CCNU was selected as the nitrosourea in a combination chemotherapy protocol to be described later, primarily because of its ease of administration.

Two reported phase III trials of CCNU as postoperative therapy in patients bearing malignant gliomas have shown it to have little or no advantage with or without concurrent radiotherapy. In the three-arm study by Weir and co-workers, patients receiving CCNU and radiotherapy concurrently had a longer period to recurrence than patients receiving either CCNU or radiotherapy alone; but when radiotherapy or CCNU, respectively, was added to the latter groups at the time of recurrence, median survival was the same in all three groups.[138] Hildebrand, reporting for the European Brain Tumor Group, studied a group of 81 patients harboring malignant gliomas who were nearly neurologically normal and not steroid-dependent after craniotomy, clearly a group with a favorable prognosis.[41] Radiotherapy was not a part of this study. The free interval (time from diagnosis to progression) was not increased by CCNU, but responses were observed in 4 of 16 patients in the operation-only group when CCNU was administered at the time of progression. A comparable study with BCNU has not been reported, but the European experience raises the possibility that survival might be similar whether BCNU is administered from the time of diagnosis or started at the time of recurrence. A projection of the authors' phase II experience with BCNU in comparison with the Brain Tumor Study Group's phase III studies suggests that this may be true despite the well-known advantage of instituting treatment when the tumor burden is low. Perhaps BCNU is more effective against larger tumors with a smaller growth fraction, a possibility suggested by experience with the intracerebral glioma 26 and 9L rat models.

Procarbazine

Procarbazine (PCB), a methyl hydrazine analog, is rapidly oxidized to a lipophilic azo derivative and enters brain.[50,89] Like the nitrosoureas it probably functions as a cell cycle–nonspecific agent. Procarbazine has the advantage of oral administration. Most patients experience nausea and vomiting during the first few days of each course, but rarely does this require stopping chemotherapy. Like the nitrosoureas procarbazine depresses the bone marrow, leukopenia being more pronounced than thrombocytopenia. The nadir for white blood cells usually occurs in the latter part of the 30-day period of administration, but low counts may persist for four to six weeks after the drug is stopped. Because it is a monoamine oxidase inhibitor, procarbazine may produce a psychotic reaction, and in one of three patients with this complication treatment was discontinued. Among 43 patients receiving the drug, 4 developed a skin rash, but treatment was continued without secondary complications. Other investigators have encountered severe skin reactions requiring that drug treatment be discontinued.[120]

In the one phase II trial reported, the response rate was 52 per cent (14 of 27 patients) for a median duration of six months. In this study procarbazine was administered at a single dose of 150 mg per square meter per day for 30 days. The dose was escalated in 50-mg increments at the beginning of each course to minimize nausea and vomiting. The course was repeated (with appropriate dose modification) after a rest period of 30 days.[56,151]

Procarbazine is an active drug with potential for combination chemotherapy because it has no recognized cross-resistance with the nitrosoureas. The Brain Tumor Study Group phase III study of procarbazine indicated activity comparable to that of BCNU.[131]

Vinca Alkaloids (Vincristine and Vinblastine Sulfate)

Vincristine (VCR), a drug used widely in the treatment of tumors outside the central nervous system, has shown limited activity against astrocytomas and medulloblastomas.[9,59,126,144] Rosenstock, Evans, and Schut recently reported responses in 8 of 16 children harboring recurrent low- and high-grade astrocytomas and medulloblastomas.[107] They encountered minimal toxic effects on a schedule of 1.5 mg per square meter weekly for 12 weeks with treatment on alternate weeks thereafter. Vincristine is cell cycle–specific, causing metaphase arrest. Although it does not cross the blood-brain barrier, it exhibits peripheral neurotoxicity that is monitored easily and has little or no effect on the bone marrow. As a

cell cycle–specific agent that spares the bone marrow, vincristine offers some attraction as one component of multiple-drug protocols. In the authors' experience it did not enhance the effectiveness of BCNU, but it is one of three drugs in an effective combination (procarbazine, CCNU, and vincristine) to be described later.[28]

Vinblastine sulfate, also acting as a cell cycle–specific agent, has not been investigated in depth, in part because of its toxicity. Reports have suggested slight activity when it is administered by arterial infusion.[143] The paucity of evidence supports further clinical investigation of this agent.

Other Agents

Methotrexate

A lipid-insoluble and highly ionized molecule, methotrexate (MTX) does not cross normal brain capillaries, and with unimportant exceptions it has been administered by intrathecal (intraventricular) injection and infusion.[147] Its safety and effectiveness in the treatment of meningeal leukemia have led to clinical trials in solid tumors and meningeal carcinomatosis.* Behaving as a cell cycle–specific agent, methotrexate expresses its primary toxicity by bone marrow depression. Serious central neurotoxicity has been associated with elevated levels of the drug in cerebrospinal fluid.

Clinicians will continue to use intrathecal methotrexate. Its greatest value appears to be in the treatment of meningeal carcinomatosis.[123,155] One of the authors (C.W.) has suggested intrathecal methotrexate as a substitute for spinal axis irradiation in the initial treatment of medulloblastoma with the purpose of sparing the spinal bone marrow. The treatment of recurrent medulloblastomas is severely compromised because of radiation-induced spinal bone marrow depletion, and if adjuvant chemotherapy is to be administered in customary doses, some means must be devised for circumventing conventional spinal irradiation.

5-Fluorouracil

A cell cycle–specific agent, 5-fluorouracil (5-FU) has favorable pharmacokinetic

---

* See references 7, 85, 123, 147, 155.

characteristics, and although it has not emerged from a phase II trial as an active drug in man, in the 9L rat model, when administered 3 to 15 days after a single dose of BCNU, 5-FU achieved long-term survival and an occasional cure. This finding supports the kinetic strategy of using a cell cycle–specific agent in a rapidly proliferating tumor with a large growth fraction, following an effective tumor reduction (e.g., the 99.9 per cent cell kill produced by this dose of BCNU.[106] In a current phase II study the authors are evaluating 5-FU in a continuous 72-hour infusion (equal to the cell cycle time of malignant gliomas) at a dose of 1000 mg per square meter per day administered two weeks after a single dose (180 to 200 mg per square meter) of BCNU.[46] 5-FU has been well tolerated and adds little to the bone marrow depression of BCNU. It is hoped that laboratory experience can be duplicated clinically by extending the duration of response, although it is doubtful that 5-FU will improve the frequency of response attained with BCNU alone.

Hydroxyurea

Another cell cycle–specific agent, hydroxyurea (HU), has been used in conjunction with adjuvant irradiation in the treatment of malignant gliomas, and that experience has been summarized by Irwin, reporting for the Western Cooperative Oncology Group.[49] The results of this study suggest some activity, and because of the advantages of oral administration and little toxicity, hydroxyurea has potential as a cell cycle–specific component of drug combinations.

Dianhydrogalactitol

Dianhydrogalactitol (DAG) is a remarkably effective drug against the murine ependymoblastoma.[33,67] Levin has investigated its pharmacokinetic behavior in tumor-bearing animals, and the agent is entering phase II trials. Although it has not shown activity in malignant astrocytomas, one striking response was observed in a patient with recurrent medulloblastoma, suggesting that the drug deserves further consideration.

Epipodophylotoxin

This agent has shown limited activity in one phase II trial, and despite a difficult dose schedule, it may prove to be a useful drug under special circumstances.[125]

Mithramycin

Mithramycin exhibited activity in preliminary phase II trials, but in the only phase III study it was ineffective.[134]

COMBINATION CHEMOTHERAPY

The present thrust in the treatment of cancer is the concurrent (or sequential) use of multiple therapeutic modes, i.e., operation, radiotherapy, chemotherapy, and immunotherapy. For some time it has been evident that few advanced cancers will be cured by single chemotherapeutic agents, and the superiority of combination chemotherapy has been an established fact. A detailed consideration of the strategy behind combinations of two or more drugs is beyond the scope of this chapter, but a few examples will illustrate the reasoning behind this approach using: (1) drugs with different or complementary oncolytic modes of action, e.g., BCNU and procarbazine; (2) drugs with differing toxicity, e.g., BCNU and vincristine; or (3) drugs that exploit the kinetic susceptibility of a tumor cell population (cell cycle–nonspecific and cell cycle–specific activity), e.g., BCNU and 5-FU.

A relatively small number of drug combinations have been investigated. Two of these, procarbazine, CCNU, and vincristine (PCV) and BCNU–5 fluorouracil, have shown activity against recurrent malignant gliomas, achieving remissions in over 80 per cent of patients with median times to further tumor progression of 24 to 28 weeks.[38,62a,71a,71b] An unpublished trial of cyclophosphamide, CCNU, and vincristine indicated little activity of this combination, probably attributable to the failure of the active species of cyclophosphamide to reach the central nervous system. Two combinations are described, one to illustrate a principle, and the other to report a highly active combination that may be improved by modification of doses and dose schedule.

BCNU–Procarbazine

The logic of combining the two most effective single agents in a phase II trial was inescapable because these drugs have no pharmacological similarities. It was anticipated that cells resistant to one might be susceptible to the other. In the original protocol the two drugs were administered together in proportionately reduced doses. Among 65 patients treated, 45 harbored malignant gliomas. In the latter group the unequivocal response rate was 30 per cent for a median duration of 34 weeks, and the probable response rate was 17 per cent for a median duration of 20 weeks. Of interest, 16 patients who received no prior treatment fared as well as those patients who had undergone operation or radiotherapy or both prior to chemotherapy. These results were no better than those achieved by either agent used alone and were inferior to the response with PCV combined therapy.

When the disappointing results of this study were known, the combination was explored in the laboratory by using a matrix design. As described earlier, this study showed that the combination was decidedly more effective than either drug alone, but only when the dose of BCNU was relatively large, the dose of procarbazine was relatively small, and the procarbazine was administered four to eight days following BCNU. Further, separation of the drugs by an interval reduced toxicity and permitted the use of larger doses.[71] The BCNU-procarbazine combination has not been reintroduced as a revised phase II protocol, but this is a promising study that should be pursued.

PCV (Procarbazine, CCNU, and Vincristine)

These three drugs were selected for specific reasons. The theoretical basis for combining a nitrosourea and procarbazine was indicated earlier. Although CCNU has been somewhat less effective than BCNU, in a multiple-drug protocol the advantage of a single oral dose over three daily intravenous infusions was decisive. To these two cell cycle–nonspecific agents, vincristine was added as a cell cycle–specific drug of limited but unquestioned value with the objective of retarding repopulation of the tumor by cycling surviving cells. In the original 28-day schedule (PCV[1.]) CCNU was given on day 1, procarbazine on days 1 to 14, and vincristine on days 1 and 8. In the authors' initial phase II study the unequivocal response rate was 44 per cent, and with the addition of a probable response (stable disease) rate of 16 per cent the overall response rate was 60 per cent for a median duration of seven months. PCV[1.] was strikingly active against recurrent medulloblastomas, with seven unequivocal responses and four probable responses in a group of 12 evaluable patients. The impaired bone marrow reserve in these patients, all of whom had received spinal irradiation, compromised treatment, and in the majority of cases therapy had to be discontinued at a time when the tumor remained responsive to greatly reduced (25 per cent of calculated) doses.

The PCV[1.] protocol has been revised to incorporate the information obtained by Levin, as was described earlier. In the new protocol (PCV[3.]) the dose of CCNU is increased, an interval separates the administration of CCNU and procarbazine, and the cycle is six weeks rather than four weeks. The schedule for PCV[3.] is shown in Table 96–11. Limited experience with this new schedule indicates less toxicity, and this alone is an advantage. PCV[1.] is an effective and easily administered drug combination, and in the authors' experience it has been the treatment of choice for medulloblastomas. PCV[3] is comparable to BCNU–5-fluorouracil in activity and length of remission produced.[61a,70a]

Shapiro and Young modified the preceding schedules as follows: CCNU (50 mg per square meter) and vincristine (1 mg per square meter) on days 1 and 15, and procarbazine (75 mg per square meter) on days 1 to 28 followed by a period of 28 days without treatment. They treated recurrent malignant gliomas with results comparable to the authors', but of greater interest was a group of 17 patients in whom radiotherapy and PCV were adjunctive to operation. The projected survival of the latter patients exceeds 51 weeks: 9 patients were still living at 29 to 82 weeks at the time the report was made. Their experience reinforces the favorable impression of this drug combination.

TABLE 96-11   SCHEDULE FOR PCV (PROCARBAZINE, CCNU, VINCRISTINE) PHASE II STUDY

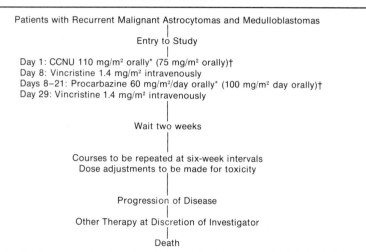

Patients with Recurrent Malignant Astrocytomas and Medulloblastomas

Entry to Study

Day 1: CCNU 110 mg/m² orally* (75 mg/m² orally)†
Day 8: Vincristine 1.4 mg/m² intravenously
Days 8–21: Procarbazine 60 mg/m²/day orally* (100 mg/m² day orally)†
Day 29: Vincristine 1.4 mg/m² intravenously

Wait two weeks

Courses to be repeated at six-week intervals
Dose adjustments to be made for toxicity

Progression of Disease

Other Therapy at Discretion of Investigator

Death

* Dose for malignant astrocytomas.
† Dose for medulloblastomas.

RADIOSENSITIZERS

Although not strictly within the scope of chemotherapy, radiosensitizers should be mentioned briefly. Sano and co-workers reported beneficial results from using bromuridine in conjunction with postoperative radiotherapy, but the difficulties encountered in maintaining a continuous carotid arterial infusion for many weeks excludes this form of therapy from widespread adoption.[115,116] Because of the interest in hydroxyurea generated by Irwin and collaborators, the authors are engaged in an ongoing phase III study (Western Cooperative Oncology Group) comparing radiotherapy plus BCNU with and without hydroxyurea administered during radiotherapy.[49] The hydroxyurea has been well tolerated. Too few patients have been accrued to permit a preliminary analysis of survival.

Urtasun and co-workers recently reported impressive results in a two-arm phase III study of glioblastomas, one group of patients receiving postoperative radiotherapy alone and the other group receiving high-dosage metronidazole (Flagyl) during the course of radiotherapy.[129] On the basis of this report Levin, Wara, Phillips, and Wilson have designed a phase III study in which (1) radiotherapy plus BCNU will be compared with (2) radiotherapy plus PCV. This study, conducted by the Northern California Oncology Group, is nearing completion. No report has been published.

STEROIDS (GLUCOCORTICOIDS)

Today a detailed account of the value of steroids in the management of patients with brain tumors seems unnecessary. This information is available in an excellent review by Gutin.[37] Certain principles and observations, however, are pertinent to the use of steroids in patients undergoing chemotherapy, and, briefly, these are:

1. The antiedema effect of steroids is dose-dependent, and high dosages (up to and occasionally above 100 mg of Decadron per day) will produce responses not observed at lower dosages.[100]

2. Large doses are well tolerated and associated with few serious complications.

3. In the patient harboring a tumor, maintenance of initial clinical improvement induced by steroids will require continuous administration.

4. In the patient receiving a steroid and an oncolytic drug concurrently, improvement in neurological function and brain scans (radionuclide and CT) can be considered evidence of drug responsiveness only when improvement occurs while the patient is receiving the same dose of steroid.

5. To minimize steroid side effects in a steroid-dependent patient, periodic attempts should be made to reduce the maintenance dose in small increments. This is true particularly in the early postoperative period, following completion of radiotherapy, and during the course of successful chemotherapy.

6. Steroids have shown direct oncolytic activity in an animal model, and anecdotal evidence suggests that they may have a similar effect in man.[36] A current Brain Tumor Study Group protocol failed to show antineoplastic activity of methyl prednisolone.

SELECTION OF DRUGS FOR SPECIFIC PROBLEMS

Recommendations for the choice of drugs in specific situations are indicated in Table 96–12. Only those tumors for which an effective drug or drug combination has been identified have been selected. Certain tumors are conspicuously absent either because therapy has been ineffective or because experience with a particular tumor is limited.

IMMUNOTHERAPY

No clinical study has shown the value of immunotherapy for brain tumors. With the present state of knowledge, it is predictable

TABLE 96–12   RECOMMENDED CHEMOTHERAPY FOR SPECIFIC TUMORS

TUMOR	DRUG(S)
Malignant glioma	
Recurrent after radiotherapy	BCNU; PCV; procarbazine, BCNU-5FU
Untreated (except by surgery)	Radiotherapy plus BCNU
Ependymoma, recurrent	BCNU
Medulloblastoma, recurrent*	PCV; procarbazine
Metastatic melanoma	PCV
Meningeal carcinomatosis	Intrathecal methotrexate; PCV
Metastatic hypernephroma	Radiotherapy plus dianhydrogalactitol

* The Children's Cancer Study Group and the Radiation Therapy Oncology Group are currently evaluating the efficacy of CCNU, procarbazine, and vincristine as adjuvant therapy.

that further definition of the complex immune mechanisms related to central nervous system tumors will precede informative trials of clinical immunotherapy. This therapeutic modality has exciting potential because it is highly specific and nontoxic. Undoubtedly, progress in the field will go forward more rapidly as immunotherapy is applied successfully to nonneural tumors.

Acknowledgment: This work was supported in part by NIH Cancer Center Grant CA 13525 and NIH Grants CA 15435, CA 15515, CA 15203, and CA 19992. V.L. is the recipient of ACS Faculty Research Award 155.

REFERENCES

1. Ariel, I. M.: Intra-arterial chemotherapy for metastatic cancer to the brain. Amer. J. Surg. *102*:647, 1961.
2. Ausman, J. I., and Levin, V. A.: Intra- and extravascular distribution of standard drug molecules in brain tumor and brain. *In* Drake, C. G., and Duviosin, R. eds.: Fourth International Congress of Neurological Surgery, 1969. International Congress Series No. 193. New York, Excerpta Medica Foundation, 1970, p. 41.
2a. Baker, D.: Unpublished results.
3. Barker, M., Hoshino, T., Gurcay, O., et al.: Development of an animal brain tumor model and its response to therapy with 1,3-bis (2-chloroethyl)-1-nitrosourea. Cancer Res., *33*:976–986, 1973.
4. Baum, E. S., Koch, H. F., Corby, D. G., and Plunket, D. C.: Intrathecal methotrexate. Lancet, *1*:649, 1971.
5. Benson, J. W., Kiehn, C. L., and Holden, W. D.: Cancer chemotherapy by arterial infusion. Arch. Surg., *87*:125, 1963.
6. Bering, E. A., Jr., Wilson, C. B., and Norrell, H. A., Jr.: The Kentucky conference on brain tumor chemotherapy. J. Neurosurg., *27*:1, 1967.
7. Bleyer, W. A.: Current status of intrathecal chemotherapy for human meningeal neoplasms. *In* Modern Concepts in Brain Tumor Therapy. Proceedings of National Cancer Institute Symposium, Atlanta, Ga. February 26–28, 1976. Washington, D.C., Department of Health, Education, and Welfare, 1977.
8. Boldrey, E. B., and Sheline, G.: Delayed transitory clinical manifestations after radiation treatment of intracranial tumors. Acta Radiol. (Ther.), *5*:5–10, 1965.
9. Braham, J., Sarova-Pinhas, I., and Goldhammer, Y.: Glioma of the brain treated by intravenous vincristine sulphate. Neurochirurgia (Stuttgart), *12*:195–200, 1969.
10. Broder, L. E., and Rall, D. P.: Chemotherapy of brain tumors. *In* Bingham, W. G., Jr., ed.: Recent Advances in Brain Tumor Research.

Progress in Experimental Tumor Research. Vol 17. Basel, Karger, 1972, pp. 373–399.

11. Brodie, B. B., Kurz, H., and Schanker, L. S.: The importance of dissociation constant and lipid-solubility in influencing the passage of drugs into the cerebrospinal fluid. J. Pharmacol. Exp. Ther., *130*:20, 1960.

12. Bunge, R. P., and Settlage, P. H.: Neurological lesions in cats following cerebrospinal fluid manipulation. J. Neuropath. Exp. Neurol., *61*:471, 1957.

13. Chirigos, M. A., Humphreys, S. R., and Goldin, A.: Effectiveness of cytoxan against intracerebrally and subcutaneously inoculated mouse lymphoid leukemia L1210. Cancer Res., *22*:187–195, 1962.

14. Clark, E. E., and Hattner, R. S.: Brain scintigraphy in recurrent medulloblastoma. Radiology, *119*:633–636, 1976.

15. Crafts, D. C., and Wilson, C. B.: Animal models of brain tumors. *In* Brain Tumor Therapy. National Cancer Institute monograph 46. 1977, pp. 11–17.

16. Crafts, D. C., Levin, V. A., and Nielsen, S. L.: Intracarotid BCNU: A toxicity study in monkeys. Cancer Treat. Rep., *60*:541–547, 1976.

17. Crafts, D. C., Levin, V. A., Edwards, M. S., et al.: Chemotherapy of recurrent medulloblastoma with combined procarbazine, CCNU and vincristine. J. Neurosurg., *49*:589–592, 1978.

18. Davis, P. L., and Shumway, M. H.: Thio-TEPA in treatment of metastatic cerebral malignancy. J.A.M.A., *175*:714, 1961.

19. Dean, M. R. E., Newton, K. A., and Swann, G. F.: Percutaneous intra-arterial chemotherapy in the treatment of intracranial neoplasms: A review of 36 cases. Brit. J. Radiol., *40*:828, 1967.

20. DeWys, W. D., and Fowler, E. H.: Report of vasculitis and blindness after intracarotid injection of 1,3-bis (2-chloroethyl)-1-nitrosourea (BCNU; NSC-409962) in dogs. Cancer Chemother. Rep., *57*:33, 1973.

21. Engeset, A., Brennhovd, I., and Stovner, J.: Intra-arterial infusions in cancer chemotherapy. A technique for testing drug distribution. Lancet, *1*:1382, 1962.

22. Espiner, H. J., Vowles, K. D. J., and Walker, R. M.: Cancer chemotherapy by intra-arterial infusion. A preliminary report concerning tumors of the head and neck. Lancet, *1*:177, 1962.

23. Feind, C. R., Herter, F., and Markowitz, A.: Improvements in isolation head perfusion. Amer. J. Surg., *106*:777, 1963.

24. Fenstermacher, J. D., and Johnson, J. A.: Filtration and reflection coefficients of the rabbit blood-brain barrier. J. Physiol. (London), *211*:341–346, 1970.

25. Fenstermacher, J. D., Rall, D. P., Patlak, C. S., et al.: Ventriculocisternal perfusion as a technique for analysis of brain capillary permeability and extra cellular transport in capillary permeabilty. *In* Proceedings of the Alfred Benzon Symposium 11. Copenhagen, Munksgaard, 1969, pp. 483–490.

26. Fewer, D.: Specific agents in brain tumor chemotherapy. *In* Fewer, D., Wilson, C. B., and Levin, V. A., eds.: Brain Tumor Chemotherapy, Springfield, Ill., Charles C Thomas, 1976.

27. Fewer, D., Wilson, C. B., Boldrey, E. B., et al.: Phase II study of 1-(2-chloroethyl)-3-cyclohexyl-1-nitrosourea (CCNU; NSC-79037) in the treatment of brain tumors. Cancer Chemother. Rep., *56*:421–427, 1972.

28. Fewer, D., Wilson, C. B., Boldrey, E. B., et al.: The chemotherapy of brain tumors: Clinical experience with carmustine (BCNU) and vincristine. J.A.M.A., *222*:549–552, 1972.

29. Freeman, J. E., Johnston, P. G. B., and Voke, J. M.: Somnolence after prophylactic cranial irradiation in children with acute lymphoblastic leukemia. Brit. Med. J., *4*:523–525, 1973.

30. French, J. D., West, P. M., Von Amerongen, F. K., and Magoun, H. W.: Effects of intracarotid administration of nitrogen mustard on normal brain and brain tumors. J. Neurosurg., *9*:378, 1952.

31. Garfield, J., and Dayan, A. D.: Postoperative intracavitary chemotherapy of malignant gliomas. J. Neurosurg., *39*:315, 1973.

32. Gehan, E. A., and Walker, M. D.: Prognostic factors for patients with brain tumors. *In* Modern Concepts in Brain Tumor Therapy. Proceedings of National Cancer Institute Symposium, Atlanta, Ga., February 26–28, 1976. Washington, D. C., Department of Health, Education and Welfare, 1977.

33. Geran, R. I., Congleton, G. F., Dudeck, L. E., et al.: A mouse ependymoblastoma as an experimental model for screening potential antineoplastic drugs. Cancer Chemother. Rep., *4*:53–87, 1974.

34. Gray, J. W.: Cell cycle analysis from computer synthesis of deoxyribonucleic acid histograms. J. Histochem. Cytochem., *22*:642–650, 1974.

35. Greenhouse, A. H., Neuberger, K. T., and Bowerman, D. L.: Brain damage after intracarotid infusion of methotrexate. Arch. Neurol. (Chicago), *11*:618, 1964.

36. Gurcay, O., Wilson, C., Barker, M., et al.: Corticosteroid effect on transplantable rat glioma. Arch. Neurol., *24*:266–269, 1971

37. Gutin, P. H.: Corticosteroid therapy in patients with brain tumors. *In* Modern Concepts in Brain Tumor Therapy. Proceedings of National Cancer Institute Symposium, Atlanta, Ga., February 26–28, 1976. Washington, D. C., Department of Health, Education, and Welfare, 1977.

38. Gutin, P. H., Wilson, C. B., Kumar, A. R. V., et al.: Phase II study of procarbazine, CCNU and vincristine combination chemotherapy in the treatment of malignant brain tumors. Cancer, *35*:1398–1404, 1975.

39. Handel, S. F., Powell, M. R., Wilson, C. B., et al.: Scintiphotographic evaluation of response of brain neoplasms to systemic chemotherapy. J. Nucl. Med., *12*:292–296, 1971.

40. Heby, O., Marton, L. J., Wilson, C. B., et al.: Polyamine metabolism in a rat brain tumor cell line: Its relationship to the growth rate. J. Cell Physiol., *83*:511–521, 1975.

41. Hildebrand, J.: Discussion. *In* Modern Concepts in Brain Tumor Therapy. Proceedings of National Cancer Institute Symposium, Atlanta, Ga. February 26–28, 1976. Washington, D.C.,

Department of Health, Education, and Welfare, 1977.

42. Hirano, A., Becher, N., and Zimmerman, H.: Pathological alterations in the cerebral endothelial cell barrier to peroxidase. Arch. Neurol., *20*:300, 1969.

43. Hochward, G. M., Wald, A., and Malhan, C.: The sink action of cerebrospinal fluid volume flow. Arch. Neurol., *3*:339–344, 1976.

44. Hockey, A. A., and Mealey, J., Jr.: Effects of intracisternal vinblastine in dogs. Surg. Forum, *16*:427, 1965.

45. Hommes, O. R., and Leblond, C. P.: Mitotic division of neuroglia in the normal adult rat. J. Comp. Neurol., *129*:269–278, 1967.

46. Hoshino, T.: Therapeutic implications of brain tumor cell kinetics. *In* Modern Concepts in Brain Tumor Therapy. Proceedings of National Cancer Institute Symposium, Atlanta, Ga., February 26–28, 1976. Washington, D.C., Department of Health, Education, and Welfare, 1977.

47. Hoshino, T., Barker, M., Wilson, C. B., et al.: Cell kinetics of human gliomas. J. Neurosurg., *37*:15–26, 1972.

48. Hoshino, T., Wilson, C. B., Rosenblum, M. L., et al.: Chemotherapeutic implication of growth fraction and cell cycle time in glioblastoma. J. Neurosurg., *43*:127–135, 1975.

49. Irwin, L.: Discussion. *In* Modern Concepts in Brain Tumor Therapy. Proceedings of National Cancer Institute Symposium, Atlanta, Ga., February 26–28, 1976. Washington, D.C., Department of Health, Education, and Welfare, 1977.

50. Kabra, P. M., Levin, V. A., and Weinkam, R.: Effectiveness of nitrosoureas as a function of their lipid solubility in the chemotherapy of experimental rat brain tumors. Cancer Chemother. Rep., *58*:787–792, 1974.

51. Koo, A. H., Fewer, D., Wilson, C. B., et al.: Lack of correlation between clinical and angiographic findings in patients with brain tumors under BCNU chemotherapy. J. Neurosurg., *37*:9–14, 1972.

52. Korr, H., Schultze, B., and Mauer, W.: Autoradiographic investigations of glial proliferation in brain of adult mice. J. Comp. Neurol., *160*:477–490, 1975.

53. Kramer, S.: Hazards of therapeutic irradiation of central nervous system. Clin. Neurosurg. *15*:301–318, 1968.

54. Kricheff, I. I., Lin, J. P., and Phy, N.: Some aspects of computed tomography of the head. *In* Modern Concepts in Brain Tumor Therapy. Proceedings of National Cancer Institute Symposium, Atlanta, Ga., February 26–28, 1976.

55. Kumar, A. R. V., Hoshino, T., Wheeler, K. T., et al.: Comparative rates of dead tumor cell removal from brain, muscle, subcutaneous tissue and peritoneal cavity. J. Nat. Cancer Inst., *52*:1751–1755, 1974.

56. Kumar, A. R. V., Renaudin, J., Wilson, C. B., et al.: Procarbazine hydrochloride in the treatment of brain tumors: Phase 2 study. J. Neurosurg., *40*:365–371, 1974.

57. Lampert, P., Tom, M. I., and Rider, W. D.: Disseminated demyelination of the brain following

60Co (gamma) radiation. Arch. Path. (Chicago), *68*:322–330, 1959.

58. Lampksin, B. C., Higgins, G. R., and Hammond, D.: Absence of neurotoxicity following massive intrathecal administration of methotrexate. Cancer, *20*:1780, 1967.

59. Lassman, L. P., Pearce, G. W., and Gang, J.: Sensitivity of intracranial gliomas to vincristine sulfate. Lancet, *1*:296–297, 1965.

60. Levin, V. A.: Pharmacological principles of brain tumor chemotherapy. Adv. Neurol. *15*:315–325, 1976.

60a. Levin, V. A.: Unpublished results.

61. Levin, V. A., and Chadwick, M.: Distribution of 5-fluorouracil-2-14C and its metabolites in a murine glioma. J. Natl. Cancer Inst., *49*:1577, 1972.

62. Levin, V. A., and Kabra, P. M.: Effectiveness of nitrosoureas as a function of their lipid solubility in the chemotherapy of experimental rat brain tumors. Cancer Chemother. Rep., *58*:787–792, 1974.

62a. Levin, V. A., and Wilson, C. B.: Chemotherapy: The agents in current use. Sem. Oncol., *2*:63–67, 1975.

63. Levin, V. A., and Wilson, C. B.: Pharmacological considerations in brain tumor chemotherapy. *In* Fewer, D., Wilson, C. B., and Levin, V. A., eds.: Brain Tumor Chemotherapy. Chapter 3. Springfield, Ill., Charles C Thomas, 1976.

64. Levin, V. A., and Wilson, C. B.: Nitrosoureas: Clinical and experimental considerations in the treatment of brain tumors. *In* Hellman, K., and Connors, T. A., eds.: Chemotherapy. Vol. 7. New York, Plenum Press, 1977, pp. 277–283.

65. Levin, V. A., Fenstermacher, J. D., and Patlak, C.: Sucrose and insulin space measurements of cerebral cortex in four mammalian species. Amer. J. Physiol., *219*:1528, 1970.

66. Levin, V. A., Freeman-Dove, M., and Landahl, H. D.: Permeability characteristics of brain adjacent to tumors in rats. Arch. Neurol. (Chicago), *32*:785–791, 1975.

67. Levin, V. A., Freeman-Dove, M. A., and Marothen, C. E.: Dianhydrogalactitol (NSC-132313): pharmacokinetics in normal and tumor-bearing rat brain and antitumor activity against three intracerebral rodent tumors. J. Nat. Cancer Inst., *56*:535–539, 1976.

68. Levin, V. A., Kabra, P. M., and Freeman-Dove, M. A.: Pharmacokinetics of intracarotid artery 14C-BCNU in the squirrel monkey. J. Neurosurg., *48*:587–593, 1978.

69. Levin, V. A., Clancy, T. P., Ausman, J. I., et al.: Uptake and distribution of 3H-methotrexate by the murine ependymoblastoma. J. Nat. Cancer Inst., *48*:875, 1972.

70. Levin, V. A., Crafts, D. C., Horman, D. M., et al.: Criteria for evaluating patients undergoing chemotherapy for malignant brain tumors. J. Neurosurg., *47*:329–335, 1977.

71. Levin, V. A., Crafts, D. C., Wilson, C. B., et al.: BCNU (NSC–409962) and procarbazine (NSC–77213) treatment for malignant brain tumors. Cancer Treat. Rep., *60*:243–249, 1976.

71a. Levin V. A., Edwards, M. S., Wright, D. C., et al.: Modified Procarbazine, CCNU, and vincristine combination chemotherapy (UCSF

PCV #3) in the treatment of malignant brain tumors. Cancer Treat. Rep., *64*:237–241, 1980.

71b. Levin, V. A., Hoffman, W. F., Pischer, T. L., et al.: BCNU-5-fluorouracil combination in the treatment of recurrent malignant brain tumors. Cancer Treat. Rep., *62*:2071–2079, 1978.

72. Lewis, P. D.: The fate of the subependymal cell in the adult rat brain, with a note on the origin of microglia. Brain, *91*:721–736, 1968.

73. Lloyd, J. W., Hughes, J. T., and Davies-Jones, G. A. B.: Relief of severe intractable pain by barbotage of cerebrospinal fluid. Lancet, *1*:354, 1972.

74. Mahaley, M. S., Jr., and Woodhall, B.: An evaluation of plasma levels of alkylating agents during regional chemotherapeutic perfusions. J. Surg. Res., *1*:285, 1961.

75. Mahaley, M. S., Jr., and Woodhall, B.: Regional chemotherapeutic perfusion and infusion of brain and face tumors. Ann. Surg., *166*:266, 1967.

76. Mark, V. H., Kjellberg, R. N., Ojemann, R. G., and Soloway, A. H.: Treatment of malignant brain tumors with alkylating agents. Neurology (Minneap.), *10*:772, 1960.

77. Marton, L. J.: Polyamines and brain tumors, *In* Modern Concepts in Brain Tumor Therapy. Proceedings of National Cancer Institute Symposium, Atlanta, Ga., February 26–28, 1976. Washington, D.C., Department of Health, Education, and Welfare, 1977.

78. Marton, L. J., Heby, O., Levin, V. A., et al.: The relationship of polyamines in cerebrospinal fluid to the presence of central nervous system tumors. Cancer Res., *36*:973–977, 1976.

79. Matsutani, M., and Hoshino, T.: Analysis of tumor growth in recurrent malignant gliomas. Brain Nerve (Tokyo), *27*:277–281, 1975.

80. Mealey, J., Jr.: Treatment of malignant cerebral astrocytomas by intra-arterial infusion of vinblastine. Cancer Chemother. Rep. *20*:121, 1962.

81. Moss, G.: Total perfusion of brain with cancer chemotherapeutic agents. Neurology (Minneap.), *15*:531, 1965.

82. Nelsen, T. S., Eigenbrodt, E. H., and Bagshaw, M. A.: Low-flow fail-safe intra-arterial infusion. Arch. Surg. (Chicago), *87*:640, 1963.

83. Nelson, J. S. R., and Schiffer, L. M.: Autoradiographic detection of DNA polymerase containing nuclei in sarcoma 180 ascites cells. Cell Tissue Kinet., *6*:45–54, 1973.

84. Newton, K. A.: The distribution of dyes and fluorescent substances by the blood stream within tumors. Brit. J. Radiol., *38*:224, 1965.

85. Newton, W. A., Jr., Sayers, M. P., and Samuels, L. D.: Intrathecal methotrexate (NSC–740) therapy for brain tumors in children. Cancer Chemother. Rep., *52*:257–261, 1968.

86. Nordman, E., and Rekonen, A.: Interpretation of 99mTc-pertechnetate scintigraphy after irradiation of brain tumours. Int. J. Nucl. Med. Biol., *2*:25–29, 1975.

87. Norrell, H., and Wilson, C. B.: Brain tumor chemotherapy with methotrexate given intrathecally. J.A.M.A., *201*:15, 1967.

88. Okeda, R., and Shibata, T.: Radiation encephalopathy—an autopsy case and some comments on the pathogenesis of delayed radionecrosis of central nervous system. Acta Path. Jap., *23*:867–883, 1973.

89. Oliverio, V. T.: Pharmacologic disposition of procarbazine. *In* Proceedings of the Chemotherapy Conference on Procarbazine, March 13, 1970. Washington, D. C., Department of Health, Education, and Welfare, 1971.

90. Ommaya, A. K.: Subcutaneous reservoir and pump for sterile access to ventricular cerebrospinal fluid. Lancet, *2*:983, 1963.

91. Ommaya, A. K., Rubin, R. C., Henderson, E. S., et al.: A new approach to the treatment of inoperable brain tumors. Med. Ann. D.C., *34*:455, 1965.

92. Owens, G., Javid, R., and Belmusto, L.: Chemotherapy of glioblastoma multiforme. *In* deVet, A. V., ed.: Proceedings of the Third International Congress of Neurological Surgery, 1965. International Congress Series, No. 110. New York, Excerpta Medica Foundation, 1966, pp. 752–755.

93. Owens, G., Javid, R., Belmusto, L., et al.: Intra-arterial vincristine therapy of primary gliomas. Cancer, *18*:756, 1965.

94. Owens, G., Javid, R., Tallon, M., et al.: Arterial infusion chemotherapy of primary gliomas. A report of thirty cases. J.A.M.A., *186*:802, 1963.

95. Perese, D. M., Day, C. E., and Chardack, W. M.: Chemotherapy of brain tumors by intra-arterial infusion. J. Neurosurg., *19*:215, 1962.

96. Pizzo, P. A., Bleyer, W. A., Poplack, D. G., et al.: Reversible dementia temporally associated with intraventricular therapy with methotrexate in a child with acute myelogenous leukemia. J. Pediat., *88*:131–133, 1976.

97. Pool, J. L.: Management of recurrent gliomas. Clin. Neurosurg., *15*:265–287, 1968.

98. Rall, D. P., and Zubrod, C. G.: Mechanisms of drug absorption and excretion: Passage of drugs in and out of the central nervous system. Ann. Rev. Pharmacol., *2*:109, 1962.

99. Ransohoff, J., and Weiss, J.: Cerebrospinal fluid sterols in the evaluation of patients with gliomas. *In* Modern Concepts in Brain Tumor Therapy. Proceedings of National Cancer Institute Symposium, Atlanta, Ga., February 26–28, 1976. Washington, D.C., Department of Health, Education, and Welfare, 1977.

100. Renaudin, J., Fewer, D., Wilson, C. B., et al.: Dose dependency of Decadron in patients with partially excised brain tumors. J. Neurosurg., *39*:302–305, 1973.

101. Rider, W. D.: Radiation damage to the brain—a new syndrome. J. Canad. Ass. Radiol., *14*:67–69, 1963.

102. Ringkjob, R.: Treatment of intracranial gliomas and metastatic carcinomas by local application of cytostatic agents. Acta Neurol. Scand., *44*:318, 1968.

103. Rosenblum, M. L., Knebel, K. D., Vasquez, D. A., et al.: In vivo clonogenic tumor cell kinetics following 1,3-bis(2-chloroethyl)-1-nitrosourea brain tumor therapy. Cancer Res., *36*:3718–3725, 1976.

104. Rosenblum, M. L., Knebel, K. D., Wheeler, K. T., et al.: Development of an in vitro colony formation assay for the evaluation of in vivo

chemotherapy of a rat brain tumor. In Vitro, 11:264–273, 1975.

105. Rosenblum, M., Reynolds, A. F., Smith, K. A., et al.: Chloroethylcyclohexyl nitrosourea (CCNU) in the treatment of malignant brain tumors. J. Neurosurg., 39:306–314, 1973.

106. Rosenblum, M., Wheeler, K. T., Wilson, C. B., et al.: In vitro evaluation of in vivo brain tumor chemotherapy with 1,3-bis(2-chloroethyl)-1-nitrosourea. Cancer Res., 35:1387–1391, 1975.

107. Rosenstock, J. G., Evans, A. E., and Schut, L.: Response to vincristine of recurrent brain tumors in children. J. Neurosurg., 45:135–141, 1976.

108. Rubin, R. C., Larson, R., and Rall, D. P.: 8-Azaguanine (NSC-749). I. Preclinical toxicity studies and a preliminary report on intrathecal perfusion therapy for patients. Cancer Chemother. Rep., 50:283, 1966.

109. Rubin, R., Owens, E., and Rall, D.: Transport of methotrexate by the choroid plexus. Cancer Res., 28:689, 1968.

110. Rubin, R. C., Ommaya, A. K., Henderson, E. S., et al.: Cerebrospinal fluid perfusion for central nervous system neoplasms. Neurology (Minneap.), 16:680, 1966.

111. Rubinstein, L. J.: Tumors of the Central Nervous System. Washington, D.C., Armed Forces Institute of Pathology, 1972, p. 351.

112. Rubinstein, L. J.: Correlation of animal brain tumor models with human neuro-oncology. In Modern Concepts in Brain Tumor Therapy. Proceedings of National Cancer Institute Symposium, Atlanta, Ga., February 26–28, 1976. Washington, D.C., Department of Health, Education, and Welfare, 1977.

113. Rush, B. F., Jr., Horie, N., and Klein, N. W.: Intra-arterial infusion of the head and neck. Anatomic and distributional problems. Amer. J. Surg., 110:510, 1965.

114. Saiki, J. H., Thompson, S., Smith, F., and Atkinson, R.: Paraplegia following intrathecal chemotherapy. Cancer, 29:370, 1972.

115. Sano, K., Hoshino, T., and Nagai, M.: Radiosensitization of brain tumor cells with a thymidine analogue (bromouridine). J. Neurosurg., 28:530–538, 1968.

116. Sano, K., Hoshino, T., Nagai, M., et al.: Studies on a radiosensitizer (5-bromo-2'-deoxyuridine) in the treatment of malignant brain tumors. Neurol. Medicochir. (Tokyo), 8:227, 1966.

117. Schiffer, L. M.: Personal communication. 1976.

118. Schiffer, L. M., Markoe, A. M., and Nelson, J. S. R.: Evaluation of the PDP index as a monitor of growth fraction during chemotherapy. In ERDA Series NTIC: The Cell Cycle in Malignancy and Immunity. Springfield, Va., 1975, pp. 459–472.

119. Shapiro, W. R., and Ausman, J. I.: The chemotherapy of brain tumors: A clinical and experimental review. In Plum, F., ed.: Recent Advances in Neurology. Philadelphia, F. A. Davis, 1969 pp. 150–235.

120. Shapiro, W. R., and Young, D. F.: Chemotherapy of malignant glioma with lomustine alone and lomustine combined with vincristine sulfate and procarbazine hydrochloride. Arch. Neurol. (Chicago), 33:394, 1976.

121. Shapiro, W. R., and Young, D. F.: Treatment of malignant glioma. Arch. Neurol., (Chicago), 33:494–500, 1976.

122. Shapiro, W. R., Chernik, N. L., and Posner, J. B.: Necrotizing encephalopathy following intraventricular instillation of methotrexate. Arch. Neurol. (Chicago), 28:96, 1973.

123. Shapiro, W. R., Young, D. F., and Posner, J. B.: Treatment of leptomeningeal neoplasm with intraventricular methotrexate (MTX) and arabinosylcytosine (ara-C). In Proceedings of American Association for Cancer Research. A.A.C.R. Abstracts 759, 1975.

124. Shuttleworth, E. C., Jr.: Barrier phenomena in brain tumors. In Bingham, W. G., Jr., ed.: Recent Advances in Brain Tumor Research. Progress in Experimental Tumor Research, Vol. 17. Basel, S. Karger, 1972, pp. 279–290.

125. Skylansky, B. D. Mann-Kaplan, R. S., Reynolds, A. F., Jr., et al.: 4-Demethyl-epipodophyllotoxin-D-thenylidene-glucoside (PTG) in the treatment of malignant intracranial neoplasms. Cancer, 33:460–467, 1974.

126. Smart, C. R., Ottoman, R. E., and Rochlin, D. B.: Clinical experience with vincristine (NSC-67574) in tumors of the central nervous system and other malignant diseases. Cancer Chemother. Rep., 52:733–741, 1968.

127. Swann, G. F.: Recent advances in neuroradiology. Postgrad. Med. J., 37:385, 1961.

128. Tucker, L. L., Jr., and Talley, R. W.: Prolonged intra-arterial chemotherapy for inoperable cancer: A technique. Cancer, 14:493, 1961.

129. Urtasun, R. C., Chapman, J. D., Band, P., et al.: Phase I study of high-dose metronidazole: A specific in vivo and in vitro radiosensitizer of hypoxic cells. Radiology, 117:129–133, 1975.

130. Verity, G. L.: Tissue tolerance: Central nervous system. Radiology, 91:1221–1225, 1968.

131. Walker, M. D.: Brain tumor study group: A survey of current activities. In Modern Concepts in Brain Tumor Therapy. Proceedings of National Cancer Institute Symposium, Atlanta, Ga., February 26–28, 1976. Washington, D.C., Department of Health, Education, and Welfare, 1977.

132. Walker, M. D., and Hurwitz, B. S.: BCNU (1,3-bis(2-chloroethyl)-1-nitrosourea, NSC 409962) in the treatment of malignant brain tumor: A preliminary report. Cancer Chemother. Rep., 54:263–271, 1970.

133. Walker, M. D., Dalgard, D. W., and Hurwitz, B. S.: The toxicity of intrathecal drugs and their ionic content. Proc. Amer. Ass. Cancer Res., 10:97, 1969.

134. Walker, M. D., Alexander, E., Jr., Hunt, W. E., et al.: Evaluation of mithramycin in the treatment of anaplastic gliomas. J. Neurosurg., 44:655–667, 1976.

135. Watkins, E.: Chronometric infusor—an apparatus for protracted ambulatory infusion therapy. New Eng. J. Med., 269:850, 1963.

136. Watkins, E., Jr., and Sullivan, R. D.: Cancer chemotherapy by prolonged arterial infusion. Surg. Gynec. Obstet., 118:3, 1964.

137. Waxman, A. D., Siemsen, J. K., Wolfstein, R. S., et al.: Evaluation of postcraniotomy patients by radionuclide scan. J. Neurosurg., 43:471–476, 1975.

138. Weir, B., Band, P., Urtasun, R., et al.: Radio-

therapy and CCNU in the treatment of high grade, supratentorial astrocytomas. J. Neurosurg., *45*:129–135, 1976.

139. Weiss, S. R., and Raskind, R.: Pathologic findings in brain tumors treated with local methotrexate. Unpublished observations.

140. Wheeler, G. P., Bowdon, B. J., Grimsley, J. A., et al.: Interrelationships of some chemical, physicochemical, and biological activities of several 1-(2-haloethyl)-1-nitrosureas. Cancer Res., *34*:194–200, 1974.

141. Wheeler, K. T., Deen, D. F., Wilson, C. B., et al.: BCNU–Modification of the in vitro radiation response in 9L brain tumor cells of rats. Int. J. Radiat. Oncol. Biol. Phys., *2*:79–88, 1977.

142. Wheeler, K. T., Rosenblum, M. L., Williams, M. E., et al.: Absence of recovery from BCNU-induced sublethal and potentially lethal damage in rat brain tumor cells: In vitro and in vivo. Brit. J Cancer, submitted for publication.

143. Wilson, C. B.: Chemotherapy of brain tumors by continuous arterial infusion. Surgery, *55*:640–653, 1964.

144. Wilson, C. B.: Medulloblastoma. Current views regarding the tumor and its treatment. Oncology, *24*:273–290, 1970.

145. Wilson, C. B.: Chemotherapy of brain tumors. Adv. Neurol., *15*:361–367, 1976.

146. Wilson, C. B., and Hoshino, T.: Principles of tumor cell population kinetics and and their application to brain tumors: A review. J. Neurosurg., *42*:123–131, 1975.

147. Wilson, C. B., and Norrell, H. A., Jr.: Brain tumor chemotherapy with intrathecal methotrexate. Cancer *23*:1038–1044, 1969.

148. Wilson, C. B., Boldrey, E. B., and Enot, K. J.: 1,3-bis(2-chlorethyl)-1-nitrosourea (NSC-409962) in the treatment of brain tumors. Cancer Chemother. Rep., *54*:273–281, 1970.

149. Wilson, C. B., Crafts, D., and Levin, V.: Brain tumors: Criteria of response and definition of recurrence. *In* Modern Concepts in Brain Tumor Therapy. Proceedings of National Cancer Institute Symposium, Atlanta, Ga., February 26–28, 1976. Washington, D.C., Department of Health, Education, and Welfare, 1977.

150. Wilson, C. B., Wheeler, K., Levin, V. A., et al.: Brain tumor chemotherapy: Translation of laboratory experiments into clinical trials. Arch. Neurol. (Chicago), *33*:394, 1976.

151. Wilson, C. B., Gutin, P., Kumar, A. R. V., et al.: Single agent chemotherapy of brain tumors: A five-year review. Arch. Neurol. (Chicago), *33*:739–744, 1976.

152. Wilson, G. H., Byfield, J., and Hanafee, W. N.: Atrophy following radiation therapy for central nervous system neoplasms. Acta Radiol. (Ther.) (Stockholm), *11*:361–368, 1972.

153. Woodhall, B., and Mahaley, M. S., Jr.: Isolated perfusion in treatment of advanced carcinoma. Amer. J. Surg., *105*:624, 1967.

154. Woodhall, B., Hall, K., Mahaley, S., Jr., and Jackson, J.: Chemotherapy of brain cancer: Experimental and clinical studies in localized hypothermic cerebral perfusion. Ann. Surg., *150*:640, 1959.

155. Young, D. F., Shapiro, W. R., and Posner, J. B.: Treatment of leptomeningeal cancer. Neurology (Minneap.), *25*:370, 1975.

97

RADIATION THERAPY OF BRAIN TUMORS

Operative resection, radiation therapy, chemotherapy, and combinations thereof are utilized in the treatment of intracranial tumors. An operation may be the definitive treatment or primarily for decompression and biopsy to precede radiation therapy. Chemotherapy, in the treatment of primary tumors of the central nervous system, is at present largely restricted to the role of a palliative or an adjunct to operative and irradiation treatment. To select the appropriate therapy for a given patient requires knowledge of both the biological behavior of the specific tumor and the value of each treatment modality, used singly or in combination.

X-rays and gamma-rays, which consist of photons, are used in radiotherapy of central nervous system tumors. Other types of irradiation, e.g., protons, alpha particles, neutrons, and pi-mesons, are being investigated but are not ready for routine clinical application.* Both x-rays and gamma-rays are part of the electromagnetic spectrum, and their physical properties are similar. They are absorbed exponentially in tissue, and their biological effect is mediated through the production of charged ions and free radicals in the target material. The actual distribution of energy deposited in the target material, hence the volume affected, will vary with the energy of the radiation, the size of the radiation source, the dimensions and shape of the treatment beam, the use of filters, the source-to-target distance, and the collimation system.

Modern radiation therapy given with curative intent is largely limited to mega-voltage irradiation, i.e., employs a source with an energy greater than one million electron volts. Megavoltage, compared with kilovoltage, irradiation has the advantages of greater penetration, less absorption in bone, less side scatter, and reduced dosage to skin and subcutaneous tissues. A ^{60}cobalt radiation source gives gamma-rays of 1.17 and 1.33 Mev. Linear accelerators in common use produce x-rays ranging from 4 to 25 Mev. The larger the radiation source, the greater will be the penumbra. Longer distances between source and tissue reduce the divergence of the beam within the tissue. In general, linear accelerators have more sharply defined radiation beams than do ^{60}cobalt machines. In addition to the collimation system built into each machine, special radiation shielding blocks, wedge filters, and tissue compensating filters are utilized to shape the large dose volume and to protect sensitive normal tissues.

The biological basis of radiation therapy is complex. The intent, of course, is to destroy the tumor with a radiation dose that is tolerated by whatever normal tissue must be included in the irradiated volume. Even when the radiation equipment and treatment planning are optimal, i.e., include the best selection of treatment fields, rotation, protective radiation blocks, tissue compensating filters, and the like, some normal tissue is virtually always included. The success of treatment thus depends upon many interrelated factors: (1) careful treatment planning designed to limit the dosage to noncritical structures, (2) the inherent sensitivity of the irradiated normal and tumor cells, (3) the total number of various cell types present, (4) the ability of normal

---

* See references 14, 26, 31, 46, 51, 55.

G. E. SHELINE AND W. M. WARA

cells to migrate into and tumor cells to me-tastasize out of the irradiated volume, (5) the repopulation capability of normal cells in proportion to that of tumor cells, (6) rear-rangement of cells in the cell cycle between radiation fractions, (7) the relative ability of tumor and normal cells to repair sublethal radiation damage between treatment frac-tions, and (8) the oxygen tension and time required for reoxygenation of hypoxic tumor cells—hypoxia may decrease radio-sensitivity by threefold. While each of these factors when studied experimentally has been shown to be important, the extent to which each influences a particular clini-cal situation usually is unknown. In prac-tice, the radiation therapist, after selecting the approach that gives the best physical distribution of absorbed dose, tends to apply the maximum dose consistent with an acceptable risk for critical normal struc-tures. Certain tumors known to be particu-larly radiosensitive may be treated with a smaller dose, but in general, it is the sensi-tivity of normal tissues that limits radiation therapy.

RADIATION TOLERANCE OF THE CENTRAL NERVOUS SYSTEM

The radiation dose–time fractionation regimens employed in patients with brain tumors, especially with the large doses used for malignant gliomas, carry a degree of risk. Although currently available data are inadequate to determine with precision the rate of injury associated with a given treatment regimen, a number of factors are known to influence the risk. The larger the daily dose, the total dose, or the volume of brain irradiated, the greater the risk. Cer-tain anatomical structures are more radio-sensitive than others. The lens of the eye is particularly sensitive.[29] The functional defi-cit varies with the part of the brain injured. A small area of necrosis in the brain stem might be fatal, whereas a similar lesion in a frontal lobe might pass unnoticed. The im-mature central nervous system, particularly before myelination is well advanced, is thought to be more sensitive than the adult brain.[4] Experience indicates that there is small risk of clinically significant injury to the brain if the total dose does not exceed 5000 to 5500 rads and individual daily frac-tions are no more than 180 to 200 rads.[22] Such dose fractionation schemes are used for treatment of relatively benign tumors of the central nervous system. Larger doses, with increased risk, are used for the more malignant gliomas in which, without radical therapy, early death is virtually assured. For children less than 18 to 24 months of age the dose should be reduced by about 10 per cent. Bloom, Wallace, and Henk have arbitrarily chosen 3 years as the age below which the dose is reduced from 5000 rads in seven weeks to 4000 to 4500 rads in six to seven weeks.[4]

The adverse effects of irradiation of the central nervous system may be considered in three groups, depending upon the time of appearance of symptoms. The reactions that appear during the course of radiation therapy are thought to be due to cerebral edema.[19] With modern conventionally frac-tionated radiotherapy, i.e., daily fractions not in excess of about 200 rads, such reac-tions are infrequent and when they occur are usually easily reversible with adreno-corticosteroid therapy. Onset of the second type of reaction comes within a few weeks to three or four months after completion of the radiation.[5] This type is probably due to temporary demyelination. It usually mimics the original symptoms and signs from the tumor, occurs in about 20 to 25 per cent of patients, is transient in nature, and requires no therapy. If treatment is needed, corti-costeroids generally suffice. This reaction is an important one to recognize because it is not indicative of tumor recurrence and should not result in a premature alteration of the treatment regimen.

The third group of reactions is far more serious. Onset may be any time from a few months up to five or ten years after irradia-tion.[19] This type of reaction is insidious in onset, and may progress to scarring or ne-crosis that causes functional impairment or even death. The pathological mechanism is not well understood, but the phenomenon probably is due to an alteration of the vas-cular supply to the brain. Fortunately, with conventional radiotherapy this complica-tion is infrequent. Kramer and associates reviewed the literature from 1937 to 1967 and found only 57 cases of proved brain ne-crosis from radiation therapy.[22] In only 5 of 57 patients was the tumor dose below 7000 rads. It is possible that the risk is greater than this review implies, since radiation necrosis of the brain may well be underreported; most patients who die after therapy for a brain tumor are assumed to have had a recurrence of the tumor, and frequently postmortem examination is not performed. It must, however, be kept in mind that in a clinical situation the acceptable risk from radiation therapy must be related to the prognosis that attends either inadequate or no irradiation.

PRIMARY TUMORS

Astrocytoma

There are numerous reports in the literature regarding the use of radiation therapy for treatment of astrocytomas. Some authors have indicated that radiation therapy was of significant value, whereas others have questioned its usefulness.* Most reported data are inconclusive because control groups of nonirradiated patients are not included or because radiotherapy was inadequate. There has been no prospective randomized controlled study to test the efficacy of irradiation therapy for these relatively differentiated astrocytomas.

Leibel and co-workers reviewed a series of patients with astrocytomas who were treated between 1942 and 1967 (Table 97–1).[24] Craniotomy with attempted operative removal of the tumor was carried out in each patient. Excluding those who died in the postoperative period, there were 122 patients. These were separated into three groups. The first included 14 patients in whom the surgeon thought the tumor to

---

* See references 6, 24, 25, 41, 52.

have been completely resected; none received radiotherapy. The second consisted of 37 with incomplete resection, but no postoperative radiation therapy. The third group included 71 patients with incomplete resection and postoperative irradiation.

To date there has been no recurrence among the 14 nonirradiated patients who had total resection of the astrocytoma. These tumors were mostly cystic cerebellar astrocytomas in children. The only death occurred in an elderly patient who died of congestive heart failure twelve years postresection. After complete resection, postoperative radiation therapy is not needed.

For patients with an incompletely resected astrocytoma, the five-year survival rate without irradiation was 19 per cent compared with 46 per cent when irradiation was given. At 20 years approximately one fourth of those irradiated were living without recurrence, but all nonirradiated patients had died. It appears that for patients with an incompletely resected astrocytoma, postoperative radiation therapy increases the disease-free interval and controls the disease for at least 20 years in about 25 per cent. It is thought that the 15- and 20-year survival rates for irradiated patients would have been greater had those treated during the 1940s and early 1950s been treated as aggressively as those irradiated more recently.

When the survival rates for incompletely resected astrocytomas were reviewed according to the degree of malignancy as determined histologically, a beneficial effect of postoperative radiation therapy was again evident (Table 97–2). For patients with grade I tumors, the five-year recurrence-free survival rate was 58 per cent with irradiation and 25 per cent without.

TABLE 97–1   SURVIVAL RATES IN ASTROCYTOMA ACCORDING TO THERAPY*

| INTERVAL (YEARS) | TOTAL RESECTION | | INCOMPLETE RESECTION | | | |
| | | | No Irradiation | | Plus Irradiation | |
	Per Cent	Patients at Risk	Per Cent	Patients at Risk	Per Cent	Patients at Risk
1	100	14	51	37	80	71
3	100	14	27	37	59	71
5	100	14	19	37	46	71
10	100	12	11	37	35	54
15	89	9	4	28	25	32
20	88	8	0	19	23	26

* Modified from Leibel, S., Sheline, G., Wara, W., et al.: The role of radiation therapy in the treatment of astrocytomas. Cancer, 35:1551–1557, 1975.

TABLE 97–2　FIVE-YEAR SURVIVAL RATE IN INCOMPLETELY EXCISED ASTROCYTOMA*

| | PER CENT OF PATIENTS SURVIVING | |
	Grade I	Grade II
Not irradiated	25	0
Irradiated	58	25

* Modified from Leibel, S., Sheline, G., Wara, W., et al.: The role of radiation therapy in the treatment of astrocytomas. Cancer, 35:1551–1557, 1975.

For those with grade II tumors it was 25 per cent with and zero without.

It is the authors' policy to irradiate any incompletely excised astrocytoma. Treatment is started as soon as the patient has recovered from the operation and the wound is well healed. Administered in daily fractions of approximately 180 rads, the total tumor dose is 5000 to 5500 rads, depending upon the age of the patient and the grade of the tumor.

Malignant Glioma

The literature on malignant gliomas is confused by the fact that two different classification systems are widely used. Even worse, the terminology of the two systems is often intermingled. One system classifies according to the apparent histological degree of malignancy, with grade I being the least and grade IV the most malignant.[17] The other classifies according to the presumed cell of origin.[39] For present purposes, lesions variously termed malignant astrocytoma, undifferentiated astrocytoma, or astrocytoma grade III are considered as a single group termed malignant astrocytoma. Tumors diagnosed as astrocytoma grade IV or glioblastoma multiforme, as defined by the criteria of Rubinstein, are grouped under the title glioblastoma multiforme.[39] On the basis of this nomenclature, the weighted average survival rates for patients treated by operation alone or by resection plus postoperative radiation therapy were calculated for patients reported from four different institutions (Table 97–3).[21,42,48,52] In these four reports it was possible to distinguish both the type of glioma and which patients did or did not receive radiation therapy.

The survival rate of patients with malignant astrocytomas was improved—up to at least five years—by the addition of postoperative radiation therapy. At five years the weighted average survival rates for the four series of patients were <2 per cent (1 of 63) with resection only and 16 per cent when irradiation therapy was added. The average five-year survival rate for patients reported by Kramer and by Sheline, who used a minimum radiation dose of at least 5000 rads, was 20 per cent.[21,42] Thus, while the outlook for patients with malignant astrocytomas is dismal, it is not hopeless and aggressive radiation therapy is indicated. The authors use doses of 6000 rads, at the rate of 180 per day to very generous fields that usually include the entire brain. Kramer has used either 6000 rads to the whole brain or 5000 rads to the whole brain plus an additional 1500 rads to the identified tumor volume.

With glioblastoma multiforme, postresection radiation therapy improves the survival rate for at least one year and possibly

TABLE 97–3　SURVIVAL RATES IN MALIGNANT GLIOMA*

| | SURVIVAL RATE (PER CENT) | | | NO. OF PATIENTS AT RISK |
	1 Year	3 Years	5 Years	
Malignant astrocytoma				
Resection only	12	7	2	63
Resection plus radiation therapy	40	27	16	128
Glioblastoma multiforme				
Resection only	8	0	0	145
Resection plus radiation therapy	24	6	0	90

* Data from combined series: Kramer, S.: Radiation therapy in the management of malignant gliomas. In Seventh National Cancer Conference Proceedings. Philadelphia, J. B. Lippincott Co., 1973, pp. 823–826. Sheline, G.: Conventional radiation therapy of gliomas. In Recent Results in Cancer Research. Gliomas. Current Concepts in Biology. Diagnosis and Therapy. New York, Springer-Verlag, 1975, pp. 123–234. Stage, W., and Stein, J.: Treatment of malignant astrocytomas. Amer. J. Roentgen., 120:7–18, 1974. Uihlein, A., Colby, M., Layton, D., et al.: Comparison of surgery and surgery plus irradiation in the treatment of supratentorial gliomas. Acta Radiol., 5:67–78, 1966.

for two or three years after treatment. In each of the four series of patients included in Table 97–3, however, the five-year survival rate was zero regardless of whether the patients were or were not irradiated. At present there are numerous organized studies in which combinations of postoperative radiation therapy and various chemotherapeutic agents are being investigated.

Medulloblastoma

In children, the medulloblastoma, which generally arises in the midline of the cerebellum, accounts for 15 to 20 per cent of intracranial tumors. The so-called "arachnoidal cerebellar sarcoma" of adults is probably a variant of the medulloblastoma.[40] Medulloblastomas frequently invade the subarachnoid space and metastasize throughout the entire cerebrospinal axis. McFarland and co-workers reported a 33 per cent incidence rate for metastases within the central nervous system; 94 per cent of these occurred along the spinal canal, whereas only 6 per cent were intracranial.[28] Had many of these patients not received radiation therapy to the entire cerebrospinal axis, the metastasis rate would undoubtedly have been higher. Thus in treating the medulloblastoma, one must direct therapy to the whole central nervous system.

Without radiation therapy, the outlook for the patient with medulloblastoma is similar to that for glioblastoma multiforme. The disease is nearly always fatal, and the postoperative course is short. With operation alone, Davidoff reported an average survival of 13 months.[10] His only long-term survivor had five operative procedures and died sixty-three months following the diagnosis.

The medulloblastoma usually is considered to be one of the more radioresponsive of tumors that arise within the central nervous system. Nevertheless, even in patients who have received radiation therapy both at the primary site and along the spinal axis, there has been a high rate of failure. These failures have gradually led radiation therapists to increase the dose administered, and it is now general practice to give the maximum dose that can be tolerated by the brain and cord. Jenkin made a survey of twenty institutions that participated in the

Children's Cancer Study Group.[16] Approximately two thirds of the fifteen investigators responding to his questions advocated doses of 5000 to 5500 rads to the primary tumor site and doses of 3500 to 4000 rads to the remainder of the central nervous system. Six of the fifteen responders use a smaller dose to the primary tumor, and five use a reduced dose to the spinal cord. Bloom, Wallace, and Henk recommended doses of 4500 to 5000 rads to the primary tumor site, including the upper cervical spine, and 2000 to 2500 rads to the remainder of the spine.[4] The authors use doses of 5500 to the primary tumor site, 4500 to the remainder of the brain, and 4000 to the spine. The doses are reduced 10 or 15 per cent for patients under 2 or 3 years of age. The brain is treated with daily fractions of 170 to 180 rads, and the spine with 160 rads. Irradiation of the entire central nervous system requires multiple treatment fields, and great care must be taken not only to avoid skip areas between fields but also to avoid overlapping radiation beams. With these large doses, overlap in the cord would almost certainly lead to transverse myelopathy.

Five-year survival rates for patients who received radiation therapy to the entire central nervous system are presented in Table 97–4. The larger series presented by Bloom, Wallace, and Henk and by McFarland and co-workers had five-year survival rates of around 30 per cent.[4,28] Kramer and

TABLE 97–4 SURVIVAL RATES IN MEDULLOBLASTOMA TREATED BY RADIATION OF ENTIRE CENTRAL NERVOUS SYSTEM

SOURCE	NO. OF PATIENTS	5-YEAR SURVIVAL RATE (PER CENT)
Bloom, Wallace, and Henk*	69	32[a]
McFarland et al.†	23	30
Kramer‡	6	50
Sheline§	8	63[b]

[a] Forty per cent for patients completing therapy.
[b] Actually 88 percent survived 5 years but 2 were known to have recurrence.

* The treatment and prognosis of medulloblastoma in children. Amer. J. Roentgen., 105:43–62, 1969.
† Medulloblastoma—a review of prognosis and survival. Brit. J. Radiol., 42:198–214, 1969.
‡ Radiation therapy in the management of brain tumors in children. Ann. N.Y. Acad. Sci., 159:571–584, 1969.
§ Radiation therapy of tumors of the central nervous system in childhood. Cancer, 35:957–964, 1973.

Sheline, who used more aggressive radiation therapy, i.e., larger doses, reported survival rates of 50 per cent or better.[20, 43] Whether the better results will continue as more patients are treated is unknown.

Most patients exhibit an improvement, often marked, during or shortly after completion of the radiation therapy. Improvement frequently begins within a few days following operative decompression, whether this is done by subtotal removal of the primary tumor or by shunting of the cerebrospinal fluid. The improvement usually is maintained unless the tumor recurs. Bloom, Wallace, and Henk reported that 18 of 22 children who survived five years were leading active lives without serious disability.[4] The authors' experience has been similar.

The radiation doses used for treatment of medulloblastoma retard bone growth, with consequent shortening of the spine. They may produce varying degrees of pituitary deficiency; growth hormone production in children appears to be particularly sensitive to irradiation.[35]

Ependymoma

Ependymomas, like medulloblastomas, are sensitive to irradiation. Most cannot be completely excised, and postoperative radiation therapy is required. Table 97–5 presents five-year survival rates for two operative series.[9,37] It also gives results for patients who received postoperative radiation therapy with doses of 4500 rads or more.[7,32] With operation alone, Cushing had a 20 per cent five-year survival rate.[9] Ringertz and

Reymond reported a 27 per cent five-year survival rate, but two of their nine patients living at five years had recurrent tumor from which they died within the next six months.[37] In patients who received postoperative radiotherapy, Bouchard and Peirce had 58 per cent five-year and 50 per cent 10-year recurrence-free survival rates.[7] The 5- and 10-year recurrence-free survival rates for irradiated patients (dose ≥ 4500 rads) of Phillips, Sheline, and Boldrey were 87 per cent and 62 per cent, respectively.[32] Other authors have reported similar survival rates for irradiated and nonirradiated patients. It may be concluded that radiation therapy is of value in the treatment of ependymomas and should be given whenever the operative resection is not total.

The major problem in the irradiation of ependymomas relates to the portion of the central nervous system that needs to be treated. Some radiotherapists believe that all ependymomas, like medulloblastomas, require irradiation of the entire cerebrospinal axis, while others contend that such extensive irradiation is not always necessary. Certainly some ependymomas do seed within the cerebrospinal fluid pathways. Irradiation of the entire system with therapeutic doses is, however, a major procedure and may be attended with significant morbidity. The question is whether the frequency of metastases justifies giving large doses of irradiation to the whole head and spine of all patients or whether a subset of patients at high risk can be identified.

Svien, Gates, and Kernohan found spinal arachnoid implants at autopsy in 6 of 19 patients.[49] In each of the six patients with implants the primary tumor had been in the

TABLE 97–5 SURVIVAL RATES IN EPENDYMOMA TREATED BY OPERATIVE RESECTION OR RESECTION PLUS RADIATION

SOURCE	TREATMENT	SURVIVAL RATE (PER CENT)	
		5 Years	10 Years
Cushing*	Resection	20	
Ringertz and Reymond†	Resection	27[a]	
Bouchard and Peirce‡	Resection plus irradiation[b]	58	50
Phillips, Sheline, and Boldrey§	Resection plus irradiation[b]	87	62

[a] Twenty-one per cent recurrence-free.

[b] Tumor dose ≥4500 rads.

* Intracranial Tumors: Notes Upon a Series of Two Thousand Verified Cases with Surgical Mortality Percentages Pertaining Thereto. Springfield, Ill., Charles C Thomas, 1932.

† Ependymomas and choroid plexus papillomas. J. Neuropath. Exp. Neurol., 8:355–380, 1949.

‡ Radiation therapy in the management of neoplasms of the central nervous system with a special note in regard to children: Twenty years' experience, 1939–1958. Amer. J. Roentgen., 84:610–628, 1960.

§ Therapeutic considerations in tumors affecting the central nervous system. Ependymomas. Radiology, 83:98–105, 1964.

fourth ventricle and the neoplasm was less than well differentiated, i.e., grade II or higher. In a subsequent report, Svien, Mabon, Kernohan, and Craig stated that none of 162 patients with ependymoma had clinical evidence of spinal metastases.[50] Fokes and Earle reported 14 instances of seeding from 127 patients whose material was reviewed at the Armed Forces Institute of Pathology.[12] All 14 instances of spinal seeding occurred among the 60 patients examined at autopsy. Obviously the extent of the disease at the time of autopsy in a patient whose therapy has failed may differ from that present at the time of diagnosis when treatment decisions are being made. In 70 patients with intracranial ependymomas, Kricheff and associates reported only one case of seeding and that was found at autopsy.[23] Barone and Elvidge reported no evidence of seeding in 47 patients with intracranial ependymomas.[2] Phillips and co-workers reported two instances of seeding among 42 patients.[32] The overall incidence of seeding from ependymomas is hardly sufficient to justify routine treatment of the entire central nervous system.

Table 97–6 presents information on clinically evident spinal seeding from ependymomas. These data were taken from reports in which both the location and the grade of malignancy of the ependymoma could be ascertained.[3,18,43,50] Only one of 48 supratentorial lesions showed evidence of seeding, and this was among the 23 high-grade ependymomas. Of the infratentorial primaries, 27 per cent with high-grade lesions and 4 per cent with low-grade lesions seeded. These data may imply a falsely high rate, since some cases of seeding were diagnosed late in the course of the disease, e.g., five of the seven patients with seeding reported by Kim and Fayos already had recurrent intracranial disease.[18] It seems clear that patients with high-grade, malignant posterior fossa ependymomas need therapy to the entire central nervous system. Whether other ependymomas require more than generous local field irradiation is doubtful.

Oligodendroglioma

Oligodendrogliomas are relatively rare and information regarding radiation therapy of these tumors is scarce. The available evidence, however, does suggest that for the incompletely resected oligodendroglioma, postoperative radiation therapy via a portal encompassing the tumor with an adequate margin is beneficial. Excluding patients who died shortly after operation, the weighted average five-year survival rate for a pooled group of patients treated by operation alone was 35 per cent.[1,11,45] In comparison, the five-year survival rate for patients given postoperative radiation therapy was 63 per cent.[7,36,45] Since only patients who survived the postoperative period were included in the calculation, the difference in survival rates appears significant. Ten-year survival data are even more limited; combining the cases of Bouchard and Peirce and Sheline and co-workers, 2 of 8 nonirradiated patients survived without recurrence for 10 years, whereas 7 of 14 who received radiotherapy were without recurrence for 10 to 20 years.

Brain Stem Tumors

Because of their location, intrinsic tumors of the brain stem often are treated with radiation without biopsy. Frequently they respond favorably. Of 27 children with brain stem tumors treated by the authors, 19 (71 per cent) showed distinct improvement after radiation therapy.[44] Ten of 24 (41 per cent) and 5 of 15 (33 per cent) were living without evidence of recurrence at 5 and 10 years, respectively. The remainder either failed to respond or developed a recur-

TABLE 97–6 CLINICAL SPINAL SEEDING FROM EPENDYMOMAS*

Location and Grade	Fraction Seeding	
Supratentorial		
High grade	1 of 23	
Low grade	0 of 14	1 of 48
Grade unknown	0 of 11	
Infratentorial		
High grade	9 of 34	11 of 83
Low grade	2 of 49	

* Pooled data from: Bloom, H.: Treatment and prognosis of intracranial tumors in children. Presented at the 27th Annual Midwinter Radiological Conference at the Los Angeles Radiological Society, Los Angeles, California, February 2, 1974. Svien, H., Mabon, R., Kernohan, J., and Craig, M.: Ependymoma of the brain—pathologic aspects. Neurology, 3:1–13, 1953. Sheline, G.: Radiation therapy of brain tumors. Cancer, 39:873–881, 1977. Kim, Y., and Fayos, J.: Intracranial ependymomas. Radiology, 124:805–808, 1977.

rence, usually within 12 to 18 months, and died shortly thereafter.

Pineal and Suprasellar Tumors

Suprasellar tumors and those occurring in the region of the pineal gland form a rare group of midline cerebral tumors. The majority are of germ cell origin, with germinomas accounting for over 50 per cent of all lesions found in the region of the pineal.[39] Teratoma, choriocarcinoma, embryonal carcinoma, and tumors of the pineal parenchyma occur but are less frequent. Because of the high operative mortality rate associated with lesions in this location and the fact that complete resection is rarely possible, these tumors usually have been irradiated without biopsy. With recent advances in operative techniques, more patients now reach the radiation oncologist with a histological diagnosis. Since the histological type influences the therapy, a histological diagnosis is of value if it can be obtained without causing undue morbidity or death.

Table 97–7 shows the results obtained by irradiation of pineal and suprasellar tumors. Most tumors included in this table were not subjected to biopsy. The average control rate for all patients was 65 per cent. Because the reported incidence of spinal metastases is low, averaging around 10 per cent, and there is morbidity associated with irradiation of the entire spinal axis, it is not necessary to irradiate the spinal cord routinely. Generous fields should be used to cover the known tumor and the ventricular system. The total tumor dose is 4500 to 5000 rads with daily fractions of 180 rads. If a diagnosis of germinoma has been established, the dose probably can be reduced.

Meningioma

Published data on the use of radiation therapy in the treatment of meningiomas are controversial; some authors have advocated irradiation, while others have thought it of little or no value. The authors' experience with radiation therapy of meningiomas is summarized in Table 97–8.[54] Eighty-four patients were thought to have had total or complete operative resection of the tumor and did not receive radiation therapy. Of these, 49 have been observed longer than five years and 23 longer than 10 years. There has been no recurrence.

Ninety-two patients had subtotal resection: 58 were not irradiated, while the other 34 received postoperative radiotherapy. The 5- and 10-year recurrence-free survival rates for those whose tumors were incompletely resected and not irradiated were 14 per cent (3 of 22) and 10 per cent (1 of 10), respectively. Patients with incomplete resection but who received postoperative irradiation had 78 per cent and 77 per cent 5- and 10-year survival rates. These data suggest that, as with other incompletely resected tumors, postoperative irradiation delays or prevents recurrence.

TABLE 97–7   RESULTS OF RADIATION THERAPY IN PINEAL AND SUPRASELLAR TUMORS

AUTHOR	PATIENTS WITHOUT DISEASE	RISK PERIOD
Rubin and Kramer*	6 of 8	19 months
Maier and Dejong†	7 of 10	16 months
Simson et al.‡	5 of 7	3–18 years
Bradfield and Perez§	8 of 16	3–18 years
Mincer et al.‖	8 of 12	4–14 years
Wara et al.¶	9 of 13	5–19 years
	43 of 66 (65%)	

* Ectopic pinealoma: A radiocurable neuroendocrinologic entity. Radiology, 85:512–523, 1965.

† Pineal body tumors. Amer. J. Roentgen., 99:826–832, 1967.

‡ Suprasellar germinomas. Cancer, 22:533–544, 1968.

§ Pineal tumors and ectopic pinealomas. Analysis of treatment and failures. Radiology, 103:399–406, 1972.

‖ Pinealoma. A report of twelve irradiated cases. Cancer, 37:2713–2718, 1976.

¶ Radiation therapy for pineal tumors and suprasellar germinomas. Radiology, 124:221–223, 1977.

TABLE 97–8   SURVIVAL RATES IN MENINGIOMAS*

EXTENT OF RESECTION	RECURRENCE-FREE SURVIVAL RATES	
	>5 Years	>10 Years
Complete—not irradiated	39 of 49 (10)	19 of 23 (4)
Incomplete—not irradiated	3 of 22 (3)	1 of 10 (2)
irradiated	14 of 18 (0)	10 of 13(0)

( ) = dead of intercurrent disease without recurrence of the meningioma.

* Patients were treated at the University of California at San Francisco.

INTRACEREBRAL METASTASES

Radiation therapy of metastatic disease within the central nervous system is almost invariably performed for palliation. The signs and symptoms present will vary depending upon the location, number, and size of the metastases. According to Posner, about 12 per cent of cancer patients who undergo autopsy have intracerebral metastases, and in about two thirds of these the metastases are multiple.[33] Since most patients with cerebral metastases have a short life expectancy, median survival on the order of a few months, the autopsy-determined incidence of multiplicity is nearly representative of the situation existing at the time cerebral lesions become symptomatic.

As advocated by Ransohoff, selected patients may benefit from operative excision.[34] According to Ransohoff the lesion should be single, insofar as can be demonstrated, and operatively accessible. He believes that the patient whose central nervous system metastasis has occurred in the absence of other known metastases and whose primary cancer has been locally controlled is the best candidate for excision. Using such selection criteria and with the addition of postoperative radiotherapy to the whole brain, Ransohoff reported a 10 per cent operative mortality rate, a median survival time between 6 and 12 months, and a 38 per cent survival rate for one year or longer. Whether these relatively good results are due to the combined therapy or to selection of patients with the most favorable disease is unknown.

Hendrickson summarized the results of radiation therapy alone in over 1000 patients entered into a national cooperative study by members of the Radiation Therapy Oncology Group.[13] There was no selection, i.e., all patients referred with brain metastasis were included. Whole brain irradiation was given in five fractions per week but with varying daily and total doses. The treatment regimens ranged from 10 treatments of 300 rads each to 20 of 200 each. Partial or complete relief of convulsions and headache was achieved in 85 per cent of the patients. Mentation and motor function partially or completely recovered in more than 70 per cent. The median survival time for the entire group was 15 weeks, and this did not vary significantly between the different treatment regimens. The median survival time, however, did vary with the state of neurological function. The median survival for patients initially able to work and with minimal neurological signs was 30 weeks. Patients who required hospitalization had a median survival of approximately five weeks. Unfortunately, larger radiation doses were not tested nor was the duration of control of central nervous system symptoms reported.

For metastatic disease the authors irradiate the entire intracranial contents, whether single or multiple metastases have been demonstrated and whether or not a metastasis had been operatively excised. The dose fractionation scheme is varied according to the condition of the patient. A patient with advanced disease and short life expectancy is treated with 10 fractions of 300 rads each or even with 5 of 400 each. On the other hand, a patient in good general condition and who appears to have a relatively slowly progressing cancer is treated with more conventional fractionation, 200 rads per day to a total of around 5000 rads; this is done on the unproved assumption that the smaller fractions and greater total may be better tolerated and the improvement longer lasting.

Leukemia of the Central Nervous System

A special circumstance of metastatic disease occurs in the child with acute lymphoblastic leukemia. With systemic chemotherapy, the majority of children with this disease go into bone marrow remission, but since the chemotherapy does not uniformly penetrate the meninges, without further treatment of the central nervous system approximately 50 per cent of these patients develop overt meningeal leukemia. Therefore, after bone marrow remission has been achieved, either craniospinal irradiation (2400 rads) or cranial irradiation (2400 rads) with coincident intrathecal methotrexate is given to eradicate microscopic foci of meningeal disease. Such adjuvant therapy has reduced the incidence of meningeal leukemia to less than 10 per cent.[15]

The treatment regimen for gross meningeal leukemia is currently under investigation. This disease carries a grave prognosis.

Present therapy combines craniospinal irradiation in large doses with repeated intrathecal drug administrations prolonged over time. A similar treatment regimen is utilized in the lymphoma patient with meningeal disease.

REFERENCES

1. Bailey, P., and Bucy, P.: Oligodendrogliomas of brain. J. Path. Bact. *32*:735–751, 1929.
2. Barone, B., and Elvidge, A.: Ependymomas, a clinical survey. J. Neurosurg., *33*:428–438, 1970.
3. Bloom, H.: Treatment and prognosis of intracranial tumors in children. Presented at the 27th Annual Midwinter Radiological Conference at the Los Angeles Radiological Society, Los Angeles, California, February 2, 1974.
4. Bloom, H., Wallace, E., and Henk, J.: The treatment and prognosis of medulloblastoma in children. Amer. J. Roentgen., *105*:43–62, 1969.
5. Boldrey, E., and Sheline, G.: Delayed transitory clinical manifestations after radiation treatment of intracranial tumors. Acta Radiol. [Ther.], *5*:5–510, 1967.
6. Bouchard, J.: Central nervous system. *In* Fletcher, J., ed.: Textbook of Radiotherapy. 2nd Ed. Philadelphia, Lea & Febiger, 1973, pp. 336–418.
7. Bouchard, J., and Peirce, C.: Radiation therapy in the management of neoplasms of the central nervous system with a special note in regard to children: Twenty years' experience, 1939–1958. Amer. J. Roentgen., *84*:610-15—628, 1960.
8. Bradfield, J., and Perez, C.: Pineal tumors and ectopic pinealomas. Analysis of treatment and failures. Radiology, *103*:399–406, 1972.
9. Cushing, H.: Intracranial Tumors: Notes Upon a Series of Two Thousand Verified Cases with Surgical Mortality Percentages Pertaining Thereto. Springfield, Ill., Charles C Thomas, 1932.
10. Davidoff, L.: A thirteen year follow-up study of a series of cases of verified tumors of the brain. Arch. Neurol. Psychiat., *44*:1246–1261, 1940.
11. Earnest, F., Kernohan, J., and Craig, W.: Oligodendrogliomas: Review of 200 cases. Arch. Neurol. Psychiat., *63*:964–976, 1950.
12. Fokes, E., Jr., and Earle, K.: Ependymomas: Clinical and pathological aspects. J. Neurosurg., *30*:585–594, 1969.
13. Hendrickson, F.: Radiation therapy of metastatic tumors. Seminars Oncol., *2*:43–46, 1975.
14. Hussey, D., Fletcher, G., and Caderao, J.: Experience with fast neutron therapy using the Texas A & M variable energy cyclotron. Cancer, *34*:65–77, 1974.
15. Hustu, H., Aur, R., Veroza, M., et al.: Prevention of central nervous system leukemia by irradiation. Cancer, *32*:585–597, 1973.
16. Jenkin, R.: Personal communication, 1974.
17. Kernohan, J., and Sayre, G.: Astrocytomas. *In* Tumors of the Central Nervous System. Fascicle 35, Washington, D.C., Armed Forces Institute of Pathology, 1952, pp. 22–42.
18. Kim, Y., and Fayos, J.: Intracranial ependymomas. Radiology, *124*:805–808, 1977.
19. Kramer, S.: The hazards of therapeutic irradiation of the central nervous system. Clin. Neurosurg., *15*:301–318, 1968.
20. Kramer, S.: Radiation therapy in the management of brain tumors in children. Ann. N.Y. Acad. Sci., *159*:571–584, 1969.
21. Kramer, S.: Radiation therapy in the management of malignant gliomas. *In* Seventh National Cancer Conference Proceedings. Philadelphia, J. B. Lippincott Co., 1973, pp. 823–826.
22. Kramer, S., Southard, M., and Mansfield, C.: Radiation effect and tolerance of the central nervous system. Front. Rad. Ther. Oncol., *6*:332–345, 1972.
23. Kricheff, I., Becker, M., Schneck, S., and Taveras, J.: Intracranial ependymomas. A study of survival in 65 cases treated by surgery and irradiation. Amer. J. Roentgen., *91*:167–175, 1964.
24. Leibel, S., Sheline, G., Wara, W., et al.: The role of radiation therapy in the treatment of astrocytomas. Cancer, *35*:1551–1557, 1975.
25. Lindgren, M.: Roentgen treatment of gliomata. Acta Radiol., *40*:325–334, 1953.
26. Lloyd, D., Reading, D., Purrott, R., et al.: Expansion of a negative pi-meson peak to cover a range of depths useful for radiotherapy. Brit. J. Radiol., *51*:41–45, 1978.
27. Maier, J., and Dejong, D.: Pineal body tumors. Amer. J. Roentgen., *99*:826–832, 1967.
28. McFarland, D., Horwitz, H., Saenger, E., and Bahr, G.: Medulloblastoma—a review of prognosis and survival. Brit. J. Radiol., *42*:198–214, 1969.
29. Merrian, G., Jr., and Focht, E.: Radiation dose to the lens in treatment of tumors of the eye and adjacent structures. Possibilities of cataract formation. Radiology, *71*:357–369, 1958.
30. Mincer, F., Meltzer, J., and Botstein, C.: Pinealoma. A report of twelve irradiated cases. Cancer, *37*:2713–2718, 1976.
31. Parker, R., Berry, H., Gerdes, A., et al.: Fast neutron beam radiotherapy of glioblastoma multiforme. Amer. J. Roentgen., *127*:331–335, 1976.
32. Phillips, T., Sheline, G., and Boldrey, E.: Therapeutic considerations in tumors affecting the central nervous system. Ependymomas. Radiology, *83*:98–105, 1964.
33. Posner, J.: Management of central nervous system metastases. Seminars Oncol., *4*:81–91, 1977.
34. Ransohoff, J.: Surgical management of metastatic tumors. Seminars Oncol., *2*:21–27, 1975.
35. Richards, G., Wara, W., Grumbach, M., Kaplan, S., Sheline, G., and Conte, F.: Delayed onset of hypopituitarism: Sequelae of therapeutic irradiation of central nervous system, eye, and middle ear tumors. J. Pediat., *89*:553–559, 1976.
36. Richmond, J.: Malignant tumours of the central nervous system. *In* Raven, R., ed.: Cancer 5. London, Butterworth & Co., 1959, pp. 375–389.
37. Ringertz, N., and Reymond, A.: Ependymomas and choroid plexus papillomas. J. Neuropath. Exp. Neurol., *8*:355–380, 1949.
38. Rubin, P., and Kramer, S.: Ectopic pinealoma: a radiocurable neuroendocrinologic entity. Radiology, *85*:512–523, 1965.
39. Rubinstein, L.: Tumors of the Central Nervous System. 2nd Series, Fascicle 6. Washington,

D.C., Armed Forces Institute of Pathology, 1972.

40. Rubinstein, L., and Northfield, D.: The medulloblastoma and the so-called "arachnoidal cerebellar sarcoma." Brain, *87*:379–412, 1964.

41. Schultz, M., Wang, C., Zinniger, G., and Tefft, M.: Radiotherapy of intracranial neoplasms. Progr. Neurol. Surg. *2*:318–370, 1968.

42. Sheline, G.: Conventional radiation therapy of gliomas. *In* Recent Results in Cancer Research. Gliomas. Current Concepts in Biology. Diagnosis and Therapy. New York, Springer-Verlag, 1975, pp. 123–234.

43. Sheline, G.: Radiation therapy of tumors of the central nervous system in childhood. Cancer, *35*:957–965, 1973.

44. Sheline, G.: Radiation therapy of brain tumors. Cancer, *39*:873–881, 1977.

45. Sheline, G., Boldrey, E., Karlsberg, P., and Phillips, T.: Therapeutic considerations in tumors affecting the central nervous system. Oligodendrogliomas. Radiology, *82*:84–89, 1964.

46. Sheline, G., Phillips, T., Field, S., et al.: Effects of fast neutrons on human skin. Amer. J. Roentgen., *111*:31–41, 1971.

47. Simson, L., Lampe, I., and Abell, M.: Suprasellar germinomas. Cancer, *22*:533–544, 1968.

48. Stage, W., and Stein, J.: Treatment of malignant astrocytomas. Amer. J. Roengten., *120*:7–18, 1974.

49. Svien, H., Gates, E., and Kernohan, J.: Spinal subarachnoid implantation associated with ependymoma. Arch. Neurol. Psychiat., *62*:847–856, 1949.

50. Svien, H., Mabon, R., Kernohan, J., and Craig, M.: Ependymoma of the brain—pathologic aspects. Neurology, *3*:1–13, 1953.

51. Tobias, C.: Pretherapeutic investigations with accelerated heavy ions. Radiology, *108*:145–158, 1973.

52. Uihlein, A., Colby, M., Layton, D., et al.: Comparison of surgery and surgery plus irradiation in the treatment of supratentorial gliomas. Acta Radiol., *5*:67–78, 1966.

53. Wara, W., Fellows, C., Sheline, G., et al.: Radiation therapy for pineal tumors and suprasellar germinomas. Radiology, *124*:221–223, 1977.

54. Wara, W., Sheline, G., Newman, H., et al.: Radiation therapy of meningiomas. Amer. J. Roentgen., *123*:453–458, 1975.

55. Withers, H.: Biological basis for high-LET radiotherapy. Radiology, *108*:131–137, 1973.

98

TUMORS OF THE
SELLA AND
PARASELLAR AREA
IN ADULTS

PITUITARY ADENOMAS

Embryology, Anatomy, and Structures of the Normal Pituitary Gland

Before closure of the anterior neuropore, which occurs in human gestation at the 20-somite stage (ovulation age: 26 days), a small ectodermal diverticulum called Rathke's pouch appears in the roof of the stomodeum, immediately in front of the buccopharyngeal membrane.[78,186] As the fetus develops, this pouch extends in front of the notochord and toward the diencephalon, gradually narrowing at its attachment to the pharyngeal roof as it elongates. Simultaneously, a downward growth—the infundibulum—develops from the floor of the diencephalon. During a later stage of gestation, the infundibulum gives rise to the stalk and the posterior lobe (pars nervosa) of the hypophysis. Its cells become pituicytes, which seem to have glial properties, and nerve fibers that later will carry neurosecretory material grow into the posterior lobe from the supraoptic and paraventricular nuclei.

Rathke's pouch and the infundibulum continue to grow toward one another until, during the final stages of fetal development, Rathke's pouch loses its attachment to the pharyngeal roof by the rupture of its original epithelial stalk. Remnants of this stalk, which are lobules of moderately differentiated epithelial cells, remain in this region throughout adulthood.[17] In the adult, some of these remnants form the pharyngeal hy-

pophysis, which is located in the roof of the epipharynx, immediately at the vomero-sphenoidal articulation. This microscopically small organ contains either active cells that produce growth hormone or inactivated squamous epithelium; very rarely, a craniopharyngioma or a pituitary adenoma originates from the pharyngeal hypophysis.[15,145,151]

After contact is established between Rathke's pouch and the infundibulum, Rathke's pouch undergoes great modification. The cells of its anterior wall proliferate and gradually compress the lumen of the pouch, which narrows to a cleft during fetal development. This cleft can usually be found in children, but it disappears before adulthood, leaving only a few small cysts.[186] The posterior part of Rathke's pouch, which is in direct contact with the pars nervosa and constitutes the pars intermedia, never develops, but remains thin. Beginning in the fetal period and continuing throughout childhood and adult life, its mucoid cells may slowly and progressively invade the posterior lobe. Tubular serous gland rests develop in the pars intermedia and adjacent pars nervosa in 49 per cent of men and 78 per cent of women.[181]

Cell proliferation in the anterior wall of Rathke's pouch produces the pars anterior of the hypophysis. The upper part of the pars anterior extends along the ventral aspect of the stalk and into the angle between the stalk and the chiasm. This extension is termed "pars tuberalis," although in humans it has no relation to the median em-

A. M. LANDOLT AND C. B. WILSON

inence of the tuber cinereum as it does in other mammals such as the cat. The pars tuberalis usually encircles the lower part of the hypophyseal stalk where nests of squamous cells, which occasionally contain keratinous entities that imitate microcraniopharyngiomas, may form. These squamous cell accumulations, which appear with advancing age and are more likely to be identified in older persons, have been found during autopsy in as few as 24 per cent and as many as 70 per cent of specimens.[48,135]

The first cells containing electron-dense hormone granules are visible under the electron microscope at 7.5 to 9 weeks of gestation.[45] During the following weeks, four distinct cell types can be differentiated, each characterized by a specific type of secretory granule. When grown in tissue culture, cells from the human fetal hypophysis taken during the tenth to the nineteenth weeks of gestation secrete somatotropic (growth) hormone (STH), thyroid-stimulating hormone (TSH), prolactin (PRL), follicle-stimulating hormone (FSH), and luteinizing hormone (LH) into the culture fluid. At this stage of gestation, the level of hormone production in pituitary cultures can be influenced by hypothalamic releasing factors.[66]

Adult Adenohypophysis

The normal adult adenohypophysis resembles a horizontally positioned kidney in shape, if the neurohypophysis is disregarded. It is yellowish orange, in contrast to the cherry-shaped posterior lobe and its stalk, which are whitish pink. Its diameters are 12 to 15 mm transversely, 8 to 10 mm sagittally, and 5 to 7 mm vertically. It occupies about 75 per cent of the normal sella, although the variations are quite considerable in this respect, and its average weight is 0.6 to 0.7 gm.[22] The hypophysis of a nonpregnant woman is about 100 mg heavier than that of a man; during pregnancy, its weight increases to an average of 0.8 to 1.0 gm.[186]

The pituitary is surrounded by the sphenoid bone on its anterior, inferior, and posterior surfaces; by the cavernous sinus on its lateral surfaces; and by the diaphragma sellae and the chiasmatic cistern and its contents on its superior surface. The configurations of these structures vary to a certain extent among normal individuals, and these variations must be taken into account by both the diagnostic radiologist and the surgeon in evaluating the patient who harbors a parasellar mass.

Sphenoid Bone

The sphenoid bone consists of the sphenoid body, the two alae magnae, the two alae parvae, and the pterygoid processes (Fig. 98–1). The sphenoid body contains the pituitary fossa, which is delineated in front by the tuberculum sellae and the transversely oriented chiasmatic sulcus. The limbus sphenoidalis separates the chiasmatic sulcus from the planum sphenoidale. The dorsum sellae and its two posterior clinoid processes form the posterior wall of the sella. The bony floor that separates the sella from the underlying sphenoid sinus extends from the tuberculum sellae in front to the base of the dorsum in back. The sphenoid sinus varies considerably in size, shape, and internal structure among adults, but three main types can be classified according to the extent to which the sphenoid bone is pneumatized (Fig. 98–2).[77] The *conchal type* sinus does not extend into the sphenoid body. It is small, and is separated from the sella turcica by spongy bone of up to 10 mm thickness. The conchal type is found in children, but in only 3 per cent of adults. The *presellar type,* which is found in 11 per cent of adults, does not penetrate beyond a plane perpendicular to the planum sphenoidale through the tuberculum sellae. For this reason, the anterior wall of the sella does not bulge into the sphenoid sinus in the presellar type as it does in the *sellar type.* The sellar type occurs in 86 per cent of adults; the thickness of the floor is 1 mm or less in 72 to 82 per cent, and even less than 0.5 mm in 40 per cent, of specimens.[12,183] In this type, the sinus can extend into the upper clivus, and occasionally it extends into the dorsum sellae (Fig. 98–3).

The sphenoid sinus is divided by a sagittal septum that is rarely located exactly at the midline, but is usually displaced toward one side or the other. The cavity is frequently subdivided by additional minor septae. The carotid arteries bulge into the superolateral wall of the sinus in 71 per cent of cases.[183] These arteries are usually covered by bone, but no bone separates the artery from the sinus mucosa in 4 per cent of

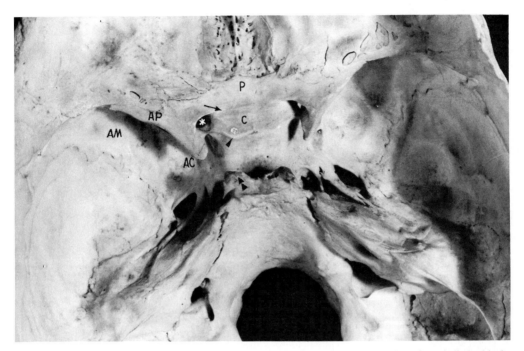

Figure 98–1 Topography of the sphenoid bone as seen from the vertex. The pituitary fossa is limited in front by the tuberculum sellae (*arrowhead*) and in the back by the dorsum sellae and the two posterior clinoid processes (*double arrowhead*). The limbus sphenoidalis (*arrow*) separates the planum sphenoidale (P) in front from the chiasmatic sulcus (C), which leads toward the optic foramen (*asterisk*). AP, ala parva; AM, ala magna; AC, anterior clinoid process. (Courtesy of Prof. S. Kubik, Department of Anatomy, University of Zurich, Switzerland.)

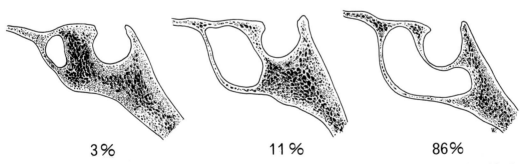

3%   11%   86%

Figure 98–2 Variations in extension of the sphenoid sinus into the body of the sphenoid bone found in the adult: The conchal type is seen in 3 per cent, the presellar type in 11 per cent, and the sellar type in 86 per cent of the normal adult population.

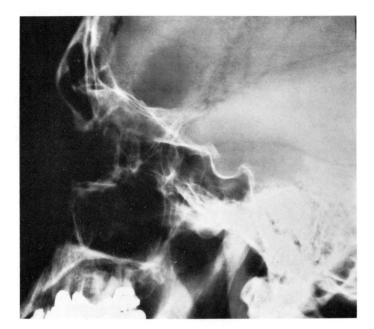

Figure 98–3 Lateral radiograph of a normal skull with a large sphenoid sinus extending into the dorsum sellae in a 61-year-old man.

cases. Two openings in the anterior wall of the sphenoid sinus connect the sinus with the nasal cavity. These foramina, right and left, are separated by the sphenoid rostrum.

The anatomy of the sellar region can be determined from lateral x-rays; the projections must be taken on a strictly perpendicular axis, which can be aligned easily by superposing the anterior clinoid processes.

The sellar floor usually appears as a single line of uniform thickness, and the anatomical landmarks can easily be seen. When the ligaments between the anterior clinoid, the middle clinoid (lateral to the tuberculum sellae), and the posterior clinoid processes have calcified, they are visible on the radiographs (Fig. 98–4).[94] Frontal projections are more difficult to analyze because the

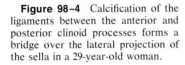

Figure 98–4 Calcification of the ligaments between the anterior and posterior clinoid processes forms a bridge over the lateral projection of the sella in a 29-year-old woman.

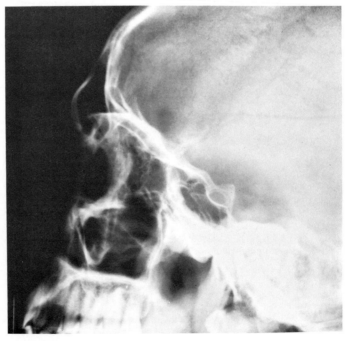

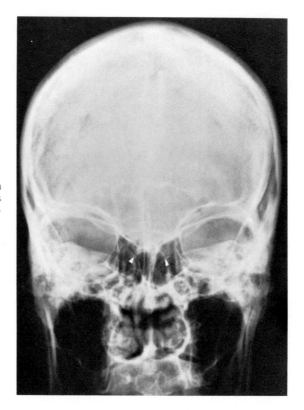

Figure 98–5 Radiograph of a normal skull in the anteroposterior projection. The sellar floor is visible behind the overlying ethmoid sinuses (*arrowheads*).

overlying structures of the ethmoid sinuses and the nose obscure the sellar region (Fig. 98–5).

In comparison with the information provided by x-ray projections, more precise anatomical data can be obtained from frontal tomograms, in which the sellar floor is seen extending between the two carotid sulci (Fig. 98–6). The floor is usually flat or slightly convex (bulging upward), but occasionally may be concave. It is most often symmetrical, although a slight asymmetry is not necessarily anomalous.[94,176] The sellar floor should be uniformly thick throughout; focal thinning of the floor, even in the absence of focal bulging, strongly suggests the presence of a microadenoma.

Cavernous Sinuses

The cavernous sinuses are situated lateral to both the sella and the sphenoid sinus, and extend down to the floor of the middle cranial fossa (Fig. 98–7). The carotid artery passes in the interior of the sinus, which is subdivided into several channels by numerous septae. The sixth nerve runs lateral to the artery. The oculo-

motor and trochlear nerves are situated in the upper lateral wall of the cavernous sinuses, whereas the first and the second di-

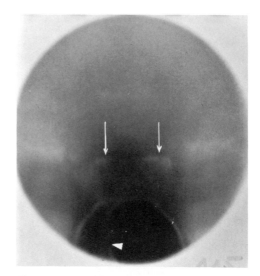

Figure 98–6 Frontal tomogram of a normal sella with a flat sellar floor in a 23-year-old woman. The septum of the sphenoid sinus is asymmetrical (*arrowhead*). The posterior clinoid processes are visible (*arrows*).

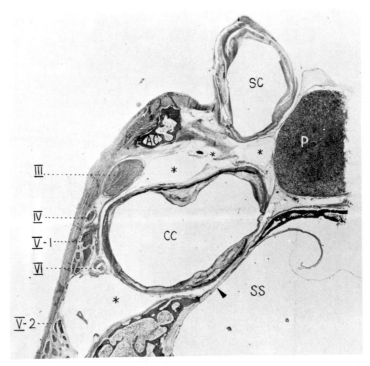

Figure 98–7 Histological section through the cavernous sinus near the tip of the anterior clinoid process (AC) shows the topography of the oculomotor (III), trochlear (IV), ophthalmic (V-1), mandibular (V-2) and abducens (VI) nerves. The cavernous (CC) and supraclinoid (SC) portions of the internal carotid artery show atheromatous vessel wall changes. Note the intimate relation of the carotid artery with the pituitary (P). There is no bone interposed between the sphenoid sinus (SS) and the carotid in this case (*arrowhead*). The cavernous sinus consists of four different venous channels (*asterisks*). (Courtesy of Prof. S. Kubik, Department of Anatomy, University of Zurich, Switzerland.)

visions of the trigeminal nerve are in the middle and inferior lateral wall. Although the average distance between the two carotid arteries in the cavernous sinus is 12 to 14 mm, the carotid siphons may be quite tortuous, swinging medially to within 4 mm of one another, or coursing laterally to an intercarotid distance of 23 mm. The intercavernous venous connections can traverse the anterior surface of the pituitary gland (76 to 85 per cent of cases) or the posterior surface (37 per cent of cases) or both.*

Diaphragma Sellae

The diaphragma sellae extends between the tuberculum and the dorsum sellae. The diaphragm is usually thick at its periphery and thinner toward its center. The shape of the diaphragm and the diameter of its central opening vary widely among individuals (Fig. 98–8).[22,183,197] As a rule, the subarach-

noid space of the chiasmatic cistern has only very narrow extensions below the diaphragm, but if the diaphragm does not cover the upper surface of the pituitary gland, these extensions of the subarachnoid space may enlarge into the sella, forming an "empty" sella.[53] When this is the case, the sella is usually enlarged, and pituitary tissue is spread out along its walls, the bulk of the tissue lying characteristically on the floor and the base of the dorsum sellae.

Optic Chiasm

The optic chiasm, shown in Figure 98–9, is located wholly over the diaphragm in only 12 per cent of cases; ordinarily it projects over only part of the diaphragm and part of the dorsum sellae (79 per cent).[197] Only rarely does the chiasm occupy the prefixed position (5 per cent), in which a part of the chiasm is situated over the chiasmatic sulcus and the remaining part rests on the diaphragm, or the postfixed position (4 per cent), in which it rests

---

* See references 12, 85, 168, 183.

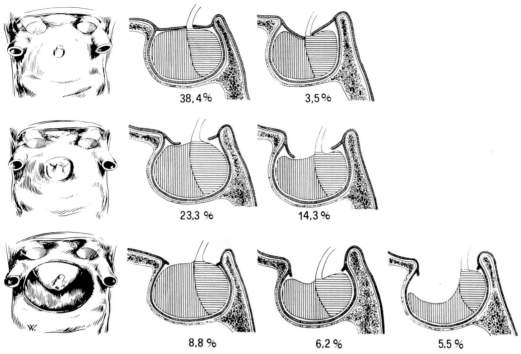

Figure 98–8   Variation and respective frequencies of the shape of the diaphragma sellae, the diameter of its central opening, and the size of the extension of the suprasellar cistern into the sella.

on and behind the dorsum sellae. The distance between the diaphragm and the basal surface of the chiasm may be very slight, the two surfaces being separated only by interposed arachnoid, or it may be as great as 10 mm.

Circle of Willis

The circle of Willis is heptagonal in shape and embraces the optic chiasm, the infundibulum, the tuber cinereum, the corpora mamillaria, and the posterior perforated space. Only the very large and tortuous posterior communicating arteries are in proximity to the sella and the optic tract.[197] The anterior cerebral artery usually crosses the optic nerves immediately in front of the optic chiasm, but frequently one artery or both lie in apposition to the chiasm (Fig. 98–10). The relation of the artery to the chiasm is not fixed. In cases of tumor growth, the artery can move forward or, more often, backward, which stretches the small feeding vessels that run to the chiasm from the internal carotid and anterior cerebral arteries.[11,41,143]

Blood Supply

The blood supply to the pituitary comes from three sources and is distributed by way of three vascular beds that are not connected by adequate anastomoses.[143,226,227] The inferior hypophyseal artery, which arises from the carotid artery within the cavernous sinus, supplies the posterior lobe and the immediately adjacent portion of the anterior lobe. The superior hypophyseal arteries, of which there are usually two or three on either side, branch from the internal carotid artery immediately after it has emerged from the dura mater at the medial side of the anterior clinoid process. They supply the inferior aspects of the optic nerves and the chiasm, forming a plexus at the base of the stalk. From this area, some of the vessels run freely within the subarachnoid space to the pituitary (loreal or trabecular arteries), while others enter the interior of the stalk. An interruption of the superior hypophyseal arteries during stalk section will cause large infarcts in the central part of the anterior pituitary gland.[39] The very small inferior and anterior capsular arteries, which also arise directly from

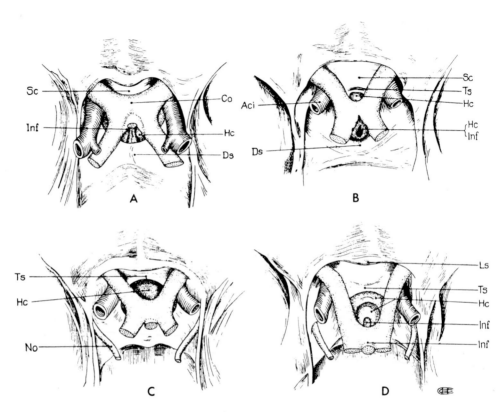

Figure 98–9   Variations of the relation between the optic chiasm and the sella turcica. *A*. A portion of the optic chiasm is located on the chiasmatic sulcus, the remaining portion rests upon the diaphragma sellae; this type is found in 5 per cent of autopsy cases. *B*. The optic chiasm is wholly located over the diaphragma sellae; this type is found in 12 per cent of autopsy cases. *C*. The optic chiasm is located almost wholly over the diaphragma sellae, and a small proportion projects onto the dorsum sellae; this type is found in 79 per cent of autopsy cases. *D*. The optic chiasm is located on and behind the dorsum sellae; this type is found in 4 per cent of autopsy cases. Sc, sulcus chiasmatis; Inf, infundibulum; Co, chiasma opticum; Hc, hypophysis cerebri; Ds, dorsum sellae; Aci, arteria carotis interna; Ts, tuberculum sellae; No, nervus oculomotorius; Ls, limbus sphenoidalis. (From Schaeffer, J. P.: Some points in the regional anatomy of the optic pathway, with special reference to tumors of the hypophysis cerebri and resulting ocular changes. Anat. Rec., *28*:243–279, 1924. Reprinted by permission.)

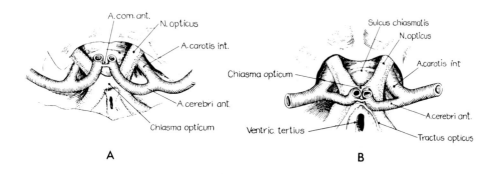

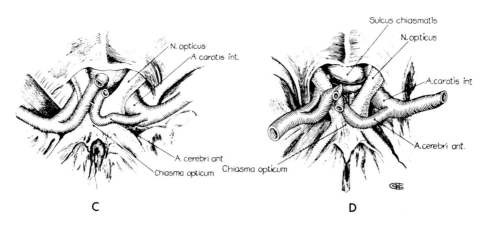

Figure 98–10 Variations of the anterior cerebral arteries in relation to the optic chiasm. *A*. Both anterior cerebral arteries cross the optic nerves immediately in front of the chiasm. *B*. Both anterior cerebral arteries are so placed that pressure could readily be brought to bear upon the uncrossed visual fibers. *C*. The right anterior cerebral artery cuts the optic chiasm in the sagittal plane, and the left artery comes in contact only with the optic nerve. It is apparent that the right artery might interrupt the chiasmal fibers. *D*. The right anterior cerebral artery has a chiasmal relation and the left crosses the optic nerve well in advance of the chiasm. (From Schaeffer, J. P.: Some points in the regional anatomy of the optic pathway, with special reference to tumors of the hypophysis cerebri and resulting ocular changes. Anat. Rec., *28*:243–279, 1924. Reprinted by permission.)

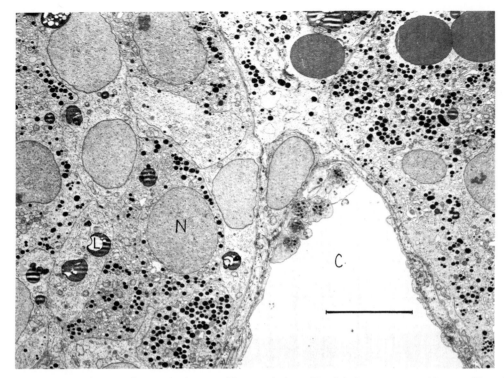

Figure 98–11   Electron micrograph of a normal human pituitary. Two lobules are separated by a capillary, C. They consist of tightly accumulated secretory cells containing round nuclei, N; lipid droplets, L; and innumerable black secretory granules. Scale 1 μ.

the internal carotid, supply only a small area at the margin of the gland. The venous drainage from the pituitary leads first to capsular veins, and from there directly into the cavernous and intercavernous sinuses.

Microscopic Anatomy

Histological sectioning reveals that the anterior lobe is composed of a network of branching lobules, which are composed of epithelial cells that are surrounded by a thin layer of connective tissue, and interjacent sinusoids. Although these lobules contain only three types of cell—eosinophilic, basophilic, and chromophobic—according to much of the literature, Romeis demonstrated at least six types of cell that can be differentiated with more sophisticated staining methods using up to four different dyes.[7,65,87,177,186] Each of four of these cell types produces a separate hormone. The fifth, a specific cell type that has distinct staining properties, produces the two gonadotropic hormones, follicle-stimulating hormone (FSH) and luteinizing hormone (LH). The sixth delineates the small colloid follicles. During their secretory cycle, these cells accumulate and release their secretory products, and correspondingly undergo changes in their affinity to dyes. These alterations are evident, for example, in the chromophilic cell, which becomes chromophobic as its cytoplasmic secretory granules are depleted.

Electron micrographs of the human hypophysis show that the lobules of the anterior lobe are packed with secretory cells that are characterized by secretory granules of different sizes and electron densities (Fig. 98–11). Several authors have suggested that the size of the granules within a cell may indicate the specific tropic hormone that it contains, but more recent observations suggest that the granules within cells belonging to the same category may be larger when at rest than during their phase of secretory activity.*

In addition to the granule-containing, hormone-producing cells, the hypophysis also contains an ungranulated cell type that forms the margin of the colloid-containing follicles. This is the only true chromophobe

---

* See references 12, 56, 88, 130, 167, 171, 195.

cell. It does not seem to have secretory properties.

At the present time, cell types in the normal and adenomatous pituitary gland can be unequivocally identified by means of immunohistological techniques. The hormone granules within the cells are coupled to a marker (fluorescein or peroxidase, rarely ferritin) through the action of a specific antihormone antibody, after which they can be specifically identified by either light or electron microscopy.* The evidence obtained by these methods has confirmed that, with the exception of two hormones (FSH and LH), which are produced by the gonadotropic cell, each pituitary hormone —prolactin, somatotropin, thyrotropin, corticotropin, and melanocyte-stimulating hormone (MSH)—is produced by an individual, specific cell type.

Pathology of Pituitary Adenomas

Historical Background

Pituitary adenomas are the only true primary adenomas of the cranial cavity and, for this reason, belong to the class of epithelial neoplasms. In 1839, Bressler mentioned three cases of "pituitary cancer."[18] During the latter part of the nineteenth century, the interest in pituitary tumors increased as descriptions of acromegaly appeared in the literature.[62,138,213] These neoplasms were considered an acromegalic enlargement of the hypophysis resulting from an unknown growth-stimulating factor until Gubler, in 1900, and Fraenkel and colleagues, in 1901, reported that the pituitary adenoma represented the primary lesion causing abnormal growth throughout the body.[59,69]

Staining Properties of Adenomas

Dott and collaborators in 1925 and Erdheim in 1926 correlated the staining properties of the adenoma that were seen in histological sections with certain clinical syndromes.[44,48] Dott differentiated the chromophobic adenomas, which he associated with various degrees of pituitary insufficiency, from the eosinophilic adenomas that cause signs of hypophyseal hyperfunc-

tion (acromegaly and gigantism). Shortly thereafter, in 1928, Bailey and Cushing described a mixed-type adenoma that contained a mixture of eosinophil and chromophobe cells, and that produced simultaneous signs of increased and decreased pituitary function, as represented by acromegalic dyspituitarism.[5] The clinical significance of the basophilic adenoma was first recognized by Cushing in 1932.[35]

Erdheim's scheme for classifying adenomas was similar to that of Dott and his colleagues, but it included the "pregnancy-cell adenoma," which had been first described by Kraus.[44,48,115] Although later authors rejected the validity of the "pregnancy-cell adenoma," it is now known to be a prolactinoma and is beginning to receive increased attention (see the section on endocrine-active adenomas).[104,230]

Architectural Classification of Adenomas

Three architectural types of pituitary adenomas have been differentiated on the basis of the distribution of connective tissue and blood vessels observed in histological sections of the tumor (Figs. 98–12 to 98–14).[104,161] The frequency of occurrence for each type has been reported by Nurnberger and Korey.[161] The *diffuse type* (54 per cent) has little stroma and few blood vessels dispersed among uniform cells that lack any specific architectural arrangement. The structure of the *sinusoidal type* (31 per cent) is similar to that of the normal pituitary gland, except that it has more cells per lobule, and all the cells are of the same type; the septa between the irregular lobules in this type are often incomplete. The third variety, the *papillary type* (15 per cent), displays centrally located capillaries with some connective tissue, and the adenoma cells, occasionally four to five layers deep, radiate away from this core. This type can be mistaken for an ependymoma. Many adenomas do not have a uniform structure, but comprise two or occasionally all three types, with one type predominating.

From the neurosurgeon's perspective, the architectural classification has only a limited value because it distinguishes no anamnestic, clinical, or prognostic differences. The surgeon differentiates adenomas on a pragmatic basis: The diffuse-

---

* See references 65, 102, 140, 147, 155, 156.

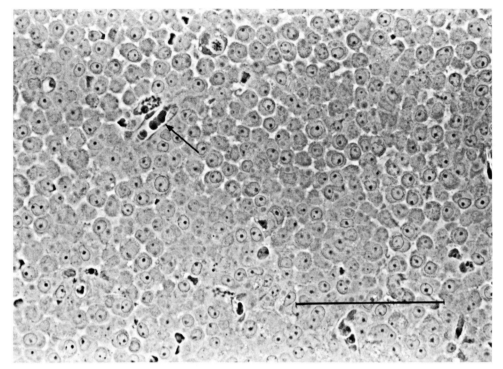

Figure 98–12 A diffuse adenoma obtained from a patient suffering from acromegaly shows a dense accumulation of uniform cells with only a few interposed capillaries (*arrow*) and no collagenous stroma. Phase-contrast micrograph of osmium-fixed, plastic-embedded tissue. Scale 100 μ.

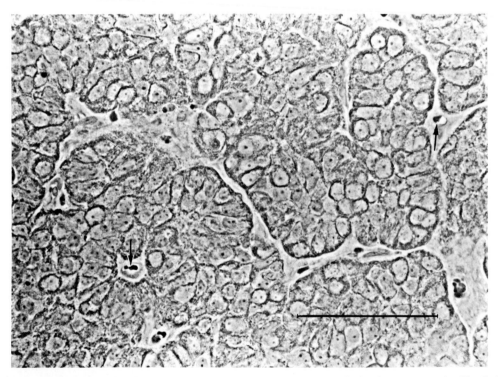

Figure 98–13 Sinusoidal-type adenoma tissue obtained from a patient suffering from acromegaly. The finely granular cells form irregular lobules with interposed connective tissue and capillaries (*arrows*). Phase-contrast micrograph of osmium-fixed, plastic-embedded biopsy. Scale 100 μ.

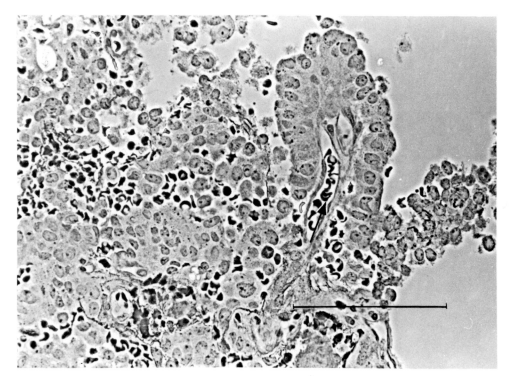

Figure 98–14   Papillary-type adenoma without endocrine activity. The adenoma cells radiate away from a central capillary (*arrow*). Phase-contrast micrograph of osmium-fixed, plastic-embedded tissue. Scale 100 μ.

type adenoma is soft and can be removed easily by suction, whereas the sinusoidal type may have almost the same consistency as the normal gland, which makes its selective removal more difficult. In the sinusoidal type, normal tissue can be differentiated from adenomatous tissue only by the difference in color; the adenoma is paler and is grayish pink, whereas the normal gland is yellowish orange.

Secretory Properties of Adenomas

After Romeis observed that the normal pituitary contains more than three different cell types, various additional findings were reported that indicated that the eosinophil-basophil-chromophobe classification was an inadequate scheme for differentiating pituitary adenomas.[186] Forbes and colleagues reported that the amenorrhea-galactorrhea syndrome is caused by prolactin-secreting eosinophilic or chromophobic adenomas.[58] (See also Chapter 25.) Thyrotropic adenomas were defined as either chromophobic or basophilic. Chromophobic and amphophilic (staining with acid as well as with alkaline dyes) adenomas were differen-

tiated in extremely rare cases of hypergonadotropism. When the experiments of McCormick and Halmi clearly demonstrated that improved fixation and staining techniques could show the presence of stainable granules in almost every one of their series of 145 unselected pituitary adenomas, the designation "chromophobe" adenoma lost its original significance.[144] These descriptions of new hormone entities that augmented Romeis's observations rendered the former nomenclature obsolete, since the relation between histological findings and clinical observations that had been established ceased to have any meaning.

Even the earliest ultrastructural examinations of pituitary adenoma biopsies, which were undertaken in the early 1960's, revealed secretory granules in all specimens examined, regardless of whether or not the patient had signs of endocrine hyperfunction (Figs. 98–15 through 98–17).* The release of the secretory granule contents into the intercellular space is visible in

---

* See references 57, 74, 133, 134, 164, 174, 178, 198, 217.

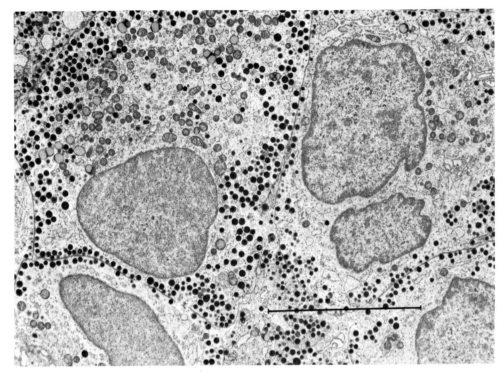

Figure 98–15   Electron micrograph of a pituitary adenoma with dense intracellular accumulation of black secretory granules obtained from a patient suffering from acromegaly. Scale 10 μ.

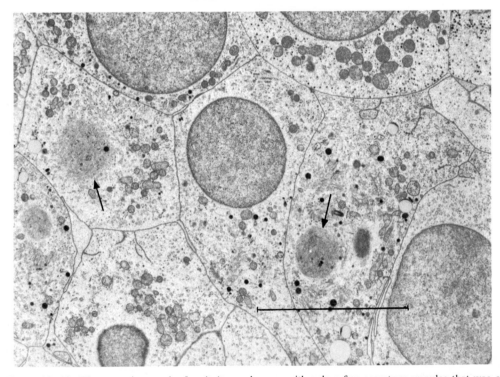

Figure 98–16   Electron micrograph of a pituitary adenoma with only a few secretory granules that was obtained from a patient suffering from acromegaly (compare with Figure 98–15). The arrows point to intracytoplasmic
aggregations of filaments that are typical for acromegaly. Scale 10 μ.

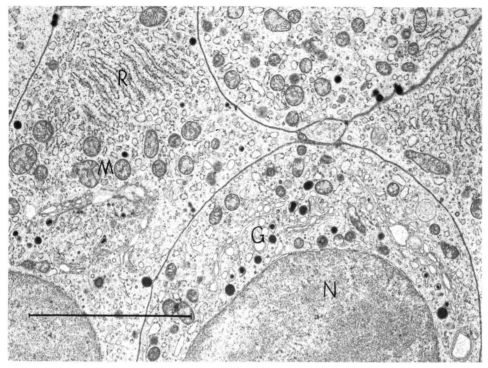

Figure 98–17 Electron micrograph of prolactinoma cells that demonstrate active hormone synthesis. N, cell nucleus; G, Golgi apparatus; R, rough-surfaced endoplasmic reticulum; M, mitochondria. The black secretory granules vary in size and shape. Scale 5 μ.

all but a very few cases of pituitary adenomas (Fig. 98–18). The membrane of the hormone granule fuses with the cell membrane, and an opening develops at the point of contact through which the contents of the granule spill into the intercellular space, where they are quickly dissolved.[51] This process is called exocytosis.

The number and size of the granules stored in the interior of the adenoma cells vary from case to case, even within one nosological group, such as acromegaly (cf. Figs. 98–15 and 98–16). As several authors have noted, hormone identification cannot be determined on the basis of granule size, since the granules usually are larger in cells containing many granules than they are in cells that have only a few granules.[118] For example, one comparative immunohistological examination revealed that growth hormone can be identified in all biopsy specimens that have cells containing a great variety of granule sizes, provided that all the biopsies have been obtained from acromegalic patients.[124] A comparison of the morphological findings with the results of radioimmunological hormone determinations

showed that the size and number of granules in the adenoma cells depend on the rate of granule formation and exocytosis rather than on the nature of the hormone that the cell contains.[118] Certain morphological features of the granules may, however, provide an insight into the secretory activity of the adenoma.[120]

Functional Terminology

Neither light nor electron microscopy provides a reliable means by which to determine the hormone type of a given adenoma. Only immunohistological techniques can provide an accurate determination, and the results obtained can be correlated easily with both clinical and endocrinological data. These three forms of data constitute the basis for the functional classification of hypophyseal adenomas described in Table 98–1.

The first group of adenomas in the authors' classification system produces signs of endocrine hyperfunction that become apparent either on clinical examination or endocrinological testing. The second group

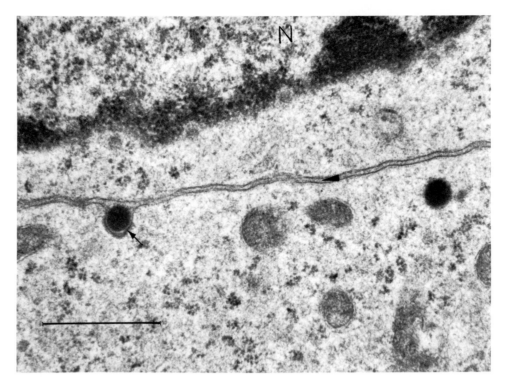

Figure 98-18 Extrusion by exocytosis of a prolactin granule from a prolactinoma cell (*arrow*). The arrowhead indicates intercellular space. N, cell nucleus. Scale 0.1 μ.

produces the signs of a space-occupying lesion, and hormone determinations yield values that are either within or below normal limits. These neoplasms are designated "adenomas without endocrine activity," or "endocrine-inactive adenomas."

TABLE 98-1 FUNCTIONAL CLASSIFICATION OF HUMAN PITUITARY ADENOMAS

PITUITARY ADENOMAS	ESTIMATED FREQUENCY (PER CENT)
Adenomas with signs of endocrine activity	
Somatotropic adenomas: acromegaly, gigantism	25
Prolactinomas	35
Corticotropic adenomas: Cushing's, Nelson's syndromes	5
Thyrotropic adenomas (rare)	< 1
Gonadotropic adenomas (rare)	< 1
Adenomas producing several hormones: STH–PRL, ACTH–PRL, PRL–TSH	10
Adenomas lacking signs of endocrine activity (no endocrine hypersecretion)	
Oncocytomas	5
Adenomas producing small amount of normal hormones: STH, PRL	5
Adenomas producing abnormal substances	15

Endocrine-Active Adenomas

SOMATOTROPIC ADENOMAS. The adenoma that causes either acromegaly or gigantism was once reported to occur most frequently of all the adenomas characterized by endocrine activity. Cushing reported that their incidence was 28 per cent of all pituitary adenomas; Tönnis and colleagues, 28 per cent; Bailey, 25 per cent; Grant, 14 per cent; and Kernohan and Sayre, 11 per cent.[4,36,68,104,208] Since the rediscovery of the prolactin-producing adenoma, however, this is no longer the case.

The round or polygonal cells of the somatotropic adenoma are either densely or sparsely granulated, and on this basis, they correspond respectively to the eosinophil and chromophobe in the terminology of light microscopists (cf. Figs. 98–15 and 98–16). Spherical, intracytoplasmic aggregates of filaments are characteristic of this type of adenoma, but are found only in about 55 per cent of cases.[23,178] Tubular inclusions in the perinuclear cistern of the endothelial cells of the adenoma are found in 30 per cent of cases associated with acromegaly, and in only 2 per cent of other adenoma types; one case has been reported in which these inclusions were associated with a thyrotropic adenoma.[32,112,127]

PROLACTINOMAS. Prolactinomas were considered rare until the radioimmunological blood prolactin assay became available (see Chapter 25). Initially, it was thought that prolactinomas were responsible only for the amenorrhea-galactorrhea syndrome.[58] However, a systematic examination of the blood from patients whose seemingly "inactive" adenomas produced amenorrhea but no galactorrhea in the women, and impotency but only one case of gynecomastia in the men, revealed that prolactin levels were elevated (up to 1950 ng per milliliter, normal upper limit 15 ng per milliliter) in 30 to 60 per cent of the patients.[95,126] This new entity was anticipated in the work of Peillon and collaborators, who showed that stimulating certain adenomas with estrogens caused headaches, progressive visual deficits, and histological signs of tumor proliferation with interstitial hemorrhage.[170]

Ultrastructural examination of prolactinomas, which stain with erythrosin, reveals a cellular composition similar to that seen in acromegaly, with a wide variation in the number and size of the stored secretory granules (cf. Fig. 98–17).* The exocytosis of secretory granules not only occurs on the cell walls oriented toward the nearest capillary, as it does in the normal pituitary, but it also is observed frequently on the whole cell circumference. It is this phenomenon that Horvath and Kovacs have termed "misplaced exocytosis."[93] The presence of prolactin in these secretory granules can be observed by both light and electron microscopy.[111,126] The rare instances of dystropic intra-adenomatous calcification in pituitary adenomas occurs only in prolactinomas.[125]

CORTICOTROPIC ADENOMAS. These adenomas manifest their presence by either Cushing's disease or Nelson's syndrome.[35,158] The clinical features are discussed in Chapter 25.

Although features of the adenoma that produces Cushing's disease differ somewhat from those that produce Nelson's syndrome, both types contain cells that have a large number of moderately electron-dense, ACTH-containing granules. In Cushing's

syndrome, chronically elevated levels of glucocorticoids in the blood—which may be of either endogenous or exogenous origin—produce a perinuclear hyalin halo in both normal and neoplastic corticotrophs. These changes, which were described by Crooke in 1935, can be observed in about 55 per cent of Cushing's adenomas; however, Crooke's cells do not occur in the adenoma of Nelson's syndrome because, in this condition, the glucocorticoid levels achieved by replacement therapy are normal.[30,118,193]

THYROTROPIC ADENOMAS. The two types of thyrotropic adenomas can be differentiated clinically.[118] The type that is associated with hyperthyroidism does not respond well to thyrostatic treatment.[148] The other type occurs in patients who have had long-standing hypothyroidism and is probably caused by chronic hypothalamic stimulation of the pituitary. These adenomas exhibit no characteristic staining behavior under the light microscope unless specifically designed procedures are used.[132]

GONADOTROPIC ADENOMAS. These are extremely rare; nine cases have been reported in the literature.[31,61,64,202,224] Follicle-stimulating hormone production was observed in four of the adenomas, and was combined with luteinizing hormone production in three others, and with prolactin production in one additional case. One adenoma secreted only luteinizing hormone.

About 10 per cent of the endocrine-active adenomas secrete two hormones at the same time. Galactorrhea caused by accompanying prolactin secretion is not unusual in women suffering from acromegaly, and secretion of prolactin in combination with adrenocorticotropin, thyrotropin, or luteinizing hormone has been observed.[40,122] The prolactin found in these patients could originate from two sources: The adenoma, which produces only growth hormone, presses on the pituitary stalk circulation, impeding the flow of blood. Disconnected from its source of hypothalamic inhibition, the remaining normal pituitary gland is free to produce excess prolactin. Alternatively, prolactin and growth hormone can be secreted by the adenoma itself. It has not been established yet whether both hormones are secreted by the same cell type, or whether there are two cell lines, each one of which is responsible for the production of one specific hormone, al-

---

* See references 87, 118, 126, 169, 185, 209.

though the evidence favors the former hypothesis.

Endocrine-Inactive Adenomas

This type of adenoma, which originally was termed the "chromophobe" adenoma, once represented the largest group; a frequency of occurrence ranging from 72 to 89 per cent has been reported.[36,104,208] As modern techniques have supplied more precise endocrinological data, the number of adenomas that manifest no endocrine hyperfunction and that produce only signs of a mass accompanied by either no endocrine disturbance or various degrees of hypopituitarism, has decreased to only 25 per cent of all pituitary adenomas (see Table 98–1).[97] Several subtypes of the endocrine-inactive adenoma can be differentiated.

ONCOCYTOMAS. These tumors composed of cells containing a shrunken nucleus and a swollen, finely granular cytoplasm that stains with eosin, were first identified in locations other than the pituitary by Hamperl.[79] Only recently have they been described in the pituitary gland.[110,123] Oncocytomas represent about 5 per cent of pituitary adenomas. Their cytoplasm is filled with abnormal, metabolically defective mitochondria that have a strong affinity to eosin, even though they lack secretory granules.[197] Because oncocytomas seem to be unable to secrete hormones as a consequence of their metabolic defect, they represent the prototype of the original "chromophobe" adenoma, in spite of their eosinophilia. They may originate from the normally occurring oncocytes in the unaltered pituitary gland or from neoplastic oncocytes, which occasionally are seen in other types of adenomas; some authors have suggested that they may originate from the tubular serous gland rests connected to the intermediate lobe.[150,167,201]

In most endocrine-inactive adenomas, the process of formation and release of hormone granules takes place just as it does in the endocrine-active group; however, there are fewer cytoplasmic secretory granules, and their diameters are usually smaller, in the inactive group. Histoimmunology has afforded the means to differentiate among the adenomas in this group. About one fourth of them, or about 5 per cent of all adenomas, show a positive reaction with either growth hormone or prolactin antibodies, even though they are not associated with signs of acromegaly or an elevation of corresponding hormones in the blood.[107,229] On the basis of this evidence, it must be assumed that these adenomas produce growth hormone or prolactin, but only in amounts that are too small to produce elevated blood levels and clinical manifestations.[196]

The true nature of the remaining 15 per cent of the endocrine-inactive adenomas has not been established. Possibly these neoplasms produce abnormal substances that fail to react with the specific antibody used in radioimmunoassay and immunohistological study, or perhaps these substances are not recognized by the biological receptor.

Gross Pathology

Microscopic, subclinical adenomas and hyperplasias have been found in 10 to 25 per cent of routine autopsies performed on patients who had no antemortem evidence of an endocrine disorder.[28,187] The assumption that pituitary adenomas originate from these entities is substantiated by the similar age distribution among the patients who have incidental microlesions and those who have the larger, clinically observed adenomas.[153] Before the patient becomes aware of an endocrine disturbance and seeks medical help, the responsible adenoma usually has grown to a diameter of 3 to 5 mm.

Microadenomas

The microadenomas (diameter by definition less than 10 mm) that can be clinically detected all lie entirely within the sella turcica but, with few exceptions, deform the surrounding bony structures of the sella and diaphragm to some extent. Small adenomas in the anterior lobe have no demonstrable capsule. What appears to be a capsule encasing the larger adenomas is actually a condensation and tangential rearrangement of the normal lobules surrounding the adenoma. Under the microscope, the boundary between the normal gland tissue and the neoplastic tissue may appear quite sharp, or it may be poorly defined (Figs. 98–19 and 98–20). Corticotropic adenomas are often more poorly defined than the other adenomas. A

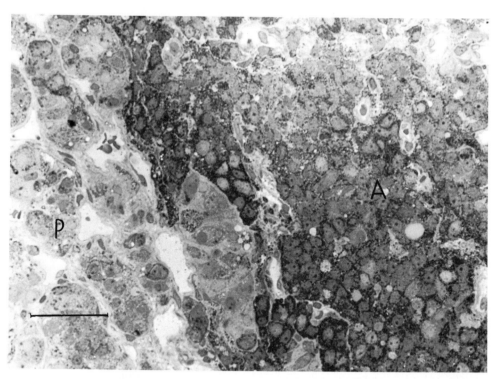

Figure 98–19 Sharp boundary between the adenoma (A) and the normal pituitary tissue (P) in a biopsy obtained from an acromegalic patient. Osmium fixation, plastic embedding, toluidine blue staining. Scale 100 μ. (From Landolt, A. M.: Progress in pituitary adenoma biology. Results of research and clinical applications. *In* Krayenbühl, H., ed.: Advances and Technical Standards in Neurosurgery. Vol. 5. Wien, New York, Springer-Verlag, 1978, pp. 3–49. Reprinted by permission.)

"pseudocapsule" only occasionally forms from the remaining connective tissue after the secretory cells of the compressed normal pituitary have disappeared.

The different types of hypersecreting microadenomas are located in preferential sites within the remaining normal pituitary gland. The somatotropic and lactotropic (prolactin-producing) microadenomas are usually situated in the laterobasal part of the gland. Somatotropic growths occupy a lateral position in a more anterior site. The microadenomas associated with Cushing's disease often lie in the central core of the remaining gland, but may occupy the posterior lobe or lateral wing of the anterior lobe. Hardy has reported a single thyrotropic microadenoma located in the central area near the surface of the gland.[81] This distribution of secreting adenomas is not surprising, since it coincides with the preferential distribution of the corresponding cells in the normal gland.[7,75]

Further growth of the microadenoma occurs first within the sella and causes the sella to enlarge. The floor bulges downward into the sphenoid sinus. The dorsum sellae may become thin on only one side at first, but in time it becomes uniformly thinned and undercut. These changes result in a *ballooned sella,* the presence of which indicates that the adenoma is no longer in the microadenoma stage. At this time, the cavernous and intercavernous sinuses are compressed, but the dura forming the lateral walls of the sella turcica is much more resistant to pressure from the adenoma than are the floor and the diaphragm, and is displaced only slightly.

Extrasellar Expansion and Invasion

As the adenoma continues to grow, it expands into the extrasellar spaces. At first, it is usually expansive, and only later becomes invasive, but there is no rule by which to predict when the invasion of the surrounding structures will begin.[72] Extrasellar expansion occurs most often in an upward direction. The diaphragm bulges and

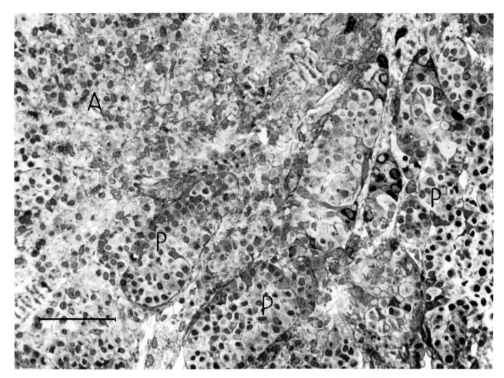

Figure 98–20 Invasion of adenoma cells (A) between lobules of the normal anterior pituitary (P) in a patient suffering from Nelson's syndrome. Osmium fixation, plastic embedding, toluidine blue staining. Scale 100 μ. (From Landolt, A. M.: Progress in pituitary adenoma biology. Results of research and clinical applications. *In* Krayenbühl, H., ed.: Advances and Technical Standards in Neurosurgery. Vol. 5. Wien, New York, Springer-Verlag, 1978, pp. 3–49. Reprinted by permission.)

becomes thin; although surgeons approaching a pituitary adenoma transcranially often refer to the diaphragm as "tumor capsule," this is a misnomer. The adenoma pushes the chiasm up against the anterior cerebral and anterior communicating arteries, stretching them until they are taut, and their restrictive force may produce a notch in the chiasm. The resulting deformation of the chiasm is thought to cause the bitemporal hemianopia that afflicts patients during this stage of tumor development.[190] Further growth ultimately leads to compression of the anterior part of the third ventricle, and eventually the tumor may extend to the foramen of Monro.

The adenoma can reach through clefts that are normally quite narrow, and after traversing a restricted passageway, it may enlarge considerably. Four superior extensions in the suprasellar space are recognized: The adenoma usually reaches out between the optic nerves in front of a post-fixed chiasm and, in the case of the *subfrontal extension*, extends along the floor of the anterior cranial fossa. This tumor extension may produce deformities of one or both anterior horns of the ventricles. The *lateral extension* may pass between the chiasm above and the carotid artery below, or alternatively, it may extend between the carotid above and the upper edge of the cavernous sinus below, usually compressing the oculomotor nerve. The *posterior extension* reaches over the dorsum sellae into the interpeduncular fossa and may eventually grow down along the clivus (see Fig. 98–32).[72,104,230] The *inferior extensions* grow into the sphenoid sinus and eventually may occupy this area completely. The bony floor of the sella may disappear entirely, but the periosteum and the sinus mucosa remain intact.

Invasive adenomas are found in about 5 per cent of all cases. The growth of invasive tumors may be either localized or generalized.[96,230] As the tumor traverses the dura of the sellar floor, the downward invasive growth may completely destroy the sphenoid sinus and extend into the nasal cavity.

Growth in a more posterior direction culminates in destruction of the clivus and further extradural growth into the posterior cranial fossa. Lateral invasion into the cavernous sinus causes disturbances of the third, fourth, fifth, and sixth cranial nerves —the third nerve is the one most frequently affected—and may cause papilledema and ipsilateral exophthalmus (Fig. 98–21). The tumor may then progress from the sinus on an extradural route to the floor of the middle cranial fossa and may invade the temporal lobe after traversing the dural barrier a second time. Invasion of the dura and arachnoid of the diaphragm gives the tumor direct access to the subarachnoid space, where it may give rise to metastases.

All types of endocrine-active adenomas are capable of invasive growth, but ACTH-secreting tumors seem to be relatively more inclined to exhibit this behavior. Although invasiveness has been considered a sign of malignancy, Bailey suggested that invasiveness alone was not a sufficient criterion by which to define malignancy.[4,96,159]

Metastasis

Metastases are an undisputed sign of malignancy. Although the pituitary gland may be the site of metastases from extracranial cancer (most frequently breast cancer, but also bronchial, prostatic, intestinal, uterine, and pharyngeal cancers), pituitary neoplasms rarely metastasize to other areas of the body. When metastases from the pituitary do occur, they do so by way of the subarachnoid space (48 per cent), the lymphatic system and the bloodstream (44 per cent), or both simultaneously (8 per cent).[118] The likelihood of subarachnoid spread is greater in patients who have undergone operative treatment of an adenoma.

Most metastases from the pituitary have been found in the liver (72 per cent) and lymph nodes (18 per cent), but they have been noted in bone, kidney, bladder, uterus, vagina, heart, and lung as well. Metastatic spread occurs relatively more often in association with corticotropic

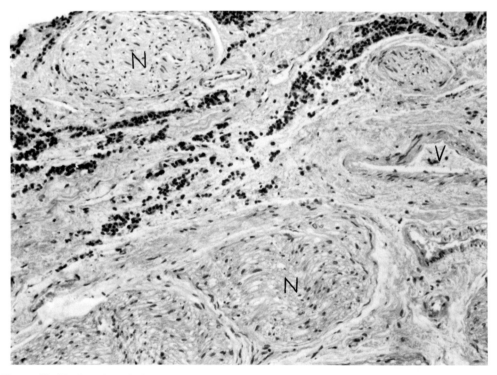

Figure 98–21 Invasion of adenoma cells between the nerve fiber bundles (N) and blood vessels (V) of the cavernous sinus in a patient suffering from amenorrhea-galactorrhea syndrome. Autopsy material, formalin fixation, paraffin embedding, hematoxylin-eosin staining. (Courtesy of Prof. C. Hedinger, Department of Pathology, University of Zurich, Switzerland.)

adenomas (20 per cent) than with acromegaly (12 per cent) or "inactive" adenomas (68 per cent). Because these inactive adenomas were considered chromophobes at the time of this series, prolactin levels in the blood were not determined.[118]

Histological studies of metastatic pituitary tumors and invasive adenomas have revealed an abnormal cellular pattern exhibiting such features as polymorphism of cells and nuclei, multiple nucleoli, greater numbers of mitoses, and an absence of stainable granules.* Because all these features have been observed in strictly localized lesions, however, their presence is not necessarily a proof of malignancy.[5,19,159,184] The authors' experience and a review of the reported cases have led to the conclusion that histological techniques do not afford a reliable means by which to characterize the biological behavior of a tumor.

Tumors of the Neurohypophysis

The neurohypophysis is the secondary site of astrocytomas and ependymomas spreading from the diencephalon and third ventricle. It is the primary site of the granular cell myoblastoma (choristoma), of which 21 cases have been described.[118] The neurohypophyseal tumor was first described by Lüthy and Klingler in 1951.[136] This type of tumor consists of large round or oval cells and spindle-shaped cells. The nuclear structure of these cells is dense, and their cytoplasm contains many small granules that produce positive histochemical reactions for protein, lipids, and polysaccharides that are positive to the periodic acid–Schiff (PAS) stain. Electron microscope studies show that these granules are lysosomal in nature. Neurohypophyseal tumors seem to originate from microscopic "choristomas," which have been found in 1.8 to 17 per cent of routine autopsies.[135,203]

Etiology of Pituitary Adenomas

In theory, pituitary adenomas could arise either spontaneously or in response to peripheral (target organ) or central (hypothalamic) disorders. The origin is an important factor to consider in determining appropri-

---

* See references 3, 44, 52, 60, 86, 96, 104, 105, 142, 223.

ate therapy because selective extirpation of a pituitary adenoma that is produced by hypothalamic stimulation must be accompanied by treatment to correct the basic regulatory disorder, or there is risk of a second adenoma's developing. Secondary pituitary tumors that arise in association with hypothyroidism can be treated by the addition of an adequate amount of thyroid hormone, which causes these tumors to regress to the extent that compression of the optic chiasm is relieved.[131] The enlarged pituitary produces abnormal amounts of thyrotropic hormone, and the mass represents hyperplastic rather than neoplastic thyrotropin-secreting cells that remain responsive to inhibition and stimulation by hypothalamic and peripheral factors.[70]

Prolactinomas can be easily induced in experimental animals by the administration of large doses of estrogens.[47,63] The dosages used for contraceptive purposes in humans, however, are about 100 to 500 times as small as those used in experimental animals, and there is as yet no proof that these dosage levels are capable of inducing pituitary adenomas in humans. Our observations of women in whom prolactinomas were found after they discontinued the use of birth-control pills are inconclusive. Since most of these women had complained of menstrual irregularities before they began using the drug, it is not clear whether they harbored the prolactinomas before they began using the contraceptive, or whether the growth of the prolactinomas was stimulated by the drug. Nonetheless, it is clear that the higher dosages of estrogens used for therapeutic purposes are capable of stimulating a pre-existing prolactinoma.[170]

The number of prolactin cells may be increased in the normal gland surrounding a prolactinoma, just as the number of corticotropic cells may be increased in the para-adenomatous tissue in patients who have Cushing's or Nelson's disease. This finding has suggested to some that a hypothalamic factor may initiate these adenomas.[194]

The normal pituitary readily reacts to extrapituitary stimuli induced by either diffuse or nodular hyperplasia; this reaction causes the pituitary enlargement that takes place during pregnancy.[49] A similar reaction occurs after partial destruction of the pituitary gland; however, because the nodular hyperplasias in partially destroyed glands are fully hypothalamodependent, they cannot be considered "adenomas."[116] An occasional "subclinical microadenoma," the origin of which can be compared to that of the functional hyperplasias, may become independent of hypothalamic influence, begin to grow, and produce abnormal amounts of one or more hormones.[28] The loss of hypothalamic dependence may be gradual, as it is in cases of acromegaly, for example. During glucose tolerance tests, adenomas in acromegalic patients may respond with a decrease in growth hormone production, may show no reaction at all, or paradoxically, may produce an increase of the hormone. It seems reasonable to propose that subclinical microadenomas remain under hypothalamic inhibitory control, whereas autonomous, enlarging pituitary adenomas have, to varying degrees, escaped from hypothalamic influence. Clearly, not every subclinical microadenoma will eventually develop into an autonomous pituitary adenoma during the host's lifetime.

Symptoms and Findings in Pituitary Adenomas

Clinical and Endocrine Findings

The clinical and endocrine findings in patients suffering from pituitary adenomas are caused either by hypersecretion or hyposecretion of one or several pituitary hormones. This aspect is discussed in detail in Chapter 25.

Neurological and Ophthalmological Findings

Subjective Complaints

The incidence of visual loss, which was the most critical presenting symptom cited in earlier neurosurgical series of patients harboring pituitary adenomas, has diminished considerably, now that successful treatment of pituitary endocrine disorders has become common practice and neurosurgeons no longer limit operative intervention to decompression of the visual pathways. Increasingly often, patients are being referred for treatment at a very early stage, when the intrasellar microadenoma is manifested by only endocrine disturbances.[120]

Visual loss usually develops slowly over a period of months, sometimes even years. Many middle-aged patients who harbor endocrine-inactive adenomas first receive a prescription for glasses because of suspected presbyopia. Some patients describe a slowly growing, curtainlike shadow that obscures the temporal parts of the visual field.

Frontal, temporal, occipital, or generalized headaches can accompany a pituitary adenoma at any stage, and constitute a symptom in 20 per cent of patients.[141] They are more frequently a symptom in acromegalic patients, and especially in acromegalic women; Hardy and colleagues reported this symptom in 11 of 24 women who were acromegalic.[83] These headaches are not related to the size of the adenoma, but rather to the presence or absence of increased somatotropic hormone production. Photophobia, a rare symptom of acromegaly, was first described by Cushing in 1912; it has also been seen in a patient harboring a craniopharyngioma.[33,216]

Objective Findings

The most obvious ocular signs of pituitary adenomas are pallor of the optic discs and bitemporal field defects. The degree of pallor is not necessarily related to the extent of visual loss. Atrophic excavation of the disc is an unfavorable prognostic sign.

The characteristic field deficit associated with pituitary adenomas is bitemporal hemianopia, which may involve the peripheral field, the central field, the paracentral field, or any combination of the three. Approximately 70 per cent of patients exhibit partial or complete bitemporal field defects, and the remaining 30 per cent show homonymous defects, central scotomas, or irregular and unclassifiable defects.[216,221] The bitemporal field involvement usually affects the upper temporal quadrant first, and then the lower temporal quadrant. The nasal fields are affected only in a late stage of tumor development, when they show a progressive, concentric contraction, leaving a paracentral rest before the eye becomes blind.[37] The finding of a bilateral central scotoma indicates that the tumor is pressing from behind toward the chiasm, since the macular fibers, which decussate in the posterior part of the chiasm, are damaged in this situation.[215] This type of posterior chiasmal compression is most likely to occur in patients who have a prefixed chiasm.

Papilledema is observed only rarely, and never occurs while the adenoma is confined to the sella: Nurnberger and Korey found only seven cases of papilledema among their 117 patients; one patient had a cavernous sinus syndrome, and the others had tumors that had expanded subfrontally.[161] Proptosis usually is a sign of vascular stasis in the cavernous sinus or extension of the tumor through the superior orbital fissure.

Extraocular muscle palsies reportedly occur in about 10 per cent of patients.[216,221] The third cranial nerve is most frequently affected, followed by the sixth and the fourth nerves. Although an extraocular muscle palsy seldom signifies a pituitary adenoma, it indicates that the tumor has either compressed or, less often, invaded the cavernous sinus. A temporal extension of the adenoma that has grown over the superior edge of the cavernous sinus may cause an oculomotor palsy (cf. Fig. 98–32).

Neurological manifestations of pituitary adenomas involving structures other than the visual system are extremely rare. An extension into the interpeduncular cistern and subsequent compression of a cerebral peduncle can cause hemiparesis in the late stage of the disease. Seizures have been reported to occur in 1 to 10 per cent of patients and tend to occur in association with temporal lobe involvement.[6,86,161]

Neuroradiological Examination

The neuroradiological examination permits the surgeon to differentiate four stages in the evolution of pituitary adenomas: microadenomas, adenomas with sellar enlargement, locally invasive and destructive adenomas, and paninvasive adenomas.[83,137,146,176] A careful evaluation of skull radiographs and frontal and lateral tomograms of the sellar region can provide the necessary diagnostic information in the majority of cases; microadenomas can be detected only with tomography.

Skull Radiographs and Tomograms

In patients harboring microadenomas, routine skull radiographs may show a double sellar floor but are otherwise unremarkable; the calculated volume of the sella is still normal at this stage. Frontal tomographic studies reveal either focal bulging, atrophy, or a lateral slope of the sella floor (Fig. 98–22). A comparison of lateral cuts taken on an axis at identical distances from the midline will show differences in the

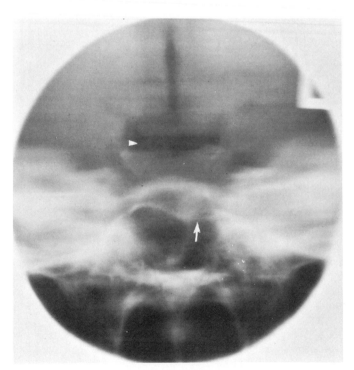

Figure 98–22 Unilateral depression of the sellar floor (*arrow*) in a 21-year-old woman who had a prolactinoma measuring 8 mm in diameter. Note normal suprasellar cistern (*arrowhead*). Frontal pneumotomogram.

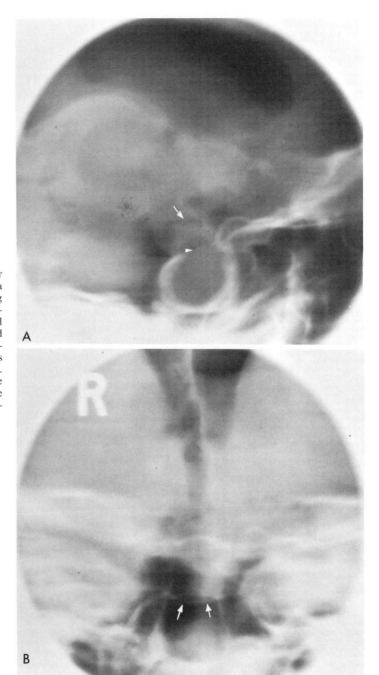

Figure 98–23 *A*. Intrasellar adenoma causing ballooned sella in a 16-year-old man suffering from gigantism. There is no suprasellar extension. Note normal configuration of the anterior third ventricle (*arrow*). Pneumotomogram. The diaphragma sellae is marked by an arrowhead. *B*. Frontal pneumotomogram of the same adenoma. The floor of the sella is thinned and shows a symmetrical bulging (*arrows*).

contour of the sella. The dorsum sellae may be normally thinned and concave at the midline, and when focal enlargement of the sella is in the midline and is limited to the mid-dorsum, its significance is questionable. These changes are, of course, more pronounced when the adenoma has reached a diameter greater than 10 mm. Tumors with a diameter of less than 3 mm cannot be localized with radiological methods.

Progressive intrasellar growth results in a typical ballooned sella and a more symmetrically concave sellar floor (Fig. 98–23). The dorsum sellae is thinned and lengthened, and the posterior clinoid processes disappear. The anterior clinoid processes usually remain normal, however, until the tumor has become much larger. The cortical layer of bone surrounding the sella is usually thinned, but it remains intact during the early phases of this stage. The sellar volume increases beyond its normal size (240 to 1092 cu mm).[42]

Adenomas that have become locally extensive or locally invasive may produce a more or less enlarged sella, and local tumor herniations can be seen particularly well if they extend into the sphenoid sinus, as shown in Figure 98–24; however, similar deformities can be produced by the normal carotid bulge or by aneurysms.[176] Invasive growth is apparent if it extends into the bone of the dorsum sellae and the cranial end of the clivus; in these situations, the dorsum sellae may become separated from the clivus.

The sella is usually greatly enlarged by adenomas that have become diffusely invasive, and its contours can be distinguished only with difficulty if at all. In these cases, the sellar floor is missing, and the sphenoid sinus is partially or completely filled with soft tissue. The dorsum sellae is usually missing, and the upper part of the clivus is destroyed (Fig. 98–25). The anterior clinoid processes are thinned and may be deflected upward.

Information regarding the size, shape, and localization of suprasellar and lateral extensions of pituitary adenomas can be obtained only from contrast studies, including pneumoencephalography, arteriography, and venography, or from computed tomographic studies.

Pneumoencephalography

The pneumoencephalogram is the most valuable radiographic examination available for the detection and delineation of pituitary tumors.[9] Tomography of the air-filled basal cisterns must be performed in every case of a suspected or proved pituitary adenoma. Microadenomas can tilt the diaphragma sellae, either with or without a complementary depression of the sellar floor. These changes will be apparent in frontal tomograms; however, the relation between the diaphragm and the optic chiasm often is not evident. The position of the diaphragm at the entrance of the sella establishes that the adenoma either is localized within the sella or has a suprasellar component.

Adenomas that have suprasellar and parasellar extensions cause deformations of the basal cerebrospinal fluid cisterns, and may cause changes in the contour of the lateral and third ventricles. Small suprasellar extensions can be seen as soft masses of tissue that extend in a more or less semicircular fashion into the chiasmatic cistern above the entrance of the sella (Fig. 98–26). Larger tumors may have subfrontal and retroclival extensions. Constriction of the adenoma at the level of the diaphragma sellae can produce a dumbbell-shaped tumor that is evident in frontal and lateral tomograms (cf. Fig. 98–32). Suprasellar exten-

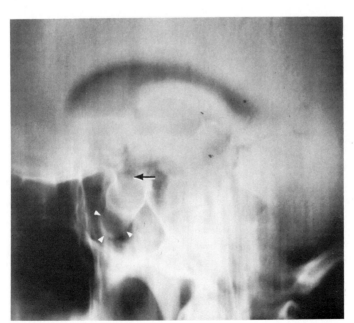

Figure 98–24 Focal growth of a pituitary adenoma herniating into the sphenoid sinus (*arrowheads*), as seen in a lateral view of a pneumotomogram obtained from a 20-year-old acromegalic woman. The arrow points to the normally positioned diaphragma sellae.

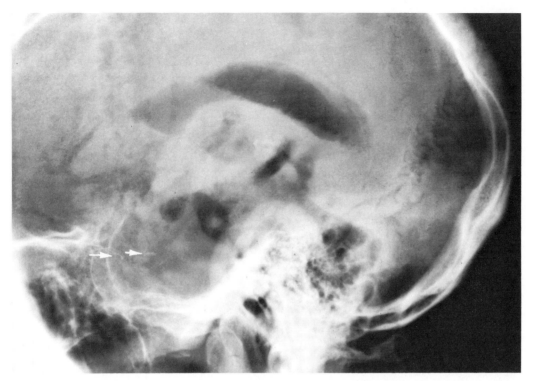

Figure 98–25 Lateral view of a pneumoencephalogram obtained from a 49-year-old man suffering from an invasive pituitary adenoma. The whole sella is destroyed and the adenoma extends into the sphenoid sinus. The cranial part of the clivus can no longer be seen. The arrows point to the destroyed anterior clinoid processes.

sions of moderate size can compress the anterior part of the third ventricle. The supraoptic and infundibular recesses are blunted at first and later disappear. In lateral views, the anterior third ventricle has a round indentation instead of the normal recesses. Larger tumors cause an amputation of the basal part of the third ventricle, which is apparent in frontal views (Fig. 98–26B). The temporal horn of the lateral ventricle is displaced laterally and superiorly in extensions reaching into the middle cerebral fossa, whereas superior temporal extensions can compress the frontal horn (Fig. 98–27).[72]

Angiography

Although angiography does not delineate the relation of the pituitary adenoma to the surrounding structures that are directly pertinent to the neurosurgical evaluation, angiograms must be obtained in evaluating endocrine-inactive tumors because it is essential to rule out the presence of an aneurysm in these cases. Many suprasellar

extensions are not apparent angiographically.[9] Larger adenomas cause an elevation of the first segment of the anterior cerebral artery and a straightening and elevation of the supraclinoid portion of the internal carotid artery (the opening of the siphon) (Fig. 98–28). Lateral extensions displace the cavernous portion of the carotid laterally, but this can be seen better in retrograde cavernous sinus venograms using basal projections.

Precise delineation of the blood supply and circulation in a pituitary adenoma is possible with the use of magnification-subtraction angiography. A posterior pituitary blush can be seen in 96 per cent of normal angiograms. Baker was able to demonstrate the normal meningohypophyseal trunk from which the inferior hypophyseal artery arises, and reported finding a tumor blush in over 80 per cent of his patients who had pituitary adenomas.[8] The authors have been unable to reproduce his results and have rarely seen circulation within a pituitary adenoma, except very occasionally in larger tumors.

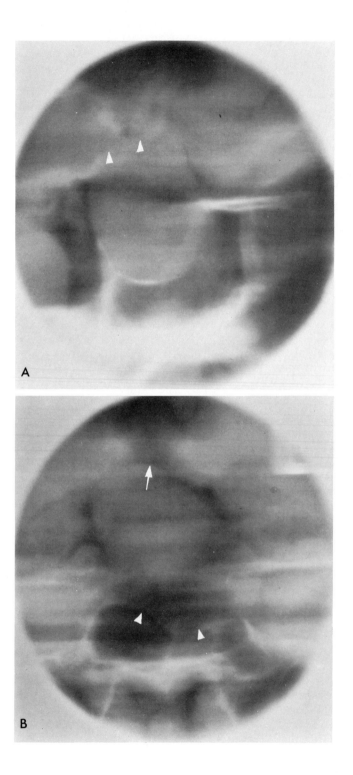

Figure 98–26 *A*. Lateral pneumotomogram of a large intrasellar and suprasellar prolactinoma in a 58-year-old man. Note the indentation of the anterior third ventricle (*arrowheads*). *B*. Frontal pneumotomogram of the same prolactinoma. The floor of the sella is thinned and asymmetrical (*arrowheads*). The third ventricle is indented by the suprasellar polycyclic tumor extension (*arrow*).

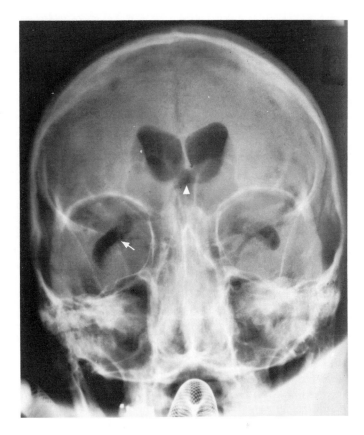

Figure 98–27 Paninvasive prolactinoma in a 47-year-old woman. Note the large suprasellar extension with compression of the third ventricle (*arrowhead*) and the tilting of the right temporal horn (*arrow*) caused by a temporal extension of the adenoma. Beginning hydrocephalic enlargement of both lateral ventricles.

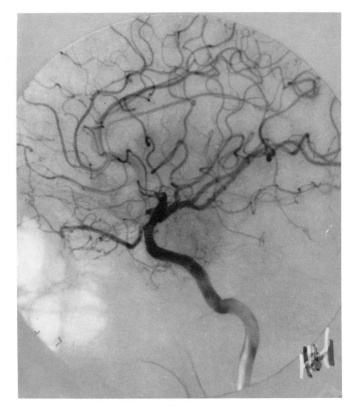

Figure 98–28 Lateral view of an internal carotid arteriogram showing elevation of the supraclinoid internal carotid artery—''opening of the siphon.'' Note the fine pathological vessels in the region of the adenoma. (Courtesy of Dr. Hoi Sang U, Department of Neurological Surgery, University of California School of Medicine, San Francisco, California.)

Computed Tomography

Computed tomography (CT) can delineate the suprasellar cistern in 85 per cent of routine normal examinations.[154] The cistern appears as a five- or six-pointed star in the CT images (Fig. 98–29). It is delineated by the frontal aspect of the pons, the medial aspect of the hippocampal uncus, and the posterior-basal aspect of the frontal lobe. The dorsum sellae may appear in its center. Contrast infusion can demonstrate the basilar and supraclinoid carotid arteries. Cerebrospinal fluid density can usually be demonstrated above, but not within, the sella by this procedure.

Only pituitary adenomas with suprasellar extensions can be demonstrated by using the computed tomography units that are now available. Before administration of contrast material, most pituitary adenomas with suprasellar extensions appear as slightly mottled masses that have inhomogeneously increased densities. Some adenomas may have the same density as the surrounding brain, but the absence of the suprasellar cistern in these cases raises the suspicion of suprasellar extension. Ade-

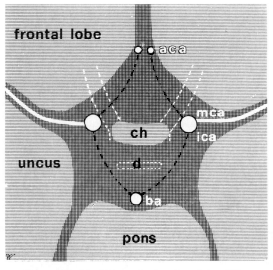

Figure 98–29 Schematic drawing of the different structures that can be visualized by computed tomography through the suprasellar cistern. The frontal lobe, uncus, and pons delineate a pentagon that contains the chiasm (ch), dorsum sellae (d), internal carotid artery (ica), middle cerebral artery (mca), anterior cerebral artery (aca), and basilar artery (ba).

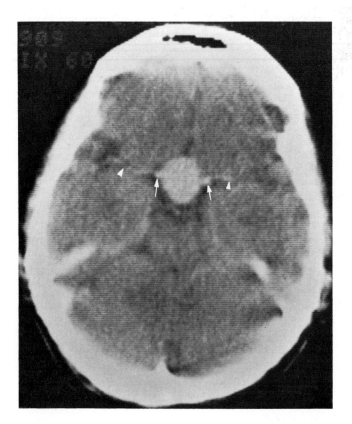

Figure 98–30 Computed tomography with contrast enhancement of a suprasellar extension of a pituitary adenoma. The arrows point to the internal carotid arteries, the arrowheads to the middle cerebral arteries.

nomas almost always show contrast enhancement with a homogeneous or mottled blush (Fig. 98–30). Cyst formation can be demonstrated (Fig. 98–31). At its present stage of technological development, computed tomography is not a substitute for pneumoencephalography, however, because it does not supply all the anatomical details necessary either for planning and performing an operation or for directing irradiation.

Treatment

Every decision regarding the treatment of pituitary adenomas must have two objectives: to decompress the nervous structures, particularly the visual pathways, affected by the adenoma; and to achieve complete and lasting restoration of normal hormone secretion. For endocrine-active adenomas, these objectives can be achieved only if all of the pathological tissue is excised. The patient's condition is not truly "ameliorated" merely by decreasing the abnormal hormone secretion, because the endocrine disease persists, despite a certain reduction in its activity. Three basically different methods of treatment can be used, alone or in combination, to treat pituitary adenomas (Table 98–2).

TABLE 98–2   METHODS OF TREATMENT OF PITUITARY ADENOMAS

OPERATIVE PROCEDURES
Transcranial extirpation
  Paramedian subfrontal approach
  Pterional approach
  Subtemporal approach
Transsphenoidal extirpation
  Sublabial transseptal transsphenoidal approach
  Transantral transsphenoidal approach
  Transethmoidal transsphenoidal approach
Stereotaxic destruction (either transcranial or transnasal)
  Cryodestruction
  High-frequency coagulation
RADIOTHERAPY
Percutaneous high-voltage irradiation
Heavy-particle irradiation
Stereotaxic isotope implantation
MEDICAL TREATMENT WITH ANTISECRETORY DRUGS
Bromocriptine

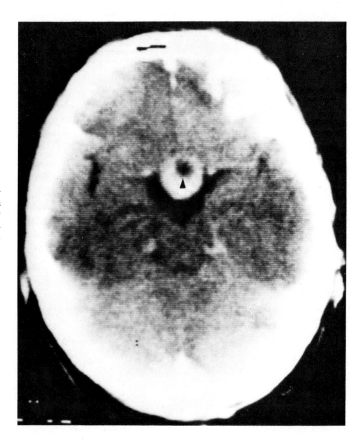

Figure 98–31 Computed tomogram after contrast enhancement of a suprasellar enlargement of a pituitary adenoma with an eccentrically located intra-adenomatous cyst (*arrowhead*).

Operative Removal

In the descriptions of the procedures for resection of pituitary tumors that follow, it is assumed that the patient is left-hemisphere dominant and the surgeon is right-handed. Modification of the customary approach from the right side is reserved for unusual situations, such as extension of the tumor into the left anterior or middle fossa, operation for recurrence after earlier right-sided craniotomy, and right-hemisphere dominance.

Transcranial Approaches

Pituitary tumors can be operated on by way of three intracranial approaches, each of which offers certain advantages in particular situations. These approaches provide different exposures of the sella and suprasellar structures. The paramedian subfrontal and pterional approaches are alternative routes to the sella, whereas the subtemporal approach has a very specific indication.

PARAMEDIAN SUBFRONTAL APPROACH. The first pituitary adenoma operation was performed by Sir Victor Horsley in 1889 using the paramedian subfrontal procedure.[92] In making this approach, the surgeon arrives at the sella in a direct line from the crista galli across the planum sphenoidale to the tuberculum sellae. A forehead scar can be avoided by making a two-thirds coronal scalp incision.

The critical exposure is obtained by correct placement of the anterior-medial burr hole in the four-hole, frontotemporal osteoplastic bone flap. This burr hole, or trephine, should be placed so that it crowds the midline. If the right frontal sinus is small, the burr hole is placed far forward above the sinus, but ordinarily it is placed so that it enters the sinus. Care must be taken to close the sinus and to achieve a watertight closure of the dura. The posterior-medial burr hole, which is made at or behind the hairline, need not be placed so near the midline; 2 cm from the sagittal sinus is the most common site.

The right olfactory tract is interrupted behind the olfactory bulb, which is left intact. The frontal lobe is gently elevated as the retractor is advanced down the midline toward the tuberculum sellae. At this point in the procedure, the surgeon has both optic nerves in full view and has a field of vision passing in a plane across the top of the dorsum sellae. Before proceeding further, the surgeon may wish to drill off the tuberculum sellae and enter the anterior aspect of the sella across the sphenoid sinus in the manner described by Rand, in order to diminish the depth of retraction required.[179] In the case of a prefixed chiasm, this approach is essential to obtain adequate exposure of an intrasellar tumor; however, the opening in the sphenoid sinus must be closed with special care because of the danger of postoperative rhinorrhea.

As a rule, it is possible to anticipate a prefixed chiasm, either by the pattern of visual field involvement, which classically is bitemporal hemianopic scotoma, or by attention to the distance from the air-filled, preoptic recess to the tuberculum sellae. In these instances, another approach is selected.

The suprasellar component of the tumor is located between the laterally displaced optic nerves. It is covered by the stretched dura and arachnoid, which are often incorrectly designated a "capsule." At the interface of the tumor with compressed, nonneoplastic pituitary tissue, the "pseudocapsule," if one is present, consists of the compressed vascular and delicate connective tissues remaining after the normal adenohypophyseal cells have atrophied as a consequence of pressure from the tumor. The dura covering the sphenoid bone and cavernous sinuses forms the interface between the tumor and the sella proper, and the tissue covering the suprasellar surface of the tumor consists of the thinned, stretched sellar diaphragm and thickened arachnoid. Consequently, "extracapsular" removal of a large pituitary adenoma is anatomically impossible.[10,80]

After aspiration for a cystic component of the mass, the exposed surface of the tumor is coagulated with bipolar forceps and excised. The tumor, which is usually soft, is loosened with spoons and curets, and then is removed with a sucker and pituitary rongeur. If the "capsule" is adhering to the optic nerves and chiasm, forceful separation risks impairing the precarious blood supply to these structures. If a retrochiasmal nodule is present, it should be removed, leaving the adherent "capsule" attached to the tuberal region and pituitary stalk. In the case of a large sella, a dental mirror is useful for identifying remnants of tumor that are not in the field of direct vision. Perfect hemostasis can and must be obtained with bipolar coagulation and temporary packing of the sella. Silver clips can be applied to the undersurface of the "capsule" if desired. If the chiasm and optic nerves have not been separated from the tumor, the surgeon can avoid subsequent retraction of the nerves into the empty sella by placing a piece of temporalis muscle within the sella. Closure is routine, although special attention should be given to any openings into the frontal sinuses.

PTERIONAL APPROACH. The pterional approach described by Adson in 1918 is still commonly used, although modern operative techniques require a less extensive dural exposure than originally was necessary.[1,103,228] This approach offers the surgeon a shorter route to the pituitary than is possible in the transfrontal procedure. An approach made along the right sphenoid wing is advantageous in that it spares the olfactory tract and requires less elevation of the frontal lobe. It has a decided disadvantage, however, in that it requires a lateral exposure of the tumor either across the optic nerve or between the optic nerve and carotid artery; consequently, the surgeon's view of the left optic nerve and the interior of the sella is compromised. A prefixed chiasm cannot obstruct access to the adenoma in the pterional procedure, as it can in the subfrontal procedure.

A unilateral skin incision is made behind the hairline, and the bone flap is placed laterally. After the frontotemporal bone has been removed, the greater sphenoid wing is rongeured down to the roof of the orbit. The dura is then opened, and the surgeon can easily approach along the posterior edge of the sphenoid wing to the carotid, the chiasm, and the adenoma.

SUBTEMPORAL APPROACH. As an alternative to the paramedian subfrontal procedure, Horsley proposed the subtemporal approach, which would avoid the operative difficulties presented by the frontal bridging veins.[92] Caton and Paul, who first used his procedure, were not successful in reaching the tumor with this approach, and Cushing's attempts were successful in only two of eight cases.[24,34]

The preceding subfrontal approaches are suitable for tumors that can be removed through the triangular space bounded by the tuberculum sellae, the optic nerves, and the chiasm, but they are not suitable if the suprasellar mass lies behind the chiasm, extends above and behind the dorsum sellae, and elevates the midportion of the third ventricular floor. This anatomical configuration, which is more typical of craniopharyngiomas than of pituitary adenomas, can be identified accurately by pneumoencephalography. The preoptic recess, although it is often reduced to a slit, approximates the tuberculum sellae, and the superior surface of the tumor is capped by a crescent-shaped third ventricle. This situation calls for a subtemporal exposure.

The subtemporal approach requires a slack brain and a temporal craniectomy carried down to the floor of the middle fossa. A laterally situated bone flap permits the surgeon to approach the tumor either beneath the anterior temporal lobe or along the inferior aspect of the sphenoid wing. Unless the bulk of the tumor lies far into the posterior area, a retrochiasmal suprasellar extension of a pituitary adenoma can be removed more easily and with less risk by the transsphenoidal route. A suprasellar retrochiasmal mass can be removed by the subtemporal approach, but this direct lateral exposure severely restricts access into the sella. In addition, while it is effective in decompressing the optic chiasm, a subtemporal exposure precludes total removal of both intrasellar and suprasellar components of an encapsulated tumor such as a craniopharyngioma.

When a retrochiasmal tumor has displaced the optic chiasm superiorly and rostrally—not only when the chiasm is prefixed initially but also when the optic nerves have been foreshortened by the retrochiasmal mass—the rostral floor of the third ventricle and the lamina terminalis are brought into apposition, displaced superiorly and rostrally, and thinned. Given this situation, the surgeon who has made a subfrontal approach can enter the lamina terminalis to expose the tumor above and behind the chiasm and between the laterally displaced optic tracts. Forewarned of a retrochiasmal mass, some surgeons will elect a subtemporal approach, whereas others will elect a subfrontal paramedian approach through the lamina terminalis, particularly when total excision of a presumed craniopharyngioma may prove necessary. When a retrochiasmal mass is encountered unexpectedly during a subfrontal operation, inspection through the lamina terminalis is safer than strong retraction of the optic chiasm.

Transsphenoidal Procedures

All approaches to the pituitary from the inferior side are directed through the sphenoid sinus. The first successful transnasal operation was performed by Schloffer in 1907.[200] He reflected the patient's nose toward one side, resected the whole septum and the turbinates, and removed the adenoma through the opened sphenoid sinus. A great many modifications of this procedure have been developed.*

Cushing, in 1914, combined the most effective features of several transsphenoidal approaches, and designed the sublabial transseptal approach that is still used today.[34] Although Cushing himself later discontinued his use of this approach because it did not afford a sufficiently clear view of sources of bleeding, the procedure was reintroduced in 1958 by Guiot, who used loupes and an illuminated speculum designed by Dott to obtain a better view of the field.[71] Only since the development of the surgical microscope and televised radiofluoroscopy has the procedure been rendered entirely safe.[73,80,84,222]

The transethmoidal and transantral approaches are variations of the transsphenoidal approach that enable the surgeon to minimize the intranasal damage and to avoid an injury to the septum that may lead to atrophic rhinitis.[26,77,163,205]

SUBLABIAL TRANSSEPTAL TRANSSPHENOIDAL APPROACH. The patient is treated with nose drops containing Bacitracin for two or three days before the operation. Systemic antibiotics are no longer considered necessary because almost all cultures obtained from the sinus mucosa removed intraoperatively are either sterile or grow only normal respiratory flora.

The transsphenoidal procedure is carried out with the patient in a semi-sitting position. The head is held by pin fixation, and is turned to face the surgeon, who stands at the patient's right. A fluoroscopic image intensifier is positioned at an angle that will provide a collimated lateral view of the

sella on a television monitor. If the tumor extends above the sella, then air is introduced through a lumbar subarachnoid catheter to fill the third ventricle and suprasellar cisterns.

An antiseptic scrub solution is used to cleanse the nasal passages and the upper gingival and labial mucosa. If a graft is required, the right lateral thigh is disinfected. The nasal and labial submucosal tissues are infiltrated with epinephrine (1:200,000) in lidocaine (0.5 per cent), after which a horizontal incision is made high on the gingiva between the canine teeth. The soft tissues are lifted upward to expose the lower half of the piriform aperture, which is then enlarged by removing the maxillary rim both laterally and inferiorly.

A submucosal plane is developed along the nasal floor and septum, and the mucosa is reflected laterally by advancing a self-retaining speculum down the nasal septum to the sphenoidal rostrum. The anterior nasal spine is removed. The cartilaginous part of the nasal septum is either cut at its base and subluxated laterally so it can be replaced at the end of the operation, or else it is removed. The posterior osseous part of the septum and the adherent cartilage are removed. The rostrum of the sphenoid is opened with a rongeur or an air drill. Punches are used to enlarge the opening into the sinus, after which the sphenoid sinus mucosa is reflected, removed, and submitted for culture. Fluoroscopic monitoring and a direct view of the field maintained with the operating microscope (300-mm objective, 12.5 × eyepiece) guide all subsequent maneuvers.

The anterior wall of the sella is perforated with an air drill; then, with small punches, bone is removed from the tuberculum sellae superiorly to the floor inferiorly, and laterally to the medial edge of each cavernous sinus. Venous bleeding is controlled with tiny pledgets of oxidized cellulose (Surgicel). Bipolar forceps are used to coagulate the exposed dura around its periphery, and the dura is excised to permit maximal exposure of the sellar contents.

Intrasellar adenomas. The various types of intrasellar adenomas reside in individual preferential sites throughout the sellar region. These tumors seldom exceed a diameter of 2 cm. Tumors having a diameter of 5 mm or less are seldom visible at the

---

* See references 46, 76, 90, 98, 109; for review cf. 89.

exposed surface. Polytomograms usually are useful in determining the position of the tumor because signs of focal bulging and thinning in the sella provide a guide to the neighboring adenoma. If the location of the tumor is not apparent, incisions are extended into the gland. In the cases of adenomas secreting growth hormone and prolactin, vertical incisions are made in the lateral wings of the gland. A midline vertical incision may disclose the adenoma in patients who have small ACTH-secreting adenomas, but the tumors associated with Cushing's disease may be found occupying any of a variety of positions within the sella.

Adenomas are individually distinct and, while their consistency and color may vary, they can be unequivocally distinguished from normal anterior pituitary tissue. Although differentiation from the posterior lobe may be difficult, confirmation by frozen section is decisive. Multiple incisions into the anterior pituitary have not produced detectable impairment of the glandular function.

There is little problem in the exposure of larger intrasellar tumors, except in the case of certain prolactin-secreting adenomas that occupy the lateral angle at the base of the dorsum sellae and frequently burrow into the body of the sphenoid bone. Adequate exposure of these tumors requires removal of the ipsilateral sellar floor and subjacent cancellous sphenoid bone. All gross tumor is removed under 16× to 25× magnification. Because the boundary between the tumor and the normal gland is distinct, it is not necessary to obtain frozen sections of grossly normal tissues.

When the tumor is confined to the sella, and if the cavity does not communicate with the subarachnoid space, Gelfoam soaked in absolute alcohol is packed into the cavity repeatedly for a total exposure to alcohol of 6 to 10 minutes to destroy any remaining microscopic nests of tumor cells. The alcohol does penetrate the exposed surface of the normal gland, but the depth of penetration seems to be negligible, and the authors have observed no detrimental effect on pituitary function.

The extent to which the remaining cavity is packed varies, depending on the position of the tumor's superior surface in relation to the sellar diaphragm. If removal of the tumor has exposed the diaphragm or arach-

noid, fascia lata is placed over this surface and held in place with fat and Surgicel, the latter serving to hold the mobile fat in position. Alternatively, fat without fascia is used to fill the cavity; the removal of muscle will result in a painful thigh, and the use of fat has proved equally satisfactory. In the event of frank leakage of cerebrospinal fluid, a second piece of fascia lata is placed over the anterior dural opening before the sella is closed with a piece of septal cartilage. A piece of cartilage carved to cover the sellar opening is slipped inside the dural edges in the case of larger tumors or, in the case of smaller tumors, is placed extradurally beneath the bone edges. After the anesthesiologist has briefly elevated intrathoracic pressure to verify adequate exclusion of cerebrospinal fluid, the cartilage graft and surrounding bone are covered with a thin layer of biological adhesive.

Adenomas with suprasellar extension. The lumbar spinal subarachnoid catheter, which is used to inject air at the start of the operation, is retained by the anesthesiologist to control the position of the suprasellar tumor and the diaphragma sellae. The entire surface of the suprasellar capsule must be in the surgeon's field of vision. When the tumor is of modest suprasellar proportions, this presents no problem because the capsule is forced into the sella by the slightly increased intracranial pressure associated with general anesthesia. If the suprasellar capsule does not descend as the intrasellar tumor is removed, however, which is sometimes the case after pneumoencephalography, the anesthesiologist can inject small increments of normal saline into the subarachnoid catheter until intracranial pressure forces the suprasellar tumor into the operative field. Occasionally, the capsule falls to the bottom of the excavated sella, obscuring the posterior extension of the tumor above and behind the dorsum sellae. In this situation, withdrawal of cerebrospinal fluid will elevate the capsule, affording the surgeon a view of any tumor remaining in a posterior-superior direction. A dental mirror is used to inspect all surfaces of the cavity remaining after the removal of larger tumors and, when used adeptly, can provide an excellent view of otherwise inaccessible areas.

Two or more silver clips are attached to the midportion of the suprasellar capsule; they serve both as a fluoroscopic guide to avoid excessive packing of the sella and as a marker to follow in the postoperative period—to determine the presence of a hematoma at first, and the regrowth of tumor later on.

Bacitracin solution is used often during the operation to irrigate the operative field. After the final irrigation, the speculum is removed, the sublabial incision is closed with catgut sutures, and both nasal cavities are packed gently with petrolatum gauze coated with Bacitracin ointment. Patients are instructed to use an aqueous nasal ointment for two to three months.

Adenomas with extension into the sphenoid sinus. Surprisingly often, small nodules of tumor perforate the dura and bone and come to lie within the sphenoid sinus— or, rarely, within the body of the sphenoid bone—covered only by mucosa. These small extensions can be removed cleanly and easily, but it is difficult, sometimes impossible, to remove massive extensions into the sinus completely, and the deficient sellar walls can make the proper orientation problematical.

TRANSANTRAL TRANSSPHENOIDAL APPROACH. The sella is exposed through the maxillary and the inferior ethmoid sinuses by incising the buccal mucosa over the anterior wall of the maxillary sinus, removing the underlying bone, and resecting the medial bony wall of the sinus to expose the lateral soft nasal wall, which is mobilized to increase the operative field. A lower ethmoidectomy is then performed. The anterior wall of the sphenoid sinus is exposed and opened, after which the surgeon proceeds with the maneuvers described earlier.

The large operative cavity, with the exception of the intrasellar portion, which is filled with muscle, is plugged with gauze. The gauze is successively removed between the sixth and ninth postoperative days.

TRANSETHMOIDAL TRANSSPHENOIDAL APPROACH. The eyelids on the side to be operatively exposed are sutured together. A semicircular skin incision is then made around the medial angle of the eye, passing the lateral edge of the nasal bone. The periosteum is separated from the underlying bone, care being taken that neither the periorbita nor the trochlea is injured when the eye is reflected laterally to expose the lamina papyracea of the ethmoid cells. The ethmoid cells are opened anteriorly, and the lacrimal sac is displaced laterally. The lateral mucosa of the nasal cavity is then exposed and displaced medially—the ethmoidal arteries must be avoided—to expose the frontal wall of the sphenoid sinus. The posterior part of the nasal septum is removed together with the rostrum of the sphenoid. The operation then proceeds in the manner already described.

The cavity is filled with gauze at the end of the procedure. The gauze is led out through the nasal cavity and is removed during the first week after operation. The periosteum and the skin are sutured, and the eyelids are opened.

Stereotaxic Operations

Stereotaxic procedures are discussed in Chapter 146.

Radiotherapy

There are three radiotherapy methods that can be applied to pituitary adenomas. High-voltage percutaneous radiotherapy involves the use of local doses of 4000 rads delivered over a period of four to five weeks; larger doses can cause radiation necrosis of the hypothalamus.[29,113] Heavy-particle treatment yields better results than conventional megavoltage irradiation, but the facilities for this procedure are not widely available.[108,128] Interstitial Curie therapy, the third method of pituitary radiotherapy, which involves implanted radioactive gold, yttrium, or iridium seeds, is discussed in detail in Chapter 99.[139,152]

Medical Treatment

The medical treatment of patients suffering from pituitary adenomas has two goals: first, to restore sufficient secretion of pituitary trophic hormones either by the replacement of the pituitary hormone itself (growth hormone, antidiuretic hormone), or by a substitution of the hormones of the pituitary-dependent glands (glucocorticoids, thyroid hormone, androgens, estrogens); and second, the inhibition of abnormal pituitary hormone secretion (prolactin, growth hormone) by bromocriptine. Details regarding the medical treatment of these patients are discussed in Chapter 25.

Indications and Contraindications for the Different Methods of Treatment

Each patient who harbors a pituitary adenoma must be evaluated individually to determine the most appropriate method of treatment. None of the treatments available will give optimal results in every patient, and each method has its advantages and disadvantages. However, open operative procedures performed under the operating microscope afford a more selective separation of the adenoma tissue from the normal gland and other surrounding structures than any other technique. In addition, pathological tissue specimens of good quality can be obtained only during open procedures. Blind procedures—and all stereotaxic operations and radiotherapeutic procedures are blind, in the sense that they do not visualize and direct treatment selectively to the target tissue—must occasionally either fail to obliterate an extension of the adenoma or cause damage to the normal pituitary gland and hypothalamus. Radiotherapy is reserved for cases in which either operation is precluded by the patient's medical condition or the tumor cannot be totally removed.

The choice of either the transcranial or the transsphenoidal operation depends entirely on the growth pattern and extension of the adenoma. Specific indications strictly dictate the decision to use one or the other approach. In Guiot's series, the transsphenoidal procedure was absolutely indicated for 28 per cent of his patients, and the transcranial approach for 10.5 per cent; for 61.5 per cent of his patients, either procedure would provide a satisfactory approach to the adenoma, although the transsphenoidal operation was preferred because it involves lower mortality rates and less morbidity (Table 98–3).[72] The absolute indications for transcranial procedures are: subfrontal extension, dumbbell suprasellar extension, large suprasellar extension with a small sella, temporal extension, and retroclival extension (Fig. 98–32). The absolute indications for transsphenoidal operations are: intrasellar microadenoma, sphenoidal extension, prefixed chiasm (suggested by paracentral scotoma), cerebrospinal fluid rhinorrhea, pituitary apoplexy, cystic adenomas, invasion of the clivus, and advanced age of the patient.[72,221]

The sublabial transseptal operation is generally preferred to the transethmoidal operation because it provides a more advantageous angle between the line of approach and the planum sphenoidale, and affords the surgeon a more direct view of the suprasellar space (Fig. 98–33). In addition, since the sublabial operation is a direct midline approach, the surgeon's view of small tumors is equally good on both sides of the sella; this is not so in transantral and transethmoidal procedures. An added disadvantage of transantral operations is that they seem to produce considerable blood loss.[106]

Because radiotherapy does not promptly lower the secretory level of the particular hormone produced by an active adenoma, it is the procedure of choice only when the objective is to diminish the size of the tumor by nonoperative means. Postoperative radiotherapy is used routinely for all cases in which the surgeon has been unable to remove all neoplastic tissue or in which the postoperative endocrinological studies demonstrate a residual excess hormone secretion.*

The incidence of recurrent adenomas is lower in patients who have undergone postoperative irradiation than in those who have not. Henderson, in a five-year follow-up of Cushing's patients whose pituitary adenomas were treated by means of transcranial operation, found recurrences in 12.9 per cent of those who had undergone postoperative irradiation and in 42.5 per cent of those who had not.[86]

A residual increased prolactin secretion can also be treated with bromocriptine, which restores normal prolactin values in a large percentage of cases. Patients who are suspected of harboring an adenoma because of elevated prolactin levels, but whose sellar tomograms reveal no apparent abnormality, may be treated with bromocriptine if pregnancy is desired.[16]

The use of all stereotaxic procedures—including cryosurgery, high-frequency coagulation, implantation of radioactive material, and proton-beam irradiation—must be restricted to adenomas that are confined to the sella or that have only small extrasellar extensions.[108,152,180] The scar tissue that has formed in patients who have undergone radiotherapy (particularly the implantation

---

* See references 2, 50, 72, 153, 211, 221.

TABLE 98-3 MORTALITY AND MORBIDITY RATES IN TRANSCRANIAL AND TRANSSPHENOIDAL PITUITARY OPERATIONS

	APPROACH (PER CENT)		
	Transcranial	Transsphenoidal	AUTHORS
Mortality rate	1.2–16	0.4–2	Fager et al.* Guiot† Hardy et al.‡ Kautzky and Lüdecke§ Laws et al.‖ Mundinger and Riechert¶ Ray and Patterson** Svien and Colby†† Wilson and Dempsey‡‡
Reoperations for suspected hematoma	3–4	0.6–1.2	Guiot† Svien and Colby†† Wilson and Dempsey‡‡
Cerebrospinal fluid rhinorrhea	rare	2.5–6.4	Guiot† Nicola§§ Ray and Patterson** Wilson and Dempsey‡‡
Visual function loss	6–7	0.4–3.2	Fager et al.* Guiot† Laws et al.‖ Tönnis et al.‖‖ Wilson and Dempsey‡‡
Postoperative epilepsy	3–4	—	Svien and Colby‡‡
Psychiatric changes	14–22 41–48 after additional x-ray therapy	—	Fischer et al.¶¶

* Indications for and results of surgical treatment of pituitary tumors by the intracranial approach. In Kohler, P. O., and Ross, G. T., eds.: Diagnosis and treatment of pituitary tumors. Amsterdam/New York, Excerpta Medica/American Elsevier, 1973, pp. 146–155.
† Transsphenoidal approach in surgical treatment of pituitary adenomas: General principles and indications in non-functioning adenomas. In Kohler, P. O., and Ross, G. T., eds.: ibid, pp. 159–178.
‡ Acromégalie-gigantisme: Traitement chirurgical par exerese transsphenoidale de l'adénome hypophysaire. Neuro-chirurgie (Paris), suppl 2, 19:1–184, 1973.
§ Experiences with transsphenoidal approach to the hypophysis. In Kuhlendahl, H., et al., eds.: Modern Aspects of Neurosurgery. Vol 4. Amsterdam/New York, Excerpta Medica/American Elsevier, 1973, pp. 135–141.
‖ Transsphenoidal decompression of the optic nerve and chiasm. J. Neurosurg., 46:717–722, 1977.
¶ Hypophysentumoren, Hypophysektomie. Stuttgart, Georg Thieme Verlag, 1967, pp. 224–227.
** Surgical experience with chromophobe adenomas of the pituitary gland. J. Neurosurg., 36:726–729, 1971.
†† Treatment for chromophobe adenoma. Springfield, Ill., Charles C Thomas, 1967, pp. 1–107.
‡‡ Transsphenoidal microsurgical removal of 250 pituitary adenomas. J. Neurosurg., 48:13–22, 1978.
§§ Transsphenoidal surgery for pituitary adenomas with extrasellar extension. Progr. Neurol. Surg., 6:142–199, 1975.
‖‖ Bericht über 264 operierte Hypophysenadenome. Acta Neurochir. (Wien), 3:113–130, 1953.
¶¶ Psychische Spätfolgen nach operativer Behandlung von Hypophysentumoren. Arch. Psychiat. Nervenkr., 210:387–406, 1968.

of radioactive material) more than one year before an open operation may make the procedure more difficult. Since it is usually difficult to separate the adenomatous tissue from the normal gland in these patients, a radical hypophysectomy must be used to treat the adenoma.[83,120]

Results of Treatment

General Considerations

The results of different forms of treatment depend mainly on the preoperative size and the growth characteristics of the tumor.[72,81,83] The best results are obtained in treating intrasellar microadenomas (stage I). Hormone secretions can be restored to normal in most of these cases, and complications usually do not occur. Large, circumscribed adenomas (stage II) are more difficult to treat, but the outcome usually is favorable in terms of restoration of both vision and normal endocrine function. The function of the normal gland, however, is endangered considerably more at this stage of tumor development than it is in stage I. The outcome in treating stage III adenomas is determined by the extent to which the invasive growth can be localized in this group. Adenomas that have reached the stage of paninvasive growth (stage IV) cannot be cured by operation, and the endocrine disease usually continues. The degree to which percutaneous radiotherapy can shrink these lesions is variable and unpredictable.

It is almost impossible to draw any statistical comparison between the results of the various therapeutic procedures that have been outlined. Certain methods, such as proton-beam irradiation and stereotaxic operations, are used to treat only intrasellar lesions that are likely to respond favorably to therapy and that can be treated with equal success by using open operative methods. The statistics regarding operative therapy, however, reflect not only results with these tumors but also the results with the additional proportion of large tumors that are more likely to have an unfavorable outcome and are treated only by open procedures. The bias is particularly evident in the data on transcranial operations, which represent several series compiled decades ago and which usually include tumors that cannot be managed satisfactorily by other methods.

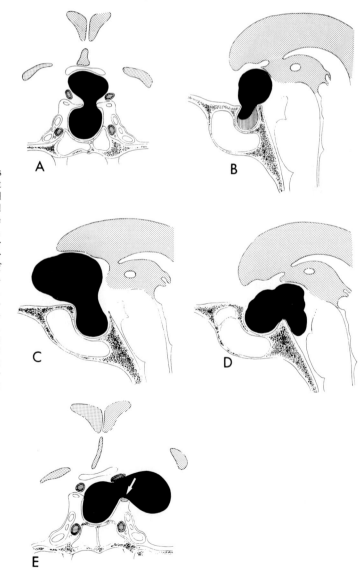

Figure 98–32 Configurations of pituitary adenomas that must be operated on by a transcranial approach. *A*. Dumbbell-shaped adenoma with narrow neck at the level of the sella entrance. *B*. Adenoma with large suprasellar extension and small intrasellar portion without enlargement of bony aperture of sella. *C*. Adenoma with subfrontal extension. *D*. Adenoma with retrosellar expansion without destruction of dorsum sellae and upper clivus. *E*. Adenoma with extension into the middle cerebral fossa; the arrow marks the site of the possible compression of the oculomotor nerve, which can occur without invasion of the cavernous sinus.

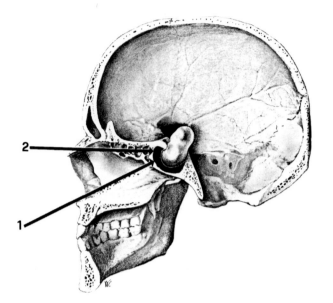

Figure 98–33 Schematic representation of the difference in the angle of approach of the sublabial transseptal (1) and the transethmoidal (2) approaches. The sublabial procedure allows visualization of suprasellar tumor extensions.

Visual Results

In a recent series, improvement and often restoration of normal vision was achieved in 42.6 to 83 per cent of the patients undergoing a transcranial procedure, and in 71.7 to 81 per cent of the patients treated by the transsphenoidal approach.[129] In another series, conventional radiotherapy alone resulted in improvement in 61 per cent. A careful comparison between patients treated with either operation or radiotherapy alone has shown that both forms of therapy are effective. Although radiotherapy was about 15 to 30 per cent less effective than operation, Svien and Colby favored radiotherapy because none of the irradiated patients died as a result of treatment.[204] Antisecretory medical treatment occasionally ameliorates visual field defects and oculomotor disturbances, but only a few cases in which this treatment was successful have been reported.[120,212]

Endocrinological Results

Acromegaly

The endocrinological results obtained in the therapy of acromegaly depend mainly on the size of the adenoma and the stage to which it has progressed. Hardy and colleagues achieved a cure by transsphenoidal operations in 76 per cent of their patients who had enclosed adenomas (stages I and II), but in only 55 per cent of those who had locally invasive adenomas (stage III); no cures were achieved in patients having stage IV adenomas.[84] Similar results were reported by U and colleagues.[211] In another series, a comparison of the growth hormone levels in acromegalic patients before and after operation revealed normal postoperative somatotropin levels (less than 5 ng per milliliter) in 2 of 8 patients treated with craniotomy, and in 13 of 19 patients treated with transsphenoidal procedures.[122]

High-voltage radiotherapy lowered somatotropic hormone levels to below 5 ng per milliliter in only 5 of 16 patients reported by Gordon and Roth.[67] Proton-beam irradiation has proved more effective; 48 per cent of the 118 patients treated by Kjellberg and Kliman had normal posttreatment levels.[108] The data reported by Lawrence and colleagues indicate that the levels decrease rather slowly after heavy-particle treatment.[128] Normal values (less than 5 ng per milliliter) were achieved in 30 per cent of his patients within two years, in 68 per cent within six years, and in 95 per cent within eight years. Stereotaxic implantation of [90]yttrium seeds lowered fasting somatotropin levels to less than 5 ng per milliliter in 15 of 50 patients in a first series, 6 of 9 patients in a second series, and 6 of 8 patients in a third series.[27,100,225] Stereotaxic cryosurgery brought levels to normal (less than 4 ng per milliliter) postoperatively in 20 of 32 patients (with death of 3 patients) in one group and in 1 of 3 patients in another.[27,180]

Medical treatment with bromocriptine is effective in restoring prolactin levels to normal in the majority of patients who had hyperprolactinemia.[206] Although bromocriptine is less effective in treating acromegalic patients, Sachdev and colleagues reported that dosages of 20 to 60 mg per day reduced the somatotropic hormone level to less than 5 ng per milliliter in 4 of 21 patients.[192]

Prolactinoma

Prolactinomas can be treated by operation, cryotherapy, conventional radiotherapy, or bromocriptine. In young women suffering from amenorrhea or amenorrhea-galactorrhea as a consequence of hypophyseal microadenomas, successful therapy will restore normal prolactin levels, and consequently will also restore normal menstrual cycles and the ability to become pregnant.

Antunes and colleagues reported normal postoperative prolactin levels in six of seven patients who underwent transsphenoidal operations, in one of four patients who had transsphenoidal operations and postoperative radiotherapy, and in none of nine patients who had radiotherapy only.[2]

Preoperative prolactin levels have a prognostic value. Transsphenoidal micro-operative procedures resulted in normal postoperative prolactin levels (less than 25 ng per milliliter) in 78 per cent of 142 patients whose preoperative values were below 200 ng per milliliter, but in only 16 per cent of 113 patients with preoperative values above 200 ng per milliliter (Table 98–4).* Preoperative prolactin levels do not necessarily correlate with the size of the adenoma.[25] The adenoma's size, therefore, may not be the primary determinant of the results of operation—additional factors are involved.[121] Hyperplasia of functionally blocked prolactin cells is present in the normal hypophysis adjacent to the prolactinoma in about half the patients who harbor these tumors.[121,194] Because a reactivation of secretory activity may occur in this region after the adenoma is removed, any residual hyperprolactinemia does not necessarily indicate that removal of the adenoma tissue has been incomplete. In this situation, reoperation or postoperative radiotherapy is not appropriate. Antisecretory drugs must be used. Medical treatment with daily doses of 2.5 to 12 mg of bromocriptine reduces elevated prolactin levels in the majority of patients who have hyperprolactinemia.[175]

Cushing's Disease

Corticotropic adenomas causing Cushing's disease can be treated best either by

---

* See references 2, 25, 83, 122, 207, 220.

TABLE 98–4 ENDOCRINE RESULTS OF PROLACTINOMA OPERATION

| | POSTOPERATIVE PROLACTIN LEVEL | | | |
| | In Patients With Preoperative Level Greater Than 200 ng/ml | | In Patients With Preoperative Level Less Than 200 ng/ml | |
SERIES	Elevated	Normal	Elevated	Normal
Antunes et al.*	18	0	4	9
Chang et al.†	3	0	9	10
Hardy et al.‡	16	11	5	48
Tindall et al.§	8	3	6	20
Werder et al.//	23	1	2	8
Landolt¶	27	3	5	16
Total	95 (84%)	18 (16%)	31 (22%)	111 (78%)

The difference between the two groups is significant ($p < .01$).

* Prolactin secreting pituitary tumors. Ann. Neurol., 2:148–153, 1977.
† Detection, evaluation, and treatment of pituitary microadenomas in patients with galactorrhea and amenorrhea. Amer. J. Obstet. Gynec., 128:356–363, 1977.
‡ Prolactin-secreting pituitary adenomas: Transsphenoidal microsurgical treatment. In Robyn, C., and Harter, M., eds.: Progress in Prolactin Physiology and Pathology. Amsterdam, Elsevier–North Holland Biomedical Press, 1978, pp. 361–370.
§ Transsphenoidal microsurgery for pituitary tumors associated with hyperprolactinemia. J. Neurosurg., 48:849–860, 1978.
// Treatment of patients with prolactinomas. J. Endocr. Invest., 1:47–58, 1978.
¶ Landolt, A. M.: Unpublished data.

transsphenoidal micro-operative stereotaxic intervention or by Bragg peak proton
irradiation, since the majority of these
tumors are still in the microadenoma stage
at the time the disease is diagnosed.[108,128,172]
Hardy reported eight cures among 10 patients, and Tyrrell and colleagues reported
remissions in 17 of 18 patients.[8,210] Dalton,
who routinely performed total hypophysectomies for these adenomas because of their
known tendency to invasive growth,
achieved complete remissions in 11 of 14
patients who were followed for one to eight
years.[38] Proton-beam irradiation effected
total remissions in 63 per cent of the patients reported by Kjellberg and Kliman.[108]
Mundinger had remissions in 12 of 13 patients who received [90]yttrium implanta-
tions.[152]

Nelson's Syndrome

The therapy undertaken for patients who
have Nelson's syndrome must be more aggressive than that used for those who have
Cushing's disease because their adenomas
are usually larger and have more aggressive
growth characteristics.[173,188] Operation and
proton irradiation are the most effective
modes of therapy against these adenomas,
but the results are inferior to those obtained
in Cushing's disease. Wilson and co-workers reported favorable operative results in
only 4 of 19 patients, whereas Kjellberg and
Kliman realized complete remissions in 8 of
their 11 patients who were treated with proton-beam irradiation.[108,173]

Complications

In addition to the complications that can
be attributed to anesthesia, prolonged bed
rest, concomitant medical problems, and
endocrine disturbances (hypopituitarism,
diabetes insipidus, inappropriate antidiuretic hormone secretion), each therapeutic
procedure can produce its own specific pattern of complications (Table 98–5). If one
of these complications is encountered, appropriate steps, such as reopening of the
wound or emergency operation, must be
considered.

Special Entities

Pituitary Apoplexy

Pituitary apoplexy, which was first described by Bleibtreu in 1905, is characterized by the sudden onset of hemorrhage,
which may or may not involve spillage into
the subarachnoid space; by necrosis in the
interior of a pituitary adenoma; or by both
of these signs.[14] Large portions of the adenoma are usually necrotic. Asymptomatic,
old, hemorrhagic cysts have been found in
6.8 per cent of a recent series of 282
adenomas, but apoplectic hemorrhages
occurred in only 3.5 per cent.[122] There is

TABLE 98–5 POTENTIAL COMPLICATIONS ASSOCIATED WITH METHODS OF TREATMENT

INTRACRANIAL OPERATIONS
Intracranial hematoma
Wound infection
Low-pressure hydrocephalus
Damage to cranial nerves
Cerebrospinal fluid rhinorrhea

Brain edema
Meningitis
Cerebrovascular insults
Epileptic seizures
Personality changes (frontal lobe damage)

TRANSSPHENOIDAL OPERATIONS
Intra- and extrasellar hematoma
Meningitis
Sinusitis
Damage to teeth

Cerebrospinal fluid rhinorrhea
Cranial nerve palsies
Atrophic rhinitis

STEREOTACTIC PROCEDURES
Intratumoral bleeding
Meningitis

Cerebrospinal fluid rhinorrhea
Cranial nerve damage

RADIOTHERAPY
Tumor swelling (requires emergency operation)
Delayed radiation necrosis of hypothalamus, pituitary, and optic nerves

MEDICAL TREATMENT WITH BROMOCRIPTINE
Nausea
Vomiting
Stomach burning

(These disappear after discontinuation of medication or reduction of dosage; cf. Chapter 25.)

some evidence that pituitary apoplexy more frequently accompanies the adenomas of acromegaly than other adenomas; in nonacromegalic patients, it may be the first clinical symptom noted.[21,189]

The apoplectic hemorrhage is probably a consequence of the stretched diaphragma sellae compressing the trabecular arteries that supply the tumor from above. The resulting ischemia leads to an infarction, followed by bleeding into the infarcted area. The bleeding may be precipitated by head trauma, radiation therapy, or anticoagulation.[189] Stimulation of a prolactinoma by large doses of estrogen frequently gives rise to intra-adenomatous hemorrhages that may be gross or microscopic.[170]

Patients experiencing apoplectic hemorrhage notice first a sudden, excruciating headache located mainly in the bifrontal area. They may remain alert, or they may develop dullness, confusion, and stupor that may progress to coma. Symptoms and signs of meningismus are common. Unilateral, or more often bilateral, ophthalmoplegia or paresis of the third and fourth cranial nerves is typical. Acute loss of visual acuity and visual field defects occur less frequently. Visual impairment is always an alarming sign; occasionally a patient may be rendered blind. There may be impairment of trigeminal function, and rarely hemiplegia or hemiparesis can occur.[189]

Skull radiographs reveal an enlarged sella in almost every case. Typically, spinal fluid pressure is elevated, and the bloody or xanthochromic fluid has an increased protein content.[189]

The typical clinical findings, including bilateral cranial nerve signs and evidence of an enlarged sella on the plain skull x-ray, virtually establish the presence of pituitary apoplexy. The differential diagnosis must, however, exclude the presence of an aneurysm of the circle of Willis, especially in the posterior communicating and basilar arteries.

Emergency parenteral substitution of steroids in large doses may be necessary to obviate acute adrenal insufficiency and consequent cardiovascular failure. Medical conditions must be treated before an operation is undertaken. Transsphenoidal evacuation of the hematoma is the treatment of choice because it causes the least additional trauma to the damaged optic system. The hemorrhagic cyst is easily evacuated, and the remaining adenomatous tissue can be removed by suction. After operative treatment, the prognosis in terms of survival and recovery of visual function is usually good if the patient regains consciousness promptly and if cardiovascular shock can be treated successfully. Even severe visual disturbances can be reversed if decompression of the optic chiasm can be achieved within a few days after the apoplectic hemorrhage.[122]

Empty Sella Syndrome

The "empty sella" described by Busch is often an incidental finding in routine autopsies.[22] In this condition, the diaphragma sellae has a large opening, and the remaining normal pituitary tissue is usually flattened and forms only a thin layer of tissue on the floor of the sella. The posterior lobe is much less deformed and bulges in front of the dorsum sellae. The sella is usually moderately enlarged. Most patients who have an empty sella are asymptomatic and need neither medical nor surgical care. Because radiographic evidence of an enlarged sella may be wrongly attributed to the presence of a neoplasm, and may lead to an unnecessary operation or radiotherapy, a correct diagnosis is essential. It is useful to distinguish the "primary" empty sella syndromes, which appear spontaneously, from the "secondary" syndromes, which appear following operative or radiotherapeutic procedures.[219]

Primary Empty Sella

Several factors may contribute to the development of a primary empty sella. First, there is a large opening in the diaphragm. Second, the subarachnoid space, which normally extends only slightly below the diaphragm, expands. Third, expansion may follow pituitary atrophy that occurs, for example, as a consequence of repeated hyperplasias during previous pregnancies, or it may follow pituitary infarcts or be a consequence of increased cerebrospinal fluid pressure.[55,162] The syndrome occurs more frequently in women than in men and is often associated with arterial hypertension and obesity.

Many patients (64 per cent) who harbor pituitary adenomas complain of headaches but are otherwise asymptomatic.[157] This statistic may well be a matter of selection, however, because it is less likely that skull radiographs, which often reveal the sellar enlargement initially, will be performed on persons who do not have headaches. Trigeminal neuralgia was found in 2 of 31 patients in a series reported by Neelon and colleagues.[157] Although spontaneous cerebrospinal fluid rhinorrhea is a rare complication, it is an urgent one that requires operative intervention.[20,149,166,218] Visual deficits may occur if the optic nerves and chiasm are displaced into the sella; this rare complication occurs only in patients who have a secondary empty sella in which optic nerves adherent to a suprasellar "capsule" are drawn into an evacuated sella. Papilledema reportedly occurs in 8 per cent, and visual field defects (mainly enlargement of the blind spot) in 16 per cent of cases.[55]

In the series reported by Neelon and colleagues, 20 of the 26 patients who had radiographically proved empty sellas did not have endocrine abnormalities, 4 had partial hypopituitarism, and only 1 had complete hypopituitarism.[157] The one patient in this series who had pituitary hyperfunction suffered from acromegaly. The coexistence of a partially empty sella with an endocrine-active microadenoma has also been observed in patients with prolactinomas, acromegaly, or Cushing's disease.[43]

Radiographs reveal an enlargement or deformity of the sella or both in 90 per cent of the patients who have the empty sella syndrome; in 85 per cent, the volume of the sella is above the norm (240 to 1092 cu mm).[42,157] In this syndrome, the sella is often ballooned; but asymmetries in the configuration of the floor occur less frequently than they do in conjunction with adenomas. The contour of the floor is typically smooth and gently curved. In contrast to the "open" configuration seen with intrasellar masses, which tend to straighten the curve of the dorsum and separate the clinoid process, the empty sella maintains a normal "closed" configuration. The cortical bone of the floor is usually intact and does not have focal areas of destruction or atrophy.

Pneumoencephalography remains the definitive diagnostic study for the empty sella syndrome.[99] This procedure must be done with special care, since air is not readily seen in the sella unless lateral tomograms are taken with the patient's head in an overhanging position (Fig. 98–34). The radiograph may or may not show a marginal, crescent-shaped mass of soft tissue representing the remaining normal gland, and the position of an accompanying microadenoma may or may not be outlined.[43]

Operative treatment of the empty sella is mandatory whenever the patient has rhin-

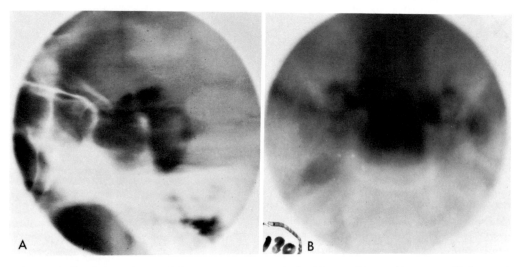

Figure 98–34 *A.* Lateral view of the pneumotomogram obtained from a 40-year-old woman suffering empty sella syndrome. Note the extension of the air-filled suprasellar cistern into the interior of the sella. *B.* Frontal view of the pneumotomogram obtained from the same patient showing the symmetrical excavation of the sellar contents.

orrhea or a demonstrated secretory microadenoma. The authors prefer the transsphenoidal approach. In patients who have rhinorrhea, the site of the cerebrospinal fluid leak is usually readily seen opening through the dura and the defective sellar floor into the sphenoid sinus; it is typically located low on the anterior wall. If a microadenoma is present, it is removed in the usual manner after the dura is opened. Closure requires a special technique: A piece of thigh muscle that is the same size as the sella is inserted between a large and a small piece of cartilage, which has been obtained from the nasal septum. A 3-0 silk suture is threaded twice through the three pieces. The muscle and the smaller piece of cartilage are then brought into the interior of the sella; the larger piece of cartilage remains outside, apposed to the sella floor (Fig. 98–35). Traction is applied on the suture and pulls the two pieces of cartilage together, at the same time squeezing the muscle out to form a tight seal. The sphenoid sinus must be filled with additional muscle tissue. A tube for continuous lumbar cerebrospinal fluid drainage is left in place for seven days.[119] This procedure is also effective treatment in the rare case of trigeminal neuralgia accompanying an empty sella, since it deflects the cerebrospinal fluid pulsations from the nerves in their parasellar course.

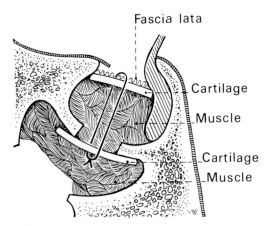

Fascia lata

Cartilage

Muscle

Cartilage

Muscle

Figure 98–35 Plastic closure of an empty sella opened from below. The two pieces of cartilage inside and outside of the sella are pulled together by a tightly knotted ligature, which causes an expansion of the interposed piece of muscle tissue that seals the cerebrospinal fluid fistula tightly. (From Landolt, A. M.: Therapeutic aspects of the empty sella syndrome. *In* Glaser, J. S., ed.: Neuro-Ophthalmology. Vol. 9. St. Louis, C. V. Mosby Co., 1977, pp. 229–235. Reprinted by permission.)

Secondary Empty Sella

Successful treatment of pituitary adenomas and functional hypophysectomies usually lead to the development of an asymptomatic secondary empty sella. If the chiasm has become fixed to the "capsule," however, complete transsphenoidal removal of an adenoma may cause the diaphragm and the attached chiasm to descend into the sella, stretching the optic pathways and, in some cases, resulting in recurrent visual disturbances. A careful neuroradiological examination will disclose the true nature of the condition. This situation can be corrected by repositioning the diaphragm from below and filling the sella with pieces of bone and cartilage.[165] When the diaphragm and tumor "capsule" do not descend spontaneously into the sella after complete removal of the adenoma, bone should be implanted in the sella to prevent this condition. Additional discussion of the empty sella syndrome is given in Chapter 100.

NONPITUITARY NEOPLASMS

With the exception of meningiomas and craniopharyngiomas, nonpituitary tumors are seldom encountered in and around the sella. Suprasellar gliomas involving the rostral third ventricle and chordomas are discussed in Chapters 82 and 89. In the discussion of the operative management of nonpituitary neoplasms that follows, more detailed attention is given to meningiomas and craniopharyngiomas than to the tumors that are less common to the sellar region. Inevitably, some areas of the discussion may seem redundant within this text, but the inclusion of those tumors that also arise in other intracranial sites is helpful in formulating an overview of the tumors that occupy parasellar locations.

Parasellar Meningiomas

This discussion is confined to the meningiomas that arise from the tuberculum sellae, the anterior clinoid process, the diaphragma sellae, and the dorsum sellae. The meningiomas of the inner sphenoid wing and those arising from the anterior clinoid process can be distinguished, if somewhat arbitrarily, because of the larger size of the inner-third meningiomas at the time of diagnosis and the characteristic lateral extension of the pterional tumors. Meningiomas originating from the anterior clinoid process produce monocular visual loss while they are still very small, and it is this symptom that first directs attention to the presence of the tumor. The majority of clinoidal meningiomas are 2 cm in diameter or smaller at the time of operation.

Large meningiomas arising from the cribriform plate and the planum sphenoidale may encroach upon the sella at a late stage, but they are more appropriately considered subfrontal, rather than parasellar, tumors. Similarly, tumors originating from the infratentorial aspect of the dorsum sellae are included with the clivus meningiomas, and tumors occupying the incisura, the floor of the middle fossa, and the optic canal are not considered parasellar for present purposes.

In the past, exploration of the optic nerves and chiasm was undertaken when a progressive monocular or binocular visual loss was otherwise unexplained and the diagnostic studies gave negative results. Today, because of the sophistication and accuracy of neuroradiological diagnostic techniques, exploratory craniotomy for unexplained visual loss is no longer necessary. For the tumors under consideration, neuroradiological procedures now can establish the diagnosis with respect to the location and size of the tumor, and often can establish the nature of the tumor as well.

The minimum essential radiographic evaluation of a suspected parasellar tumor requires 2-mm polytomography in both frontal and lateral projections, selective carotid and vertebral angiography, and a CT scan performed with contrast enhancement. If the size of the tumor is not revealed by a diffuse angiographic blush, then pneumoencephalography with polytomographic cuts will define even tumors measuring no more than a few millimeters. The same information can be obtained by CT scanning of tumors enhanced by contrast, although this procedure provides less satisfactory information regarding the anatomical relationships of the tumor.

Polytomography may disclose a subtle erosion of the bone, but the most typical finding is a sharply localized area of hyperostotic bone. Meningiomas arising from the anterior clinoid process and tuberculum may extend into the optic canal, in which case thin-section (1-mm) polytomographic cuts through the entire length of the optic canal and the anterior clinoid process will reveal expansion of the cranial aspect of the canal and, at times, adjacent hyperostosis. Erosion and hyperostosis can involve the tuberculum, the anterior clinoid process, and the tip of the dorsum sellae together with its posterior clinoid processes. The only tumor that does not produce these changes in the bone is the rare meningioma that arises from the diaphragma sellae. Occasionally, mottled calcification can be seen within heavily psammomatous meningiomas; calcification does not exclude the presence of a calcified prolactinoma.[125]

If a parasellar meningioma, situated laterally, does not cross the midline, and if the tumor does not occupy the tuberculum, the surgeon may prefer to make a pterional approach. The authors, however, prefer a paramedian subfrontal exposure for the majority of parasellar meningiomas, the only exception being those tumors that are confined to the anterior clinoid process.

Unless the neuroradiological studies indicate that the tumor originates from the tip of the dorsum sellae, the surgeon may be surprised to encounter the pituitary stalk in front of, and displaced forward by, the meningioma. The rare parasellar meningiomas that arise from the diaphragm are situated variably, but intimately, in relation to the stalk. As a rule, these are relatively small tumors, 2 cm or less, that are intimately related to the optic nerves and chiasm, and that often displace, and sometimes surround, the carotid arteries, the posterior communicating arteries, and the pituitary stalk.

Since the hyperostotic bone of parasellar meningiomas seldom contains tumor cells, the tumor's point of origin can be obliterated by destroying the dura, for which one of two techniques may be used. Cutting cautery can be used precisely with the aid of magnification and selection of the smallest wire loops, but this technique can injure the surrounding structures, either directly or by the transmission of heat. Unless the tumor has an unusually tough consistency, the use of cutting loops is unnecessary. The authors prefer to use bipolar coagulation and to excise the tumor in a piecemeal fashion, despite the additional time that this procedure requires. Bipolar forceps are used to grasp and char tiny bites of tumor, and the charred fragments are then removed with a fine pituitary rongeur. When bleeding from the surface of the tumor becomes troublesome, the tumor should be attacked at the dural attachment through which it derives its blood supply.

If the tumor extends into the cranial end of the optic canal, the canal should be unroofed with a high-speed air drill before an attempt is made to extract the tongue of tumor.

Craniopharyngiomas

Because craniopharyngiomas occur more frequently among the pediatric age group, they are discussed in detail in Chapter 84. The discussion in this chapter is concerned with craniopharyngiomas occurring in adults.

In adults, craniopharyngiomas generally are detected at an earlier stage of development than they are in children. In contrast to the majority of craniopharyngiomas, which originate in the suprasellar region, the primarily intrasellar tumors that produce only hypopituitarism can be diagnosed while they are still small and confined to the sella, regardless of the patient's age. There are no consistent histological differences between the craniopharyngiomas found in children and those found in adults, although the tumors in adults are somewhat more likely to be solid. Skull radiographs show calcification in the craniopharyngiomas of 81 per cent of the children and 40 per cent of the adults.[91] More recent evidence obtained with computed tomography, which is a more sensitive technique, indicates that areas of calcification can be seen in the majority of adult craniopharyngiomas.

Total operative removal of adult craniopharyngiomas is difficult, and in the authors' experience, only a minority of them can be extirpated safely. Unless the tumor is calcified to the point of being rocklike, however, decompression of the optic nerves and chiasm can be achieved with solid as well as with cystic tumors.

The three transcranial approaches to the craniopharyngioma are the subfrontal, the subtemporal, and the transventricular approaches. When preoperative studies suggest that total removal is a reasonable pos-

sibility—and assuming that the tumor is not primarily retrochiasmal—the authors prefer a paramedian subfrontal exposure. As in the case of pituitary adenomas, when the mass lies behind the chiasm, the tumor should be approached either subtemporally or through the lamina terminalis. Craniopharyngiomas that originate within and are confined to the third ventricle are quite rare. These tumors should be removed by a transventricular approach through the anterior corpus callosum.

The transsphenoidal approach is ideally suited to the removal of craniopharyngiomas that are either largely or entirely confined to an expanded sella. In the case of a cystic tumor that either occupies or extends into the sella, an alternative to attempted total removal is fenestration. In performing fenestration, a wide opening is made from the sphenoid sinus into the cyst, and the intervening sinus mucosa, sellar floor, dura, and tumor capsule are removed. The risk of fenestration is that a cerebrospinal fluid–sphenoid fistula may be created by opening into the subarachnoid space. If the sella is expanded forward and downward into the sphenoid sinus, however, and if the floor of the sella is thinned at the proposed site of fenestration, the surgeon can be reasonably certain that the tumor is in immediate apposition to the dura of the sella and that any intrasellar extension of the subarachnoid space has been obliterated. Fenestration affords the continued drainage of fluid from the cystic cavity into the sphenoid sinus and nasopharynx.

Despite belief to the contrary, craniopharyngiomas are radiosensitive.[114,117] If the operation has accomplished only incomplete removal of the tumor or drainage of its cystic component by transcranial aspiration or transsphenoidal fenestration, it should be followed by irradiation. In recent years, when the requisite conditions have been satisfied, the authors have been inclined to perform fenestration and follow it with radiotherapy, regardless of the patient's age.

Germinoma

Suprasellar germinomas preferentially affect children, whereas pineal germinomas have a predilection for women. The suprasellar germinoma presents a predictable clinical triad of hypothalamic hypopituitarism, diabetes insipidus, and involvement of the optic chiasm. Diabetes insipidus is often the initial abnormality, and this condition may precede other manifestations by many months or several years. In the past, suprasellar germinomas were incorrectly named "ectopic pinealomas." Their histological features are identical to those of testicular seminomas, ovarian dysgerminomas, and pineal germinomas. The suprasellar germinoma, like its counterpart in the pineal gland, is an atypical teratoma in which germinoma is the dominant teratomatous tissue.[191]

Pneumoencephalography and computed tomography reveal this tumor as a mass occupying varying areas of the suprasellar cistern and anterior part of the third ventricle. Although the clinical triad provides strong evidence regarding the nature of the tumor, the diagnosis requires histological verification unless characteristic tumor cells are recovered from the cerebrospinal fluid. The tumor can be seen through a small frontotemporal craniotomy. In most cases, it appears as a soft gray tumor mass involving the tuberal region of the pituitary stalk. If tumor is not apparent, the anterior portion of the third ventricle should be exposed by opening the lamina terminalis. Because this is a radiocurable neoplasm, any attempt at radical removal is ill-advised; because the tumor is liable to seed through the cerebrospinal fluid, the surgeon should obtain tissue for diagnosis and proceed no further.

Other Tumors

Other tumors located within and in immediate proximity to the sella do not occur frequently enough to either permit or justify detailed descriptions in this context.

Tumors of the neurohypophysis are exceedingly rare.[191] Pilocytic astrocytomas may originate from pituicytes in the posterior lobe, but their histological features are not unique to this region. More characteristic is the *choristoma,* a tumor considered to be of astrocytic origin. This rare tumor has been reviewed by Landolt.[118] Operative extirpation and postoperative radiotherapy produced improvement of vision and a survival of 22 years.

Congenital tumors may occupy the sella,

the parasellar subarachnoid cisterns, or the third ventricle. Although the pineal gland is the most common site of intracranial *teratomas,* the sella and the suprasellar region are the next most common sites. Parapituitary teratomas usually are primarily intrasellar and most often are benign and encapsulated. They lend themselves to operative removal unless they contain malignant elements. *Dermoids* virtually never occur within the sella, although massive frontal fossa dermoids may encroach upon the suprasellar cistern. Most frequent among the congenital tumors is the *epidermoid,* which occurs most often in the parasellar region, and next most often in the area behind the cerebellopontine angle. The majority of parasellar epidermoids occupy the middle fossa, often entering the temporal horn through the choroidal fissure. Epidermoids also arise in the suprasellar cistern and the third ventricle. Their cure requires removal of the epithelial capsule. The irritating contents of these frequently cystic tumors can produce a severe sterile meningitis. In treating an epidermoid, the addition of hydrocortisone to the fluid used for irrigation may decrease the inflammatory meningeal response. Epidermoids can mimic craniopharyngiomas, but ordinarily both gross and microscopic differences are distinctive, in spite of the histogenetic relationships that exist.[214]

Tumors either arising from or involving the sphenoid bone can encroach upon the sellar and parasellar structures. Among these uncommon entities are *primary tumors of the sphenoid sinus; nasopharyngeal carcinomas; metastatic tumors,* those from the breast ranking first; *giant cell tumors; aneurysmal bone cysts; chondromas;* and *fibrous dysplasia of the sphenoid bone. Histiocytosis* may infiltrate the hypothalamus, infundibulum, and neurohypophysis, and in the absence of recognized extracranial disease, craniotomy may be required to establish the diagnosis.

NONNEOPLASTIC MASSES

Inflammatory Lesions

The only inflammatory lesion affecting the sellar region is the *pituitary abscess,* and even this entity is rare (cf. the review of Domingue and colleagues).[43] The majority of pituitary abscesses occur in association with pituitary adenomas; these abscesses may also appear in some patients who present with meningitis and an enlarged sella. Although transsphenoidal drainage is the procedure of choice for treating pituitary abscesses, postoperative cerebrospinal fluid rhinorrhea is a potential complication.

Tuberculous and mycotic *granulomas* may involve the parasellar area, and when the correct diagnosis cannot be established by simpler means, a subfrontal exploration may be necessary.

Noninflammatory Lesions

Simple *cysts* and cysts of Rathke's cleft origin may occupy the sella and may mimic an endocrine-inactive pituitary adenoma.[43] Simple drainage of these cysts, preferably by a transsphenoidal approach, and treatment of the cyst epithelium with absolute alcohol in order to destroy the cyst lining appears to be adequate treatment. Even in the case of simple drainage without treatment with alcohol, recurrence is unlikely despite the cyst's lining having been left intact.

Arachnoid cysts occur within the sella, but more often occur in the suprasellar and parasellar spaces. Because arachnoid cysts found within the sella have either no opening or only a minute connection into the chiasmatic cistern, air does not enter the cyst at the time of pneumoencephalography. When the arachnoid cyst occupies the suprasellar space, it should be treated by creating a large window between the cyst and an adjacent large subarachnoid cistern. Although arachnoid that forms the cyst wall is left behind, recurrence is unusual.

Finally, sphenoid *mucoceles, encephaloceles,* and *aneurysms* may encroach upon sellar and parasellar structures. Aneurysms can mimic many of the common neoplastic and nonneoplastic processes in and around the sella. In spite of the sophistication of nonangiographic diagnostic techniques, there are very few situations—other than that of an intrasellar secreting pituitary tumor—in which the surgeon should approach a mass without having first performed preoperative carotid and vertebral angiography. Clearly, exceptions can and should be made, but only when an aneurysm can be excluded beyond reasonable doubt and when the relationship of parasellar arteries to the mass is not an issue.

REFERENCES

1. Adson, A. W.: Hypophysial tumors through the intradural approach. J.A.M.A., *71*:721–726, 1918.
2. Antunes, J. L., Housepian, E. M., Frautz, A. G., Holub, D. A., Hui, R. M., Carmel, P. W., and Quest, D. O.: Prolactin secreting pituitary tumors. Ann. Neurol., *2*:148–153, 1977.
3. Bailey, O. T., and Cutler, E. C.: Malignant adenomas of the chromophobe cells of the pituitary body. Arch. Path. (Chicago), *29*:368–399, 1940.
4. Bailey, P.: Tumors of the hypophysis cerebri. *In* Penfield, W., ed.: Cytology and Cellular Pathology of the Nervous System. New York, Paul B. Hoeber Inc., 1932, pp. 905–951.
5. Bailey, P., and Cushing, H.: Studies in acromegaly. VII. The microscopical structure of the adenomas in acromegalic dyspituitarism (fugitive acromegaly). Amer. J. Path., *4*:545–563, 1928.
6. Bakay, L.: The results of 300 pituitary adenoma operations (Prof. Herbert Olivecrona's series). J. Neurosurg., *7*:240–255, 1950.
7. Baker, B. L.: Functional cytology of the hypophysial pars distalis and pars intermedia. *In* Knobil, E., and Sawyer, W. H., eds.: Handbook of Physiology. Vol. 4: 1, Section 7, Endocrinology. Washington, American Physiological Society, 1974, pp. 45–80.
8. Baker, H. L., Jr.: The angiographic delineation of sellar and parasellar masses. Radiology, *104*:67–78, 1972.
9. Bentson, J. R.: Relative merits of pneumographic and angiographic procedures in the management of pituitary tumors. *In* Kohler, P. O., and Ross, G. T., eds.: Diagnosis and Treatment of Pituitary Tumors. Amsterdam, New York, Excerpta Medica–American Elsevier, 1973, pp. 86–99.
10. Bergland, R. M.: Pathological considerations in pituitary tumors. Progr. Neurol. Surg., *6*:62–94, 1975.
11. Bergland, R., and Ray, B. S.: The arterial supply of the human optic chiasm. J. Neurosurg., *31*:327–334, 1969.
12. Bergland, R. M., and Torack, R. M.: An ultrastructural study of follicular cells in the human anterior pituitary. Amer. J. Path., *57*:273–297, 1969.
13. Bergland, R. M., Ray, B. S., and Torack, R. M.: Anatomical variations in the pituitary gland and adjacent structures in 225 human autopsy cases. J. Neurosurg., *28*:93–99, 1968.
14. Bleibtreu, L.: Ein Fall von Akromegalie (Zerstörung der Hypophyse durch Blutung). München. Med. Wschr., *52*:2079–2080, 1905.
15. Bock, E.: Beitrag zur Pathologie der Hypophyse. Virchow. Arch., *252*:98–112, 1924.
16. Boyd, A. E., III, Reichlin, S., and Turksay, R. N.: Galactorrhea-amenorrhea syndrome:

Diagnosis and therapy. Ann. Intern. Med., *87*:165–175, 1977.

17. Boyd, D. J.: Observations on the human pharyngeal hypophysis. J. Endocr., *14*:66–77, 1956.

18. Bressler, H.: Die Krankheiten des Kopfes und der Sinnesorgane. Vol. 1: Die Krankheiten des Gehirns und der äussern Kopfbedeckungen. Berlin, Verlag d. Voss'schen Buchhandlung, 1839, pp. 295–296.

19. Brion, S., and Fanjoux, J.: Histologie. *In* Guiot, G., ed.: Adénomes Hypophysaires. Paris, Masson & Cie, 1958, pp. 142–156.

20. Brisman, R., Hughes, J. E., and Mount, L. A.: Cerebrospinal fluid rhinorrhea and the empty sella. J. Neurosurg., *31*:538–543, 1969.

21. Brougham, M., Heusner, A. P., and Adams, R. D.: Acute degenerate changes in adenomas of the pituitary body—with special reference to pituitary apoplexy. J. Neurosurg., *7*:421–439, 1950.

22. Busch, W.: Die Morphologie der Sella turcica und ihre Beziehungen zur Hypophyse. Virchow. Arch. [Path. Anat.], *320*:437–458, 1951.

23. Cardell, R. R., and Knighton, R. S.: The cytology of a human pituitary tumor: An electron microscopic study. Trans. Amer. Microsc. Soc., *85*:58–78, 1966.

24. Caton, R., and Paul, F. T.: Notes of a case of acromegaly treated by operation. Brit. Med. J., *2*:1421–1423, 1893.

25. Chang, R. J., Keye, W. R., Young, J. R. Wilson, C. B., and Jaffe, R. B.: Detection, evaluation, and treatment of pituitary microadenomas in patients with galactorrhea and amenorrhea. Amer. J. Obstet. Gynec., *128*:356–363, 1977.

26. Chiari, O.: Ueber eine Modification der Schlofferschen Operation von Tumoren der Hypophyse. Wien. Klin. Wschr., *25*:5–6, 1912.

27. Conway, L. W., O'Foghludha, F. T., and Collins, W. F.: Stereotactic treatment of acromegaly. J. Neurol. Neurosurg. Psychiat., *32*:48–59, 1969.

28. Costello, R. T.: Subclinical adenoma of the pituitary gland. Amer. J. Path., *12*:205–215, 1936.

29. Crompton, M. R., and Layton, D. D.: Delayed radionecrosis of the brain following therapeutic x-radiation of the pituitary. Brain, *84*:85–101, 1961.

30. Crooke, A. C.: A change in the basophil cells of the pituitary gland common to conditions which exhibit the syndrome attributed to basophil adenoma. J. Path. Bact., *41*:339–349, 1935.

31. Cunningham, G. R., and Huckins, C.: An FSH and prolactin secreting pituitary tumor: Pituitary dynamics and testicular histology. J. Clin. Endocr., *44*:248–253, 1977.

32. Curé, M., Trouillas, J., Lhéritier, M., Girod, C., and Rollet, J.: Inclusions tubulaires dans une tumeur hypophysaire, Nouv. Presse Méd., *1*:2309–2311, 1972.

33. Cushing, H.: The Pituitary Body and Its Disorders. Clinical States Produced by Disorders of the Hypophysis Cerebri. Philadelphia, J. B. Lippincott Co., 1912, pp. 140–143.

34. Cushing, H.: Surgical experiences with pituitary disorders. J.A.M.A., *63*:1515–1525, 1914.

35. Cushing, H.: The basophil adenomas of the pituitary body and their clinical manifestations (pituitary basophilism). *In* Papers Relating to the Pituitary Body, Hypothalamus and Parasympathetic Nervous System. Springfield, Ill., Charles C Thomas, 1932.

36. Cushing, H.: "Dyspituitarism": Twenty years later. With special consideration of the pituitary adenomas. Arch. Intern. Med. (Chicago), *51*:487–557, 1933.

37. Cushing, H., and Walker, C. B.: Distortions of the visual field in cases of brain tumor (chiasma lesions, with special reference to bitemporal hemianopsia). Brain, *37*:341–400, 1914.

38. Dalton, G.: Transsphenoidal hypophysectomy for pituitary tumors. Proc. Roy. Soc. Med., *67*:885–889, 1974.

39. Daniel, P. M., and Prichard, M. M. L.: Studies of the hypothalamus and the pituitary gland with special reference to the effects of transsection of the pituitary stalk. Acta Endocr. (Kobenhavn), Suppl. 201, *80*:1–216, 1975.

40. Davidoff, L. M.: Studies in acromegaly. III. The anamnesis and symptomatology in one hundred cases. Endocrinology, *10*:461–483, 1926.

41. Dawson, B. H.: The blood vessels of the human optic chiasm and their relation to those of the hypophysis and hypothalamus. Brain, *81*:207–217, 1958.

42. DiChiro, G., and Nelson, K. B.: The volume of the sella turcica. Amer. J. Roentgen., *87*:989–1008, 1962.

43. Domingue, J. N., Wing, S. D., and Wilson, C. B.: Pituitary adenomas in partially empty sellas. J. Neurosurg., *48*:23–28, 1978.

44. Dott, N. M., Bailey, P., and Cushing, H.: A consideration of the hypophysial adenomata. Brit. J. Surg., *13*:314–366, 1925.

45. DuBois, P.: Données ultrastructurales sur l'antéhypophyse d'un embryon humain à la huitième semaine de son développement. C. R. Soc. Biol. (Paris), *162*:689–692, 1968.

46. Eiselsberg, A. von: Operations upon the hypophysis. Ann. Surg., *52*:1–14, 1910.

47. el Etreby, M. F., and Günzel, P.: Prolaktinzell-Tumoren im Tierexperiment und beim Menschen. Arzneimittelforschung, *23*:1768–1790, 1973.

48. Erdheim, J.: Pathologie der Hypophysengeschwülste. Ergebn. Path., *21/II*:482–561, 1926.

49. Erdheim, J., and Stumme, E.: Über die Schwangerschaftsveränderung der Hypophyse. Beitr. Path. Anat., *46*:1–132, 1909.

50. Fager, C. A., Poppen, J. L., and Takaoka, Y.: Indications for and results of surgical treatment of pituitary tumors by the intracranial approach. *In* Kohler, P. O., and Ross, G. T., eds.: Diagnosis and Treatment of Pituitary Tumors. Amsterdam, New York, Excerpta Medica–American Elsevier, 1973, pp. 146–155.

51. Farquhar, M. G.: Origin and fate of secretory granules in cells of the anterior pituitary gland. Trans. N.Y. Acad. Sci., *23*:346–351, 1961.

52. Feiring, E. H., Davidoff, L. M., and Zimmerman, H. M.: Primary carcinoma of the pituitary. J. Neuropath. Exp. Neurol., *12*:205–223, 1953.

53. Ferner, H.: Die Hypophysenzisterne des Menschen und ihre Beziehung zum Entstehungs-

mechanismus der sekundären Sellarweiterung. Z. Anat. Entwicklungsgesch, *121*:407–416, 1960.

54. Fischer, P.-A., Schmidt, G., and Wanke, K.: Psychische Spätfolgen nach operativer Behandlung von Hypophysentumoren. Arch. Psychiat. Nervenkr., *210*:387–406, 1968.

55. Foley, K. M., and Posner, J. B.: Does pseudotumor cerebri cause the empty sella syndrome? Neurology (Minneap.), *25*:565–569, 1975.

56. Foncin, J. F.: Morphologie ultra-structurale de l'hypophyse humaine. Neurochirurgie, *17*: suppl, 1:10–24, 1971.

57. Foncin, J. F., and Le Beau, J.: Étude en microscopie optique et électronique d'une tumeur hypophysaire à fonction adrénocorticotrope. C. R. Soc. Biol. (Paris), *157*:249–252, 1963.

58. Forbes, A. P., Henneman, P. H., Griswald, G. C., and Albright, F.: A syndrome characterized by galactorrhea, amenorrhea and low urinary FSH: Comparison with acromegaly and normal lactation. J. Clin. Endocr., *14*:265–271, 1954.

59. Fraenkel, A., Stadelmann, E., and Benda, C.: Klinische und anatomische Beiträge zur Lehre von der Akromegalie. Deutsch. Med. Wschr., *27*:513–517, 536–539, 564–566, 1901.

60. Frazier, C. H.: A series of pituitary pictures. Commentaries on the pathologic, clinical and therapeutic aspects. Arch. Neurol. Psychiat. (Chicago), *23*:656–695, 1930.

61. Friend, J. N., Judge, D. M., Sherman, B. M., and Sauten, R. J.: FSH-secreting pituitary adenomas: Stimulation and suppression studies in two patients. J. Clin. Endocr., *43*:650–657, 1976.

62. Fritzsche, C. F., and Klebs, E.: Ein Beitrag zur Pathologie des Riesenwuchses. Klinische und pathologisch-anatomische Untersuchungen. Leipzig, F. C. W. Vogel, 1884.

63. Furth, J., Ueda, G., and Clifton, K. H.: The pathophysiology of pituitaries and their tumors: Methodological advances. *In* Husch, H., ed.: Methods in Cancer Research. Vol. 10. New York, Academic Press, 1973, pp. 201–277.

64. Geller, S., Ayme, Y., Kandelman, M., Grisoli, F., and Scholler, R.: Micro-adénome hypophysaire à LH. Ann. Endocr. (Paris), *37*:281–282, 1976.

65. Girod, C.: Histochemistry of the adenohypophysis. *In* Graumann, W., and Neuman, K., eds.: Handbuch der Histochemie, Vol. VIII Supplements, part 4. Stuttgart, G. Fischer, 1976, pp. 1–325.

66. Goodyer, C. G., St. George Hall, C., Guyda, H., Robert, F., and Giroud, C. J-P.: Human fetal pituitary in culture: Hormone secretion and response to somatostatin, luteinizing hormone releasing factor, thyrotropin releasing factor and dibutyrylcyclic AMP. J. Clin. Endocr., *45*: 73–85, 1977.

67. Gordon, P., and Roth, J.: The treatment of acromegaly by conventional pituitary irradiation. *In* Kohler, P. O., and Ross, G. T., eds.: Diagnosis and Treatment of Pituitary Tumors. Amsterdam, New York, Excerpta Medica–American Elsevier, 1973, pp. 230–233.

68. Grant, F. C.: Surgical experience with tumors of the pituitary gland. J.A.M.A., *136*:668–671, 1948.

69. Gubler, R.: Ueber einen Fall von acuter, maligner Akromegalie. Korresp.-Bl. Schweiz. Ärz., *30*:761–771, 1900.

70. Guinet, G., Tournaire, J., Orgiazzi, J., and Robert, M.: Amenorrhée-galactorrhée; image radiologique d'adénome hypophysaire; hyperthyréostimuline freinable. Ann. Endocr. (Paris), *33*:376–389, 1972.

71. Guiot, G.: Adénomes Hypophysaires. Paris, Masson & Cie, 1958.

72. Guiot, G.: Transsphenoidal approach in surgical treatment of pituitary adenomas: General principles and indications in non-functioning adenomas. *In* Kohler, P. O., and Ross G. T., eds.: Diagnosis and Treatment of Pituitary Tumors. Amsterdam, New York, Excerpta Medica–American Elsevier, 1973, pp. 159–178.

73. Guiot, G., Rougerie, J., Brian, S., and Hertzog, E.: L'utilisation des amplificateurs de brillance en neuro-radiologie et dans la chirurgie stereotaxique. Ann. Chir. (Paris), *12*:689–695, 1958.

74. Gusek, W.: Vergleichende licht- und elektronenmikroskopische Untersuchungen menschlicher Hypophysenadenome bei Akromegalie. Endokrinologie, *42*:257–283, 1962.

75. Halmi, N. S.: The current status of human pituitary cytophysiology. New Zeal. Med. J., *80*:551–556, 1974.

76. Halstead, E. A.: Remarks on the operative treatment of tumors of the hypophysis with the report of two cases operated on by an oro-nasal method. Surg. Gynec. Obstet., *10*:494–502, 1910.

77. Hamberger, C. A., Hammer, G., Norlen, G., and Sjogren, B.: Transantrosphenoidal hypophysectomy. Arch. Otolaryng. (Chicago), *74*:2–8, 1961.

78. Hamilton, W. J., Boyd, J. D., and Mossmann, H. W.: Human Embryology, Prenatal Development of Form and Function. 3rd Ed. Baltimore, Williams & Wilkins Co., 1962.

79. Hamperl, H.: Über das Vorkommen von Onkocyten in verschiedenen Organen und ihren Geschwülsten. Virchow. Arch. [Path. Anat.], *298*:327–375, 1937.

80. Hardy, J.: Transsphenoidal microsurgery of the normal and pathological pituitary. Clin. Neurosurg., *16*:185–216, 1969.

81. Hardy, J.: Transsphenoidal surgery of hypersecreting pituitary tumors. *In* Kohler, P. O., and Ross, G. T., eds.: Diagnosis and Treatment of Pituitary Tumors. Amsterdam, New York, Excerpta Medica–American Elsevier, 1973, pp. 179–194.

82. Hardy, J., and Wigser, S.: Transsphenoidal surgery of pituitary fossa tumors with televised radiofluoroscopic control. J. Neurosurg., *23*: 612–619, 1965.

83. Hardy, J., Beauregard, H., and Robert, F.: Prolactin-secreting pituitary adenomas: Transsphenoidal microsurgical treatment. *In* Robyn, C., and Harter, M., eds.: Progress in Prolactin Physiology and Pathology. Amsterdam, Elsevier–North Holland Biomedical Press, 1978, pp. 361–370.

84. Hardy, J., Robert, F., Somma, M., and Vezina, J. L.: Acromégalie-gigantisme: Traitement

chirurgical par exérèse transsphenoidale de l'adénome hypophysaire. Neurochirurgie (Paris), suppl. 2, *19*:1–184, 1973.

85. Harris, F. S., and Rhoton, A. L., Jr.: Anatomy of the cavernous sinus. A microsurgical study. J. Neurosurg., *45*:169–180, 1976.

86. Henderson, W. R.: The pituitary adenomata: A follow-up study of the surgical results in 338 cases (Dr. Harvey Cushing's series). Brit. J. Surg., *26*:811–921, 1939.

87. Herlant, M.: The cells of the adenohypophysis and their functional significance. Int. Rev. Cytol., *17*:299–382, 1964.

88. Herlant, M.: Introduction. *In* Tixler-Vidal, A., and Farquhar, M. G., eds.: The Anterior Pituitary. New York, Academic Press, 1975, pp. 1–19.

89. Heuer, G. J.: The surgical approach and treatment of tumors and other lesions about the optic chiasm. Surg. Gynec. Obstet., *53*:489–518, 1931.

90. Hirsch, O.: Endonasal method of removal of hypophyseal tumors. With report of two successful cases. J.A.M.A., *55*:772–774, 1910.

91. Hoff, J. T., and Patterson, R. H., Jr.: Craniopharyngiomas in children and adults. J. Neurosurg., *36*:299–302, 1972.

92. Horsley, V.: On the technique of operations on the central nervous system. Brit. Med. J., *2*:411–423, 1906.

93. Horvath, E., and Kovacs, F. K.: Misplaced exocytosis. Distinct ultrastructural features in some pituitary adenomas. Arch. Path. (Chicago), *97*:221–224, 1974.

94. Howe, H. S.: Normal and abnormal variations in the pituitary fossa. Neurol. Bull., *2*:233–238, 1919.

95. Jacobs, L. S., and Daughaday, W. H.: Pathophysiology and control of prolactin secretion in patients with pituitary and hypothalamic disease. *In* Pasteels, J. L., and Robyn, C., eds.: Human Prolactin. Amsterdam, New York, Excerpta Medica–American Elsevier, 1973, pp. 189–205.

96. Jefferson, G.: The Invasive Adenomas of the Anterior Pituitary. Liverpool, University Press of Liverpool, 1954.

97. Joplin, G. F., Jackson, R. A., Arnot, R. N., Burke, C. W., Doyle, F. H., Harsoulis, P., Lewis, P. D., Macerlean, D. P., Marshall, J. C., Noorden, S. van, and Fraser, T. R.: The effect of yttrium-90 implantation on endocrine function and visual fields in patients with "functionless" pituitary tumours, with biopsy and radiological findings. Clin. Endocr., *4*:139–163, 1975.

98. Kanavel, A. B.: Removal of tumors of the pituitary body by an infranasal route. J.A.M.A., *53*:1704–1707, 1909.

99. Kaufman, B., Pearson, O. H., and Chamberlin, W. B.: Radiographic features of intrasellar masses and progressive, asymmetrical non-tumorous enlargements of the sella turcica, the "empty" sella. *In* Kohler, P. O., and Ross, G. T., eds.: Diagnosis and Treatment of Pituitary Tumors. Amsterdam, New York, Excerpta Medica–American Elsevier, 1973, pp. 100–125.

100. Kaufman, B., Pearson, O. H., Shealy, C. N., Chernak, E. S., Samaan, N., and Storaasli, J. P.: Transnasal-transsphenoidal yttrium-90 pituitary implantation in the treatment of acromegaly. Radiology, *86*:915–920, 1966.

101. Kautzky, R., and Lüdecke, D.: Experiences with transsphenoidal approach to the hypophysis. *In* Kuhlendahl, H., Brock, M., Le Vay, D., and Weston, T. J., eds.: Modern Aspects of Neurosurgery. Vol 4. Amsterdam, New York, Excerpta Medica–American Elsevier, 1973, pp. 135–141.

102. Kawarai, Y., and Nakane, P. K.: Localization of tissue antigens on the ultrathin sections with peroxidase-labeled antibody method. J. Histochem. Cytochem., *18*:161–166, 1970.

103. Kempe, L. G.: Operative Neurosurgery. Vol. 1: Cranial, Cerebral, and Intracranial Vascular Disease. New York, Springer-Verlag, 1968, pp. 79–87.

104. Kernohan, J. W., and Sayre, G. P.: Tumors of the pituitary gland and infundibulum. *In* Atlas of Tumor Pathology. Section X, fascicle 36. Washington, Armed Forces Institute of Pathology, 1956.

105. King, A. B.: The diagnosis of carcinoma of the pituitary gland. Bull. Johns Hopk. Hosp., *89*:339–353, 1951.

106. Kinnman, J.: Acromegaly—An ultrastructural analysis of 51 adenomas and a clinical study in 80 patients treated by transanthrosphenoidal operation. Kungl. Boktryckeriet. Stockholm, P. A. Norstedt & Söners, 1973, pp. 1–226.

107. Kirsch, W. M., and Nakane, P. K.: A histochemical examination of pituitary adenomas with enzyme-labelled antibodies. *In* Carrea, R., Ishii, S., and Le Vay, D., eds.: Fifth International Congress of Neurological Surgeons, Intl. Congr. Series No. 293. Amsterdam, Excerpta Medica, 1973, p. 35.

108. Kjellberg, R. N., and Kliman, B.: Bragg peak proton hypophysectomy for hyperpituitarism and neoplasms. Progr. Neurol. Surg., *6*:295–325, 1975.

109. Kocher, T.: Ein Fall von Hypophysis-Tumor mit operativer Heilung. Deutsch. Z. Chir., *100*:13–37, 1909.

110. Kovacs, K., and Horvath, E.: Pituitary "chromophobe" adenoma composed of oncocytes. A light and electron microscopic study. Arch. Path. (Chicago), *95*:235–239, 1973.

111. Kovacs, K., Horvath, E., Pritzker, K. P. H., and Schwartz, M. L.: Pituitary growth hormone cell adenoma with cytoplasmic tubular aggregates in the capillary endothelium. Acta Neuropath. (Berlin), *37*:77–79, 1977.

112. Kovacs, K., Horvath, E., Corenblum, B., Sirek, A. M. T., Penz, G., and Ezrin, C.: Pituitary chromophobe adenomas consisting of prolactin cells—A histologic, immunocytochemical and electron microscopic study. Virchow. Arch. [Path. Anat.], *366*:113–123, 1975.

113. Kramer, S.: Indication for, and results of, treatment of pituitary tumors by external radiation. *In* Kohler, P. O., and Ross G. T., eds.: Diagnosis and Treatment of Pituitary Tumors. Amsterdam, Excerpta Medica, 1973, pp. 217–229.

114. Kramer, S., Southard, M., and Mansfield, C. M.:

Radiotherapy in the management of craniopharyngiomas: Further experiences and late results. Amer. J. Roentgen., *103*:44–52, 1968.

115. Kraus, E. J.: Die Beziehungen der Zellen des Vorderlappens der menschlichen Hypophyse zueinander unter normalen Verhältnissen und in Tumoren. Beitr. Path. Anat., 58:159–210, 1914.

116. Landolt, A. M.: Regeneration of the human pituitary. J. Neurosurg., 39:35–41, 1973.

117. Landolt, A. M.: Can craniopharyngiomas be treated by radiotherapy (histologic and ultrastructural considerations)? *In* Bushe, K. A., Spoerri, O., and Shaw, J., eds.: Progress in Paediatric Neurosurgery. Stuttgart, Hippokrates Verlag, 1974, pp. 232–236.

118. Landolt, A. M.: Ultrastructure of human sella tumors—correlation of clinical findings and morphology. Acta Neurochir. (Wien), suppl. 22:1–167, 1975.

119. Landolt, A. M.: Therapeutic aspects of the empty sella syndrome. *In* Glaser, J. S., ed.: Neuro-Ophthalmology. Vol 9. St. Louis, C. V. Mosby Co., 1977, pp. 229–235.

120. Landolt, A. M.: Progress in pituitary adenoma biology. Results of research and clinical applications. *In* Krayenbühl, H., ed.: Advances and Technical Standards in Neurosurgery. Vol. 5. Wien, New York, Springer-Verlag, 1978, pp. 3–49.

121. Landolt, A. M.: Biology of pituitary adenomas. *In* Faglia, G., Giovanelli, M. A. and MacLeod, R. M., eds.: Pituitary Microadenomas. New York, Academic Press, 1980, pp. 107–122.

122. Landolt, A. M.: Unpublished data.

123. Landolt, A. M., and Oswald, U. W.: Histology and ultrastructure of an oncocytic adenoma of the human pituitary. Cancer, 31:1099–1105, 1973.

124. Landolt, A. M., and Rothenbühler, V.: The size of growth hormone granules in pituitary adenomas producing acromegaly. Acta Endocr. (Kobenhavn), 84:461–469, 1977.

125. Landolt, A. M., and Rothenbühler, V.: Pituitary adenoma calcification. Arch. Path. Lab. Med., 101:22–27, 1977.

126. Landolt, A. M., Rothenbühler, V., and Kistler, G.: Morphology of chromophobe adenoma. *In* Fahlbusch, R., and Werder, K. V., eds.: Treatment of Pituitary Adenomas. Stuttgart, Georg Thieme Verlag, 1978, pp. 154–171.

127. Landolt, A. M., Ryffel, V., Hosbach, H. O., and Wyler, R.: Ultrastructure of tubular inclusions in endothelial cells of pituitary adenomas associated with acromegaly. Virchow. Arch. [Path. Anat.], 370:129–140, 1976.

128. Lawrence, J. H., Linfoot, J. A., Born, J. L., Tobias, C. A., Chong, C. Y., Okerlund, M. O., Manuvgian, E., Garcia, J. F., and Connell, G. M.: Heavy particle irradiation of the pituitary. Progr. Neurol. Surg., 6:272–294, 1975.

129. Laws, E. R., Jr., Trautmann, J. C., and Hollenhorst, R. W.: Transsphenoidal decompression of the optic nerve and chiasm. J. Neurosurg., 46:717–722, 1977.

130. Lederis, K.: A preliminary report on the ultrastructure of human neurohypophysis. J. Endocr., 27:133–135, 1963.

131. Linquette, M., Fossatti, P., and Derrien, G.: Les adénomes hypophysaires réactionels à des désordres hormonaux périphériques. Actualités Endocr., 13:247–256, 1973.

132. Linquette, M., Fossatti, P., May, J. P., Decoulx, M., and Fourlinnie, J. C.: Adénome hypophysaire à cellules thyréotropes avec hyperthyréoidie. Ann. Endocr. (Paris), 30:731–740, 1969.

133. Luse, S. A.: Ultrastructural characteristics of normal and neoplastic cells. Progr. Exp. Tumor Res., 2:1–35, 1961.

134. Luse, S. A.: Electron microscopy of brain tumors. *In* Fields, W. S., and Sharkey, P. C., eds.: The Biology and Treatment of Intracranial Tumors. Springfield, Ill., Charles C Thomas, 1962, pp. 75–103.

135. Luse, S. A., and Kernohan, J. W.: Granular-cell tumors of the stalk and posterior lobe of the pituitary gland. Cancer, 8:616–622, 1955.

136. Lüthy, F., and Klingler, M.: Der Tumorettentumor des Hypophysenhinterlappens. Schweiz. Z. Allg. Path., 14:721–729, 1951.

137. Mahmoud, M. E. S.: The sella in health and disease. Brit. J. Radiol., suppl. 8:1–100, 1958.

138. Marie, P.: Sur deux cas acromégalie. Rev. Méd., 6:297–333, 1886.

139. Marshall, J. C., Noorden, S. van, and Fraser, T. R.: The effect of yttrium-90 implantation on endocrine function and visual fields in patients with "functionless" pituitary tumours, with biopsy and radiological findings. Clin. Endocr., 4:139–163, 1975.

140. Marshall, M., Jr.: Localization of adrenocorticotropic hormone by histochemical and immunochemical methods. J. Exp. Med., 94:21–30, 1951.

141. Martins, A. N.: Pituitary tumors and intrasellar cysts. *In* Vinken, P. J., and Bruyn, G. W., eds.: Handbook of Clinical Neurology. Vol. 17, Tumours of the Brain and Skull, part II. Amsterdam, New York, Elsevier–North Holland Publishing Co., 1974, pp. 375–439.

142. Martins, A. N., Hayes, G. J., and Kempe, L. G.: Invasive pituitary adenomas. J. Neurosurg., 22:268–276, 1965.

143. McConnell, E. M.: The arterial blood supply of the human hypophysis cerebri. Anat. Rec., 115:175–203, 1953.

144. McCormick, W. F., and Halmi, N. S.: Absence of chromophobe adenomas from a large series of pituitary tumors. Arch. Path. (Chicago), 92:231–238, 1971.

145. McPhie, J. L., and Beck, J. S.: The histological features and human growth hormone content of the pharyngeal pituitary gland in normal and endocrinologically-disturbed patients. Clin. Endocr., 2:157–173, 1973.

146. Metzger, J., and Fischgold, H.: Radiologie—correlations radio-ophthalmogiques. *In* Guiot, G., ed.: Adénomes Hypophysaires. Paris, Masson & Cie, 1958, pp. 92–127.

147. Moriarty, G. C., and Halmi, N. S.: Electron microscopic study of the adrenocorticotropin-producing cell with the use of unlabelled antibody and the soluble peroxidase complex. J. Histochem. Cytochem., 20:590–603, 1972.

148. Mornex, R., Tommasi, M., Cure, M., Farcot, J., Orgiazzi, J., and Rousset, B.: Hyperthyroidie

associée à un hypopuitarisme au cours de l'évolution d'une tumeur hypophysaire sécrétant TSH. Ann. Endocr. (Paris), *33*:390–396, 1972.

149. Mortara, R., and Norrell, H.: Consequences of a deficient sellar diaphragm. J. Neurosurg., *32*:565–573, 1970.

150. Mosca, L., and Vassallo, G.: Morfologica dei tumori ipofisari nell'uomo. Atti Congr. Naz. Soc. Ital. Endocr., *13*:340–401, 1972.

151. Müller, W.: Über die Ranchendachhypophyse. Acta Neurochir. (Wien), suppl. *3*:128–133, 1955.

152. Mundinger, F.: Interstitial Curie-therapy in treatment of pituitary adenomas and for hypophysectomy. Progr. Neurol. Surg., *6*:326–379, 1975.

153. Mundinger, F., and Riechert, T.: Hypophysentumoren, Hypophysektomie. Stuttgart, Georg Thieme Verlag, 1967, pp. 224–227.

154. Naidich, T. P., Pinto, R. S., Kushner, M. J., Lin, J. P., Kricheff, I. I., Leeds, N. E., and Chase, N. E.: Evaluation of sellar and parasellar masses by computed tomography. Radiology, *120*:91–99, 1976.

155. Nakane, P. K.: Application of peroxidase-labelled antibodies to the intracellular localization of hormones. Acta. Endocr. (Kobenhavn) suppl., *153*:190–204, 1971.

156. Nakane, P. K., and Pierce, G. B.: Enzyme-labeled antibodies: Preparation and application for localization of antigens. J. Histochem. Cytochem., *14*:929–931, 1966.

157. Neelon, F. A., Goree, J. A., and Lebovitz, H. E.: The primary empty sella: Clinical and radiographic characteristics and endocrine function. Medicine (Balt.), *52*:73–92, 1973.

158. Nelson, D. H., Meakin, J. W., Dealy, J. R., Matson, D. D., Emerson, K., and Thorn, G. W.: ACTH-producing tumor of the pituitary gland. New Eng. J. Med., *259*:161–164, 1958.

159. Newton, T. H., Burhenne, H. J., and Palubinskas, A. J.: Primary carcinoma of the pituitary. Amer. J. Roentgen., *37*:110–120, 1962.

160. Nicola, G.: Transsphenoidal surgery for pituitary adenomas with extrasellar extension. Progr. Neurol. Surg., *6*:142–199, 1975.

161. Nurnberger, J. I., and Korey, S. R.: Pituitary Chromophobe Adenomas. Neurology, Metabolism, Therapy. New York, Springer Publishing Co., 1955, pp. 1–282.

162. Obrador, S.: The empty sella and some related syndromes. J. Neurosurg., *36*:162–168, 1972.

163. Oehlecker, F.: Zur Trepanation des Türkensatels bei Tumoren der Hypophyse und der Gehirnbasis. Arch. Klin. Chir., *121*:490–511, 1922.

164. Olivier, L., Porcile, E., Brye, C., and Racadot, J.: Étude de quelques adénomes hypophysaires chez l'homme en microscopie électronique. Bull. Ass. Anat. (Nancy), *127*:1258–1265, 1965.

165. Olson, D. R., Guiot, G., and Derome, P.: The symptomatic empty sella: Prevention and correction via the transsphenoidal approach. J. Neurosurg., *37*:533–537, 1972.

166. Ommaya, A. K., DiChiro, G., Baldwin, M., and Pennybaker, J.: Nontraumatic cerebrospinal fluid rhinorrhea. J. Neurol. Neurosurg. Psychiat., *31*:214–225, 1968.

167. Paiz, C., and Hennigar, G. R.: Electron microscopy and histochemical correlation of human anterior pituitary cells. Amer. J. Path., *59*:43–73, 1970.

168. Parkinson, D.: A surgical approach to the cavernous portion of the carotid artery. Anatomical studies and case report. J. Neurosurg., *23*:474–483, 1965.

169. Peake, G. T., McKeel, D. W., Jarett, L., and Daughaday, W. H.: Ultrastructural, histologic and hormonal characterization of a prolactin-rich human pituitary tumor. J. Clin. Endocr., *29*:1383–1393, 1969.

170. Peillon, F., Vila-Porcile, E., Olivier, L., and Racadot, J.: L'action des oestrogènes sur les adénomes hypophysaires chez l'homme. Documents histopathologiques en microscopie optique et électronique et apport de l'expérimentation. Ann. Endocr. (Paris), *31*:259–270, 1970.

171. Pelletier, G.: Classification et physiopathologie des tumeurs hypophysaires. Un. Méd. Can., *100*:1779–1783, 1971.

172. Pitts, L. H.: Personal communication, 1977.

173. Pitts, L. H.: Personal communication, 1978. Cf. Wilson, C. B., Tyrrell, J. B., Fitzgerald, P. A., and Pitts, L.: Neurosurgical aspects of Cushing's disease and Nelson's syndrome. *In* Tindall, G. T., and Collins, W. F.: Clinical Management of Pituitary Tumors. New York, Raven Press, 1979, pp. 229–238.

174. Porcile, E., Brye, C. de, and Racadot, J.: Données ultrastructurales concernant une tumeur adénohypophysaire humaine. J. Microscopie, *3*:49, 1964.

175. Pozo, E. del, and Flückiger, E.: Prolactin inhibition: Experimental and clinical studies. *In* Pastells, J. L., and Robyn, C., eds.: Human Prolactin. Amsterdam, New York, Excerpta Medica–American Elsevier, 1973, pp. 291–301.

176. Pribram, H. W., and Boulay, G. H. du: Sella turcica. *In* Newton, T. H., and Potts, D. G., eds.: Radiology of the Skull and Brain. Vol. 1, Book 1: The Skull. St. Louis, C. V. Mosby Co., 1971, pp. 357–405.

177. Purves, H. D.: Cytology of the adenohypophysis. In Harris, G. W., and Donovan, B. T., eds.: The Pituitary Gland. Vol. 1. London, Butterworth & Co., Ltd., 1966, pp. 147–232.

178. Racadot, J., Olivier, L., Porcile, E., Brye, D. de, and Klotz. H. P.: Adénome hypophysaire du type "mixte" avec symptomatologie acromégalique. II. Étude au microscope optique et au microscope électronique. Ann. Endocr. (Paris), *25*:503–507, 1964.

179. Rand, R. W.: Transfrontal Transsphenoidal Craniotomy in Pituitary and Related Tumors using Microneurosurgery. St. Louis, C. V. Mosby Co., 1969, pp. 74–86.

180. Rand, R. W., Heuser, G., and Adams, D. A.: Ten-year experience with stereotaxic cryohypophysectomy. Progr. Neurol. Surg., *6*:252–271, 1975.

181. Rasmussen, A. T.: The incidence of tubular glands and concretions in the adult human hy-

pophysis cerebri. Anat. Rec., *55*:139–169, 1933.

182. Ray, B. S., and Patterson, R. H.: Surgical experience with chromophobe adenomas of the pituitary gland. J. Neurosurg., *36*:726–729, 1971.

183. Renn, R. F., and Rhoton, A. L.: Microsurgical anatomy of the sellar region. J. Neurosurg., *43*:288–298, 1975.

184. Robert, F.: L'adénome hypophysaire dans l'acromégalie-gigantisme. Étude macroscopique, histologique et ultrastructurale. Neurochirurgie, *19*: suppl. 2:117–162, 1973.

185. Robert, F., and Hardy, J.: Prolactin-secreting adenomas. A light and electron microscopical study. Arch. Path. (Chicago), *99*:625–633, 1975.

186. Romeis, B.: Hypophyse. *In* Möllendorff, M. von, ed.: Handbuch der mikroskopischen Anatomie des Menschen. Vol. 6, part 3. Berlin, Julius Springer, 1940.

187. Roussy, G., and Oberling, R.: Contribution à l'étude des tumeurs hypophysaires. Prèsse Méd., *41*:1799–1804, 1933.

188. Rovit, R. L., and Berry, R.: Cushing's syndrome and the hypophysis. A reevaluation of pituitary tumors and hyperadrenalism. J. Neurosurg., *23*:270–292, 1965.

189. Rovit, R. L., and Fein, J. M.: Pituitary apoplexy: A review and reappraisal. J. Neurosurg., *37*:280–288, 1972.

190. Rucker, C. W., and Kernohan, J. W.: Notching of the optic chiasm by overlying arteries in pituitary tumors. Arch. Ophthal. (Chicago), *51*:161–170, 1954.

191. Russell, D. S., and Rubinstein, L. J.: Pathology of Tumours of the Nervous System. 4th Ed. Baltimore, Williams & Wilkins Co., 1977.

192. Sachdev, Y., Gomez-Pan, A., Turnbridge, W. M. G., Duns, A., Weightman, D. R., Hall, R., and Goolamali, S. K.: Bromocriptine therapy in acromegaly. Lancet, *2*:1164–1168, 1975.

193. Saeger, W.: Fine structure of corticotrophic cells and of pituitary adenomas in Cushing's syndrome. Acta Endocr. (Kobenhavn) suppl., *173*:28, 1973.

194. Saeger, W.: Die Morphologie der para-adenomatösen Adenohypophyse. Virchow. Arch. [Path. Anat.], *372*:299–314, 1977.

195. Salazar, H., MacAulay, M. A., Charles, D., and Prado, M.: The human hypophysis in anencephaly. I. Ultrastructure of the pars distalis. Arch. Path. (Chicago), *87*:201–211, 1969.

196. Sasaki, R., Misumi, S., Fujii, T., Takeda, F., and Yamamoto, K.: Quantitative measurement of the ability of human growth hormone. Neurol. Med. Chir. (Tokyo), *15*:7–11, 1975.

197. Schaeffer, J. P.: Some points in the regional anatomy of the optic pathway, with special reference to tumors of the hypophysis cerebri and resulting ocular changes. Anat. Rec., *28*:243–279, 1924.

198. Schelin, U.: Chromophobe and acidophil adenomas of the human pituitary gland. Acta. Path. Microbiol. Scand., suppl. 158, 1962.

199. Schiefer, H. G., Hübner, G., and Kleinsasser, O.: Riesenmitochondrien aus Onkocyten menschlicher Adenolymphome. Isolierung, morphologische und biochemische Untersu-

chungen. Virchow. Arch. Zellpath., *1*:230–239, 1968.

200. Schloffer, H.: Erfolgreiche Operation eines Hypophysentumors auf nasalem Wege. Wien. Klin. Wschr., *20*:621–624, 1907.

201. Schochet, S. S., Jr., McCormick, W. F., and Halmi, N. S.: Salivary gland rests in the human pituitary. Light and electron microscopical study. Arch. Path. (Chicago), *98*:193–200, 1974.

202. Snyder, P. J., and Sterling, F. H.: Hypersecretion of LH and FSH by a pituitary adenoma. J. Clin. Endocr., *42*:544–550, 1976.

203. Sternberg, C.: Ein Choristom der Neurhypophyse bei ausgebreiteten Oedemen. Zbl. Allg. Path., *31*:585–591, 1921.

204. Svien, H. J., and Colby, M. Y., Jr.: Treatment for chromophobe adenoma. Springfield, Ill., Charles C Thomas, 1967. pp. 1–107.

205. Svien, H. J., and Litzow, T. J.: Removal of certain hypophyseal tumors by the transantral-sphenoid route. J. Neurosurg., *23*:603–611, 1965.

206. Thorner, M. O., Chait, A., Aitken, M., Benker, G., Bloom, S. R., Mortimer, C. H., Sanders, P., Stuart Mason, P., and Bessen, G. M.: Bromocriptine treatment of acromegaly. Brit. Med. J., *2*:299–303, 1975.

207. Tindall, G. T., McLanahan, C. S., and Christy, J. H.: Transsphenoidal microsurgery for pituitary tumors associated with hyperprolactinemia. J. Neurosurg., *48*:849–860, 1978.

208. Tönnis, W., Oberdisse, K., and Weber, E.: Bericht über 264 operierte Hypophysenadenome. Acta Neurochir. (Wien), *3*:113–130, 1953.

209. Trouillas, J., Curé, M., Heritier, M. L., Girod, C., Pallo, D., and Touraire, J.: Les adénomes hypophysaires avec amenorrhée-galactorrhée ou galactorrhée isolée. Lyon Méd., *236*:359–375, 1976.

210. Tyrrell, J. B., Brooks, R. M., Fitzgerald, P. A., Cofoid, P. B., Forsham, P. H., and Wilson, C. B.: Cushing's disease: Selective transsphenoidal resection of pituitary microadenomas. New Eng. J. Med., *298*:753–758, 1978.

211. U, H. S., Wilson, C. B., and Tyrrell, J. B.: Transsphenoidal microhypophysectomy in acromegaly. J. Neurosurg., *47*:840–852, 1977.

212. Vaidya, R., Aloorkar, S., and Sheth, A.: Therapeutic regression of putative pituitary hyperplasia and/or microadenoma with CB 154. Fertil. Steril., *28*:362, 1977.

213. Verga, A.: Casa sinolare di prosopectasia. Reale Instituto Lombardo di Scienze e Lettere. Rendiconti. Classe di Scienze Matematiche e Naturali, *1*:111–117, 1864. Republished in Atti Accad. Med. Lombard., *19*:1363–1379, 1964.

214. Vivo, R. E. del, Armenise, B., and Regli, R.: Varieta formali e problemi istogenetici del craniofaringioma. Arch. De Vecchi, *38*:1–79, 1962.

215. Walsh, F. B., and Ford, F. R.: Central scotomas —their importance in topical diagnosis. Arch. Ophthal. (Chicago), *24*:500–534, 1940.

216. Walsh, F. B., and Hoyt, W. F.: Clinical Neuro-Ophthalmology. 3rd Ed. Vol. 3. Baltimore, Williams & Wilkins Co., 1969, pp. 2130–2156.

217. Wechsler, W., and Hossmann, K. A.: Elektronenmikroskopische Untersuchungen chromophober Hypophysen-Adenome des Menschen. Zbl. Neurochir., 26:105–122, 1965.

218. Weiss, M. H., Kaufman, B., and Richards, D. E.: Cerebrospinal fluid rhinorrhea from an empty sella: transsphenoid obliteration of the fistula. J. Neurosurg., 39:674–676, 1973.

219. Weiss, S. R., and Raskind, R.: Non-neoplastic intrasellar cysts. Int. Surg., 51:282–288, 1969.

220. Werder, K., Fahlbusch, R., Landgraf, R., Pickardt, C. R., Rjosk, H. K., and Scriba, P. C.: Treatment of patients with prolactinomas. J. Endocr. Invest., 1:47–58, 1978.

221. Wilson, C. B., and Dempsey, L. C.: Neuro-ophthalmology and transsphenoidal removal of pituitary adenomas. In Smith, J. L., ed.: Neuro-Ophthalmology Update. New York, Masson & Cie, 1977, pp. 221–226.

222. Wilson, C. B., and Dempsey, L. C.: Transsphenoidal microsurgical removal of 250 pituitary adenomas. J. Neurosurg. 48:13–22, 1978.

223. Wise, B. L., Brown, H. A., Naffziger, H. C., and Boldrey, E. B.: Pituitary adenomas, carcinomas, and craniopharyngiomas. Surg. Gynec. Obstet., 101:185–193, 1955.

224. Woolf, P. D., and Schenk, E. A.: An FSH-producing tumor in a patient with hypogonadism. J. Clin. Endocr., 38:561–568, 1974.

225. Wright, A. D., Hartog, M., Paller, H., Tevaar-werk, G., Doyle, F. H., Arnot, R., Joplin, G. F., and Fraser, T. R.: The use of yttrium-90 implantation in the treatment of acromegaly. Proc. Roy. Soc. Med., 63:221–223, 1970.

226. Xuereb, G. P., Prichard, M. M. L., and Daniel, P. M.: The arterial supply and venous drainage of the human hypophysis cerebri. Quart. J. Exp. Physiol., 39:199–217, 1954.

227. Xuereb, G. P., Prichard, M. M. L., and Daniel, P. M.: The hypophysial portal system of vessels in man. Quart. J. Exp. Physiol., 39:219–230, 1954.

228. Yasargil, M. G. Fox, J. L., and Ray, M. W.: The operative approach to aneurysms of the anterior communicating artery. In Krayenbühl, H., ed.: Advances and Technical Standards in Neurosurgery. Vol. 2. Vienna, Springer-Verlag, 1975, pp. 115–128.

229. Zimmerman, E. A., Defendini, R., and Frantz, A. G.: Prolactin and growth hormone in patients with pituitary adenomas: A correlative study of hormone in tumor and plasma by immunoperoxidase technique and radioimmunoassay. J. Clin. Endocr., 38:577–585, 1974.

230. Zülch, K. J.: Biologie und Pathologie der Hirngeschwulste. In Olivecrona, H., and Tönnis, W., eds.: Handbuch der Neurochirurgie. Vol. 3. Berlin-Göttingen-Heidelberg, Springer-Verlag, 1956.

99

RADIATION THERAPY
OF PITUITARY TUMORS

Virtually all tumors of the pituitary gland arise in the anterior lobe. The anterior lobe, or pars anterior, is derived from Rathke's pouch and is epithelial in origin.[17] The tumors vary in size from a few millimeters, the so-called "microadenomas" detected primarily because of endocrine hypersecretion, to several centimeters in diameter. They may compress the remaining pituitary gland, causing hypopituitarism, or extend from the sella turcica to displace or invade adjacent structures. The optic chiasm and nerves are the structures most frequently impaired. Erosion through the floor of the sella into the sphenoid sinus or nasopharynx, or invasion of the brain or cavernous sinuses may occur.

Treatment of pituitary tumors presents an interesting challenge to endocrinologists, radiation therapists, and neurosurgeons. The goal of therapy is to destroy or remove the tumor, to relieve the compression of the pituitary gland and extrapituitary structures, and to control excessive hormone production. Ideally, the therapy should have no associated mortality, nor should it cause hypopituitarism or result in injury to adjacent structures such as the optic chiasm. Although medical suppression is occasionally used, definitive therapy usually is operative removal by craniotomy or the transsphenoidal approach, or radiation therapy, or both.

Radiation therapy may take one of several forms. These include implantation of radioactive sources into the tumor, external irradiation with cyclotron-produced particle (e.g., proton) beams, or external irradiation with high-energy photons (x- or gamma-rays). Radionuclide implantation and proton beam therapy are limited to selected cases and are techniques available only in a few centers throughout the world. On the other hand, conventional megavoltage photon radiotherapy is generally applicable to all pituitary tumors and is widely available.

While a detailed discussion of the technical aspects of conventional radiotherapy is not presented here, a few general comments are in order. Over the years a number of different techniques have developed. Treatment via bilateral opposed fields, the simplest and earliest technique, yields a dosage pattern in which the temporal lobes of the brain receive a larger dose than the pituitary. Since the dose-response curve for pituitary adenomas indicates that the maximum safe dose should yield the highest control rate, the dose to temporal lobes limits the applicability of this technique. The use of three treatment portals, one coronal and two wedged bilateral opposed fields, gives a better dose distribution and still can be applied to relatively large volumes. Various types of rotational beam therapy have been developed in recent years and are now widely utilized. For tumor volumes less than 5 or 6 cm in diameter the authors currently use bilateral coronal 110-degree arcs with moving wedge filters. This technique has been made practical by computer calculation of dosimetry. When larger treatment volumes are necessary, three- or two-field techniques are used. For adenomas, a dose of 4500 rads calculated at the 95 per cent isodose line is given in about five weeks. The daily dose should not exceed 200 rads; larger total doses or daily fractions cause complications at an unacceptable rate when used for adenomas (e.g., optic nerve damage).[1]

G. E. SHELINE AND W. M. WARA

Craniopharyngiomas, which are discussed later, are treated by similar techniques but with a moderately larger dose.

Major complications can ensue from external irradiation given to the pituitary-hypothalamic area, especially when the patient is a growing child. Several isolated instances of pituitary hormone deficiencies have been reported in children who have received relatively large doses of irradiation.[8,26,40] Now many centers have reported a significant incidence of growth hormone deficiency after moderate doses (4000 to 5000 rads).* The exact site and incidence of such radiation injury remains uncertain at the present time; however, clinicians must be aware of this entity and carefully assess endocrinological function in patients who may be potentially at risk.

Older reviews usually classified pituitary adenomas as chromophobic ("nonfunctional"), eosinophilic (with gigantism or acromegaly), or basophilic (Cushing's disease). Recent information derived from electron microscopy, immunoperoxidase staining, radioimmunoassay, and the new hormone assays require a different approach to classification.[31] For example, adenomas associated with acromegaly often appear chromophobic by light microscopy but prove to have eosinophilic granules when studied by the newer techniques. With current techniques, many tumors previously thought "nonfunctional" have been found to be endocrinologically active. Thus, emphasis is shifting from the classification based on tinctorial staining and routine light microscopy to one based on function and extension of the pituitary tumor.

"NONFUNCTIONING" CHROMOPHOBE ADENOMAS

A substantial body of data has accumulated regarding the entity previously called "nonfunctioning chromophobe" adenoma. It is now known that many, probably a third or more, of these adenomas secrete prolactin, and this group should be restudied so that the endocrinologically active can be appropriately separated from the truly nonfunctional lesions. Such studies are in

progress, but in the meantime, treatment decisions must be based on information available.

As a group these tumors tend to be large, and pressure-induced defects such as decreased visual fields or hypopituitarism usually lead to the diagnosis. Occasionally the diagnosis is fortuitous and due to the finding of sellar expansion on a skull film taken for some unrelated reason, usually trauma. When symptomatic, about 95 per cent of patients have visual field deficits at the time of diagnosis. Many of these lesions erode into the sphenoid sinus, and 2 or 3 per cent of patients present with extension through the sella into the nasopharynx. Hypopituitarism is common.[38] These tumors tend to grow slowly, and recurrence may become evident only after 5 to 10 or more years. Thus, final assessment of treatment results requires long observation periods.

It is the consensus that particularly in the presence of major visual field deficits, most of these adenomas should be treated by conservative operative resection with decompression of the optic chiasm followed by radiation therapy.[18,36] The resection permits biopsy confirmation of the diagnosis and, more importantly, provides the most reliable and rapid decompression of the optic apparatus. In terms of initial response to treatment, operation alone is the equivalent of operation plus radiation therapy. If, however, radiation therapy is withheld, the recurrence rate after 5 or 10 years is high. Sheline reported a 5-year determinate control rate of 43 per cent for resection alone versus a 95 per cent rate for resection plus radiation therapy. At 10 years these rates were 11 and 82 per cent, respectively.[36]

In selected patients with small lesions and minimal visual field defects or with medical contraindication to operative management, radiation therapy alone may provide adequate therapy. In such patients the response rate and the five-year control rate appear to be as good as with resection plus radiation therapy.[7,13,29,36] Whether these results will hold up over longer follow-up intervals is not known. Additionally, patients with exceptionally large invasive tumors in whom attempted resection carries a rather high risk of morbidity and death with little chance of improving visual defects should be treated primarily by radiation therapy.[18,36] In these patients the basic intent of therapy is prevention of further growth and visual deterioration.

---

* See references 12, 28, 30, 33, 34, 35.

ACROMEGALY

Before the availability of a reliable human growth hormone (HGH) assay, the diagnosis of acromegaly was based on clinical findings such as bone and soft-tissue overgrowth and measurement of effects on target organs such as adrenal glands, thyroid, and gonads.[9,10] The diagnosis tended to be established relatively late in the course of the disease. Field defects were present in 17 of 37 (46 per cent) of the patients reported by Sheline, Goldberg, and Feldman.[39] Once the diagnosis was established, unless large field deficits were present, the accepted treatment was external radiation therapy. In the presence of large visual field defects, initial operative decompression was favored. The radiation therapy regimen gradually evolved into a course of daily treatments of 180 to 200 rads carried to a total of 4000 to 5000 rads. Smaller doses yielded lesser control rates and larger doses were associated with an increase in complications from the irradiation. With radiotherapy, the control rate was about 70 to 80 per cent and recurrences were rare. Of necessity, evaluation was based on lack of further growth and reversal of endocrine abnormalities associated with the target organs. Minor visual field defects often reversed, and decrease in the soft-tissue overgrowth sometimes occurred.[2,39]

With availability of the human growth hormone assay in the mid-1960's, it became apparent that in the first months following radiation therapy there was little or no decrease in growth hormone level. Other methods of therapy such as implantation of radioactive sources into the pituitary, heavy particle irradiation, transsphenoidal cryohypophysectomy (TCH), and transsphenoidal microsurgery (TMS), soon supplanted conventional radiation therapy.[11,22,23] Levin reported a series of 50 consecutive patients treated by transsphenoidal cryohypophysectomy.[23] At diagnosis these patients had small tumors and none had significant extension outside the sella. Diagnosis was established by a growth hormone level above 10 ng per milliliter or one that was not suppressed after glucose administration. Seventy-six per cent developed normal growth hormone levels within a matter of days after operation. There were no operative deaths, but

postoperatively permanent adrenal insufficiency occurred in 12 per cent, hypothyroidism in 10 per cent, and diabetes insipidus in 4 per cent. Preliminary data suggest that transphenoidal micro-operative removal of the tumor is similarly effective and as safe as cryohypophysectomy. The late recurrence rates for transsphenoidal cryohypophysectomy and transsphenoidal microsurgery are as yet unestablished. It should be noted that both methods require a high level of skill and experience; in nine previously untreated acromegalic patients who received transsphenoidal microsurgery, Atkinson and co-workers had one case of hypothyroidism and hypoadrenalism, one case of unilateral blindness, and one death.[3]

In 1970 Roth and associates reported a group of 20 acromegalic patients in whom pre- and postirradiation human growth hormone assays were done who were treated by conventional external irradiation.[32] The growth hormone levels decreased slowly after irradiation: by one to two years the mean decrease was 51 per cent; two and a half years after therapy, the mean decrease was 76 per cent. Because of the minimal side effects, they advocated restoration of conventional irradiation for treatment of acromegaly. Lawrence, Pinsky, and Goldfine described 12 patients, 9 of whom achieved normal growth hormone levels after irradiation.[21] The three failures were among the six patients with initial growth hormone levels of 50 ng per milliliter or higher. Sheline and Wara reported similar results with no significant complications.[38]

At the present time, it appears that conventional external irradiation therapy, heavy-particle irradiation therapy, transsphenoidal cryohypophysectomy, and transsphenoidal microsurgery yield about the same control rates. The rates of survival after heavy-particle irradiation are shown in Figure 99–1. The return of growth hormone levels to the normal range occurs within a matter of days following the operative procedures, but requires from months to several years after irradiation. Whether the rapid decrease of growth hormone justifies the operative complications is not clear. If gross tumor remains after resection, however, or if the growth hormone level is still elevated, postoperative irradiation is indicated. Recent data indicate that the majority of the operative failures can be salvaged by conventional radiation therapy.[37]

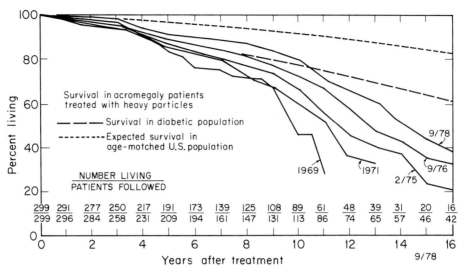

Figure 99–1 Survival after heavy-particle irradiation. (Courtesy of J. H. Lawrence, Donner Laboratory, Berkeley, California.)

CUSHING'S DISEASE

Cushing's disease, bilateral adrenal hyperplasia secondary to excess pituitary adrenocorticotropic hormone (ACTH) production, must be carefully distinguished from other causes of Cushing's syndrome. Adrenal tumors are treated by operative resection. Treatment of Cushing's disease requires control of excessive cortisone production by both adrenal glands. This may be accomplished by bilateral adrenalectomy or reduction of ACTH excretion by the pituitary gland. Bilateral total adrenalectomy is effective but leaves the patient dependent upon steroid replacement therapy. Bilateral subtotal adrenalectomy, while less likely to cause hypoadrenalism, often fails to control the excessive corticosteroid production.

Although in the past demonstrable pituitary tumors have been found in only about 10 per cent of patients with Cushing's disease, polytomography and micro-operative techniques have shown that the large majority of these patients do have pituitary adenomas. While a few are large enough to expand the sella and be evident on ordinary skull roentgenograms, most are only a few millimeters in diameter. Careful transsphenoidal selective excision, particularly of the "micro" adenomas, less than 1 cm in diameter, appears to give a high control rate with relatively little morbidity.[11,41] If the preliminary data are substantiated with a larger number of patients, transsphenoidal resection will probably prove to be the best method of therapy. Skill is required to identify and excise these small lesions without producing hypopituitarism or other operative morbidity. Whether recurrence will be a problem is as yet unestablished.

Cushing's disease can be controlled in about half the patients by conventional external irradiation therapy with virtually no complications. Heuschele and Lampe gave a dose of 4000 rads to the pituitary in four to four and a half weeks and had complete remission in 10 to 16 patients.[14] The average time to evidence of biochemical improvement was about five months. Clinical improvement became evident in about seven months. Orth and Liddle found that of 44 patients with Cushing's disease, 23 per cent were cured by conventional irradiation and another 29 per cent were sufficiently improved that no other therapy was required.[27] There were no complications. Bilateral adrenalectomy was used for radiation failures. Edmonds and co-workers, using less strict criteria of control, reported that 9 of 15 patients had complete biochemical remission after external radiation therapy.[6] Edmonds noted that the response to irradiation may require many months and recommended that adrenalectomy for radiation failure should be delayed at least one year if the clinical situation permits. Irradiation-induced reduction of pituitary function, whether the function is due to a normal pituitary or a pituitary adenoma, requires a relatively long time.

Thus in Cushing's disease due to a microadenoma of the pituitary, transsphenoidal resection gives a good control rate with relatively little morbidity, but the late recurrence rate is unknown. Radiation therapy with a control rate of about 50 per cent has very few associated complications but often requires months before being effective. In case of adenomas not readily controlled by microdissection, it is recommended that radiation therapy to the pituitary be tried before resorting to adrenalectomy.

HYPERPROLACTINEMIA

Prolactin-secreting pituitary adenomas may be large and involve adjacent structures or may be small and identifiable only by their functional activity and polytomography of the sella. Robert and Hardy reported on a comparison of light and electron microscopy in 25 prolactin-secreting adenomas associated with amenorrhea, with or without galactorrhea.[31] Fourteen were described as microadenomas (i.e., less than 10 mm in diameter), while seven had supersellar extension and four extended into the sphenoid sinus. By electron microscopy, all 25 tumors contained secretory granules; by light microscopy, approximately two thirds would have been called chromophobe adenomas.

In contrast to the small prolactin-secreting adenomas, some prolactin-producing tumors are of substantial size, expanding the sella and compressing or invading adjacent structures. As mentioned earlier, at least one third of the pituitary tumors previously considered "nonsecretory" or "nonfunctional" chromophobe adenomas that presented with expanded sellae, visual field deficits, extension into the sphenoid or cavernous sinus, and hypopituitarism were actually prolactin-secreting tumors. Frequently, such lesions cannot be completely resected without excessive morbidity, regardless of whether the resection is performed by a transsphenoidal or transcranial approach. These tumors should be treated as recommended for the large, so-called "nonfunctioning chromophobe" adenomas, namely, by conservative operative removal with decompression of the optic chiasm followed by a full course of external radiation therapy.

CRANIOPHARYNGIOMA

Craniopharyngiomas are derived from Rathke's pouch and may be intrasellar, extrasellar, or both. They are not endocrinologically functional, but may have compressive features similar to adenomas arising from the anterior lobe of the pituitary. The behavior and need for treatment of these tumors vary. While congenital in origin, some of them may be diagnosed late in life or as an incidental finding at postmortem examination. Symptomatic craniopharyngiomas are often discovered earlier, the majority being diagnosed during childhood. They are indolent, slowly expanding tumors, but even with conservative operative removal, morbidity and mortality rates have been considerable. Radical operations in these patients have led to severe morbidity and many deaths.* In other series, including those of Bloom, Kramer and coworkers, and McKissock and Ford, conservative subtotal operative removal plus postoperative radiotherapy has yielded control rates at least comparable to those of radical operations but with reduced morbidity.[5,19,26] Bloom has reported 5- and 10-year survival rates of 85 and 72 per cent, respectively, for cases treated by irradiation following aspiration or biopsy.[5] He cautions that prolonged follow-up will be necessary to assess final results, but it appears that both survival and quality of life are improved.

Recently Lichter and associates reported 8 of 17 (47 per cent) of patients treated only by operation had a recurrence. In comparison, only 2 of 10 patients (20 per cent) who had a partial operative removal followed by irradiation had a recurrence.[24] Radiotherapy on these patients was done via the coronal arc technique described earlier with total tumor doses of 5000 to 6000 rads, depending upon age of the patient and amount of residual tumor. There were no deaths, and morbidity was limited to partial pituitary dysfunction in one patient. Although the available information is limited, it appears that the greatest likelihood of

---

* See references 4, 15, 16, 25, 26.

control with minimal morbidity is achieved by limited operative removal followed by irradiation.

REFERENCES

1. Aristizabal, S., Caldwell, W., and Avila, J.: The relationship of time-dose fractionation factors to complications in the treatment of pituitary tumors by irradiation. Int. J. Radiat. Oncol. Biol. Phys., 2:667–673, 1977.
2. Arner, B., Lindgren, M., and Lindquist, B.: Results of roentgen treatment of acromegaly. A clinical review. Acta Endocr., 29:575–586, 1958.
3. Atkinson, R., Becker, A., Martins, A., Schaaf, M., Dimond, R., Wartofsky, L., and Earll, J.: Acromegaly: Treatment by transsphenoidal microsurgery. J.A.M.A., 233:1279–1283, 1975.
4. Bartlett, J.: Craniopharyngiomas—a summary of 85 cases. J. Neurol. Neurosurg. Psychiat., 34:37–41, 1971.
5. Bloom, H.: Combined modality therapy for intracranial tumors. Cancer, 35:111–120, 1975.
6. Edmonds, M., Simpson, W., and Meakin, J.: External irradiation of the hypophysis for Cushing's disease. J. Canad. Med. Ass., 107:860–862, 1972.
7. Emmanuel, I.: Symposium on pituitary tumours (3) Historical aspects of radiotherapy, present treatment technique and results. Clin. Radiol., 17:154–160, 1966.
8. Fuks, Z., Glatstein, E., Marsa, G., Bagshaw, M., and Kaplan, H.: Long-term effects of external radiation on the pituitary and thyroid glands. Cancer, 37:1152–1161, 1976.
9. Glick, S., Roth, J., Yalow, R., and Berson, S.: Immunoassay of human growth hormone in plasma. Nature (Lond.), 199:784–787, 1963.
10. Greulich, W., and Pyle, S.: Radiographic Skeletal Development of the Hand and Wrist. Stanford, Calif., Stanford University Press, 1959.
11. Hardy, J.: Transsphenoidal surgery of hypersecreting pituitary tumors. In, Kohler, P., and Ross, G. I., eds.: Diagnosis and Treatment of Pituitary Tumors. New York, American Elsevier [Amsterdam, Excerpta Medica], 1973, pp. 179–194.
12. Harrop, J., Davies, T., Capra, L., and Marks, V.: Hypothalamic-pituitary function following successful treatment of intracranial tumors. Clin. Endocr., 5:313–321, 1976.
13. Hayes, T., Davis, R., and Raventos, A.: The treatment of pituitary chromophobe adenomas. Radiology, 98:149–153, 1971.
14. Heuschele, R., and Lampe, I.: Pituitary irradiation for Cushing's syndrome. Radiol. Clin. (Basle), 36:27–31, 1967.
15. Kahn, E., Gosch, H., Seeger, J., and Hicks, S.: Forty-five years experience with the craniopharyngiomas. Surg. Neurol., 1:5–12, 1973.
16. Katz, E.: Late results of radical excision of craniopharyngiomas in children. J. Neurosurg., 42:86–90, 1975.
17. Kernohan, J., and Sayre, G.: Tumors of the Central Nervous System. Fascicle 35. Washington,

D.C., Armed Forces Institute of Pathology, 1952, pp. 17–42.
18. Kramer, S.: Radiation therapy in the management of malignant gliomas. In Seventh National Cancer Conference Proceedings. American Cancer Society. Philadelphia, J. B. Lippincott Co., 1973, pp. 823–826.
19. Kramer, S.: Radiation therapy in the management of craniopharyngiomas. In Deeley, T., ed.: Modern Radiotherapy and Oncology—Central Nervous System Tumors. London, Butterworth & Co., 1974, pp. 204–223.
20. Larkins, R., and Martin, F.: Hypopituitarism after extracranial irradiation: Evidence for hypothalamic origin. Brit. Med. J., 1:152–153, 1973.
21. Lawrence, A., Pinsky, S., and Goldfine, I.: Conventional radiation therapy in acromegaly: A review and reassessment. Arch. Intern. Med., 128:369–377, 1971.
22. Lawrence, J., Linfoot, J., Born, J., Tobias, C., Chong, C., Okerlund, M., Manougian, E., Garcia, J., and Connell, G.: Heavy particle irradiation of the pituitary. Progr. Neurol. Surg., 6:272–294, 1975.
23. Levin, S., Schneider, V., Rubin, A., Hofeldt, F., Becker, N., Adams, J., Seymour, R., and Forsham, P.: Rapid metabolic responses and lasting effects of cryohypophysectomy for acromegaly. In Abstracts, IV International Congress of Endocrinology, Washington, D.C. Amsterdam, Excerpta Medica, 1972, p. 135.
24. Lichter, A., Wara, W., Sheline, G., Townsend, J., and Wilson, C.: The treatment of craniopharyngiomas. Int. J. Radiat. Oncol. Biol. Phys., 2:675–683, 1977.
25. Matson, D., and Crigler, J.: Management of craniopharyngioma in childhood. J. Neurosurg., 30:377–390, 1969.
26. McKissock, W., and Ford, R.: Results of treatment of the craniopharyngiomas (abstract). J. Neurol. Neursosurg. Psychiat., 29:475–479, 1966.
27. Orth, D., and Liddle, G.: Results of treatment in 108 patients with Cushing's syndrome. New Eng. J. Med., 285:243–247, 1971.
28. Perry-Keene, D., Connelly, J., Young, R., Wettenhall, H., and Martin, F.: Hypothalamic hypopituitarism following external radiotherapy for tumours distant from the adenohypophysis. Clin. Endocr., 5:373–380, 1975.
29. Pistenma, D., Goffinet, D., Bagshaw, M., Hanbery, J., and Eltringham, J.: Treatment of chromophobe adenomas with megavoltage irradiation. Cancer, 35:1574–1582, 1975.
30. Richards, G., Wara, W., Grumbach, M., Kaplan, S., Sheline, G., and Conte, F.: Delayed onset of hypopituitarism: Sequelae of therapeutic irradiation of central nervous system, eye and middle ear tumors. J. Pediat., 89:553–559, 1976.
31. Robert, G., and Hardy, J.: Prolactin-secreting adenomas. A light and electron microscopical study. Arch Path. (Chicago), 99:625–633, 1975.
32. Roth, J., Gorden, P., and Brace, K.: Efficacy of conventional pituitary irradiation in acromegaly. New Eng. J. Med., 282:1385–1391, 1970.
33. Samaan, J., Bakdash, M., Cadero, J., Cangir, A., Jesse, R., Jr., and Ballantyne, A.: Hypopituitarism after external irradiation—evidence for both hypothalamic and pituitary origin. Ann. Intern. Med., 83:771–777, 1975.

34. Shalet, S., Beardswell, C., Morris-Jones, P., and Pearson, D.: Pituitary function after treatment of intracranial tumors in children. Lancet, 2: 104–107, 1975.
35. Shalet, S., Beardswell, C., Pearson, D., and Morris-Jones, P.: The effect of varying doses of cerebral irradiation on growth hormone production in childhood. Clin. Endocr., 5:287–290, 1976.
36. Sheline, G.: Treatment of chromophobe adenomas of the pituitary gland and acromegaly. *In* Kohler, P., and Ross, G. I., eds.: Diagnosis and Treatment of Pituitary Tumors. New York, American Elsevier [Amsterdam, Excerpta Medica], 1973, pp. 201–216.
37. Sheline, G., and Drake, K.: Unpublished data, 1977.
38. Sheline, G., and Wara, W.: Radiation therapy of acromegaly and nonsecretory chromophobe adenomas of the pituitary. *In* Seydel, H., ed.: Tumors of the Nervous System. New York, John Wiley & Sons, 1975.
39. Sheline, G., Goldberg, M., and Feldman, P.: Pituitary irradiation for acromegaly. Radiology, 76:70–75, 1961.
40. Tan, B., and Kunaratnam, N.: Hypopituitary dwarfism following radiotherapy for nasopharyngeal carcinoma. Clin. Radiol., 17:302–304, 1961.
41. Wilson, C.: Personal communication, 1977.

100

EMPTY SELLA SYNDROME

Visual field defects, enlargement of the sella turcica, and pituitary dysfunction have been the traditional hallmarks of intrasellar tumors. Although therapeutic decisions in the past have rested primarily on these "cardinal signs," there is increasing awareness that nontumorous conditions often mimic intrasellar tumors. The empty sella turcica is a common cause of nontumorous sellar enlargement and is often misdiagnosed (Table 100–1). Its clinical course is usually uneventful, and therapeutic intervention is rarely required. Although the clinical features of the empty sella turcica do not allow it to be clearly distinguished from pituitary tumor, certain aspects of its clinical setting often suggest the diagnosis. Furthermore, the proper application of pneumoencephalography is often diagnostic and can distinguish this condition from neoplastic enlargement of the sella.

DEFINITION

In the broadest sense of the term, "empty sella" refers to any communicating extension of the subarachnoid space into the pituitary fossa. The term "empty sella syndrome" extends this definition to include a remodeling or flattening of the pituitary gland against the sellar floor and usually a remodeling and enlargement of the sella itself. On gross anatomical inspection, these features give the impression that the sella is empty. The normal intrasellar contents—namely, the globular pituitary, its stalk, and the dural coverings and blood vessels—are distorted and may appear to be absent (Fig. 100–1).

ETIOLOGY

An empty sella may exist for one of two reasons: incomplete anatomical formation of the diaphragma sellae, which allows the arachnoid to herniate directly into the pituitary fossa as shown in Figure 100–2, or collapse of the suprasellar arachnoid (and occasionally other structures) into the sella after the intrasellar contents have been reduced in volume by an operation or irradiation or have undergone infarction and necrosis (Fig. 100–3).[14,21] These two conditions, one developmental and the other pathological, give rise to the clinical syndromes referred to respectively as the "primary" (or "idiopathic") and "secondary" empty sella syndromes (Table 100–2).

PRIMARY (IDIOPATHIC) EMPTY SELLA SYNDROME

The dural reflections that form the diaphragma sellae provide a complete covering that is penetrated only by the infundibular stalk, but anatomical variations in the diaphragma are frequent. They have been described and classified by Busch and include: type I, a funnel-shaped depression of the diaphragma sellae; type II, incomplete closure of the diaphragma sellae around the hypophyseal stalk; and type III, a wide defect in the diaphragma such that only a peripheral ring of tissue measuring 2 mm or less in width is present, which leaves the pituitary gland completely exposed and covered only with arachnoid (type III A), associated with symmetrical or eccentric indentation of the pituitary gland by the

---

S. F. HODGSON, R. V. RANDALL, AND E. R. LAWS

TABLE 100–1   CAUSES OF ENLARGED SELLA TURCICA

Neoplasm
Empty sella
  Primary
  Secondary
Arachnoid cyst
Granuloma
Aneurysm
Increased intracranial pressure

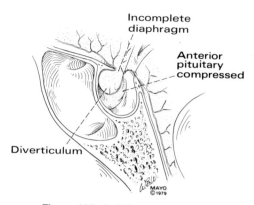

Figure 100–2   Primary empty sella.

herniating arachnoid pouch (type III B), or with complete remodeling or flattening of the pituitary gland (type III C).[8] Defects extensive enough to be associated with flattening of the pituitary have been demonstrated in 5.5 to 6.7 per cent of autopsy series.[3,8] In the study by Bergland and associates, the occurrence of a subarachnoid space that lies within the sella exceeded 20 per cent, and anatomical defects in the diaphragma sellae of 5 mm or more were demonstrated in as many as 39 per cent of consecutive autopsy cases without pituitary disease.[3] Anatomical defects in the diaphragma occur six times as often in women as in men, a sexual predominance that most likely explains the greater number of female patients seen with the empty sella syndrome.[24] It has been suggested that the high frequency of the empty sella among females may reflect changes in the sella due to transient enlargement of the pituitary during pregnancy.[33,48] That the sella actually enlarges during pregnancy has been refuted, however.[39]

Defects in the diaphragma may not be the only requirement for the formation of an empty sella, because wide openings are seen that are unpenetrated by the subarachnoid space. Erosion and remodeling of bony structures within the calvarium have long been known to occur in association with states of increased intracranial pressure. Normal variations in cerebrospinal fluid pressure transmitted to the intrasellar subarachnoid space are also thought to be of importance in the remodeling of the pituitary gland and its surrounding bony structures.[15] Increased cerebrospinal fluid pressure has been reported in the primary empty sella syndrome and is usually found in association with pseudotumor cerebri, hypertension, congestive heart failure, and the hypoventilation-obesity (pickwickian) syndrome.[17,23,33,43]

Furthermore, it is thought that in such cases the extent of sellar enlargement and remodeling may be more or less directly related to the degree of elevation of cerebrospinal fluid pressure. Normal pulsatile

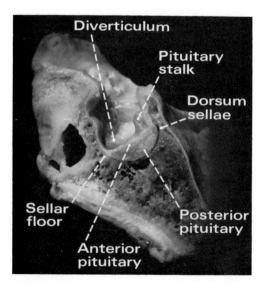

Figure 100–1   Gross anatomy of empty sella turcica.

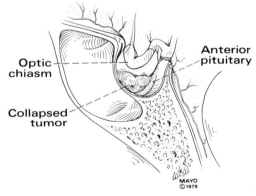

Figure 100–3   Secondary empty sella.

TABLE 100–2 CAUSES OF EMPTY SELLA SYNDROME

Primary (idiopathic) empty sella syndrome
Secondary empty sella syndrome
  Operative removal of sellar contents
    Therapeutic hypophysectomy
    Operation for intrasellar tumor
  Radiation therapy of sellar contents
    External radiation therapy
    Intrasellar implantation of radioactive isotopes
  Infarction of sellar contents
    Infarction of normal pituitary
    Infarction of intrasellar tumor

variations in the cerebrospinal fluid pressure transmitted through the incompetent diaphragma are thought to result in a globular remodeling of the sella, which initially remains normal in size, whereas prolonged elevation of the pressure may eventually cause expansion of the sella and remodeling of the pituitary gland.[23] The remodeled pituitary is most often reduced in size, flattened, and located in a posterior and inferior position along the sellar floor. The dorsum and the sellar floor may be thinned or eroded. Erosions of the sellar floor may penetrate the roof of the sphenoid sinus, and formation of a communicating sinus at this site probably explains the occurrence of cerebrospinal fluid rhinorrhea in some patients with the empty sella syndrome. It has also been suggested that increased cerebrospinal fluid pressure, perhaps augmented by transient increases due to straining, coughing, or sneezing, results in the reestablishment of patency of the vestigial craniopharyngeal duct and allows cerebrospinal fluid within the sella to enter the nasal passages.[6] Although sellar remodeling is generally symmetrical, it is important to emphasize that asymmetrical remodeling also occurs, often in association with eccentrically located septa within the sphenoid sinus that merge with the inferior aspect of the sellar floor.

Clinical and Laboratory Findings

The majority of patients with the primary empty sella syndrome are middle-aged, obese, multiparous, and often hypertensive women. Presenting complaints may be nonspecific (for example, headache, "sinus trouble," fatigue) or may reflect a state of increased intracranial pressure and the conditions that give rise to it. Impairment of vi-

sion occurs infrequently, but visual field defects have been demonstrated.[33] In patients with the primary empty sella syndrome, visual field defects are usually associated with increased intracranial pressure. Cases have been reported in which significant field defects were found in the presence of normal intracranial pressures, however, and presumably in these cases the defects were caused by prolapse of the optic nerves and chiasm into the empty sella.[7,12] Cerebrospinal fluid rhinorrhea may occur and is often complicated by bacterial meningitis.[6,22,33,43–45] Except for the occasional discovery of visual field defects and increased cerebrospinal fluid pressure and rhinorrhea, the neurological evaluation is unrevealing. Electroencephalographic findings have been nonspecific, but experience with electroencephalography in this entity has been limited.[4]

Roentgenographically demonstrated enlargement of the sella is most often an incidental and unexpected finding in those patients with nonspecific complaints. Although sellar enlargement is usually indicative of pituitary tumor, several roentgenographic characteristics of the expanded but empty sella help to differentiate these two conditions. Lateral roentgenograms characteristically reveal the empty sella to be modestly enlarged (Fig. 100–4). Its contour is symmetrical and rounded or globular, so the walls are smoothly curved. The clinoid processes are not displaced, and the dorsum sellae is not straightened, in contrast to changes often seen with expanding intrasellar tumors.[33] Erosion of the bony margins is rarely conspicuous. It must be re-emphasized that remodeling of the sellar floor, though usually symmetrical, is not always so, and a "double floor" contour may be seen on lateral projections.

Anteroposterior projections usually demonstrate a flat or concave sellar floor, but lateral sloping is present when remodeling is asymmetrical. Spiral tomograms confirm the findings seen on standard x-ray films of the head and differentiate changes more commonly associated with intrasellar neoplasm, such as discrete areas of erosion or distortion.

Pneumoencephalography used to be the only practical way to visualize an empty sella (Fig. 100–5). Bilateral carotid angiography with magnification and subtraction techniques is not helpful in the diag-

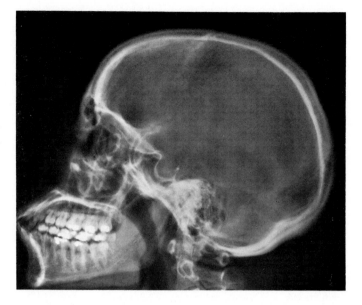

Figure 100–4 Primary empty sella. Lateral roentgenogram of head demonstrates rounded or "globular" symmetrical sellar enlargement.

nosis, but this technique can reveal a small adenoma coexisting with an empty sella. A residual drop of intraspinal contrast medium that has found its way into the intrasellar cistern may identify an empty sella (Fig. 100–6).

Usually, an empty sella can be readily diagnosed by means of the new-generation computed tomographic scanners. In making the diagnosis, the authors use these criteria: (1) an area of low attenuation (CSF) extends from the suprasellar cistern to below the level of the diaphragm into the sella in coronal views and (2) after injection of contrast medium, the pituitary stalk may be seen to extend down to a flattened pituitary gland in the bottom of the sella in coronal views (Fig. 100–7); and (3) the optic chiasm lies lower than usual and may dip below the level of the diaphragm of the sella in coronal and axial views (Fig. 100–8). Cisternography with metrizamide is an alternative method for demonstrating an empty sella (Fig. 100–9).

In general, the primary empty sella syndrome does not cause significant clinical endocrine syndromes, and tests of end-organ and pituitary-hypothalamic function are usually normal.[21,22,33,35,38] There are many published exceptions to this generalization, but they are virtually impossible to interpret because the information given does not permit clear separation of primary from secondary types of the empty sella

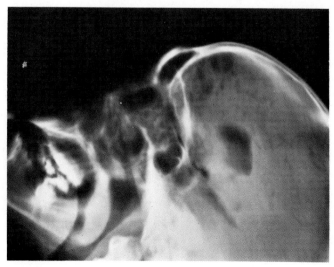

Figure 100–5 Primary empty sella. Pneumoencephalogram taken in "brow-up" position. Air is seen within sella turcica.

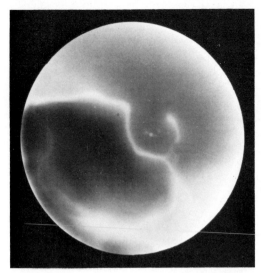

Figure 100-6 Primary empty sella. Contrast material from previous myelogram can be seen lying within the intrasellar subarachnoid space. Sella is of normal size.

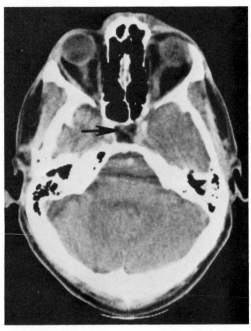

Figure 100-8 Primary empty sella (axial view). Low-lying optic chiasm (*arrow*) extends downward partway into the empty sella.

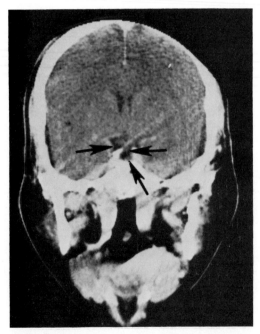

Figure 100-7 Primary empty sella (coronal view). Area of low attenuation (cerebrospinal fluid) extends from suprasellar cistern (*left arrow*) downward into the sella. The contrast-enhanced pituitary stalk (*right superior arrow*) courses downward to the flattened pituitary gland (*right inferior arrow*).

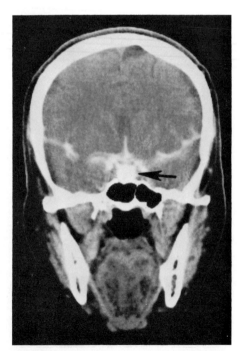

Figure 100-9 Primary empty sella (coronal view). Metrizamide outlines the empty sella (*arrow*).

syndrome; and as is seen later, pituitary function may be compromised in the secondary empty sella syndrome. In these reports, conclusions pertaining to abnormal pituitary endocrine function rely primarily on incomplete or indirect supporting data and leave open the possibility that incidental coexisting endocrine disease is present or that antecedent changes in the pituitary —for example, infarction—have predisposed the sella and the pituitary to both emptiness and malfunction.[9]

These objections notwithstanding, a limited number of well-documented cases suggest that endocrine abnormalities can occur in the primary empty sella syndrome, and panhypopituitarism, galactorrhea with and without increased serum prolactin levels, amenorrhea, and hypogonadotropism have been described.* More often, reported endocrine abnormalities have consisted of minor variations in the biochemical responses of the pituitary to various provocative tests that have not been associated with observable clinical manifestations.† Evidence of pituitary hyperfunction and the empty sella syndrome usually indicates the incidental coexistence of a pituitary adenoma—a not surprising association when one considers the common nature of the empty sella syndrome and the fact that the pituitary, although distorted in shape, usually remains histologically and functionally normal and retains its susceptibility to other pathological processes.[9,30,40] Other associated conditions have been reported and appear to have occurred by chance. They include the Achard-Thiers syndrome, the Foster Kennedy syndrome, virilization, renal tubular acidosis (with galactorrhea), and a single case of diabetes insipidus.[1,2,12,31,36]

Clinical Course and Management

The clinical course of the primary empty sella syndrome is uneventful, and patients whom the authors have observed up to 10 years have had no evidence of overt endocrine or neurological disease. Rarely, cerebrospinal fluid rhinorrhea may occur after the initial diagnosis, and radiological evidence of progressive remodeling of the sella has been observed.[20] Long-term follow-up is meager, and virtually no longitudinal information is available concerning the few patients considered to have neuroendocrine manifestations. Until such data become available, all patients with the primary empty sella syndrome should undergo periodic reassessment. The reassessment should include inquiry regarding signs and symptoms of endocrinopathy, cerebrospinal fluid rhinorrhea, or increased intracranial pressure, and standard roentgenograms of the head with polytomographic and anteroposterior and lateral views of the sella for comparison of sellar size and contour. Examination should include evaluation of the optic fundi and assessment of the visual fields. The extent of endocrine testing may be limited to static measurements of pituitary-dependent end-organ function. More precise evaluation of the pituitary-hypothalamic interrelationships may be accomplished by provocative testing with either thyrotropin-releasing hormone (to test the response of thyroid-stimulating hormone and prolactin) or insulin-induced hypoglycemic stimulation (to test the response of growth hormone, adrenocorticotropic hormone, and corticosteroids).[38]

Treatment

The uncomplicated primary empty sella turcica syndrome requires no treatment. Cerebrospinal fluid rhinorrhea, symptomatic and severe increases in intracranial pressure, and the development of significant visual field defects are the three indications for operative intervention, which is discussed in the section on treatment of secondary empty sella syndrome.

SECONDARY EMPTY SELLA TURCICA

The appearance of visual field defects after ablation of pituitary tumors by operation or irradiation has traditionally been considered prima facie evidence of tumor recurrence or enlargement. Colby and Kearns first drew attention to the fact that destruction of the pituitary was infrequently followed by visual field defects that were not caused by expanding tumor but

---

* See references 2, 5, 10, 11, 22, 25, 32, 33, 37, 41, 42.

† See references 2, 9, 16, 18, 33, 35, 44.

were instead related to a sella rendered "empty" by the ablative process.[11] The term "secondary empty sella syndrome" has been applied to this situation, and the "secondary empty sella" now refers to any sella in which the contents have become recessed or completely evacuated and into which suprasellar structures have descended, including arachnoid and subarachnoid space, pituitary stalk, scar tissue, optic chiasm, or part of the hypothalamus and third ventricle.

Secondary empty sella turcica may occur for various reasons, as listed in Table 100–2), among them operative removal of intrasellar structures; external radiotherapy of or radioactive yttrium or gold implantation in the pituitary or intrasellar lesions; and spontaneous infarction or necrosis of pituitary tumors.*

Doyle and McLachlan have stated that approximately 20 per cent of untreated patients with acromegaly have extension of the subarachnoid space ranging from 2 to 8 mm in depth below the expected position of the diaphragma.[13] It is not clear from their statement whether this is a normal variation expected on the basis of the findings in normal persons reported by Bergland and associates or whether this is in some way related to the presence of acromegaly or the growth hormone–producing pituitary tumor.[3]

Observations at operation and autopsy have indicated two possible mechanisms for production of visual field defects in the secondary empty sella syndrome. (1) The optic apparatus may become entrapped in thickened arachnoid or scar tissue and be displaced downward as the scar tissue contracts. (2) The optic chiasm may also be pushed inferiorly by herniation of brain tissue into the sella. Severe angulation of the optic nerves and chiasm and segmental necrosis of these structures have been observed.[21,29]

Impairment of the visual fields may occur within a few months to several years after the removal of intrasellar contents. Characteristically, the field defects are asymmetrical and variable. They may be unilateral or bilateral, concentric or eccentric. Visual field constrictions, segmental defects, bitemporal hemianopsia, and central sco-

tomas have all been described.[21] The irregular nature of the field defects may be the sole clinical clue to the presence of the secondary empty sella syndrome. The symptoms are limited to declining vision occasionally associated with headache and are otherwise not remarkable. X-ray films of the head generally are unchanged from early postoperative films, but postoperative remodeling is occasionally seen.

The diagnosis of the secondary empty sella syndrome is usually made by pneumoencephalography, which is indicated when visual field defects occur at any time after operation or radiotherapy. Omission of pneumoencephalography may lead to serious diagnostic error, an unnecessary operation, or inappropriate exposure of the sella and the displaced optic apparatus to radiotherapy. Occasionally, scar tissue and adhesions prohibit the entrance of air into the sella, and the diagnosis is finally made by operative exploration.

Treatment

For patients who have postoperative or postirradiation visual field defects that are small and peripheral, follow-up at frequent intervals by tangent screen perimetry and roentgenograms of the head will suffice as long as the condition remains stable. Central scotomas and evidence of progression are indications for early operative exploration.

The operative approach to the empty sella may be by craniotomy or via the transsphenoidal route and is identical to that used for pituitary tumor.[26,27] When accurate preoperative diagnosis has been possible, the transsphenoidal approach is usually the safer and more effective. In the case of visual loss due to prolapse of the optic nerves and chiasm, the empty sella is packed with muscle or fat and a "chiasmapexy" is accomplished.[46,47]

If the indication for operation is cerebrospinal fluid rhinorrhea from an empty sella, the transsphenoidal approach usually is effective.[28] The site of the cerebrospinal fluid communication is identified, and the sella is packed with muscle or fat to obliterate the leak. The sphenoid sinus usually is packed as well.

Increased intracranial pressure may be associated with, and may in some cases

---

* See references 21, 28, 30, 31, 34, 42.

produce, the empty sella syndrome. In the case of a medically intractable, symptomatic increase in intracranial pressure that is not caused by tumor or meningitis, operative intervention may be required. A lumboperitoneal shunt usually is effective in controlling increased intracranial pressure and is preferable to bilateral subtemporal decompression.

In the authors' series of 375 patients operated upon for sellar and parasellar disease and managed primarily by the transsphenoidal micro-operative approach, 12 patients had an empty sella. In three patients the condition was misdiagnosed as pituitary adenoma; these patients had not undergone pneumoencephalography. Two of the three had galactorrhea; one of these had only a typical empty sella, and the other had a pituitary microadenoma and an empty sella. Two other patients had secondary empty sellas with visual field changes; one of these had undergone craniotomy for a craniopharyngioma, and the other was an acromegalic patient who had been treated previously with stereotaxic thermocoagulation for a pituitary adenoma. Two patients had chiasmal visual field defects produced by intrasellar arachnoid cysts with suprasellar extension. Two patients presented with cerebrospinal fluid rhinorrhea through an empty sella. All these patients were managed with a transsphenoidal procedure. An additional patient had severe enough symptoms and signs of increased intracranial pressure to require a lumboperitoneal shunt.

Indications for an aggressive therapeutic approach to the empty sella syndrome are rare and well circumscribed. Emphasis must be placed on a high degree of alertness, accuracy of diagnosis, and diligent follow-up with endocrinological and radiological evaluation.

REFERENCES

1. Banerjee, T., and Meagher, J. N.: Foster Kennedy syndrome, aqueductal stenosis and empty sella. Amer. Surg., *40*:552–544, 1974.
2. Bar, R. S., Mazzaferri, E. L., and Malarkey, W. B.: Primary empty sella, galactorrhea, hyperprolactinemia and renal tubular acidosis. Amer. J. Med., *59*:863–866, 1975.
3. Bergland, R. M., Ray, B. S., and Torack, R. M.: Anatomical variations in the pituitary gland and adjacent structures in 225 human autopsy cases. J. Neurosurg., *28*:93–99, 1968.
4. Berke, J. P., Buxton, L. F., and Kokmen, E.: The "empty" sella. Neurology (Minneap.), *25*:1137–1143, 1975.
5. Bernasconi, V., Giovanelli, M. A., and Papo, I.: Primary empty sella. J. Neurosurg., *36*:157–161, 1972.
6. Brisman, R., Hughes, J. E. O., and Mount, L. A.: Cerebrospinal fluid rhinorrhea and the empty sella. J. Neurosurg., *31*:538–543, 1969.
7. Buckman, M. T., Husain, M., Carlow, T. J., et al.: Primary empty sella syndrome with visual field defects. Amer. J. Med., *61*:124–128, 1976.
8. Busch, W.: Die Morphologie der Sella turcica and ihre Beziehungen zur Hypophyse. Virchow. Arch. [Path. Anat.], *320*:437–458, 1951.
9. Caplan, R. H., and Dobben, G. D.: Endocrine studies in patients with the "empty sella syndrome." Arch. Intern. Med. (Chicago), *123*:611–619, 1969.
10. Coenegracht, J. M., de Bie, J. P. A. M., Coene, L. N. M., et al.: Deficiency of gonadotropin-releasing factor in a patient with hydrocephalus internus. J. Neurosurg., *43*:239–243, 1975.
11. Colby, M. Y., Jr., and Kearns, T. P.: Radiation therapy of pituitary adenomas with associated visual impairment. Proc. Staff. Meet. Mayo. Clin., *37*:15–24, 1962.
12. Dahlstrom, R., and Acers, T. E.: Chiasmatic arachnoiditis and empty sella: Report and discussion of a case. Ann. Ophthal., *7*:73–76, 1975.
13. Doyle, F., and McLachlan, M.: Radiological aspects of pituitary-hypothalamic disease, Clin. Endocr., *6*:53–81, 1977.
14. Drury, M. I., O'Loughlin, S., and Sweeney, E.: Houssay phenomenon in a diabetic. Brit. Med. J., *2*:709, 1970.
15. Du Boulay, G. H., and El Gammal, T.: The classification, clinical value and mechanism of sella turcica changes in raised intracranial pressure. Brit. J. Radiol., *39*:422–442, 1966.
16. Faglia, G., Ambrosi, B., Beck-Peccoz, P., et al.: Disorders of growth hormone and corticotropin regulation in patients with empty sella. J. Neurosurg., *38*:59–64, 1973.
17. Foley, K. M., and Posner, J. B.: Does pseudotumor cerebri cause the empty sella syndrome? Neurology (Minneap.), *25*:565–569, 1975.
18. Gabriele, O. F.: The empty sella syndrome. Amer. J. Roentgen., *104*:168–170, 1968.
19. Ganguly, A., Stanchfield, J. B., Roberts, T. S., et al.: Cushing's syndrome in a patient with an empty sella turcica and a microadenoma of the adenohypophysis. Amer. J. Med., *60*:306–309, 1976.
20. Grossman, C. B.: Dynamic roentgenographic changes in the empty sella syndrome. Radiology, *116*:341–344, 1975.
21. Hodgson, S. F., Randall, R. V., Holman, C. B., et al.: Empty sella syndrome. Report of 10 cases. Med. Clin. N. Amer., *56*:897–907, 1972.
22. Jordan, R. M., Kendall, J. W., and Kerber, C. W.: The primary empty sella syndrome: Analysis of the clinical characteristics, radiographic features, pituitary function and cerebrospinal fluid adenohypophysial hormone concentrations. Amer. J. Med., *62*:569–580, 1977.
23. Kaufman, B.: The "empty" sella turcica: A manifestation of the intrasellar subarachnoid space. Radiology, *90*:931–941, 1968.

24. Kaufman, B., and Chamberlin, W. B., Jr.: The ubiquitous "empty" sella turcica. Acta Radiol. [Diagn.] (Stockholms), *13*:413–425, 1972.

25. Kleinberg, D. L., Noel, G. L., and Frantz, A. G.: Galactorrhea: A study of 235 cases, including 48 with pituitary tumors. New Eng. J. Med., *296*:589–600, 1977.

26. Laws, E. R., Jr., and Kern, E. B.: Complications of trans-sphenoidal surgery. Clin. Neurosurg., *23*:401–416, 1976.

27. Laws, E. R., Jr., Trautmann, J. C., and Hollenhorst, R. W., Jr.: Transsphenoidal decompression of the optic nerve and chiasm: Visual results in 62 patients. J. Neurosurg., *46*:717–722, 1977.

28. Leclereq, T. A., Hardy, J., Vezina, J. L., et al.: Intrasellar arachnoidocele and the so-called empty sella syndrome. Surg. Neurol., *2*:295–299, 1974.

29. Lee, W. M., and Adams, J. E.: The empty sella syndrome. J. Neurosurg., *28*:351–356, 1968.

30. Login, I., and Santen, R. J.: Empty sella syndrome: Sequela of spontaneous remission of acromegaly. Arch. Intern. Med. (Chicago), *135*:1519–1521, 1975.

31. Matisonn, R., and Pimstone, B.: Diabetes insipidus associated with an empty sella turcica. Postgrad. Med. J., *49*:274–276, 1973.

32. Mortara, R., and Norrell, H.: Consequences of a deficient sellar diaphragm. J. Neurosurg., *32*:565–573, 1970.

33. Neelon, F. A., Goree, J. A., and Lebovitz, H. E.: The primary empty sella: Clinical and radiographic characteristics and endocrine function. Medicine (Balt.), *52*:73–92, 1973.

34. Obrador, S.: The empty sella and some related syndromes. J. Neurosurg., *36*:162–168, 1972.

35. Ridgway, E. C., Kourides, I. A., Kliman, B., et al.: Thyrotropin and prolactin pituitary reserve in the "empty sella syndrome." J. Clin. Endocr., *41*:968–973, 1975.

36. Shore, R. N., DeCherney, A. H., Stein, K. M., et al.: The empty sella syndrome: Virilization in a 59-year-old woman. J.A.M.A., *227*:69–70, 1974.

37. Shreefter, M. J., and Friedlander, R. L.: Primary empty sella syndrome and amenorrhea. Obstet. Gyne., *46*:535–538, 1975.

38. Snyder, P. J., Jacobs, L. S., Rabello, M. M., et al: Diagnostic value of thyrotrophin-releasing hormone in pituitary and hypothalamic diseases: Assessment of thyrothrophin and prolactin secretion. Ann. Intern. Med., *81*:751–757, 1974.

39. Sones, P. J., and Heinz, E. R.: The sella turcica and multiparity: With comments on the effects of pseudotumor cerebri. Brit. J. Radiol., *45*:503–506, 1972.

40. Sutton, T. J., and Vezina, J. L.: Co-existing pituitary adenoma and intrasellar arachnoid invagination. Amer. J. Roentgen., *122*:508–510, 1974.

41. Thomas, H. M., Jr., Lufkin, E. G., Ellis, G. J., III, et al.: Hypogonadotropism and "empty sella": Improvement in 2 cases with clomiphene citrate. Fertil. Steril., *24*:252–259, 1973.

42. Verdy, M., Lalonde, J.-L., Durivage, J., et al: Acromégalie et selle turcique vide. Un. Med. Canada, *104*:249–252, 1975.

43. Weisberg, L. A., Housepian, E. M., and Saur, D. P.: Empty sella syndrome as complication of benign intracranial hypertension. J. Neurosurg., *43*:177–180, 1975.

44. Weisberg, L. A., Zimmerman, E. A., and Frantz, A. G.: Diagnosis and evaluation of patients with an enlarged sella turcica. Amer. J. Med., *61*:590–596, 1976.

45. Weiss, M. H., Kaufman, B., and Richards, D. E.: Cerebrospinal fluid rhinorrhea from an empty sella: Transsphenoidal obliteration of the fistula; technical note. J. Neurosurg., *39*:674–676, 1973.

46. Welch, K., and Stears, J. C.: Chiasmapexy for the correction of traction on the optic nerves and chiasm associated with their descent into an empty sella turcica: Case report. J. Neurosurg., *35*:760–764, 1971.

47. Wood, J. H., and Dogali, M. D.: Visual improvement after chiasmapexy for primary empty sella turcica. Surg. Neurol., *3*:291–294, 1975.

48. Zatz, L. M., Janon, E. A., and Newton, T. H.: The enlarged sella and the intrasellar cistern. Radiology, *93*:1085–1091, 1969.

101

PSEUDOTUMOR CEREBRI

Causes of increased intracranial pressure (intracranial hypertension) unassociated with a tumor or mass are numerous. The definition of a syndrome encompassing all such causes is dangerous because it tends to reassure the physician rather than stimulate him to pursue those conditions that are treatable and to try to understand the pathophysiological changes underlying the problem. Table 101–1 lists a number of non-mass conditions in which intracranial hypertension may be seen. Included in this group are disorders that are surgically or medically treatable, and there are those in which, as a result of the complications of the underlying medical illness, an operatively treatable process exists (e.g., subdural hematoma in metabolic illness associated with a bleeding diathesis). Certainly some of the conditions manifest systemic signs of illness unassociated with any feature of neurological impairment. Moreover, the intracranial contents may not be involved in the disease process at the time of clinical presentation, as the severity of the problem may be less than that needed to cause intracranial hypertension.

There remains a group of patients in whom intracranial hypertension exists in a benign form. It is this category of conditions that has been called benign intracranial hypertension or pseudotumor cerebri or, as first labeled by Quincke in 1897, serous meningitis.[84] Arbitrarily classified as a group, such patients exhibit papilledema (or a bulging fontanel in the infant) but demonstrate no evidence of overt neurological impairment except for the nonspecific signs of intracranial hypertension such as a sixth nerve palsy. A noteworthy exception to this rule is the occasional presence of impaired visual acuity or visual field defect. Such patients have neither seizures nor alteration of mental function. Diagnostic studies exclude ventricular dilatation as the cause of intracranial hypertension, and the cerebrospinal fluid pressure is elevated; there is, however, no other abnormality in protein, sugar, or cellular constituents.

The uniformity linking such patients, the syndrome, therefore may be considered a negative concept. Laboratory studies fail to demonstrate a mass lesion, an infectious or inflammatory state, or obstruction or distortion of the midline ventricular system; and on the basis of clinical presentation and the absence of convulsions, focal signs of neurological impairment, or mental changes, are excluded nonapparent toxic, metabolic, degenerative, or demyelinating conditions.

In some patients, the syndrome may represent a response to some exogenous factor whose elimination is promptly followed by a resolution of the signs and symptoms of intracranial hypertension. In others, symptomatic therapy is offered to keep the intracranial pressure in a range that will not threaten vision until the inciting cause or mechanism disappears. Table 101–2 presents diseases, exogenous factors, and endogenous physiological alterations that have been considered causally related to pseudotumor cerebri.

SIGNS AND SYMPTOMS

In general, the severity of signs and symptoms associated with pseudotumor cerebri is less than that noted in patients who suffer from a mass process causing in-

TABLE 101–1 INTRACRANIAL HYPERTENSION UNASSOCIATED WITH A MASS

CAUSES	PRESUMED PATHOPHYSIOLOGY
Ventricular dilatation, hydrocephalus 　Developmental anomaly 　Post meningitis 　Post intracranial hemorrhage 　Post acquired aqueductal stenosis 　Basilar neoplastic or granulomatous (e.g., sarcoid) meningitis	Obstruction of ventricular system outflow or blockage of cerebrospinal fluid pathways
Hypertensive encephalopathy	Arteriolar constriction, vascular permeability
Metabolic disorders 　Chronic uremia 　Diabetic ketoacidosis	Vascular permeability, intracellular swelling caused by metabolic derangement
Intoxication 　Heavy metals (lead, arsenic) 　Kepone	Vascular permeability, intracellular swelling caused by metabolic derangement
Infections 　Bacterial 　　Septic cerebral emboli 　　Meningitis 　　Brucellosis 　Viral 　Parasitic	Vascular permeability, direct toxic action of infectious agent or its products on cerebral intracellular metabolism causing cell swelling
Demyelinating or degenerative disease 　Multiple sclerosis 　Schilder's disease	Perivascular inflammatory reaction causing vascular permeability
Cardiorespiratory disorders 　Congestive heart failure 　Chronic pulmonary disease 　　Cor pulmonale 　　Pulmonary hypoventilation	Hypercarbia causing arterial dilatation and increased permeability, obstruction of intracranial venous outflow
Vascular disorders 　Infarction 　Inflammatory vasculitis (including granulomatous disease) 　Serum sickness, allergic reaction	Vascular permeability, swelling of cells deprived of metabolic needs
Miscellaneous causes 　Status epilepticus 　Trauma	Vascular permeability, cellular swelling secondary to physiological insult; exhaustion from exceeding metabolic capacity, disruption of structural integrity
Increased cerebrospinal fluid protein caused by spinal tumor or parainfectious polyneuritis	Occlusion of sites of cerebrospinal fluid reabsorption by high protein content

tracranial hypertension. Symptoms such as headache, dizziness, nausea, vomiting, tinnitus, blurred vision, diplopia, and vague paresthesias are described. In addition to the lesser severity of the symptoms in contrast to that described by the tumor patient, there is also a greater fluctuation in the day-to-day complaints and an absence of lethargy. On the other hand, the mild nature of the early symptoms may misguide the patient to not seek medical attention until significant visual complaints occur, sometimes with overnight abruptness. In the author's experience, 10 per cent of patients observed with this syndrome suffered irreversible impairment of visual function. This includes five patients with significant deficits: permanent decrease in acuity of greater than 20/100 in each eye in three, an altitudinal hemianopia in one, and complete amaurosis in the fifth patient. The incidence of permanent visual impairment in patients with this syndrome may be as high as 22 per cent.[54]

Additional signs implying dysfunction of the visual system include temporary hemianopia and quadrantanopia, sluggishly reactive pupils, and in those with grossly impaired vision, optic atrophy.

Signs of neurological impairment in the infant include a bulging anterior fontanel. In the older child and adult, papilledema is the common sign. Occasional confusion occurs when a patient with pseudopapilledema is examined because of a headache complaint. Appropriate techniques distinguishing this congenital anomaly from papilledema will decide the correct diagnosis.

Abducens nerve palsy and facial nerve palsy are noted as nonspecific signs of intracranial hypertension, particularly in children.[17] Gait imbalance or mild ataxia is not infrequently seen but is often related to the complaint of dizziness.

TABLE 101–2　MECHANISMS CAUSALLY RELATED TO PSEUDOTUMOR CEREBRI

CAUSES	AGE RANGE (Years)	SEX F	SEX M	AUTHORS
Intracranial venous drainage obstruction				
Mastoiditis and lateral (sigmoid) sinus obstruction	3–5	3	13	Greer and Berk[43]
Extracerebral mass lesions	5–41	3	3	Mones[74]
Congenital atresia or stenosis of venous sinuses	5 wk–10 yr	0	3	Kinal[60]
				Greer[39]
Head trauma	4–5	1	1	Kinal[61]
Cryofibrinogenemia	23	0	1	Dunsker et al.[22]
Polycythemia vera	41	0	1	Loman and Dameshek[69]
Paranasal sinus and pharyngeal infections	2–24	5	6	Symonds[95]
Cervical or thoracic venous drainage obstruction				
Intrathoracic mass lesions and postoperative obstruction of venous return	4 mo–44 yr	2	4	Hooper[47]
				Fitz-Hugh et al.[28]
				Boruchow et al.[10]
Endocrine dysfunction				
Pregnancy	16–37	8	0	Greer[34,35]
Menarche	11–14	10	0	Greer[36]
Marked menstrual irregularities	10–30	7	0	Greer[37]
Oral contraceptives	19–24	2	0	Shenk[89]
				Buchheit et al.[13]
Obesity	19–43	26	0	Patterson et al.[80]
				Greer[38]
Withdrawal of corticosteroid therapy	3¼–19	1	5	Greer[34,35]
Addison's disease	3–23	3	2	Walsh[97]
				Boudin et al.[11]
				Jefferson[53]
Hypoparathyroidism	27–36	3	1	Sugar[94]
"Catch-up" growth after deprivation, treatment of cystic fibrosis, correction of heart anomaly	3–6 mo	3	0	DiLiberti and O'Brien[20]
				Capitanio and Kirkpatrick[14]
				Bray and Herbst[12]
Hematological disorders				
Acute iron deficiency anemia	15–29	3	0	Schwaber and Blumberg[88]
				Ikkala and Laitinen[51]
				Stoebner et al.[93]
Pernicious anemia	22	1	0	Murphy and Costanzi[75]
Thrombocytopenia	14–50	3	1	Watkins et al.[98]
Wiskott-Aldrich syndrome	7	0	1	Greer[39]
Vitamin metabolism				
Chronic hypervitaminosis A	15–21	2	2	Gerber et al.[32]
				Greer[39]
				Feldman and Schlezinger[25]
Acute hypervitaminosis A	2–7½ mo	1	4	Marie and See[71]
Hypovitaminosis A	115½ mo	2	1	Cornfield and Cook[18]
				Bass and Fisch[5]
Cystic fibrosis and hypovitaminosis A	5½ mo	0	1	Abernathy[1]
Vitamin D–deficiency rickets	7 mo	0	1	Hochman and Mejlszenkier[46]
Drug reaction				
Tetracycline	4 mo–24 yr	0	2	Greer[39]
				Koch-Weser and Gilmore[64]
Perhexiline maleate	40–60	2	1	Stephens et al.[91]
Nalidixic acid	6 mo	0	1	Borens and Sundstrom[9]
Sulfamethoxazole	14 mo–4½ yr	1	1	Ch'ien[15]
Indomethacin	10	1	0	Konomi et al.[65]
Penicillin	9	1	0	Schmitt and Krivit[87]
Prophylactic antisera	11–34	0	6	Kennedy[59]
Miscellaneous				
Galactosemia	9–19 days	0	3	Huttenlocher et al.[50]
Galactokinase deficiency				
Sydenham's chorea	8	1	0	Chun et al.[16]
Sarcoidosis	5–27	3	1	Allison[3]
Roseola infantum	5–11 mo	0	2	Oski[79]
Hypophosphatasis	3 mo	1	0	Fraser et al.[31]
Paget's disease				Knaggs[63]

Certain specific signs and symptoms related to the cause of pseudotumor are discussed with the etiological interpretation.

ETIOLOGY

Obstruction of Intracranial Venous Drainage

Mastoiditis

Prior to the era of antibiotic therapy, chronic mastoiditis was a common cause of pseudotumor cerebri as a consequence of the contiguous spread of the inflammatory response to the sigmoid and lateral sinus. As a result of occlusion of this draining venous sinus, intracranial hypertension would ensue as a consequence of the increased hydrostatic pressure within the entire venous system exceeding that necessary to permit absorption of cerebrospinal fluid. In addition, increased volume of blood within the cranial vault contributed to the elevated pressure.

Obviously, total obstruction of intracranial venous drainage does not occur, since this is incompatible with life. In experiments with dogs, ligation of the major cranial venous draining vessels results in intracranial hypertension and ventricular dilatation or intracranial hypertension without hydrocephalus for as long as six months.[7,44]

In man, ligation of some intracranial venous structures may be performed with impunity in the course of a craniotomy, since collateral channels are ubiquitous. There are noteworthy exceptions; for example, ligation of the posterior half of the superior sagittal sinus causes brain infarction. In any event, obstruction of the major channel of intracranial venous drainage via the internal jugular veins may be relieved by collateral run-off through diploic and scalp veins that drain into the external jugular vein or via superficial cortical veins extending forward into the orbital and facial veins, as well as the venous system at the base of the skull through vertebral and pterygoid veins.

Children aged 5 to 12 years represent the largest group of patients who suffer from pseudotumor cerebri caused by chronic mastoiditis and obstruction of the lateral and sigmoid sinus (otitic hydrocephalus). Often a history of recurrent or recent mid-dle ear infections is obtained, but this may not necessarily be the case. The middle ear infection may have occurred months previously, and no particular sign or complaint such as mastoid tenderness, decreased auditory acuity, or change in the appearance of the tympanic membrane may be noted. Fever is absent.

Anatomical variations of the intracranial venous draining pattern, in part, determine the nature of the intracranial complications of chronic mastoiditis when they occur. Brain abscess, cortical thrombophlebitis, and simple obstruction of the sigmoid sinus in the retromastoid region are the problems encountered. In 39 per cent of humans examined at autopsy, the greatest volume of blood leaving the cranial vault goes via the right jugular vein. This includes that which comes from the cortical surfaces bilaterally and the right subcortical area via the superior sagittal sinus and the right lateral and sigmoid sinus. The left lateral and sigmoid sinus and the left jugular vein drain the deep portions of the brain, primarily the left hemisphere. In 13 per cent, the situation is reversed insofar as it is the left jugular that drains the majority of the intracranial volume. This separation of the draining venous system indicates an absence of a true hemodynamic confluence of the major sinuses at the torcular Herophili. It helps explain the findings of pseudotumor cerebri in 15 children observed by this author in whom the right mastoid was affected in 13 and the left in 2.

Skull roentgenograms and special views of the mastoid regions confirm the presence of intracranial hypertension as well as the mastoiditis. Brain scan and computed tomography exclude the presence of a mass. The electroencephalogram is mildly abnormal in about half the cases, occasionally revealing slowing in that portion of the brain adjacent to the affected mastoid region, implying some cerebral involvement, although the cerebrospinal fluid does not indicate the presence of any inflammatory reaction.

The cerebral angiogram is the most critical test, establishing the diagnosis of venous sinus occlusion and helping to exclude the presence of a mass lesion and ventricular dilatation. In order to be certain of the venous drainage pattern, four-vessel catheterization and injection are most appropriate (Fig. 101–1). A prolonged arterial and cap-

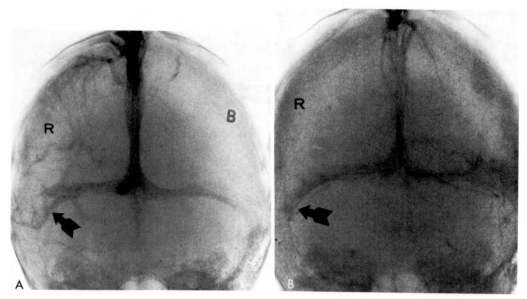

Figure 101–1 Pseudotumor cerebri caused by mastoiditis and right lateral sinus occlusion in a 9-year-old child. *A*. Venous sinus phase of carotid arteriogram. Arrow points to occluded sinus. *B*. Venous sinus phase of vertebral arteriogram.

illary phase, irregularity of the affected sinus indicating thrombosis, and prominent collateral veins are to be expected, the definitive picture being represented by the obstruction of dye in the affected sinus and the absence of filling of the internal jugular veins.

Retrograde venography via the jugular vein obviously is not adequate to prove the diagnosis. Moreover, this procedure caused seizures in animals that underwent prior ligation of the torcular Herophili.[44]

Mastoidectomy, in addition to antibiotics, is the treatment of choice. It has been argued that antibiotics alone would be adequate. In many cases, they will have already been administered; in one instance, dosage equivalent to that offered for meningitis was given for four days after the diagnosis of mastoiditis and lateral sinus obstruction was established, but papilledema worsened and the persistently elevated intracranial pressure led to the need for mastoidectomy.

During mastoidectomy, sterile granulation tissue, rather than frank pus, is encountered overlying the sigmoid sinus. Debridement will permit the compressed sinus to expand, and blood will flow into the jugular vein. A thrombus may be palpated in the sinus, giving rise to the consideration of a thrombectomy or distal ligation of the jugu-

lar vein to prevent embolization to the heart. Thrombectomy is not easily accomplished successfully, and the ligation approach would eliminate the benefits of spontaneous recanalization. Furthermore, in none of the author's cases in which the jugular vein was not ligated did embolization occur. Anticoagulant therapy is contraindicated because of the fear of intracranial venous bleeding.

The expectation is that mastoidectomy and debridement will facilitate the recanalization of the thrombosed sinus and allow collateral venous channels to develop, thereby facilitating intracranial venous drainage. Lumbar puncture performed periodically to reduce intracranial hypertension is suggested as a temporizing measure until this vascular reaction takes place.

In the author's experience, 13 of 16 children had resolution of all signs and symptoms of increased pressure within three weeks after mastoidectomy. In two, the pressure remained elevated for at least six months after the procedure, although papilledema and symptoms of intracranial hypertension disappeared within a two-month period postoperatively. The last child improved within four months; however, a sudden increase in intracranial pressure was the presumed cause of the overnight appearance of amaurosis bilaterally. It was assumed that rethrombosis of the sinus had taken place, but no additional studies were permitted; two years later he is still blind, albeit without other symptoms of increased pressure.

Other Causes of Intracranial Venous Sinus Obstruction

Neoplasia disseminated to the skull is another cause of intracranial hypertension when the major draining venous sinuses are blocked.[74] The lesion, such as neuroblastoma, remains extracerebral and is often radiosensitive, thereby offering a treatment approach that will alleviate the intracranial hypertension, although the underlying disease is most often fatal.

Congenital atresia or stenosis of the primary venous sinus channels is another uncommon cause of intracranial hypertension. One 10-year-old boy presented with a cosmetic disfigurement caused by prominent veins on the forehead, which represented the collateral route for intracranial venous drainage.[39] Arteriography demonstrated atresia of the lateral sinuses. Although he showed symptoms of neither intracranial hypertension nor papilledema nor embarrassment of vision, the cerebrospinal fluid pressure was 300 mm of water. Hydrocephalus was not present.

In contrast to this child, two of four infants under 10 months of age with congenital atresia of major draining venous sinuses exhibited hydrocephalus.[60]

This ability to tolerate intracranial hypertension implies a physiological adjustment that is possible if the abnormality evolves slowly and the pressure is only modestly elevated. Furthermore, the presence of ventricular dilatation only in infants as a result of venous occlusion implies a greater vulnerability of the brain or ventricular cavity in this age group.

Lastly, intracranial venous sinus obstruction following trauma has been described as a cause of pseudotumor cerebri.[61] Dural sinus venography defined this problem in a patient who sustained a fracture that incited a thrombosis in the underlying venous sinus, causing intracranial hypertension without other sequelae. Treatment was supportive, and resolution of the intracranial hypertension occurred.

Systemic Disease and Intracranial Venous Sinus Thrombosis

In most instances in which a generalized disease is associated with intracranial venous thromboses, the clinical features reflect hemorrhage or infarction. Intracranial hypertension may accompany such instances of venous thrombosis occurring in children suffering from marasmus, a hyperosmolar state, or certain hemoglobinopathies.[26,30,89]

On the other hand, a benign state of intracranial hypertension has been described in a patient suffering from cryofibrinogenemia wherein obstruction (thrombosis?) at the junction of the right transverse sinus and the jugular vein was presumed to be the cause.[22] A thecoperitoneal shunt benefited the patient after subtemporal decompression, corticosteroids, and acetazolamide were unsuccessful. The patient subsequently died with midbrain infarction and, on autopsy, showed total occlusion of the posterior end of the superior sagittal sinus, the straight sinus, and both lateral sinuses.

Less well-documented instances of intracranial hypertension related to systemic illness leading to venous sinus thrombosis include cases of polycythemia vera and paranasal and pharyngeal infections that caused retrograde venous thrombosis.[69,95]

Neck and Thoracic Obstruction of Cranial Venous System

Neck operations for thyroid or parathyroid disease cause pseudotumor cerebri as a result of incidental ligation of the major draining jugular vein.[28] This is a temporary phenomenon that resolves spontaneously in less than four weeks.

Mediastinal mass lesions and mediastinitis may result in intracranial hypertension as well, owing to obstruction of the superior vena cava.[47] An operatively induced thrombosis of the superior vena cava has also led to pseudotumor cerebri following repair of congenital heart disease. In this case, the superior vena cava was anastomosed to the right pulmonary artery.[10] Reoperation was necessary, since collateral channels do not develop under these circumstances.

Endocrine Dysfunction

In the previously described conditions, occlusion of intracranial venous drainage has been invoked as the mechanism for pseudotumor cerebri. Other causes have been delineated. The mechanism for the development of the intracranial hypertension remains obscure, however. It is on the basis of similar historical or physical features that groups of patients have been defined who fit the description of the syndrome. In some, a physiological aberration is inferred.

The preponderance of females presenting with pseudotumor cerebri in all series (eight females to one male) in itself suggests an endocrine relationship; however, no specific chemical or hormonal factors have been uncovered.

The appearance of pseudotumor cerebri during the early months of pregnancy, in girls entering menarche, in women with marked menstrual irregularities, and in those taking oral contraceptive medication implies a relationship between hormonal status and intracranial hypertension.[13,34-36,97] A hormonal factor is also inferred as the cause of pseudotumor in the obese woman.[38,80] This last group constitutes the largest single category of patients suffering from this syndrome. It is not related to alveolar hypoventilation, and the obese man only rarely may have pseudotumor cerebri; however, no data reflecting the results of endocrine function in the obese woman with pseudotumor cerebri can explain the cranial process. The abnormal metapyrone stimulation test result suggesting a disturbance in the pituitary-adrenal axis in the obese woman with pseudotumor cerebri may be explained as an effect of the intracranial hypertension rather than as a pathogenesis of the syndrome itself.[78] Additional endocrinological studies in obese women, in estrogen-treated women, and in those given oral contraceptive drugs have not revealed a significant abnormality of adrenocortical function.[21,81]

Nevertheless, adrenocortical dysfunction itself has been considered the cause of pseudotumor cerebri in certain instances, for example, in Addison's disease.[11,53,97] A more common relationship between adrenocortical dysfunction and pseudotumor cerebri is observed in patients, particularly children, who after receiving long-term corticosteroids orally or topically have had the dosage tapered or discontinued.[34,35] This would support a relationship between adrenocortical insufficiency and intracranial hypertension. In vivo studies in adrenalectomized animals, as well as in vitro cerebral tissue experiments from such animals, support the concept of an increased brain volume in adrenocortical insufficiency.[19,24,67]

An inference might be made that adrenocortical hormone therapy is appropriate in those instances of frank adrenal insufficiency. In the author's experience with children having pseudotumor in association with corticosteroid therapy withdrawal, replacement therapy has not been necessary, since spontaneous remission occurred in six children within three weeks after they became symptomatic. It is also the author's belief that, in those other patients with pseudotumor cerebri and presumed endocrine dysfunction, corticosteroid therapy has not proved to be of value. Moreover, in the obese woman such therapy would enhance the obesity and prolong the signs and symptoms of the pseudotumor problem, if not worsen it.

Neuroradiological studies including CT scans, arteriograms, pneumoencephalograms, and ventriculograms are normal in patients with pseudotumor cerebri related to presumed endocrine dysfunction (Fig. 101-2). Even in the woman experiencing pseudotumor cerebri in association with the use of oral contraceptive drugs, no abnormality is noted. Cerebral arteriography with particular attention to the intracranial venous drainage system identifies no obstruction, although in light of the relationship between oral contraceptives and the tendency for vascular occlusion, this might have been presupposed.[41,42,98] Cerebrospinal fluid profiles are normal. Treatment of the intracranial hypertension in pregnant women and girls entering menarche is supportive, the approach being repeated lumbar punctures until the syndrome resolves in two or three weeks. It is infrequent that a recurrence of pseudotumor cerebri is noted in subsequent pregnancies.[77]

Unfortunately, the relatively rapid resolution of signs and symptoms with symptomatic treatment did not occur in women with pseudotumor cerebri who exhibited

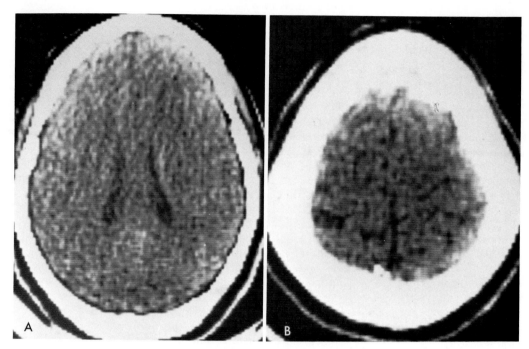

Figure 101–2 *A*. Computer-assisted tomogram of a 17-year-old obese woman with pseudotumor cerebri. Ventricles are "narrow." *B*. Higher cut on the scan demonstrates normal sulcal pattern.

marked irregularity in menstrual function. In this group there was a persistence of the syndrome's features, and an unpredictable fluctuation in the intracranial hypertension was observed. Sometimes the condition was favorably affected by the appearance of normal menstrual bleeding, while at other times being adversely affected by the normal period. A prolonged course over several months' time was not unusual. Five of seven women in this group noted a significant weight gain during the premenstrual phase when symptoms of pseudotumor cerebri were most evident.[36,37] Diuretics, including acetazolamide, did not prevent the appearance of the signs and symptoms nor did they shorten the prolonged intermittent course. No specific ovarian hormone treatments were efficacious either. It is because of the irregularity in the course of such women and the concern that sudden irreversible visual impairment may ensue that a neurosurgical shunting procedure is advocated as a prophylactic measure. One such patient, for example, underwent a series of lumbar puncture treatments over an 85-day period only to be readmitted on the ninetieth day with visual impairment of four hours' duration. Despite subtemporal de-

compression and continued lumbar punctures, the visual deficit persisted. Had a shunting procedure been performed earlier, it is conceivable that this would not have occurred.

Stringent weight reduction and supportive therapy in the form of serial lumbar punctures is the most effective means of treating the obese woman with pseudotumor cerebri. Although exacerbations of the signs and symptoms did occur in some obese women, this was correlated with a failure to maintain weight control, and improvement coincided with a return of weight reduction.

Hypoparathyroidism is a specifically treatable cause for pseudotumor cerebri.[94] Again, no theory is offered to explain the intracranial hypertension nor why vitamin D may produce a resolution of the intracranial process. The rapid gain in weight seen in nutritionally deprived children who receive nourishment may be accompanied by intracranial hypertension.[14] This same phenomenon may be witnessed in the child who is being treated for cystic fibrosis and after successful operative intervention in children with patent ductus arteriosus.[12,20]

Hematological Disorders

An association between certain hematological disorders and pseudotumor cerebri has been made in a small group of patients. Pseudotumor cerebri and acute iron deficiency anemia, or chlorosis, have been described in the adolescent.[51,88] The absence of any change in mental function would exclude cerebral edema related to anoxia as the cause of the intracranial hypertension. Although transfusion is curative, in one instance the signs and symptoms of pseudotumor disappeared within seven days of the institution of oral iron therapy before there was any significant rise in hemoglobin concentration.[93] Iron replacement, rather than the restoration of the hemoglobin level, was inferred to be the cause of the resolution of the intracranial hypertension. Interestingly, the patient was obese and short (188 pounds and 62 inches tall), thereby suggesting that perhaps the cause as well as the resolution of pseudotumor was related to some other endocrine process.

Isolated case reports of pseudotumor in association with pernicious anemia, thrombocytopenia, and the Wiskott-Aldrich syndrome also do not provide a satisfactory explanation for the intracranial hypertension.[39,69,75,99] Once again, the absence of mental changes makes the likelihood of cerebral hypoxia on an ischemic basis remote.

In these instances, correction of the underlying disorder plus supportive therapy in the form of serial lumbar punctures was adequate to restore the intracranial pressure to normal in less than one month.

Vitamin Metabolism

Pseudotumor cerebri occurring as a rare complication of pernicious anemia and hypoparathyroidism represents two instances in which vitamin deficiency is considered to play a role in the appearance of intracranial hypertension—deficiency of B_{12} and D respectively. Vitamin D–deficiency rickets is another rare disorder in which this particular vitamin has been related to the syndrome.[46] The nature of the condition may, however, be more readily attributable to the phenomenon of pseudotumor cerebri related to the "catch-up" growth phenomenon seen after recovery from deprivation in infants.

More commonly, vitamin A has been involved as cause of pseudotumor cerebri. The ingestion of increased amounts, usually given to treat acne, over a period of months has resulted in intracranial hypertension in the adolescent and young woman.[25,32,39] Associated signs such as alopecia and cheilosis are noted. Elevated vitamin A blood levels confirm the diagnosis; the history, however, is usually sufficient to understand the problem, and treatment by vitamin withdrawal is all that is needed.

Accidental ingestion of an overdose of vitamin A by the pre–school aged child is a rare cause of pseudotumor cerebri; however, the irritability and other signs of neurological dysfunction described in such patients would suggest a toxic encephalopathy rather than a benign state of intracranial hypertension. In one case, resolution of signs and symptoms occurred spontaneously after several days.[71]

Vitamin A deficiency in infants treated with the so-called hypoallergenic diets or as a result of malabsorption as in cystic fibrosis has resulted in a bulging anterior fontanel and intracranial hypertension.[1,5,18,58] This resolves shortly after the administration of the vitamin.

Vitamin A deficiency is a known cause of intracranial hypertension in the calf and, in the rabbit, serves as an experimental model for this problem. Both an obstruction to the flow of cerebrospinal fluid and an increased production of the fluid have been considered pathogenetic mechanisms.[48,102] No interpretation for the intracranial hypertension in hypervitaminosis states has been offered.

Drug Reaction

Allergic or toxic responses to drugs in susceptible patients, particularly infants and children, have resulted in pseudotumor cerebri. These drugs have included tetracycline, nalidixic acid, sulfamethoxazole, perhexiline maleate, and indomethacin.*

In other children, again, the features of a toxic encephalopathy appear in association

---

* See references 9, 15, 39, 64, 65, 91.

with intracranial hypertension, implying a process that may not be benign. Such a state has been described after injections of penicillin or prophylactic antisera.[59,87]

Removal of the offending substance is the critical therapy. Other supportive measures should be added.

Miscellaneous Causes

Among the miscellaneous causes of pseudotumor cerebri are included galactokinase deficiency and galactosemia.[50] It is hypothesized that impaired galactose metabolism results in the cerebral accumulation of a nondiffusable alcohol (dulcitol), which attracts water by osmosis.

Sydenham's chorea, roseola infantum, hypophosphatasia, sarcoidosis, and Paget's disease are other conditions in which pseudotumor cerebri is said to occur.[3,16,31,63,79] In these patients, the relationship of the systemic process and the intracranial hypertension is somewhat tenuous and may be interpreted as an effect of a toxic process on the brain. As described previously, the relationship of these as well as other conditions or diseases and the appearance of intracranial hypertension is not discussed, since the process does not fit the arbitrary definition of a benign state of intracranial hypertension. Nevertheless, it should be noted that, when all the aforementioned conditions have been considered and excluded as a known cause of something known to be associated with pseudotumor cerebri, there remains approximately 15 to 20 per cent of all patients experiencing this syndrome who cannot be placed in any known category.

DIAGNOSTIC EVALUATION

The evaluation of an alert patient with papilledema but no localizing neurological signs must be approached with an understanding of historical and clinical features that indicate the condition is pseudotumor cerebri. Noninvasive diagnostic studies include the electroencephalogram, which in the adult patient with pseudotumor is usually normal. In children the incidence of abnormal tracings may approach 60 per cent; there is, however, no consistent pattern of electroencephalographic abnormality.[8] It is suggested that this merely represents a difference between the immature and adult brains in their response to intracranial hypertension. Under experimental conditions, intracranial hypertension induced by placing lamp black in the cisterna magna of animals, leading to hydrocephalus, results in diffuse slow wave activity. Intracranial hypertension caused by the intrathecal administration of distilled water, on the other hand, produces no change in the electroencephalogram.[92]

Plain skull roentgenograms are routinely performed, which may identify skull erosion or thickening, mastoiditis, and abnormal calcification as well as signs of increased pressure. Computer-assisted tomography reassures the physician that neither a mass nor ventricular dilatation exists. Narrow ventricles are noted occasionally. When air encephalography was done routinely either by burr hole ventriculography or via the lumbar route, approximately 20 per cent of patients demonstrated narrow lateral ventricles. The CT scan also reveals a sulcus pattern over the convexity that appears normal (see Fig. 101–2).

Following this study, it is recommended that four-vessel carotid arteriography be performed if the nature of the problem is not apparent and especially if venous occlusive disease is a strong possibility. In other words, in the obese female or in such conditions as hypervitaminosis A, when a likely cause for the pseudotumor cerebri is apparent, arteriography is not necessary.

The lumbar puncture is the last neurodiagnostic test usually performed for diagnostic as well as therapeutic purposes. This author does not recommend the performance of a unilateral Queckenstedt test. In that test, compression of the jugular vein ipsilateral to sigmoid sinus occlusion induces no rise in cerebrospinal fluid pressure, whereas compression of the contralateral jugular vein does cause a rise in pressure. The results are unreliable and the test is potentially dangerous.

Gross measurement of the relative volume of cerebrospinal fluid, as determined by the Ayala index (fluid removed × fluid pressure/opening pressure), revealed a value implying increased cerebrospinal fluid volume 63 per cent of the time it was measured and normal volume 37 per cent of the time.[4] Cerebrospinal fluid protein in the lumbar sac was less than 20 mg per 100 ml in 43 of 65 patients.

Another test designed to assess the function of cerebrospinal fluid mechanisms in pseudotumor cerebri involves the intrathecal injection of radioactive iodinated serum albumin. In one study, patients with this syndrome revealed a delay in absorption over the convexity of the hemispheres as well as delay in the appearance of the radioactivity in the blood.[6] In one of these patients, upon resolution of the signs and symptoms of pseudotumor cerebri, the results of the radioactive study reverted to normal. In another study of 10 patients with pseudotumor, 4 demonstrated a delayed flow of the radiopharmaceutical but only 1 had a prolonged parasagittal accumulation.[52]

Another test, involving a constant infusion manometric technique, revealed a severely abnormal bulk absorption capacity in the one patient with pseudotumor cerebri so studied.[49] This type of test is concerned with the controlling physiological parameters related to the regulation of intracranial hypertension. One element concerned with regulation of intracranial hypertension is the compliance factor, which has to do with the distention of meningeal membranes and the compression of the vascular tree. The second major element is the resistance factor, which controls the reduction of cerebrospinal fluid volume by shunting fluid through the arachnoid villi. In animal experiments, small-volume short-duration infusions of artificial cerebrospinal fluid revealed that the regulation of fluid volume by means of outflow resistance factors is the major mechanism for protecting the brain against the effects of increasing intracranial pressure.[70] In animals with induced intracranial hypertension, the ultrastructural changes of the arachnoid villi revealed increased vacuole formation and increased transcellular channels as well as a diminished apposition of endothelial cell interdigitations.

From these studies it can be inferred that the cerebrospinal fluid compartment is larger than normal in pseudotumor cerebri. It is not established whether this phenomenon is related to a defective cerebrospinal fluid absorptive mechanism or one overburdened because of excess production. Except for patients with obstruction of intracranial venous outflow, in whom it might be presupposed that because of an increase in the pressure of the superior sagittal sinus the normal gradient between the sinus and the subarachnoid space is reversed, the nature of the intracranial hypertension has not been established. At the time of a decompression procedure or exploratory craniotomy or even when burr hole ventriculography is performed, a frequent observation is the distended subarachnoid space overlying the brain, which appears to be wet ("weeping brain"). This is in contrast to the tight, tense, swollen brain seen in patients suffering from intracranial hypertension accompanying a mass lesion or hydrocephalus.

Additional support for the concept of a defective cerebrospinal fluid absorptive capacity relates to that group of patients who have experienced pseudotumor cerebri after corticosteroid therapy has been tapered or withdrawn. Acute corticosteroid withdrawal in the rat resulted in increased resistance to cerebrospinal fluid outflow.[55] In the dog being given corticosteroids, there was observed a slight decrease in cerebrospinal fluid absorption, but when the steroids were withdrawn, absorption was significantly reduced and there was an increased resistance to flow.[56]

Impaired cerebrospinal fluid absorption, possibly at the arachnoid villi, remains an attractive hypothesis for the cause of intracranial hypertension in many patients with pseudotumor cerebri. Agenesis of arachnoid granulations has been described in infants who demonstrate hydrocephalus.[33,45] It is conceivable that the age of the patient and the duration of the intracranial hypertension are the factors that cause ventricular dilatation. In the adult patient with persistent pseudotumor cerebri, there does occur a gradual enlargement of the ventricular cavity, as reflected in repeat pneumoencephalography a year or more after onset of symptoms in two patients followed by this author. Computed tomography will help define such changes in ventricular size with time.

Regional blood flow studies using radioactive techniques have also contributed to our understanding of this syndrome.[72] In pseudotumor cerebri, regional cerebral blood volume is increased while the regional cerebral blood flow is slightly decreased. This increase in blood volume is presumed to be a response to the basic process of intracranial hypertension in which cerebral vasodilatation reflects an attempt of the cerebral vasculature to keep the cerebral blood flow constant. Following lumbar puncture in two patients, there was only a minor decrease in regional cerebral blood volume and no change in cerebral blood flow. Since intracranial hypertension may result from vascular engorgement, an interpretation consistent with those instances of pseudotumor cerebri associated with venous sinus obstruction, consideration might be given to this increased blood volume mechanism as at least one reason why the raised intracranial pressure occurs. In other words, this may be one of the fundamental causes of the intracranial hypertension rather than just a response to the raised pressure. On the other hand, direct observation of the brain and arteriography do not provide any confirmatory evidence for this vascular engorgement theory.

The results of diagnostic tests thus far have brought to mind the possibilities that the basic intracranial process contributing to the intracranial hypertension is an excess of cerebrospinal fluid or a state of vascular engorgement. The last consideration concerns the brain itself. Is there reason to believe that cerebral edema or swelling exists? As stated, a variety of diseases of endogenous, as well as exogenous, origin may result in cerebral edema. This may occur as a consequence of alteration in the intracranial vascular integrity leading to an increased brain capillary permeability or vasogenic edema; or edema may be caused by a breakdown of the cellular elements' metabolism, leading to swelling of neurons, glia, and endothelial cells accompanied by a concomitant decrease in the brain's extracellular space (cytotoxic edema).[27] There are several indirect lines of evidence against cerebral edema, either vasogenic or cytotoxic, being the cause of the intracranial hypertension. As we know cerebral edema from other clinical conditions associated with it, it is characterized by findings of neurological impairment, including alterations in mental status as well as other evidence of deranged function. The electroencephalogram is diffusely slow. At the time of lumbar puncture, the cerebrospinal fluid volume is decreased. In pseudotumor cerebri, however, the patient is clinically normal, the electroencephalogram is usually normal, and the cerebrospinal fluid

volume is increased. Moreover, brain biopsy specimens obtained at the time of subtemporal decompression did not reveal brain edema.[38]

SPECIAL PROBLEMS OF DIFFERENTIAL DIAGNOSIS

Two areas of special concern in the differential diagnosis of pseudotumor cerebri are the empty sella syndrome and, in the young infant, the full anterior fontanel.

The empty sella syndrome is commonly seen in the obese woman who presents with headaches and menstrual irregularities and whose routine skull roentgenograms demonstrate an enlarged sella turcica. In contrast with the obese women patients with pseudotumor cerebri who have papilledema and increased intracranial pressure, and whose x-rays define an enlarged sella turcica, this group of obese women does not have papilledema or documented increased intracranial pressure.[29] The enlarged empty sella is thought to represent an extension of the subarachnoid space into the sella. Pneumoencephalography in such patients reveals a flattened pituitary gland against the sella floor. The concept offered is that intermittent or subacute intracranial hypertension induces the herniation of the subarachnoid tissue through an incompetent diaphragma sellae. The obese woman with the empty sella syndrome may not have papilledema because pressure on the optic nerves in the region of the sella occludes the subarachnoid pathways leading to the optic discs. When such patients also have increased intracranial pressure, the treatment approach is obviously identical to that offered the obese woman with pseudotumor cerebri. In the absence of intracranial hypertension, the obese patient with the empty sella syndrome should be treated by dietary restriction, although there is no evidence that this is beneficial. The empty sella syndrome is discussed in greater detail in Chapter 100.

The second problem sometimes confused with pseudotumor cerebri exists in the infant with a full or wide open anterior fontanel. As previously described, there are infants with pseudotumor cerebri caused by disordered vitamin metabolism and certain drugs; Table 101–3 is a list of conditions in which a full fontanel may be mistaken for a

TABLE 101–3 CONDITIONS CAUSING LARGE ANTERIOR FONTANELS IN YOUNG INFANTS

CHROMOSOMAL ANOMALIES
 Down's syndrome
 13 Trisomy
 18 Trisomy

POLYGENIC ANOMALIES
 Achondroplasia
 Apert's syndrome
 Cleidocranial dysostosis
 Familial megalencephaly
 Pyknodysostosis
 Kenny's syndrome
 Hallermann-Streiff syndrome
 Russell-Silver syndrome
 Other chondromalacias

TOXIC OR METABOLIC CONDITIONS
 Aminopterin insult in utero
 Athyrotic hypothyroidism
 Malnutrition
 Osteogenesis imperfecta

state of increased intracranial pressure during early infancy.[82] Excluded from this list is the very common state encountered in a febrile infant in which a bulging fontanel represents a true state of intracranial hypertension related in some way to the extracranial infectious process. This has been attributed to osmolar shifts, a toxic effect, or the results of inappropriate antidiuretic hormone secretion and has been termed meningismus.

TREATMENT OF PSEUDOTUMOR CEREBRI

Operative treatment to correct the intracranial hypertension is available for patients with mastoiditis causing lateral sinus obstruction and other forms of intracranial venous sinus obstruction. Similarly, in patients who are acutely anemic from blood loss, those suffering from disturbance of vitamin metabolism, and others who experience the symptoms of intracranial hypertension following drug therapy, the treatment approach is specific.

To help facilitate the resolution of signs and symptoms and particularly in those patients for whom specific therapy is unavailable, decompressive procedures are appropriate to prevent visual impairment. Even in the absence of specific therapy, the effect of a single lumbar puncture and other diagnostic procedures improved the patient's

symptoms in 33 per cent of the author's series and, whether coincidentally or not, was followed shortly thereafter by the disappearance of pseudotumor cerebri (Table 101–4). Serial lumbar punctures were another approach used in the patient with persistent symptoms. At the time of lumbar puncture, fluid was removed in sufficient quantity to lower the pressure to normal. The frequency of these treatments was based on the patient's status. In the past, when intracranial hypertension persisted despite serial lumbar punctures done over an arbitrary period (days to weeks), subtemporal decompression was performed. In many instances, this procedure did not resolve the intracranial hypertension problems, and repeated lumbar punctures were necessary as well following operation.

It should be stressed that, in most instances, a beneficial response would occur merely by the passage of time, and active neurosurgical intervention may prove to be both unwarranted and hazardous. As specific examples of the dangers of operation four patients in the author's series who underwent subtemporal decompression experienced contralateral partial seizures with simple motor components and complex symptoms beginning 6 to 12 months after operation. These developments were attributable to the effects of trauma to the temporal lobe, which herniated through the decompression site. In addition, one other patient exhibited otorrhea as a complication of such an operation.

TABLE 101–4 RESULTS OF DECOMPRESSIVE PROCEDURES IN PSEUDOTUMOR CEREBRI*

THERAPY	NO. OF PATIENTS	COMPLI-CATIONS
Single lumbar puncture or air encephalography only	42	0
Serial lumbar punctures (four or more)	26	0
Serial lumbar punctures followed by thecoperitoneal shunts	3	0
Serial lumbar punctures and subtemporal decompression	21	3
Subtemporal decompression	24	2
Exploratory craniotomy	4	1 (died)

* One hundred and twenty cases of pseudotumor cerebri treated at J. Hillis Miller Health Center, Gainesville, Florida, and Columbia Presbyterian Medical Center, New York, N.Y.

The current approach is to perform a thecoperitoneal shunt after serial lumbar punctures prove to be of only temporary benefit. This procedure is to be considered early in the course of evaluation and treatment of the patient when specific treatment is unavailable and the risks of sudden visual impairment are evident because of the unpredictability of the patient's problems; such would be the case, for example, in the woman with marked menstrual irregularities. The ventriculoperitoneal shunt is not advocated because of the danger of cerebral trauma and the problems of shunt tube patency where the ventricular cavities are narrow.

Drug therapy including corticosteroids, acetazolamide, and oral and intravenous osmolar loads have been used from time to time in patients who are refractory to other forms of supportive treatment. The arguments for the use of corticosteroids as well as its lack of value are buttressed by animal experiments and clinical trials. On the advocacy side are certain studies showing that corticosteroid treatment appeared to lessen the severity of brain edema when a cerebral hemisphere was exposed to air, when psyllium seeds were implanted in the brain, and in situations in which blood vessel permeability was induced by trauma.[23,66,68,83,85] On the other hand, in the animal brain made edematous with triethyl tin, the positive effect of corticosteroids was apparent only if the drug was given before the edema was induced.[96] Focusing on the question of spinal fluid formation and flow as the mechanism involved with the intracranial hypertension, it has been shown that intravenous corticosteroids reduce cerebrospinal fluid flow to about 50 per cent within an hour, whereas in dogs, orally administered corticosteroids produce a reduction of cerebrospinal fluid absorption.[56,86] Clinical experience in patients with pseudotumor cerebri gives conflicting results as well. In certain, but not all, children in one series, corticosteroids were said to be of value in reducing the pressure.[101] According to another report, continuous monitoring of intracranial pressure in two obese women patients treated with large doses of corticosteroids did not demonstrate any lowering of cerebrospinal fluid pressure.[54] Personal experience has not convinced the author that the use of corticosteroids is of any value except in those instances in which a presumed state of adrenal insufficiency exists; moreover, as stated, in the obese patient it often prolongs the problem by maintaining the patient's weight.

Acetazolamide, a carbonic anhydrase inhibitor, reduces the rate of cerebrospinal fluid formation by 50 per cent; however, when it was used for periods up to two months in two of the author's patients, no beneficial effects were witnessed and the intracranial hypertension persisted.[57,62]

Oral hyperosmolar agents and dehydrating drugs, including oral urea 1.0 gm per kilogram per day, oral glycerol 1.0 to 1.5 gm per kilogram per day, hydroflumethiazide 100 mg on alternate days, and chlorthalidone 200 mg on alternate days, have been used with some success in patients with pseudotumor.[54] The effectiveness of such agents cannot be attributed to a difference between osmolarity values in the plasma and the brain, and it is difficult to understand the benefits on the basis of dehydration unless it is accompanied by weight reduction that is maintained beyond the initial period of diuresis in the obese patient with pseudotumor cerebri. Oral glycerin has been advocated in the treatment of pseudotumor cerebri.[2,76] Its rapid metabolism, however, eliminates its effect as an agent useful in inducing osmolar changes in the brain, and it has not been shown to be of value in the one patient with persistent intracranial hypertension who was so treated and evaluated by the author. Again, it should be stressed that a beneficial response reported after the administration of such drugs during the early phase of pseudotumor cerebri is not a valid interpretation of drug effect, since diagnostic procedures alone, including at least one lumbar puncture, are often all that is needed to resolve the intracranial hypertension.

FOLLOW-UP ASSESSMENT

Eleven per cent of patients in the author's series continued to demonstrate increased intracranial pressure when lumbar punctures were performed five or more months after admission. All had regression of their signs and symptoms of intracranial hypertension (papilledema, headache, and the like) prior to the five-month period, and the lumbar punctures were performed because the recorded pressure at the time of the previous study was elevated (greater than 200 mm of cerebrospinal fluid). It is implied by this observation that in the asymptomatic period a physiological state exists in which the compliance of the meninges is altered or the rate of cerebrospinal fluid production and absorption is adjusted to the point of clinical tolerance for the patient with pseudotumor cerebri. This new physiological state is represented by an increased cerebrospinal fluid pressure.

In those patients with persistent symptoms, repeat neurodiagnostic studies are performed at varying periods, seeking a different specifically treatable cause for the intracranial hypertension that may have been missed the first time. In a group of patients with pseudotumor cerebri that was reported earlier, subsequent studies had revealed the presence of tumors three to nine months after initial evaluation in four patients.[103] The fact that neither cerebral arteriography nor brain scanning were available at that time makes such studies out of date for comparison.

In the author's series, long-term assessment of about 50 patients with pseudotumor cerebri was possible for a period of 18 months to 14 years. In the others, it was less than a year. In only one patient was a tumor (chemodectoma) recognized one year after initial evaluation. Computed tomography was not available at that time.

REFERENCES

1. Abernathy, R. S.: Bulging fontanel as presenting sign in cystic fibrosis. Amer. J. Dis. Child., 130:1360–1362, 1976.
2. Absolon, M. J.: Unusual presentation of benign intracranial hypertension. Early treatment with oral glycerol. Brit. J. Ophthal., 50:683–688, 1966.
3. Allison, J. R., Jr.: Sarcoidosis. Southern Med. J., 57:27–32, 1964.
4. Ayala, G.: Die Physiopathologie der Mechanik des Liquor cerebrospinalis und des Rachidealquotieten. Mschr. Psychiat. Neurol., 58:65–101, 1925.
5. Bass, M. H., and Fisch, G. R.: Increased intracranial pressure with bulging fontanel. Neurology (Minneap.), 11:1091–1094, 1961.
6. Bercaw, B. L., and Greer, M.: Transport of intrathecal 1311 RIHSA in benign intracranial hypertension. Neurology (Minneap.), 20:787–790, 1970.
7. Bering, E. A., Jr., and Salibi, B.: Production of hydrocephalus by increased cephalic-venous pressure. Arch. Neurol. Psychiat., 81:693–698, 1959.
8. Bodensteiner, J., and Matsuo, F.: EEG in benign intracranial hypertension J. Neurol. Sci., 34:1007–1010, 1977.
9. Borens, L. O., and Sundstrom, B.: Intracranial hypertension in a child during treatment with nalidixic acid. Brit. Med. J., 2:744–745, 1967.
10. Boruchow, I. B., Bartley, T. D., Elliott, L. P., and Schiebler, G. L.: Late superior vena cava syndrome after superior vena cava–right pulmonary artery anastomosis. New Eng. J. Med., 281:646–650, 1969.
11. Boudin, G., Funck-Brentano, J. L., and Gayno, M.: Maladie d'Addison par aplasie surrenale et syndrome para-biermerien. Bull. Soc. Méd. Hôp. Paris, 66:1736–1740, 1956.
12. Bray, P. F., and Herbst, J. J.: Psuedotumor cerebri as a sign of "catch-up" growth in cystic fibrosis. Amer. J. Dis. Child., 126:78–79, 1973.
13. Buchheit, W. A., Burton, C., Burritt, H., and Shaw, D.: Papilledema and idiopathic intracranial hypertension. New Eng. J. Med., 280:938–942, 1969.
14. Capitanio, M. A., and Kirkpatrick, J. A.: Widening of the cranial sutures: A roentgen observation during periods of accelerated growth in patients treated for deprivation dwarfism. Radiology, 92:53–59, 1969.
15. Ch'ien, L. T.: Intracranial hypertension and sulfamethoxazole. Letter to the Editor. New Eng. J. Med., 283:47, 1970.
16. Chun, R. W. M., Smith, N. J., and Forster, F. M.: Papilledema in Sydenham's chorea. Amer. J. Dis. Child., 101:641–643, 1962.
17. Chutorian, A. M., Gold, A. P., and Braum, C. W.: Benign intracranial hypertension and Bell's palsy. New Eng. J. Med., 296:1214–1215, 1977.
18. Cornfield, D., and Cook, R. E.: Vitamin A deficiency: Case report. Unusual manifestation in a 5½ month old baby. Pediatrics, 10:33–38, 1952.
19. Davenport, V. D.: Relation between brain and plasma electrolytes and electroshock seizure thresholds in adrenalectomized rats. Amer. J. Physiol., 156:322–327, 1949.
20. DiLiberti, J., and O'Brien, M. L.: Pseudotumor cerebri following patent ductus arteriosus ligation. J. Pediat., 87:489, 1975.
21. Dunkelman, S. S., Fairhurst, B., Plager, J., and Waterhouse, C.: Cortisol metabolism in obesity. J. Clin. Endocr., 24:832–841, 1964.
22. Dunsker, S. B., Torres-Reyes, E., and Peden, J. C.: Pseudotumor cerebri associated with idiopathic cryofibrinogenemia. Arch. Neurol. (Chicago), 23:120–127, 1970.
23. Eisenberg, H. M., Barlow, C. F., and Lorenzo, A. V.: Effect of dexamethasone on altered brain vascular permeability. Arch. Neurol. (Chicago), 23:18–22, 1970.
24. Elliott, K. A. C., and Yrarrazaval, S.: An effect of adrenalectomy and cortisone on tissue permeability in vitro. Nature (London), 169:416–417, 1952.
25. Feldman, M. H., and Schlezinger, N. S.: Benign intracranial hypertension associated with hypervitaminosis A. Arch. Neurol. (Chicago), 22:1–7, 1970.
26. Finberg, L.: Pathogenesis of lesions in the nervous system in hypernatremic states. Pediatrics, 23:40–45, 1959.

27. Fishman, R. A.: Brain edema. New Eng. J. Med., *293*:706–711, 1975.
28. Fitz-Hugh, G. S., Robins, R. B., and Craddock, W. D.: Increased intracranial pressure complicating unilateral neck dissection. Laryngoscope, 76:893–906, 1966.
29. Foley, K. M., and Posner, J. B.: Does pseudotumor cerebri cause the empty sella syndrome? Neurology (Minneap.), *25*:565–569, 1975.
30. Ford, F. R.: Diseases of the Nervous System in Infancy, Childhood and Adolescence. 4th Ed. Springfield, Ill., Charles C Thomas, 1960, p. 889.
31. Fraser, D., Yendt, E. R., and Christie, F. H. E.: Metabolic abnormalities in hypophosphatasia. Lancet, *1*:286, 1955.
32. Gerber, A., Raab, A. P., and Sobel, A. E.: Vitamin A poisoning in adults. Amer. J. Med., *16*:729–745, 1955.
33. Gilles, F. H., and Davidson, R. I.: Communicating hydrocephalus with deficient dysplastic parasagittal arachnoidal granulations. J. Neurosurg., *35*:421–426, 1971.
34. Greer, M.: Benign intracranial hypertension. II. Following corticosteroid therapy. Neurology (Minneap.), *13*:439–441, 1963a.
35. Greer, M.: Benign intracranial hypertension. III. Pregnancy. Neurology (Minneap.), *13*:670–672, 1963b.
36. Greer, M.: Benign intracranial hypertension. IV. Menarche. Neurology (Minneap.), *14*:569–573, 1964a.
37. Greer, M.: Benign intracranial hypertension. V. Menstrual dysfunction. Neurology (Minneap.), *14*:668–673, 1964b.
38. Greer, M.: Benign intracranial hypertension. VI. Obesity. Neurology (Minneap.), *15*:382–388, 1965.
39. Greer, M.: Benign intracranial hypertension in children. Pediat. Clin. N. Amer., *14*:819–830, 1967.
40. Greer, M.: Management of benign intracranial hypertension (pseudotumor cerebri). Clin. Neurosurg., *15*:161–174, 1968.
41. Greer, M.: Uncommon causes of stroke: Diseases of the vessel wall. Geriatrics, *32*:28–41, 1977.
42. Greer, M.: Uncommon causes of stroke: Intravascular components. Geriatrics, *33*:51–56, 1978.
43. Greer, M., and Berk, M. S.: Lateral sinus obstruction and mastoiditis. Pediatrics, *31*:840–844, 1963.
44. Guthrie, T. C., Dunbar, H. S., and Karpell, B.: Ventricular size and chronic increased intracranial venous pressure in the dog. J. Neurosurg., *33*:407–414, 1970.
45. Gutierrez, Y., Friede, R. L., and Kaliney, W. J.: Agenesis of arachnoid granulations and its relationship to communicating hydrocephalus. J. Neurosurg., *43*:553–558, 1975.
46. Hochman, H. I., and Mejlszenkier, J. D.: Cataracts and pseudotumor cerebri in an infant with vitamin D–deficiency rickets. J. Pediat., *90*:252–254, 1977.
47. Hooper, R.: Hydrocephalus and obstruction of the superior vena cava in infancy. Clinical study of the relationship between cerebrospinal fluid pressure and venous pressure. Pediatrics, *28*:792–799, 1961.
48. Howell, J. M., and Thompson, J. M.: Lesions associated with the development of ataxia in chicks. Brit. J. Nutr., *21*:741–750, 1967.
49. Hussey, F., Schanzer, B., and Katzman, R.: A simple constant infusion manometric test for measurement of CSF absorption. Neurology (Minneap.), *20*:665–680, 1970.
50. Huttenlocher, P., Hillman, R. E., and Hsia, Y. E.: Pseudotumor cerebri in galactosemia. J. Pediat., *76*:902–905, 1970.
51. Ikkala, E., and Laitinen, L.: Papilledema due to iron deficiency anemia. Acta Haemat. (Basel), *29*:368–370, 1963.
52. James A. E., Harbert, J. C., Joffer, P. B., and Deland, F. H.: CSF imaging in benign intracranial hypertension. J. Neurol. Neurosurg. Psychiat., *37*:1053–1058, 1974.
53. Jefferson, A.: A clinical correlation between encephalopathy and papilledema in Addison's disease. J. Neurol. Neurosurg. Psychiat., *19*:21–27, 1956.
54. Jefferson, A., and Clark, J.: Treatment of benign intracranial hypertension by dehydrating agents with particular reference to the measurement of the blind spot area as a means of recording improvement. J. Neurol. Neurosurg. Psychiat., *39*:627–639, 1976.
55. Johnston, I.: Reduced CSF absorption syndrome. Lancet *2*:418–420, 1973.
56. Johnston, I., Gilday, D. L., and Hendrick, E. B.: Experimental effects of steroids and steroid withdrawal on fluid absorption. J. Neurosurg., *42*:690–695, 1975.
57. Katzman, R., and Pappius, H. M.: Brain Electrolytes and Fluid Metabolism. Baltimore, Williams & Wilkins Co., 1973.
58. Keating, J. P., and Feigin, R. D.: Increased intracranial pressure associated with probable vitamin A deficiency in cystic fibrosis. Pediatrics, *46*:41–46, 1970.
59. Kennedy, F.: Certain nervous complications following the use of therapeutic and prophylactic sera. Amer. J. Med. Sci., *177*:555–559, 1929.
60. Kinal, M. E.: Hydrocephalus and the dural venous sinuses. J. Neurosurg. *19*:195–201, 1962.
61. Kinal, M. E.: Traumatic thrombosis of dural venous sinuses in closed head injuries. J. Neurosurg., *27*:142–145, 1967.
62. Kister, S. J.: Carbonic anhydrase inhibition. VI. The effect of acetazolamide on cerebrospinal fluid flow. J. Pharmacol. Exp. Ther., 117 (1956) 402–405.
63. Knaggs, R. L.: Leontiasis ossea. Brit. J. Surg., *11*:347–349, 1924.
64. Koch-Weser, J., and Gilmore, E. B.: Benign intracranial hypertension in an adult after tetracycline therapy. J.A.M.A., *200*:345–347, 1967.
65. Konomi, H., Imai, M., Nihei, K., Kamoshita, S., and Tada, H.: Indomethacin causing pseudotumor in Bartter's syndrome. New Eng. J. Med., *298*:855, 1978.
66. Lee, J. C., and Olozewski, J.: Permeability of cerebral blood vessels in healing of brain wounds. Neurology (Minneap.), *9*:7–14, 1959.
67. Leiderman, P. H., and Katzman, R.: Effect of adrenalectomy, desoxycorticosterone and cortisone and brain potassium exchange. Amer. J. Physiol., *175*:271–275, 1953.

68. Lippert, R. G., Suien, H. J., Grindlay, J. H., et al.: The effect of cortisone on experimental cerebral edema. J. Neurosurg., *17*:583–589, 1960.

69. Loman, J., and Dameshek, W.: Increased intracranial venous and cerebrospinal fluid pressure in polycythemia. Trans. Amer. Neurol. Ass., *70*:84, 1944.

70. Mann, J. D., Butler, A. B., Rosenthal, J. E., Maffeo, C. J., Johnson, R. N., and Bass, N. H.: Regulation of intracranial pressure in rat, dog and man. Ann. Neurol., *3*:156–165, 1978.

71. Marie, J., and See, G.: Acute hypervitaminosis A of the infant. Its clinical manifestation with benign acute hydrocephalus and pronounced bulge of the fontanel: A clinical and biological study. Amer. J. Dis. Child., *87*:731–736, 1954.

72. Mathew, N. T., Meyer, J. S., and Ott, E. O.: Increased cerebral blood volume in benign intracranial hypertension. Neurology (Minneap.), *25*:646–649, 1975.

73. Metcalf, M. G., and Beaven, D. W.: Plasma-corticosteroid levels in women receiving oral contraceptive tablets. Lancet, *2*:1095–1096, 1963.

74. Mones, R. J.: Increased intracranial pressure due to metastatic disease of venous sinuses. Neurology (Minneap.), *15*:1000–1007, 1965.

75. Murphy, R. E., and Costanzi, J. J.: Pseudotumor cerebri associated with pernicious anemia. Ann. Intern. Med., *70*:777–782, 1969.

76. Newkirk, T. A., Tourtelotte, W. W., and Reinglass, J. L.: Prolonged control of intracranial pressure with glycerin. Arch. Neurol. (Chicago), *27*:95–96, 1972.

77. Nickerson, C. W., and Kirk, R. F.: Recurrent pseudotumor cerebri in pregnancy. Report of 2 cases. Obstet. Gynec., *26*:811–813, 1965.

78. Oldstone, M. B. A.: Disturbance of pituitary-adrenal interrelationships in benign intracranial hypertension. J. Clin. Endocr., *26*:1366–1369, 1966.

79. Oski, F. A.: Roseola infantum. Amer. J. Dis. Child., *101*:376–378, 1961.

80. Patterson, R., Depasquale, N., and Mann, S.: Pseudotumor cerebri. *Medicine* (Balt.), *40*:85–99, 1961.

81. Plager, J. E., Schmidt, K. G., and Stanbetz, W. J.: Increased unbound cortisol in plasma of estrogen-treated subjects. J. Clin. Invest., *43*:1066–1072, 1964.

82. Popich, G. A., and Smith, D. W.: Fontanels: Range of normal size. J. Pediat., *80*:749–752, 1972.

83. Prados, M., Strowgen, M. A., and Feindel, W.: Studies on cerebral edema. II. Reaction of brain to exposure to air; physiologic changes. Arch. Neurol. Psychiat., *54*:290–300, 1945.

84. Quincke, H.: Uber Meningitis serosa und verwandte Zustande. Deutsch. Z. Nervenheilk., *9*:149–168, 1897.

85. Rouit, R. L., and Hagan, R.: Effects of dexamethasone on abnormal permeability of blood-brain-barrier following cerebral injury in cats. Surg. Forum, *16*:442–444, 1965.

86. Sato, O., Hara, M., Asai, T., Ryuichi, T., and Kageyama, N.: The effect of dexamethasone phosphate on the production rate of CSF in the spinal subarachnoid space of dogs. J. Neurosurg., *39*:480–484, 1973.

87. Schmitt, B. D., and Krivit, W.: Benign intracranial hypertension associated with delayed penicillin reaction. Pediatrics, *43*:50–53, 1969.

88. Schwaber, J. R., and Blumberg, A. G.: Papilledema associated with blood loss anemia. Ann. Intern. Med., *55*:1005–1007, 1961.

89. Shenk, E. A.: Sickle cell trait and superior longitudinal sinus thrombosis. Ann. Intern. Med., *60*:465–470, 1964.

90. Sidell, A. D., and Daly, D. D.: The electroencephalogram in cases of benign intracranial hypertension. Neurology (Minneap.), *11*:413–417, 1961.

91. Stephens, W. P., Eddy, J. D., Parsons, L. M., and Snigh, S. P.: Raised intracranial pressure due to perhexiline maleate. Brit. Med. J., *1*:21, 1978.

92. Stewart, W. A.: Electroencephalographic changes associated with different forms of experimentally produced increased intracranial pressure. Bull. Johns Hopk. Hosp., *69*:240–265, 1941.

93. Stoebner, R., Kiser, R., and Alperin, J. B.: Iron deficiency anemia and papilledema; rapid resolution with oral iron therapy. Amer. J. Dig. Dis., *15*:919–922, 1970.

94. Sugar, O.: Central neurological complications of hypoparathyroidism. Arch. Neurol. Psychiat., *70*:86–107, 1953.

95. Symonds, C. P.: Hydrocephalus and focal cerebral symptoms in relation to thrombophlebitis of the dural sinuses and cerebral veins. Brain, *60*:531–550, 1937.

96. Taylor, J. M., Levy, W. A., Herzog, I., and Scheinberg, L. C.: Prevention of experimental cerebral edema by corticosteroids. Neurology (Minneap.), *15*:667–674, 1965.

97. Walsh, F. B.: Papilledema associated with increased intracranial pressure in Addison's disease. Arch. Ophthal. (Chicago), *47*:86, 1952.

98. Walsh, F. B., Clark, D. B., Thompson, R. S., and Nicholson, D. H.: Oral contraceptives and neuro-ophthalmologic interest. Arch. Ophthal. (Chicago), *74*:628–640, 1965.

99. Watkins, C. H., Wagener, H. P., and Brown, R. W.: Cerebral symptoms by choked optic discs in types of blood dysergasia. Amer. J. Ophthal., *24*:1374–1383, 1941.

100. Weinman, C. G., McDowell, F. H., and Plum, F.: Papilledema in poliomyelitis. Arch. Neurol. Psychiat., *66*:722–727, 1951.

101. Weisberg, L. A., and Chutorian, A. M.: Pseudotumor cerebri of childhood. Amer. J. Dis. Child., *131*:1243–1248, 1977.

102. Witsel, E. W., and Hunt, G. M.: The ultrastructure of the choroid plexus in hydrocephalic offspring from vitamin A deficient rabbits. J. Neuropath. Exp. Neurol., *21*:250–262, 1962.

103. Zuidema, G. D., and Cohen, S. J.: Pseudotumor cerebri. J. Neurosurg., *11*:433–441, 1954.

102

SPINAL CORD
TUMORS IN ADULTS

Although spinal cord tumors have been written about for many centuries, most of the knowledge of their treatment has been gained in the last 100 years. In 1888, Horsley and Gowers reported the first successful removal of an intradural extramedullary tumor.[35] In 1907 Elsberg reported the first successful operation on an intramedullary tumor.[16] In 1919 Dandy introduced air myelography, and in 1921 Sicard and Forestier introduced positive contrast myelography.[13,54] The next major development in the operative treatment of spinal cord tumors was Greenwood's introduction of bipolar coagulation in 1940, followed the next year by his successful total extirpation of an intramedullary tumor, which resulted in complete neurological recovery and freedom from recurrence for 35 years.[26,27] Operations on spinal cord tumors were further advanced by Malis's modification and improvement of the bipolar coagulation unit and by Kurze's introduction of the operative microscope in 1964.[39,41]

INCIDENCE

Tumors of the spinal cord and its coverings occur relatively rarely. The true incidence in the general population is difficult to determine, since most of the statistics have been accumulated from large neurosurgical units that attract central nervous system problems. Two studies, however, are of importance in defining the true incidence of spinal cord tumors. The first is Kurland's 1958 study of the incidence of central nervous system tumors in the population of Rochester, Minnesota.[38] During a 10-year period, 12 intraspinal tumors were diagnosed in a population of 30,000 people; during the same period, 50 intracranial neoplasms were discovered, giving a ratio of approximately four intracranial neoplasms to one spinal neoplasm and an incidence of 12.9 spinal cord tumors per 100,000 population. A second important study was a survey of tumors of the central nervous system in Iceland during a 10-year period, 1954 to 1963, by Guomundsson.[31] During this period, the population of Iceland ranged from 152,000 to 187,314; 234 brain tumors and 27 spinal cord tumors were diagnosed. These figures give a ratio of approximately nine intracranial tumors to one spinal tumor and an incidence of 1.1 spinal tumors per 100,000 population. Nittner, in 1976, suggested that approximately one fifth of central nervous system tumors occurred in the spinal cord.[45] In a composite study of 23,620 tumors of the central nervous system, there were 18,735 of the brain and 4885 of the spinal canal.

In large collections of spinal cord tumors, the most common are neurilemmomas, meningiomas, ependymomas, and astrocytomas (Table 102–1). The vast majority are benign. In Nittner's review of 4885 spinal cord tumors collected from the literature in 1976, there were 649 intramedullary glial tumors exclusive of ependymomas, 126 ependymomas, 1129 neurolemmomas, 1088 meningiomas, 370 sarcomas, 305 angiomas, 323 metastases, and 895 miscellaneous tumors.[45] Approximately 16 per cent of spinal cord tumors are intramedullary, the remainder being extramedullary. In Slooff and associates' review of 1322 tumors of the spinal cord at Mayo Clinic, 29 per cent were neurilemmomas, 25.5 per cent were meningiomas, 22 per cent were gliomas,

TABLE 102–1 CHARACTERISTICS OF MOST COMMON SPINAL CORD TUMORS

CHARACTERISTIC	NEURILEMMOMA	MENINGIOMA	EPENDYMOMA	ASTROCYTOMA
Incidence (fraction of spinal cord tumors)	One quarter	One fifth	One eighth	One twelfth
Sex	Equal	Four fifths female	Three fifths male	Equal
Spinal level	Half thoracic	Two thirds thoracic	Half lumbar	Half thoracic
Treatment	Total excision	Total excision	Total excision	Subtotal excision plus radiation therapy
Prognosis	Excellent	Excellent	Good	Good to poor depending on degree of malignancy

11.9 per cent were sarcomas, 6.2 per cent were vascular tumors, 4 per cent were chordomas, and 1.4 per cent were epidermoids (Fig. 102–1).[55]

SURGICAL ANATOMY

The spinal cord is an ovoid neural structure that lies within the vertebral canal and extends from the foramen magnum to the intervertebral disc level between L1 and L2. On occasion, it may reach only to the body of T12, or it may extend to the lower body of L2 in the adult. The spinal cord extends to L3 at birth. The cord has a tendency to be more caudally located in women and in the colored races.[2] The cord moves with changes in position; the conus medullaris rises with flexion and descends with extension. The spinal cord is cylindrical but somewhat flattened dorsoventrally so that its width is always greater than its dorsoventral diameter. Its greatest width in the cervical enlargement has a transverse diameter of 13 to 14 mm; in the lumbar enlargement, 11 to 13 mm; and in the thoracic portion, about 10 mm.

Usually there are 31 pairs of spinal nerves in man, but the number may vary, particularly if there is variation in the number of vertebrae. The first pair of spinal nerves exits from the vertebral column between the atlas and the skull, and each remaining cervical nerve exits above the vertebra corresponding in number except for the eighth cervical segment, which leaves above the T1 vertebra. Beginning with the first thoracic nerve, all the remaining spinal nerves exit below the vertebra of their number. There are 8 cervical, 12 thoracic, 5 lumbar, 5 sacral, and 1 coccygeal paired groups.

All the spinal nerves have a dorsal root ganglion except, usually, the first cervical root and the coccygeal nerves. Occasion-

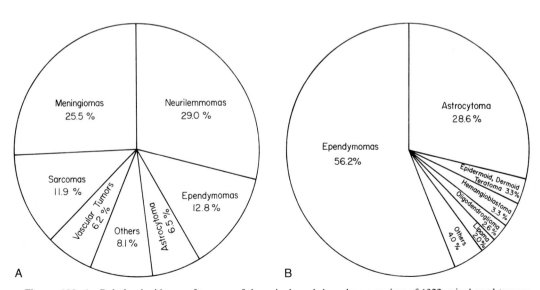

A   B

Figure 102–1 Relative incidence of tumors of the spinal cord, based on a review of 1322 spinal cord tumors reported from the Mayo Clinic.

ally, the first cervical root will have a small rudimentary ganglion or share the ganglion with the spinal accessory nerve; however, variations may be found at any level of the cord with absence of the nerve root or duplication of ganglia. The spinal cord segment C1 and the first cervical vertebra are at the same level. As one descends the vertebral levels, the cord levels become progressively higher than the corresponding vertebral levels so that the lower border of the T12 segment overlaps the upper part of the body of the eleventh thoracic vertebra and is opposite the spine of the tenth. The fifth lumbar segment of the cord lies in the interspace between the twelfth thoracic and the first lumbar vertebrae.

The cord is surrounded by dense fibrous tissue called pia mater; the longitudinal fibers midway between the ventral and dorsal roots extend laterally to attach to the dura mater and suspend the cord laterally. These attachments are called dentate ligaments, and there are 21 such attachments extending from the most superior, between the vertebral artery and the twelfth cranial nerve, to the lowest, between the twelfth thoracic root and the first lumbar root. The pia mater also forms the filum terminale, which runs from the posterior inferior aspect of the conus medullaris to its insertion on the dorsal surface of the coccyx. The pia mater also contains the blood vessels of the spinal cord.

Thirty-one pairs of radicular artery branches penetrate the vertebral canal through the intervertebral foramen. They are of three types: (1) the proper radicular branches, which end within the roots or on the dura mater before reaching the spinal cord; (2) the pia mater radicular branches, which do not penetrate beyond the arterial system surrounding the spinal cord; and (3) the spinal branches, which are the only ones that vascularize the spinal cord. Of the 31 radicular branches, 7 or 8 at the most really participate in the vascularization of the spinal cord.[40] The spinal cord is made up of three large arterial areas, the superior or cervicothoracic area, the intermediate or midthoracic area, and the lower or thoracolumbar area. The superior or cervicothoracic area includes the cervical cord and the first two or three thoracic segments. It receives blood primarily from the anterior spinal artery descending from the vertebral

artery and rarely extending below the fourth cervical segment, from a branch of the intertransverse foraminal portion of the vertebral artery, and from a branch of the costocervical trunk. The intermediate or midthoracic area of the cord extends from T3 to T8 and usually receives its vascularization from a single artery situated at approximately T7. The lower or thoracolumbar area includes the last three or four thoracic segments and the lumbar enlargement. This area receives its supply usually from a single artery coming from one of the last dorsal or first lumbar arteries. It has been called the ramus magnus radicularis anterior of Adamkiewicz and usually enters between T9 and T12. An anastomotic loop of the conus medullaris has been described and receives supply from vessels coming from the cauda equina and from the great artery of Adamkiewicz.

PATHOPHYSIOLOGY OF SPINAL CORD TUMORS

Space-occupying lesions of the spinal canal usually produce symptoms by involving long tracts of the spinal cord and by involving nerve roots. In 1923, Oppenheim classified the three clinical stages of spinal cord compression.[42] The first stage is characterized by root pain and segmental sensory or motor disturbances. The second stage is a Brown-Séquard syndrome, or incomplete transsection syndrome, and the third stage is complete transsection.

Usually, the first sign of compression of the spinal cord long tracts is a disturbance of motor function. If it is gradual in onset, spasticity results; if the onset is acute, there is a flaccid paresis. In typical cases, the patient first complains of fleeting or slowly progressive weakness of the extremities described as an increasing tiredness or fatigue. This progresses to spastic paresis. Slow-growing tumors, such as meningiomas and neurilemmomas, often produce spastic paresis. Rapidly progressive neoplasms, such as metastatic tumors, may result in an acute transsection syndrome with flaccid paresis and loss of reflexes. Sensory long tracts of the spinal cord may be involved individually or collectively. Progressive lesions that cause transsection of the cord usually involve the posterior columns initially and cause disorders of epicritic superficial cutaneous sensation. Later, there is a disturbance of function of the anterolateral tracts with loss of feeling of pain and temperature. Compression of the dorsal surface of the cord, which is more common in meningiomas and neurilemmomas, usually involves all modalities of superficial sensation, position, and vibration. This finding on examination usually indicates an extramedullary tumor.

Intramedullary tumors sometimes produce bilateral disassociative sensory disturbances with isolated damage to the anterolateral tracts. There is a disturbance of pain and temperature senses, but touch and position senses are intact. Clinically, sensory disturbances usually start in the distal part of the lower extremities and slowly extend proximally to the level of the lesion. At first, patients often complain only of paresthesias and numbness. Objective sensory disturbances do not appear until late. Damage of the sensory tracts of the cord may produce painful dysesthesias far removed from the affected level of the cord. These dysesthesias, called funicular pain, may present as deep, nonspecific pain in a limb. As presenting symptoms, sensory disturbances predominate with intramedullary tumors, motor symptoms with meningiomas, and root symptoms with neurilemmomas. The first sign of root damage is usually unilateral pain at the level of the dermatome of the root. The pain may be worse at night, particularly while the patient is supine, or with the Valsalva maneuver. The root pain may be mild and of relatively short duration if loss of conduction through the root occurs early. In addition to pain, there may be hypesthesia in the dermatome as well as fasciculations, which are characteristic of extramedullary lesions, and eventually paresis and amyotrophy.

Soft tumors may cause deformation of the spinal cord before producing symptoms, whereas firm or hard tumors produce symptoms earlier and may actually cause contusion of the cord with spine motion. Contrecoup compression of the cord is quite common, particularly in meningiomas. Even ventral meningiomas produce more posterior column signs because the dorsal cord is pushed against the hard bone, giving rise to vascular compression and early ischemia of the long tracts.

High cervical cord tumors usually present with neck pain and headache in the greater occipital nerve distribution. Frequently there is stiffness and postural abnormality of the head combined with severe pain on any neck motion. With the development of long tract signs, respiratory weakness and distress and early involvement of the diaphragm may be manifest in intercostal breathing and the use of accessory muscles of respiration.

Lower cervical cord tumors frequently produce pain in the arm or shoulder, and mimic the symptoms of cervical disc disease. Lower motor neuron signs in combination with long tract signs may be indistinguishable from those in cervical spondylosis with myelopathy.

In thoracic cord tumors it is difficult to localize the level of disturbance. Funicular pain and long-tract motor disturbances are quite common, and root symptoms may be three or more vertebrae below the cord level involved. The Beevor's sign (upward movement of the umbilicus with contraction of the abdominal muscles), showing integrity of the T9 and T10 motor roots as opposed to absence of the T11 and T12 roots, sometimes is of help in localization. If the sensory deficit is complete, it quite accurately indicates the location of the tumor, and if it is severe, the accompanying motor weakness may not be reversible.

Tumors of the conus medullaris and cauda equina are distinguished by early loss of bladder and bowel control with symmetrical saddle anesthesia. Pain occurs late in conus lesions, whereas cauda equina lesions produce pain early and sphincter involvement late. Extradural tumors of the conus in particular produce early bladder dysfunction. In contrast, intramedullary tumors of the conus may not directly involve the lower lumbosacral segments and may not affect sphincter control despite a rather extensive neurological disturbance.

SPECIAL DIAGNOSTIC TESTS

The special tests for diagnosis of spinal cord tumors are plain spinal roentgenograms, tomograms, spinal tap, myelography, spinal angiography, and total body scanning (computer-assisted tomography).

Roentgenography

The first special test performed for the diagnosis of spinal cord tumor should be the plain spine roentgenogram. The most common roentgenographic change caused by spinal cord tumors is widening of the interpeduncular distance, which is seen in both intramedullary and extramedullary tumors (Fig. 102–2). Other commonly seen bony changes are widening of neural foramina and scalloping of the vertebral bodies (Figs. 102–3 and 102–4). Intraspinal calcification is rarely seen on plain films but may be seen with the use of tomography. The loss of a pedicle and evidence of bone destruction or blastic changes of the vertebral body are quite common in malignant extradural lesions.

Lumbar Puncture

In the evaluation of a patient suspected of having a spinal cord tumor, a spinal tap should not be performed before myelography. A spinal tap may precipitate a cord

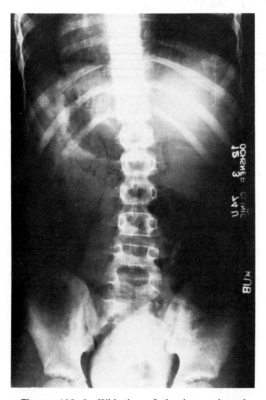

Figure 102–2 Widening of the interpeduncular distance.

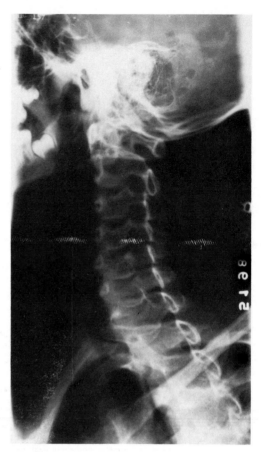

Figure 102–3 Enlargement of the neural foramina at C4–C5, as seen in nerve sheath tumors.

shift and incarceration requiring an emergency operative procedure before the lesion has been adequately localized. In addition, a spinal tap may cause a collapse of the subarachnoid space. In this situation, a second tap for myelography may be technically unsatisfactory because of subdural or epidural injection of the contrast agent. If the spinal tap is done before myelography, a Queckenstedt test should be performed to indicate whether a total block is present. If there is no block, then spinal fluid may be removed for analysis. Extremely high protein levels (as high as several grams) and xanthochromic fluid may be found if a tumor is present. When a cauda equina tumor is suspected and a satisfactory spinal puncture cannot be done in the lumbar area, a lateral C1–C2 spinal tap should be done and Pantopaque injected at this level. The spinal needle should be placed either below or above the suspected location of the lesion. If the patient has a total block, a

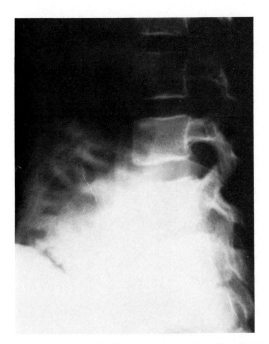

Figure 102–4   Scalloping of the bodies of the third and fourth lumbar vertebrae seen in ependymoma.

lateral C1 puncture can be done, and Pantopaque can be run down from above to demonstrate the top of the lesion and verify that there is no other lesion above the area of block. This information is particularly important in cases of von Recklinghausen's disease.

Myelography

Myelography is the most important special test in the diagnosis of spinal cord tumors. It indicates not only the level and size of the tumor when the subarachnoid space is not blocked, but also the lower border of the tumor and the need for immediate operation when a block is complete. For a myelogram of a patient suspected of having a spinal cord tumor, either the cervical or the lumbar route may be used. For the lumbar route the needle should be placed below the level of the lesion if that lesion is thought to lie within the cauda equina. If the lesion is thought to be higher, the needle is usually placed at the third lumbar interspace. The puncture is made, but no fluid is removed from the subarachnoid space until a Queckenstedt test has been performed. This test is performed by compressing both jugular veins. The test is neg-

ative when a rapid rise in pressure with compression is followed by a rapid fall in pressure with release. A rapid rise and a delayed fall may mean that the bevel of the needle is in a partially subarachnoid and partially subdural location. A positive result of the Queckenstedt test is either a very slow rise and fall or no rise of cerebrospinal fluid in the manometer. In this case, only 1 or 2 ml of contrast material is inserted. With the patient head-down, the canal is then fluoroscopically inspected until the block is visualized. If the block is complete, the needle is removed without removing a specimen of spinal fluid. At this point, it frequently is valuable to remove the needle and place the patient in a supine position. A lateral C1 subarachnoid puncture may be done and 1 or 2 ml of contrast material inserted in the cervical subarachnoid space. The contrast material is then run down to the top of the block to determine its extent and to rule out multiple lesions. If a complete block is present, the level of the block and the tumor should be marked either with a metal skin marker or by injecting a small amount of methylene blue dye in the spinous process at the level of the lesion. If the Queckenstedt test is negative, a specimen of spinal fluid may be taken for analysis for protein and cells before insertion of contrast material. Contrast material should be added in sufficient quantity to outline the tumor mass. After the fluoroscopic examination, the contrast material should be removed.

Extramedullary intradural tumors characteristically have an intradural convexity at the caudal end (Fig. 102–5). A crosstable lateral view will show the anterior-posterior relationship to the cord (Fig. 102–6). The exact position of an extramedullary intradural tumor is exceedingly important, since the spinal dura should never be opened in an area where pressure might displace the cord or cause herniation through the dural incision. If the tumor is laterally placed, the dura should be opened over the tumor. If the tumor is anteriorly placed, a proper approach is via a large lateral and anterior bony removal. On myelography, extradural lesions are usually distinguished by a paintbrush ending, tapering gradually on each side above and below the point of maximum encroachment (Fig. 102–7). If the extradural lesion produces a partial block, there is usually an hourglass type of

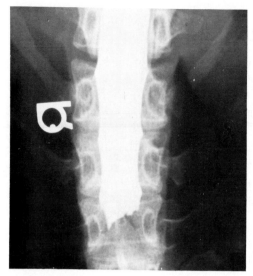

Figure 102–5 Crescent-shaped defect of a ventrally placed meningioma.

defect (Fig. 102–8). Intramedullary tumors usually do not cause spinal block but rather a fusiform enlargement of the spinal cord shadow (Fig. 102–9). Occasionally, centrally placed anterior extramedullary lesions may simulate intramedullary lesions by flattening the cord. This is particularly true of cervical spondylosis or anterior disc rupture.

Spinal Angiography

Spinal angiography has not been widely used for diagnosing spinal cord tumors, but it is particularly helpful in hemangioblastomas, arteriovenous malformations, and occasionally a meningioma (Fig. 102–10). It is also of help when a lesion occurs in an area where the major radicular arteries are expected. The location of the dominant radicular artery can be known preoperatively and its interruption during removal of a tumor can be avoided.

Radioisotope Scanning, Electromyography, and Computed Tomography

The use of radioisotope scanning and electromyography has been of little value in the diagnosis of spinal cord tumors. Total body scanning can provide a quite adequate

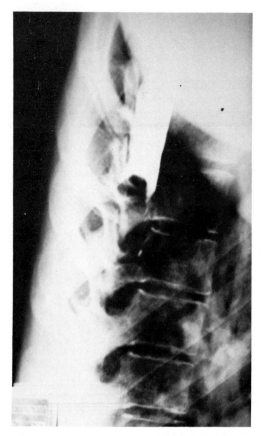

Figure 102–6 Capping of a dorsally placed nerve sheath tumor.

diagnosis if the lesion is calcified, but is usually of less help if the lesion is noncalcified. It is expensive and ordinarily will not be needed as a supplement to the tests already discussed. With the upgrading of the machines and matrices in the future, however, total body scanning will doubtless play an important role in the diagnosis of spinal cord tumors.

NEURILEMMOMAS AND NEUROFIBROMAS

Spinal neurilemmomas and neurofibromas are the most common spinal cord tumors (cf. Fig. 102–1A). They constitute 16 to 30 per cent of all spinal tumors in reported series.[17,24,37,45] Approximately 72 per cent are intradural and extramedullary, 14 per cent are extradural, 13 per cent are dumbbell, and 1 per cent are intramedullary.[45] They occur most frequently in the thoracic, next most frequently in the

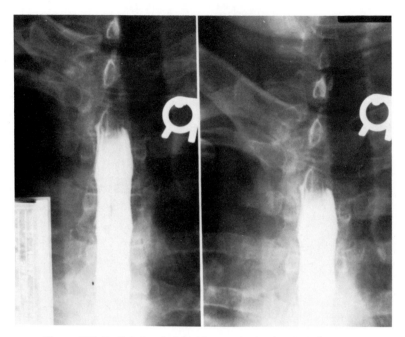

Figure 102–7 Paintbrush defect in an extradural metastatic cancer.

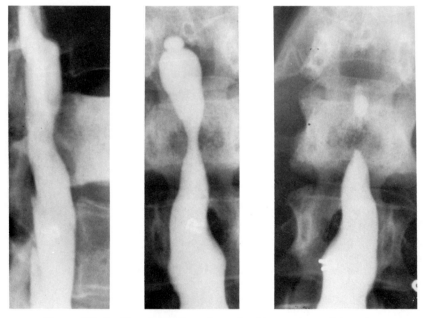

Figure 102–8 Hourglass defect of extradural hemangioma of the spine.

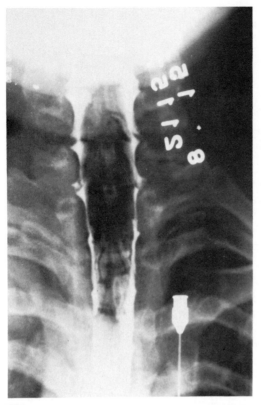

Figure 102–9   Fusiform defect in intramedullary ependymoma.

with the least neurological deficit before operation, but recovery has been reported in some cases of complete transsection syndromes. The operative mortality rate is reported as 0 to 7 per cent.[45] Radiation therapy is not indicated in these benign tumors.

MENINGIOMAS

Meningiomas are the second most common spinal cord tumor, making up approximately 22 per cent of all spinal cord tumors. They occur in women approximately 80 per cent of the time and predominantly affect patients in the fourth, fifth, and sixth decades of life. They may occur anywhere in

cervical, and least often in the lumbar segments. They have no particular sex predilection and occur primarily in the fourth and fifth decades. They commonly produce nerve root symptoms early and long tract signs later.

Neurilemmomas and neurofibromas of the spinal canal generally produce radiological changes. The diagnostic features on plain roentgenograms are widening of the interpeduncular distance in approximately half the cases and enlargement of the intervertebral foramen. They rarely calcify. When neurilemmomas extend as hourglass tumors, they may produce a typical and sharply defined soft tumor mass in the paraspinous position. Enlargement of the intervertebral foramina, however, may be a dysplastic sign of von Recklinghausen's disease of bone without the presence of a neurofibroma. On myelography neurilemmomas are revealed by spinal cord deviation and a capping defect in the contrast column (Fig. 102–11).

The treatment of neurilemmomas is total extirpation. The results are best in patients

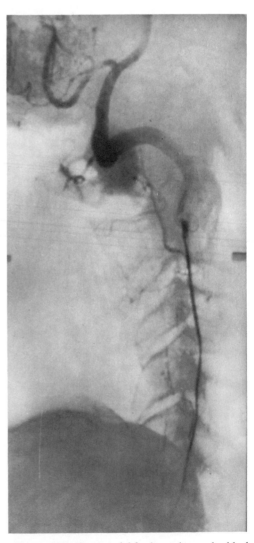

Figure 102–10   Arterial feeder and vascular blush of a C1 meningioma.

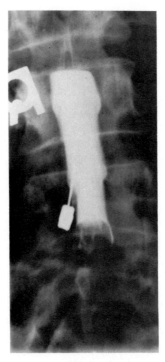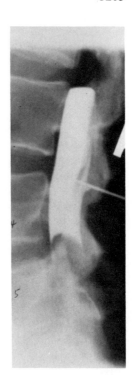

Figure 102–11 Capping defect of a cauda equina nerve sheath tumor.

the spinal canal, but approximately two thirds occur in the thoracic region. They frequently are attached to the insertion of the dentate ligament and extend dorsally or ventrally.

Spinal meningiomas rarely undergo malignant change. Melanotic meningiomas of the spinal cord are rare, and a recent review by Scott and co-workers suggests that these usually do not act as malignant tumors and that long-term survivals have been reported.[53] Most meningiomas are intradural and extramedullary; 15 per cent are extradural. Multiple meningiomas are rare but may be seen in von Recklinghausen's disease or in an occasional isolated occurrence. Meningiomas usually produce symptoms by first involving the motor long tracts.

On plain roentgenograms calcification or erosion of a pedicle or vertebral body is not commonly seen. Bony reaction is produced in approximately 30 per cent of the cases, but it may be difficult to visualize without tomograms. The myelographic picture is similar to that of neurilemmomas. A vascular stain may be seen on spinal angiography (see Fig. 102–10).

The treatment of spinal meningiomas is excision. The results are slightly less favorable than in removal of neurilemmomas but still are excellent. The operative mortality rates range from 0.9 to 12 per cent.[45] Radiation therapy and chemotherapy for benign meningiomas are not indicated.

EPENDYMOMAS

Ependymomas constitute roughly 13 per cent of all spinal cord tumors, with the cauda equina ependymoma being by far the most common type (see Fig. 102–1B). Of 169 cases of spinal ependymoma analyzed by Slooff and associates, 99 (56.5 per cent) were situated at the level of the cauda equina, and 70 (43.5 per cent) were totally intramedullary.[55] Spinal ependymomas show a predilection for the male sex and usually produce symptoms in the mid-thirties. The two most common initial symptoms are pain and weakness of a limb. The legs are far more commonly involved than the arms, and the pain may be local vertebral pain or a radicular type. Sphincter disturbances are particularly common in cauda equina ependymomas. Fincher's syndrome, the sudden onset of subarachnoid hemorrhage with acute sciatica, is a rare example of acute onset in cauda equina ependymomas and may be precipitated by pregnancy or by trauma.[21]

Ependymomas gave rise to bony alterations in the spine in 15 per cent of Slooff and co-workers' patients and in 36 per cent of those with intramedullary tumors reported by Guidetti and Fortuna.[30,55] An increase in interpeduncular distance was the most common and valuable sign, the next being scalloping of the bodies of the vertebrae. Calcification of an ependymoma is exceedingly rare. In intramedullary ependymomas, myelography demonstrates diffuse widening of the cord shadow over a number of vertebral levels (see Fig. 102–9). The combination of air and positive contrast will fail to show any cord collapse as seen in hydromyelia. Cauda equina ependymomas appear as loculated masses (Fig. 102–12).

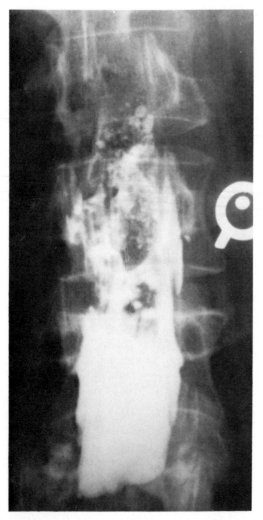

Figure 102–12 Multiloculated cauda equina ependymoma.

Total excision is the treatment of choice for ependymomas. Guidetti and Fortuna reported 20 cases of ependymomas with 16 total removals, 3 subtotal removals, and 1 myelotomy with biopsy.[30] Some ependymomas, particularly the giant ependymomas that penetrate dura, erode bone, and enter the soft tissue, are unresectable; with the use of an operative microscope and microbipolar coagulation, however, most ependymomas can be safely removed (cf. Fig. 102–5). Horrax and Henderson, in 1939, and Fischer and Tommasi, in 1976, have reported total removal of ependymomas extending from the medulla oblongata to the conus medullaris with good functional results.[22,34] Recent operative mortality rates range from 0 to 10.9 per cent.[22]

Most authors prefer not to irradiate tumors that apparently have been totally removed.[22,28,42,56] For subtotally removed tumors, particularly if they are histologically aggressive or malignant, radiation therapy is indicated. Intrathecal methotrexate may be helpful as an adjunct to radiation therapy for patients whose spinal fluid contains malignant cells.

ASTROCYTOMAS

Spinal astrocytomas are less common than ependymomas. Slooff and co-workers reported 86 astrocytomas among 291 gliomas of the cord (29.5 per cent).[55] Well-differentiated astrocytomas show a predilection for the male, whereas malignant astrocytomas and glioblastomas have an equal sex incidence. Microcysts or large syrinxes are associated with these tumors. The symptoms of astrocytomas, usually produced by involvement of long tracts, are commonly unilateral or bilateral paresis with dissociated sensory loss and sphincter disturbances in the thoracolumbar area.

The most common x-ray finding is widening of the interpeduncular distances over several segments, which is characteristic of all intramedullary lesions. Myelographic characteristics are the same as those of intramedullary ependymomas.

The classic treatment of astrocytomas of the cord has been bony decompression with aspiration of cysts and radiation therapy. This treatment was used because it was believed that these tumors were impossible to remove. Recently, however, Stein totally removed intramedullary astrocytomas in three cases, and in Malis' experience with 20 astrocytomas, two apparently complete removals were obtained.[42,56] At the present time, adequate statistics are not available for comparison of the results of subtotal removal with those of subtotal removal followed by radiation therapy, particularly in well-differentiated tumors. Drainage of tumor cysts may be accomplished percutaneously.[8,58]

METASTATIC TUMORS

Primary tumors are the most prevalent in patients under 50 years of age, while metastatic carcinomas are more prevalent in patients over 50 years of age. Metastatic tumors of the spinal cord usually occur in the 50- to 70-year age group and are more common in men than in women. The percentage of symptomatic spinal cord tumors that are metastatic is difficult to ascertain. Torma reported on 250 histologically verified malignant extradural tumors of the spinal cord and column.[57] He states that extradural malignant tumors constitute 20 to 30 per cent of all spinal tumors. In this series of 250 tumors, 170 (68 per cent) were metastatic, 40 (16 per cent) were diffuse lymphomas or myelomas, 24 (9.6 per cent)

were primary osteogenic sarcomas or chordomas, and 16 (6.4 per cent) were primary nonosteogenic tumors. In the author's practice, over half of all spinal cord tumors have been metastatic.

The most common metastatic tumors to the spine are from lung, breast, prostate, and kidney and from sarcomas and lymphomas (Table 102–2). They occur most frequently in the thoracic area. Of 127 metastatic spinal tumors reported by Chade, 59 were localized in the epidural space, 24 to the vertebral body, and 44 to the epidural space and vertebra; 5 were intradural, and 2 were intramedullary.[11] The clinical picture is a short history of root pain and localized back pain followed rapidly by progressive long-tract signs.

X-ray evidence frequently is present with both osteolytic and osteoblastic changes with or without pathological compression fractures. If the patient's primary tumor is known and he has not developed motor weakness, treatment is dexamethasone plus radiation therapy. If motor signs are present, then decompressive laminectomy followed by radiation therapy is the treatment of choice. Operative decompression usually is useless if paraplegia is complete, particularly if it has occurred over a very short period of time. Decompression is probably also contraindicated for patients who are in poor general condition with widespread metastases, particularly metas-

TABLE 102–2 METASTATIC TUMORS OF THE SPINE: TOTALS OF FOUR REPORTED SERIES

	WHITE ET AL* 1971	CHADE† 1968	AULD AND BUERMAN‡ 1966	VIETH AND ODOM§ 1965	TOTALS NUMBER	TOTALS PER CENT
Lung	31	27	16	14	88	17
Breast	37	23	2	15	77	16
Prostate	23	19	8	7	57	11
Kidney	13	25	5	5	48	9
Cancer of unknown site	9	16	8	11	44	8
Sarcoma	24	0	2	6	32	6
Lymphoma	27	0	3	0	30	6
Gastrointestinal tract	11	10	3	6	30	6
Thyroid	8	20	0	0	28	6
Melanoma	8	0	0	4	12	2
Others	26	18	10	10	64	13
					510	100

* White, W. A., Patterson, R. H., Jr., and Bergland, R. M.: Role of surgery in the treatment of spinal cord compression by metastatic neoplasm. Cancer, 27:558–561, 1971.
† Chade, H. O.: Metastasen der Wirbelsäule und des Rückenmarks. Schweitz. Arch. Neurol. Neurochir. Psychiat., 102:257–287, 1968.
‡ Auld, A. W., and Buerman, A.: Metastatic spinal epidural tumors. Arch. Neurol. (Chicago), 15:100–108, 1966.
§ Vieth, R. G., and Odom, G. L.: Extradural spinal metastases and their neurosurgical treatment. J. Neurosurg., 23:501–508, 1965.

tases involving the liver. The results of treatment of epidural metastatic cancer vary with the particular tumor type, the poorest being obtained when the primary tumors are lung cancer and melanoma and the best being obtained in the lymphomas. Good results are obtained with breast, kidney, and thyroid cancers.

SPINAL LIPOMAS

Ehni and Love stated that spinal lipomas account for 1 per cent of primary spinal tumors and that two fifths are extradural and three fifths, intradural.[15] These statistics have been supported by more recent reports.[25,50] The sexual incidence is equal.

In intradural spinal lipomas, the symptoms begin in the first 30 years of life, with the most usual onset being around puberty. Pregnancy and large weight gain may precipitate symptoms. The most common area of involvement is the thoracic spine, and the next most common, the cervical area. The tumors frequently extend over four or five segments of the cord, usually lie in the pia, and cavitate the posterior column, being juxtamedullary but subpial. Occasionally they may be multiple and may be associated with other tumors such as dermoids and teratomas. They are frequently associated with bony abnormalities of the spine, particularly spina bifida occulta, and with subcutaneous lipomas at the same level (Fig. 102–13). The treatment is operative decompression in which the pia over the tumor is split and the tumor is subtotally removed. Some total removals have been performed, but because of the fibrous adhesions between the mass and the cord, there is usually little or no dissection plane and attempts at removal may produce further cord injury. After operation, the patient's total body fat should be reduced and an optimal body weight maintained. Even with subtotal removal, long symptom-free survival is common, the longest reported being 33 years.[55]

Extradural lipomas affect primarily the middle and lower thoracic segments. The highest peak of onset is in the forties, and the history of symptoms is usually short. These tumors adhere loosely to the dura and frequently can be removed, but they may be angiolipomas or fibrolipomas. They have no characteristic x-ray appearance.

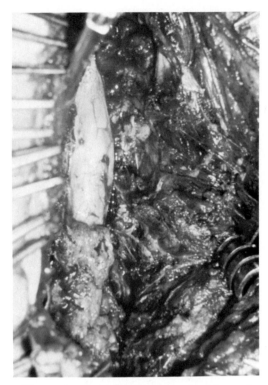

Figure 102–13 Epidural and intradural lipoma involving the cauda equina and conus.

HEMANGIOBLASTOMAS

Hemangioblastomas make up approximately 1 per cent of spinal cord tumors. There is no sex preference. Symptoms usually begin in the thirties. They are most often single and most frequently located in the cervicothoracic cord. Sixty per cent of them are intramedullary. Syringomyelia is associated in two thirds of cases, and Lindau's disease is present in one third. On myelography, meningeal varicosities are seen in 48 per cent of the cases, and spinal angiography is diagnostic (Fig. 102–14). The treatment is total removal. Total excision is usually possible without increasing the neural deficit if the operative microscope and microsurgical techniques are used. It is important, however, not to enter these lesions but rather to work about their periphery.

DERMOIDS, EPIDERMOIDS, AND TERATOMAS

These tumors make up 1 to 2 per cent of all spinal cord tumors and are of congenital

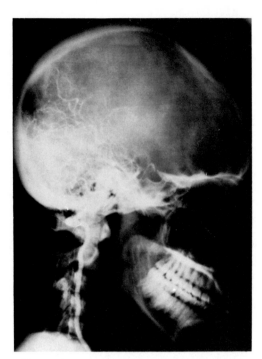

Figure 102–14 Intramedullary vascular blush of a hemangioblastoma at C3.

origin. They occur predominantly in the lumbosacral area, involving the conus and cauda equina; they may, however, occur anywhere in the spinal canal (Fig. 102–15). They are usually associated with other congenital defects; spina bifida and dermal sinus tracts are the most common associated lesions, but hypertrichosis, skin pigmentation, and cutaneous angiomas are also found.

The treatment of these tumors is operative, optimal therapy being total resection. Because they usually adhere firmly to the cauda equina and to the conus, total removal frequently is not possible without producing severe neurological damage. It is extremely important to protect against spillage of the contents of these tumor cysts to prevent chemical arachnoiditis. If the capsule of the cyst is thin, the complete contents should be evacuated through a small needle into a syringe before total excision rather than risking entering the cyst and spilling the contents. Even subtotal resection, however, will arrest progression of neurological deficits for many years. If the symptoms progress, reoperation is indicated. Teratomas, particularly those in the sacrococcygeal region, have a predisposition to malignant change. Therefore, ther-

apy of teratomas is frequently operation plus radiation therapy and chemotherapy.

CHORDOMAS

Chordomas have been said to make up approximately 1 per cent of spinal cord tumors.[55] They are most common in the sacrococcygeal area (approximately half the tumors). The second most frequently affected region is the cervical area, particularly near the atlas and axis. Approximately one third occur in the base of the skull, and the remainder in other areas of the spine.

These tumors usually produce localized back pain; root irritation and cord compression occur late and develop slowly. Men are affected twice as often as women. Roentgenograms of the spine usually show both destruction of bone with sparing of the bony cortex and new bone formation.

The chordoma is a slow, progressive, malignant growth, and the treatment of choice is total removal. This is usually not obtainable because of the large size of the lesion before diagnosis and because of the difficulty of achieving a complete resection.

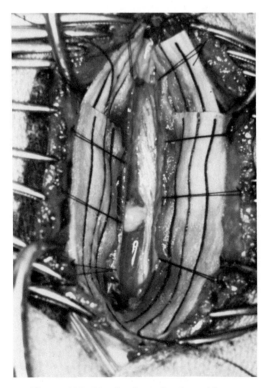

Figure 102–15 Cauda equina dermoid cyst.

No documented case of cure of chordoma has been reported. Many patients have gone five years tumor-free, only to have recurrence of tumor. Apparently cured chordomas should be considered to be in a stationary phase, not cured.

A transoral or anterior cervical approach gives the best access to tumors at the C1 and C2 level. An attempt at total resection of the involved bone with associated anterior or posterior fusion is the treatment of choice. Frequently, radiation therapy also will be required.

Sacrococcygeal chordomas are best reached via a combined posterior neurosurgical and anterior colorectal approach. Total resection of the tumor is desirable. If total removal of a chordoma is to be accomplished, an en bloc resection of the lesion is necessary so that normal tissue margins are present. The en bloc resection frequently requires the total removal of one or two vertebral bodies and the insertion of a long strut interbody graft for stability. Grafting is not necessary, however, at the sacral level. Although chordomas rarely metastasize, distant metastases have occurred, particularly after operative intervention.

OPERATIVE TREATMENT OF SPINAL CORD TUMORS

Prognosis

The morphological and histological characteristics and the location of the tumor, and rate of progression of symptoms are the factors that determine whether or not operative treatment will be successful. When progression of symptoms is slow, even when paresis is complete or nearly complete, recovery can be expected after careful removal of the tumor. When progression of symptoms is rapid, either early or late in the course of the disease, emergency decompression is necessary to prevent permanent neurological deficit. If paralysis is nearly complete only 24 hours after it began, a significant degree of improvement following operation is unlikely. If paralysis is acute and has been complete for 24 to 48 hours, the chance of recovery is nil. By contrast, paralysis that develops slowly over several weeks may be 75 per cent complete, and yet a complete recovery can

be obtained. Recovery is most dramatic when long-tract signs are predominant, but not so with anterior horn cell loss.[27]

Intramedullary Tumors

Successful operation on intramedullary tumors is dependent upon the histological type and the extent of the lesion, optical magnification, good illumination, and microinstrumentation and coagulation.

For operations on tumors involving the cervical spinal cord, the sitting position offers technical advantages. The safety of the sitting position can be improved with Doppler ultrasonic monitoring of the heart sounds, a right atrial catheter, a pressure suit, positive-pressure ventilation, and intra-arterial pressure monitoring to help in the detection and treatment of air embolism. The prone position is used for dealing with thoracic and lumbar lesions.

The bony decompression should be made beyond the margins of the lesion both cephalad and caudad (Fig. 102–16). During the extradural portion of the operation hemostasis should be excellent so that the intradural portion is not hampered by blood

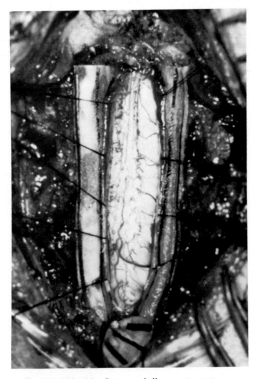

Figure 102–16　Intramedullary astrocytoma.

staining the field. A myelotomy of the full extent of the lesion should be made in the thinnest area of the dorsal cord. Care should be taken to stay away from the dorsal root entry zone. If the tumor is associated with a cyst or hematoma cavity, the cyst should be only partially decompressed so that the partially filled cyst may be used to develop a cleavage plane between the tumor and the surrounding cord.

For removal of intramedullary tumors, the binocular operative microscope is superior to optical loupes (Fig. 102–17). The size of the patient and the depth of the wound will dictate the focal length of the objective used. In the cervical area, a 250-mm lens is usually adequate; however, in the thoracic and lumbar areas, frequently a 300-mm, and sometimes a 400-mm, lens will be necessary. Five- to ten-power magnification is usually used. The use of a diploscope or a scope with a binocular side arm is advantageous because it allows the assistant to be of greater help.

Ependymomas frequently have a thin pseudocapsule. It is important to try to save the capsule because the chances of finding a correct plane of dissection are re-duced if the tumor itself is entered directly. Sometimes the dissection plane will be difficult to develop at one end of the tumor but easy at the other; the surgeon should work from the easiest dissection plane first. When the tumor is gently lifted from the cord, the small ventral feeding vessels are stretched, then coagulated, and divided with microscissors. If, when either ependymomas or astrocytomas are dissected, there is no identifiable cleavage plane between tumor and cord, a subtotal removal will be necessary. The concept of total removal at any cost is dangerous and should be condemned. Again, if the dissection plane cannot be maintained, a subtotal removal should be performed. If the tumor has been totally removed, the dura should be closed. If, however, there is any question of inadequate decompression, then the dura should be left open with a piece of Gelfoam covering the dural defect. The use of dural substitutes complicates the procedure, but adds little to the amount of arachnoiditis present if one has to reoperate.

Dexamethasone has proved helpful in reducing operative complications. It should be started before the operation and continued for approximately five to seven days afterward.

Intradural Extramedullary Tumors

Removal of intradural extramedullary tumors is often most rewarding. Operations to remove these tumors have been facilitated by the operative microscope with its excellent light source as well as microinstrumentation and coagulation. Optical loupes, however, are adequate in most cases. The focal length of the objective is determined by the depth of the wound. Magnification used is usually in the 5-power range.

Neurilemmomas usually are easily removed because they are located, for the most part, on the dorsal root, displacing the cord laterally and slightly ventrally (Fig. 102–18). The tumor is easily approached by dividing the nerve root or rootlets to which it is attached and then using traction on the tumor to draw it away from the cord. The adhesions between the tumor and cord are divided by sharp dissection. If a large radicular artery is associated with the root, care is taken to preserve the artery.

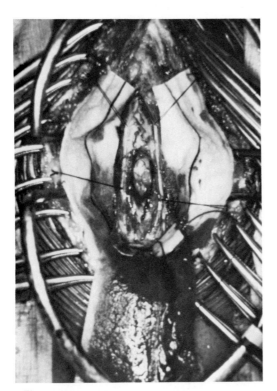

Figure 102–17 Postremoval of intramedullary hemangioblastoma.

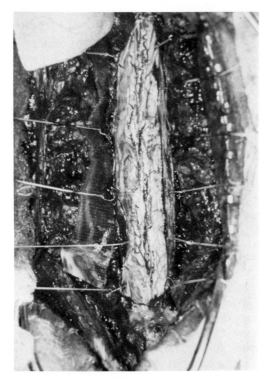

Figure 102–18 Lateral and ventral displacement of the cord by a nerve sheath tumor.

The intradural portion of a dumbbell neurilemmoma that is both extra- and intradural should be removed first to prevent inadvertent injury to the cord. If a transthoracic removal of the extradural tumor is necessary, the dural defect in the root sleeve is repaired to prevent a cerebrospinal fluid pleural fistula from forming. Following the total removal of neurilemmomas, the dura is easily closed.

In operating upon meningiomas, one must remove the entire dural attachment of the tumor to avoid recurrence. There is a high risk of recurrence when electrocautery is used to coagulate the point of attachment. Dorsal and dorsolateral meningiomas are usually quite easy to remove (like the neurilemmomas); however, anterior and anterolateral tumors are more difficult. Wide lateral bone removal, to the point of costotransversectomy, is necessary to remove some anterior lesions. Care should be taken to avoid compression or trauma to the cord. Anterior lesions frequently require division of one or more nerve roots and dentate ligaments at the level of and above and below the tumor to provide adequate room for removal. These ventral tumors are best removed in a piecemeal fashion by using sharp dissection, suction, and microbipolar coagulation. Following the piecemeal removal of the tumor, the dural attachment should be removed with a relatively generous fragment of normal-appearing dural cuff. Dural defects can be repaired with lumbodorsal fascia, and ventral defects that cannot be sewed may be closed by simply inserting a piece of fascia or a small thin layer of Gelfoam between the cord and the bone.

Extradural Spinal Cord Tumors

The commonest extradural tumor of the spine is metastatic cancer. The essentials of operation for epidural tumors are decompression of the cord in the metastatic tumors and gross total removal of those tumors that are not metastatic. The use of bipolar coagulation is a great help, since frequently these tumors are extremely vascular. Adequate decompression may produce vertebral instability, which may be corrected by anterior or posterior bone grafts or a combination of both. Acrylic struts and Harrington rods are also valuable in unstability problems.

RADIATION THERAPY

Radiation therapy has been used primarily in the treatment of intramedullary gliomas, extradural metastatic carcinomas, and other malignant tumors. A good statistical analysis of the effect of radiation therapy on the various gliomas affecting the spinal cord is not available. Most authors seem to believe that, if an ependymoma or an astrocytoma has been totally removed, irradiation should not be given. In the case of partially removed tumors, particularly the well-differentiated astrocytomas and ependymomas, some groups simply watch the patient, and if there is recurrence, reoperate and remove more tumor. Others use postoperative irradiation after subtotal removal of these tumors. This second course appears to be logical, since in the brain these tumors have been shown to be radiosensitive, and if radiation therapy is to be most effective, it should be applied when the tumor population is smallest. Using supervoltage irradiation, either with cobalt or

SPINAL CORD TUMORS IN ADULTS

SPINAL CORD TUMORS IN ADULTS 3213

with linear accelerator, treatment is usually given in a tumor dose of 4500 to 5000 rads over a period of five to six weeks.

CHEMOTHERAPY

At the present time, the use of chemotherapy for spinal cord tumors should be considered experimental. The one exception is the intradural implant for lymphoma, medulloblastoma, and ependymoma, in which intrathecal methotrexate, 0.5 mg per kilogram, not exceeding a total dose of 25 mg, is of value.

REFERENCES

ibliography
1. Arendt, A.: Ependymoma. In Vinken, P. J., and Bruyn, G. W., eds.: Handbook of Clinical Neurology. Vol. 20. Amsterdam, North Holland Publishing Co.; New York, American Elsevier Co., Inc., 1976, pp. 323–352.
2. Ariel, I. M., and Verdu, C.: Chordoma: An analysis of twenty cases treated over a twenty-year span. J. Surg. Oncol., 7:27–44, 1975.
3. Arseni, C., and Maretsis, M.: Tumors of the lower spinal cord associated with increased intracranial pressure and papilledema. J. Neurosurg., 27:105–110, 1967.
4. Bailey, I. C.: Dermoid tumors of the spinal cord. J. Neurosurg., 33:676–681, 1970.
5. Barone, B. M., and Elvidge, A. R.: Ependymomas. A clinical survey. J. Neurosurg. 33:428–438, 1970.
6. Bouchard, J.: Role of radiation therapy in the management of spinal cord and other lesions. In Radiation Therapy of Tumors and Diseases of the Nervous System. Philadelphia, Lea & Febiger, 1966, pp. 207–217.
7. Bouchard, J.: Radiation Therapy of Tumors and Diseases of the Nervous System. Philadelphia, Lea & Febiger, 1966.
8. Booth, A. E., and Kendall, B. E.: Percutaneous aspiration of cystic lesions of the spinal cord. J. Neurosurg., 33:140–144, 1970.
9. Browne, T. R., Adams, R. D., and Roberson, G. H.: Hemangioblastoma of the spinal cord: review and report of five cases. Arch. Neurol. (Chicago), 33:435–441, 1976.
10. Calogero, J. A., and Moossy, J.: Extradural spinal meningiomas: Report of four cases. J. Neurosurg., 37:442–447, 1972.
11. Chade, H. O.: Metastatic tumours of the spine and spinal cord. In Vinken, P. J., and Bruyn, G. W., eds.: Handbook of Clinical Neurology. Vol. 20. Amsterdam, North Holland Publishing Co.; New York, American Elsevier Co., Inc., 1976, pp. 415–434.
12. Crosby, E. C., Humphrey, T., and Tauer, E. W.: Correlative Anatomy of The Nervous System. New York, Macmillan Publishing Co., 1962.
13. Dandy, W. E.: The diagnosis and localization of spinal cord tumors. Ann. Surg., 81:223–254, 1925.
14. Dhermain, P. M.: Place de la radiothérapie dans le traitement des tumeurs médullaires intradurales et extra-durales. Société Francaise de Radiologie Médicale 52–62 Nov. 1969.
15. Ehni, G., and Love, J. G.: Intraspinal lipomas: Report of cases; review of the literature and clinical and pathological study. Arch. Neurol. Psychiat., 53:1–28, 1945.
16. Elsberg, C. A.: Some aspects of the diagnosis and surgical treatment of tumors of the spinal cord, with a study of the end results in a series of 119 operations. Ann. Surg., 81:1057–1073, 1925.
17. Elsberg, C. A.: Surgical Diseases of the Spinal Cord, Membranes and Nerve Roots: Symptoms, Diagnosis and Treatment. New York, Paul B. Hoeber, 1941.
18. Epstein, B. S., Epstein, J. A., and Postel, D. M.: Tumors of spinal cord simulating psychiatric disorders. Dis. Nerv. Syst., 32:741–743, 1971.
19. Fager, C. A.: Indications for neurosurgical intervention in metastatic lesions of the central nervous system. Med. Clin. N. Amer., 59:487–494, 1975.
20. Farmilo, R. W., McAuley, D. L., and Osborne, D. R. S.: Papilloedema and spinal cord tumours. New Zeal. Med. J., 80:100–104, 1974.
21. Fincher, E. F.: Spontaneous subarachnoid hemorrhage in intradural tumors of the lumbar sac: A clinical syndrome. J. Neurosurg., 8:576–584, 1951.
22. Fischer, G., and Tommasi, M.: Spinal ependymomas. In Vinken, P. J., and Bruyn, G. W., eds.: Handbook of Clinical Neurology. Vol. 20. Amsterdam, North Holland Publishing Co.; New York, American Elsevier Co., 1976, pp. 353–388.
23. Fornasier, V. L., and Horne, J. G.: Metastases to the vertebral column. Cancer, 36:590–594, 1975.
24. Gautier-Smith, P. C.: Clinical aspects of spinal neurofibromas. Brain, 90:359–394, 1967.
25. Giuffre, R.: Spinal lipomas. In Vinken, P. J., and Bruyn, G. W., eds.: Handbook of Clinical Neurology. Vol. 20. Amsterdam, North Holland Publishing Co.; New York, American Elsevier Co., Inc., 1976, pp. 389–414.
26. Greenwood, J. Jr.: Surgical removal of intramedullary tumors. J. Neurosurg., 26:276–282, 1967.
27. Greenwood, J., Jr.: Spinal cord tumors. In Youmans, J. R., ed.: Neurological Surgery. Vol. 3. Philadelphia-London-Toronto, W. B. Saunders Co., 1973, pp. 1514–1534.
28. Greenwood, J., Jr.: Personal communication, 1976.
29. Guidetti, B.: Intramedullary tumours of the spinal cord. Acta Neurochir. (Wien), 17:7–23, 1967.
30. Guidetti, B., and Fortuna, A.: Surgical treatment of intramedullary hemangioblastoma of the spinal cord. J. Neurosurg., 27:530–540, 1967.
31. Guomundsson, K. R.: A survey of tumours of the central nervous system in Iceland during the 10-year period 1954–1963. Acta Neurol. Scand., 46:538–552, 1970.
32. Hall, A. J., and Mackay, N. N. S.: The results of laminectomy for compression of the cord or cauda equina by extradural malignant tumour. J. Bone Joint Surg., 55-B:497–505, 1973.
33. Horcajada, J., and Salah, S.: Zur Klinik und

Therapie der spinalen Meningeome. Erfohrungen mit 83 Fällen. Acta Neurochir. (Wien), 28:291–304, 1973.

34. Horrax, G., and Henderson, D. G.: Encapsulated intramedullary tumor involving the whole spinal cord from medulla to conus. Complete enucleation with recovery. Surg. Gynec. Obstet., 68:814–819, 1939.

35. Horsley, V., and Gowers, W. R.: A case of tumour of the spinal cord. Trans. Roy. Med. Chir. Soc. Glasg., 70:377, 1888.

36. Hurth, M.: Les hemangioblastomes intrarachidiens. Neurochirurgie, 21:suppl. 1:1–136, 1975.

37. Iraci, G., Peserico, L., and Salar, G.: Intraspinal neurinomas and meningiomas. A clinical survey of 172 cases. Int. Surg., 56:289–303, 1971.

38. Kurland, L. T.: The frequency of intracranial and intraspinal neoplasms in the resident population of Rochester, Minnesota. J. Neurosurg., 15:627–641, 1958.

39. Kurze, T.: Microtechniques in neurological surgery. Clin. Neurosurg., 11:128–137, 1964.

40. Lazorthes, G., Gouaze, A., Zader, J. O., Santini, J. J., Lazorthes, Y., and Burdin, P.: Arterial vascularization of the spinal cord: Recent studies of the anastomotic substitution pathways. J. Neurosurg., 35:253–262, 1971.

41. Malis, L. T.: Bipolar coagulation in microsurgery. In Donaghy, R. M. P., and Yasargil, M. G. eds.: Conference on Micro-Vascular Surgery, Stuttgart, 1967. St. Louis, C. V. Mosby Co., 1967, pp. 126–129.

42. Malis, L. T.: Personal communication, 1976.

43. Marsa, G. W., Goffinet, D. R., Rubinstein, L. J., and Bagshaw, M. A.: Megavoltage irradiation in the treatment of gliomas of the brain and spinal cord. Cancer, 36:1681–1689, 1975.

44. Maurice-Williams, R. S., and Lucey, J. J.: Raised intracranial pressure due to spinal tumours: 3 rare cases with a probable common mechanism. Brit. J. Surg., 62:92–95, 1975.

45. Nittner, K.: Spinal meningiomas, neurinomas, and neurofibromas and hourglass tumours. In Vinken, P. J., and Bruyn, B. W., eds.: Handbook of Clinical Neurology. Vol. 20. Amsterdam, North Holland Publishing Co.; New York, American Elsevier Co., Inc., 1976, pp. 177–322.

46. Paillas, J. E., Alliez, B., and Pellet, W.: Primary and secondary tumours of the spine. In Vinken, P. J., and Bruyn, G. W., eds.: Handbook of Clinical Neurology. Vol. 20. Amsterdam, North Holland Publishing Co.; New York, American Elsevier Co., Inc., 1976, pp. 19–54.

47. Pool, J. L.: The Surgery of spinal cord tumors. Clin. Neurosurg., 17:310–330, 1969.

48. Puito, R. S., Lui, J. P., Firooznia, H., and Lefleur, R. S.: The osseous and angiographic features of vertebral chordomas. Neuroradiology, 9:231–241, 1975.

49. Rand, R. W.: Microneurosurgery. St. Louis, C. V. Mosby Co., 1969.

50. Rogers, H. M., Long, D. M., Chou, S. N., and French, L. A.: Lipomas of the spinal cord and cauda equina. J. Neurosurg., 34:349–354, 1971.

51. Runnels, J. B., and Hanbery, J. W.: Spontaneous subarachnoid hemorrhage associated with spinal cord tumor. J. Neurosurg., 40:252–254, 1974.

52. Salah, S., Horcajada, J., and Perneczky, A.: Spinal neurinomas–a comprehensive clinical and statistical study of 47 cases. Neurochirurgia (Stuttgart), 18:77–84, 1975.

53. Scott, M., Ferrara, V. L., and Peale, A. R.: Multiple melanotic meningiomas of the cervical cord. J. Neurosurg., 34:555–559, 1971.

54. Sicard, J. A., and Forestier, J.: Méthode radiographique d'exploration de la cavité épidurale par le lipiodol. Rev. Neurol. (Paris), 28:1264. 1921.

55. Slooff, J. L., Kernahera, J. W., and MacCarty, C. S.: Primary Intramedullary Tumors of the Spinal Cord and Filum Terminale. Philadelphia and London, W. B. Saunders Co., 1964.

56. Stein, B. M.: Personal communication, 1976.

57. Torma, T.: Malignant tumors of the spine and spinal extradural space. Acta Surg. Scand., suppl. 225:1–176, 1957.

58. Westberg, G.: Gas myelography and percutaneous puncture in the diagnosis of spinal cord cysts. Acta Radiol. [Diagn.] (Stockholm), suppl. 252:7–67, 1966.

59. Wood, E. H., Berue, A. S., and Taveros, J. M.: The value of radiation therapy in the management of intrinsic tumors of the spinal cord. Radiology, 63:11–24, 1954.

60. Yasargil, M. G.: Microsurgery Applied to Neurosurgery. Stuttgart, Georg Thieme, 1969.

103

SPINAL CORD
TUMORS IN CHILDREN

Physicians who deal with the neurological problems of infancy and childhood work in an environment in which many things are not what they appear to be. This may be owing to the difficulty in communication with patients, even those who have learned to talk, who have difficulty in relating to the descriptive terms of adult life. Fear of illness, of pain, and even of death, in children as young as 3 to 4 years, will make the pediatric patient falsify or deny symptoms, and as a result, the diagnosis and treatment of disease of the central nervous system in the young requires patience, wisdom, and good detective instincts.

This chapter is based on experience with 80 spinal cord tumors occurring in a pediatric age group. Many authors have stated that the ratio of spinal cord tumors to brain tumors is 1:5 or even 1:20.[2-4,6,7,9] The 80 spinal cord tumors in this series were seen during an interval in which there were approximately 827 tumors of the brain treated at the same institution. Thus, the ratio of spinal cord to brain tumors is approximately 1:10.

In order to simplify discussion, the tumors have been classified into five major categories: congenital, or developmental, tumors; intrinsic, or primary, spinal cord tumors; blood-borne metastases; cerebrospinal fluid–borne metastases; and tumors compressing by direct extension.

INCIDENCE

In the author's series of 80 patients, there were 51 males and 29 females. The sex incidence is approximately the same as that for intracranial neoplasms.

As seen in Table 103–1, the preponderance of males to females is conspicuous in congenital tumors and in those tumors producing compression by direct extension. In the other three categories, there was no significant sexual predelection.

The greatest number of cases occurred between the ages of 1 and 3 years, and this also would fit with the large number of congenital tumors whose appearance is heralded only by either failure of the patient to achieve significant milestones in ambulation and control of bladder and bowel, or by regression of already acquired achievement levels (Fig. 103–1). Prior to 1 year of age, it is difficult to detect subtle changes in spinal cord function.

Figure 103–2 serves to illustrate the position, not only in segmental level but also in cross section according to diagnosis. The random scattering of mass lesions from the medullary-cervical junction to the sacral level and from the extradural space to the intramedullary area is peculiar to this age group.

SYMPTOMS

The development of symptoms in the majority of cases was slow and subtle, and the disease often was undetected over long periods of time. Most of the patients had symptoms lasting at least three months before definitive diagnosis was made, many had them for 9 and 12 months before they suggested a working diagnosis, and a small group had symptoms for more than a year prior to medical treatment (Table 103–2).

The number and variety of erroneous first diagnoses clearly illustrate the difficul-

---

E. B. HENDRICK

**TABLE 103–1 SEX INCIDENCE
IN RELATION TO TUMOR TYPE**

CLINICAL CLASSIFICATION	MALE	FEMALE
Congenital tumors	17	7
Intrinsic cord tumors	8	6
Blood-borne metastases	5	6
Cerebrospinal fluid–borne metastases	8	4
Tumors compressing by direct extension	12	6
Total	51	29

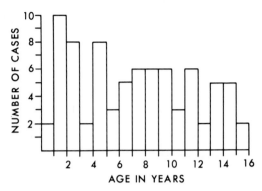

Figure 103–1 Age incidence of intraspinal tumors (number of cases per year of age).

ties of clinical assessment in a pediatric age group. In approximately one third of the patients, a diagnosis was made initially that was entirely out of keeping with the symptoms and signs, and led to a confused clinical diagnostic and therapeutic course (Table 103–3).

Regardless of the ultimate pathological diagnosis or the final anatomical location of the lesion, the most common symptom in

these children was weakness of the lower extremities and trunk (Fig. 103–3). Next in frequency were complaints of back pain of a diffuse nature and of root pain. Bladder and bowel symptoms predominated in the younger age group, and complaints sugges-

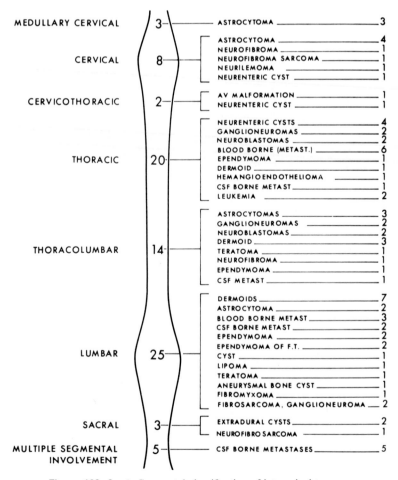

A

Figure 103–2 *A*. Segmental classification of intraspinal tumors.

Illustration continued on opposite page

TABLE 103-2 DURATION OF INITIAL SYMPTOMS PRIOR TO DEFINITIVE DIAGNOSIS

MONTHS	NUMBER OF PATIENTS
0 to 3	36
3 to 6	5
6 to 9	12
9 to 12	20
12 plus	7

TABLE 103-3 ERRONEOUS FIRST DIAGNOSES

Guillain-Barré-syndrome (2)
Amyotonia congenita (2)
Idiopathic scoliosis (2)
Manipulation by chiropractor (2)
Cerebral palsy
Parasagittal lesion
Scheuermann's disease
Hemiagenesis of sacrum
Poliomyelitis
Functional disorder
Hip disease
Subarachnoid hemorrhage
Muscle spasm
Friedreich's ataxia
Cerebral atrophy
Sciatic neuritis
Froin's syndrome
Dwarfism
Fecal impaction
Anal stenosis
Encephalopathy
Demyelinating disorder
Communicating hydrocephalus

tive of general malaise confused the picture in at least 25 per cent of the patients.

The abnormalities detected on physical examination, however, suggested in more than 75 per cent of the cases that the central nervous system and, in particular, the spinal cord was involved (Fig. 103–4). Hyporeflexia or hyperreflexia, motor weakness, and sensory disturbance accompanied by muscle wasting, sphincter involvement, and local tenderness of the spine as well as spinal postural deformity predominated and were present in almost every case. Three patients with diffuse intradural tumor breakdown presented with meningitis, and two with secondary tumors presented with papilledema. This, however, was most unusual.

The five pathological categories into which spinal cord masses have been divided notwithstanding, it is obvious on consideration of the symptoms and signs that any spinal mass, congenital or neoplastic, can be responsible for any or all of the diagnostic clues. One, therefore, cannot distin-

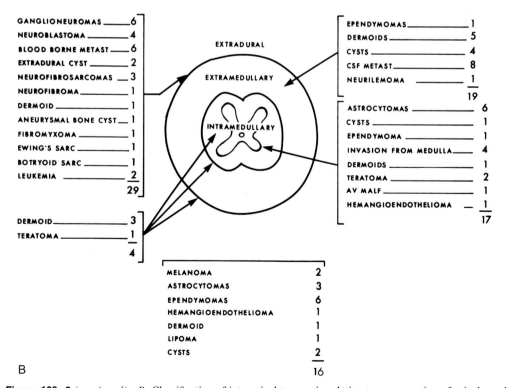

Figure 103–2 (*continued*) B. Classification of intraspinal tumors in relation to cross section of spinal canal.

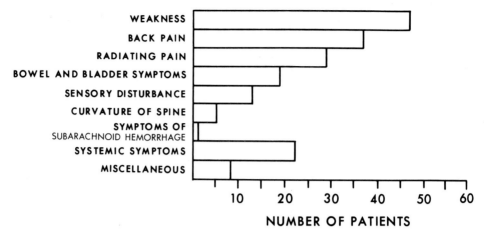

Figure 103–3   Symptoms of intraspinal tumor. Muscle weakness, usually of lower extremities, and back pain suggest a spinal lesion in the pediatric patient.

guish between the various categories of neoplasia or mass lesion on the basis of signs and symptoms alone.

Congenital tumors are often suggested by the cutaneous stigmata that may be present. These include the subcutaneous lipoma, the abnormal hairy patch in the midline, capillary hemangiomas, sacral dimples or sinus tracts, and unusual skin pigmentation such as café-au-lait spots. While the presence of these cutaneous manifestations does suggest an underlying spina bifida and possible congenital abnormality, many of the intraspinal lesions of a congenital nature were at locations far distant from the cutaneous stigmata, and indeed, many existed in patients with no skin manifestations.

INVESTIGATION

Careful and complete x-ray examination of the spine is the single most effective and most easily performed diagnostic procedure after the clinical examination (Table 103–4). Plain roentgenograms showed the tumor in 55 cases (69 per cent). Abnormalities seen on the plain x-ray varied from spina bifida at or adjacent to the level of the lesion to erosion of the pedicles over one or two segments and widening of the spinal canal that indicated the presence of a longstanding space-occupying lesion. In other studies, enlargement of the vertebral foramina with erosion of pedicles at one level suggested extension into the extradural space from an extradural lesion in the ret-

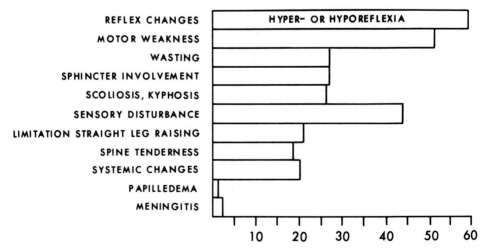

Figure 103–4   Clinical signs of spinal tumor. Changes in power, sensation, and reflexes predominate.

TABLE 103–4 RADIOGRAPHIC INVESTIGATION OF SPINAL CORD TUMORS IN CHILDREN

PLAIN ROENTGENOGRAMS
Positive	55	
Negative	14	
	12	Cerebrospinal fluid–borne metastases
	1	Ependymoma
	1	Dermoid
Unknown	10	

MYELOGRAMS (LUMBAR, CISTERNAL)
Positive	63	
Negative	0	
Not done	14	
	6	Cerebrospinal fluid–borne metastases
	1	Presence of meningitis
	1	Infected dermoid
	1	Dermoid
	4	Not necessary
	1	Cyst—neglect

rothoracic or retroperitoneal area. Erosion of the bodies of the vertebrae was an unusual and rather unreliable diagnostic sign.

Myelography, initially performed with the standard method using iophendylate and more recently with metrizamide, and computed tomography demonstrated the tumor in all patients on whom they were performed. The myelogram is the definitive investigation in spinal cord tumors and is essential to satisfactory operative treatment of these lesions. The levels of the intraspinal neoplasms and their extent can only be determined in this manner.

OPERATIVE TREATMENT

The obvious treatment of intraspinal mass lesions is laminectomy and meticulous excision, aided more recently by the use of the operative microscope. Operative procedures in the very young, particularly the infant, cannot be performed with the same elan, or perhaps careless disregard for the future, with which they might be undertaken in an adult patient. Extensive and radical removal of the neural arches with lateral involvement of the articular facets will produce crippling kyphosis and scoliosis as the child grows. Indeed, if it is superimposed on an already unstable spinal musculature, marked damage can result. Many of these patients will need Harrington or Dwyer reconstructive procedures.

Spinal cord operations in the pediatric age group are most easily and satisfactorily

performed with the patient in the prone position on a well-upholstered operative frame that produces support at the iliac crest and lower part of the pelvis and across the shoulders, allowing the abdomen and lower part of the chest to hang free. Small infants are mainly abdominal breathers, and compression of the abdomen during an operation results in increased bleeding in the operative site and some not inconsiderable difficulty with anesthesia. The need for meticulous hemostasis becomes obvious when dealing with small patients whose proportional blood loss, compared with an adult's, is of great importance.

The techniques for removal of mass lesions, either extradural, intradural, extramedullary, or intramedullary, are not different from those described by other authors for dealing with spinal cord tumors in general.

Postoperatively, children recover from their systemic disabilities more rapidly than adults, although the recovery from neurological deficits does not seem to vary from age group to age group.

Continual and close follow-up should be done postoperatively on all pediatric patients with intraspinal lesions, not only to detect recurrence of the primary problem but to begin early treatment of any skeletal abnormalities occurring as a result of either the presence of the original mass lesion or the procedure required to remove the mass.

RESULTS

All patients in this series have been followed for a minimum of six years, and many have been followed for 20 to 23 years. The results of treatment are set forth in Table 103–5.

An excellent result is no evidence of clinical radiological recurrence of the initial disease at follow-up. The patient is neurologically intact.

A good result is no evidence of recurrence of the initial problem but some persistent neurological deficit.

A fair result is persistence of neurological deficit with evidence of the presence of the original disease. A poor result is no improvement or progression of the initial disease with major neurological deficit and resulting in the death of the patient.

TABLE 103–5   RESULTS OF TREATMENT OF SPINAL CORD TUMORS IN CHILDREN

CLINICAL CLASSIFICATION	TUMOR	NUMBER	SPINAL SEGMENT	RESULTS
Developmental or congenital tumors	Dermoids	11	Lumbosacral	Excellent
	Teratoma	3	Thoracolumbar	Good
	Lipoma	1		
	Neurenteric and teratomatous cysts	7	Upper thoracic	Excellent
	Extradural cysts	2	Sacral	Excellent
Intrinsic or primary cord tumors	Astrocytoma	9	Cervical	Excellent 50% Fair 50%
	Ependymoma	6	Filum terminale Thoracolumbar	Good Excellent
	Arteriovenous malformation	1	Thoracic	Excellent
Blood-borne metastases	Primary malignant tumor	9	Thoracic	Poor
Cerebrospinal fluid–borne metastases	Glioma	7	Multiple	Poor
	Melanoma	2	Sacral	Poor
	Ependymoma	2	Basal regions	Good
Tumors compressing by direct extension	Neuroblastoma	5	Thoracic	Excellent 50% Poor 50%
	Ganglioneuroma	5	Thoracic	Excellent
	Neurofibroma	1	Cervical	Excellent
	Schwannoma	1		
	Neurofibrosarcoma	3	Variable	Poor
	Bone tumors	3	Thoracic	Varied

Developmental or Congenital Tumors

The congenital lesions invariably present with associated developmental anomalies of the vertebral bodies and arch, including such dysraphic defects as fused bodies or hemivertebrae, agenesis of the sacrococcygeal area, diastematomyelia, congenital widening of the interpedicular space, and various cutaneous abnormalities.[5,8] While the mass lesions themselves produce neurological deficit, the majority of the signs and symptoms occur with growth either in the period between 1 and 4 years or in the adolescent growth spurt. The problems are usually a result of fixation or compression of the cord at a specific level. The majority of the lesions classified as dermoids according to the lumbosacral segment and the total excision gave an excellent result. The neurenteric or teratoma cyst developing from the canal of Kovalevsky and occurring in the upper thoracic area also yielded excellent results because of the facility with which they could be removed. Operations on teratomas and lipomas with their diffuse lobulation among the roots and extensive attachments to the spinal cord itself produce less satisfactory results, mainly because of the inability to remove the lesions entirely.

Intrinsic or Primary Spinal Cord Tumors

These lesions are not associated with a rapid growth pattern. They manifest themselves as a result of changes produced by pressure on previously normal structures.[1] The plain x-rays show erosion of pedicles and flattening of the interpedicular distance, scalloping of the posterior aspects of the vertebral body, but rarely any associated developmental defect of the bone. Myelograms have been invaluable in dealing with this particular group of patients. The results are dependent upon the extent of the lesion, its location, the presence or absence of a cystic component, particularly in the cervicothoracic area, and the ability of the surgeon to excise it satisfactorily. Postoperative radiation has had unsatisfactory results. While these patients do not die of their disease, their existence with paraplegia or quadriplegia has devastating effects on the individual and the family.

Blood-Borne Metastases

A secondary metastatic development of intradural metastases occurs primarily in the thoracic region, owing to the "watershed" effect of the spinal cord circulation at that point. The most common sources of these metastases are Ewing's sarcoma and neuroblastoma. The results are extremely poor, the death of the individual occurring usually as a result of a primary tumor shortly after the initiation of general treatment.

Cerebrospinal Fluid–Borne Metastases

This is an unusual group of cases in which the malignant gliomas had spread from other areas, producing spinal cord symptoms in an individual whose intracranial symptoms had improved or disappeared. The ependymomas that did occur in this group yielded good results with a satisfactory response to radiation and chemotherapy. The other nine tumors including seven gliomas and two melanomas ended with a poor result.

Tumors Producing Compression by Direct Extension

In this particular group of tumors, which have characteristics peculiar to the pediatric age group, the results will vary according to the age at which the diagnosis is made and treatment is carried out. Neuroblastoma, when treated in the infant under the age of 18 months or indeed 1 year, carries an extremely good prognosis as compared with the same tumor treated at a later age. The excellent results were in the infants, and the poor results in the older children. Ganglioneuromas, being benign tumors, were most often readily accessible because they presented as extensions of posterior thoracic mass lesions. The results were excellent. The sarcomas, as one might expect with malignant tumors, led to poor results. Bone tumors, including Ewing's sarcoma, are unpredictable in their course. No patient had an excellent result.

SUMMARY

Operative treatment of tumors of the spinal cord in childhood is rewarding, particularly in patients under 7 years of age. Greater care in the handling of soft tissues and bony structures during the operative procedure results in a major improvement in the long-term skeletal growth and neurological function of the individuals.

Improvements in diagnostic radiology, with more precise localization and greater ability to follow the patient during the postoperative course without major invasion of the body cavities, has improved the handling of secondary complications.

Improvements in radiation and chemotherapy have also changed the outlook for children with the more malignant tumors. A review of spinal cord tumors in the pediatric age group 10 years from now will probably reveal much higher survival and neurological recovery rates, particularly among the patients with sarcomas and carcinomas.

REFERENCES

1. Arseni, C., and Samitca, D. C.: Primary intraspinal tumours in children and adolescents. J. Neurosurg., 40:631–638, 1974.
2. Gerlich, J. G., Jensen, H., Koos, W., and Kraus, H.: Paediatrische Neurochirurgie. Stuttgart, Georg Thieme Verlag, 1967, pp. 647–662.
3. Harwood-Nash, D. C., and Fitz, C. R.: Neuroradiology in Infants and Children. Vol. 3. St. Louis, C. V. Mosby Co., 1976, pp. 1167–1227.
4. Ingraham, F. D., and Matson, D. D.: Neurosurgery of Infancy and Childhood. 2nd Ed. Springfield, Ill., Charles C Thomas, 1961.
5. Matson, D. D., and Tachdjian, M. O.: Intraspinal tumours in infants and children: Review of 115 cases. Postgrad. Med., 34:279–285, 1963.
6. Milhorat, T. H.: Paediatric Neurosurgery. Philadelphia, F. A. Davis, 1978.
7. Raud, R. W., and Raud, C. W.: Intraspinal Tumours of Childhood. Springfield, Ill., Charles C Thomas, 1960.
8. Schey, W. L.: Vertebral malformations and associated somatico-visceral abnormalities. Clin. Radiol., 27:341–353, 1976.
9. Till, K.: Paediatric Neurosurgery. Oxford, Blackwell Scientific Publications, 1975.

104

RADIATION THERAPY OF TUMORS OF THE SPINAL CORD

Radiation therapy plays an important role in the treatment of tumors that arise within the spinal cord or meninges and those that secondarily involve the cord by extension from a vertebra or metastasis from a distant primary carcinoma. Most of these lesions cannot be totally resected; hence, the definitive treatment is radiation therapy. The operation is important, however, to establish the diagnosis, to provide rapid decompression of the cord if necessary, and to remove the bulk of tumor.

The basic principles for treating primary tumors of the spinal cord are similar to those for treating brain tumors of similar histological type. Control of a primary tumor means control of the patient's disease, whereas failure may mean death or severe neurological disability, depending upon tumor site and type. Therefore, these tumors should be treated aggressively; with most tumors this means with a radiation dose that carries some risk to the spinal cord from the irradiation itself. Since treatment of metastatic tumors causing compression of the spinal cord generally is palliative only, these lesions are often treated more rapidly but with a smaller total dose. Treatment of metastases depends upon location of the tumor, extent of the neurological injury, and the general status of the patient; for example, a patient with a slowly progressive malignant tumor deserves a different treatment than would be appropriate for a patient whose early death from other metastases is imminent.

Although the risk of radiation injury to the spinal cord associated with a particular treatment technique is not well quantitated, guidelines are available: radiation sensitivity increases with the length of cord irradiated, the size of the individual daily dose, and the total dose given.[1,5,9,12] There is also indication that the thoracic portion of the cord is more sensitive than the cervical or lumbar portions. According to Kramer, who has suggested that the functional tolerance of the cord is 10 to 15 per cent lower than that of the brain, a total dose of 5000 rads given in 25 fractions over a total of five weeks carries an acceptable risk for the cervical and lumbar cord, and for the thoracic cord that total should be reduced by about 10 per cent.[7,8] Using daily fractions of 180 rads and a total of 5000 to 5500 rads, the authors have not observed permanent cord injury, but this treatment regimen does carry a low risk of cord damage.[19] For an individual patient, the risk from the treatment must be balanced against the anticipated sensitivity of the specific tumor to the radiation and the risk from the tumor if it remains uncontrolled.

Radiation injury to the cord is manifest in two ways. The onset of symptoms from the syndrome of lesser import appears from a few weeks to three or four months after completion of radiation therapy. The initial symptom is usually a sensation of tingling in the lower extremities elicited by flexion of the cervical spine (Lhermitte's sign). It is thought to be due to a transient demyelination and usually is self-limited, disappearing without treatment after a few months. The second form of radiation injury may appear any time from a few months to several years post-treatment. It is probably due to a combination of radiation-induced fibrosis and interference with the vascular supply of the cord. This type of injury is

W. M. WARA AND G. E. SHELINE

generally progressive and tends to be permanent. It may result in complete transverse necrosis with loss of both sensory and motor function below the level of injury.[3,5,8]

PRIMARY SPINAL CORD TUMORS

Primary intraspinal tumors are relatively uncommon, constituting about 15 per cent of tumors arising within the central nervous system. Schwannomas, meningiomas, and gliomas occur with about equal frequency and together account for three fourths of spinal tumors.[18] Approximately two thirds of the gliomas are ependymomas, the majority of which are in the filum terminale.

Published data on the treatment of spinal cord tumors are difficult to interpret, and treatment decision frequently must be based on inference from brain lesions of similar histological type.

While a few of the primary tumors are totally resectable, e.g., some ependymomas of the filum terminale, the majority are not and require radiation therapy. In general, if total operative removal is possible without excessive neurological complications, it

should be attempted; if removal is complete, operation alone constitutes adequate treatment.[4,20] Depending upon tumor type, radiation therapy may extend the recurrence-free interval or be curative.

Table 104-1 shows the results of treatment of ependymomas of the spinal cord. The extent of operative resection of the ependymomas in the patients of Wood and co-workers and of Schuman and co-workers was not stated, but probably the patients they irradiated had not had complete tumor resection.[15,20] The remainder of the data in this table relate to patients in whom only a biopsy or an incomplete resection was performed and in whom long-term control may be presumed to be due to the irradiation. All seven of the nonirradiated patients of Schuman and associates and of Barone and Elvidge had recurrence of ependymoma. For these patients with non-irradiated tumors Schuman's group reported a median symptom-free interval of three years; and Barone and Elvidge, an average survival of two and a half years. With irradiation, Schuman and co-workers reported, three of three patients were without recurrence at five years, and Barone and Elvidge had four of eight alive (time after treatment unstated) with an average survi-

TABLE 104-1   EPENDYMOMAS OF THE SPINAL CORD

AUTHOR	RADIOTHERAPY	RESULTS	
		No Evidence of Disease	"Alive"
Wood et al.*	Multiple courses 1000–3000 R	12 of 15 5 yr	
	Multiple courses 1000–3000 R	9 of 9 12 yr	
Schuman et al.†	None	0 of 4 "Median symptom-free interval" 3 yr	
Scott‡	1700–3700 R	3 of 3 5 yr	
Slooff et al.§	2500–5000 R	3 of 3 12–23 yr	
	Spinal cord None		
	Some		9 of 23 (39%)
	Filum terminale		16 of 26 (61%)
	None		4 of 11 (36%)
	Some		11 of 17 (65%)
Barone and Elvidge‖	None		0 of 3 (Avg. surv. 2.5 yr)
	Some		4 of 8 (Avg. surv. 9.5 yr)
Schwade et al.¶	~5000 R	12 of 12 3 yr	
	~5000 R	5 of 6 5 yr (1 patient lost)	

* The value of radiation therapy in the management of intrinsic tumors of the spinal cord. Radiology, 63:11–22, 1954.
† The biology of childhood ependymomas. Arch. Neurol., 32:731–739, 1975.
‡ Infiltrating ependymomas of the cauda equina. J. Neurosurg., 41:446–448, 1974.
§ Primary Intramedullary Tumors of the Spinal Cord and Filum Terminate. Philadelphia. W. B. Saunders Co., 1964. No data regarding radiation therapy dose, etc.
‖ Ependymomas—A clinical survey. J. Neurosurg., 33:428–438, 1970. Incompletely removed tumors. No data regarding radiation therapy dose, etc.
¶ Management of primary spinal cord tumors. Int. J. Radiat. Oncol. Biol. Phys. 4:389–393, 1978.

Osteoma

Osteomas are the most common benign bone neoplasms of the skull and facial structures. They present as circumscribed, slowly enlarging outgrowths of bone on either the inner or outer table of the skull, typically being detected in young adults and more commonly in females than in males (Fig. 105–1). They are most common in the paranasal sinuses and the mastoid cells. The roentgenographic appearance is that of a fairly well-defined, smoothly homogeneous bony density that extends outward and, when examined tangentially, appears domelike.[25,58] There is no erosion, as might be seen in meningioma, but the appearance of a spongy osteoma may suggest bone erosion. Osteomas may be of varying density, depending on their degree of ossification.[11] Tangential views demonstrate preservation of the diploë, an aid in differentiating this lesion from meningioma. In addition, osteomas do not produce the increase in size of the vascular channels of the skull that is

so often seen with meningioma. Multiple osteomas of the calvaria, paranasal sinuses, and mandible form part of the triad (with soft-tissue tumors of the skin and colonic polyposis) of Gardner's syndrome.[13]

Occasionally an osteoma may arise from the inner table and project into the cranial cavity (Fig. 105–2). In this location, its differentiation from meningioma bone becomes more difficult, but tangential views should establish a lack of invasion into the diploë.

Microscopically the tumor is by definition a nidus of osteoid tissue in a background of osteoblastic connective tissue and is completely enclosed by reactive bone. Some individuals have stated that an osteoma represents a reaction to infection, but Lichtenstein does not believe this to be true.[44] Histological differentiation from fibrous dysplasia is difficult, but smooth, homogeneous, and sharply defined sclerotic nodules are unusual in the calvaria in fibrous dysplasia.

The treatment of these lesions usually is

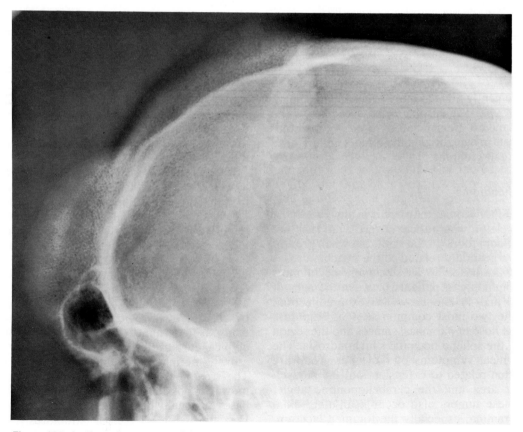

Figure 105–1   Extensive osteoma of the spongy type. The lesion extends from the level of the frontal sinus to the coronal suture. The inner table is intact and uninvolved.

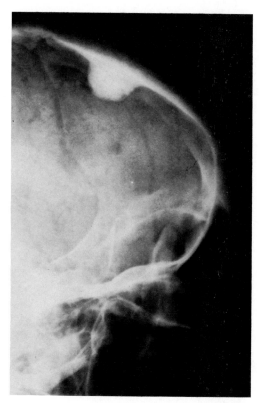

Figure 105–2 Osteoma arising from inner table. The lesion is quite dense and homogeneous, and there is thickening of the adjacent inner table. The diploë and outer table are not involved.

quite simple. They may be removed by operation, and the type of removal depends upon the size of the tumor and its location. A small circumscribed lesion may be removed totally, leaving the inner table intact. In such cases, plastic repair is not necessary. Larger lesions may require craniotomy and the removal of a sizable bone flap, in which case, a cranioplasty is indicated. In the experience of the authors, the tumor can be removed from the bone flap, and the flap autoclaved and then replaced primarily.

Fibroma

Fibromas of the skull are extremely rare. Dandy has reported one case of a nonossifying fibroma arising in the diploë in the parietal region.[23] Some authors have reported ossifying fibromas that characteristically occur in the frontal region, but the exact histological definition of such lesions appears to be difficult, and other individuals

classify these tumors as manifestations of fibrous dysplasia.[42]

Giant Cell Tumor

The benign giant cell tumor of the skull is an extremely rare lesion. It is more typically a tumor of long bones and occurs in persons aged 20 through 40, without sex predilection. Giant cell tumors do frequently occur in the jaw; when encountered in the skull, they are generally related to the endochondral bone of the base. Roentgenographic findings for such lesions in the skull have not been reported in detail, but the primary abnormality appears to be a sharply demarcated area of bone destruction.[46]

Lichtenstein grades these tumors into three categories according to their apparent degree of malignancy. Strict correlation between the microscopic appearance, the initial clinical behavior, and the eventual outcome is not possible, however, and there is apparently considerable overlap between benign and malignant forms.[44]

If at all possible, total excision is the treatment of choice. Irradiation results in a sizable incidence of sarcomatous degeneration.

Hemangioma

Hemangiomas constitute about 10 per cent of the benign tumors of the skull and are three times as frequent in females as in males. About two thirds of all hemangiomas of bone are located in the skull or the vertebral column. The most common clinical symptom is headache, which has been attributed to involvement of the pericranium. The tumor grows between the tables of the skull; only rarely is the dura involved.

There are basically two types of these lesions, cavernous and capillary. The cavernous hemangiomas are the most common and are generally found in the frontal or parietal regions. The capillary forms are quite rare. They are destructive and are associated with a large soft-tissue component that may cause compression of the underlying brain.[64]

Characteristically, hemangioma of the skull presents radiographically as an irregularly marginated, somewhat circular area of decreased density that has a honeycombed

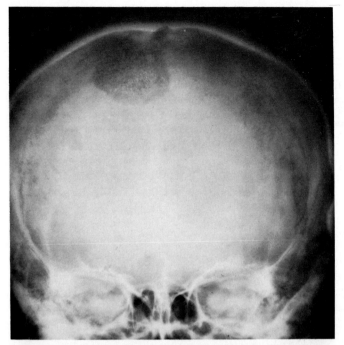

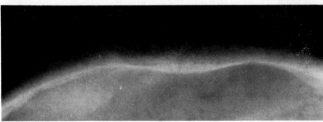

Figure 105–3 Hemangioma of the skull. The tumor arises in the diploë (*lower photo*) and expands that layer. Note the honeycombed appearance on both projections. The margins of this somewhat circular radiolucency are well defined but not sclerotic.

appearance (Fig. 105–3). The lesion typically occurs in the diploë. Trabeculae are widely separated and tend to radiate peripherally. The margins are well defined, and occasionally one may see a thin margin of bony condensation. The degree of radiolucency is frequently less than that of other lytic processes. On tangential views, the diploë is usually expanded, with some erosion of the outer table and a vertical orientation of the trabeculae within the lesion. The inner table typically is well preserved. The pattern of involvement is similar to that of childhood anemias, but the lesion is smaller, more localized, and not as thick.

On operative exploration, the hemangioma appears as a hard blue-domed mass lying beneath an intact pericranium. En bloc removal or curettage is curative. Although radiation has been advocated as a method of treatment by some, there is no good evidence for its value. Differentiation of this lesion from meningioma depends on the demonstration of an intact inner table and the lack of hyperostosis.

Dermoid and Epidermoid Tumors

Dermoid and epidermoid tumors of the cranium are characteristically supraorbital or anterior temporal in location and also are common near the vertex. These tumors may, however, occur anywhere in the calvaria. It is now generally held that these embryonal rests are differentiated according to whether dermal elements are evident or not.[59] Their clinical and radiographic presentations are identical. A typical lesion presents as a swelling on the surface of the skull. Frequently, it has been present for many years. Matson states that these lesions feel rubbery, are nontender, and may be either movable or fixed to the skull, usually with a connection to the overlying skin. The midline lesions over the bridge of the nose or near the torcular are of particular importance because of the great frequency with which they are associated with an intracranial extension that may involve the major venous sinuses or the cerebellum or both.[45]

Plain skull roentgenograms reveal a sharply defined lytic lesion usually arising in the diploë but involving all tables of the skull (Fig. 105–4).[25,58] The margins are sclerotic and may appear somewhat scalloped or lobulated. The lesion may have a cystic character with resultant thickening of the vault that is visible when viewed tangentially.

Epidermoid and dermoid tumors probably arise in the diploë and expand in all directions. Continuous desquamation within the tumor produces expansion that compresses adjacent bone, producing the sclerotic margins. These tumors must be differentiated from other sharply defined calvarial defects such as foramina of emissary veins, pacchionian granulations, and encephaloceles. Dermoid and epidermoid tumors have a tendency to become infected, and a surrounding area of osteomyelitis is not uncommon. True teratomas of the calvarium do occur, but there is nothing diagnostic about their appearance preoperatively unless some unusual structure is contained within them.

The treatment of these lesions is operative. The small laterally placed lesions without significant intracranial extension or evidence of infection may be removed en bloc, and a careful search may be made for a sinus tract or other evidence of intracranial extension. Curettage of the bony margins will usually result in adequate healing. When a midline lesion is approached near the bridge of the nose or near the torcular, it is extremely important to drape the patient appropriately so that a full-scale anterior or posterior fossa exploration can be

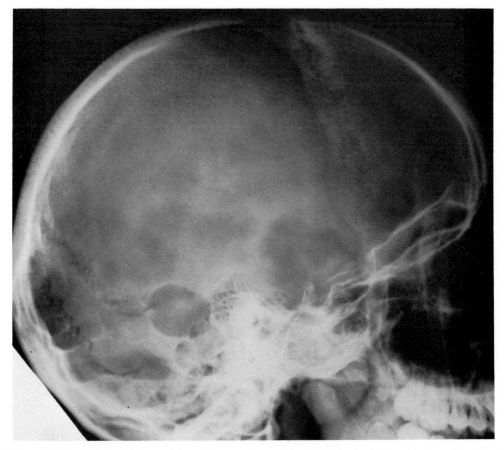

Figure 105–4 Epidermoid tumor of the skull presenting as a sharply defined radiolucent lesion with a sclerotic margin in the posterior temporal region.

performed if necessary. Because of the frequent involvement of the large venous sinuses, the intracranial extensions must be followed carefully and preparations for sinus repair made before the procedure is started.[45]

Malignant Primary Neoplasms

Chondrosarcoma

Primary chondrosarcomas of the skull are very rare.[61] These lesions may occur as a result of malignant degeneration in a preexisting chondroma, but such an occurrence is also rare. Chondrosarcoma is a tumor of adult life and generally occurs around the base of the skull. The history is frequently quite long and not very dramatic. Pain or the occurrence of a mass is usually the major complaint. These tumors may attain a considerable size before they are discovered, and metastases are frequent. Roentgenograms demonstrate destruction of bone with irregular, poorly defined margins (Fig. 105–5).[47] Only the location at the base of the skull and the occasional demonstration of stippled calcifications adjacent to the area of bone destruction serve to distinguish this tumor from carcinomatous metastasis, lymphoma, or myeloma.

Radical resection is the treatment of choice, and if the lesion can be totally excised, a cure may be effected. Supplemental radiation therapy may be of value, especially if total removal is impossible.

Osteogenic Sarcoma

Osteogenic sarcoma is the most common primary malignant tumor of bone. Even so, it is quite rare in the skull, and Vandenberg was able to find only seven cases involving the skull in a large series of bone tumors.[61] In general this is a disease of persons between the ages of 15 and 25, though there is a second modest peak in older patients with advanced Paget's disease. An occasional case occurs as a late result of radiotherapy.[2]

These tumors grow rapidly, and the history is usually quite short. Pain and local swelling are common complaints, and early metastasis is frequent, characteristically to the lungs. From a radiographic standpoint, osteosarcoma usually presents as a large lytic area with poorly defined margins.[25,33] One may see radiating bony spicules in a "sunray" appearance adjacent to the advancing margin of the osteolytic process, but this is less frequent in the skull than in the long bones. The spiculation is usually associated with thickening of the calvaria at the advancing edge, owing to subperiosteal extension. Calcification or ossification within the lytic tumor mass is most unusual.[20,32]

Osteosarcomas are extremely vascular and are sometimes referred to as bony aneurysms. Microscopically, they exhibit extreme variability, with foci of new bone formation, necrosis, hemorrhage, telangiectasia, or a frankly sarcomatous stroma. Lichtenstein makes the statement that no two of these tumors are exactly alike.[44]

Osteogenic sarcoma arising from preexisting Paget's disease of the skull is more frequent than primary osteosarcoma. Esti-

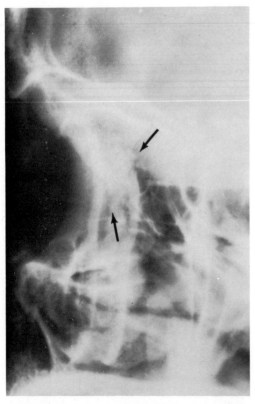

Figure 105–5 Chondrosarcoma in the cribriform plate region. Note the absence of the cribriform plate anteriorly with a soft-tissue mass destroying bone and filling the anterior ethmoid cells (*arrows*).

mates of the frequency of sarcomatous degeneration in osteitis deformans range between 10 and 15 per cent. Radiographically, there is rapid progression of lysis within the thickened and irregularly dense bone involved by Paget's disease. The entire thickness of the calvarium is destroyed as the lesion advances.[32]

Radical resection is the treatment of choice. Supervoltage irradiation therapy is usually employed in conjunction with operative therapy.

The five-year survival rate probably is no greater than 10 per cent with any form of treatment.

Fibrosarcoma

Fibrosarcoma may arise from periosteum, scalp, or dura.[18] Although early roentgenographic changes suggest thinning of the outer table by an overlying soft-tissue mass, there is often complete destruction of all tables of the skull over a wide area in later stages of the disease. Because of this rapid growth, the margins of the lytic process are irregular (Fig. 105–6). The differential diagnosis includes a multiplicity of processes that produce bone destruction and an accompanying soft-tissue mass. Carcinomatous metastases tend to be smaller and multiple, while meningioma rarely causes an extracranial soft-tissue mass and then only very late, long after other signs have suggested the diagnosis. Osteogenic sarcoma without bone production at its periphery cannot be differentiated radiographically from fibrosarcoma, but microscopic examination of the latter demonstrates sarcoma cells in a fibrous stroma without new bone formation. A combination of radical resection and irradiation appears to be the treatment of choice. The process is less inexorable than the osteogenic sarcoma, and long-term survivors are on record.

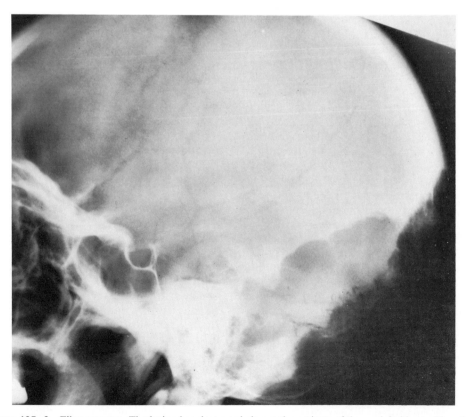

Figure 105–6 Fibrosarcoma. The lesion has destroyed almost the entirety of the occipital bone. The advancing edge is scalloped in some areas and grossly irregular in others. Histologically, there were few mitoses, but the relentless clinical course suggested that this was a fibrosarcoma rather than a fibroma.

Chordoma

Chordomas arise from notochordal remnants in the clivus and produce destruction of the basisphenoid.[37] These tumors, which present mainly in the third and fourth decades of life, are slow growing, and adjacent undestroyed portions of the basisphenoid may show a sclerotic appearance.[25] As the tumor enlarges, adjacent portions of the base of the posterior and middle cranial fossae including the sphenoid wings and petrous tips are destroyed. It is not uncommon to see enlargement of the superior orbital fissure with destruction of the adjacent greater sphenoid wing at the time of initial diagnosis. Forward extension may result in complete destruction of a portion of the clivus; lateral skull x-rays will then reveal a soft-tissue mass in the nasopharynx. Taveras and Wood estimate that calcification with a coarse stippled appearance occurs in these slow-growing tumors in about one third of cases.[58] The differential diagnosis includes chondroma, chondrosarcoma, meningioma, and metastasis to the clival region. Calcification, if present in a destructive lesion in a younger individual, would militate against metastasis. Angiography is usually required for more definitive diagnosis as well as for localization of tumor extension.

The treatment of chordoma in the clival region is a frustrating endeavor, usually palliative but not curative. Operative exploration and biopsy, via a suboccipital approach for the lower and a subtemporal-transtentorial approach for the upper clival chordoma, will establish the diagnosis. Although decompression of the brain stem can be accomplished by radical removal of the tumor, cranial nerve deficits usually are not improved by the operation. A decompressive procedure certainly prolongs the period of survival, but ultimately the tumor will recur.

Radiation therapy as a form of palliative treatment for clival chordoma remains controversial. There is no good evidence that it retards the tumor growth; when radical operative removal is deemed too risky, however, it is still an acceptable form of treatment. It is essential, nevertheless, that a histological diagnosis be made before such therapy is instituted.

Frequently, a combined approach, i.e., extensive operative removal of the tumor followed by radiation therapy, appears to be the preferred treatment.

SECONDARY TUMORS OF THE SKULL

Benign Secondary Neoplasms

Meningioma

The pathological description and classification of meningiomas have been the source of considerable debate over the years, and to some extent this debate continues today. The classic monograph of Cushing and Eisenhardt still constitutes a primary reference on this subject.[22] Meningiomas are tumors of late adult life; they are rare, but not unknown, in childhood. One third to one half occur in the parasagittal region. Parasagittal, convexity, sphenoid wing, and posterior fossa meningiomas account for 80 per cent of all intracranial meningiomas.[58] A detailed description of the diagnostic and therapeutic aspects of meningiomas is given in Chapter 92. Because of the difficulties in differential diagnosis that may occur, however, a description of the effects of these tumors upon the skull is given here.

In 1907, Spiller noted that localized thickening of the skull was associated with a tumor of the meninges, and by 1925 had described this hyperostosis in detail.[56,58] Cushing described eight types of characteristic involvement of bone by underlying meningioma: (1) scarcely any change in the bone, though evidence of increased vascularity may be present; (2) thinning of the bone by pressure from beneath without tumor invasion; (3) definite internal hyperostosis; (4) local bony thickening with increase in thickness of the diploë, internal hyperostosis, and a palpable external tumor; (5) a mound of ivory-like bone on the external aspect of the skull with associated en plaque extension of the tumor internally; (6) marked hyperostosis, both internally and externally; (7) an external mass of tumor between the galea and skull; and (8) the entire hyperostotic area largely replaced by the tumor.[22] It is not unusual for meningioma cells to invade adjacent bone and provoke an osteoblastic response. In fact, this hyperostosis is the most common specific sign of intracranial meningioma on plain skull radiographs (Fig. 105–7A).[34] The

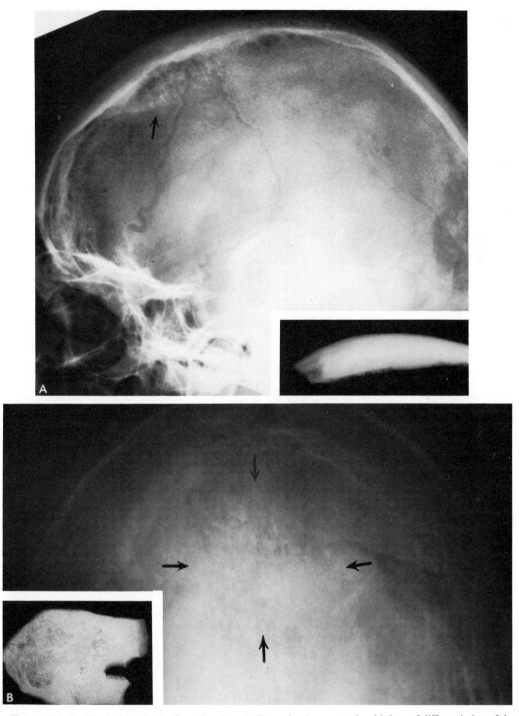

Figure 105–7 Meningioma in the frontal region. *A*. Extensive hyperostosis with loss of differentiation of the tables of the skull (see inset photo of excised specimen) and a brush border on the internal aspect at the site of tumor attachment (*arrow*). Note enlarged bony grooves of middle meningeal artery branches supplying the tumor. *B*. Frontal projection demonstrates a fenestrated appearance likely due to vascular channels permeating the involved bone.

inner table is almost always most severely involved, with thickening that may have a brush border. Commonly, the blastic response extends into the diploë, which may actually be obliterated. The outer table is less frequently involved, but an occasional lesion presents as a hard mass composed of thickened outer table bulging under the scalp. The margins of the lesion, when viewed en face, are rather poorly defined. Tangential views are most valuable in demonstrating extension of the process through the diploë and defining the extent of involvement most accurately. Less frequently, sclerosis may be intermixed with small irregular areas of osteolysis. Meningioma bone is highly vascular, and enlarged arterial channels may be visualized penetrating through the bone. En face, these have a distinctive fenestrated appearance

(Fig. 105–7*B*). Enlarged meningeal arteries supplying the tumor produce large tortuous vascular grooves on the inner table. An increase in the size of the foramen spinosum is said to be a frequent sign of meningioma (owing to an enlarged middle meningeal artery), but asymmetry of the two foramina spinosa is not unusual in normal individuals; this sign is of little value in the diagnosis of meningioma.

Bony involvement by meningioma is found in a high percentage of cases of convexity, cribriform plate, sphenoid ridge, and planum sphenoidale lesions (Fig. 105–8). Differentiation from fibrous dysplasia may be particularly difficult at the base of the skull, although fibrous dysplasia involving the base is frequently a bilateral and somewhat symmetrical process, while such a pattern in meningioma is exceedingly

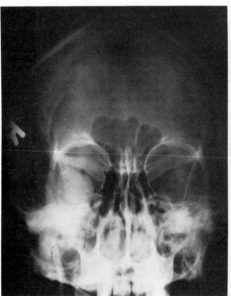
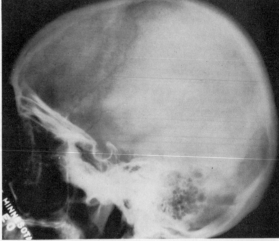
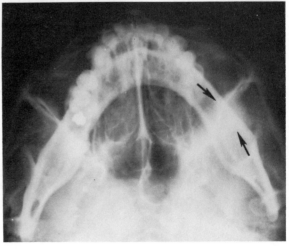
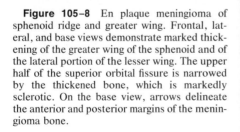

Figure 105–8 En plaque meningioma of sphenoid ridge and greater wing. Frontal, lateral, and base views demonstrate marked thickening of the greater wing of the sphenoid and of the lateral portion of the lesser wing. The upper half of the superior orbital fissure is narrowed by the thickened bone, which is markedly sclerotic. On the base view, arrows delineate the anterior and posterior margins of the meningioma bone.

rare. In addition, fibrous dysplasia occurs chiefly in the first three decades of life, much earlier than the peak incidence of meningioma. Angiography often aids in the differentiation, the external carotid circulation being only mildly enlarged and prominent in an area of fibrous dysplasia, while it is usually quite markedly enlarged when meningioma involves the bone.

There is no correlation between the size of the area of bony involvement and the size of the adjacent intracranial tumor.[25] Lesions along the sphenoid ridge and those involving the anterior wall and floor of the middle cranial fossa frequently are en plaque. In this situation, almost the entirety of the tumor consists of bony thickening. In other cases, particularly in convexity meningiomas, there may be a very large soft-tissue tumor with considerable displacement of adjacent brain and relatively minimal bony involvement.

Meningioma arising adjacent to bone may occasionally cause erosion and destruction of the bone without provoking an osteoblastic response. The areas of involvement show poorly defined margins, and if viewed tangentially, may exhibit a greater degree of involvement of inner table than of outer table. Differentiation from metastasis, myeloma, or even acute inflammation in the case of a solitary lytic area may, however, be impossible on plain skull roentgenograms; angiography will resolve the problem. The treatment of meningioma is considered in detail in Chapter 92. It should be emphasized, however, that prior to operative removal of bone, angiography is mandatory to delineate possible intracerebral extension. It should be noted that a meningioma involving bone is invariably quite vascular. Successive removal of the tumorous bone by rongeur with constant application of bone wax for hemostasis is the preferred technique of excision. It is important to drape the area generously and to be prepared to find intracranial extension as well as to perform cranioplasty if such is required. If there is suspicion of intracranial extension, the dura under the meningioma bone should be incised for inspection of the underlying brain.

Glomus Jugulare Tumor

These tumors are discussed in Chapter 107.

Malignant Secondary Tumors

Metastatic Carcinoma

The majority of metastatic lesions involving the skull arise from carcinomas of the breast and lung. Bone metastases from a wide spectrum of malignant neoplasms are similar in appearance and so may be discussed in general as osteoblastic or osteoclastic in type. In the osteoblastic form there is sclerosis and thickening due to bone reaction around the malignant infiltrate. Osteoclastic metastases are characterized by absorption and destruction of bone resulting in radiolucency. Osteoblastic metastases are characteristically produced by carcinoma of the prostate, carcinoma of the breast, carcinoma of the urinary bladder, and occasionally by hypernephroma. Rarely, almost any metastatic neoplasm may present in this fashion. Osteoclastic or osteolytic lesions are much more frequent and may be found in all of the foregoing as well as in carcinomas of the lung, uterus, gastrointestinal tract, and thyroid and in malignant melanoma.[25,58]

Osteoclastic metastases to the skull typically present as multiple radiolucencies with ill-defined margins (Fig. 105–9). The size and degree of radiolucency of the multiple lesions vary in the same patient. The larger lesions tend to be more radiolucent since they have destroyed the entire thickness of the skull. Lesions less than 5 mm in diameter frequently are confined to the diploë. The radiographic appearance of these lesions may closely simulate that of multiple myeloma. Acute osteomyelitis is also an important consideration in the differential diagnosis, especially in the case of a solitary metastasis. In general, the degree of overlying soft-tissue swelling with small metastatic lesions is minimal compared with that with osteomyelitis.

Osteoblastic metastases may present as areas of slightly increased density without radiolucency (Fig. 105–10). The areas of involvement show slight thickening on tangential projections and usually are poorly marginated. The multiplicity of the lesions tends to make this picture quite distinctive. In the case of carcinoma of the breast, one may see mixed lucent and sclerotic lesions that can simulate meningioma but are, of course, multiple and often quite extensive (Fig. 105–9B). Rarely metastases from

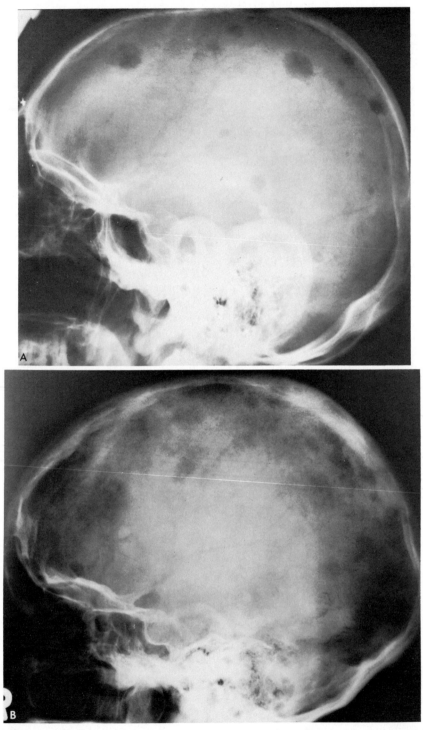

Figure 105–9 Carcinomatous metastases to the skull. *A*. Metastatic carcinoma of the lung. Multiple radiolucent lesions of varying size and radiolucency. Many of the lesions show a beveled edge, indicating that one table is
involved to a greater extent than the other. The margins are irregular and without sclerosis. *B*. Metastatic carcinoma of the breast. Diffuse involvement with an intermixed osteolytic and osteoblastic picture.

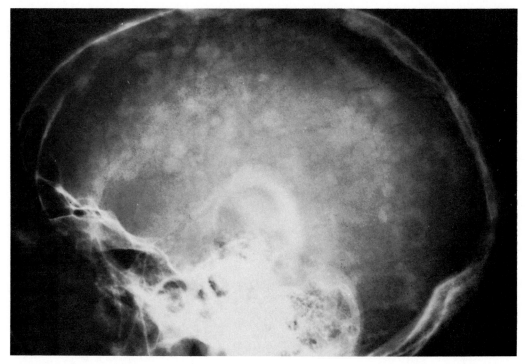

Figure 105–10   Osteoblastic metastases to the skull in a patient with carcinoma of the prostate. The calvaria is riddled with sclerotic lesions, which lie mainly in the diploë.

other sources may produce this mixed lytic-blastic picture.

Metastases may affect any portion of the skull, not only the calvaria, where they are relatively easy to detect, but also the base.[48] In particular, a frequent site of involvement is the region of the dorsum sellae, where such destruction may mimic the demineralization of chronically increased intracranial pressure. Early in the process the metastatic lesion is likely to be more extensive than the erosions of intracranial hypertension. Larger metastatic lesions tend to destroy the upper clivus and adjacent medial portions of the petrous tips, findings that would be unusual in intracranial hypertension but may resemble those of chordoma.

The treatment of the skull metastases is correlated with treatment of the primary disease. In general, this will be local radiation therapy or systemic and local chemotherapy. Occasionally biopsy of a skull lesion will be necessary for diagnosis, and if this is the case, complete excision of the individual lesion should be attempted and followed by the appropriate systemic treatment.

Neuroblastoma

Neuroblastoma is one of the most common tumors of childhood, and the skull is a frequent site of metastasis. Diffuse nodular radiolucencies simulating the appearance of metastatic carcinoma are common (Fig. 105–11).[25] These lesions are highly vascular and elevate the periosteum as they spread, producing the appearance of radial bone spiculation that extends out into the soft tissues and frequently is visible only under a bright light. A similar process takes place on the inner aspect with extension of tumor in an extradural plane and invasion of the sutures resulting in pronounced sutural diastasis.[12] The dura acts as a barrier to deeper spread. When tangential views are studied under a bright light, the degree of calvarial thickening with radial spiculation may be quite striking, particularly in the frontal and occipital regions. While spontaneous resolution of these tumors into more benign forms occasionally occurs with maturation, involvement of the skull is a poor prognostic sign. Metastasis to the facial bones and orbits occurs frequently, and patients often present initially with periorbital

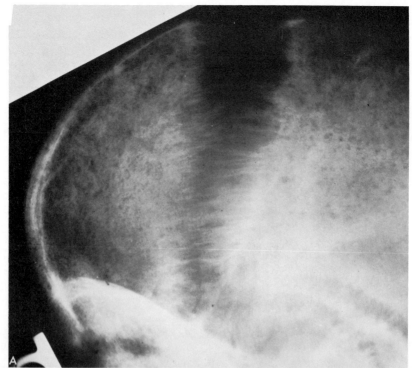

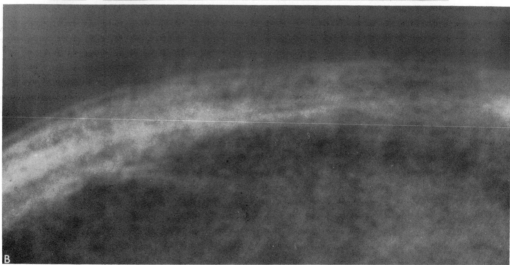

Figure 105–11   Neuroblastoma metastatic to the skull. *A*. Marked separation of sutures. The cranial bones are diffusely involved by tiny radiolucent lesions representing hematogenous metastasis. Note spiculated bone extending outward from the outer table in the frontal region, a manifestation of periosteal elevation. *B*. Magnification view of the nodular radiolucencies and radial bone spiculation.

ecchymoses and an associated abdominal mass. When the teeth or sinuses are involved, an associated osteomyelitis is quite common.

These tumors are quite sensitive to orthovoltage or supervoltage ionizing radiation, and local irradiation is the therapy of choice.

Ewing's Tumor

This sarcoma of childhood was originally described by Lücke in 1866, but was defined in such detail by Ewing that it is now associated with his name. Ewing's tumor is rarely primary in the skull, but metastasis to the skull is frequent. The most common complaint is pain, usually intermittent in character and quite often more severe at night. Later in the course of the disease a mass may appear, and there frequently is a history of spontaneous fluctuation in the size of the mass with increasing pain during periods of enlargement. Associated anemia, leukocytosis, and fever are very common.

The appearance of the lesion is not characteristic from a radiographic standpoint. Typically, there is destruction of bone with irregular poorly defined margins and an overlying soft-tissue mass. There may be minor periosteal reaction that suggests an inflammatory lesion, but bone destruction is the dominant feature. Ewing's sarcoma should be considered in the differential diagnosis of any bone lesion resembling osteomyelitis. The earliest destructive changes apparently involve the diploë with the formation of small radiolucent areas.[38,63]

The cellular structure of the tumor is characteristic. The lesion is composed of compact, strikingly uniform cells with indistinct borders and large prominent nuclei. The greatest problems occur in differentiating this tumor from reticulum cell sarcoma and from neuroblastoma with skeletal metastases.[44] This differentiation is quite important because of the difference in prognosis between Ewing's tumor and reticulum cell sarcoma primary in bone. Regardless of the type of therapy, the five-year survival rate with Ewing's sarcoma is less than 5 per cent. These tumors are initially quite radiosensitive, so radiation therapy is the treatment of choice. Recurrences are common, and the prognosis is not good with any kind of treatment.

Reticulum cell sarcoma may be confused histologically with Ewing's sarcoma.[57] The differentiation is quite important because reticulum cell sarcoma has a much better prognosis for survival. Lichtenstein discusses the pathological differentiation of reticulum cell sarcoma from metastatic neu-

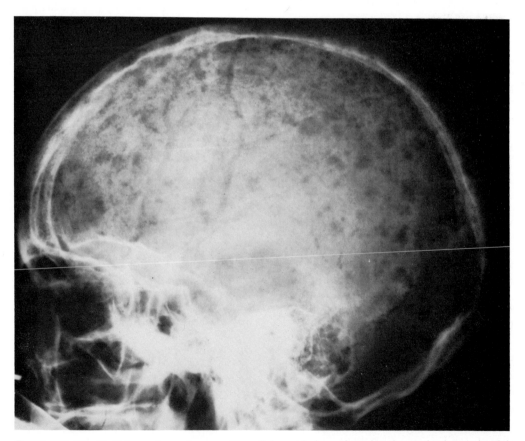

Figure 105–12 Multiple myeloma. Innumerable radiolucent lesions of varying size predominantly involving diploë, but with spread to inner and outer tables. The radiographic appearance of metastatic carcinoma may be identical.

roblastoma and from Ewing's sarcoma in considerable detail.[44] Willis has pointed out the dangers of accepting a diagnosis of Ewing's sarcoma on clinical and roentgeno-graphic grounds alone and advocates bi-opsy in all cases.[63]

Myeloma

Multiple myeloma is a common disease affecting males more frequently than fe-males and generally occurring between the ages of 40 and 60. The most usual pre-senting symptoms are pain, weight loss, pathological fracture in a long bone or ver-tebra, and a palpable tumor. Seventy per cent of patients have anemia. Associated findings are hypercalcemia, hyperglobulin-emia, and Bence Jones proteinuria. The diagnosis can usually be made by biopsy of a lesion or examination of the bone mar-row. The skull is commonly affected, but any bone may be involved. In terminal stages of the disease, it is not uncommon for almost every bone in the body to show evidence of tumor.

Skull radiographs reveal multiple sharply defined punched-out radiolucent areas in-volving all tables with no evident surround-ing sclerosis (Fig. 105–12). The lesions ap-pear in great number, involving wide areas of the calvaria. Since the disease begins (in the skull) in the diploë, small lesions may involve only this layer, but there will al-ways be other calvarial lesions involving all tables on the same film.[25] A rather unusual presentation is that of a solitary myeloma that may attain a diameter of 2 to 3 cm be-fore other lesions are recognized. Gen-erally, the multiple radiolucencies vary in diameter from 2 to 10 mm. Multiple mye-loma must be differentiated from metastatic carcinoma (the radiographic appearance may be identical) and from lymphoma.

Irradiation of the skull lesions is a possi-ble mode of therapy, but chemotherapy of the systemic disease is preferable.

Leukemia

Leukemias in childhood often present with skeletal involvement associated with anemia and fever, and such lesions fre-quently suggest infection. Calvarial lesions are rare. They present as ill-defined areas of rarefaction that are not as dramatic as those seen in myeloma and may demonstrate pe-ripheral periosteal new bone in a manner similar to neuroblastoma.[25] Calvarial de-posits in adult leukemias are almost un-known.

It is possible to obtain symptomatic reso-lution of skull lesions by low-dosage irra-diation, but chemotherapy of the primary disease is now more effective, and radiation is only employed as a supplement for symp-tomatic relief.

Lymphoma

Bone pain is one of the earliest indica-tions of skeletal involvement in Hodgkin's disease, but bony changes often cannot be demonstrated radiographically until late in the course of the disease.[21] In less aggres-sive cases, sclerotic margins surrounding irregular areas of lysis may be seen, and an occasional patient will show intermixture of lytic and blastic components similar to those of some metastatic carcinomas. The skull is sixth in order of frequency of bony involvement, with vertebrae, sternum, and pelvis being the most common sites. Occa-sionally an associated extradural tumor mass (detectable by angiography) may re-quire removal because of brain com-pression.

The more aggressive lymphomas (lym-phosarcoma, reticulum cell sarcoma) rarely involve the skull. The radiographic picture of multiple radiolucencies of varying size with ill-defined ragged edges simulates that of metastatic carcinoma. These lymphoma-tous processes are highly sensitive to radia-tion.[25]

Nasopharyngeal and Paranasal Sinus Carcinomas Involving the Skull

Neoplasms arising from structures of the head and neck may spread to involve the skull directly. The most common neo-plasms to involve bone by direct extension are carcinomas of the nasopharynx and paranasal sinuses. Carcinoma at the base of the skull, either within the sphenoid sinus or the nasopharynx, involves the sphenoid bone by direct extension. If the sphenoid is well pneumatized, the soft-tissue mass may be outlined radiographically within the cav-ity of the sphenoid sinus (Fig. 105–13). With further extension, the entire bony margin of the sella may be destroyed as well as other bony structures adjacent to the base of the skull (e.g., pterygoid plates). Typically, a patient presents with pain, signs of cranial nerve involvement, and minimal, if any, evidence of bone destruction on plain skull films. In these cases tomography is often very helpful.[29,35] The presence of a soft-tissue mass in the nasopharynx is easily diagnosed on lateral skull films in an adult in whom the normal soft-tissue thickness of the nasopharynx is only a few millimeters. Under age 30, however, the nasopharynx may normally be much thicker. A base view of the skull (vertical submental projection) may demonstrate destruction of bone and a soft-tissue mass encroaching upon the air shadow of the nasopharynx.

Most paranasal sinus cancers are associated with invasion of the bone by the time they become symptomatic. When these neoplasms are discovered in the frontal or ethmoid sinuses, it has been common practice to consider them inoperable, and radiation therapy has been the treatment of choice. As operative procedures for cancer have become more extensive, there has been an increasing interest in the treatment of these lesions by radical resection. Ketcham, Van Buren, and their collaborators have had extensive experience with lesions of this type.[40]

NONNEOPLASTIC TUMORS SIMULATING SKULL NEOPLASMS

Traumatic Lesions

Cephalhematoma

Cephalhematoma of the newborn results from a subperiosteal hemorrhage. It has been estimated that this occurs in 1.5 per cent of all live births, and it is said to be more common in children with high birth weights and in forceps delivery.[27] Cephalhematomas are most common in the parietal convexities. Since the periosteum is tightly attached at sutural margins, the soft-tissue mass is delimited by these margins. The majority of these tumors disappear without treatment in two weeks to three months.

The lesion is usually best demonstrated on tangential views. During the first three to four days only a soft-tissue mass is seen,

but toward the latter part of the first week of life calcific edges are seen arising from the sutural margins and projecting into the soft tissues of the scalp. This shell-like calcification progressively increases in both length and thickness until the mass is completely bridged, usually within two weeks (Fig. 105–14).[58] Simultaneously, there is a gradual process of resorption of the inner table of the involved portion of the skull. This process of remodeling with creation of new inner and outer tables continues over a period of weeks to years. Usually, however, it is complete within one to two months. Residual bony thickening and asymmetry (cephalhematoma deformans) is the exception but, if present, may have a cystic appearance simulating that of fibrous dysplasia or epidermoid tumor. A review of the patient's history and any available previous skull radiographs should aid in this differentiation. If such a deformation occurs, simple removal of the lesion is curative. Cranioplasty may be utilized if necessary.

Intradiploic Cyst

A second type of traumatic defect that occurs characteristically in the newborn and in young children is the intradiploic cyst.[27] This apparently results from hemorrhage into the diploë (intradiploic hematoma). The lesion presents as a swelling that is usually otherwise asymptomatic. The characteristic radiographic appearance is that of a radiolucent round or oval defect in the diploic space with a very fine sclerotic margin. Such lesions rarely need treatment; if it is necessary to obliterate them for cosmetic reasons, simple curettage is adequate.

Leptomeningeal Cyst

Linear skull fractures in children may occasionally lead to extensive resorption of bone. Leptomeningeal cyst is probably the result of a dural tear at the time of skull fracture. A small projection of arachnoid herniates through the dural tear and becomes entrapped in the fracture. Persistent pulsation of the cerebrospinal fluid leads to formation of a communicating cyst. The expanding cyst gradually erodes adjacent bone, producing a lytic defect with scalloped margins (Fig. 105–15).[58] It is impor-

Text continued on page 3250

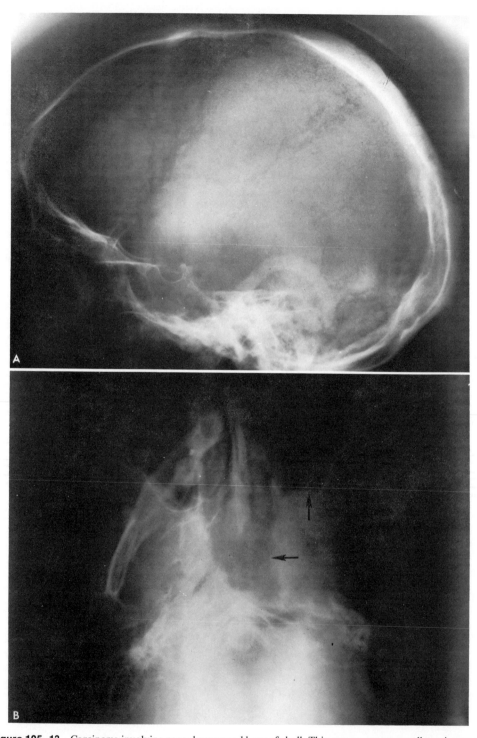

Figure 105–13   Carcinoma involving nasopharynx and base of skull. This was a squamous cell carcinoma originally primary in the lip with direct invasion into soft tissues of the cheek and jaws. *A.* Lateral view of skull shows
soft-tissue mass in the sphenoid sinus with area of bone destruction at the upper margin of the clivus. *B.* Soft-tissue
mass in nasopharynx with invasion into body and left greater wing of sphenoid, clivus, and posterior portion of left
maxillary antrum. Note destruction of left pterygoid plates and foramen ovale (*arrows*).

Illustration continued on opposite page

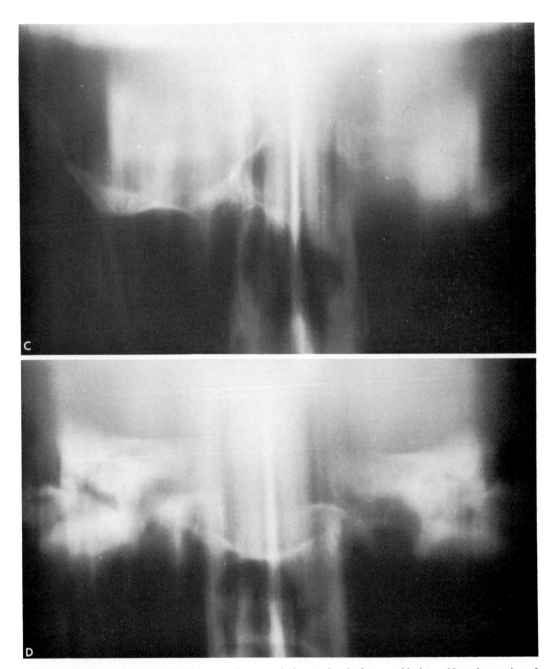

Figure 105–13 (*continued*) *C*. Tomogram in coronal plane at level of pterygoid plates. Note destruction of left pterygoid plates and of body and greater wing of sphenoid bone on the left. *D*. Tomogram at level of jugular foramina showing destruction of medial wall of the left jugular foramen.

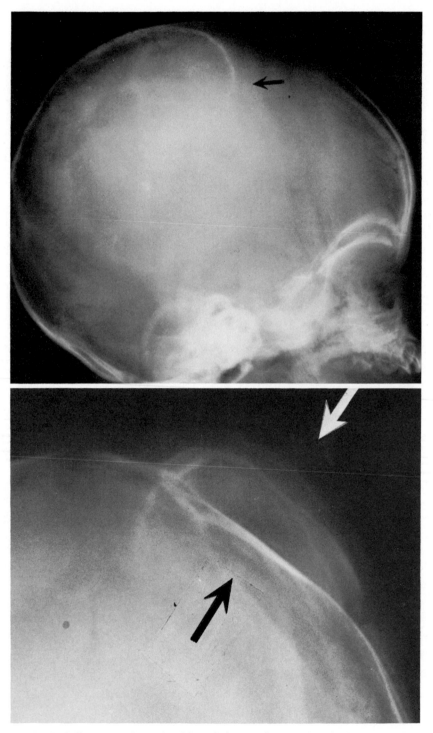

Figure 105–14 Cephalhematoma. Lateral and frontal views made at age 6 weeks demonstrate complete calcific bridging of the hematoma with remodeling of bone already in progress. Arrows show margins of lesion.

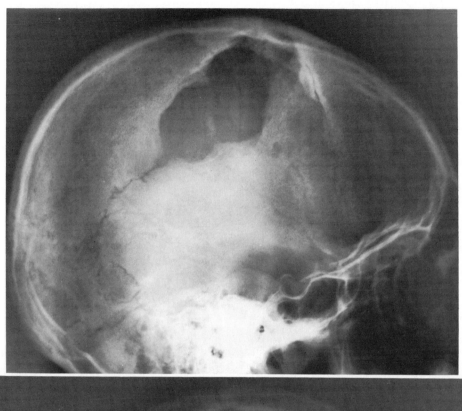

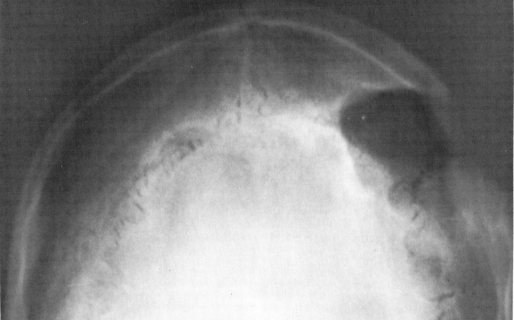

Figure 105–15   Leptomeningeal cyst. Lateral and frontal views in a 15-year-old boy who had sustained a fissure fracture of the skull at age 8 months. Note the scalloped margins of the defect. On the frontal view, note eversion of the bony margins due to the expanding pulsatile cyst.

tant to realize that the lesion expands not only between the fracture edges but also deep to the inner table and thus may cause atrophy of underlying cerebral tissue.[14] Since this complication is much more frequent in infancy and early childhood, skull fractures in children should be carefully followed radiographically until the fracture line is healed. If serial roentgenograms demonstrate progressive widening of the fracture line with undulating margins, the diagnosis of leptomeningeal cyst appears likely. Pneumoencephalography, angiography, or even direct puncture of the palpable portion of the calvarial defect will confirm the diagnosis.

Occasionally, these cysts also cause expansion between tables of the bony skull. Although these lesions are much more common in children, the process may occur following a skull fracture in an adult. If the lesion is progressive and large enough to warrant treatment, excision of the cyst and repair of the dural laceration are curative. An occasional defect is large enough to require cranioplasty.

Additional discussion of post-traumatic cysts is given in Chapter 64.

Fibrosing Osteitis

This process also follows fracture and presents as a soft depression in the skull or as a localized area of bone destruction. There is no leptomeningeal cyst demonstrable in these cases, but the roentgenographic appearance of the two is identical. Exploration reveals resorption of bone and replacement with fibrous scar.[27] If the defect is sufficiently large, cranioplasty may be warranted.

Radiation Necrosis

Radiation necrosis of the skull probably occurs with greater frequency than reports in the literature would suggest. Although radiation necrosis likely develops earlier in craniotomy flaps, the majority of such cases have been described in patients who have not undergone craniotomy. Unless complicated by frank osteomyelitis, the diagnosis is usually made on routine follow-up examination. The typical radiographic appearance is one of multiple small areas of decreased density with relative decrease in density of the entire skull surrounding these areas in a pattern suggestive of the radiation therapy fields. The process is usually asymptomatic, and cases have been followed for many years in which there was no significant change in the appearance of the skull. Because of the asymptomatic nature of the problem, it is very difficult to determine exactly when this process appears, but published cases and personal experience suggest that it occurs several years after irradiation. The moth-eaten appearance must be differentiated from metastatic carcinoma, multiple myeloma, and osteomyelitis. Correlation with radiation portals will generally establish the diagnosis. Healing may take place slowly over many years with a gradual replacement by irregularly sclerotic bone. Rarely, osteogenic sarcoma or malignant giant cell tumor may arise on a matrix of radiation necrosis.[2]

Vascular Impressions in the Skull

Normal vascular structures as well as vascular tumors of the scalp, dura, and brain may cause impressions on the skull that simulate tumors of the calvaria. Pacchionian granulations often produce localized areas of calvarial thinning with slightly lobulated margins that can simulate lytic lesions, either benign or malignant. Tangential views reveal thinning of the inner table and diploë, which are invaginated by the arachnoid granulation. Large granulations may erode the outer table as well. Although these radiolucencies are typically clustered in the parasagittal region, they also commonly occur in the occipital squamosa and occasionally in more lateral portions of the frontal and parietal bones.

Cirsoid Aneurysms

Cirsoid aneurysms of the scalp may produce thinning of the outer table of a lobulated nature. Examination of the soft tissues under a bright light will reveal a soft-tissue mass adjacent to the area of bone thinning. External carotid angiography will establish the diagnosis and delineate the arteries supplying the malformation. Similar bone changes due to superficial cortical or dural arteriovenous malformations are occasionally noted on the inner table aspect.[55] Curvilinear calcifications adjacent to the area of bone thinning and enlarged vascular channels leading to this region may suggest the diagnosis, but angiography (internal and external carotid) is required for diagnosis.

Sinus Pericranii

Sinus pericranii is a congenital defect involving the skull in which the intracranial sinuses, usually the superior sagittal sinus in the frontal region, are connected with the extracranial space through abnormal emissary vessels. The lesion is characterized by a soft fluctuant swelling that is increased in size when the head is in a dependent position.[17] Radiographically, the midline location of a smooth sharply marginated round defect may also suggest this entity, but differentiation from epidermoid tumor or eosinophilic granuloma usually requires angiography.

Defects Secondary to Intracranial Disease

Erosions of the skull suggesting bone neoplasms may also occur with other primary intracranial lesions besides meningioma. Rarely, a slow-growing intracerebral glioma will significantly erode adjacent bone. Characteristically, the inner table is first involved, and subsequently, the diploë and the outer table. Such a lesion presents as an area of radiolucency with poor margination. Similar erosions may be seen in areas where the skull is normally thin (e.g., floor and anterior walls of the middle cranial fossa, orbital roofs, temporal squamosa), where they are due to long-standing increased intracranial pressure.[58] Differentiation from metastasis, meningioma, or tumors invading from adjacent structures usually requires angiography.

Metabolic Diseases Affecting the Skull

A multiplicity of metabolic abnormalities may cause radiographic changes in the skull that may mimic neoplastic processes. Such changes are important to recognize, for they may be the first clue to the correct diagnosis of the systemic disease.

Hyperparathyroidism

Hyperparathyroidism with resulting increased parathyroid hormone secretion results in marked abnormalities of metabolism of calcium and phosphorus. Blood calcium levels are generally elevated and blood phosphorus levels are usually lowered. Balance studies indicate an increased loss of both calcium and phosphorus from the body. Bone changes are ubiquitous. In the skull there are wide areas of granular osteoporosis; this porous bone gives the calvaria a woolly appearance (Fig. 105–16A). Larger areas of porosis may coalesce (osteitis fibrosa cystica of von Recklinghausen) into "brown tumors," which appear radiographically as sharply defined lytic areas; the surrounding osteoporotic matrix generally establishes the diagnosis (Fig. 105–16B).[10,25] In the healing stages of hyperparathyroidism, patchy irregular sclerosis of the calvaria may be seen.[58] The diagnosis is usually not difficult, since these sclerotic lesions are superimposed on the diffuse granular osteoporosis typical of the disease. Patchy sclerosis may also be seen in patients with secondary hyperparathyroidism due to renal failure.[65]

Pseudohypoparathyroidism

Pseudohypoparathyroidism is a congenital dysplasia of bony structures with hypocalcemia that does not respond to parathyroid hormone. As part of the bony dysplasia, there is often a diffuse increase in thickness and density of the calvaria. The process is generalized, involving the entire skull, and is usually associated with other manifestations of the syndrome (short metacarpals and metatarsals, accelerated bony maturation, soft-tissue calcification).[26]

Acromegaly

The bony changes in acromegaly secondary to acidophilic adenoma of the pituitary include enlargement of the mandible with increase in the angle subtended by the body and ramus, prominence and enlargement of the paranasal sinuses, and thickening and sclerosis of the calvaria with obliteration of the diploic space.[58]

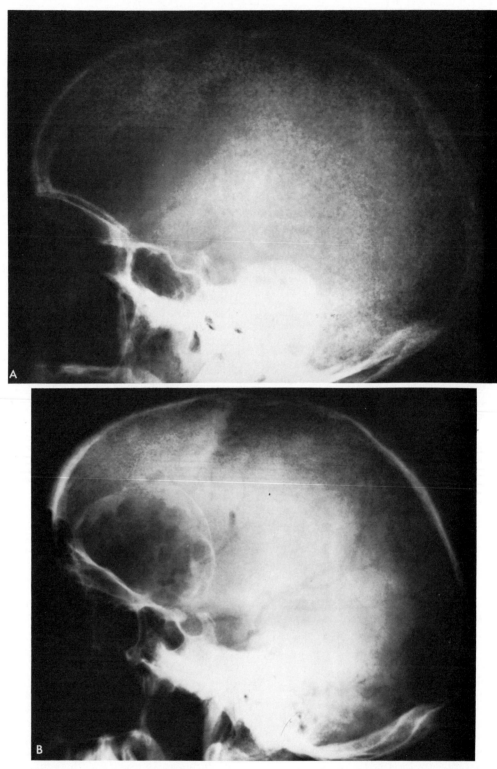

Figure 105-16   Hyperparathyroidism. *A.* Diffuse granular osteoporosis giving the skull a ''salt and pepper'' appearance. *B.* ''Brown tumor'' in inferior frontal region. Corrective therapy had already been instituted in this case, so the granular appearance of the skull is not as impressive as in the patient depicted in *A.*

Hypervitaminosis A

In the infant, hypervitaminosis A may result in cortical hyperostosis of multiple bones, including the skull, that is similar to Caffey's disease.[8,9]

Hypervitaminosis D

The radiographic hallmark of hypervitaminosis D is metastatic calcinosis in soft tissues (especially kidneys), arterial walls, and hyaline cartilage.[16] These calcifications may occur in the dura, and Edeiken and Hodes state that premature calcification of the falx is the most consistent sign of hypervitaminosis D.[26] On occasion, these dural calcifications may be difficult to differentiate from neoplasms of the inner table. The calvaria may become quite dense, although long bones may exhibit mild demineralization. When vitamin D is discontinued, the metastatic calcification is resorbed.

Vitamin D Deficiency

Vitamin D deficiency results in rickets, and in advanced stages the diagnosis presents little difficulty. The head is squared and enlarged. There is a rather symmetrical diffuse hyperostosis of the skull, predominantly in the frontal regions.[58] The base is less frequently involved, and the thickening tends to taper near the sutures. Because the involved bone is soft and malleable, abnormalities of shape and contour may occur, the most common of which is thinning and flattening of the occipital bone, generally termed craniotabes. These areas of bony deformity are characteristic and do not present a problem in differential diagnosis. Sutures and fontanelles widen and are easily compressible. Following administration of vitamin D, healing begins, and considerable thickening of the calvaria with permanent deformity may result.[7]

Secondary (Renal) Rickets

Secondary (renal) rickets, which accompanies chronic renal disease of childhood, may cause similar changes, but in addition, thickening of the calvaria with patchy areas of sclerosis in a mottled pattern similar to that described in healing of hyperparathyroidism may be seen. These areas of thickening and sclerosis must be differentiated from Paget's disease.[65]

Fluorine Intoxication

Chronic fluorine intoxication may result in an increase in thickness and density of the skull, which usually is rather generalized. There may be proliferation of very dense cortical bone, and the disease may be difficult to differentiate from other hyperostotic processes. Long bones, ribs, and vertebrae are also involved with diffuse cortical sclerosis and thickening.[5]

Osteomyelitis of the Skull

Infections of the skull may be quite difficult to differentiate from a number of other lesions and so must be included in a discussion of tumors of the skull. Extension from an infected paranasal sinus or an adjacent inflammatory process in the scalp and direct contaminating trauma are the most common causes. Hematogenous spread from a distant infection is less common. As with osteomyelitis elsewhere in the skeleton, radiographic changes often lag behind clinical signs and symptoms.[31] Earliest changes are seen as small nodular radiolucencies in the outer table or diploë. The base of the skull is rarely involved, but when it is, the process is especially serious. In young children the sutures of the skull tend to limit the disease, but this is not true in adults. The osteomyelitis may remain localized or it may spread contiguously or via the diploic veins.[58] As the disease progresses, the bone acquires a moth-eaten appearance with coalescence of smaller areas of lysis into larger lesions, and frequently there is a surrounding area of visible edema and swelling that is sometimes designated as "Pott's puffy tumor" (Fig. 105–17). With time, poorly defined sclerosis is seen at the margins of the lytic process, but periosteal new bone formation is almost unknown. Unlike other osseous structures, the skull has such a rich blood supply that the formation of sequestra (areas of dead bone, which become quite dense) is uncommon.[25] The radiographic appearance of cured osteomyelitis may remain stable, or endosteal bone regeneration may occur.

Tuberculous, luetic, and other low-grade chronic bacterial infections may be demonstrated by a poorly defined patchy sclerosis (Fig. 105–18).[25] Circumscribed areas of lysis may be present but are not dominant. While involved areas of bone are usually

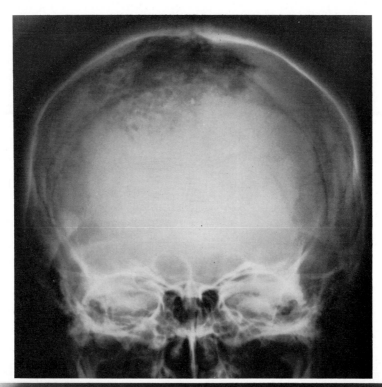

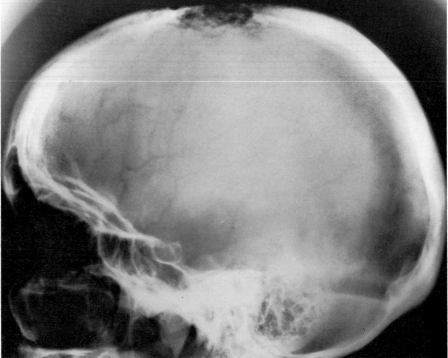

Figure 105–17 Osteomyelitis of the skull, frontal and lateral views. Three months earlier, a sebaceous cyst of the scalp had been excised. The wound became infected. Coalescent nodular radiolucencies are characteristic. Note the absence of either marginal sclerosis or sequestra.

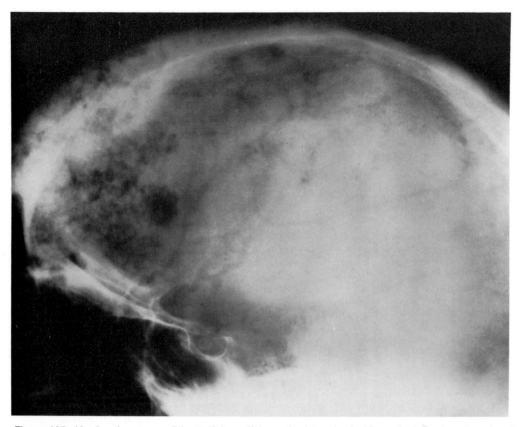

Figure 105–18 Luetic osteomyelitis. Nodular radiolucencies intermixed with poorly defined patchy sclerosis suggest a chronic inflammatory process of bone.

sclerotic and thickened, soft-tissue thickening may be minimal or absent. A number of fungal infections including actinomycosis, coccidioidomycosis, and blastomycosis have been reported with radiographic appearances similar to tuberculosis or lues, and granulomatous lesions from *Echinococcus* and *Trichinella* have been reported. Yaws and leprosy may also be present with lesions similar to those of other granulomatous diseases.

Miscellaneous Lesions Affecting the Skull

Osteopetrosis

Osteopetrosis (Albers-Schönberg disease) is a rare familial disorder of bone characterized by diffuse increase in density and thickness of cortical bone throughout the body.[62] There is complete loss of differentiation of the tables of the skull (Fig. 105–19). The foramina of the skull are fre-

quently encroached upon; optic atrophy is a frequent but late occurrence in this disease. Views of the optic foramina and of the foramina at the base of the skull should always be obtained in evaluation of patients with suspected osteopetrosis. In childhood, the process may not be completely manifest and the bones of the vault may be normal.[25] Usually, however, the base of the skull shows increased density. A similar involvement of the skull may be seen in progressive diaphyseal dysplasia (Engelmann's disease). This may be differentiated from osteopetrosis by examination of the long bones in which increased density of the cortex is not so marked or homogeneous and is accompanied by abnormal tubulation, which is not generally seen in osteopetrosis.[50] Also to be considered in this category is hyperostosis corticalis generalisata (Van Buchem's disease), a rare familial disorder that causes diffuse thickening and sclerosis of the calvaria with narrowing of foramina resulting in cranial nerve deficits.[60] The hyperostosis is most prominent

veal an irregularly marginated rarefaction without surrounding eburnation (Fig. 105–22). On tangential views, the margins of the lesion are often beveled owing to differences in degree of involvement of inner and outer tables.[25,58] Actively progression lesions do not show sclerosis of the margins, but bandlike sclerosis may be seen during healing, which may occur spontaneously or following relatively small doses of radiation. Involvement of orbital margins may occasionally result in a dense sclerosis in the healing phase. The solitary lucent lesion may be confused with epidermoid, myeloma, and metastatic carcinoma, but the age of the patient and the lack of symptoms aid in the differential diagnosis.

Radiation therapy can be curative, but because of the difficulties with the differential diagnosis, complete surgical excision is preferable. The lesions heal readily after curettage, and radiation therapy for a solitary lesion may be unnecessary unless the dura has been involved. Matson points out

the importance of obtaining a radiographic bone survey to evaluate the possibility of generalized histiocytosis.[45]

Multiple lesions of the skull in histiocytosis are commonly associated with widespread skeletal involvement. The lesions become confluent as they expand. More lesions are found in the frontal bone than in any other skeletal component. Soft tumor masses may be palpable over the eroded areas after perforation of the outer table. When the lesion occurs adjacent to the orbit, proptosis may develop because of the mass or because of venous obstruction. Lesions invading brain parenchyma are extremely rare. The erosions have distinct and clear-cut but irregular edges and have been described as maplike. The areas of bone destruction may be extremely large, and destruction may eventually involve the paranasal sinuses and facial bones.[25,58] Following diagnostic biopsy, low-dosage radiation therapy is the treatment of choice for localized bony lesions, but corticosteroids

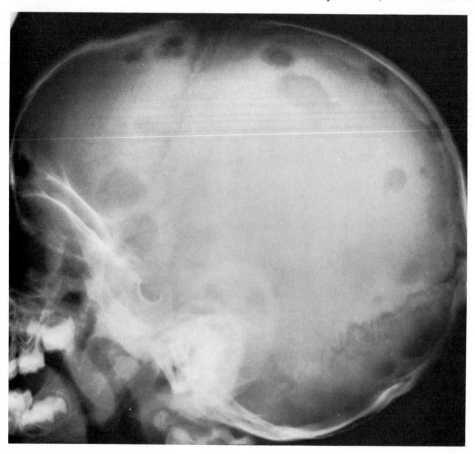

Figure 105–22 Histiocytosis X. Numerous radiolucent lesions with beveled margins scattered throughout the skull in a young infant.

are frequently necessary for treatment of systemic involvement.

Mucocele

A mucocele is an encapsulated fluid collection within a paranasal sinus, formed by outlet obstruction of the sinus ostium and characterized by expansion of the involved sinus with thinning of its walls and compression of adjacent structures. Its contents are almost always mucoid rather than serous and are usually sterile. A mucocele may become infected, in which case it is better designated a pyocele. These lesions are most common in the frontoethmoidal area. In the frontal region, there is frequently associated soft-tissue swelling overlying the frontal sinus. Mucocele is one of the more common causes of unilateral exophthalmos. These masses erode bone, but their slow growth allows formation of new sclerotic bony walls with characteristic encroachment on the bony orbit. Osteoma in the frontal sinus is frequently coexistent with a frontoethmoidal mucocele.[52] Although the sphenoid sinus is not a common site of involvement, sphenoid mucocele may simulate an intrasellar tumor with destruction of the walls of the sella, soft-tissue mass in the sphenoid sinus, and enlargement of the superior orbital fissure (Fig. 105–23).[6] Differentiation from intrasellar neoplasm is important because of the high incidence of postoperative meningitis following direct attack on a sphenoid mucocele; tomography and angiography may be of some aid in this regard.

Complete removal of these lesions is usually possible and is curative. Though they are sterile, it is very important to avoid spilling the contents intracranially, for severe chemical meningitis may occur. In this respect, it is important to obtain lateral tomograms in frontoethmoidal mucoceles to ascertain whether the lesion has broken through the posterior wall of the frontal sinus into the cranial cavity, a factor that greatly increases the possibility for intracranial spill. Some favor a transnasal approach to the sphenoid mucocele.

Anemias of Infancy and Childhood

Infants with severe anemia may utilize the diploë as a major source of red blood cell production. Resultant skull changes may be important in the differential diagnosis of skull tumors. These diseases are of historical interest, changes suggestive of anemia having been described in the skulls of pre-Columbian Peruvian and North American Indians as well as in the Mayans of the Yucatan. The abnormalities are most striking in thalassemia (Cooley's anemia), in which overgrowth of the bone marrow causes generalized widening of the diploë with resultant atrophy of the outer table. The trabeculae of the diploë are stretched and assume a radial striated pattern (Fig. 105–24). The striations are perpendicular to the inner table, which remains intact. Occasionally, the changes are asymmetrical. The tremendous enlargement of the marrow prevents pneumatization of the maxillary sinuses. The occipital bone inferior to the internal occipital protuberance is often spared, since there is usually no marrow in this location. Tubular bones also show expansion of medullary spaces, most evident in the metacarpals, metatarsals, and phalanges. The homozygous form carries a poor prognosis, with few patients surviving childhood, but heterozygous individuals are less severely affected and have a better prognosis.[19]

Similar changes are seen in iron deficiency anemia, but the involvement is generally less extensive, and facial bones and long bones are rarely involved. Sickle cell disease and hereditary spherocytosis (familial hemolytic anemia) also exhibit less severe calvarial changes. Infants with cyanotic congenital heart disease may present with marked thickening of the diploë and a pattern similar to that just described, owing to erythroid hyperplasia.[36,53]

If a child survives into adult life, the thickened skull may persist while changes in the long bones tend to disappear. The characteristic atrophy of the outer table with preservation of the inner table, however, serves to differentiate this process from other hyperostotic lesions.

Neuroectodermal Dysplasias

While bone involvement in generalized neurofibromatosis is quite common, most of these defects require no differentiation from skull neoplasms. The abnormalities of bone in neurofibromatosis are usually limited to absence of bones (especially the posterior wall of the orbit) and the erosive ef-

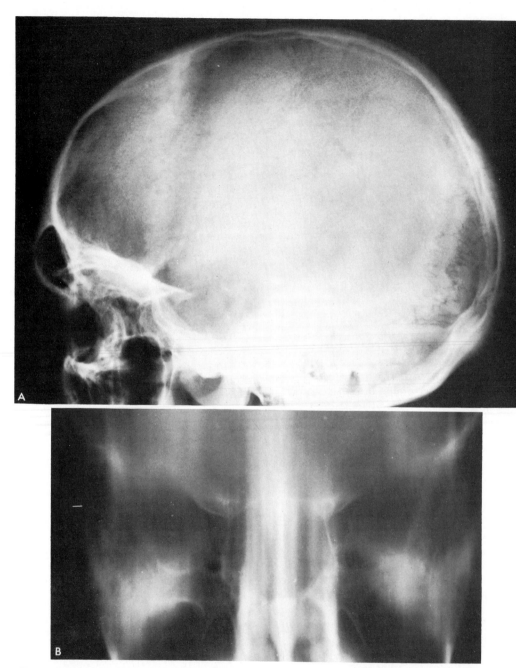

Figure 105–23 Mucocele of the sphenoid sinus. *A.* Destruction of the walls of the sella turcica simulating a pituitary neoplasm. Note soft-tissue density projecting into posterior ethmoid region. The posterior clinoids are displaced superiorly and posteriorly. *B.* While plain films failed to demonstrate the bony walls of the mucocele, tomograms revealed the walls to be intact but extremely thin.

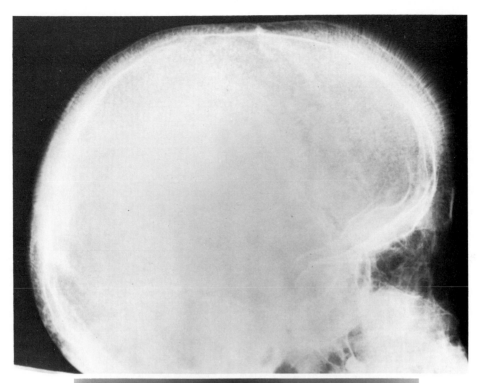

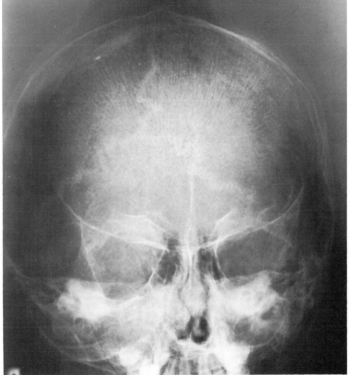

Figure 105–24   Thalassemia (Cooley's anemia) with expansion of the diploë. Note characteristic radial striations of diploic trabeculae. The frontal and maxillary sinuses are poorly developed because of the bony overgrowth.

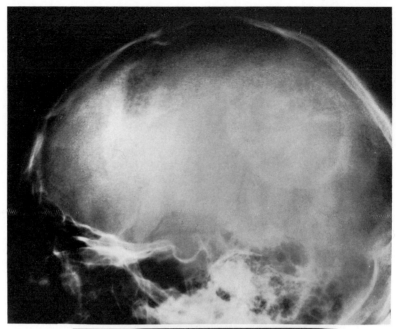

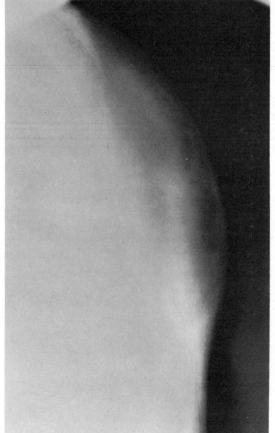

Figure 105–25 Fibrous dysplasia of the cystic type. The lesion in the left parietal bone is sharply marginated and, on tangential view, projects outward. The inner table is preserved.

fects of tumors.[4,30] Jaffe has described sharply marginated ovoid or round defects in the region of the lambdoid sutures in patients with neurofibromatosis that may be confused radiographically with epidermoid tumor. This is apparently a result of bone dysplasia in generalized neurofibromatosis.[39]

Although osteosclerotic nodules in the inner table have been described in tuberous sclerosis, such findings are extremely rare. These small ill-defined densities may be confused with the peripheral calcified glial nodules, which are so typical of this disease, unless tangential roentgenograms are obtained.

Fibrous Dysplasia

Fibrous dysplasia is a disease of young people from childhood through the third decade with a higher incidence in males than in females. The process may be monostotic or polyostotic.[28] This interesting disease of unknown etiology may present with isolated involvement of the skull or less commonly as part of a generalized process involving multiple osseous structures.[26] The roentgenographic patterns are generally classified into three groups: cystic, sclerotic, and mixed.[42]

The cystic variety is seen as a radiolucent widening of the diploic layer with thinning of the outer table and relatively less involvement of the inner table (Fig. 105–25). The margins of this radiolucent process are sharply defined with a sclerotic rim simulating the appearance of epidermoid tumor. These lesions, however, are usually larger than epidermoid tumors. The cystic variety occurs mainly in the cranial vault.

The sclerotic lesions produce a diffuse, often bilaterally symmetrical thickening of the floor of the anterior and middle cranial fossae (Fig. 105–26). The lesions usually involve a portion of or all of the sphenoid bone and its wings. There may be resultant foraminal encroachment, but cranial nerve

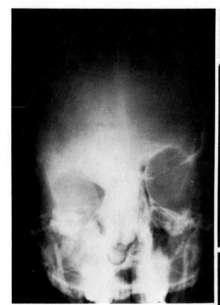
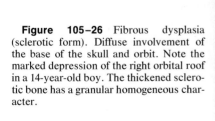
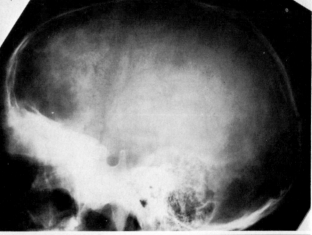
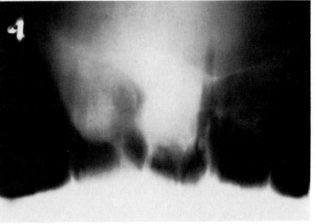

Figure 105–26 Fibrous dysplasia (sclerotic form). Diffuse involvement of the base of the skull and orbit. Note the marked depression of the right orbital roof in a 14-year-old boy. The thickened sclerotic bone has a granular homogeneous character.

deficits are unusual. This process may simulate the appearance of meningioma, especially if the lesion is unilateral. In general, the sclerotic form of fibrous dysplasia appears more homogeneous than meningioma bone, but in many cases accurate radiological differentiation cannot be made without angiography.

The mixed form is the least common of the three varieties. It simulates the cystic variety in that it occurs mainly in the vault, the diploë is widened, and the outer table is thinned. Intermixed with the expanded lucent areas, however, are patches of increased density similar to those seen in Paget's disease but more sharply defined. The process is generally fairly localized, unlike the more diffuse nature of Paget's disease.

Histologically, lesions of fibrous dysplasia appear as multiple areas of fibrous tissue contained within islands of bone with evidence of both blastic and clastic activity. Leeds and Seaman have reviewed the natural history of fibrous dysplasia in 15 patients followed over periods varying from 6 to 39 years.[42] Only 2 of the 15 patients showed any progression of their bony involvement, the other lesions remaining stable and unchanged. Generally, no treatment is advised unless orbital compression or involvement of neural foramina is evident. The lesions rarely undergo sarcomatous degeneration, and if an active increase in size or local inflammation becomes apparent, then total excision of the lesion with cranioplasty is the treatment of choice. It must be remembered that the area of fibrous dysplasia is extremely vascular, and blood loss during such an operative procedure is likely to be considerable. The process must be differentiated from osteogenic sarcoma and fibrosarcoma. When localized, it has also been designated as ossifying fibroma, though some authors feel this is a separate pathological process.

Osteitis Fibrosa Disseminata

In 1937, Albright and associates described a related syndrome that they termed osteitis fibrosa disseminata.[1] The disease is characterized by polyostotic fibrous dysplasia, an unusual pigmentation of the skin, and endocrine disturbance, especially precocious puberty in females, without hyperparathyroidism. The bony le-

sions of Albright's syndrome tend to be unilateral, but they do not present special radiographic features that distinguish them from fibrous dysplasia without extraosseous involvement.

REFERENCES

1. Albright, F., Butler, A. M., Hampton, A. O., and Smith, P.: Syndrome characterized by osteitis fibrosa disseminata, areas of pigmentation and endocrine dysfunction, with precocious puberty in females: report of five cases. New Eng. J. Med., *216*:727, 1937.
2. Berg, N. Landberg, T., and Lindgren, M.: Osteonecrosis and sarcoma following external irradiation of intracerebral tumors. Acta Radiol. Ther. (Stockholm), *4*:417–436, 1966.
3. Berkman, Y. M., and Blatt, E. S.: Cranial and intracranial cartilaginous tumors. Clin. Radiol., *9*:327–333, 1968.
4. Binet, E. F., Kieffer, S. A., Martin, S. H., and Peterson, H. O.: Orbital dysplasia in neurofibromatosis. Radiology, *93*:829–833, 1969.
5. Bishop, P. A.: Bone changes in chronic fluorine intoxication; roentgenographic study. Amer. J. Roentgen., *35*:577–585, 1936.
6. Bloom, D. L.: Mucoceles of the maxillary and sphenoid sinuses. Radiology, *85*:1103–1109, 1965.
7. Bromer, R. S.: Rickets. Amer. J. Roentgen., *30*:582–589, 1933.
8. Caffey, J.: Infantile cortical hyperostoses. J. Pediat., *29*:541–559, 1946.
9. Caffey, J.: Chronic poisoning due to excess of vitamin A. Amer. J. Roentgen., *65*:12–25, 1951.
10. Camp, J. D.: Osseous changes in hyperparathyroidism; roentgenologic study. J.A.M.A., *99*:1913–1917, 1932.
11. Camp, J. D.: Tumors of the scalp and skull and their significance as revealed by roentgenograms. Med. Clin. N. Amer., *25*:1103, 1941.
12. Carter, T. L., Gabrielsen, T. E., and Abell, M. R.: Mechanism of split cranial sutures in metastatic neuroblastoma. Radiology, *91*:467–470, 1968.
13. Chang, C. H., Piatt, E. D., Thomas, K. E., and Watne, A. L.: Bone abnormalities in Gardner's syndrome. Amer. J. Roentgen., *103*:645–652, 1968.
14. Chorobski, J., and Davis, L.: Cyst formation of skull. Surg., Gynec. Obstet., *58*:12–31, 1934.
15. Christensen, F. C.: Bone tumors: Analysis of 1,000 cases with special reference to location, age, and sex. Ann. Surg., *81*:1074–1092, 1925.
16. Christensen, W. R., Liebman, C., and Sosman, M. C.: Skeletal and periarticular manifestations of hypervitaminosis. Amer. J. Roentgen., *65*:27–41, 1951.
17. Cohn, I.: Sinus pericranii (Stromeyer), report of a case; review of the literature. Surg. Gynec. Obstet., 614–624, 1926.
18. Conley, J., Stout, A. P., and Healey, W. V.: Clinicopathologic analysis of eighty-four patients with an original diagnosis of fibrosarcoma of the head and neck. Amer. J. Surg., *114*:564–569, 1967.

19. Cooley, T. B., Witwer, E. R., and Lee, P.: Anemia in children with splenomegaly and peculiar changes in bones; report of cases. Amer. J. Dis. Child., *34*:347–363, 1927.

20. Coventry, M., and Dahlin, D. C.: Osteogenic sarcoma: A critical analysis of 430 cases. J. Bone Joint Surg., *48A*:1, 1966.

21. Craver, L. F., and Copeland, M. M.: Changes in bone in Hodgkin's granuloma. Arch. Surg., *28*:1062–1086, 1934.

22. Cushing, H., and Eisenhardt, L.: Meningiomas: Their Classification, Regional Behavior, Life History and Surgical End Results. Springfield, Ill., Charles C Thomas, 1938.

23. Dandy, W. E.: Dean Lewis Practice of Surgery, Vol. XII. Hagerstown, Md., W. F. Prior Co., 1932.

24. Dickson, D. D., Camp, J. D., and Ghormley, R. K.: Osteitis deformans: Paget's disease of the bone. Radiology, *44*:449–470, 1945.

25. DuBoulay, G. H.: Principles of x-ray diagnosis of the skull. New York, Butterworth & Co., Ltd., 1965.

26. Edeiken, J., and Hodes, P. J.: Roentgen Diagnosis of Diseases of Bone. Baltimore, Williams & Wilkins Co., 1967.

27. Epstein, J. A., and Epstein, B. S.: Deformities of the skull surfaces in infancy and childhood. J. Pediat., *70*:636–647, 1967.

28. Feiring, W. E., Feiring, H., and Davidoff, L. M.: Fibrous dysplasia of the skull. J. Neurosurg., *8*:377–397, 1951.

29. Fletcher, G. H., and Million, R. R.: Malignant tumors of the nasopharynx. Amer. J. Roentgen., *93*:44–55, 1965.

30. Friedman, M. M.: Neurofibromatosis of bone. Amer. J. Roentgen., *51*:623–630, 1944.

31. Furstenberg, A. C.: Osteomyelitis of skull: Osteogenetic processes in repair of cranial defects. Ann. Otol., *40*:996–1012, 1931.

32. Garland, L. H.: Osteogenic sarcoma of the skull. Radiology, *45*:45–48, 1945.

33. Geschickter, C. F.: Primary tumors of the cranial bones. Amer. J. Cancer, *26*:155–180, 1936.

34. Gold, L. H. A., Keiffer, S. A., and Peterson, H. O.: Intracranial meningiomas. A retrospective analysis of the diagnostic value of plain skull films. Neurology (Minneap.), *19*:873–878, 1969.

35. Gosepath, J., and Reisner, K.: On the clinical picture of malignant nasopharyngeal tumors with special reference to tomography with multidimensional spread. Z. Laryng. Rhinol. Otol. *47*:409–429, 1968.

36. Grinnan, A. G.: Roentgenologic bone changes in sickle-cell and erythroblastic anemia; report of 9 cases. Amer. J. Roentgen., *34*:297–309, 1935.

37. Haas, G. M.: Chordoma of cranium and cervical portion of spine: Review of literature with report of cases. Arch. Neurol. (Chicago), *32*:300–327, 1934.

38. Jaffee, H. L.: Tumors and Tumorous Conditions of the Bones and Joints. Philadelphia, Lea & Febiger, 1958.

39. Jaffe, N.: Calvarial bone defects involving the lambdoid suture in neurofibromatosis. Brit. J. Radiol., *38*:23–27, 1965.

40. Ketcham, A. S., Wilkins, R. H., Van Buren, J. M., and Smith, R. R.: A combined intra-cranial facial approach to the paranasal sinuses. Amer. J. Surg., *106*:698–703, 1963.

41. Knighton, R. S., and Fox, J. DeW.: Diagnosis and treatment of eosinophilic granuloma of skull. J.A.M.A., *162*:1294–1297, 1956.

42. Leeds, N., and Seaman, W.: Fibrous dysplasia of the skull and its differential diagnosis. Radiology, *78*:570, 1962.

43. Lichtenstein, L.: Histiocytosis X. Integration of eosinophilic granuloma of bone, "Letterer-Siwe disease" and "Schuller-Christian disease" as related manifestations of a single nosologic entity. A.M.A. Arch. Path., *56*:84–102, 1953.

44. Lichtenstein, L.: Bone Tumors. 3rd Ed. St. Louis, C. V. Mosby Co., 1965.

45. Matson, D. D.: Neurosurgery of Infancy and Childhood. Springfield, Ill., Charles C Thomas, 1969.

46. McNerney, J. C.: Giant cell tumors of bones of the skull. J. Neurosurg., *6*:169, 1949.

47. Minagi, H., and Newton, T. H.: Cartilaginous tumors of the base of the skull. Amer. J. Roentgen., *105*:308–313, 1969.

48. Moore, A. B.: A roentgenologic study of metastatic malignancy of bones. Amer. J. Roentgen., *6*:589–593, 1919.

49. Moore, S.: Hyperostosis Cranii. Springfield, Ill., Charles C Thomas, 1955.

50. Neuhauser, E. B. D., Schwachman, H., Wittenborg, M., and Cohen, J.: Progressive diaphyseal dysplasia. Radiology, *51*:11–22, 1948.

51. Olsen, T. G.: Sarcoidosis of the skull. Radiology, *80*:232–235, 1963.

52. Pool, J. L., Potanos, J. N., and Krueger, E. G.: Osteomas and mucoceles of the frontal paranasal sinuses. J. Neurosurg., *19*:130–135, 1962.

53. Powell, J. W., Weens, H. S., and Wenger, N. K.: The skull roentgenogram in iron deficiency anemia and in secondary polycythemia. Amer. J. Roentgen., *95*:143–147, 1965.

54. Rowbotham, G. F.: Neoplasms that grow from the bone forming elements of the skull. A survey of 20 cases. Brit. J. Surg., *45*:123–134, 1957.

55. Rumbaugh, C. L., and Potts, D. G.: Skull changes associated with intracranial arteriovenous malformations. Amer. J. Roentgen., *98*:525–534, 1966.

56. Spiller, W. G.: Hemicraniosis and cure of brain tumor by operation. J.A.M.A., *49*:2059, 1907.

57. Strange, V. M., and DeLorimier, A. A.: Reticulum cell sarcoma primary in skull; report of 3 cases. Amer. J. Roentgen., *71*:40–50, 1954.

58. Taveras, J. M., and Wood, E. H.: Diagnostic Neuroradiology. Baltimore, Williams & Wilkins Co., 1964.

59. Toglia, J. U., Netsky, M. G., and Alexander, E., Jr.: Epithelial (epidermoid) tumors of the cranium. Their common nature and pathogenesis. J. Neurosurg., *23*:384–393, 1965.

60. Van Buchem, F. S. B., Hadders, H. N., Hansen, J. F., and Woldring, M. G.: Hyperostosis corticalis generalisata. Report of seven cases. Amer. J. Med., *33*:387–397, 1962.

61. Vandenberg, H. J., Jr., and Coley, B. L.: Primary tumors of the cranial bones. Surg., Gynec. Obstet., *90*:602–612, 1950.

62. Vidgoff, B., and Bracher, G. J.: Osteopetrosis, report of a case. Amer. J. Roentgen., *44*:197–202, 1940.

63. Willis, R. A.: Metastatic neuroblastoma in bone, presenting the Ewing sarcoma with a discussion of "Ewing's sarcoma." Amer. J. Path., *16*:317–331, 1940.

64. Wyke, B. D.: Primary hemangioma of the skull: A rare cranial tumor. Amer. J. Roentgen., *61*:302–316, 1949.

65. Zimmerman, H. B.: Osteosclerosis in chronic renal disease. Amer. J. Roentgen., *88*:1152–1169, 1962.

106

NEUROSURGICAL ASPECTS OF CRANIOFACIAL NEOPLASIA

Neoplasms that arise in the marginal areas between routine neurosurgical and otolaryngological operative sites may be dilemmas for both disciplines. Indeed, in the past, many malignant paranasal sinus tumors were considered unresectable because of their proximity to, encroachment upon, or actual penetration into the cranial cavity. Management by excision of neoplasms in certain areas deep in the face and skull base is possible only with the combination of transcranial and transfacial approaches. As a result, a comprehensive understanding of the anatomical relationships between the deep facial structures and the floor of the cranial cavity is fundamental to the cooperative effort of the neurosurgeon and the otolaryngologist for the resection of these lesions.

ANATOMY

Maxillary Sinus

The maxillary sinus is a cavitation of the maxilla that is best envisaged as a box with an opening on its supramedial aspect that permits drainage through the lateral nasal wall into the middle meatus of the nose. The floor of the sinus is made up laterally by the maxillary alveolar bone and upper teeth, and medially by a small portion of the lateral roof of the oral cavity (Fig. 106–1). The anterior and lateral faces of the maxillary sinus are covered by the muscles of facial expression. The roof of the sinus is mainly made up by the floor of the orbit, but medially it has a common wall with the floor of the ethmoid sinus. Posteriorly a thin plate of bone separates the maxillary sinus from the pterygomaxillary space (Fig. 106–2). Contained within this space is the second division of the trigeminal nerve, which has reached this position by traversing the sphenoid bone through the foramen rotundum from the middle cranial fossa. Also contained within this space is a very important autonomic nerve that joins the maxillary nerve to subserve secretory motor and vasomotor functions to the nasal mucosa and lacrimal gland. This nerve, the vidian nerve or nerve of the pterygoid canal, traversing a canal of the same name from the foramen lacerum to the pterygomaxillary space, thus provides a route for tumor spread to the medial aspect of the middle fossa. From the neurosurgical point of view, the pterygomaxillary space can be thought of as being deep to the medial aspects of the middle fossa in the region of the foramina ovale and rotundum, and this is the area in which tumors that have spread to the pterygomaxillary space will make their appearance by eroding the intervening bone.

Ethmoid Sinus

The ethmoid sinuses are a labyrinth of small paranasal spaces that separate the medial wall of the orbit from the lateral wall of the nose (see Fig. 106–1 and Fig. 106–3).

G. CORKILL AND P. DONALD

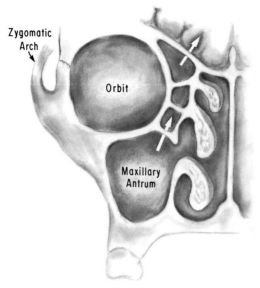

Figure 106-1 Coronal section of the head showing the relationship of the maxillary sinus and the ethmoid sinuses. Arrows indicate the route of intracranial spread of neoplasms from these cavities.

The roof of the sinus, the fovea ethmoidalis, is the floor of the anterior cranial fossa. The roof is extremely thin and extends to the region of the optic foramen. The cribriform plate forms an interconnecting bridge between the sinuses. The ethmoid block is narrower and shorter anteriorly than posteriorly. From the neurosurgical perspective, it is this area around the midline of the anterior fossa, ranging from the optic nerves posteriorly to in front of the cribriform plate anteriorly, that is the site of intracranial extension of tumors arising in the ethmoid sinuses. Operative management in this area will consist of monoblock resection without undue hazard to neurological structures other than the olfactory tracts.

Frontal Sinus

The frontal sinus is a pneumatization of the central portion of the vertical process of

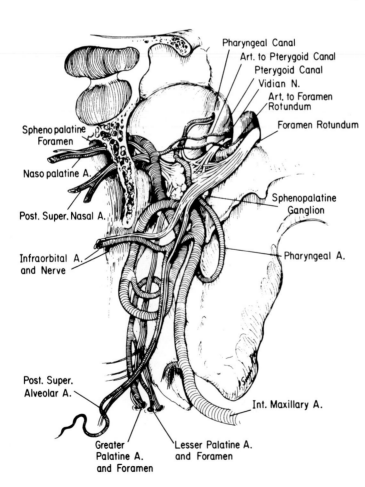

Figure 106-2 Contents of the pterygopalatine fossa. (From Morgenstein, K. M.: Surgery of the pterygopalatine fossa, *In* English, G. M., ed.: Otolaryngology. Hagerstown, Md., Harper & Row, 1976, Chapter 39, p. 3. Reprinted by permission.)

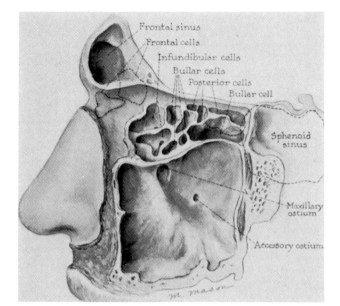

Figure 106-3 Parasagittal section through the head illustrating the ethmoid block. Note the various cell groups. (From Van Alyea, O. E.: Nasal Sinuses. Baltimore, The Williams & Wilkins Co., 1951. Reprinted by permission.)

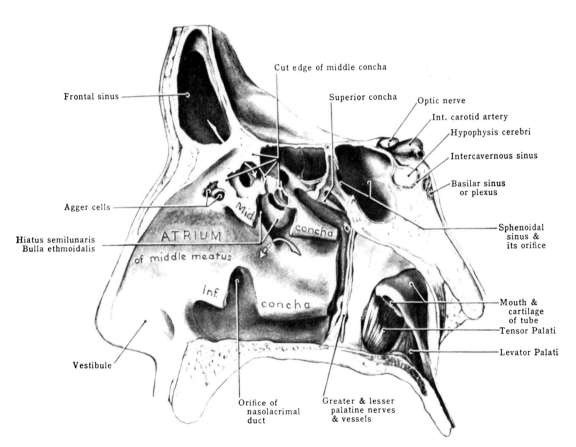

Figure 106-4 Parasagittal section through the head illustrating the frontal sinus, its drainage into the nose, and its relationship to the anterior cranial fossa. (Reproduced by permission from J. C. B. Grant's An Atlas of Anatomy, 7th Ed., copyright © 1978, The Williams & Wilkins Company.)

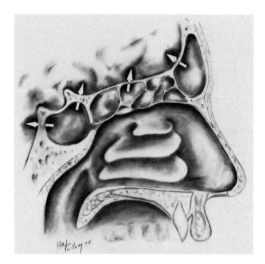

Figure 106–5 Parasagittal section through the head demonstrating the routes of spread of paranasal sinus neoplasms into the cranial cavity.

the frontal bone. The posterior wall of the sinus is extremely thin, permitting easy extension of a neoplasm into the anterior fossa (Fig. 106–4). In addition, lesions in the anterior ethmoid cells may pass superiorly through the floor of the frontal sinus and thence into the anterior fossa (Fig. 106–5). The frontonasal ducts permit access to tumor arising from the nasal cavities into the sinus and thence into the anterior fossa. This region is familiar to the neurosurgeon because of its frequent involvement in trauma, and he will have no difficulty in visualizing how posterior extensions of frontal sinus tumors will impinge upon intracranial contents.

Infratemporal Fossa

The infratemporal fossa lies on the lateral aspect of the skull deep to the zygomatic arch, the masseter muscle, and the ramus of the mandible. It contains mainly the body of the temporalis muscle. This space has direct continuity with the pterygomaxillary space through the pterygomaxillary fissure (Fig. 106–6). Tumors arising in the maxillary sinus or the nasopharynx can extend to the pterygomaxillary space and through the fissure into the infratemporal fossa. The portion of the sphenoid bone separating this space from the middle fossa is thin, permitting easy penetration by neoplasm. In contrast to tumors arising in the maxillary sinus, which will make their ap-

pearance in the medial aspect of the middle fossa, tumors arising from this space will encroach upon the lateral aspects of the middle fossa if they invade the intracranial space.

Nasopharynx

The nasopharynx is located at the posterior limit of the nasal cavities and is in continuity with them through the choanae. The roof is the clivus, the posterior wall the body of Cl, and the lateral walls, the eustachian tube and superior constrictor muscle (Fig. 106–7). Neoplasms in this location reach the cranial cavity by two main routes: (1) direct extension laterally through the foramen lacerum into the cavernous sinus; and (2) lateral growth through the eustachian tube into the temporal bone, giving access to the middle fossa through the tegmen tympani and tegmen mastoideum. If the tumor grows laterally it may reach the pterygomaxillary space and reach the cranial fossa by two additional routes. The first is through the foramina that empty into this space, and the second is by further lateral extension into the infratemporal fossa and then superiorly through the greater wing of the sphenoid into the middle fossa.

Temporal Bone

The superior aspect of the petrous part of the temporal bone is the floor of the middle fossa. The posterior aspect of the bone is the anterior part of the posterior fossa (Fig. 106–8). Entry to the temporal bone is provided by the eustachian tube, the jugular foramen, the carotid canal, and the stylomastoid foramen (Fig. 106–9). Lesions of the parotid gland can spread to the external auditory canal through the cartilaginous portion via the lymphatic channels of Santorini. Paragangliomas can enter the bone through its vascular foramina.

Primary neoplasms of the external auditory canal, middle ear, and mastoid easily penetrate the tegmen tympani and tegmen mastoideum to invade the middle fossa. Neoplasms of the statoacoustic and facial nerves can extend to the cranial cavity either by the internal auditory canal or by penetration through the thin roof of the mastoid air cell system.

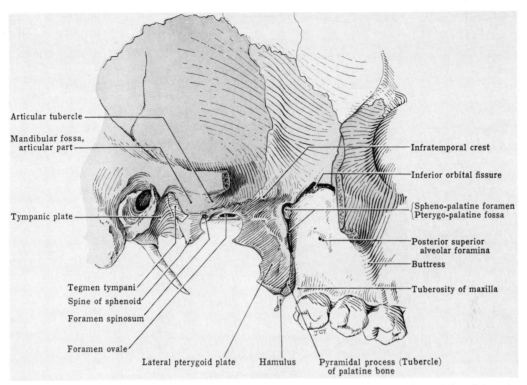

Figure 106–6 Infratemporal fossa. (Reproduced by permission from J. C. B. Grant's An Atlas of Anatomy, 7th Ed., copyright © 1978, The Williams & Wilkins Company.)

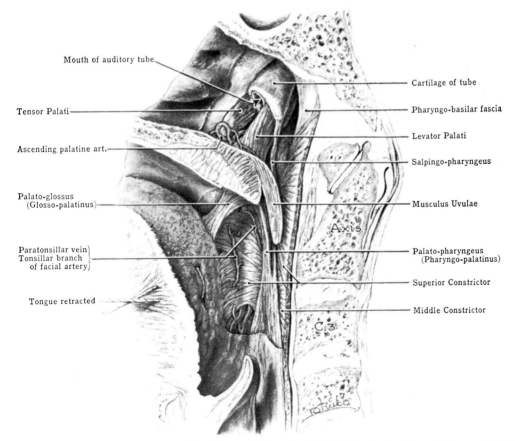

Figure 106–7 Nasopharynx. (Reproduced by permission from J. C. B. Grant's An Atlas of Anatomy, 7th Ed., copyright © 1978, The Williams & Wilkins Company.)

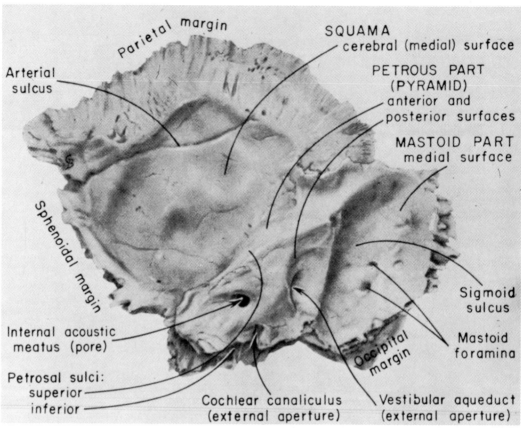

Figure 106–8   Medial view of the right temporal bone showing its relationships to the middle and posterior cranial fossae. (From Anson, B. J., and Donaldson, J. A.: Surgical Anatomy of the Temporal Bone and Ear. 2nd Ed. Philadelphia, W. B. Saunders Co., 1973, p. 6. Reprinted by permission.)

BASIC CONCEPTS

Basically a craniofacial operation for cancer is a combined effort by the neurological surgeon and the otorhinolaryngologist to remove tumors through a craniotomy and a transfacial approach. The reluctance of neurosurgeons to participate in such a venture is understandable when one considers the risk of potential intracranial infection that is posed by the transfacial approach. Contamination of the field by intraoral, nasal, and paranasal contents is an unavoidable problem during the exposure of most of these tumors. Reduction of bacterial flora in the mouth is achieved by preparing the oral cavity with Betadine. Trimming the nasal vibrissae and scrubbing the nasal vestibule with antiseptic partially sterilize the nose. The interposition of an antibiotic-soaked towel between the craniotomy and the facial incisions helps to further isolate the cranial cavity from the upper aerodigestive tract until the final moments of delivery of the specimen and during the initial stages of closure. The use of prophylactic antibiotics before, during, and following operation is the final step in prophylaxis. In the authors' experience of 25 cases, postoperative infection has been a problem in only one, that of a patient who died of a brain abscess three months postoperatively. Quite probably, her abscess was related to an unobliterated cavity between the frontal bone and the brain. Scrupulous avoidance of dead space in subsequent cases has eliminated this problem. Once the diagnosis has been made and the necessary tests have been performed, the neurosurgeon and the otorhinolaryngologist should discuss the plans of each for the incisions and dissection. It is mutually beneficial to be present for one another's part of the operation. Both surgeons must be present for the delivery of the specimen and the initial steps of the closure. The postopera-

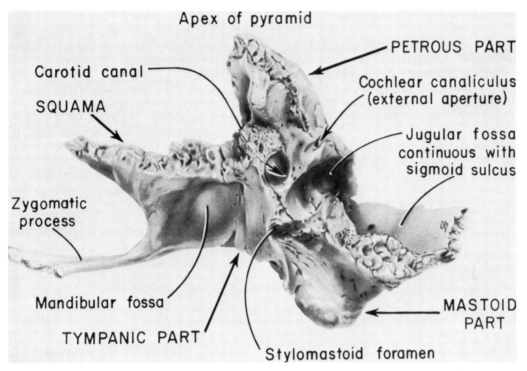

Apex of pyramid

PETROUS PART

Carotid canal

Cochlear canaliculus
(external aperture)

SQUAMA

Jugular fossa
continuous with
sigmoid sulcus

Zygomatic
process

Mandibular fossa

MASTOID
PART

TYMPANIC PART

Stylomastoid foramen

Figure 106–9 Base view of the temporal bone demonstrating the foramina that provide access for tumor to the intracranial cavity. (From Anson, B. J., and Donaldson, J. A.: Surgical Anatomy of the Temporal Bone and Ear. 2nd Ed. Philadelphia, W. B. Saunders Co., 1973, p. 9. Reprinted by permission.)

tive management, although a shared responsibility, falls primarily on the neurosurgeon initially, as the most important early complications usually are intracranial.

DISEASE ENTITIES

Esthesioneuroblastoma

This rare neoplasm arises in the nasal vault or the superior nasal meatus. It has its origin in neural crest cells rather than, as earlier thought, from the esthesioneuroblast, the stem cell of olfactory epithelium.[5,15]

In macroscopic appearance, this tumor is an encapsulated firm, brown to pinkish, lobulated mass, usually without evidence of ulceration. Microscopic appearance is characterized by neuroblasts and neurocytes in proportions that vary from lesion to lesion. Other features include fibrillar material, pseudorosettes, and true rosettes. Classification according to cellular maturation and rosette formation, such as that of Mendelhoff, has no bearing on clinical be-

havior or prognosis.[15] Certain ultrastructural appearances have made possible a definitive differentiation of this lesion from the sarcomas or poorly differentiated epithelial neoplasms.[12] The electron microscopic findings of neurites and secretory granules is diagnostic of esthesioneuroblastoma. These granules can be made to fluoresce in a histochemical test using formaldehyde fumes. The biogenic amines within the granules are responsible for this reaction. Judge and co-workers state that this test is even more diagnostic than electron microscopy.[11] The histological pattern of the tumor appears benign, but the local recurrence rate and the 20 per cent metastatic spread belie this histological interpretation.[21] The mode of spread is superiorly through the cribriform plate and laterally via the ethmoid sinuses through the fovea ethmoidalis to the anterior fossa. Metastases are to cervical lymph nodes, lungs, and the skeletal system.

Clinical Presentations

Presenting symptoms include nasal obstruction, epistaxis, anosmia, and purulent drainage. If the tumor is large, the nose may be swollen. On intranasal examination, however, there is invariably a brownish-red polypoid lesion. There is a definite capsule and usually no evidence of invasion. The lesion is often mistaken for an inflammatory nasal polyp. Extensive tumors may produce proptosis and a mass effect in the region of the inferior orbital fissure. Preliminary sinus x-rays are essential, augmented by coronal plane tomography. These studies will show the extent of bony erosion and possible evidence of intracranial invasion. The diagnosis is established by biopsy, which can be done under local anesthesia in a clinic setting.

Treatment

The operative excision is done through a lateral rhinotomy (Fig. 106–10). An external ethmoidectomy is performed, and the lesion is excised from the nasal vault. These tumors are relatively radioresistant and tend to recur early if treated with even high-dosage radiation therapy. Moreover, if they are so treated, operating later for recurrence through an irradiated field is fraught with difficulty and accompanied by a high complication rate. Neurosurgical treatment will be necessitated by any intracranial extension. The usual sites of penetration are the cribriform plate and the fovea ethmoidalis. The penetration will be suggested by defects in the floor of the anterior fossa as evidenced by tomography. The performance of air studies may be considered but probably will not be useful unless the tumor extension is particularly large. A CT scan may suggest but cannot exclude intracranial extension.

Since the olfactory tract will be sacrificed, the preoperative discussion should inform the patient that he will have anosmia. The combined operative approach calls for neurosurgical exposure of the floor of the anterior fossa and immobilization extradurally of the frontal lobes as in the pro-

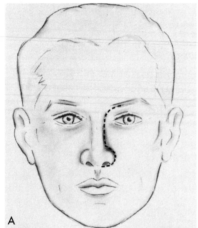

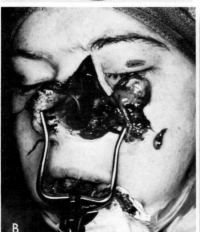

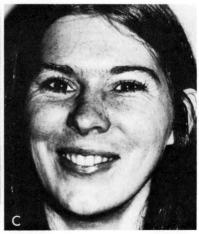

Figure 106–10 *A*. Lateral rhinotomy incision. *B*. Esthesioneuroblastoma being excised through a lateral rhinotomy incision. *C*. Appearance of the patient six months after combined operative and radiation therapy.

cedure for the repair of a cerebrospinal fluid fistula of the cribriform plate region. The aim is to facilitate an en bloc resection of the affected bone in this area of the base of the brain. If the tumor has extended through the dura, a macroscopic resection of the tumor should still be performed. A dural graft should follow.

If the dura over the area involved with the tumor can be retracted, then resection of the tumor from below by the otorhinolaryngologist can be accomplished. Interposing a sponge between the dura and the brain will make the removal of the bone safer. An alternative is for the neurosurgeon to tap out with a chisel the involved portion of the anterior midline fossa from above. From this position, however, he cannot see the extent of the tumor in the sinus, and therefore the former technique is preferred.

Results

Approximately 160 cases of esthesioneuroblastoma have been reported in the world literature. The most extensive review was by Skolnik and co-workers, who in 1966 reviewed the 97 cases in the literature at that time.[21] They found the five-year survival rate to be 52 per cent, but 50 per cent of the patients who died had local recurrences. The craniofacial approach was used in very few of these cases. Schenck and Ogura reported on eight cases in their experience in 1972.[19] They recommended resection followed by radiation, but did not use the combined approach for the resection. Cantrell and associates reported on 12 cases and had their best results with craniofacial excision and preoperative irradiation.[5]

Carcinoma of the Paranasal Sinuses

The poor prognosis of malignant diseases in the paranasal sinus areas was, in the past, often related to their proximity to the floor of the cranial cavity. The use of combined craniofacial operations has, however, revolutionized the treatment of these lesions.

Although the etiology of carcinomas of the head and neck area remains obscure, these lesions seem quite definitely to be re-lated to heavy cigarette smoking and excessive alcohol ingestion. An increased incidence of ethmoid sinus carcinoma was found by Acheson and associates in hardwood furniture workers.[1] Also, a large number of patients who contracted maxillary sinus carcinoma were found to have had a history of chronic sinusitis.[3,16]

Malignant neoplasms of the paranasal sinuses are most commonly squamous cell in type, with adenocarcinomas as the next largest group (Fig. 106–11).[3] Squamous cell tumors run the gamut of differentiation usually seen in other sites. The most common adenocarcinoma is the adenoid cystic variety. Microscopically, squamous cell carcinoma appears as sheets and islands of cells rich in eosinophilic cytoplasm with hyperchromatic nuclei of highly variable size and shape. There are frequent mitotic figures. The demonstration of desmosomes and the presence of pearls of keratin material are characteristic of the most differentiated type. As differentiation becomes more anaplastic the disappearance of squamous pearls, the diminution of cytoplasm, and the absence of desmosomes become more apparent. The most anaplastic of the squamous cell carcinomas are frequently indistinguishable from poorly differentiated adenocarcinomas and sarcomas of similiar differentiation. The adenoid cystic carcinoma is characterized by a monotonous array of cells comprising scant cytoplasm and highly hyperchromatic nuclei arranged in sheets and cords with frequent circular cystic spaces, which give it its name.

The carcinomatous process within the sinus expands it and then erodes through its walls, extending into adjacent sinuses as well as fissures and foramina, which eventually leads to breakthroughs into the interior confines of the cranial vault. There appears to be an unusual propensity for sinus neoplasms to extend into adjacent sinus cavities. This propensity may be the result of the often exceeding thinness of the walls that separate one cavity from the next and the fact that, once this cavity is gained, there is no local tissue resistance.

Signs and Symptoms

Maxillary Sinus

The symptoms of maxillary sinus neoplasms are often ascribed by the patient to

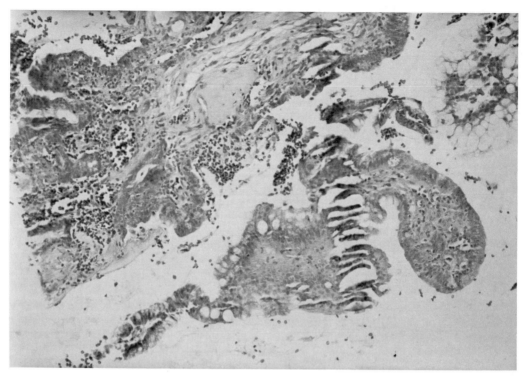

Figure 106–11   Adenocarcinoma of ethmoid sinus.

adjacent structures. Swelling extending through the floor may cause the patient to complain of an ill-fitting denture, loose teeth, an ulcerating mass in the hard palate, or even the presence of an antraoral fistula (Fig. 106–12). Extension through the anterior wall presents as numbness over the cheek and adjacent portion of the nose due to involvement of the infraorbital nerve. Swelling of the cheek and, eventually, ulceration through the facial skin are seen in advanced cases. Involvement of the medial wall of the sinus, which is also the lateral wall of the nose, may result in tumor presenting as a mass occupying the nasal fossa. Nasal obstruction, epistaxis, foul purulent discharge, and even swelling of the nasal framework are commonly encountered symptoms in lesions with this extension. Superior extension can result in proptosis, as shown in Figure 106–13, epiphora from involvement of the nasolacrimal duct, and if posterior superior involvement ensues, paralysis of the eye and blindness.

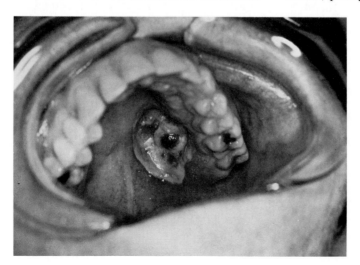

Figure 106–12 Adenocarcinoma of left maxillary sinus presenting as a mass in the palate.

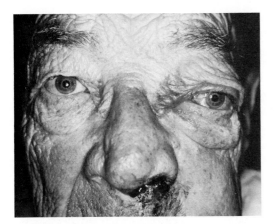

Figure 106-13 Squamous cell carcinoma of the left maxillary and ethmoid sinuses.

Posterior extensions will result in ablation of the function of the second division of the fifth cranial nerve as it crosses the pterygomaxillary space.

Ethmoid Sinus

Lesions of the ethmoid sinuses often are occult and often do not become apparent until they erode into the nose or the orbit or present with neurological signs from extension into the cranial cavity. The erosion into the nose often appears as a benign nasal polyp. Orbital extension will cause proptosis and lateral displacement of the globe. These tumors may present as predominantly neurosurgical problems due to upward extension that involves various cranial nerves. Unilateral anosmia, visual field defects, decreased visual acuity, and ophthalmoplegia may be early manifestations of upward extensions of this tumor.

Radiographic evidence of extension of disease is best seen with coronal plane tomography (Fig. 106–14).

Sphenoid Sinus

The sphenoid sinus is rarely involved with primary neoplasm; extension from the ethmoid sinuses is not uncommon, however. Symptoms relating to involvement of the sphenoid sinus are due to the effect on structures adjacent to it: the pituitary, the contents of the cavernous sinuses, the optic chiasm, and the superior orbital fissure.

Radiologically, extensive erosion of the pituitary fossa with or without an associated mucocele as a cause may raise the

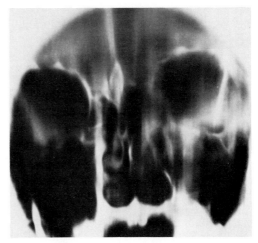

Figure 106-14 Coronal plane tomogram showing extensive bony destruction of the medial and superior orbital walls by an extensive squamous cell carcinoma of the ethmoid sinuses.

suspicion of intrasellar disease such as neoplasms and parasellar disease such as neoplasms and aneurysms. The predominant age groups for these lesions are the same as for the sinus tumor.

Treatment of Malignant Sinus Tumors

Unless they are very small the treatment for these lesions usually involves combining an operation and radiation therapy. Because of the 27 per cent incidence of retropharyngeal lymph node involvement, postoperative radiation therapy is strongly advised.[10] If central extension is encountered irradiation must be delayed until the area of resection has healed.

For the maxillary sinus, the traditional Weber-Ferguson incision is made, exposing the maxilla to facilitate a total maxillectomy and orbital exenteration (Fig. 106–15). This operative approach is followed by combined intracranial and extracranial excision of the floor of the anterior fossa and any involved adjacent dura and frontal lobe. A lateral rhinotomy incision gives access to tumors in the ethmoid bloc (Fig. 106–16). Neurosurgical participation involves resection of portions of the floor of the anterior fossa by a standard bicoronal approach (Fig. 106–17). An antibiotic-soaked sponge should be interposed between the retracted frontal lobes and the floor. Exposure can be further aided by intraoperative lumbar spinal fluid drainage. This exposure will enable the otorhinolaryngologist working from

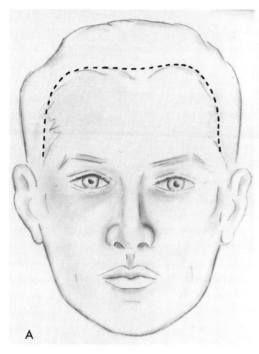

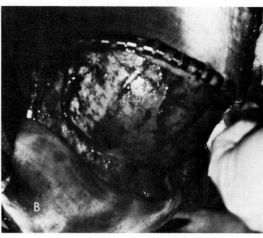

Figure 106–15 *A.* Coronal incision outlined. *B.* Coronal incision with the scalp covered with an antibiotic-soaked wrapping, which is sometimes called Cushing's veil.

below to make the definitive dissection without damaging the brain.

Defects in the dura are due to extension of the tumor. Excision of the tumor, the involved dura, and silent subfrontal cortex of the brain should be accomplished and the dura repaired with a graft (Fig. 106–18). Fascia lata is preferred for repairing the dural defect, since inorganic material may promote a long-lasting infection. In the absence of overt preoperative sinus infection, however, acrylic may be used, or the defect may be repaired by a procedure from below. Reflection of a periosteal flap from

the floor of the anterior fossa and the anterior wall of the anterior fossa and use of a nasal septal cartilage flap are also useful procedures when needed for repair of such defects.

Postoperatively, the possibility of a cerebrospinal fluid leak is a significant consideration. Specimens from the patient's nasopharynx should be cultured. Appropriate antibiotics should be given before, during, and after the operation for any flora that are grown. If none are grown, then ampicillin usually is sufficient as a prophylactic measure. The patients should be warned against

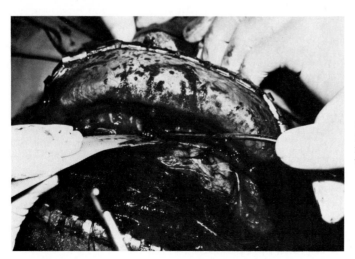

Figure 106–16 Standard bicoronal craniotomy to expose tumor in the floor of the anterior cranial fossa. The sucker on the right side of the illustration points to the tumor.

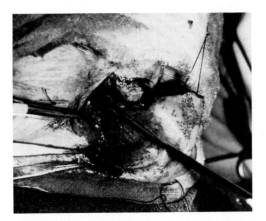

Figure 106–17 Lateral rhinotomy portion of craniofacial resection of an adenocarcinoma of the ethmoid sinus.

sneezing or raising the pressure in their mouths. The anesthesiologists should have impressed upon them the need for a clear airway. The patients are probably best nursed at a 45-degree angle rather than fully recumbent in order to minimize increased intracranial pressure, 45 degrees being optimal because the nose and forehead are then the highest part of the head. A fully erect posture will make for negative pressures in the head, tending to suck air in, and recumbent posture will tend to lead to leakage and pooling of cerebrospinal fluid in the operative area and on into the nasopharynx. In the postoperative period these patients may be anemic. Their hemoglobin should be adjusted to the normal range of values by packed cell transfusion.

Results

The largest series of cases was published in 1974 by Ketchum and associates. They analyzed 48 cases operated upon over a 14-year period. Their five-year survival rate

was 53 per cent. Serious complications were encountered in 15 patients, and minor complications were seen in 19 patients. In the former group there were six cases of meningitis; two of these patients died, and these were the only hospital deaths.[13]

Sisson and colleagues reported eight cases that were treated over a 15-year experience with no postoperative deaths and a low morbidity rate. They have three survivors free of disease at eight, four, and two years, and two cases under one year. The three remaining patients died of recurrent disease.[20]

Carcinoma of the Ear

Malignant tumors of the ear most commonly involve the auricle and are eminently amenable to local resection. Cancers of the external auditory canal, middle ear, and mastoid, however, present the greatest challenge (Fig. 106–19).

Their cause is unknown. In the external auditory canal, basal cell and squamous cell tumors are most common. The ceruminoma is a rare neoplasm that arises from the cerumen glands and behaves much like adenocarcinoma. The tumors can invade the middle ear space and extend into the eustachian tube, but more importantly, can erode the thin tegmental area of the middle ear space and mastoid to then gain entry into the middle cranial fossa.

Signs and Symptoms

The patient usually presents with a long-standing history of otorrhea. The drainage usually is thin and foul smelling, and often is tinged with blood. An important diagnostic sign is the presence of persistent pain

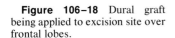

Figure 106–18 Dural graft being applied to excision site over frontal lobes.

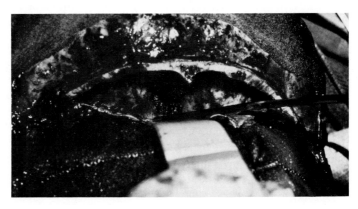

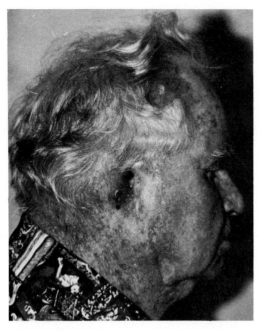

Figure 106–19   Squamous cell carcinoma of external auditory canal.

despite vigorous systemic and local treatment with antibiotics and antibiotic-steroid drops. As the disease advances, loss of hearing, vertigo, and facial nerve paralysis indicate widespread extension of disease and the necessity for rapid intervention.

Investigation should include polytomography of the temporal bone, an audiogram to assess hearing, and electronystagmography to assess the intactness of the vestibular system. Facial nerve paralysis should be investigated by direct electrical nerve stimulation studies, electromyography, and Schirmer testing. These procedures will establish the topographical and anatomical level of involvement of the nerve. Definitive diagnosis is made by biopsy.

Treatment

Resection of the temporal bone presents a formidable challenge. The bone is not only the hardest in the body, but it is also totally encircled by vascular structures.* The approach necessary to resect the tumor requires an exposure of the internal jugular vein, the internal carotid artery, the lateral and sigmoid sinuses, the superior and inferior petrosal sinuses, and the middle menin-

------

* See references 4, 6, 8, 9, 17, 18, 22.

geal artery (Fig. 106–20). The great vessels are exposed in the neck and controlled both for intraoperative safety at the time of excision of the bone and for identification of their foramina in the temporal bone's base.

Neurosurgical participation in the management of these patients consists of the extension of a craniectomy over the temporal lobe in the extradural plane posteriorly. The upper surface of the petrous bone is skeletonized just 1 cm medial to the arcuate eminence to facilitate the monoblock resection of the involved part of the temporal bone. At this stage, difficulty with bleeding from the venous structures arises, as the jugular vein is often electively occluded below. Separate ligation of the superior petrosal sinus, 5 mm proximal to its junction with the sigmoid sinus, is a decided advantage, and the ligation of the sigmoid sinus itself should be achieved by turning dural flaps above and below and incorporating them in the ligatures. When this has been accomplished the operation should be returned to the otorhinolaryngologist for completion. Retraction of the temporal lobes extradurally may be necessary to facilitate bone and tumor removal and to provide adequate exposure of the carotid artery in order to avoid injuring it.

Exposure of the block then proceeds with skeletonization of the sigmoid sinus inferiorly to the mastoid tip and deep to the facial nerve. Parotidectomy with dissection of the facial nerve is then done, and the nerve is cut at the distal end of the main trunk. The sternocleidomastoid muscle is separated from the bone as well as the posterior belly of the digastric muscle. The glenoid fossa is exposed by removal of the condylar head and neck of the mandible. The zygomatic arch is then cut across, and the definitive cuts in the temporal bone are made for en bloc resection. The defect in the squamous temporal bone is connected with a burr through the glenoid fossa to expose the bony eustachian tube canal. This bone cut is then directed inferior to the styloid process, with care taken to avoid the internal carotid artery medially. A curved osteotome cut is placed medial to the arcuate eminence and combined with cuts on the posterior surface of the petrous bone, the sigmoid sinus posteriorly being retracted, and connected to an inferior cut on the bone at the insertion of the styloid process. Gentle rocking of the osteotome

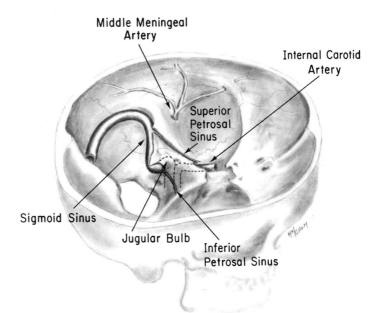

Figure 106–20 Oblique view of temporal bone with surrounding vasculature.

usually splits the bone along the carotid canal and the jugular foramen. The bone is then removed en bloc. In the age group most affected, the elderly, the dura is often attenuated and is easily torn. Tearing of the dura usually is of no consequence as long as adequate attention is paid to its repair. Special emphasis should be placed on the need to provide dural cover over area where the pia has also been violated and damaged brain is exposed. Where the pia and subarachnoid space are intact, the repair can be less meticulous. This is an important consideration in this area where dural repair is not always particularly easy. The defect is repaired with a dural graft of fat from the side of the abdomen, and the wound is closed with drains.

Postoperative care is the same as that described for the period following removal of the ethmoid and sphenoid sinus lesions.

Results

Lewis and Page reported experience of over 100 cases and had a five-year survival rate of 30 per cent.[14] Conley gave a cure rate of 25 per cent in his series of 100 cases and recommended combined radiation and operative treatment.[7] More recently, Gacek and Goodman reported a cure rate of 51.4 per cent in 37 patients who were followed for two or more years and who had either an operation alone or an operation plus radiotherapy.[8] Arena had a 41.7 per cent survival rate in 24 cases, although 2 cases had less than one year follow-up.[2]

REFERENCES

1. Acheson, E. D., Cowdell, R. H., Hadfield, E., and MacBeth, R. G.: Nasal cancer in woodworkers in the furniture industry. Brit. Med. J., 2:587–596, 1968.
2. Arena, S.: Tumor surgery of the temporal bone. Laryngoscope, 84:645–670, 1974.
3. Batsakis, J. G.: Tumors of the Head and Neck—Clinical and Pathological Considerations. Baltimore, Williams & Wilkins, 1974.
4. Campbell, E. H., Valk, B. M., and Burkland, C. W.: Total resection of the temporal bone for malignancy of the middle ear. Amer. J. Surg., 134:397–404, 1951.
5. Cantrell, R. W., Ghorayeb, B. Y., and Fitz-Hugh, G. S.: Esthesioneuroblastoma: Diagnosis and treatment. Ann. Otol., 86:760–765, 1977.
6. Conley, J.: Cancer of the middle ear. Ann. Otol., 74:555–572, 1965.
7. Conley, J.: Cancer of the ear. In Concepts in Head and Neck Surgery. New York, Grune & Stratton, 1970, pp. 69–70.
8. Gacek, R. R., and Goodman, M.: Management of malignancy of the temporal bone. Laryngoscope, 87:1622–1634, 1977.
9. Hilding, D. A., and Selker, R.: Total resection of the temporal bone for carcinoma. Arch. Otolaryng. (Chicago), 89:636–645, 1969.
10. Hilger, J. A.: Maxilloethmoidal carcinoma. Otolaryng. Clin. N. Amer., 2:543–546, 1969.
11. Judge, K. M., McGavran, M. D., and Trapukdi, S.: Fume-induced fluorescence in diagnosis of nasal neuroblastoma. Arch. Otolaryng., 102:97–98, 1976.
12. Kahn, L. B.: Esthesioneuroblastoma: A light and electron microscopic study. Hum. Path., 5:364–371, 1974.

13. Ketchum, A. S., Chretien, P. B., Shour, L., Herdt, J. R., Ommaya, A. K., and Van Buren, J. M.: Surgical treatment of patients with advanced cancer of the paranasal sinuses. *In* Anderson Hospital: Neoplasia of the Head and Neck. Chicago, Year Book Medical Publishers, Inc., 1974, pp. 187–202.

14 Lewis, J. S., and Page, R.: Radical surgery for malignant tumors of the ear. Arch. Otolaryng. (Chicago), *83*:114–119, 1966.

15. Mendeloff, J.: The olfactory neuroepithelial tumors. Cancer, *10*:944–956, 1957.

16. Montgomery, W. W.: Surgery of the Upper Respiratory System. Vol. 1. Philadelphia, W. B. Saunders Co., 1971.

17. Parsens, H., and Lewis, J. S.: Subtotal resection of the temporal bone for cancer of the ear. Cancer *7*:995–1001, 1954.

18. Ruben, R. J., Thaler, S. U., and Halzer, N.: Radiation induced carcinoma of the temporal bone. Laryngoscope, *87*:1613–1621, 1977.

19. Schenck, N. L., and Ogura, J. H.: Esthesioneuroblastoma: An enigma in diagnosis, a dilemma in treatment. Arch. Otolaryng. (Chicago), *96*:322–324, 1972.

20. Sisson, G. A., Bytell, D. E., Becker, S. P., and Ruge, D.: Carcinoma of the paranasal sinuses and cranial-facial resection. J. Laryng, *90*:59–68, 1976.

21. Skolnik, E. M., Massari, F. S., and Tenta, L. T.: Olfactory neuroepithelioma. Arch. Otolaryng. (Chicago), *84*:84–93, 1966.

22. Ward, G. E., Loch, W. W., and Lawrence, W., Jr.: Radical operation for carcinoma of the external auditory canal and middle ear. Amer. J. Surg., *82*:169–178, 1951.

107

GLOMUS JUGULARE TUMOR

The first description of the cellular base that gives origin to the glomus jugulare tumor was made by Valentine in 1840.[43] In 1905, Mönckeberg described the tumors of the carotid body, or chemodectomas.[35] Bloom reported similar tumors from other locations.[4] The first accurate description of a small mass of tissue lying in the dome of the bulb of the internal jugular vein was given by Guild in 1941. Guild also gave the mass the name glomus jugulare.[8] The structure is similar to the carotid body and other chemoreceptive organs. The first discovery of a tumor of the glomus jugulare was made by Rosenwasser in 1945.[40]

The chemodectomas resemble paragangliomas except that the latter contain chromaffin cells, whereas the chemodectomas do not. They consist of numerous rounded or ovoid hypochromatic cells arranged in alveolar-like groups within a scanty fibrous stroma. The tumor is richly supplied by blood vessels of capillary and precapillary caliber and is also richly supplied by neural elements from the glossopharyngeal nerve.

The most extensive store of information about this tumor is to be found in the otological literature. Because of the location and accessibility to operative treatment of these lesions, otologists have classified, divided, and subdivided them.[2,5,28,31,40] Many otologists have removed those that were readily accessible and have treated others with radiation. Combined otological neurosurgical ventures have been reported.[29,34] In the author's experience, these tumors do not respond to radiation. They invade the base of the skull, and their neurosurgical treatment requires intensive effort.[14]

CLASSIFICATION OF TUMORS

Glomus jugulare tumors originate from cell groups normally no larger than 0.25 to 0.5 mm in diameter. These minute bodies may lie under the mucosa of the medial wall of the middle ear and along the course of the tympanic nerve. It is likely that in some cases the neoplasm originates from these cell bodies, which would explain why in about 50 per cent of the cases reported the tumor appears to remain restricted to the middle ear. According to some otologists, the glomus jugulare, located in the adventitia of the jugular bulb, gives rise to a tumor that is much faster growing and more destructive than the one arising on the cochlear promontory. The author's observations make these conclusions most difficult to maintain. Only a thin plate of bone separates the internal jugular bulb from the tympanic cavity, and this thin plate is readily destroyed by a tumor arising either within the tympanic cavity or from the bulb of the internal jugular vein. Some tumors are confined within the jugular foramen and extend within the lumen of the internal jugular vein, reaching two thirds of the distance down the neck and even into the anastomotic veins to the external jugular vein; other tumors have an upward extension, staying completely within the sigmoid-transverse and superior and inferior petrosal sinuses. One patient (a 43-year-old woman) was treated for years for pseudotumor. Her venous sinogram was first interpreted as classic for transverse-sigmoid sinus thrombosis due to "otitic hydrocephalus.'' After some years this patient took a rapid turn for the worse, with severe papilledema, hemorrhages, and failing vision. At this time repeat sinograms revealed extension of the ''thrombosis'' over the torcular, partially occluding the transverse sinus on the opposite side and also reaching a short distance into the superior sagittal sinus. It was only when the x-ray of the base of the skull was compared with pictures taken 12 months previously that a slight enlargement of the jugular foramen was appreciated. This was seven years after the diagnosis of ''pseudotumor'' was first made. The patient had no signs relating to cranial nerves IX, X, or XI. The jugular foramen was exposed, a biopsy was taken, and the jugular bulb and part of the internal jugular vein were excised. Tumor tissue was removed from the sinus by suction. She made an uneventful recovery.

The patient just mentioned demonstrates that the tumor can stay a long time within an area where its growth follows existing channels without bony erosion and invasion. Another point can be made about this particular patient: her tumor had no outstanding arterial vascular supply. (The blood supply is the most important aspect of the author's classification system.) The patient has selective vertebral, and internal and external carotid angiography, including injection of the common carotid artery. Only one ''suspicious'' vessel of the external carotid artery could, with some hindsight, be said to be contributing to the tumor.

The criteria for classification of glomus jugulare tumors are their vascular supply and the size of the tumor.

Class 1. The small tumor of the middle ear is seen through the tympanic membrane as a bulging, reddish-blue mass. The presenting symptoms of this lesion usually are tinnitus, conductive hearing loss, facial weakness, and bleeding from the ear. The tumor can be totally removed through a transmeatal approach.

Class 2. The tumor stays totally within the lumen of the jugular bulb or may have an extension within the cranial sinus and veins in the neck.

Class 3. The tumor enlarges the jugular foramen but does not erode it. There are no clinical signs or symptoms relating to cranial nerves IX, X, and XI.

Class 4. The tumor causes enlargement of the jugular foramen and erosion of its wall, and extends to mastoid bone. There are symptoms of involvement of cranial nerves IX, X, and XI but no facial involvement. All these lesions show feeding vessels from the extracranial portion of the vertebral artery in addition to the feeding vessels from the external carotid artery. No vessels come from the intracranial portion of the vertebral artery. Even tumors that occupy the entire petrous bone, erode the dura, and invade the posterior fossa are not fed by any intrathecal vessel. These tumors have feeding vessels from the external carotid artery. Even though the tumor is still relatively small, careful subtraction angiography may make it possible to identify the ascending pharyngeal artery supplying the neoplasm. The surgeon removing these lesions must pay special attention to maintaining the facial nerve and avoiding any penetration of the bony structures of the vestibular and otic systems.

Class 5. This group includes any tumor that extends far enough into the petrous portion of the temporal bone to have involved or destroyed the function of the seventh and eighth cranial nerves and possibly also to cause signs relating to involvement of the fifth cranial nerve. The entire petrous bone may have been eroded, the tumor reaching into the posterior aspect of the cavernous sinus and into the parapharyngeal tissue of the neck. All these tumors obtain their vascular supply from the external carotid artery, the extracranial part of the vertebral artery, and the petrous portion and occasionally the proximal intracavernous portion of the internal carotid artery. Although still amenable to operative treatment, this tumor presents an added technical problem and risk because of the vascular supply from the internal carotid artery.

Class 6. In this group are lesions that have crossed the midline of the skull and have reached over the clivus and into the cavernous sinus bilaterally, revealing feeding vessels from both internal carotid arteries and thereby presenting a formidable operative undertaking. The operation was especially difficult before an embolization technique was used to block the feeding vessels of the glomus jugulare tumor.[13] In the author's experience, only tumors of this group metastasize. Besides regional lymph node involvement, metastases to the lung and the ribs have been seen. The metastatic lesions revealed the typical small nests of trabeculae of solid, tightly packed polygonal cells separated by blood channels that may range in size from capillaries to large thin-walled sinuses resembling the blood channels in a cavernous hemangioma.

DIAGNOSIS

Middle ear involvement is manifest in the majority of patients by conductive or perceptive deafness, depending on the extent of the tumor. Otorrhea—especially with a bloody discharge—pain in the ear, and tinnitus are also frequently encountered. In rare cases, a pitched bruit is heard over the mastoid process. A bluish mass may be visible through the tympanic membrane. There may be unilateral progressive paralysis of the ninth, tenth and eleventh cranial nerves; and on progression of the disease, the twelfth cranial nerve and the facial nerve are the next most frequently involved. At this later stage the patient may show signs and symptoms relating to the fifth cranial nerve. It is to be remembered that these nerves are infiltrated and compressed in their extradural course. Finally,

when the tumor forms an intracranial mass, unsteadiness of gait, nystagmus, ataxia, hemiparesis, and increased intracranial pressure will be observed.

Both carotid body and glomus jugulare tumors may contain large amounts of catecholamines that can produce severe symptoms from the cardiovascular system. High levels of metabolites in the urine have shown that large quantities of active monamines can be released from those tumors under physiological conditions.[3,9] The author has observed only one patient who was suspected of having a hormonally active glomus jugulare tumor. This patient was finally found to have a pheochromocytoma in addition to her glomus jugulare tumor. All cardiovascular symptoms disappeared after removal of the pheochromocytoma prior to removal of the glomus jugulare tumor.

Radiography and tomography of the skull usually will demonstrate enlargement of the jugular foramen and progressive erosion of the petrous and occipital bones. The erosion of the petrous bone begins from the inferomedial aspect of the jugular foramen (Fig. 107–1). In a series of six patients, the author could follow the erosion process

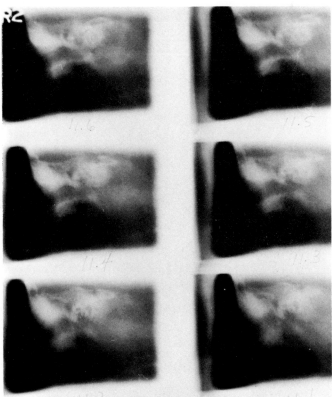

Figure 107–1 Tomography of petrous bone in glomus jugulare tumor.

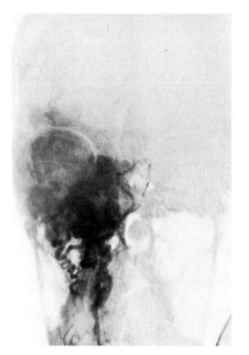

Figure 107–2 Glomus jugulare tumor. Note tumor blush occupying entire right petrous bone and reaching over midline.

over four to six years, since initially the patients refused the operation. The erosion advanced from the inferior medial aspect of the petrous portion of the jugular foramen toward the tuberculum jugulare. After the latter had been nearly destroyed, sclerosis of the mastoid, as seen in some infections, was revealed and was followed by erosion at this later stage. The erosion may destroy the entire petrous bone and a portion of the occipital bone toward the condylar process and along the lateral rim of the clivus. One patient was observed for 24 years before the widespread destruction reached the dimensions described here. Another patient who also refused operative treatment was observed for 12 years. During this time the erosion of the petrous bone reached only into the jugular tubercle. Therefore it is possible to state that the progression (growth of the tumor) is unpredictable and may be extremely slow. The opposite also may be seen. A 19-year-old woman presented with minimal widening and erosion of the jugular foramen that progressed to nearly total destruction of the petrous bone over a 12-month period. Angiography including selective common carotid views to see the ascending pharyngeal artery (an early contributing feeder), and selective ex-

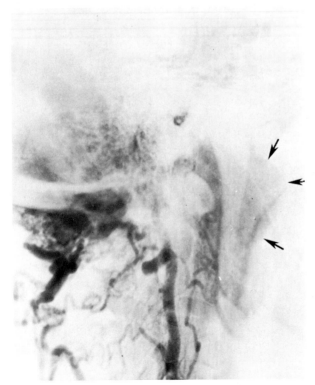

Figure 107–3 Lateral view shows tumor reaching into epipharyngeal space. Tumor is within superior portion of clivus and cavernous sinus.

ternal and internal carotid and vertebral views with subtraction films to see the important feeders coming from the petrous portion of the internal carotid artery is essential (Figs. 107–2 to 107–6).

Sagittal sinography not only will demonstrate occlusion of the sinus, mostly at the sigmoid-transverse junction level, but may also reveal even further extension of the tumor within the sinus. Ligation of the sigmoid sinus is always a part of the operative procedure, and in larger lesions, for which a combined subtemporal-suboccipital approach is required, ligation of the transverse sinus and splitting of the tentorium are part of the operative approach.

Venography to evaluate the extent of the neoplasm within the internal jugular vein is necessary in order to establish the level for ligation of the vein. Care must be taken not to break off any fragment of tumor within the lumen of the vein during the internal

jugular venography. Puncture of the vein, if no catheter study is done, should be done at the lowest level in the neck. Computed tomography will reveal the extent of the tumor in the intracranial cavity (Fig. 107–7).

CLINICAL EXPERIENCE

In the author's series there were 51 patients ranging in age from 18 to 76 years, of whom 42 were between the ages of 40 and 50. There were 40 women and 11 men. None of the 51 patients had class 1 tumors (these would have been within the domain of the otologist); 3 patients had class 2, 12 had class 3, 18 had class 4, 16 had class 5, and 2 had class 6 tumors.

Preoperative radiation therapy was given to 8 patients, but had no effect. None of the patients received selective embolization

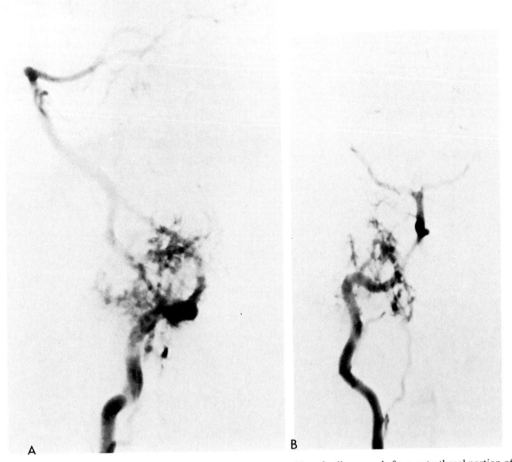

Figure 107–4 Vertebral angiogram in glomus jugular tumor. Note feeding vessels from extrathecal portion of vertebral artery. *A*. Lateral view. *B*. Anteroposterior view.

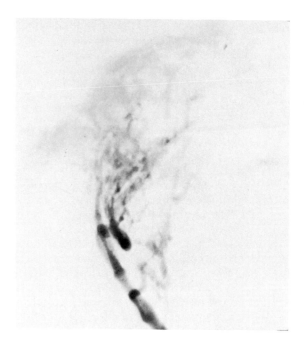

Figure 107–5 Selective external carotid angiogram (subtraction technique) in glomus jugulare tumor.

prior to operation because the procedure was not then available. The work of Hilal and others on embolization of tumor vessels appears to be the most important advance in the therapy of these lesions. It should be followed by operative excision of the tumor. Embolization would now be an essential step in the treatment of tumors belonging to classes 5 and 6.

DEATH AND MORBIDITY

Meningitis secondary to recurrent cerebrospinal fluid fistula is the prime cause of death postoperatively. Dural fistulae are most apt to occur with large lesions that destroy the dura or lesions in which the entire petrous portion of the temporal bone has to be removed, the anatomical evaginations of the dura over the jugular foramen are torn, or the internal acoustic meatus over Meckel's cave and the hypoglossal foramen are destroyed, thus leaving the dura with many openings if not severely fragmented. A dura so destroyed requires extensive grafting. Fascia lata or sheets of anterior rectus fascia were used for this purpose. All eight patients who received radiation therapy prior to operation suffered repeated breakdown of the skin and the dural graft, with resulting cerebrospinal fluid fistula and meningitis. Only one of these eight patients survived; the others died of repeated infections up to four months after the operation.

These 7 patients were among the 10 out of 51 considered to be operative fatalities. Of the remaining three deaths, one was from pulmonary embolism four days postoperatively, and the remaining two were from thrombosis of the internal carotid arteries. The latter two were the patients reported earlier who had regional lymph node, pulmonary, and bone metastases. They also developed thrombosis of the internal carotid artery related to ligation or coagulation of the feeding vessels to the tumor that came from that artery, which was the immediate cause of death in these two patients. The 41 surviving patients had no recovery in any cranial nerves that were paralyzed or without function prior to operation. Even with small lesions, if the facial nerve had total peripheral paralysis it eventually required peripheral anastomosis. All symptoms due to encroachment of the tumor on the brain stem improved. Twenty patients required ventricular peritoneal shunting. All patients in classes 5 and 6 required hospitalization for an average of 30 days.

TREATMENT

Radiation Therapy

Irradiation has no place in the treatment of glomus jugulare tumors. Not only is no beneficial effect achieved by it, but the

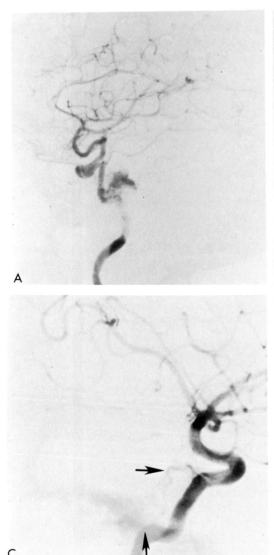

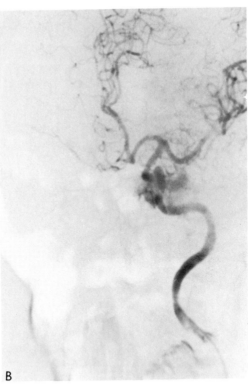

Figure 107–6 Selective internal carotid angiogram in glomus jugulare tumor. *A*. Note feeding vessels to tumor from intrapetrous portion of internal carotid artery. *B*. Subtraction film (anteroposterior view) shows feeding vessels to tumor from petrous and intracavernous section of internal carotid artery. *C*. Lateral view shows feeding vessels from intrapetrous and intracavernous portion of internal carotid artery.

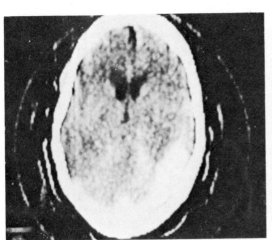

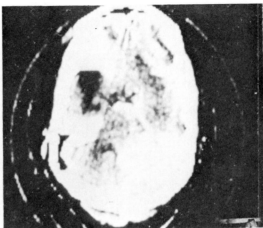

Figure 107–7 Computed tomography in right-sided glomus jugulare tumor. Note in *B* the invasion by tumor of posterior fossa, displacing the fourth ventricle.

mortality rate of seven out of the eight patients in the author's series who had received gamma radiation led to the conviction that it is contraindicated. In these patients, radiation was responsible for the breakdown of the operative area, especially where the graft would not take, and the ensuing cerebrospinal fluid fistula leading to meningitis and death. Preoperative selective occlusion of the feeding vessels with a low-viscosity silicone polymer, as reported by Hilal and Michelsen, appears the method of choice in patients in classes 5 and 6. None of the patients in this group received such therapy, however.

Selective Embolization

In addition to the foregoing series, the author has seen 12 patients who were treated by selective embolization prior to operation. Six patients received radiation therapy before embolization, the surgeon and the radiotherapist being in general agreement that the blood supply to the tumor should not be diminished in advance of radiation therapy.

There was no evidence that irradiation had any effect whatsoever except that it definitely caused necrosis and was followed by delayed healing of the operative bed in one patient.

The materials used for embolization were liquid silicone (Hidal's preparation), fragments of muscle from the patient's thigh, and particles of Gelfoam, some dipped in barium emulsion for opacification.[7,11-13,30,37]

The vessels primarily singled out for embolization were the ascending pharyngeal artery and branches of the external carotid artery, which most frequently involved the occipital artery.[22,23,25,27]

Arteries supplying the tumor that the surgeon can reach before approaching the tumor proper are best left for the surgeon to handle; these arteries include the ascending cervical artery and the deep and superficial cervical arteries (Fig. 107–8). These vessels participated especially in lesions that extended into the neck. Because of anastomosis these arteries always have with the vertebral artery in addition to supplying the tumor, their embolization carries a risk not worth taking.[21,27,39] This was learned in one patient who developed a clinical syndrome closely resembling the Wallenberg syndrome after embolization with liquefied Silastic.[16] The artery so embolized was the ascending cervical, which appeared to carry the major blood supply to the tumor after the ascending pharyngeal artery had first been eliminated by embolization. Some doubt existed whether the embolization of the ascending pharyngeal artery contributed to the neurological deficit, but chronologically the deficit occurred during embolization of that artery. This brings out the point that embolization should be done with the patient sufficiently awake for neurological status to be monitored, and this should be done by a neurologist or neurosurgeon. The embolization should be in experienced hands and should be done as close to the tumor as possible.

Another complication occurred with liquid silicon embolization of branches from the internal maxillary artery to the tumor. That patient experienced sudden excruciating pain over the first and second divisions of the fifth cranial nerve, which persisted undiminished. The procedure was immediately interrupted, and when the patient moved around he revealed truncal ataxia, dysmetria of the upper extremities on forefinger to nose test on the side of injection, rotatory nystagmus, nausea, and vomiting. The latter three symptoms disappeared within 12 to 24 hours. The patient refused any further treatment for 12 months, when the persistence of severe facial pain forced him to seek help. He submitted then to an operation for his large glomus jugulare tumor, since he was told that no attempt could be made to alleviate the facial pain without trying to remove the tumor. The tumor occupied the entire petrosal bone and bulged into the middle and posterior fossae. It was successfully removed, and a partial section of the fifth nerve root close to its entry into the pons was done. The patient was relieved of his pain but remained ataxic, and the unilateral upper extremity dysmetria persisted.

Liquid silicone, which may reach the capillary level, carries a greater risk, especially in large tumors that have a rich anastomotic network with intracranial vessels (see Fig. 107–8).* A tumor of above 5 by 5 cm should be considered a large lesion.

The vascular supply of larger tumors may also reveal shunting to the venous sinus,

---

* See references 10, 19, 20, 24, 26, 36, 38, 42.

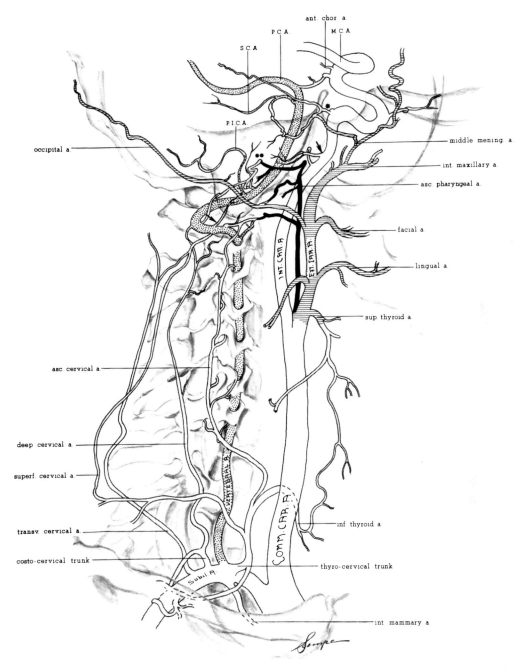

Figure 107–8 Schematic drawing of the most important supply to a glomus jugulare tumor. The shunting into the venous sinus (transverse-sigmoid sinus) often present in larger tumors is not indicated. The ascending pharyngeal artery with its enlarged tympanic branch as main supply to the tumor is shown crossing lateral to the internal carotid artery. Normally, at this level at the base of the skull, this artery stays 1 cm medial to the internal carotid artery and ends in the preclival area. The collateral network of anastomotic channels (**) between ascending pharyngeal artery and branches of the vertebrobasilar artery is frequently present in glomus jugulare tumors that bulge into the posterior fossa. Note the rather constant anastomosis of the ascending pharyngeal artery with the occipital, vertebral, and ascending cervical arteries at the C1–C2 level. Blind ending branches coming from the ascending pharyngeal artery indicate vessels supplying the tumor. The anastomotic net formed by the meningohypophyseal trunk of the intracavernous portion of the internal carotid artery (*) with the middle meningeal and intracranial arteries (superior cerebellar artery via artery of Meckel's cave) is frequently developed in large glomus jugulare tumors. Tumor vessels and angiographic blush are omitted to maintain clarity of the drawing. Vessels providing constant vascular supply to large glomus jugulare tumors from the intrapetrous portion of the internal carotid artery (*upper arrow*) and directly from extracranial vertebro-occipital section of vertebral artery (*lower arrow*) are not amenable to embolization. Note the collaterals between the ascending cervical artery, deep and superficial cervical arteries to the vertebral artery, and anastomotic branches to the ascending pharyngeal artery and their potential in supplying large glomus jugulare tumors. Ligation of these vessels close to the tumor is preferable to embolization because of the important role they may play in supplying the cord at the C1–C3 level.

which has to be considered when low-viscosity silicone embolization is being used. No bruit was observed in patients with shunting into the venous sinus, either by the patient or by the examiner.[18]

Embolization has augmented the treatment of glomus jugular tumor. A thorough knowledge of the vascular supply to the tumor must be obtained in order to distinguish which vessels can be embolized, which vessels should be left to the surgeon to ligate, and which should not be embolized because of their location and rich anastomotic collaterals to the intracranial vasculature or the systemic circulation via venous sinus pathways. The choice of material to be used for embolization will be guided by the angiographic evaluations. Small lesions under 5 by 5 cm with a lesser potential to have open collaterals to intracranial vessels are most amenable to material with the ability to penetrate to the capillary level. Larger lesions are handled with less risk by embolizing with fragments of muscle or Gelfoam. Embolization must be done as close as possible to the tumor itself and under constant monitoring of the patient's neurological status. It has been shown that at operation large tumors (above 5 by 5 cm), after even the most satisfactory embolization, bleed copiously from vessels outside the realm of embolizations, vessels coming from the vertebral artery and the intrapetrous portion of the internal carotid artery (indicated by arrows in Figure 107–8).

The author's advice to the surgeon in this situation is to continue unhesitating removal of tumor tissue to expose the parent vessel, which is usually the vertebral or, especially, the intrapetrous section of the internal carotid artery.[17]

Any hesitation, delay, or even termination of the procedure leaving tumor tissue over those sources of vascular supply carries greater risk.

Operative Therapy

Only the main technical points in the removal of tumors belonging to classes 5 and 6 are described.

The patient is placed in the park bench position with the side of the lesion up. A cardiac catheter is in place to check on air embolism. A reverse "question mark" inci-

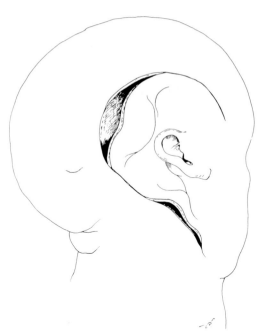

Figure 107–9 Skin incision for right-sided glomus jugulare tumor.

sion is made with the outer ear in its center (Fig. 107–9). Its inferior extent crosses the sternocleidomastoid muscle. This incision permits exposure of the feeding vessels to the tumor from the external carotid artery and ligation of the ascending pharyngeal artery. If the tumor extends into the retropharyngeal space, filling the pterygoid

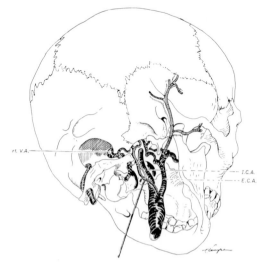

Figure 107–10 Vascular supply from extracranial arteries to right-sided glomus jugulare tumor. Note the ascending pharyngeal artery is pulled away by a blunt nerve hook. Feeding branches from vertebral artery (V.A.) and external carotid artery (E.C.A.) are shown. I.C.A., internal carotid artery.

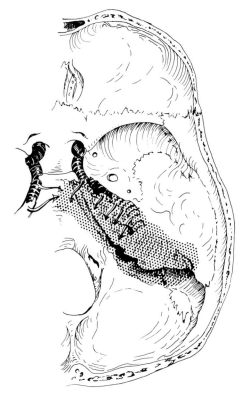

Figure 107–11 Base of skull. Stippled area shows extent of tumor. Vascular supply to tumor from internal carotid arteries (intrapetrous and intracavernous sinus section) is marked by arrows.

fossa, it is not advisable to search for the selective feeding branches of the external carotid arteries (cf. Figs. 107–3 and 107–10). Rather, one should ligate the external carotid artery. Any manipulation of the area may break up the very fragile pol-

ypous extension of the tumor reaching down within the internal jugular vein. The superior extent of the incision is then continued down to the bone, and the skin flap is reflected. The external acoustic meatus is divided and closed by a figure-8 stainless steel wire suture whose ends are brought through the skin flap so that they can be pulled out at a later date. The temporalis muscle is freed from the bone and reflected. The sternocleidomastoid muscle is freed from the mastoid process, and the arch of the atlas is exposed together with the occipital bone. The feeding vessels from the vertebral artery, which will come into view, can be identified and ligated (Figs. 107–11 and 107–12). The extent of the craniotomy and suboccipital craniectomy is seen in Figure 107–12. Additional feeders from the extracranial portion of the vertebral artery will always appear while the occipital bone and the mastoid process are being removed. During removal of the bone, again and again, the need to use bone wax will be apparent. It is useful to have the bone wax on a plate that rests on a hot water bath. The bone involved in these lesions is too fragile to withstand sufficient pressure to insert the bone wax unless the wax is slightly warm.

Figure 107–12 shows the sigmoid-transverse and superior petrosal sinuses and the dura over the temporal fossa and posterior fossa exposed. While removing the petrous bone, the surgeon will see the usual bluish, vascular, soft tumor come into view. The bone about the jugular bulb is removed,

Figure 107–12 First stage of temporal craniotomy and suboccipital craniectomy for right-sided glomus jugulare tumor (tumor classes 5 and 6). Note the removal of cranial bone over transverse sinus; exposure of vertebral artery over arch of atlas, revealing feeding branch to tumor; and external ear separated from external acoustic meatus.

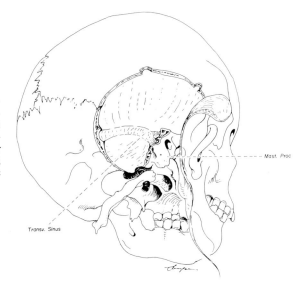

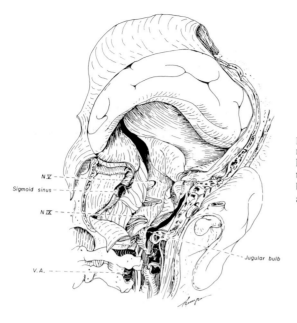

Figure 107–13 Advanced stage of operative procedure for glomus jugulare tumor. Dura over middle and posterior fossae is opened. Temporal lobe is elevated. Tentorium is split after ligation of transverse sinus. Craniectomy has exposed jugular bulb. Sigmoid sinus and jugular bulb are opened, and internal jugular vein is ligated.

permitting one, after ligation of the transverse sinus and the distal portion of the internal jugular vein, to open the sigmoid sinus, jugular bulb, and internal jugular vein for removal of intraluminal tumor tissue (Fig. 107–13). The internal jugular bulb and vein and a portion of the sinus are usually excised. Portions of the tumor are removed by suction and spoon forceps. Tumors in classes 5 and 6 usually have destroyed cranial nerves VII and VIII, and no particular effort to find or save these nerves

is made. The dominant problem with these tumors is the bleeding vessels from the petrous portion of the internal carotid artery. These feeding vessels cannot be reached until enough tumor has been removed to expose the internal carotid artery throughout its entire course to where it penetrates the foramen lacerum into the cavernous sinus. Prior to the identification and exposure of the internal carotid artery the dura over the temporal fossa and posterior fossa is opened. The transverse sinus is ligated

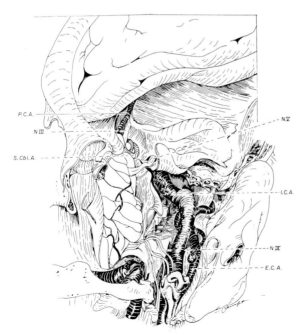

Figure 107–14 Final stage in operative removal of extensive glomus jugulare tumor. Intrapetrous section of internal carotid artery is exposed. Dura over lateral and posterior wall of posterior fossa is widely incised and partly removed, including sigmoid sinus and jugular bulb. P.C.A., posterior cerebral artery; N III, V, and IX, third, fifth, and ninth cranial nerves; S. Cbl. A., superior cerebellar artery; I.C.A., internal carotid artery; E.C.A., external carotid artery.

and divided, and the tentorium is split, permitting a complete view of the extent of the lesion as shown in Figure 107–13. The tumor may perforate the dura in several places, especially over the internal acoustic meatus and over the floor of the middle fossa. It is likely to enter the posterior fossa around the jugular foramen, over the jugular tubercle, or through the hypoglossal canal, in that order of frequency.

Exposure of the internal carotid artery is the next step. This is to be done by progressive removal of tumor tissue, which must be relatively rapid because bleeding cannot be controlled until the artery is exposed, thus revealing the feeding vessels to the tumor. Only then can these vessels be successfully clipped or occluded by bipolar coagulation. The posterior portion of the cavernous sinus usually is entered. Even so, control of the venous bleeding from this area is not a problem. It is here that the internal carotid artery has to be inspected again to identify and ligate any feeding vessels coming from it. Figure 107–14 gives a view of the large operative defect with the dura shredded in many places. The large dead space is obliterated by using the sternocleidomastoid muscle. A section of this muscle with its blood supply still attached can be rotated into the cavity. Use of the muscle in this manner not only fills a dead space but helps in hemostasis, especially with bleeding from the cavernous sinus. The dural defect is closed with fascia lata or a sheet of fascia of the anterior rectus muscle.

Acknowledgments. The author wishes to thank Marshall B. Allen, Jr., M.D., Department of Neurosurgery, and Taher A. M. El Gammal, M.D., Department of Neuroradiology, of the Medical University of Georgia, Augusta, Georgia, for roentgenological studies.

REFERENCES

1. Albernaz, J. G., and Bucy P. C.: Nonchromaffin paraganglioma of the jugular foramen. J. Neurosurg., *10*:663–671, 1953.
2. Alford, B. R., and Guilford, F. R.: A comprehensive study of tumors of the glomus jugulare. Laryngoscope, *72*:765–787, 1962.
3. Berdal, P., Braaten, M., Cappelen, C., Mylius, E. A., and Walaas, O.: Noradrenaline-adrenaline producing nonchromaffin paraganglioma. Acta Med. Scand., *172*:249–260, 1962.
4. Bloom, F.: Structure and histogenesis of tumors of the aortic bodies in dogs. Arch. Path. (Chicago), *36*:1–12, 1943.
5. Borsani, S. J.: Glomus jugulare tumors. Laryngoscope, *72*:1336–1345, 1962.
6. Denecke, H. J.: Surgery of extensive glomus jugulare tumors of the ear. Rev. Laryng. (Bordeaux), *90*:265–270, 1969.
7. Fox, A. J., and Allcock, J. M.: Successful embolization of a fistula between the ascending pharyngeal artery and internal jugular vein. Neuroradiology, *15*:149–152, 1978.
8. Guild, S. R.: A hitherto unrecognized structure, the glomus jugularis, in man. Anat. Rec., *79*:28, 1941.
9. Hamberger, C.-A., Hamberger, C. B., Wersäll, J., and Wagermark, J.: Malignant catecholamine-producing tumour of the carotid body. Acta Path. Microbiol. Scand., *69*:489–492, 1967.
10. Hayes, G. J.: External cavernous sinus fistulas. J. Neurosurg., *20*:692–700, 1963.
11. Heckster, R. E. M., Luyendik, W., and Matricali, B.: Transfemoral catheter embolization: A method of treatment of glomus jugulare tumors. Neuroradiology, *5*:208–214, 1973.
12. Hilal, S. K.: *In* Panel Discussion on Embolization Material. Neuroradiology, *16*:402–412, 1978.
13. Hilal, S. K., and Michelsen, J. W.: Therapeutic percutaneous embolization for extra-axial lesions of the head, neck, and spine. J. Neurosurg., *43*:275–287, 1975.
14. Kempe, L. G.: Operative Neurosurg. Vol. 2. Berlin, Heidelberg, New York, Springer-Verlag, 1970, pp. 72–79.
15. Kempe, L. G., VanderArk, G. D., and Smith D. R.: The neurosurgical treatment of glomus jugulare tumors. J. Neurosurg., *35*:59–64, 1971.
16. Krayenbühl, H. A.: L'Aspect angiographique de la thrombose de l'artère cérébelleuse postérieure et inférieure dans le syndrome dit de Wallenberg. Neurochirurgie, *1*:45–51, 1955.
17. Krayenbühl, H. A.: Les limites de la neurochirurgie. Med. Hyg. (Geneva), *19*:263–265, 1961.
18. Krayenbühl, H. A.: Vaskuläre Krankheiten im extrakraniellen Karotisvertebralis Bereich als ursache intrakranieller Gerausche. Munchen. Med. Wchr., *103*:2185–2187, 1961.
19. Krayenbühl, H. A.: Die Bedeutung des zerbralen Kollateralkreislaufs bei organischen Hirnleiden für deren neurochirurgische Behandlung. Schweiz. Med. Wchr., *93*:111–119, 1963.
20. Krayenbühl, H. A., and Yasargil, G.: Der subtentorielle Kollateralkreislauf im angiographischen Bild; ein pathogenetischer Beitrag zur Klinik der vasculären bulbopontinen Syndrome. Deutsch. Z. Nervenheilk., *177*:103–116, 1957.
21. Krayenbühl, H. A., Yasargil, G.: Der cerebrale kollaterale Blutkreislauf im angiographischen Bild. Acta Neurochir. (Wien), *6*:30–80, 1958.
22. Krayenbühl, H. A., and Yasargil, M. G.: The collateral circulation. *In* Cerebral Angiography. Philadelphia, J. B. Lippincott Co., 1968, pp. 165–183.
23. Lasjaunias, P., and Manelfe, C.: Arterial supply for the upper cervical nerves and the cervico-carotid anastomotic channels: Systematization of radiological anatomy. Neuroradiology, *18*:125–131, 1979.
24. Lasjaunias, P., and Moret, J.: Normal and nonpathological variations in the angiographic aspect of the arteries of the middle ear. Neuroradiology, *15*:213–219, 1978.

25. Lasjaunias, P., Théron, J., and Moret, J.: The occipital artery—anatomy—normal arteriographic aspects—embryological significance. Neuroradiology, *15*:31–37, 1978.

26. Lasjaunias, P., Moret, J., Doyon, D., and Vignaud, J.: Collatérales C_5 du siphon carotidien: Embryologie, corrélations radio-anatomique, radio-anatomie pathologique. Neuroradiology, *16*:304–305, 1978.

27. Lasjaunias, P., Moret, J., Manelfe, G., Théron, J., Hasso, T., and Seeger, J.: Arterial anomalies at the base of the skull. Neuroradiology, *13*:267–272, 1977.

28. Lederer, F. L., Skolnick, E. M., Soboroff, B. J., et al.: Nonchromaffin paraganglioma of the head and neck. Ann. Otol., *67*:305–331, 1958.

29. Leman, P., Portmann, M., Cohadon, F., et al.: Collaboration oto-neuro-chirurgicale dans l'ablation totale d'une tumeur glomique tympano-jugulaire avec extension endocrânienne. Neurochirurgie, *14*:828–820, 1968.

30. Manelfe, C., Picard, L., Bonafé, A., Roland, G., Sancier, A., and Espérance, G.: Embolisations et occlusions par ballonnets dans les processus tumoraux. Sept années d'expérience. Neuroradiology, *16*:395–398, 1978.

31. McCabe, B. F., and Fletcher, M.: Selection of therapy of glomus jugulare tumors. Arch. Otolaryng. (Chicago), *89*:156–159, 1969.

32. McMeekin, R. R., Hardman, J. M., and Kempe, L. G.: Multiple sclerosis after x-radiation: Activation by treatment of metastatic glomus tumor. Arch. Otolaryng. (Chicago), *90*:617–621, 1969.

33. Meacham, W. F., and Capps, J. M.: Intracranial glomus jugulare tumor with successful surgical removal. J. Neurosurg., *17*:157–160, 1960.

34. Michelson, R. P., and Connolly, J. E.: Removal of glomus jugulare tumor utilizing complete occlusion of the cerebral circulation. Laryngoscope, *72*:788–805, 1962.

35. Mönckeberg, I. G.: Die Tumoren der Glandula carotica. Beitr. Path. Anat., *38*:1–66, 1905.

36. Moret, J., Lasjaunias, P., Vignaud, J., and Doyon, D.: Participation de l'artère meningée moyenne à la vascularisation de la fosse postérieure. Neuroradiology, *16*:306–307, 1978.

37. Newton, H.: Embolization material; Panel discussion. Neuroradiology, *16*:402–412, 1978.

38. Parkinson, D.: Collateral circulation of cavernous carotid artery: Anatomy. Canad. J. Surg., *7*:251–268, 1964.

39. Quisling, R. G., and Seeger, J. F.: Ascending pharyngeal artery, collateral circulation simulating internal carotid artery hypoplasia. Neuroradiology, *18*:277–280, 1979.

40. Rosenwasser, H.: Carotid body tumor of the middle ear and mastoid. Arch. Otolaryng. (Chicago), *41*:64–70, 1945.

41. Rosenwasser, H.: Glomus jugulare tumors, I–VI. Arch. Otolaryng. (Chicago), *88*:29–65, 1968.

42. Rovina, M., Torrent, O., González, F., and Romere, F.: Contribution of the study of the arterial nutrition of the cervical spinal cord. Neuroradiology, *16*:375–377, 1978.

43. Valentine, G.: Ueber eine gangliöse Anschwellung in der Jacobsonschen Anastomose des Menschen. Arch. Anat. Physiol. Wissensch. Med., 287–290, 1840.

108

TUMORS OF PERIPHERAL AND SYMPATHETIC NERVES

The peripheral nervous system includes the cranial and spinal nerves and also the autonomic ganglia and nerves. The olfactory and optic tracts, being direct extensions of the central nervous system, are excluded.[11,45] Neoplasms of the peripheral nervous system develop at intracranial and intraspinal sites. Since those of cranial and spinal origin within the skull and spinal canal are discussed in other chapters, this discussion concerns only those at and distal to the neural foramina.

The tissues of the peripheral nervous system are of neuroectodermal and mesodermal origin. Disagreements as to the embryological origin of the various tumors of peripheral nerves have contributed to confusion in their classification. In this chapter, peripheral nerve tumors are separated into those of nerve sheath origin and those of neuronal, or nerve cell, origin. The nerve sheath tumors may be of neuroectodermal or mesodermal origin. The neuronal tumors are of neuroectodermal origin.

Nerve sheath tumors arise from neuroectodermal components such as Schwann cells, which form the axonal myelin sheaths, and perineurial cells, which form the perineurial sheaths of the nerve fascicles. Although perineurial cells do not produce myelin, they are histologically identical to the Schwann cells, and characteristically both have basement membranes. Most authors consider the perineurial cells to be Schwann cells.[45]

Nerve sheath tumors of mesodermal origin may arise from fibrocytes that lie in the endoneurium and throughout the nerve sheaths. Fibrocytes form the epineurium, or the external covering, of the peripheral nerve. They may be similar to Schwann cells in appearance as well as in the ability to produce fibrous tissues and collagen. They differ histologically at least in the absence of basement membranes.[45] Adipose cells, also of mesodermal origin, may be present within the nerve bundle and can give rise to benign fatty tumors.[90]

The neuronal, or nerve cell, tumors almost always arise in the ganglia of the autonomic nervous system. Rare instances of a neuronal tumor, a neuroblastoma, arising in a peripheral nerve have been reported.[70,88]

The benign tumors of Schwann cell origin are schwannomas and neurofibromas. Malignant forms are malignant schwannomas. Fibrocytes may form benign tumors resembling neurofibromas; and if malignant, they can also form neurofibrosarcomas. Nerve sheath fibrosarcomas and malignant schwannomas may, at times, be impossible to differentiate on microscopic examination. Harkin and Reed state that because of histological similarities, classification may be arbitrary.[45]

The nerve cell tumors arise primarily in the sympathetic and paraganglionic components of the autonomic nervous system. Those arising from the sympathoblasts of the sympathetic system are neuroblastomas, while the paraganglionic system gives rise to paragangliomas, the best known being the pheochromocytoma and the chemodectoma.[39]

Peripheral nerve tumors may be characterized according to structural and embryonic origins. But even then, the close resemblance of tumors of Schwann cell origin to those of fibrocyte origin makes classification difficult and sometimes arbitrary.

J. R. YOUMANS AND W. Y. ISHIDA

TUMORS OF NERVE SHEATH ORIGIN

Benign Schwannomas

Benign schwannomas are well-encapsulated tumors of Schwann cell origin. They arise in all regions of the peripheral nervous system. Usually they occur as solitary lesions, but they may be associated with von Recklinghausen's neurofibromatosis.

Because of their common Schwann cell origin, benign schwannomas and neurofibromas are sometimes classed together as "benign nerve sheath tumors" or "schwannomas."[6,23] The authors have chosen to discuss them separately because of their distinct gross, microscopic, and biological characteristics.[45]

The benign schwannoma usually displays an obvious relationship to the peripheral nerve of origin. When massive growth has occurred, however, or when the nerve of origin is small, the association with a nerve may be difficult to demonstrate. The characteristic appearance is that of an exophytic tumor that grows and causes displacement and distortion of the nerve but does not invade it. Cross-sectional examination reveals that the tumor is separated from the distorted nerve bundle by a fibrous capsule. The tumor parenchyma usually is homogeneous and solid, but cystic or hemorrhagic areas may be present.

Microscopic examination of the parenchyma verifies that the schwannoma, unlike the neurofibroma, has a clear separation of neuronal-axonal processes from tumor cells. Highly cellular Antoni type A regions consist of spindle-shaped cells with poorly visible cytoplasmic boundaries. The cells may appear very densely packed, and there may be some areas of pallisading. In other regions, less dense areas of Antoni type B tissue may appear. The cells here are more sparsely arranged and tend to align themselves in tortuous cords. Either cellular arrangement may predominate in a tumor.[45]

Infrequently, distinguishing a schwannoma from a neurofibroma histologically may be difficult. Densely cellular areas in a neurofibroma may suggest a schwannoma. Loosely arranged Antoni B areas in a schwannoma may suggest a neurofibroma. But acid mucopolysaccharide stains of the tumors usually give negative reactions in schwannomas and positive reactions in neurofibromas. Furthermore, the gross exophytic appearance of the schwannoma, contrasted with the fusiform enlargement of the nerve harboring a neurofibroma, is usually helpful in differentiating these tumors.

The nerves of origin of schwannomas are usually the sensory branches, but motor branches are involved also. The tumors usually occur in cranial and spinal nerves, but infrequently also arise in autonomic ganglia. They occur extracranially and intracranially, extraspinally and intraspinally.[21] Intraspinal tumors arise from nerve roots throughout the spinal canal. Intracranial schwannomas most frequently arise from the vestibular portion of the eighth cranial nerve, but they also arise from the oculomotor, the trochlear, and the trigeminal nerves.[5,12,53,59] In rare instances they occur on the glossopharyngeal, vagus, spinal accessory, and hypoglossal nerves.[32,38] The intracranial and intraspinal schwannomas are discussed in other chapters.

In spite of the usual distortion and compression of the adjacent nerve, most patients with benign schwannomas are remarkably asymptomatic and without neurological deficits.[24] When symptoms and neurological deficits appear, they usually are mild. Patients most frequently present because of a painless lump or because of local tenderness. When neural compression progresses with growth of a tumor, pain or weakness may prompt medical consultation. Palpation or percussion of the mass may produce pain or parethesias. Tumors lying deep in soft tissues such as the buttock or within body cavities may escape diagnosis until they have attained massive size.

The head and neck area is a relatively common location for these tumors. In this region, the lateral aspect of the neck is the most common site, with tumors arising from cervical roots, brachial plexus, cutaneous nerves, vagus nerve, and sympathetic nerves.[16,24,33] They usually present as painless, visible masses.

Schwannomas of the face are exceedingly rare. When they occur they are most often associated with the facial nerve.[3] Although usually asymptomatic, the patient may have facial weakness and pain. The majority of the tumors present superficially, distal to the stylomastoid foramen.

Often, they are misdiagnosed as tumors originating from other organs, such as the parotid gland.[60] A significant number of patients with benign facial schwannomas have multicentric tumors involving multiple nerve branches.[17] This finding underlines the importance of complete investigation of these proximal tumors, utilizing tomography if necessary to evaluate possible bony erosion as the nerves traverse bony structures.[3]

Schwannomas of the extremities, including the brachial plexus and pelvic girdle, make up another major group of peripheral nerve schwannomas.[23,24] Although these neoplasms are described as typically painless and asymptomatic, White found that 32 of 45 patients with benign schwannomas of the extremities presented with pain, tenderness, or both.[94] Nineteen had paresthesias, and one had paresis. The majority of these tumors of the extremities occur over the flexor surfaces where large nerves are situated, and usually are proximal in the extremity.[24,64]

Although the majority of schwannomas in the extremities are palpable, deeper-lying tumors of the brachial plexus or sciatic nerve may be difficult to discern. This fact can lead to their misdiagnosis as lumbar disc lesions.[23] Even if a tumor cannot be felt by the examiner, palpation of the area may produce symptoms and confirm the location of the mass.[22] Schwannomas presenting distally at the hands and wrists are often misdiagnosed as ganglion cysts.[75] These tumors have also developed in the carpal and tarsal tunnels, sometimes mimicking the classic syndromes of these areas.[65,81]

Benign schwannomas in locations other than the head, neck, and extremities make up approximately 15 to 25 per cent of the total.[24] The majority of the remaining tumors arise in the posterior mediastinum, are asymptomatic, and usually are diagnosed on routine chest x-rays.[35] They most frequently originate from spinal nerves or the sympathetic chain, but may arise from the phrenic and vagus nerves in the mediastinum.[15]

In rare cases, benign schwannomas have occurred on the trachea, in the lung, and in the heart.[9,30,69] On the trunk they may present superficially as cutaneous or breast tumors, or lie deep in the retroperitoneum as kidney and presacral masses.[56,61,67] Testimony to the fact that schwannomas can occur wherever peripheral nerves exist is their appearance within bone. Intraosseous schwannomas develop from nerves gaining entry to the marrow along with nutrient vessels. They have been described in nearly every bone in the body, but most often in the mandible and long bones.[40,95]

The operative approach to a peripheral nerve neoplasm depends on whether it is malignant or benign. If a discrete capsule is present, the neoplasm may be enucleated and examined by the pathologist. Gross inspection by the surgeon cannot rule out malignancy. If a fusiform enlargement of the nerve is present without obvious tumor tissue being visible superficially, a careful longitudinal neurolysis may be performed and a biopsy of the centrally lying tumor mass examined. In either instance, if the tumor is malignant, then radical operative resection should be considered. If the biopsy reveals the tumor to be benign, careful enucleation is the definitive treatment.

The goals of treatment are tumor resection and preservation of nerve function. Most benign schwannomas can be easily and totally enucleated without nerve damage. Following apparent total removal, recurrences are quite rare.[23,24] Even with partial resection, tumor growth is so extremely slow that most patients do not experience symptomatic regrowth. Malignant transformation of benign schwannomas rarely, if ever, occurs.[5,45] For these reasons, resection of benign tumors should not be pursued to the point of endangering vital structures. For example, if tumors involving critical nerves—as, for example, at the brachial plexus—are adherent to large vessels, they are best treated with subtotal resection. Nerve damage may be monitored during the course of the resection by intermittently measuring the nerve action potentials. This monitoring technique, along with careful micro-operative dissection, helps to preserve nerve function while allowing maximal removal of the tumor.

Neurofibroma

The neurofibroma, like the schwannoma, is a benign nerve sheath tumor of Schwann cell origin. Unlike the schwannoma, its tumor cells lie among the axonal processes and it usually is inseparable from the affected nerve bundles.[45,85] The tumor occurs both as a solitary neurofibroma and also as one of multiple tumors with von Recklinghausen's neurofibromatosis.

Solitary Neurofibroma

Solitary neurofibromas usually appear in children before the age of 10 years, and most are in the skin or subcutaneous adipose tissue. The diagnosis of a solitary neurofibroma must be made with caution, since the tumor may be the first sign of von Recklinghausen's neurofibromatosis. Examination of the solitary neurofibroma does not help in determining whether the syndrome is present.[6]

Although solitary neurofibromas usually are cutaneous, they may arise from deeper peripheral nerves. When they occur in the skin or subcutaneous tissues, they usually are painless and not associated with neurological dysfunction. They are firm, but compressible, and may be marked by slight hyper- or hypopigmentation of the overlying skin. Usually they are well circumscribed but lack the distinct capsule of schwannomas. The nerve of origin of a cutaneous neurofibroma seldom can be identified.[45] This situation can be contrasted with that of solitary neurofibromas occurring at sites other than the skin or subcutaneous fat. At noncutaneous sites, the tumors seem to be encapsulated and have a definite connection with the nerve of origin. The nerve usually enters the tumor, and on histological examination, the axons, undisplaced by the tumor mass, insinuate themselves through the tumor matrix. When occurring within a larger peripheral nerve, the clinical presentation may be similar to that of schwannomas. In spite of the intimate relationship of tumor cells to axons, most patients have no neurological deficits.

Histologically, the solitary neurofibroma consists of fusiform spindle-shaped cells that appear to be twisted and arranged in cords. The cells are loosely arrayed in an intracellular matrix consisting of collagen fibrils and mucopolysaccharide. Mast cells, lymphocytes, and fibrocytes are also present. At times, the microscopic picture may resemble that of the benign schwannoma. But the neurofibroma, unlike the schwannoma, usually reacts positively to stains for mucopolysaccharides and lacks thickened arteries or cysts.[6]

The treatment of solitary neurofibroma is operative resection. When the tumors occur in the usual cutaneous and subcutaneous locations, resection can be easily accomplished because connections to important nerves are seldom seen. If important nerves are involved, however, an attempt to spare neuronal function must be made. Even if resection of the solitary neurofibroma is partial, symptomatic recurrence usually does not occur. In the absence of von Recklinghausen's neurofibromatosis, the chance of malignant transformation is slight.[45,85]

Von Recklinghausen's Neurofibromatosis

The neurofibroma is the hallmark of von Recklinghausen's neurofibromatosis. This syndrome is a mendelian dominant phakomatosis. Its most distinctive feature is the association with neurofibromas and café au lait skin lesions. The plexiform variety of neurofibroma occurs only with von Recklinghausen's disease.

The distinguishing signs of the syndrome are the multiple widespread abnormalities of ectodermal and mesodermal origin. The true incidence of neurofibromatosis is unknown, since the majority of cases are mild and go unrecognized.

The manifestations of neurofibromatosis may be grouped into four categories.[6,45] *Central neurofibromatosis* is characterized by the absence of the peripheral manifestations of the syndrome and the presence of a number of intradural tumors, including gliomas, meningiomas, and schwannomas. Bilateral acoustic schwannomas, for example, suggest neurofibromatosis. *Peripheral neurofibromatosis* is characterized by the predominance of peripheral manifestations as evidenced by multiple cutaneous and peripheral nerve neurofibromas. *Visceral neurofibromatosis* is characterized by neurofibromas, ganglioneuromas, and schwannomas arising from the visceral autonomic system. Involvement of the genitourinary, gastrointestinal, and respiratory systems may be symptomatic. *Forme fruste* cases are those in which there is only mild expression of the syndrome, usually with superficial cutaneous abnormalities or a few neurofibromas or schwannomas.

The peripheral nerve tumors associated with neurofibromatosis are neurofibromas, schwannomas, malignant schwannomas, and less commonly, neuroblastomas and ganglioneuromas.[76] When associated with von Recklinghausen's neurofibromatosis, neurofibromas have a greater tendency toward malignant transformation than those that occur as solitary lesions.[6,23]

The plexiform neurofibroma is a morphological variant that is diagnostic of neurofibromatosis. It has a tendency to local proliferation and involvement of adjacent tissues. Approximately 3 per cent of adult patients with neurofibromatosis have plexiform tumors.[20,83] This tumor can occur in any part of the peripheral nervous system, but preferentially it involves the motor cranial nerves.[6,57] Even though it attains massive size, surprisingly few neurological deficits are noted, and operative intervention frequently is for cosmetic reasons. Disfigurement of the face with facial nerve involvement can be a major problem.[20,48,57] In unusual cases, the tumor becomes life threatening with progressive growth in the areas of the neck, tongue, and pharynx or with proximal extension into the central nervous system.[48] Resection must be performed with caution, since the still-functioning nerves usually are distorted by the tumor's infiltration and the surrounding fibrous proliferation. Although these are benign tumors, the extent of local invasion usually prevents a cure by resection.

As with the benign schwannomas, resection of neurofibromas should stop short of compromising nerve function. When critical nerves such as branches of the brachial plexus or other main trunks are involved, preservation of neural function is the main goal. The tumor, because of its intrinsic growth within a nerve, cannot be totally resected. Segmental resection of an important nerve solely to accomplish total removal of a benign tumor usually is unwarranted. Because of the possibility of malignant transformation in von Recklinghausen's disease, however, patients undergoing partial resection must be closely observed throughout their lifetimes. If a malignant tumor develops, then radical resection must be performed.[85]

Malignant Nerve Sheath Tumors

Malignant nerve sheath tumors arise from Schwann cells of neuroectodermal origin, and from fibrocytes of mesodermal origin. These tumors, similar in gross appearance, may be conveniently classified as (1) malignant schwannoma and (2) nerve sheath fibrosarcoma and malignant mesenchymoma. The confusion in terminology of primary malignant nerve sheath tumors reflects the controversy over cellular origin of clinically and grossly similar-appearing tumors. Harkin and Reed list "neurofibrosarcoma," "malignant schwannoma," "neurogenic sarcoma," "fibromyxosarcoma of nerve," "fibrosarcoma of nerve," "malignant neurinoma," "malignant peripheral glioma," "myxosarcoma of nerve sheath," "neurilemosarcoma," and "secondary malignant neuroma" as "terms used synonomously in general reference to malignant nerve sheath tumors."[45] Aside from histological differences, malignant schwannomas, nerve sheath fibrosarcoma, and malignant mesenchymomas are similar in their clinical features and are therefore discussed here as malignant schwannomas.

Malignant schwannomas arise from peripheral nerves in every anatomical region of the body. Das Gupta estimates that, over an extended follow-up period, 29 per cent of patients with neurofibromatosis developed malignant schwannomas.[23] They can also occur as solitary neoplasms in the absence of clinical neurofibromatosis.

Typically the patient presents with a superficial mass associated with pain along the course of a peripheral nerve. In the presence of neurofibromatosis, a sudden change in size of the tumor mass or its development in the peripheral nerve is highly suggestive of a malignant schwannoma. Whereas the onset of benign schwannomas usually is before age 20, the majority of patients with malignant schwannomas are older than 30 years of age.[23]

The tumor presents grossly as a fusiform enlargment of the nerve or as a lobulated mass attached to the nerve trunk. Except when arising in association with plexiform neurofibroma, the malignant schwannoma appears encapsulated as it abuts on adjacent nonneural structures. Pseudoencapsulation, the appearance of an apparently well-demarcated capsule around the tumor, results from compression of adjacent tissues by the expanding tumor mass. Histological examination of the compressed tissue will demonstrate that tumor invasion has already occurred by direct extension along fascial planes and nerve sheaths. These factors account for most local recurrences, especially following local excision of the tumor.[14]

Macroscopic examination of peripheral nerve tumors offers no consistent means of differentiating malignant from benign schwannomas. On sectioning, the tumors may appear well circumscribed, firm or soft, with areas suggesting focal necrosis or hemorrhage. Signs of neural invasion or extension of the tumor along the nerve are characteristic features of malignant schwannomas.[19] This extension may proceed over significant distances. For example, the tumor may arise in the sciatic nerve and extend proximally past the sciatic notch to form a mass in the buttock and within the pelvis. Likewise, a tumor of the vagus nerve in the neck may extend proximally to the jugular foramen. Not uncommonly, especially with brachial or lumbosacral plexus malignant schwannomas, proximal extension occurs intradurally, making many of these tumors incurable by operation. Nonneural soft-tissue sarcomas of the extremities have been shown to invade peripheral nerves and spread along their trunks.[8] Carcinoma of the head and neck has also demonstrated neural invasion of cranial nerves with proximal extension in perineurial and endoneurial spaces. Brain as well as meningeal involvement has been verified on pathological examination.[27] In all these instances of axial neuronal spread of primary nerve sheath tumor or secondary invasion by sarcoma or carcinoma, the gross external appearance of the nerve trunk may be normal. This finding demonstrates the importance of an accurate histological examination of the nerve trunk proximal and distal to the level of tumor resection. Neuronal extension of these tumors must be considered by the surgeon preoperatively so that the evaluation can include cytological examination of cerebrospinal fluid, foraminal radiography, and myelography when appropriate. [67]Gallium scanning has proved helpful in detecting malignant schwannomas or neurofibrosarcomas in neurofibromatosis.[43]

Malignant Schwannomas in Specific Sites

Head and Neck

Approximately 12 per cent of malignant schwannomas occur in the head and neck region. Most often they arise from cranial nerves, upper branches of the brachial plexus, cervical nerve roots, and the sympathetic chain. Cranial nerves that are most frequently affected appear to be the trigeminal and facial nerves. The vagus and spinal accessory nerves have also been involved in this region.[23,49] Frequently these tumors present as asymptomatic masses; they may, however, cause paresthesias and pain. Often they invade critical structures. In such cases the resection has to be limited, and this limitation contributes to the poor prognosis. The majority of the patients die within two and a half years after the diagnosis is made.[19,49]

Upper Extremities and Brachial Plexus

In the brachial plexus, these tumors typically cause pain or paresthesias in the upper extremity. The majority of patients have a palpable mass in the area of the brachial plexus. Even those who do not have a palpable mass often will have discomfort elicited by the palpation procedure.[22] There may be an intraspinal extension of the tumor, which must be considered preoperatively so that appropriate diagnostic measures can be performed.[87]

Conservative local soft-tissue excision of these brachial plexus tumors results in poor survival. To offer the patient a significant chance for cure, a radical forequarter amputation must be performed.[22,54] Although these lesions tend to be radioresistant, radiation therapy following radical excision may be beneficial.[44,87]

With malignant schwannomas in the upper extremity, primary treatment with amputation produces the highest cure rates.[23,46,54] Lesser procedures, in attempts to preserve a limb, most often result in death. In most series, these tumors show a tendency toward more proximal location in the extremity.[23]

Trunk

Malignant schwannomas occurring in the trunk are rare in patients who do not manifest von Recklinghausen's disease.[23] They occur in nearly every region of the thorax and abdomen. In the mediastinum, they present with chest discomfort and pericardial effusion.[50] Neurogenic mediastinal tumors are almost always located in the posterior mediastinum. A small number of them will prove to be malignant schwannomas, the ratio of benign to malignant schwannomas in the mediastinum being 10.8 to 1.[50] Because of their location and the late onset of symptoms, the prognosis is extremely poor.

Malignant tumors of this type arise from the sympathetic chain and vagus nerves as well as intercostal nerves.[23,50,84] In the abdomen, they present with gastrointestinal or genitourinary signs. These signs are related to the size of the tumor, which usually becomes symptomatic at a late stage of its growth. Limited operative excision results in high mortality and recurrence rates because of soft-tissue infiltration and intraneural extension. In the unusual case, a retroperitoneal malignant schwannoma may present with a typical lumbar disc syndrome, suggesting a peripheral neuropathy.[80]

Lower Extremities

The lower extremities are relatively frequently the site of malignant schwannomas, as they were in approximately 40 per cent of Das Gupta's combined series.[23] Like those in the upper extremity, the majority of the tumors are proximally located. Lesions in the buttocks and the thigh are usually associated with the sciatic and femoral nerves respectively. Unless careful examination including palpation along the course of peripheral nerves is performed, they may be misdiagnosed as a lumbar disc syndrome.

As with tumors in the upper extremity, the most difficult therapeutic decision that the surgeon must make is whether to recommend major amputation as primary treatment. Local recurrence with conservative local soft-tissue resection ranges from 30 to 60 per cent.[23,86] The recurrence rate was significantly lower in patients who were treated initially with major amputations, and the survival rate was also significantly greater. In demonstrated local recurrence of tumor following initial resection, amputation above the recurrence site is the best treatment.[86] Distant metastasis is the main cause of death in the majority of patients with tumor recurrence. Early major amputation results in fewer deaths by accomplishing total tumor resection and preventing both recurrence and distant

metastasis. Poor survival rates following amputation or major disarticulation in some series reflect the choice of radical resection only for the larger, more extensive tumors. The cure rate for malignant schwannomas in the distal portion of the extremities is high with amputation.[86]

Treatment of Malignant Schwannoma

These tumors demonstrate a propensity for two modes of extension. Like other sarcomas, they extend directly by invasion of adjacent structures and show a tendency to grow along tissue and fascial planes. They also extend axially both proximally and distally within the nerve trunk.[8,66,93] As a result of this second mode of spread, central nervous system involvement by intraneural extension of peripheral nerve tumors has occurred in most regions of the body. For example, proximal brachial plexus tumors frequently are associated with intraneural extension into the spinal subarachnoid space.[92] D'Agostino and co-workers reported seven cases of significant intraneural spread of malignant schwannoma, in three of which the patients had tumor extension from a peripheral nerve into the spinal cord.[19] When a limb is amputated as a treatment for these tumors, the proximal portion of the nerves should be studied histologically to make sure the amputation is above the tumor spread along the nerves. If tumor is found in the nerves, reamputation at a higher site is necessary.

With local excision of these tumors the recurrence rate is higher and leads to a high mortality rate from distant metastasis. This tendency for local recurrence is due to pseudoencapsulation. The apparent margins of the tumor at the time of operative exploration do not demarcate the extent of its invasion. This factor alone can contribute significantly to a recurrence rate of approximately 40 per cent after local excision.[14] Attempts to preserve adjacent blood vessels, bones, and nerves often result in subtotal tumor resection. In the absence of obvious metastases at the time of primary diagnosis, radical excision involving major amputation when possible offers the greatest chance for cure.[23,86,93]

Malignant schwannomas do not appear to metastasize frequently to the lymphatic system. Thus, the absence of tumor in lymph nodes should not suggest the absence of proximal extension of tumor along fascial planes or within nerve sheaths.

In all cases of malignant schwannoma, radical excision is the primary treatment. The extent of the resection will be determined by the anatomical site. When the tumor is in an extremity, amputation offers the greatest chance for cure. With proximal limb girdle involvement, the chance for cure is lessened. It is, however, maximized by a forequarter amputation of the upper extremity or a hemipelvectomy. Radical operation for malignant schwannoma requires a multispecialty approach in which the neurosurgeon, the orthopedic surgeon, and sometimes the general surgeon or urologist cooperate. Before a radical procedure is advised, the absence of distant metastases and central nervous system involvement must be assured. The surgeon's recommendation for radical resection must be carefully discussed with the patient, weighing the disadvantages of loss of limb and mutilation against the high risk of local recurrence and death. Radiotherapy alone is ineffective, and the course is unaltered by preoperative irradiation. Although the benefits of postoperative radiotherapy have not been proved, Das Gupta and associates recommend a dosage between 3000 and 9000 rads, depending on location and size of tumor.[24] Because of the malignant schwannoma's usual radioresistance, however, resection remains the only hope for cure.

SECONDARY NEOPLASMS OF PERIPHERAL NERVE SHEATHS

Both carcinomas and sarcomas will invade adjacent nerve sheaths.[8,27] The tumor cells infiltrate the epineurium or perineurium and extend for variable distances along the nerve, sometimes reaching the subarachnoid space of the central nervous system.[7,8] Frequently the involved nerves appear enlarged but not obviously distorted. The nerve may function normally, and the patient may be asymptomatic. Neural foraminal erosion suggests peripheral nerve involvement. Perineural extension of benign breast lesions also occurs.[41]

Extension of tumor along perineural lymphatic channels was once thought to be the mode of spread, but no histological or clinical evidence for the presence of a perineural lymphatic system exists.[58] Tumors infiltrating the nerve sheaths extend axially along the nerves in epineurial, perineurial or endoneurial planes of least resistance. Lymphatic channels may run adjacent to nerves in neurovascular bundles, but do not lie within the epineurial space. This anatomical relationship may partly explain the surprisingly low incidence of lymph node metastasis of malignant peripheral nerve tumors.[7,8]

Clinical symptoms suggesting secondary invasion of nerves by neoplasms are pain, numbness, paresthesias, and weakness. Their presence should alert the surgeon to consider and possibly explore the region, specifically seeking evidence of neural invasion. Since the perineurial extension of neoplasms may not distort the gross appearance of the nerve, a biopsy is essential to rule out the possibility of malignancy. Frequently, a recurrence following primary tumor resection may be the result of failure to detect peripheral nerve invasion at the time of the initial procedure.[27]

Perineurial invasion by carcinomas of the head and neck and by sarcomas of the extremities contribute to their high recurrence rates.[8,63,66] In the head and neck region, invasion of the perineurium and extension along cranial nerves occur most commonly with squamous cell carcinoma; however, adenocarcinoma, basal cell carcinoma, cylindromas, and lymphomas behaving in this way have also been reported.[7,27] Soft-tissue sarcomas of the extremities also are associated with perineurial extension of tumors. Evidence of peripheral nerve invasion was found in 11 of 98 extremities amputated because of soft-tissue sarcomas. In one case the tumor originating at the wrist had spread proximally to the brachial plexus.[8]

Perineurial extension allowed to progress along nerves into the cranial cavity or spinal subarachnoid space eliminates the chance for cure. Proximal extension of tumor along a branch of the trigeminal nerve may, after reaching the gasserian ganglion, progress distally again to involve other branches.[7,66] This pattern of extension has been noted in other cranial nerves and plexuses.[8,27]

PERIPHERAL NERVE CELL NEOPLASIA

The neural crest cells differentiate into the cells of neural sheath as well as the neuronal components of the peripheral nervous system. Tumors of nerve cell origin in the peripheral nervous system arise from the precursor cell, the sympathogonium, which then differentiates to the sympathoblastic and pheochromocytic lines.

The sympathoblast, with increasing degrees of differentiation, may give rise to neuroblastomas, ganglioneuroblastomas (differentiated neuroblastoma), and ganglioneuromas. Each type of neoplasm reflects progressive increase in cell maturity by its histological appearance, the clinical age of onset, and its biological activity. The neuroblastoma is predominantly a tumor of childhood. It is the least differentiated histologically and is biologically the most malignant. At the other extreme, the ganglioneuroma is a benign tumor of mature ganglion cells that tends to occur in adolescents and adults. The ganglioneuroblastoma lies between the two extremes. On microscopic examination, it has areas that resemble a neuroblastoma mixed with areas that are similar to ganglioneuroma. Its biological activity and clinical behavior are similar to those of the neuroblastoma.

The cells of the pheochromocytic line can differentiate into active pheochromocytomas or paragangliomas. Catecholamine secretion may also be found in neuroblastomas, ganglioneuroblastomas, and ganglioneuromas.[55]

Neuroblastoma

Neuroblastomas are malignant primitive neuroectodermal tumors that arise from embryonic sympathetic nervous tissue. They are found in most regions of the body.

Incidence

Of childhood neoplasms, only leukemia and brain tumors are more common than neuroblastomas. Their incidence reaches a maximum in the early years and declines in the adult years. Indeed, nearly all of them arise in childhood, with 80 per cent occurring before the age of five. They are also known to occur in fetal life. Although a rare tumor in adulthood, more than 60 such cases have been reported in the literature. When they occur in adulthood, the survival rate is low.[76]

Clinical Features

The clinical presentation usually is determined by the site of the primary tumor or its metastases and the age of the patient. When present in fetal life, a small percentage of neuroblastomas manufacture and release catecholamines that cause the mother to have palpitations, headaches, "sweats," and hypertension late in the pregnancy. Disseminated disease is demonstrated in the fetus, and sometimes there are metastases to the placenta. Congenital neuroblastoma has typical clinical features resembling erythroblastosis fetalis, with jaundice, anemia, edema, and distention of the abdomen. Sometimes this similarity to erythroblastosis fetalis leads to a delay in diagnosis. The infant frequently has liver metastases, and in about half the cases the disease is disseminated at the time of diagnosis. A unique feature of neuroblastoma in infancy is the presence of subcutaneous metastases giving the "blueberry muffin" appearance to the skin.

Despite their malignant behavior, these neoplasms show a curious ability to undergo spontaneous regression in infancy, even when there are widespread metastases. Between 62 and 70 per cent of newborns with this lesion appear to be cured with almost any form of therapy.[76] In one series of 29 spontaneous cures, the majority of patients were less than 6 months of age, and the mean age was 3 months. In addition to undergoing spontaneous cytolysis and necrosis, in rare cases the neuroblastoma may differentiate into a benign ganglioneuroma.[29]

In the neonate as well as in patients of all other ages, the most common site of the primary tumor is the abdomen, and it usually arises from the adrenal gland. This pattern accounts for 65 per cent of the tumors in children of all ages. Approximately 14 per cent are located in the chest, 4.5 per cent in the pelvis, 3.2 per cent in the neck, and 12 per cent in unknown sites.[76]

The majority of the patients do not manifest neurological deficits at the time of diagnosis. The most common findings in young children are weight loss, failure to thrive, fever, and anemia. Examination may reveal an abdominal or flank mass representing an adrenal primary tumor or a liver metastasis. Limb or joint tenderness or periorbital ecchymosis may represent metastases to long bones or bones of the oribit. Tumors presenting in the cervical region often cause neck masses, Horner's syndrome, cervical root syndromes, and rarely, vascular occlusion that sometimes involves the vena cava.[53] Thoracic lesions are almost always in the posterior mediastinum, and unless intraspinal extension or pain is manifested early, the tumors may grow to significant size while remaining asymptomatic. A small number of patients will complain of dyspnea, and some will present with a pleural effusion. Similarly, tumors in the abdomen and pelvis frequently grow to significant size before diagnosis. Enlarged abdominal girth or obvious abdominal masses accompanied by gastrointestinal or bladder symptoms may lead to the diagnosis. The majority of patients do not present initially for neurological consultation.

When neurological abnormalities are present, they usually are due to an intraspinal extension of the tumor. Pain, paresis of the extremities, or diminished sphincter control may result. In the cervical region, Horner's syndrome and arm pain may signify ganglionic involvement.

The clinical presentation of dumbbell neuroblastomas with intraspinal and extraspinal extension in children fall into two categories. Under two years of age, when the patients are unable to express themselves, approximately 50 per cent demonstrate regression in motor function. Less common clues to neurological involvement are irritability, shortness of breath, and continuous urinary dribbling. Among children over two years of age, nearly all complain of pain and a few complain of progressive paresis. In a series of 19 patients, neurological abnormalities were noted in 18. Five demonstrated flaccid paralysis, twelve had varying degrees of weakness, seven had impaired sphincter function, and five had muscle atrophy. Scoliosis was present in seven.[52]

Of 134 patients with neuroblastomas and 4 with ganglioneuroblastomas, 14 per cent had intraspinal extension of their tumors. The incidence of intraspinal extension was 32 per cent for the neuroblastomas arising in the thoracic region and originating from sympathetic ganglia, while abdominal tumors demonstrated a 10 per cent incidence.[52] These lesions account for the major neurological deficits from neuroblastoma. In intraspinal extension by dumbbell neuroblastomas as well as in the rare intra-

cranial metastasis, impingement on the central nervous system is usually by extrinsic compression rather than invasion. The spinal tumors are usually extradural in location.

Gross and Microscopic Features

These are fleshy, firm tumors, usually dark red or gray. They appear to be well demarcated, with smooth surfaces, but they also appear to be infiltrating in some areas. The primitive neuroectodermal origin is suggested by the hyperchromatic oval nuclei and the hypercellularity. The cytoplasmic borders are poorly defined. Light microscopy reveals the neuroblastoma's histological similarity to the medulloblastoma with rosette formation. Histologically, occasional areas of better-differentiated ganglion cells may suggest differentiation toward ganglioneuroblastoma.[45]

Diagnosis

The clinical presentation, especially in the presence of obvious superficial or abdominal masses, should suggest a diagnosis of neuroblastoma in the child. In the adult, because of the rarity of this tumor in this age group, the diagnosis may only be made by biopsy.

Routine chest x-rays are abnormal in almost all patients with mediastinal tumors. They may show a paravertebral mass, or an area of soft-tissue paravertebral density may appear on abdominal radiographs when there is a lumbar sympathetic or adrenal tumor.

Bone and liver scans may demonstrate metastases. Bone marrow biopsies may give histological evidence of the disease, while urinary vanillyl mandelic acid levels confirm its chemical activity.

With paravertebral masses, thorough radiographic investigation of the spine is essential. Intraspinal extension can occur without neurological signs or symptoms. Bony erosion may be present, however, and sometimes it causes foraminal enlargement. Approximately a third of patients with intraspinal involvement have scoliosis.[52] Myelography or computed tomography is essential to define such possible extension of the paravertebral mass because, although a dumbbell tumor can be removed in one operation, the intraspinal component must be removed prior to removal of the extraspinal component. Manipulation of the extraspinal component can cause swelling of the intraspinal portion and lead to further spinal cord compression and neurological deficit.[1]

Because of the tendency of neuroblastomas to infiltrate locally and to metastasize to distant areas, the total extent of the disease must be determined preoperatively. This evaluation must include a careful physical examination, nuclear scanning for metastatic disease, bone marrow biopsy, and careful radiological investigation. Appropriate therapy is determined primarily on the basis of age at diagnosis and stage of the disease. Pochedly has devised the following staging system, which is of some prognostic significance:

Stage I—Tumor confined to the organ or structure of origin.

Stage II—Tumor extending in continuity beyond the organ or structure of origin, but not crossing the midline. Ipsilateral lymph nodes may be involved.

Stage III—Tumor extending in continuity with the primary lesion beyond the midline. Regional lymph nodes may be involved bilaterally.

Stage IV—Remote disease involving the skeletal system, viscera, soft tissue, and distant lymph nodes.

Stage IV-S—Primary tumor fulfilling the characteristics of stage I or stage II, but also demonstrating remote metastatic involvement confined to liver, skin, or bone marrow, without radiographic evidence of bone metastasis.[76]

Treatment and Prognosis

The variable natural history of neuroblastoma, with its capacity for spontaneous regression in the first year of life and increasingly malignant behavior with increasing age, has complicated the determination of effective therapy. The majority of lesions do not compromise vital neurological structures and function, and therefore are managed by specialists other than neurosurgeons.

In most series, the resectable lesions are in children of less than 1 year of age. Since these children tend to do well with almost any form of treatment, it is difficult to de-termine the benefits of resection. Older children tend to manifest more widespread disease by the time of diagnosis and are more likely to have unresectable lesions. Even with partial resection in the presence of extensive disease, however, survival has been prolonged. For these reasons, radical resection is not recommended.

The roles of radiotherapy and chemotherapy are controversial. In patients with stage I, II, or IV-S disease, prolonged survival may follow any combination of surgery, radiotherapy, and chemotherapy. Thus the morbidity of each added therapeutic regimen must be weighed carefully.

The patient coming to the attention of a neurological surgeon usually will have a dumbbell tumor with intraspinal extension that causes spinal cord and nerve root compression. The recommended treatment is a laminectomy with total or subtotal tumor resection. As indicated earlier, the intraspinal tumor should be resected first. Postoperative radiotherapy is recommended. The combination of operation plus radiation gives cure rates of 60 to 70 per cent in children.[52] Chemotherapy must be considered in older patients and in all patients with stage III or stage IV disease.

Chemotherapy has been used in patients with disseminated disease. No increase in cure rate has been demonstrated; however, some survivals have been longer. Combination chemotherapy with cyclophosphamide and vincristine may offer some benefit in extending survival time in adults, but not in increasing cure rates.[28]

A patient living longer than two years following diagnosis usually can be considered cured. At present, two-year survival (or cure) rates have not been significantly altered by any of the therapeutic regimens. The main determinants of cure are the patient's age and the stage of the disease at the time of diagnosis. The present modes of therapy may alter the length of survival, but they do not dramatically affect cure rates. The child less than 1 year of age may have a 60 to 80 per cent chance of cure compared with the child between 1 and 2 years of age, whose chance of being cured is 20 to 30 per cent. Older patients have a dismal prognosis, with a 5 to 13 per cent cure rate. Patients with stages I, II, and IV-S disease at diagnosis demonstrate a 60 per cent cure rate compared with 10 per cent for those whose disease is in stages III and IV.[26,76]

Ganglioneuroblastoma

In most studies, ganglioneuroblatomas are grouped with neuroblastomas. The ganglioneuroblastoma, or differentiated neuroblastoma, appears histologically to be a more mature form of neuroblatoma. Histological examination reveals areas of primitive neuroblastoma cells combined with other areas showing prominent glial tissue and large ganglion cells.[45]

These tumors are malignant and, like neuroblastoma, tend to occur in childhood and but rarely in adulthood.[51] The gross and clinical features are similar to those of neuroblastoma. Biologically they behave like neuroblastomas, displaying the same malignant tendencies. Also, they may be endocrinologically active and produce an elevation of the urinary catecholamine levels.

Ganglioneuroblastomas are treated as neuroblastomas, since the clinical and biological activities are similar, with the distinguishing features being histological. Prognosis is poor in adults, the majority of tumors being only partially resectable because of local and distant spread. As with neuroblastomas, the prognosis is best and the cure rates are highest among infants and young children. The prognosis becomes progressively worse with increasing age.

Ganglioneuroma

Ganglioneuromas are benign tumors of the sympathetic nervous system. They are, indeed, well-differentiated, benign manifestations of the same tumor type as neuroblastoma. Neuroblastomas can differentiate into ganglioneuromas, a phenomenon that partially accounts for the spontaneous remissions in children.

The ganglioneuromas are one sixth as common as neuroblastomas. Because they tend to remain asymptomatic until attaining massive size, however, many escape early diagnosis. In contrast to neuroblastomas, which tend to occur in early childhood, ganglioneuromas are relatively uncommon in childhood. They occur predominantly in adolescence and adulthood. Most frequently they are in the mediastinum and the adrenal gland; they arise wherever sympathetic tissue is found, from the skull base to the pelvis. Rare ganglioneuromas also arise in the brain.

When they occur in the neck, Horner's syndrome usually is present, since the cervical sympathetic ganglia are involved. As the tumor grows, compression of local structures may result in arm pain or difficulty in swallowing and breathing.

Ganglioneuromas of the thoracic cavity usually occur in the posterior mediastinum. Most are symptomatic and are diagnosed on a routine chest x-ray that shows a paravertebral mass, commonly with calcification. Scoliosis may be a presenting feature. Uncommonly they may compress bronchi and result in respiratory symptoms. Dumbbell tumors may compress the spinal cord and cause paraplegia.

In the abdomen and pelvis, the majority of tumors arise from the adrenal and lumbosacral paravertebral ganglia in the retroperitoneum. There are also rare tumors of the gastrointestinal tract, arising from Meissner's and Auerbach's plexuses. Symptoms of abdominal discomfort, constipation, or diarrhea may result. Most ganglioneuromas of the abdomen and pelvis, like those in other regions, remain asymptomatic until attaining massive size.

Like their malignant counterparts of the sympathetic system, ganglioneuromas may produce catecholamines. In fact, a greater percentage of ganglioneuromas than of neuroblastomas are hormonally active.[82]

These tumors are well encased by a fibrous capsule, lobulated or oval, and firm. They are benign. With slow growth, they may become adherent to adjacent structures, and sometimes they form dumbbell tumors extending into the spinal canal. Histologically they consist of large mature ganglion cells in a surrounding matrix of fibrous connective tissue. Because ganglioneuroblastomas characteristically contain areas resembling ganglioneuromas with mature ganglion cells, an adequate biopsy must be taken. If the tumor displays rapid growth and other malignant characteristics, a higher degree of suspicion must be maintained. Invasion of a ganglion by a neurofibroma may be misinterpreted as a ganglioneuroma.[39]

Usually these tumors lend themselves to total excision. When they are dangerously adherent to such critical structures as great vessels or the spinal cord, subtotal excision is recommended. The tumors are very slow growing and rarely require further resection even after being only subtotally removed. As with other dumbbell tumors of the spine, removal of the intraspinal component is accomplished first by laminectomy. Care must be taken to avoid cord damage. When reoperation is required, usually it is because of recurring symptoms from an intraspinal tumor. Operative excision is the only effective therapy, since the tumors are quite resistant to radiation therapy and no effective chemotherapy is available. Prognosis is excellent even with partial tumor excision.

PARAGANGLIOMA

The cells of the neural crest differentiate into many components, including the sympathetic and paraganglionic systems. In the development of these systems, the primitive cells, the sympathogonia, may differentiate into ganglia and neurons to make up the sympathetic nervous system. Other primitive cells may differentiate into the paraganglia, and together with some sympathoblasts or cells destined to become sympathetic ganglia, migrate to para-axial regions, forming the paraganglionic system. The paraganglia parallel and are intimately connected with the sympathetic system extending from the head to the pelvis.

In fetal life, the numerous masses of the paraganglionic system are discrete, easily recognized, oval bodies adjacent to the great vessels and trachea in the neck and chest, and lie in para-axial regions along the entire extent of the aorta. By puberty, most have diminished in size, becoming unrecognizable on gross examination, except in the adrenal medulla.

The paraganglionic system includes the adrenal medulla and the wide network of extra-adrenal paraganglia. All components of this system maintain a network of neural connections with the sympathetic and parasympathetic systems. In the classification of the extra-adrenal paraganglionic system, Glennen and Grimley identified the following divisions on an anatomical basis: Branchiomeric and intravagal paraganglia, aorticosympathetic paraganglia, and visceral-autonomic paraganglia.[39,45] Like the adrenal medulla, most of the paraganglia have the ability to synthesize and store catecholamines. Some, like the carotid and aortic bodies, are chemoreceptors, responding to changes in acid-base balance and arterial carbon dioxide tension.

Aside from the adrenal medulla and the carotid and aortic bodies, the paraganglionic system is not well understood physiologically. Its anatomy suggests that it interacts with the rest of the autonomic system, indirectly affecting the visceral functions.[39]

Tumors of the paraganglionic system— the neurogenic tumors of the adrenal and the neuroblastoma and the pheochromocytoma—reflect its embryological origins. Neuroblastomas arise from the primitive sympathoblasts that migrated along with the embryonic paraganglion cells to their suprarenal sites. The pheochromocytoma, in Glennen and Grimley's terminology, is an "adrenal functioning paraganglioma," noting the tumor's anatomical position and endocrine status. To be more specific, a norepinephrine-secreting paraganglioma of the adrenal may be termed "norepinephrine-secreting adrenal paraganglioma."[39]

Tumors arising from chemoreceptive organs of the paraganglionic system, the carotid and aortic bodies, may be described as "carotid nonfunctioning paragangliomas." Those tumors are known classically as the chemodectomas, which may or may not be hormonally active.[39]

Paragangliomas, then, may arise wherever paraganglion tissues exist. They may or may not be catecholamine-producing and, although they are usually benign, they can also be malignant.

Pheochromocytoma

The term "pheochromocytoma" has been classically used to describe an adrenal functioning (epinephrine- and norepinephrine-secreting) paraganglioma, but it has also been applied to extra-adrenal functioning paraganglionomas.[34,39] These solid, well-circumscribed, lobular masses may occur anywhere in the paraganglionic system. They arise in the adrenal 90 per cent of the time in adults and approximately 70 per cent of the time in children.[36,47,91] Children are much more likely than adults to have bilateral tumors, as they did in 70 per cent of the cases in one series.[10]

This is a tumor predominantly of adults, but it has been reported in patients from 5 months to 82 years of age. The peak incidence is between 20 and 50 years.[91]

The pheochromocytoma usually is benign, but approximately 10 per cent are malignant. Most often, the metastases go to liver, lung, and bone.[68] The malignant tumors may grow rapidly and tend to secrete dopa and dopamine, catecholamine precursors.[91] The classic presenting symptoms and signs of pheochromocytoma are those of epinephrine and norepinephrine release. Nearly all patients have sustained or paroxysmal hypertension, but rarely blood pressure may be normal.[36,42,72] Associated common symptoms are excessive perspiration, palpitations, headaches, and paroxysmal nausea and vomiting. Syncope, seizures, and visual difficulties also may occur. These symptoms often are precipitated by physical activity and emotional stress.[62,73] In a few patients cerebral vascular accidents with hemiplegia occur prior to the diagnosis.[68] Spinal cord compression by intraspinal extension is rare.[36]

Making this diagnosis remains a major problem in the treatment of this disease. The classic symptom complex can be identified easily; many patients, however, have only mild symptoms in a setting of normal or slightly elevated blood pressure. Of hypertensive patients, approximately 0.5 per cent have pheochromocytomas.[72]

Diagnosis involves systemic screening for the presence of catecholamines or their metabolites, and preoperative tumor localization tests. During sleep, patients with pheochromocytomas have urinary excretion of norepinephrine at levels seven times as high as those of patients with essential hypertension or normotension. Plasma norepinephrine levels also have been elevated in tumor patients.[37]

The intravenous pyelogram and selective arteriogram have been utilized most frequently in the past to localize the tumors. Current use of the CT scan offers the advantages of a lower risk as well as the ability to detect bilateral and extra-adrenal tumors. Arteriography still has the advantage of demonstrating the vascular anatomy for the surgeon. Selective sampling of venous blood may be helpful in disclosing the presence and location of extra-adrenal, bilateral, or recurrent tumors too small to be detected with other studies.[25,36,37]

The treatment of pheochromocytoma is operative resection. The operative mortality rate prior to 1950 was 25 to 45 per cent, but with the use of adrenergic blockers and a better understanding of the pathophysiology of this disease, the rate has dropped to 3 per cent for smaller tumors and to 25 per cent for the more complicated ones.[4,79]

Coexistence of severe hypertensive cardiovascular disease must be recognized. Preoperatively, alpha- and beta-adrenergic blockers are utilized. Intraoperative management is critical because of blood pressure fluctuations.[18,78] Manipulation of the tumor produces striking elevations of blood pressure intraoperatively.[31] Rapid intravascular volume replacement is often needed when a precipitous drop in blood pressure occurs following removal of the tumor. Quite frequently the problem is complicated by the presence of chronic volume depletion.[78]

The prognosis following a successful resection depends on the presence or absence of malignancy, the age of the patient, and the coexistence of other diseases and association with familial related diseases. Neurofibromatosis, medullary carcinoma of the thyroid with multiple endocrine adenopathy, renal artery stenosis, and von Hippel-Lindau disease have all been associated with pheochromocytomas. In these settings, the risk of having other paragangliomas is increased.

If familial or other associated diseases are not present, the prognosis following resection of a benign pheochromocytoma is excellent. The Mayo Clinic group reported a five-year survival rate of 96 per cent.[79]

All patients with pheochromocytomas require close long-term follow-up because of the possibility of recurrences or development of other paragangliomas. The majority require ongoing antihypertensive treatment even in the absence of elevated catecholamine levels.

Chemodectoma

Paragangliomas arising from chemoreceptive tissues of the paraganglionic system are called chemodectomas. The best known are the rare carotid body chemodectomas, which typically arise at the carotid bifurcation and cause displacement of the internal and external carotid arteries. Usually the carotid body lesions present as painless lateral neck masses. Sometimes they cause neurological problems such as hoarseness, vocal cord paralysis, Horner's syndrome, and facial paresis. Also, some may be endocrinologically active and secrete catecholamines, thus creating the adrenergic picture typical of pheochromocytomas.[39]

These tumors have occurred in patients as young as 7 years and as old as 75 years, the average being 45 years.[39] Typically they are slow-growing, with symptoms present for one or two years before diagnosis; they can, however, also be aggressively malignant with metastases.

The diagnosis may be suspected because of their location at the carotid bifurcation, and is best demonstrated by subtraction angiography.[71] These are vascular tumors that usually are supplied by branches of the external carotid artery. Radionuclide perfusion scanning and CT scans may also be helpful in diagnosis.[71,74,77]

Operative resection is the best treatment available. Resection of the benign or malignant chemodectoma may require carotid segmental resection and placement of an arterial graft. Prognosis for cure is good for benign and small malignant tumors.

Some investigators state that malignant chemodectomas are relatively uncommon; others, however, disagree.[39] Of the malignant tumors, approximately 50 per cent have metastases at diagnosis, most commonly to the lymph nodes, lung, and skeleton.[77] The death rate is high with malignant chemodectomas in the presence of metastases.

Chemotherapy has been ineffective. Radiation therapy has resulted in sporadic response in malignant and recurrent tumors.[39] Operative resection is the mainstay of treatment.

REFERENCES

1. Akwari, O. E., Payne, W. S., Onofrio, B. M., Dines, D. E., and Muhm, J. R.: Dumbbell neurogenic tumors of the mediastinum: Diagnosis and management. Mayo Clin. Proc., 53:353–358, 1978.
2. Allen, R. W. Jr., Ogden, B., Bentley, F. L., and Jung, A. L.: Fetal hydantoin syndrome, neuroblastoma, and hemorrhagic disease in a neonate. J.A.M.A., 244:1464–1465, 1980.
3. Anand, C. S., Kumra, P. K., Anand, T. S., and Singh, S. K.: Facial nerve schwannoma. J. Laryng., 91:1093–1099, 1977.
4. Apgar, V., and Papper, E. M.: Pheochromocytoma: Anesthetic management during surgical treatment. Arch. Surg. (Chicago), 62:634–648, 1951.
5. Arseni, C., Dumitrescu, L., and Constantinescu, A.: Neurinomas of the trigeminal nerve. Surg. Neurol., 4:497–503, 1975.
6. Asbury, A. K., and Johnson, P. C.: Tumors of peripheral nerve. In Pathology of Peripheral

Nerve. Philadelphia, W. B. Saunders Co., 1978, pp. 206–229.
7. Ballantyne, A. J., McCarten, A. B., and Ibanez, M. L.: The extension of cancer of the head and neck through peripheral nerves. Amer. J. Surg., 106:651–667, 1963.
8. Barber, J. R., Coventry, M. B., and McDonald, J. R.: The spread of soft-tissue sarcomata of the extremities along peripheral-nerve trunks. J. Bone Joint Surg., 39-A:534–540, 1957.
9. Bartley, T. D., and Arean, V. M.: Intrapulmonary neurogenic tumors. J. Thorac. Cardiovasc. Surg., 50:114–23, 1965.
10. Bloom, D. A., and Fonkalsrud, E. W.: Surgical management of pheochromocytoma in children. J. Pediat. Surg., 9:179–184, 1974.
11. Bloom, W., and Fawcett, D. W.: A Textbook of Histology. 10th Ed. Philadelphia, W. B. Saunders Co., 1975.
12. Boggan, J. E., Rosenblum, M. L., and Wilson, C. B.: Neurilemmoma of the fourth cranial nerve. Case report. J. Neurosurg., 50:519–521, 1979.
13. Bolande, R. P.: Benignity of neonatal tumors and concept of cancer repression in early life. Amer. J. Dis. Child., 122:12–14, 1971.
14. Cantin, J., McNeer, G. P., Chu, F. C., and Booher, R. J.: The problem of local recurrence aftrer treatment of soft tissue sarcoma. Ann. Surg., 168:47–53, 1968.
15. Cavanaugh, D. G., Walker, O. M., and Treasure, R. L.: Benign schwannoma of the phrenic nerve: Case report. Milit. Med., 144:406–407, 1979.
16. Clairmont, A. A., and Conley, J. J.; Schwannomas of the cervical sympathetic nerve. Ear Nose Throat J., 57:336–339, 1978.
17. Conley, J., and Janecka, I.: Schwann cell tumors of the facial nerve. Laryngoscope, 84:958–962, 1974.
18. Daggett, P., Verner, I., and Carruthers, M.: Intraoperative management of phaeochromocytoma with sodium nitroprusside, Brit. Med. J., 2:311–313, 1978.
19. D'Agostino, A. N., Soule, E. H., and Miller, R. H.: Primary malignant neoplasms of nerves (malignant neurilemomas) in patients without manifestations of multiple neurofibromatosis (von Recklinghausen's disease). Cancer, 16:1003–1014, 1963.
20. D'Agostino, A. N., Soule, E. H., and Miller, R. H.: Sarcomas of the peripheral nerves and somatic soft tissues associated with multiple neurofibromatosis (von Recklinghausen's disease). Cancer, 16:1015–1027, 1963.
21. Danziger, J., Bloch, S., and Podlas, H.: Schwannomas of the central nervous system. Amer. J. Roentgen., 125:692–701, 1975.
22. Dart, L. H., MacCarty, C. S., Love, J. G., and Dockerty, M. B.: Neoplasms of the brachial plexus. Minn. Med., 53:959–964, 1970.
23. Das Gupta, T. K.: Tumors of the peripheral nerves. Clin. Neurosurg., 25:574–590, 1977.
24. Das Gupta, T. K., Brasfield, R. D., Strong, E. W., and Hajdu, S. I.: Benign solitary schwannomas (neurilemomas). Cancer, 24:355–366, 1969.
25. Davies, R. A., Patt, N. L., and Sole, M. J.: Localization of pheochromocytoma by selective venous catheterization and assay of plasma catecholamines. Canad. Med. Ass. J., 120:539–542, 1979.

26. DiNicola, W., Movassaghi, N., and Leikin, S.: Prognosis in black children with neuroblastoma. Cancer, 36:1151–1153, 1975.

27. Dodd, G. D., Dolan, P. A., Ballantyne, A. J., Ibanez, M. L., and Chau, P.: The dissemination of tumors of the head and neck via the cranial nerves. Radiol. Clin. N. Amer., 8:445–461, 1970.

28. Dosik, G. M., Rodriguez, V., Benjamin, R. S., and Bodey, G.: Neuroblastoma in the adult: Effective combination chemotherapy. Cancer, 41:56–63, 1978.

29. Everson, T. C., and Cole, W. H.: Spontaneous Regression of Cancer. Philadelphia, W. B. Saunders Co., 1966.

30. Factor, S., Turi, G., and Biempica, L.: Primary cardiac neurilemoma. Cancer, 37:883–890, 1976.

31. Feldman, J. M., Blaloci, J. A. Fagraeus, L., Miller, J. N., Farrell, R. E., and Wells, S. A., Jr.: Alterations in plasma norepinephrine concentration during surgical resection of pheochromocytoma. Ann. Surg., 188:758–768, 1978.

32. Fink, L. H., Early, C. B., and Bryan, R. N.: Glossopharyngeal schwannomas. Surg. Neurol., 9:239–245, 1978.

33. Fisher, R. G., and Tate, H. B.: Isolated neurilemomas of the branchial plexus. J. Neurosurg., 32:463–467, 1970.

34. Fries, J. G., and Chamberlin, J. A.: Extra-adrenal pheochromocytoma: literature review and report of a cervical pheochromocytoma. Surgery, 63:268–279, 1968.

35. Gale, A. W., Jelihovsky, T., Grant, A. F., Leckie, B. D., and Nicks, R.: Neurogenic tumors of the mediastinum. Ann. Thorac. Surg., 17:434–443, 1974.

36. Gallivan, M. V. E., Chun, B., Rowden, G., and Lack, E. E.: Intrathoracic paravertebral malignant paraganglioma. Arch. Path. Lab. Med., 104:46–51, 1980.

37. Ganguly, A., Henry, D. P., Yune, H. Y., Pratt, J. H., Grim, C. E., Donohue, J. P., and Weinberger, M. H.: Diagnosis and localization of pheochromocytoma. Amer. J. Med., 67:21–26, 1979.

38. Gayloa, G., Janis, M., and Weil, P. H.: Intrathoracic nerve sheath tumor of the vagus. J. Thorac. Cardiovasc. Surg., 49:412–418, 1965.

39. Glennen, G. G., and Grimley, P. M.: Tumors of the extra-adrenal paraganglion system. In Tumors of the Peripheral Nervous System. Washington, D.C., Armed Forces Institute of Pathology, 1974.

40. Gordon, E. J.: Solitary intraosseous neurilemmoma of the tibia. Clin. Orthop., 117:271–282, 1976.

41. Gould, V. E., Rogers, D. R., and Sommers, S. C.: Epithelial-nerve intermingling in benign breast lesions. Arch. Path. (Chicago), 99:596–598, 1975.

42. Gray, R. S., and Gillon, J.: Normotensive phaeochromocytoma with hypercalcaemia: Correction after adrenalectomy. Brit. Med. J., 1:378, 1976.

43. Hammond, J. A., and Driedger, A. A.: Detection of malignant change in neurofibromatosis (von Recklinghausen's disease) by gallium-67 scanning. Canad. Med. Ass. J., 119:352–353, 1978.

44. Handler, S. D., Canalis, R. F., Jenkins, H. A., and Weiss, A. J.: Management of brachial plexus tumors. Arch. Otolaryng. (Chicago), 103:653–657, 1977.

45. Harkin, J. C., and Reed, R. J.: Tumors of the Peripheral Nervous System. Washington, D.C., Armed Forces Institute of Pathology, 1968.

46. Herness, D., Posner, M. A., and Steiner, G.: Malignant schwannoma. Hand, 7:300–302, 1975.

47. Hodgkinson, D. J., Telander, R. L., Sheps, S. G., Gilchrist, G. S., and Crowe, J. K.: Case reports: Extra-adrenal intrathoracic functioning paraganglioma (pheochromocytoma) in childhood. Mayo Clin. Proc., 55:271–276, 1980.

48. Holt, G. R.: E.N.T. manifestations of von Recklinghausen's disease. Laryngoscope, 88:1617–1632, 1978.

49. Hutcherson, R. W., Jenkins, H. A., Canalis, R. F., Handler, S. D., and Eichel, B. S.: Neurogenic sarcoma of the head and neck. Arch. Otolaryng. (Chicago), 105:267–270, 1979.

50. Ingels, G. W., Campbell, D. C., Jr., Giampetro, A. M., Kozub, R. E., and Bentlage, C. H.: Malignant schwannomas of the mediastinum: Report of two cases and review of the literature. Cancer, 27:1190–1201, 1971.

51. Kilton, L. J., Aschenbrener, C., and Burns, C. P.: Ganglioneuroblastoma in adults. Cancer, 37:974–983, 1976.

52. King, D., Goodman, J., Hawk, T., Boles, E. T., Jr., and Sayers, M. P.: Dumbbell neuroblastomas in children. Arch. Surg. (Chicago), 110:888–891, 1975.

53. King, J. S.: Trochlear nerve sheath tumor. Case report. J. Neurosurg., 44:245–247, 1976.

54. Kline, D. G.: Comment on Richard, R. R., Siqueira, E. B., Oi, S., and Nunez, C.: Neurogenic tumors of the brachial plexus: Report of two cases. Neurosurgery, 4:66–70, 1979.

55. Kogut, M. D., and Kaplan, S. A.: Systemic manifestations of neurogenic tumors. J. Pediat., 60:694–704, 1962.

56. Kovalcik, P. J., Simstein, N. L., and Cross, G. H.: Benign neurilemmoma manifesting as a presacral (retrorectal) mass: Report of a case. Dis. Colon Rectum, 21:199–202, 1978.

57. Krueger, W., Weisberger, E., Ballantyne, A. J., and Goepfert, H.: Plexiform neurofibroma of the head and neck. Amer. J. Surg., 138:517–520, 1979.

58. Larson, D. L., Rodin, A. E., Roberts, D. K., O'Steen, W. K., Rapperport, A. S., and Lewis, S. R.: Perineural lymphatics: Myth or fact. Amer. J. Surg., 112:488–492, 1966.

59. Levinthal, R., and Bentson, J. R.: Detection of small trigeminal neurinomas. J. Neurosurg., 45:568–575, 1976.

60. Mabogunje, O. A.: Benign intraparotid neurilemoma of the facial nerve. J. Pediat. Surg., 12:577–579, 1977.

61. Majmudar, B.: Neurilemoma presenting as a lump in the breast. Southern Med. J., 69:463–464, 1976.

62. Manger, W. M., Davis, S. W., and Chu, D.: Autonomic hyperreflexia and its differentiation from pheochromocytoma. Arch. Phys. Med., 60:159–161, 1979.

63. Mark, G. J.: Basal cell carcinoma with intraneural invasion. Cancer, *40*:2181–2187, 1977.

64. Marmor, L.: Solitary peripheral nerve tumors. Clin. Orthop., *43*:183–187, 1965.

65. Menon, J., Dorfman, H. D., Renbaum, J., and Friedler, S.: Tarsal tunnel syndrome secondary to neurilemoma of the medial plantar nerve. J. Bone Joint Surg., *62-A*:301–303, 1980.

66. Mickalites, C. J., and Rappaport, I.: Perineural invasion by squamous-cell carcinoma of the lower lip: Review of the literature and report of a case. Oral Surg., *46*:74–78, 1978.

67. Miller, P. L., Tessler, A., Alexander, S., and Pinck, B. D.: Retroperitoneal neurilemmoma. Urology, *11*:619–623, 1978.

68. Modlin, I. M., Farndon, J. R., Shepherd, A., Johnston, I. D. A., Kennedy, T. L., Montgomery, D. A. D., and Welbourn, R. B.: Phaeochromocytomas in 72 patients: Clinical and diagnostic features, treatment and long term results. Br. J. Surg., *66*:456–465, 1979.

69. Nass, R. L., and Cohen, N. L.: Neurilemoma of the trachea. Arch. Otolaryng. (Chicago), *105*:220–221, 1979.

70. Nesbitt, K. A., and Vidone, R. A.: Primitive neuroectodermal tumor (neuroblastoma) arising in sciatic nerve of a child. Cancer, *37*:1562–1570, 1976.

71. O'Callaghan, J., Timperley, W. R., and Ward, P.: The CT scan and subtraction angiography in chemodectomas. Clin. Radiol., *30*:575–580, 1979.

72. Öhman, U., Granberg, P., Lindvall, N., and Sjöberg, H. E.: Pheochromocytoma: Critical review of experiences with diagnosis and treatment. Progr. Clin. Cancer, *7*:135–152, 1978.

73. Paulson, G. W., Zipf, R. E., Jr., and Beekman, J. R.: Pheochromocytoma causing exercise-related headache and pulmonary edema. Ann. Neurol., *5*:96–99, 1979.

74. Peters, J. L., Ward, M. W., and Fisher, C.: Diagnosis of a carotid body chemodectoma with dynamic radionuclide perfusion scanning. Amer. J. Surg., *137*:661–664, 1979.

75. Phalen, G. S.: Neurilemmomas of the forearm and hand. Clin. Orthop., *114*:219–222, 1976.

76. Pochedly, C.: Neuroblastoma. Littleton, Mass., Publishing Sciences Group, Inc., 1976.

77. Poster, D. S., Schapiro, H., and Woronoff, R.: Chemodectomas: Review and report of nine cases. J. Med., *10*:207–223, 1979.

78. Pratilas, V., and Pratila, M. G.: Anaesthetic management of phaeochromocytoma. Canad. Anaesth. Soc. J., *26*:253–259, 1979.

79. Remine, W. H., Chong, G. C., Van Heerden, J.

A., Sheps, S. G., and Harrison, E. G., Jr.: Current management of pheochromocytoma. Ann. Surg., *179*:740–748, 1974.

80. Richards, J. L., and Matolo, N. M.: Malignant schwannoma: Report of a case mimicking lumbar disk disease. Amer. Surg., *45*:49–51, 1979.

81. Robb, J. E.: Trigger finger due to neurilemmoma in the carpal tunnel. Hand, *10*:299–301, 1978.

82. Rosenstein, B. J., and Engleman, K.: Diarrhea in a child with a catecholamine-secreting ganglioneuroma. J. Pediat., *63*:217–226, 1963.

83. Russell, D. A., and Rubinstein, L. J.: Pathology of Tumours of the Nervous System. London, Edward Arnold, Ltd., 1959.

84. Sarin, C. L., Bennett, M. H., and Jackson, J. W.: Intrathoracic neurofibroma of the vagus nerve. Brit. J. Dis. Chest, *68*:46–50, 1974.

85. Seddon, H.: Surgical Disorders of the Peripheral Nerves. 2nd Ed. Edinburgh, London and New York, Churchill Livingstone, 1975.

86. Shiu, M. H., Castro, E. B., Hajdu, S. I., and Fortner, J. G.: Surgical treatment of 297 soft tissue sarcomas of the lower extremity. Ann. Surg., *182*:597–602, 1975.

87. Snyder, M., Batzdorf, U., and Sparks, F. C.: Unusual malignant tumors involving the brachial plexus: A report of two cases. Amer. Surg., *45*:42–48, 1979.

88. Stout, A. P.: Tumors of the peripheral nervous system. J. Missouri Med. Ass., *46*:255–259, 1949.

89. Swaiman, K. F.: Antiepileptic drugs, the developing nervous system, and the pregnant woman with epilepsy (editorial). J.A.M.A., *244*:1477, 1980.

90. Terzis, J. K., Daniel, R. K., Williams, H. B., and Spencer, P. S.: Benign fatty tumors of the peripheral nerves. Annl. Plast. Surg., *1*:193–216, 1978.

91. Van Way, C. W., III., Scott, H. W., Jr., Page D. L., and Rhamy, R. K.: Pheochromocytoma. *In* Current Problems in Surgery. Chicago, Year Book Medical Publishers, Inc., 1974.

92. Vieta, J. O., and Pack, G. T.: Malignant neurilemomas of peripheral nerves. Amer. J. Surg., *82*:416–431, 1951.

93. White, H. R., Jr.: Survival in malignant schwannoma: An 18-year study. Cancer, *27*:720–729, 1971.

94. White, N. B.: Neurilemomas of the extremities. J. Bone Joint Surg., *49-A*:1605–1610, 1967.

95. Wirth, W. A., and Bray, C. B., Jr.: Intra-osseous neurilemoma. J. Bone Joint Surg., *59-A*:252–255, 1977.

109

TUMORS OF THE SCALP

Scalp tumors can be benign or malignant. If they are malignant, they can be primary or metastatic tumors.

BENIGN TUMORS OF THE SCALP

There are as many types of tumors of the scalp as there are types of tissues present in the scalp. The most common benign tumors of the scalp would be sebaceous cysts, inclusion cysts, dermoid cysts, nevi, keratoses, lipomas, hemangiomas, lymphangiomas, and tumors of sweat gland origin. Because of the large number of glandular structures in the scalp, there are numerous tumors that derive from these structures such as syringocystadenomas and sebaceous adenomas. Other types include fibromas, e.g., neurofibromas. Vascular tumors such as aneurysms may be present. In these the mass will be pulsatile and may be accompanied by a bruit. Excising this lesion may lead to bleeding, and proximal control of the vessels or vessels involved should be assured.

The other benign lesions can usually be treated with simple excision and closure. If the defect created by excision is larger than one inch, it may be necessary to undermine the scalp and relax the galea by "ribbing" the undersurface. If this maneuver is not adequate, then closure with a skin graft or flap may be necessary.

MALIGNANT TUMORS OF THE SCALP

Malignant tumors of the scalp are not common and represent only 2 per cent of the epithelial tumors of the skin.

Malignant scalp tumors can be either primary or metastatic. Primary malignant tumors have been reviewed by Connelly.[1,2] In a series of 150 patients, 58 had melanomas, 57 had basal cell carcinomas, 24 had squamous cell carcinomas, 9 had sarcomas, and 2 had adenosarcomas. Some of these malignant growths may be associated with chronic scar, inflammation, and actinic keratoses.

Metastatic tumors have their origin in the breast, stomach, legs, kidney, prostate gland, and intestine.

Hematogenous neoplasms such as lymphomas and leukemias may be first noticed as an ulcerative lesion of the scalp (Fig. 109 –1).

Excisional biopsy of small lesions suspected of being malignant is indicated. Occasionally, histological examination will show them to be metastatic. Large undiagnosed tumors should be subjected to incisional biopsy to establish a clear diagnosis prior to embarking on a large cancer operation.

Squamous Cell Carcinoma

Squamous cell carcinomas usually are noted as an ulcerative lesion and usually arise within the skin elements themselves. These tumors of the scalp can be aggressive and will invade by direct extension and eventually be picked up by the scalp lymphatics, from which they can metastasize through the regional lymph nodes. Aggressive squamous cell carcinoma can penetrate through the bone. If this occurs, wide operative excision will include portions of the skull and occasionally portions of the underlying dura (Fig. 109–2).

Because of the proximity to the bony tis-

W. M. COCKE, JR., AND J. S. SILVERTON

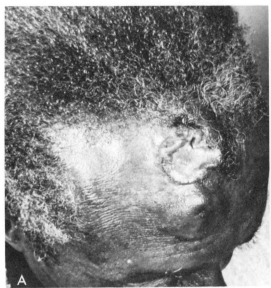
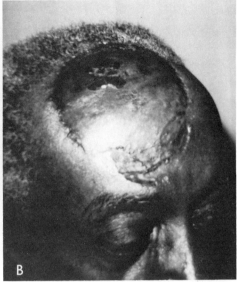

Figure 109–1 *A.* An ulcerative lesion of the frontal scalp that was thought to be a metastatic lesion of an ana-plastic nature. The patient was doing well a year after this diagnosis was made. A re-evaluation and work-up and a total excisional biopsy showed this to be a lymphoma. *B.* Postoperative result following wide excision of the tumor and reconstruction with a thick split-thickness skin graft.

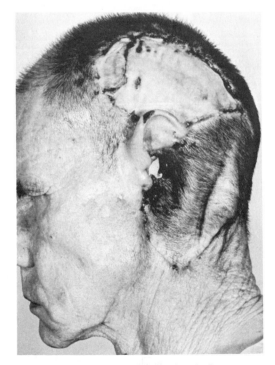

Figure 109–2 The use of a local scalp flap to cover the defect left by wide excision of a squamous cell carcinoma of the ear. Because a full thickness of skull was taken, the flap was used to cover the exposed dura. A thick split-thickness skin graft was used to cover the flap donor site on the parietal scalp.

sue, the recommended treatment for squamous cell carcinoma is wide excision and closure. If only the soft tissue is involved, the closure can be most simply done by application of a split-thickness skin graft. If bare bone or brain is exposed, however, flap closure is indicated (Fig. 109–3). The flap donor site can be closed with a split-thickness skin graft. If there is enough scalp tissue left, the best flap is from the adjacent scalp tissue. This can be elevated and rotated into position.

Basal Cell Carcinoma

Basal cell carcinoma is usually not so aggressive. It grows persistently but at a slower rate. These lesions vary widely in physical appearances, ranging from the skin-colored to the darkly pigmented, as shown in Figure 109–4, from the ulcerative to the flat, from round to eccentric. The differential diagnosis would include neuromas, sebaceous adenomas, and squamous cell carcinomas; and if pigmented, they can appear as melanomas.[3]

Small malignant lesions can be treated by electrodesiccation curettage, simple excision, or irradiation. These methods of treatment are not recommended. Most surgeons prefer to excise the lesion and send the

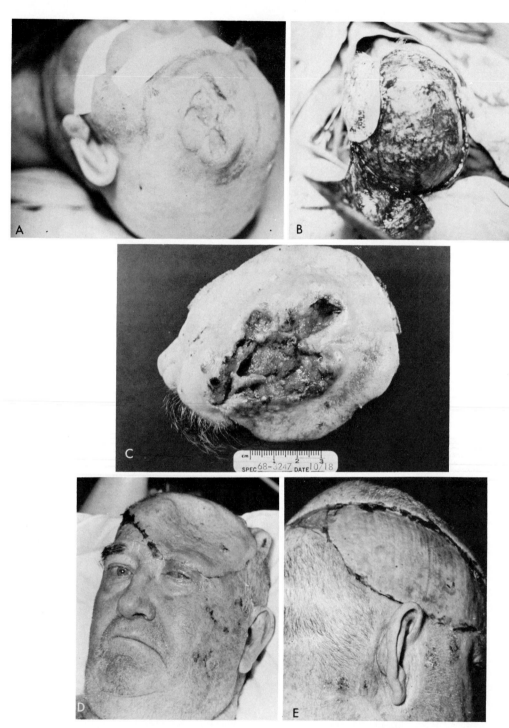

Figure 109–3 *A*. A large infiltrating squamous cell carcinoma of the frontal scalp. *B*. Operative view of the top of the patient's head. The ablative procedure was done by a combined team of neurosurgeons and plastic surgeons. *C*. The resected specimen. *D*. The postoperative status, which shows the scalp flap shifted to cover the defect over the dura. *E*. The split-thickness skin graft that was used to cover the flap donor site. This graft was taken from the thigh.

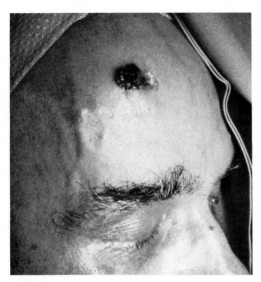

Figure 109-4 A melanotic lesion of the frontal scalp. Excisional biopsy and histological examination showed a pigmented basal cell carcinoma. A wide re-excision and closure with a split-thickness skin graft were done.

specimen to the pathologist for proper identification. Unlike the squamous cell type, basal cell carcinoma rarely involves the regional lymphatics.

The treatment for the larger lesions is operative excision. The excision should be wide enough to erradicate the tumor (Fig. 109-5). The excision may include the underlying bone and dura. Primary closure of

these large defects will be difficult, and they are usually most easily closed with a split-thickness skin graft. Many times, flap closure is necessary because of the extent of the excision and, occasionally, because of the problem of exposed bone, dura, and brain.[5] A few cases in which there has been a recurrence of basal cell carcinoma after even the most extensive radical resection have been salvaged by the use of chemosurgery.[4]

Adenocarcinoma

Adenocarcinoma arises from the skin appendages and is difficult to diagnose. The diagnosis is usually not made until the lesion has been excised and viewed histologically. Regional lymph node dissection should be considered in the presence of an aggressive sweat gland carcinoma because of the propensity to regional lymph node metastasis.

Sarcoma

Sarcomas of the scalp are rare. The initial treatment is operative resection, which must be aggressive and thorough in order to give the patient a chance for cure. An occasional sarcoma does respond to radiother-

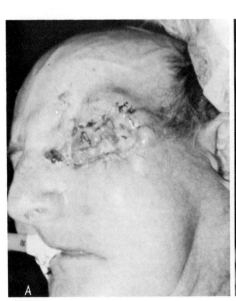
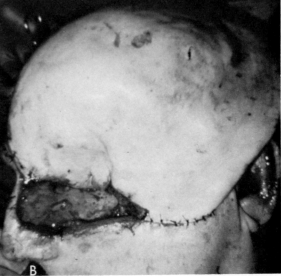

Figure 109-5 *A.* A patient with invasive basal cell carcinoma of the frontal scalp and invading the orbit and orbital contents. *B.* Following ressection of the frontal scalp, the frontal bone, a portion of the dura, the orbital contents, and the maxillary antrum, the defect was closed with the very useful and versatile scalp flap.

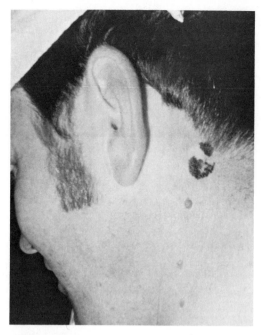

Figure 109–6 A melanotic lesion of the posterior lateral scalp area. This proved to be a malignant melanoma. The lesion was treated by wide excision and en bloc neck dissection.

apy, and if one is dealing with a tumor of which the operative ablation has not been satisfactory, a combined approach could be used.

Melanoma

Pigmented lesions of the scalp should be excised and studied histologically because if melanoma is present they are aggressive, rapidly growing, and have an extremely poor prognosis (Fig. 109–6). Melanoma usually spreads at a superficial level and laterally. The resulting local recurrence rate is as high as 25 per cent. Metastasis to regional lymph nodes is usually present in 75 per cent of the cases. The rate of survival of melanoma of the scalp is very poor.[2]

The treatment of malignant tumors of the scalp is operative with the exception of lymphomas, which respond to irradiation.

The overall five-year cure rate for carcinoma is 80 per cent, but the five-year cure rate for melanoma is only 23 per cent; if regional lymph nodes are involved, the cure rate drops to as low as 9 per cent.[1-3]

REFERENCES

1. Connelly, J. J.: Malignant tumors of the scalp: I. Analysis of 92 cases of malignant epithelial and somatic tumors of the scalp. Plast. Reconstr. Surg., *33*:1, 1964.
2. Connelly, J. J.: Malignant tumors of the scalp: II. Analysis of 58 cases of melanoma of the scalp. Plast. Reconstr. Surg., *33*:164, 1964.
3. Connelly, J.: Cancer of the Head and Neck: Treatment of Malignant Tumors of the Scalp. Washington, D.C., Butterworth & Co., 1967, pp. 99–105.
4. Mohs, F.: Chemosurgery and Cancer, Gangrene and Infections. Springfield, Ill., Charles C Thomas, 1956.
5. Rees, T. P., and Coburn, R. J.: Reconstruction of the scalp, forehead and calvaria. *In* Grabb, W. C., and Smith, J. W., eds.: Plastic Surgery, A Concise Guide to Clinical Practice. 2nd Ed. Boston, Little, Brown & Co., 1973.

Index

In this index page numbers set in *italics* indicate illustrations. Page numbers followed by (t) refer to tabular material. Drugs are indexed under their generic names when dosage or action or special use is given. The abbreviation vs. is used to indicate differential diagnosis.

Abdomen, distention of, postoperative, 1106
  ganglioneuroma of, 3310
  in head injury in children, 2093
  in multiple trauma, 2520–2521
  in thoracic spinal injury, 2346
  pain in, in cancer, 3630, 3630(t)
  of unknown origin, 3631
Abdominal cutaneous nerve syndrome, 2463
Abducens nerve, anatomy of, orbital, 3027
  clinical examination of, 20
  in infants and children, 46, 56
  in percutaneous trigeminal rhizotomy, 3569, *3571*
  palsy of, 657, *657*
  in pseudotumor cerebri, 896
  increased intracranial pressure and, 878
Ablative procedures, 3769–3786
  in refractory pain, 3763–3765
ABLB test, 697, 2974
Abnormal movement disorders, 3821–3857. See also *Dyskinesias.*
Abscess. See also names of specific abscesses.
  actinomycotic, 3399
  brain, 3343–3355
    brain scanning in, 155(t), 159
    computed tomography in, 116, *118*, 3346, *3348*, 3355
    ultrasound in, 190
  epidural, 3333
    in head injury, 1915
  spinal, epidural, vs. viral encephalitis, 3360
    extradural, 3449–3451, *3450*, *3451*
    subdural, 3451–3452, *3451*
  spinal cord, *3451*, 3452–3453, *3452*
  stitch, 1088
  subgaleal, 3328
Absence status, treatment of, 3878
Abulic trait, in normal-pressure hydrocephalus, 1424
Acceleration-deceleration injury, cervical, 2320, 2330–2332, 2338–2343, *2339*
Accident(s), care of spine in, cervical,
  thoracic, 2345
  cerebrovascular. See *Cerebrovascular accident* and *Stroke.*
Acetazolamide, cerebral blood flow and, 810(t)
  in pseudotumor cerebri, 3192
Acetylcholine, cerebral blood flow and, 808(t)
  metabolism of, 770
Achondroplasia, genetic aspects of, 1229, *1230, 1231*
  narrow spinal canal in, 2554
Acid-base balance, in multiple trauma, 2497–2500, *2498*, 2499(t)
Acid cholesteryl ester hydrolase deficiency, diagnosis of, 385(t)
Acidosis, metabolic, in multiple trauma, 2499
  respiratory, in head injury, in children, 2121
  in multiple trauma, 2500

Acoustic neuromas, 2967–3003
  angiography in, *317,* 2979–2985, *2982–2984*
  brain scanning in, 146, 150(t), 152, *153*
  computed tomography in, 122, *122,* 2976, *2977*
  diagnosis of, 2971–2992, *2974*
  operation(s) for, development of, 2968
    posterior fossa transmeatal, 2992–2997, *2992–2997*
    results of, *2998, 2999, 2999*–3000
  postoperative care in, 2997–2999
Acoustic reflex test, 700
Acrocephalopolysyndactyly, 1212–1213
Acrocephalosyndactyly, 1212–1213
Acrodysostosis, 1214
Acromegaloid appearance, vs. early acromegaly, 956
Acromegaly, 952–958
  diagnosis of, differential, 956
    potential pitfalls in, 955
  galactorrhea with, hormone secretion and, 964
  headache in, 3129
  histological study in, *3118*
  laboratory examination in, 953
  microadenoma in, 3124, *3125*
  pituitary tumor and, 952
  radiation therapy for, 3165, *3166*
  skull in, 3251
  study schedule for, 957
  treatment of, 956, 957(t)
    results of, 3146
  tumor herniation in, *3132*
Acrylic resin, cranioplasty with, 2236–2239, *2238–2240*
  advantages and complications of, 2241, *2241*
ACTH. See *Adrenocorticotropic hormone.*
Actinomycosis, 3398–3401
  meningitic, cerebrospinal fluid in, 462
Activities of daily living, in rehabilitation, 3996
Adamkiewicz, artery of, 553, *554, 556, 557, 561, 565*
Addison's disease, pseudotumor cerebri and, 3181(t)
Adenocarcinoma, ethmoid sinus, *3278,* 3279
  metastatic, tumor complexes of, *189*
  paranasal sinus, 3277
  scalp, 3319
Adenohypophysis, 935–970. See also *Anterior pituitary.*
  anatomy of, 3108
Adenoid cystic carcinoma, of paranasal sinuses, 3277
Adenoma, chromophobe, brain scanning in, *154*
  facial sebaceous, *1228*
  nonfunctioning chromophobe, radiation therapy of, 3164
  pituitary. See *Pituitary adenoma.*
Adenosine, cerebral blood flow and, 812(t)
Adenosine arabinoside, in herpes simplex encephalitis, 3363
Adenosine triphosphate, cerebral blood flow and, 812(t)

INDEX

INDEX

Brain stem (*Continued*)
  investigation of, 2776
  lesions of, coma in, 68
  responses of, in cerebral death, 755
  reticular formation of, 3466
  treatment of, 2779
  tumors of, radiation therapy of, 3102
Brain stem evoked response audiometry, 698–700, *699*
Brain tumors. See also names of specific tumors.
  biochemistry of, 2691
  biology of, 2666–2693, *2676, 2682, 2683,* 2685(t)–2687(t), *2687, 2688*
  cerebral blood flow in, 828, *829*
  chemotherapy of, 3065–3095
  classification of, 2659–2666, *2661,* 2664(t), 2759–2761, 2761(t)
  diagnostic tests for, 168(t)
  dyskinesia and, 3821
  electroencephalography in, 221, 2707
  etiological agents in, 2666–2676
  glial, 2759–2801
  grading of, 2661–2663
  growth mechanisms of, 2676–2682
  immunobiology of, 2688–2690
  incidence of, 2682–2688, *2682, 2683,* 2685(t), 2761–2762
  intracranial pressure in, increased, 889
  investigation of, 2763–2764. See also names of specific tumors.
  lymphomas as, 2836–2842
  meningeal, 2936–2966
  metastatic, 2872–2895
  neuronal, 2801–2835
  of disordered embryogenesis, 2899–2935
  operative treatment of, 2764–2765. See also names of specific tumors.
  posterior cranial fossa, in children, 2733–2758
  radiation therapy of, 3096–3106
  sarcomas as, 2845, 2855–2858
  sellar and parasellar, 3107–3155
  subarachnoid hemorrhage and, 1816
  supratentorial, in children, 2702–2732
  vascular, 2845–2855
  vs. viral encephalitis, 3360
Breast, carcinoma. See under *Carcinoma*.
Breathing. See *Respiration*.
Briquet's syndrome, "effected" pain and, 3507–3511, 3509(t), 3510(t)
Bromide psychosis, cerebral blood flow in, 829
Bromocriptine, in acromegaly, 957
  in hyperprolactinemia, 968
5-Bromo-2'-deoxyuridine, intra-arterial administration of, 3073
Bronchoscopy, fiberoptic, in atelectasis, 1019, *1019*
Bronchospasm, as postoperative complication, 1095
Brown's multitarget operation, in psychiatric disorders, 3938, *3939*
Brucellosis, cerebrospinal fluid in, 462
  intracranial hypertension in, 3180(t)
Bruising. See *Contusion*.
Bruit, carotid, asymptomatic, as indication for operation, 1567
  intracranial, in infants and children, 41, 45
BUdR, intra-arterial administration of, 3073
Burr holes, exploratory, in head injury, 1992
Burst fracture, cervical, 2319, *2320*
Butorphanol, in inappropriate secretion of antidiuretic hormone, 982

CAA 40, cerebral blood flow and, 809(t)
Caesarean section, in prevention of epilepsy, 3865
Caffeine, cerebral blood flow and, 810(t)
Calcification(s), in skull radiography, as pseudolesions, 77–80, *79,* 88, *89*
  pathological, 100, 100(t), *101–103*
  in spinal angioma, *574*

Calcification(s) (*Continued*)
  intracranial, genetic aspects of, 1227
Calcium, abnormalities of, in multiple trauma, 2501
  in cerebrospinal fluid, 450
  serum, in acromegaly, 954
Caloric test, in cerebral death, 755(t)
  of vestibular function, 683, *684*
Calvarium, defects of, 1215
Campotomy, 3829
Canavan disease, brain biopsy in, 386(t)
Cancer. See also names of specific types of cancer.
  craniofacial operation for, 3274
  endocrine treatment of, 3947
  visceral, pain in, 3627–3630
Candidiasis, 3407–3410
  meningitic, cerebrospinal fluid in, 461
Candidiosis, 3407
Candidosis, 3407
Capillary hemangioblastoma, posterior fossa, in children, 2754, *2755*
Capillary hemangioma. See *Hemangioma*.
Capsulotomy, bilateral anterior, in psychiatric disorders, 3835, 3936(t)
  vs. cingulotomy, 3936(t)
Caput succedaneum, transillumination in, 41
Carbamazepine, in afebrile seizures, 3876, 3876(t)
  in neurohypophyseal diabetes insipidus, 977
  in trigeminal neuralgia, 3558
  starting dosages of, 3877(t)
Carbenicillin, in bacterial infections, 3326
Carbon dioxide, cerebral blood flow and, 800, *800,* 801(t), 818, 830
  in acute respiratory failure, 1024
  in general anesthesia, 1123
  response to, prognosis after head injury and, 2153
Carbon monoxide poisoning, vascular ischemia in, 1542–1543, 1543(t)
Carcinoma, breast, hypophysectomy in, 3950–3952, 3984–3985
  posthypophysectomy (by craniotomy), 3984
  bronchial, hypophysectomy in, 3953
  bronchogenic, of conus, myelographic appearance of, *534*
  extracranial primary, brain scanning in, 152
  head and neck, mesencephalotomy for, 3707
    pain in, 3536–3538, *3536, 3537*
  metastatic, to skull, 3239, *3240, 3241,* 3244
  of ear, 3281, *3282, 3283*
  of scalp, 3316, *3319*
  orbital, 3059
  pancreatic, reversible nerve block in, 3655
  paranasal sinus, 3277, *3278–3281*
  prostate, hypophysectomy in, 3952–3953, 3985
Carcinogens, biological, 2675–2676, *2676*
  chemical, 2673–2675
Carcinomatosis, meningeal, cerebrospinal fluid in, 463
  chemotherapy for, 3090(t)
Cardiac arrest, in diffuse cerebral ischemia, 1540–1541
  in multiple trauma, 2492–2494
  intraoperative, 1073
  postoperative, 1097
Cardiac dysrhythmias, as postoperative complication, 1097
  in ischemic vascular disease, 1215
  intraoperative, 1072
Cardiac output, in acute respiratory failure, 1023
Cardiogenic shock, pathophysiology of, 2505
Cardiopulmonary physiology, clinical application of, formulas for, 1008(t)
  symbols in, 1007(t)
Cardiorespiratory disorders, intracranial hypertension in, 3180(t)
Cardiovascular disease, cerebrospinal fluid in, 469
Cardiovascular system, evaluation of, 1054
  in head injury in children, 2093
  in multiple trauma, 2490–2491
Carisoprodol, in histrionic personality, 3507
  in objective pain, 3489
  in psychogenic tissue tension pain, 3497

INDEX

INDEX

INDEX

INDEX

INDEX

Peripheral nerve(s) (*Continued*)
    injury of, entrapment, ischemia and pressure and, 2433–2435
        nerve conduction in, 618, 630
    in basilar skull fracture, 2251–2260
    pain of, 3534–3643
        causes of, 3636
        neuromodulation in, 3634
        rehabilitation in, 2418–2425
    lesions of, clinical examination in, 31–35, *32*, 33, 34(t)
    orbital, tumors of, 3049–3053
    receptors and, in pain, 3461–3462
    stimulators for, implantable, 3635, *3636*
    tumors of, 3299–3315
        neuronal, 3306–3311
        of Schwann cell origin, 3303–3306
    urinary bladder and sphincter, 1033–1034
Peripheral neuropathy, 3641
Peripheral paroxysmal vertigo, benign, 690
Peripheral vascular system, injuries to, in multiple trauma, 2490
    preoperative evaluation of, 1059
Peroneal nerve, electromyography of, 632
    entrapment of, 2467–2469, *2468*
    injury to, 2401–2404
        tibial nerve and, 2405–2407, *2406, 2407*
Perorbital projection, angiographic, 238, *239*
Perphenazine, in compulsive personality, 3504
    in histrionic personality, 3506, 3507
    in objective pain, 3489
    in psychogenic tissue tension pain, 3497, 3498
Personality, changes in, in supratentorial tumors in children, 2705
    compulsive, effected pain and, 3503
    constriction of, in post-traumatic syndromes, 2182
    dependent, effected pain and, 3501
    histrionic, effected pain and, 3505
Petechiae, in coma, 64(t)
Petit mal. See *Epilepsy.*
Petriellidiosis, 3401–3402
Phakomatoses, in supratentorial tumors, in children, 2704, *2705*
    nervous system neoplasia in, 1227, 1227(t)
Phantom limb pain, 2423–2424, 3637, 3637(t)
    mesencephalotomy in, 3709
    neuromodulation techniques in, 3637
Phantom target stereotaxic instrument, 3802, *3804*
Pharyngeal reflex, in cerebral death, 750
Phenacemide, in afebrile seizures, 3876(t)
Phenobarbital, in absence status, 3878
    in afebrile seizures, 3876, 3876(t)
    in febrile seizures, 3875
    in neonatal seizures, 3874
    in status epilepticus, 3878
    post–temporal lobectomy, 3889
    starting dosages of, 3877(t)
Phenol, in chronic pain syndrome, 3763
    in glycerol, administration of, 3658, *3659, 3661*
        as neurolytic agent, 3656
        results of, 3660, 3661(t)
Phenoxybenzamine, cerebral blood flow and, 809(t)
    in spastic urinary sphincter, 1045
Phenylalanine mustard, intra-arterial, 3073
Phenylephrine, cerebral blood flow and, 808(t)
    in atonic urinary sphincter, 1046
Pheochromocytoma, 3311
    glomus jugulare tumor with, 3287
Phlebitis, postoperative, 1108
Phoria, definition of, 652
Phosphatase, serum alkaline, in acromegaly, 954
Phosphate, inorganic, serum, in acromegaly, 954
Phosphocreatine, ischemia and, 777, *778*
Phosphorus, in cerebrospinal fluid, 450
Photocoagulation, in diabetic retinopathy, vs. hypophysectomy,
        3955
    vs. pituitary ablation, 3985(t)
Photophobia, in acromegaly, 3129
    in central nervous system diseases, 641(t)
Phrenic nerve, electromyography of, 632

Phycomycosis, 3423–3426
Physical therapy, 3989
Pia, formation of, 1240
Pick disease, brain biopsy in, 386(t)
Picrotoxin, cerebral blood flow and, 807, 810(t)
Pilocytic astrocytoma, 2779–2786, 3154
Pilonidal sinus, 1330
Pineal gland, in head injury, 1989
Pineal region, tumors of, 2863–2871
    angiography in, 324
    in children, 2714–2717, *2715–2717*
        in posterior fossa, 2755
    radiation therapy of, 3103, 3103(t)
Pinealoma, brain scanning in, 153
    pediatric, 162(t)
    computed tomography in, 116
Pineoblastoma, in children, 2716
Pipradol, cerebral blood flow and, 812(t)
Pitressin tannate, postcryohypophysectomy, 3979
    post–hypophysectomy by craniotomy, 3983
Pituitary abscess, 3154
Pituitary adenoma, 3107–3151
    anterior pituitary failure and, 948
    brain scanning in, 150(t), 152, *154*
    classification of, architectural, 3117, *3118, 3119*
        functional, 3121, 3122(t)
    computed tomography in, 137, *137, 138*
    corticotropic, 3123
    cryohypophysectomy in, 3978
    endocrine-active, 3122
    endocrine-inactive, 3124
    etiology of, 3128
    extrasellar expansion and invasion of, 3125
    in children, 2727–2728, *2727*
    metastasis of, 3127
    microscopic, 3124
        incidental, 969, *970*
        treatment of, 984
    pathology of, 3117, *3118–3121*, 3124, *3125, 3126*
    polysecretory, 964
    secretory properties of, 3119, *3120, 3121*
    staining properties of, 3117
    symptoms and findings in, 3129
    thyrotropic, 3123
    treatment of, 3137, 3137(t)
        complications of, 3148, 3148(t)
        medical, 3137(t), 3142
        methods of, 3143, 3144(t), *3145*
        operative, 3137(t), 3138
        radiotherapy in, 3137(t), 3142
        results of, 3144, 3147(t), 3148(t)
    ultrasound in, 190
Pituitary apoplexy, 948, 3148
Pituitary extract, posterior, cerebral blood flow and, 811(t)
Pituitary gland, 931–935
    ablation of. See *Hypophysectomy.*
    abscess of, 3154
    adenoma of, 3107–3151. See also *Pituitary adenoma.*
    anatomy of, 3107, *3109–3116*
        microscopic, 3116, *3116*
    anterior, 935–970. See also *Anterior pituitary.*
    blood supply of, 933, *934*, 3113
    embryology of, 931, *932*, 3107
    hormones of, 935–943
        deficiency of, diabetic retinopathy and, 3948–3949
            radiation therapy and, 3164
    structures adjacent to, 935, *936*
    structures of, 3107
    transsphenoidal approaches to, 3140
    tumors of. See also *Pituitary adenoma.*
        etiology of, 3128
        gonadotropin-secreting, 964
        hormone secretion and, 952
        management of, 957(t)
            early diagnosis and, 969

INDEX